ELSEVIER

evolve

To access your Student Resources, visit the web address below:

Evolve Learning Resources for *Mosby's 2006 Drug Consult for Nurses* offers the following features:

http://evolve.elsevier.com/DrugConsult/

Quarterly Drug Updates and Alerts
Abbreviated monographs on new drugs and updated information on new indications and new dosages for existing drugs. Important information about drugs recently withdrawn from the market, new drug safety information, and other news to help you provide the best possible care.

Do Not Confuse Table
A complete listing of drug names that sound alike and are often confused.

Less Frequently Used Drugs
Find vital information about drugs used less often in everyday practice.

Weblinks
Access links to places of interest on the web.

Sign-up page for the *Elsevier ePharmacology Update* newsletter
An informative, full-color, quarterly newsletter written by Evelyn Salerno, PharmD, the *Elsevier ePharmacology Update* provides current and well-documented information on new drugs, drug warnings, medication errors, and more.

Sign-up page for *Nurse Advise-ERR™ — a Medication Safety Alert!®* from the Institute for Safe Medication Practices Published monthly by the internationally recognized Institute for Safe Medication Practices (ISMP) and distributed free to students and instructors by Elsevier, *Nurse Advise-ERR™* provides tips for safe medication practice and up-to-date information on preventing medication errors.

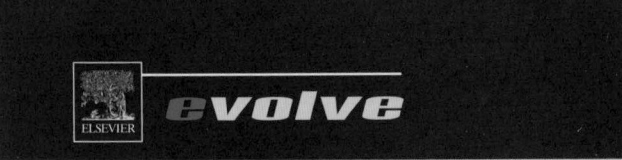

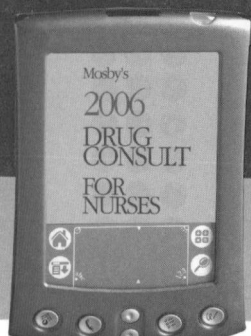

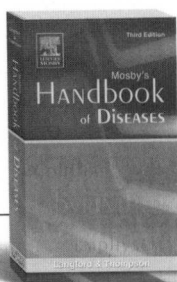

Mosby's 2006 DRUG CONSULT FOR NURSES

SPECIAL CONTRIBUTORS

Barbara B. Hodgson, RN, OCN
Cancer Institute
St. Joseph's Hospital
Tampa, Florida

Robert J. Kizior, BS, RPh
Education Coordinator
Department of Pharmacy
Alexian Brothers Medical Center
Elk Grove Village, Illinois

ELSEVIER
MOSBY

ELSEVIER
MOSBY

11830 Westline Industrial Drive
St. Louis, Missouri 63146

MOSBY'S 2006 DRUG CONSULT FOR NURSES ISBN 0-323-03466-7

NOTICE

Knowledge and best practice in this field are constantly changing. As new research and experience broaden our knowledge, changes in practice, treatment, and drug therapy may become necessary or appropriate. Readers are advised to check the most current information provided (i) on procedures featured or (ii) by the manufacturer of each product to be administered, to verify the recommended dose or formula, the method and duration of administration, and contraindications. It is the responsibility of the practitioner, relying on their own experience and knowledge of the patient, to make diagnoses, to determine dosages and the best treatment for each individual patient, and to take all appropriate safety precautions. To the fullest extent of the law, neither the Publisher nor the Authors assume any liability for any injury and/or damage to persons or property arising out or related to any use of the material contained in this book.

The Publisher

Previous edition copyrighted 2005.

International Standard Book Number 0-323-03466-7

Executive Vice President, Nursing & Health Professions: Sally Schrefer
Executive Publisher: Barbara Nelson Cullen
Executive Editor: Cindy Tryniszewski
Developmental Editor: Gina Hopf
Editorial Consultants: Karen Comerford, Doris Weinstock
Editorial Assistant: Blair Biscardi
Publishing Services Manager: Julie Eddy
Project Manager: Kelly E.M. Steinmann
Designer: Amy Buxton

Printed in the United States of America.

Last digit is the print number: 9 8 7 6 5 4 3 2 1

CONTRIBUTORS

Maryann Foley, RN, BSN
Clinical Consultant
Flourtown, Pennsylvania

Doris Greggs-McQuilkin, RN, BSN, MA
President
Academy of Medical-Surgical Nurses
Washington, D.C.

Esperanza Villanueva Joyce, EdD, RN
Dean and Professor
Our Lady of the Lake College
Baton Rouge, Louisiana

Eileen S. Robinson, RN, MSN
Continuing Education Consultant
Chadds Ford, Pennsylvania

Evelyn Salerno, BS, PharmD, RPh
Consultant Pharmacist
Editor
Elsevier ePharmacology Update
Formerly affiliated with School of Nursing
Florida International University
Clinical Assistant Professor
Nova-Southeastern College of Pharmacy
Miami, Florida

Colleen Seeber-Combs, RN, MSN
Clinical Consultant
Philadelphia, Pennsylvania

ADVISORY BOARD

Sharon Marie Abbate, RN, BSN, MSN
Assistant Professor
University of St. Francis College of Nursing
Joliet, Illinois

James D. Hoehns, PharmD, RPh, BCPS
Assistant Clinical Professor
University of Iowa College of Pharmacy
Iowa City, Iowa;
Clinical Pharmacist
Northeast Iowa Family Practice Residency Program
Waterloo, Iowa

Jeff M. Jellin, PharmD
Editor
Prescriber's Letter, and Natural Medicines Comprehensive Database
Stockton, California

Kelly W. Jones, PharmD, BCPS
McLeod Health
Florence, South Carolina

Trena L. Magers, PharmD
Clinical Pharmacy Coordinator
Provena Saint Joseph Medical Center
Joliet, Illinois

Keith M. Olsen, PharmD, FCCP, FCCM
Associate Professor
University of Nebraska Medical Center
Omaha, Nebraska

Karen Koozer Olson, RN, PhD, FNP-CS
Professor of Nursing and Graduate Program Coordinator
College of Science and Technology
School of Nursing and Health Sciences
Texas A&M University–Corpus Christi
Corpus Christi, Texas

Brenda K. Shelton, RN, MS, CCRN, AOCN
Sidney Kimmel Comprehensive Cancer Center
Johns Hopkins University
Baltimore, Maryland

Joseph P. Zbilut, RN,C, PhD, DNSc, ANP
Professor, Department of Molecular Biophysics and Physiology
Rush Medical College and Department of Adult Health Nursing
Rush College of Nursing
Chicago, Illinois

REVIEWERS

Tina R. Atkinson, RN, CRNI, ACL, PALS
Northwest Arkansas Neurosciences Center
Fayetteville, Arkansas

Arthur Briggs, RN, MS, BSN
Boston Health Care System
Brockton, Massachusetts

Tamara Brown Dolan, RN, BS
Independent Consultant
Falmouth, Massachusetts

Norma E. Hall, RN, BSN, BC
Clarian Health Partners, Inc.
Indianapolis, Indiana

Michael A. Lepsis, RN, ADN
Advance Medical Personal
Belen, New Mexico

Kate Moore, MSN, RN, CCRN, CCNS, ACNP
Air Evac EMS, Inc.
Nashville, Tennessee

Melody L. Morris, RN, BSN, EMT-P
New Hanover Regional Medical Center
Wilmington, North Carolina

FOREWORD

You may not be surprised to learn that medication errors in the United States have been linked to approximately 1,000 deaths every year. Although a multitude of factors can be attributed to the cause of serious medication errors, clearly a lack of the most up-to-date information about drug therapy plays an important role. One reason is that throughout the year the FDA is approving new drugs and releasing vital new information about drugs already on the market. What's more, many of the drugs used to treat serious conditions can also cause dangerous adverse reactions. To help keep you abreast of new drugs, recently discovered side and adverse effects, warnings, and information about dangerous drugs most likely to cause harm, you need a drug reference that's accurate, reliable, and up-to-date. You can't rely on outdated, inaccurate, or incomplete information when it comes to delivering safe patient care. You'll find that *Mosby's 2006 Drug Consult for Nurses* is a valuable resource to help you provide the highest quality of patient care related to drug therapy that you strive to achieve.

We've made *Mosby's 2006 Drug Consult for Nurses* better than ever. In addition to quickly locating all the essential information you need to know for administering thousands of generic and trade name drugs, you'll also find important updates, with the inclusion of 30 recently approved drugs by the FDA. Plus, we've added some unique features, such as practical quick-reference charts of IV infusion rates. To help prevent medication errors, we've developed a second-color icon for **High-Alert Drugs** ⚑ so that you can use extra care in administering drugs most likely to result in patient harm.

We've kept the original organization, which groups drugs by therapeutic class and then lists drugs alphabetically by generic name in each class. Organized this way, you can scan related drugs easily and compare factors that may affect their use in certain patients.

Mosby's 2006 Drug Consult for Nurses is written by the well-respected nurse and pharmacist authors Barbara B. Hodgson, RN, OCN, and Robert J. Kizior, BS, RPh. Their reputation for authoritative, clinically relevant drug information—in collaboration with our panel of expert nurse and pharmacist advisors—ensures that this drug reference book meets the highest standards for reliability and accuracy.

Armed with *Mosby's 2006 Drug Consult for Nurses*, you'll be confident that you have the latest facts for providing safe and effective drug therapy. Whether you're a student or an experienced nurse, you'll easily find the information you need and the reliability you can trust.

WHAT MAKES THIS BOOK SPECIAL

Besides providing detailed information in each drug entry, *Mosby's 2006 Drug Consult for Nurses* offers many special features designed to help make drug administration accurate and easier and safer for the patient.

KEY FEATURES

Organization by therapeutic class. By grouping drug entries within therapeutic classes, the book helps you identify drugs by clinical application and compare information about alternative drugs used for the same purpose. Each class includes an overview with key information about the drugs' therapeutic uses and mechanisms of action.

Practice-oriented nursing considerations. In every drug entry, this reference provides extensive, practice-oriented nursing considerations, putting essential drug facts directly into the context of your care.

Vital lifespan considerations. Throughout its pages, the book highlights key points related to drug therapy in pregnant, breast-feeding, pediatric, and elderly patients.

Herbal medicine section. This portion of the book includes full-length entries for the most commonly used herbs.

Handy IV compatibility chart. For everyday reference, the book features an IV Compatibility Chart that folds out for easy use and is bound into the book to prevent accidental loss.

Comprehensive appendixes. In ready-reference format, the appendixes give you easy access to additional vital drug-related information, such as the English-Spanish Drug Phrase Translator to help you provide drug therapy and teaching to Spanish-speaking patients.

UNIQUE FEATURES

Insightful illustrations. More than 20 detailed, two-color illustrations help enhance your understanding of the mechanism or site of action for selected drugs and drug classes.

Prioritized side effects. Each drug entry ranks side effects by frequency of occurrence from most common to least common. It also includes the percentage of frequency, when known. This information helps you focus your care by knowing which effects to monitor more closely.

Highlights on serious adverse reactions. In each drug entry, the book calls attention to dangerous or life-threatening reactions so that you can identify them easily and act on them promptly.

Alert icons. The pages use an *Alert* icon to spotlight critical nursing considerations that require your special attention.

Free updates. The companion website, www.evolve.elsevier.com/DrugConsult/, provides free late-breaking drug information to keep you up to date on new drugs and indications, recent warnings, withdrawals from the market, and more.

NEW TO THIS EDITION

Monographs for 30 new drugs recently approved by the FDA to provide the latest drug information.

Updated content, including interactions, precautions, alerts, patient teaching instructions, and other need-to-know information to ensure safe drug administration.

Special, **second-color icon for High-Alert Drugs** cautions you to use extra care in administering drugs most likely to cause harm.

Expanded use of the second color for icons and headings to allow you to easily identify essential information.

Five new two-color illustrations showing how and where drugs work at the cellular and tissue level.

Appendix of **drug names that sound alike and look alike** to promote safe drug administration.

Appendix of **orphan drugs** (with an introduction, list of drugs, and related websites) to inform you about drugs developed through research funded by FDA grants and that are used to treat rare chronic diseases, such as cystic fibrosis, von Willebrand's disease, and rare cancers.

Appendix for **decreasing drug errors and ensuring safe drug administration.**

Quick-reference charts of IV infusion rates for dopamine, dobutamine, nitroglycerin, norepinephrine, sodium nitroprusside, and propofol.

New appendix of **equi-analgesic dosing.** This table helps you provide better pain control for patients receiving opioid agonists by including the dosages of opioid agonists that will produce the same degree of analgesia as 10 mg of parenteral morphine given every 3 to 4 hours.

Cultural aspects of **drug therapy** appendix expanded to include **age and gender.**

HOW TO USE THIS BOOK

Mosby's 2006 Drug Consult for Nurses is divided into major sections, such as central nervous system agents, which are then divided into chapters of drugs in the same therapeutic classification, such as antianxiety agents. Each chapter introduction explains the drugs' general uses and actions (often with illustrations), lists generic drugs in the class, and identifies combination products by trade name with generic components and their strengths.

Within each chapter, detailed entries provide all the information you need about the generic drugs in the class. In every drug entry, you'll find:

Generic name, pronunciation, and trade names. Each generic drug name is listed alphabetically—and spelled phonetically—for quick identification.

Do not confuse with. This unique feature identifies generic and trade names that resemble the featured drug to help you avoid drug errors.

Category and schedule. This section lists the drug's pregnancy risk category and, when appropriate, its controlled substance schedule or over-the-counter (OTC) status.

Mechanism of action. Expanding on the chapter overview information, this section clearly and concisely details the drug's mechanism of action and therapeutic effects.

Pharmacokinetics. Under this heading, a quick-reference chart outlines the drug's route, onset, peak, and duration, when known. It's followed by a discussion of the drug's absorption, distribution, metabolism, excretion, and half-life.

Availability. This section identifies the forms that the drug comes in, for example, in tablets, sustained-release capsules, or an injectable solution. Plus, it lists the available doses and concentrations.

Indications and dosages. Here, you'll find the approved indications and routes, along with the dosage information for all age groups, including adults, elderly patients, children, neonates, and those with pre-existing conditions such as liver or kidney disease.

Off-label uses. This section brings you up to date on the off-label uses commonly seen in practice.

Contraindications. In this section, conditions that prohibit the use of the drug are listed.

Interactions. For drugs, herbal supplements, and food, this section supplies vital information about interactions with the topic drug.

Diagnostic test effects. Under this heading, you'll see a brief description of the drug's effects of laboratory and diagnostic test results, such as liver enzyme levels and electrocardiogram tracings.

IV incompatibilities and IV compatibilities. These twin sections let you know which IV drugs can't and can be given with the featured drug, whether by IV push, Y-site, or IV piggyback administration.

Side effects. Unlike other handbooks that mix common, deadly effects with rare, minor ones in a long, undifferentiated list, this book ranks side effects by frequency of occurrence as expected, frequent, occasional, and rare. Within each frequency, effects are listed by highest to lowest percentage of occurrence, when known.

Serious adverse reactions. Because serious adverse reactions are life-threatening responses that require prompt intervention, this section highlights them, apart from other side effects, for easy identification.

Nursing considerations. Using a practice-oriented format, this section presents nursing considerations in five main categories:

- *Baseline assessment* tells what to assess before giving the first dose of a drug.
- *Lifespan considerations* contains age-specific recommendations as well as information related to pregnancy and breast-feeding.
- *Precautions* alerts you to specific conditions or circumstances that call for caution when administering the drug.
- *Administration and handling* features the do's and don'ts of drug administration, with guidelines for PO, IV, IM, and other forms of the drug. It gives clear-cut instructions about how to store, prepare, and administer the drug.
- *Intervention and evaluation* describes ongoing interventions and ways to monitor the drug's therapeutic and adverse effects.
- *Patient teaching* explains exactly what to teach your patients to help them achieve the maximum therapeutic response to drugs while minimizing possible adverse effects.

Mosby's 2006 Drug Consult for Nurses is better than ever. This unique, comprehensive reference is organized to help you focus on the drugs you use in everyday practice and includes even more features to allow ready access to essential drug information. When it comes to providing quality patient care and safe drug administration, you'll need no other drug reference.

Doris Greggs-McQuilkin, RN, BSN, MA
Immediate Past President
Academy of Medical-Surgical Nurses
Washington, D.C.

ACKNOWLEDGMENTS

A technical book of this magnitude requires the dedicated commitment of many persons. Each of us appreciates the other's enduring commitment to excellence, completeness, and accuracy in compiling the information for this book. Our partnership and friendship has bridged many years and many personal challenges, and it has endured and grown with each publication. We give special thanks to Gina Hopf for her tireless efforts to develop and facilitate the format that you will see within. It has been our pleasure to work with Gina on several projects, and she continues to be an invaluable partner in our work. It has been our pleasure working with Cindy Tryniszewski, who also gave so much of her time and effort turning this project into a reality. We offer grateful acknowledgment to the editorial staff at Elsevier, who have encouraged our best efforts and who have contributed valuable ideas for content, format, and presentation. Our thanks also go to the staff at Graphic World Publishing Services for their efforts in presenting this work in an attractive and easy-to-use manner. Thanks go as well to our family and friends—personal and professional—who listen to and critique our bright ideas, make suggestions that make our work better, and provide support and encouragement at every turn.

Robert (Bob) Kizior, BS, RPh, and Barbara Hodgson, RN, OCN

BIBLIOGRAPHY

Briggs G, Freeman R, Yaffe S: *Drugs in Pregnancy and Lactation*, ed 6, Greenwood Village, Colorado, 2003, Micromedex.

Drug Facts and Comparisons, St. Louis, 2004, Facts and Comparisons.

Lacy CF, Armstrong LL, Goldman MP, et al: *Lexi-Comp's Drug Information Handbook*, ed 12, Hudson, Ohio, 2005, Lexi-Comp.

Mosby's Drug Consult 2005, ed 15, St. Louis, 2005, Mosby.

Rakel RE, Bope ET: *Conn's Current Therapy*, ed 2, Philadelphia, 2005, WB Saunders.

Takemoto CR, Hodding JH, Kraus DM: *Lexi-Comp's Pediatric Dosage Handbook*, ed 11, Hudson, Ohio, 2004, Lexi-Comp.

Trissel LA: *Handbook of Injectable Drugs*, ed 12, Bethesda, 2004, American Society of Health-System Pharmacist.

USPDI Drug Information for the Health Care Professional, 2004.

ILLUSTRATION CREDITS

Brody T, Larner J, Minneman K (eds): *Human Pharmacology: Molecular to Clinical*, ed 3, St. Louis, 1998, Mosby.

Guitierrez K (ed): *Pharmacotherapeutics: Clinical Decision Making in Nursing,* Philadelphia, 1999, WB Saunders.

Kee JL, Hayes ER (eds): *Pharmacology: A Nursing Process Approach,* ed 4, Philadelphia, 2003, WB Saunders.

Mosby's Drug Consult, 2004, ed 14, St. Louis, 2004, Mosby.

Page C, et al (eds): *Integrated Pharmacology*, ed 2, St. Louis, 2005, Mosby.

Prosser S, et al. (eds): *Applied Pharmacology for Nurses and Other Health Care Professionals*, St. Louis, 2000, Mosby.

Taylor M: *Mosby's Crash Course Pharmacology*, St. Louis, 1998, Mosby.

CONTENTS

Central Nervous System Agents

Gastrointestinal Agents

Hematologic Agents

Hormonal Agents

Immunomodulating Agents

Natural Medicines

Nutritional and Electrolyte Agents

Renal and Genitourinary Agents

Respiratory Agents

APPENDIXES

INDEX

DRUGS BY DISORDER

Generic names appear first, followed by brand names in parentheses.

Allergy
Beclomethasone (Beclovent, Vanceril)
Betamethasone (Celestone)
Brompheniramine (Dimetane)
Budesonide (Pulmicort, Rhinocort)
Chlorpheniramine (Chlor-Trimeton)
Clemastine (Tavist)
Cyproheptadine (Periactin)
Desloratadine (Clarinex)
Dexamethasone (Decadron)
Dimenhydrinate (Dramamine)
Diphenhydramine (Benadryl)
Epinephrine (Adrenalin)
Fexofenadine (Allegra)
Flunisolide (AeroBid, Nasalide)
Fluticasone (Flovent)
Hydrocortisone (Solu-Cortef)
Loratadine (Claritin)
Prednisolone (Prelone)
Prednisone (Deltasone)
Promethazine (Phenergan)
Triamcinolone (Kenalog)

Alzheimer's disease
Donepezil (Aricept)
Galantamine (Reminyl)
Memantine (Namenda)
Rivastigmine (Exelon)
Tacrine (Cognex)

Angina
Amlodipine (Norvasc)
Atenolol (Tenormin)
Diltiazem (Cardizem, Dilacor)
Isosorbide (Imdur, Isordil)
Metoprolol (Lopressor)
Nadolol (Corgard)
Nicardipine (Cardene)
Nifedipine (Adalat, Procardia)
Nitroglycerin
Propranolol (Inderal)
Timolol (Blocadron)
Verapamil (Calan, Isoptin)

Anxiety
Alprazolam (Xanax)
Buspirone (BuSpar)
Diazepam (Valium)
Doxepin (Sinequan)
Hydroxyzine (Atarax, Vistaril)
Lorazepam (Ativan)
Oxazepam (Serax)

Arrhythmias
Acebutolol (Sectral)
Adenosine (Adenocard)
Amiodarone (Cordarone, Pacerone)
Digoxin (Lanoxin)
Diltiazem (Cardizem, Dilacor)
Disopyramide (Norpace)
Dofetilide (Tikosyn)
Esmolol (Brevibloc)
Ibutilide (Corvert)
Lidocaine
Mexiletine (Mexitil)
Moricizine (Ethmozine)
Phenytoin (Dilantin)
Procainamide (Procan, Pronestyl)
Propafenone (Rythmol)
Propranolol (Inderal)
Quinidine
Sotalol (Betapace)
Tocainide (Tonocard)
Verapamil (Calan, Isoptin)

Arthritis, rheumatoid
Adalimumab (Humira)
Anakinra (Kineret)
Aspirin
Auranofin (Ridaura)
Aurothioglucose (Solganal)

Azathioprine (Imuran)
Betamethasone (Celestone)
Capsaicin (Zostrix)
Celecoxib (Celebrex)
Cyclosporine (Sandimmune)
Diclofenac (Cataflam, Voltaren)
Diflunisal (Dolobid)
Etanercept (Enbrel)
Hydroxychloroquine (Plaquenil)
Infliximab (Remicade)
Leflunomide (Arava)
Methotrexate
Penicillamine (Cuprimine)
Prednisone (Deltasone)
Valdecoxib (Bextra)

Asthma
Albuterol (Proventil, Ventolin)
Aminophylline (Theophylline)
Beclomethasone (Beclovent, Vanceril)
Budesonide (Pulmicort)
Cromolyn (Crolom, Intal)
Dexamethasone (Decadron)
Epinephrine (Adrenalin)
Flunisolide (AeroBid)
Fluticasone (Flovent)
Formoterol (Foradil)
Hydrocortisone (Solu-Cortef)
Ipratropium (Atrovent)
Levalbuterol (Xopenex)
Metaproterenol (Alupent)
Methylprednisolone (Solu-Medrol)
Montelukast (Singulair)
Nedocromil (Tilade)
Prednisolone (Prelone)
Prednisone (Deltasone)
Salmeterol (Serevent)
Terbutaline (Brethine)
Theophylline (SloBid)
Zafirlukast (Accolate)
Zileuton (Zyflo)

Attention deficit hyperactivity disorder (ADHD)
Atomoxetine (Strattera)
Desipramine (Norpramin)
Dexmethylphenidate (Focalin)
Dextroamphetamine (Dexedrine)
Imipramine (Tofranil)
Methylphenidate (Ritalin)
Pemoline (Cylert)

Benign prostatic hypertrophy (BPH)
Alfuzosin (UroXatral)
Doxazosin (Cardura)
Finasteride (Proscar)
Tamsulosin (Flomax)
Terazosin (Hytrin)

Bronchospasm
Albuterol (Proventil, Ventolin)
Bitolterol (Tornalate)
Epinephrine (Adrenalin)
Levalbuterol (Xopenex)
Metaproterenol (Alupent)
Salmeterol (Serevent)
Terbutaline (Brethine)
Theophylline (SloBid)

Cancer
Abarelix (Plenaxis)
Aldesleukin (Proleukin)
Alemtuzumab (Campath)
Alitretinoin (Panretin)
Altretamine (Hexalen)
Anastrozole (Arimidex)
Arsenic trioxide (Trisenox)
Asparaginase (Elspar)
Azacitadine (Vidaza)
BCG (TheraCys, Tice BCG)
Bevacizumab (Avastin)
Bexarotene (Targretin)
Bicalutamide (Casodex)
Bleomycin (Blenoxane)
Bortezumib (Velcade)
Busulfan (Myleran)
Capecitabine (Xeloda)
Carboplatin (Paraplatin)
Carmustine (BiCNU)
Cetuximab (Erbitux)
Chlorambucil (Leukeran)
Cisplatin (Platinol)
Cladribine (Leustatin)
Clofarabine (Clolar)
Cyclophosphamide (Cytoxan)
Cytarabine (Ara-C, Cytosar)

Dacarbazine (DTIC)
Dactinomycin (Cosmegen)
Daunorubicin (Cerubidine, DaunoXome)
Denileukin (Ontak)
Docetaxel (Taxotere)
Doxorubicin (Adriamycin, Doxil)
Epirubicin (Ellence)
Ertotinib (Tarceva)
Estramustine (Emcyt)
Etoposide (VePesid)
Fludarabine (Fludara)
Fluorouracil
Flutamide (Eulexin)
Fulvestrant (Faslodex)
Gefitnib (Iressa)
Gemcitabine (Gemzar)
Gemtuzumab (Mylotarg)
Goserelin (Zoladex)
Hydroxyurea (Hydrea)
Ibritumomab (Zevalin)
Idarubicin (Idamycin)
Ifosfamide (Ifex)
Imatinib (Gleevec)
Interferon alfa-2a (Roferon A)
Interferon alfa-2b (Intron A)
Irinotecan (Camptosar)
Letrozole (Femara)
Leuprolide (Lupron)
Lomustine (CeeNU)
Mechlorethamine (Mustargen)
Megestrol (Megace)
Melphalan (Alkeran)
Mercaptopurine (Purinethol)
Methotrexate
Mitomycin (Mutamycin)
Mitotane (Lysodren)
Mitoxantrone (Novantrone)
Nilutamide (Nilandron)
Oxaliplatin (Eloxatin)
Paclitaxel (Taxol)
Pemetrexed (Alimta)
Pentostatin (Nipent)
Plicamycin (Mithracin)
Procarbazine (Matulane)
Rituximab (Rituxan)
Streptozocin (Zanosar)
Tamoxifen (Nolvadex)
Temozolomide (Temodar)
Teniposide (Vumon)
Thioguanine
Thiotepa (Thioplex)
Topotecan (Hycamtin)
Toremifene (Fareston)
Tositumomab (Ber)
Trastuzumab (Herceptin)
Tretinoin (Vesanoid)
Valrubicin (Valstar)
Vinblastine (Velban)
Vincristine (Oncovin)
Vinorelbine (Navelbine)

Cerebrovascular accident (CVA)
Aspirin
Clopidogrel (Plavix)
Heparin
Nimodipine (Nimotop)
Ticlopidine (Ticlid)
Warfarin (Coumadin)

Chronic obstructive pulmonary disease (COPD)
Albuterol (Proventil, Ventolin)
Aminophylline (Theophylline)
Budesonide (Pulmicort)
Epinephrine (Adrenalin)
Formoterol (Foradil)
Levalbuterol (Xopenex)
Metaproterenol (Alupent)
Salmeterol (Serevent)
Theophylline (SloBid)
Tiotropium (Spiriva)

Congestive heart failure (CHF)
Amlodipine (Norvasc)
Bumetanide (Bumex)
Captopril (Capoten)
Carvedilol (Coreg)
Digoxin (Lanoxin)
Dobutamine (Dobutrex)
Dopamine (Intropin)
Enalapril (Vasotec)
Eprosartan (Teveten)
Fosinopril (Monopril)
Furosemide (Lasix)
Hydralazine (Apresoline)
Isosorbide (Isordil)
Lisinopril (Prinivil, Zestril)

Losartan (Cozaar)
Metoprolol (Lopressor)
Milrinone (Primacor)
Moexipril (Univasc)
Nitroglycerin
Nitroprusside (Nipride)
Quinapril (Accupril)
Ramipril (Altace)

Constipation
Bisacodyl (Dulcolax)
Docusate (Colace)
Lactulose (Kristalose)
Methylcellulose (Citrucel)
Milk of magnesia (MOM)
Psyllium (Metamucil)
Senna (Senokot)

Crohn's disease
Cyclosporine (Neoral)
Hydrocortisone (Cortenema)
Infliximab (Remicade)
Mesalamine (Asacol, Pentasa)
Olsalazine (Dipentum)
Sulfasalazine (Azulfidine)

Deep vein thrombosis (DVT)
Dalteparin (Fragmin)
Enoxaparin (Lovenox)
Heparin
Tinzaparin (Innohep)
Warfarin (Coumadin)

Depression
Amitriptyline (Elavil, Endep)
Bupropion (Wellbutrin)
Citalopram (Celexa)
Clomipramine (Anafranil)
Desipramine (Norpramin)
Doxepin (Sinequan)
Escitalopram (Lexapro)
Fluoxetine (Prozac)
Imipramine (Tofranil)
Maprotiline (Ludiomil)
Mirtazapine (Remeron)
Nefazodone (Serzone)
Nortriptyline (Aventyl, Pamelor)
Paroxetine (Paxil)
Phenelzine (Nardil)
Sertraline (Zoloft)
Tranylcypromine (Parnate)
Trazodone (Desyrel)
Venlafaxine (Effexor)

Diabetes mellitus
Acarbose (Precose)
Chlorpropamide (Diabinese)
Glimepiride (Amaryl)
Glipizide (Glucotrol)
Glyburide (Micronase)
Insulin
Metformin (Glucophage)
Miglitol (Glyset)
Nateglinide (Starlix)
Pioglitazone (Actos)
Repaglinide (Prandin)
Rosiglitazone (Avandia)

Diarrhea
Bismuth subsalicylate (Pepto-Bismol)
Diphenoxylate and atropine (Lomotil)
Kaolin-pectin (Kaopectate)
Loperamide (Imodium)
Octreotide (Sandostatin)
Rifaximin (Xifaxan)

Duodenal, gastric ulcers
Cimetidine (Tagamet)
Esomeprazole (Nexium)
Famotidine (Pepcid)
Lansoprazole (Prevacid)
Misoprostol (Cytotec)
Nizatidine (Axid)
Omeprazole (Prilosec)
Pantoprazole (Protonix)
Rabeprazole (Aciphex)
Ranitidine (Zantac)
Sucralfate (Carafate)

Edema
Amiloride (Midamor)
Bumetanide (Bumex)
Chlorthalidone (Hygroton)
Ethacrynic acid (Edecrin)
Furosemide (Lasix)

Hydrochlorothiazide (HydroDIURIL)
Indapamide (Lozol)
Metolazone (Zaroxolyn)
Spironolactone (Aldactone)
Torsemide (Demadex)
Triamterene (Dyrenium)

Epilepsy
Acetazolamide (Diamox)
Carbamazepine (Tegretol)
Clonazepam (Klonopin)
Clorazepate (Tranxene)
Diazepam (Valium)
Fosphenytoin (Cerebyx)
Gabapentin (Neurontin)
Lamotrigine (Lamictal)
Levetiracetam (Keppra)
Lorazepam (Ativan)
Oxcarbazepine (Trileptal)
Phenobarbital
Phenytoin (Dilantin)
Primidone (Mysoline)
Tiagabine (Gabitril)
Topiramate (Topamax)
Valproic acid (Depakene, Depakote)
Zonisamide (Zonegran)

Esophageal reflux, esophagitis
Cimetidine (Tagamet)
Esomeprazole (Nexium)
Famotidine (Pepcid)
Lansoprazole (Prevacid)
Nizatidine (Axid)
Omeprazole (Prilosec)
Pantoprazole (Protonix)
Rabeprazole (Aciphex)
Ranitidine (Zantac)

Fever
Acetaminophen (Tylenol)
Aspirin
Ibuprofen (Advil, Motrin)
Naproxen (Aleve, Anaprox, Naprosyn)

Gastritis
Cimetidine (Tagamet)
Famotidine (Pepcid)
Nizatidine (Axid)
Ranitidine (Zantac)

Gastroesophageal reflux disease (GERD)
Cimetidine (Tagamet)
Esomeprazole (Nexium)
Famotidine (Pepcid)
Lansoprazole (Prevacid)
Metoclopramide (Reglan)
Nizatidine (Axid)
Omeprazole (Prilosec)
Pantoprazole (Protonix)
Rabeprazole (Aciphex)
Ranitidine (Zantac)

Glaucoma
Acetazolamide (Diamox)
Apraclonidine (Iopidine)
Betaxolol (Betoptic)
Bimatoprost (Lumigan)
Brimonidine (Alphagan)
Brinzolamide (Azopt)
Carbachol
Carteolol (Ocupress)
Dipivefrin (Propine)
Dorzolamide (Trusopt)
Echothiophate iodide (Phospholine)
Latanoprost (Xalatan)
Levobunolol (Betagan)
Metipranolol (OptiPranolol)
Pilocarpine (Isopto Carpine)
Timolol (Timoptic)
Travoprost (Travatan)
Unoprostone (Rescula)

Gout
Allopurinol (Zyloprim)
Colchicine
Indomethacin (Indocin)
Probenecid (Benemid)
Sulindac (Clinoril)

Human immunodeficiency virus (HIV)
Abacavir (Ziagen)
Amprenavir (Agenerase)
Atazanavir (Reyataz)
Delavirdine (Rescriptor)

Didanosine (Videx)
Efavirenz (Sustiva)
Emtricitabine (Emtriva)
Enfuvirtide (Fuzeon)
Indinavir (Crixivan)
Lamivudine (Epivir)
Lopinavir/ritonavir (Kaletra)
Nelfinavir (Viracept)
Nevirapine (Viramune)
Ritonavir (Norvir)
Saquinavir (Fortovase, Invirase)
Stavudine (Zerit)
Tenofovir (Viread)
Zalcitabine (Hivid)
Zidovudine (AZT, Retrovir)

Hypercholesterolemia
Atorvastatin (Lipitor)
Cholestyramine (Questran)
Colesevelam (Welchol)
Colestipol (Colestid)
Ezetimibe (Zetia)
Fenofibrate (Tricor)
Fluvastatin (Lescol)
Gemfibrozil (Lopid)
Lovastatin (Mevacor)
Niacin (Niaspan)
Pravastatin (Pravachol)
Rosuvastatin (Crestor)
Simvastatin (Zocor)

Hyperphosphatemia
Aluminum salts
Calcium salts
Sevelamer (Renagel)

Hypertension
Amiloride (Midamor)
Amlodipine (Norvasc)
Atenolol (Tenormin)
Benazepril (Lotensin)
Bisoprolol (Zebeta)
Candesartan (Atacand)
Captopril (Capoten)
Clonidine (Catapres)
Diltiazem (Cardizem, Dilacor)
Doxazosin (Cardura)
Enalapril (Vasotec)
Eplerenone (Inspra)
Eprosartan (Teveten)
Felodipine (Plendil)
Fosinopril (Monopril)
Hydralazine (Apresoline)
Hydrochlorothiazide (HydroDIURIL)
Indapamide (Lozol)
Irbesartan (Avapro)
Isradipine (DynaCirc)
Labetalol (Normodyne, Trandate)
Lisinopril (Prinivil, Zestril)
Losartan (Cozaar)
Methyldopa (Aldomet)
Metolazone (Diulo, Zaroxolyn)
Metoprolol (Lopressor)
Minoxidil (Loniten)
Moexipril (Univasc)
Nadolol (Corgard)
Nicardipine (Cardene)
Nifedipine (Adalat, Procardia)
Nitroglycerin
Nitroprusside (Nipride)
Olmesartan (Benicar)
Perindopril (Aceon)
Pindolol (Visken)
Prazosin (Minipress)
Propranolol (Inderal)
Quinapril (Accupril)
Ramipril (Altace)
Spironolactone (Aldactone)
Telmisartan (Micardis)
Terazosin (Hytrin)
Timolol (Blocadren)
Trandolapril (Mavik)
Valsartan (Dovan)
Verapamil (Calan, Isoptin)

Hypertriglyceridemia
Atorvastatin (Lipitor)
Fenofibrate (Tricor)
Fluvastatin (Lescol)
Gemfibrozil (Lopid)
Lovastatin (Mevacor)
Niacin (Niaspan)
Pravastatin (Pravachol)
Rosuvastatin (Crestor)
Simvastatin (Zocor)

Hyperuricemia
Allopurinol (Zyloprim)
Colchicine
Probenecid (Benemid)

Hypotension
Norepinephrine (Levophed)
Phenylephrine (Neo-Synephrine)

Hypothyroidism
Levothyroxine (Levoxyl, Synthroid)
Liothyronine (Cytomel)
Thyroid

Idiopathic thrombocytopenic purpura (ITP)
Azathioprine (Imuran)
Cyclophosphamide (Cytoxan)
Danazol (Danocrine)
Dexamethasone (Decadron)
Prednisone

Insomnia
Diphenhydramine (Benadryl)
Estazolam (ProSom)
Eszopiclone (Lunesta)
Flurazepam (Dalmane)
Temazepam (Restoril)
Triazolam (Halcion)
Zaleplon (Sonata)
Zolpidem (Ambien)

Migraine headaches
Almotriptan (Axert)
Amitriptyline (Elavil, Endep)
Dihydroergotamine
Eletriptan (Relpax)
Ergotamine (Ergomar)
Frovatriptan (Frovan)
Naratriptan (Amerge)
Propranolol (Inderal)
Rizatriptan (Maxalt)
Sumatriptan (Imitrex)
Zolmitriptan (Zomig)

Multiple sclerosis (MS)
Glatiramer (Copaxone)
Interferon beta-1a (Avonex, Rebif)
Interferon beta-1b (Betaseron)
Mitoxantrone (Novantrone)
Natalizumab (Tysabri)

Myocardial infarction (MI)
Alteplase (Activase)
Aspirin
Atenolol (Tenormin)
Captopril (Capoten)
Clopidogrel (Plavix)
Dalteparin (Fragmin)
Diltiazem (Cardizem, Dilacor)
Enalapril (Vasotec)
Enoxaparin (Lovenox)
Heparin
Lidocaine
Lisinopril (Prinivil, Zestril)
Metoprolol (Lopressor)
Morphine
Nitroglycerin
Propranolol (Inderal)
Quinapril (Accupril)
Ramipril (Altace)
Reteplase (Retavase)
Streptokinase
Timolol (Blocadren)
Verapamil (Calan, Isoptin)
Warfarin (Coumadin)

Nausea
Aprepitant (Emend)
Chlorpromazine (Thorazine)
Dexamethasone (Decadron)
Dimenhydrinate (Dramamine)
Dolasetron (Anzemet)
Dronabinol (Marinol)
Droperidol (Inapsine)
Granisetron (Kytril)
Hydroxyzine (Vistaril)
Lorazepam (Ativan)
Meclizine (Antivert)
Metoclopramide (Reglan)
Ondansetron (Zofran)
Palonosetron (Aloxi)
Prochlorperazine (Compazine)
Promethazine (Phenergan)
Trimethobenzamide (Tigan)

Obsessive-compulsive disorder (OCD)
Citalopram (Celexa)
Clomipramine (Anafranil)
Fluoxetine (Prozac)
Fluvoxamine (Luvox)
Paroxetine (Paxil)
Sertraline (Zoloft)

Osteoporosis
Alendronate (Fosamax)
Calcitonin (Miacalcin)
Calcium salts
Conjugated estrogens (Premarin)
Estradiol (Estrace)
Raloxifene (Evista)
Risedronate (Actonel)
Teriparatide (Forteo)
Vitamin D

Paget's disease
Alendronate (Fosamax)
Calcitonin (Miacalcin)
Etidronate (Didronel)
Pamidronate (Aredia)
Risedronate (Actonel)
Tiludronate (Skelid)

Pain, mild to moderate
Acetaminophen (Tylenol)
Aspirin
Celecoxib (Celebrex)
Codeine
Diclofenac (Cataflam, Voltaren)
Diflunisal (Dolobid)
Etodolac (Lodine)
Flurbiprofen (Ansaid)
Ibuprofen (Advil, Motrin)
Ketorolac (Toradol)
Naproxen (Anaprox, Naprosyn)
Propoxyphene (Darvon)
Salsalate (Disalcid)
Tramadol (Ultram)

Pain, moderate to severe
Butorphanol (Stadol)
Fentanyl (Sublimaze)
Hydromorphone (Dilaudid)
Meperidine (Demerol)
Methadone (Dolophine)
Morphine (MS Contin)
Nalbuphine (Nubain)
Oxycodone (OxyFast, Roxicodone)
Ziconotide (Prialt)

Panic attack disorder
Alprazolam (Xanax)
Clonazepam (Klonopin)
Paroxetine (Paxil)
Sertraline (Zoloft)

Parkinsonism
Amantadine (Symmetrel)
Apomorphine (Apokyn)
Bromocriptine (Parlodel)
Carbidopa/levodopa (Sinemet)
Diphenhydramine (Benadryl)
Entacapone (Comtan)
Pergolide (Permax)
Pramipexole (Mirapex)
Ropinirole (Requip)
Selegiline (Eldepryl)
Tolcapone (Tasmar)

Peptic ulcer disease
Cimetidine (Tagamet)
Esomeprazole (Nexium)
Famotidine (Pepcid)
Lansoprazole (Prevacid)
Misoprostol (Cytotec)
Nizatidine (Axid)
Omeprazole (Prilosec)
Pantoprazole (Protonix)
Rabeprazole (Aciphex)
Ranitidine (Zantac)
Sucralfate (Carafate)

Pneumonia
Amoxicillin (Amoxil)
Amoxicillin/clavulanate (Augmentin)
Ampicillin (Polycillin)
Azithromycin (Zithromax)
Cefaclor (Ceclor)
Cefpodoxime (Vantin)
Ceftriaxone (Rocephin)
Cefuroxime (Kefurox, Zinacef)
Clarithromycin (Biaxin)

Co-trimoxazole (Bactrim, Septra)
Dirithromycin (Dynabac)
Erythromycin
Gentamicin (Garamycin)
Loracarbef (Lorabid)
Piperacillin/tazobactam (Zosyn)
Tobramycin (Nebcin)
Vancomycin (Vancocin)

Pneumonia, *Pneumocystis carinii*
Atovaquone (Mepron)
Clindamycin (Cleocin)
Co-trimoxazole (Bactrim, Septra)
Pentamidine (Pentam)
Trimethoprim (Proloprim)

Prostatic hyperplasia, benign
Alfuzosin (UroXatral)
Doxazosin (Cardura)
Finasteride (Proscar)
Tamsulosin (Flomax)
Terazosin (Hytrin)

Pruritus
Amcinonide (Cyclocort)
Brompheniramine (Dimetane)
Cetirizine (Zyrtec)
Chlorpheniramine (Dimetane)
Clemastine (Tavist)
Clobetasol (Temovate)
Cyproheptadine (Periactin)
Desloratadine (Clarinex)
Desonide (Tridesilon)
Desoximetasone (Topicort)
Diphenhydramine (Benadryl)
Fluocinolone (Synalar)
Fluocinonide (Lidex)
Halobetasol (Ultravate)
Hydrocortisone (Cort-Dome, Hytone)
Hydroxyzine (Atarax, Vistaril)
Prednisolone (Prelone)
Prednisone (Deltasone)
Promethazine (Phenergan)

Psychosis
Aripiprazole (Abilify)
Chlorpromazine (Thorazine)
Clozapine (Clozaril)
Fluphenazine (Prolixin)
Haloperidol (Haldol)
Lithium (Lithobid)
Olanzapine (Zyprexa)
Perphenazine (Trilafon)
Quetiapine (Seroquel)
Risperidone (Risperdal)
Thioridazine (Mellaril)
Thiothixene (Navane)
Ziprasidone (Geodon)

Reflux esophagitis (GERD)
Cimetidine (Tagamet)
Esomeprazole (Nexium)
Famotidine (Pepcid)
Lansoprazole (Prevacid)
Metoclopramide (Reglan)
Nizatidine (Axid)
Omeprazole (Prilosec)
Pantoprazole (Protonix)
Rabeprazole (Aciphex)
Ranitidine (Zantac)

Respiratory distress syndrome (RDS)
Beractant (Survanta)
Calfactant (Infasurf)
Poractant alfa (Curosurf)

Schizophrenia
Aripiprazole (Abilify)
Chlorpromazine (Thorazine)
Clozapine (Clozaril)
Fluphenazine (Prolixin)
Haloperidol (Haldol)
Lithium (Lithobid)
Olanzapine (Zyprexa)
Perphenazine (Trilafon)
Quetiapine (Seroquel)
Risperidone (Risperdal)
Thioridazine (Mellaril)
Thiothixene (Navane)
Ziprasidone (Geodon)

Smoking cessation
Bupropion (Zyban)
Clonidine (Catapres)
Nicotine (Nicoderm, Nicotrol)

Thrombosis
Dalteparin (Fragmin)
Enoxaparin (Lovenox)
Heparin
Tinzaparin (Innohep)
Warfarin (Coumadin)

Thyroid disorders
Levothyroxine (Levoxyl, Synthroid)
Liothyronine (Cytomel)
Thyroid

Transient ischemic attack (TIA)
Aspirin
Clopidogrel (Plavix)
Ticlopidine (Ticlid)
Warfarin (Coumadin)

Tremor
Atenolol (Tenormin)
Chlordiazepoxide (Librium)
Diazepam (Valium)
Lorazepam (Ativan)
Metoprolol (Lopressor)
Nadolol (Corgard)
Propranolol (Inderal)

Tuberculosis
Ethambutol (Myambutol)
Isoniazid (INH)
Pyrazinamide
Rifabutin (Mycobutin)
Rifampin (Rifadin)
Rifapentine (Priftin)
Streptomycin

Urticaria
Cetirizine (Zyrtec)
Cimetidine (Tagamet)
Clemastine (Tavist)
Cyproheptadine (Periactin)
Diphenhydramine (Benadryl)
Hydroxyzine (Atarax, Vistaril)
Loratadine (Claritin)
Promethazine (Phenergan)
Ranitidine (Zantac)

Vertigo
Dimenhydrinate (Dramamine)
Diphenhydramine (Benadryl)
Meclizine (Antivert)
Scopolamine (Trans-Derm Scop)

Vomiting
Aprepiant (Emend)
Chlorpromazine (Thorazine)
Dexamethasone (Decadron)
Dimenhydrinate (Dramamine)
Dolasetron (Anzemet)
Dronabinol (Marinol)
Droperidol (Inapsine)
Granisetron (Kytril)
Hydroxyzine (Vistaril)
Lorazepam (Ativan)
Meclizine (Antivert)
Metoclopramide (Reglan)
Ondansetron (Zofran)
Palonosetron (Aloxi)
Prochlorperazine (Compazine)
Promethazine (Phenergan)
Trimethobenzamide (Tigan)

Zollinger-Ellison syndrome
Aluminum salts
Cimetidine (Tagamet)
Esomeprazole (Nexim)
Famotidine (Pepcid)
Lansoprazole (Prevacid)
Omeprazole (Prilosec)
Pantoprazole (Protonix)
Rabeprazole (Aciphex)
Ranitidine (Zantac)

1 Aminoglycosides

amikacin sulfate
gentamicin sulfate
kanamycin sulfate
neomycin sulfate
streptomycin sulfate
tobramycin sulfate

Uses: Aminoglycosides are used to treat serious infections when other, less toxic agents aren't effective, are contraindicated, or require adjunctive therapy (such as penicillins or cephalosporins). Aminoglycosides primarily treat infections caused by gram-negative microorganisms, such as *Proteus mirabilis, Klebsiella pneumoniae, Pseudomonas aeruginosa, Escherichia coli, Serratia marcescens,* and *Enterobacter* species. They're inactive against most gram-positive microorganisms. These agents aren't well absorbed systemically from the GI tract and must be administered parenterally for systemic infections. Oral agents are given to suppress intestinal bacteria.

Action: Aminoglycosides are transported across bacterial cell membranes and are bactericidal. These drugs irreversibly bind to specific receptor proteins on bacterial ribosomes, thereby interfering with protein synthesis, preventing cell reproduction, and eventually causing cell death. (See the illustration *Sites and Mechanisms of Action: Anti-infective Agents,* page 2.)

COMBINATION PRODUCTS

NEOSPORIN GU IRRIGANT: neomycin/polymyxin B (an anti-infective) 40 mg/200,000 units/ml.
NEOSPORIN OINTMENT, TRIPLE ANTIBIOTIC: neomycin/polymyxin B (an anti-infective)/bacitracin (an anti-infective) 3.5 mg/5,000 units/400 units/g; 3.5 mg/10,000 units/400 units/g.
TOBRADEX: tobramycin/dexamethasone (a steroid) 0.3%/0.1% per milliliter or per gram.

amikacin sulfate

am-i-**kay**-sin
(Amikin)
Do not confuse amikacin or Amikin with Amicar.

CATEGORY AND SCHEDULE

Pregnancy Risk Category: C

MECHANISM OF ACTION

An aminoglycoside antibiotic that irreversibly binds to protein on bacterial ribosomes. **Therapeutic Effect:** Interferes with protein synthesis of susceptible microorganisms.

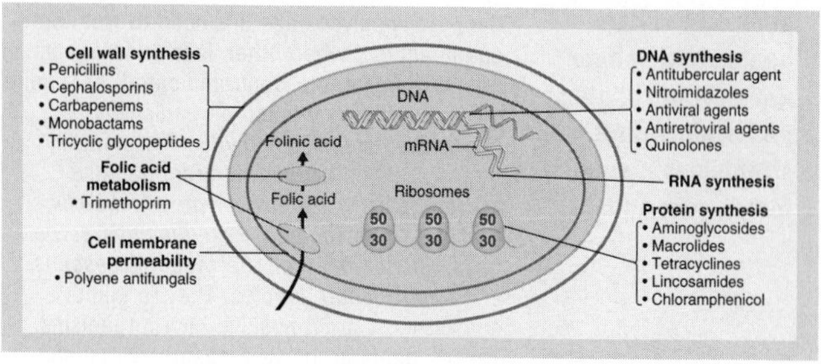

Sites and Mechanisms of Action: Anti-infective Agents

The goal of anti-infective therapy is to kill or inhibit the growth of microorganisms, such as bacteria, viruses, and fungi. To achieve this goal, anti-infective agents must reach their targets, which usually occurs through absorption and distribution by the circulatory system. When the target is reached, a drug can kill or suppress microorganisms by:

- inhibiting cell wall synthesis or activating enzymes that disrupt the cell wall, which leads to cellular weakening, lysis, and death. Penicillins (ampicillin), cephalosporins (cefazolin), carbapenems (imipenem), monobactams (aztreonam), and tricyclic glycopeptides (vancomycin) act in this way.
- altering cell membrane permeability through direct action on the cell wall, which allows intracellular substances to leak out and destabilizes the cell. Polyene antifungals (amphotericin B) work by this mechanism.
- altering protein synthesis by binding to bacterial ribosomes (50 or 30) or affecting ribosomal function, which leads to cell death or slowed growth, respectively. Aminoglycosides (gentamicin), macrolides (erythromycin), tetracyclines (doxycycline), lincosamides (clindamycin), and the miscellaneous anti-infective chloramphenicol act in this way.
- inhibiting DNA or RNA—including messenger RNA (mRNA)—by synthesis by binding to nucleic acids or interacting with enzymes required for their synthesis. Antitubercular agents (rifampin), nitroimidazoles (metronidazole), antiviral agents (acyclovir), antiretroviral agents (stavudine), and quinolones (ciprofloxacin) act like this.
- inhibiting the metabolism of folic acid and folinic acid or other cellular components that are essential for bacterial cell growth. The miscellaneous anti-infective trimethoprim has this mechanism of action.

PHARMACOKINETICS

Rapid, complete absorption after IM administration. Protein binding: 0%–10%. Widely distributed (doesn't cross the blood-brain barrier, low concentrations in CSF). Excreted unchanged in urine. Removed by hemodialysis. ***Half-life:*** 2–4 hr (increased in impaired renal function and neonates; decreased in cystic fibrosis and burn or febrile patients).

AVAILABILITY

Injection. 50 mg/ml, 250 mg/ml.

ections

sual dosage, apply

al impairment
rance greater than
. Dosage interval q12h.
learance 20–40 ml/min.
rval q24h.
clearance less than 20
Monitor levels to determine
interval.

LABEL USES
pical: Prophylaxis of minor bacte-
l skin infections, treatment of
ermal ulcer

CONTRAINDICATIONS
Hypersensitivity to gentamicin, other aminoglycosides (cross-sensitivity), or their components. Sulfite sensitivity may result in anaphylaxis, especially in asthmatic patients

INTERACTIONS
Drug

Nephrotoxic mediations, other aminoglycosides, ototoxic medications: May increase the risk of nephrotoxicity or ototoxicity.
Neuromuscular blockers: May increase neuromuscular blockade.

Herbal

None known.

Food

None known.

DIAGNOSTIC TEST EFFECTS
May increase serum creatinine, serum bilirubin, BUN, serum LDH, AST (SGOT), and ALT (SGPT) levels. May decrease serum calcium, magnesium, potassium, and sodium concentrations. Therapeutic peak serum level is 6–10 mcg/ml and trough is 0.5–2 mcg/ml. Toxic peak serum level is greater than 10 mcg/ml, and trough is greater than mcg/ml.

IV INCOMPATIBILITIES
Allopurinol (Aloprim), ampho B complex (Abelcet, AmBiso Amphotec), furosemide (Lasix heparin, hetastarch (Hespan), i bicin (Idamycin), indomethaci (Indocin), propofol (Diprivan)

IV COMPATIBILITIES
Amiodarone (Cordarone), diltia (Cardizem), enalapril (Vasotec) filgrastim (Neupogen), hydrom phone (Dilaudid), insulin, loraz (Ativan), magnesium sulfate, m azolam (Versed), morphine, multivitamins

SIDE EFFECTS
Occasional

IM: Pain, induration
IV: Phlebitis, thrombophlebitis, hypersensitivity reactions (fever, pruritus, rash, urticaria)
Ophthalmic: Burning, tearing, itc ing, blurred vision
Topical: Redness, itching

Rare

Alopecia, hypertension, weakness

SERIOUS REACTIONS
! Nephrotoxicity (as evidenced by increased BUN and serum creatini levels and decreased creatinine clearance) may be reversible if the drug is stopped at the first sign of symptoms.
! Irreversible ototoxicity (manifeste as tinnitus, dizziness, ringing or roaring in the ears, and diminished hearing), and neurotoxicity (as evidenced by headache, dizziness, lethargy, tremor, and visual disturbances) occur occasionally. The risk of these effects increases with higher dosages or prolonged

INDICATIONS AND DOSAGES
▸ UTIs

IV, IM

Adults, Elderly. 250 mg q12h.

▸ Moderate to severe infections

IV, IM

Adults, Elderly. 15 mg/kg/day in divided doses q8–12h. Maximum 1.5 g/day.
Children, Infants. 15–22.5 mg/kg/day in divided doses q8h.
Neonates. 7.5–10 mg/kg/dose q8–24h.

▸ Dosage in renal impairment

Dosage and frequency are modified based on the degree of renal impairment and serum drug concentration. After a loading dose of 5–7.5 mg/kg, the maintenance dose and frequency are based on serum creatinine levels and creatinine clearance.

CONTRAINDICATIONS
Hypersensitivity to amikacin, or other aminoglycosides (cross-sensitivity), or their components

INTERACTIONS
Drug

Nephrotoxic medications, other aminoglycosides, ototoxic medications: May increase the risk of nephrotoxicity or ototoxicity.
Neuromuscular blockers: May enhance neuromuscular blockade.

Herbal

None known.

Food

None known.

DIAGNOSTIC TEST EFFECTS
May increase serum bilirubin, BUN, serum creatinine, serum LDH, AST (SGOT) and ALT (SGPT) levels. May decrease serum calcium, magnesium, potassium, and sodium concentrations. Therapeutic peak serum level is greater than 30 mcg/ml; toxic trough serum level is greater than 10 mcg/ml.

IV INCOMPATIBILITIES
Amphotericin, ampicillin, cefazolin (Ancef), heparin, propofol (Diprivan)

IV COMPATIBILITIES
Amiodarone (Cordarone), aztreonam (Azactam), calcium gluconate, cefepime (Maxipime), cimetidine (Tagamet), ciprofloxacin (Cipro), clindamycin (Cleocin), diltiazem (Cardizem), enalapril (Vasotec), esmolol (BreviBloc), fluconazole (Diflucan), furosemide (Lasix), levofloxacin (Levaquin), lorazepam (Ativan), magnesium sulfate, midazolam (Versed), morphine, ondansetron (Zofran), potassium chloride, ranitidine (Zantac), vancomycin

SIDE EFFECTS
Frequent

IM: Pain, induration
IV: Phlebitis, thrombophlebitis

Occasional

Hypersensitivity reactions (rash, fever, urticaria, pruritus)

Rare

Neuromuscular blockade (difficulty breathing, drowsiness, weakness)

SERIOUS REACTIONS
! Serious reactions may include nephrotoxicity (as evidenced by increased thirst, decreased appetite, nausea, vomiting, increased BUN and serum creatinine levels, and decreased creatinine clearance); neurotoxicity (manifested as muscle twitching, visual disturbances, seizures, and tingling); and ototoxicity (as evidenced by tinnitus, dizziness, and loss of hearing).

NURSING CONSIDERATIONS

Baseline Assessment

- Determine the patient's history of allergies, especially to aminoglycosides and sulfites.
- Expect to correct dehydration before beginning aminoglycoside therapy.
- Establish the patient's baseline hearing acuity before beginning therapy.
- Expect to obtain a specimen for culture and sensitivity testing before giving the first dose. Therapy may begin before test results are known.

Lifespan Considerations

- Amikacin readily crosses the placenta, and small amounts are distributed in breast milk. It may produce fetal nephrotoxicity.
- Neonates and premature infants may be more susceptible to amikacin toxicity because of their immature renal function.
- Elderly patients are at increased risk for amikacin toxicity because of age-related renal impairment. They're also at increased risk for hearing loss.

Precautions

- Use amikacin cautiously in patients with 8th cranial nerve (vestibulocochlear nerve) impairment, decreased renal function, myasthenia gravis, or Parkinson's disease.

Administration and Handling

◀ALERT▶ Space amikacin doses evenly around the clock. The drug dosage is based on the patient's ideal body weight. Peak and trough serum levels are determined periodically to maintain desired serum concentrations and minimize the risk of amikacin toxicity. Therapeutic peak serum level is 20 to 30 mcg/ml; therapeutic trough serum level is 1 to 9 mcg/ml. Toxic peak serum level is greater than 30 mcg/ml; toxic trough serum level is greater than 10 mcg/ml.

IV

- Store vials at room temperature.
- Solutions normally appear clear but may become pale yellow; the yellow color doesn't affect the drug's potency. Discard the solution if a precipitate forms or dark discoloration occurs.
- Intermittent IV infusion (piggyback) is stable for 24 hours at room temperature.
- Dilute each 500 mg with 100 ml of 0.9% NaCl or D_5W.
- Infuse over 30 to 60 minutes for adults and older children. Infuse over 60 to 120 minutes for infants and young children.

IM

- Give deep IM injections slowly to minimize patient discomfort. Injections administered into the gluteus maximus are less painful than those given in the lateral aspect of the thigh.

Intervention and Evaluation

- Monitor the patient's intake and output to maintain hydration.
- Expect to monitor urinalysis results to detect casts, RBCs, WBCs, and decreased specific gravity.
- Expect to monitor peak and trough serum amikacin levels.
- Be alert for ototoxic and neurotoxic side effects.
- Assess for pain and induration at the IM injection site.
- Evaluate the IV infusion site for signs and symptoms of phlebitis, such as heat, pain, and red streaking over the vein.
- Inspect the patient's skin for a rash.
- Be alert for signs and symptoms of superinfection, particularly changes in the oral mucosa, diarrhea, and genital or anal pruritus.
- In patients with neuromuscular isorders, assess the respiratory esponse carefully.

atient Teaching

- Explain to the patient the i nce of receiving the full c mikacin treatment.
- Advise the patient that IM i ions may cause discomfort.
- Instruct the patient to notify the hysician if any hearing, visual, alance, or urinary problems occur, even if they start after therapy is completed.
- Caution the patient not to take any other drugs without first notifying the physician.
- Inform the patient that laboratory ests are an essential part of therapy.

gentamicin sulfate

jen-ta-**mye**-sin
(Alcomicin[CAN], Cidomycin[CAN], Garamycin, Genoptic, Gentak, Gentacidin)

CATEGORY AND SCHEDULE

Pregnancy Risk Category: C

MECHANISM OF ACTION

An aminoglycoside antibiotic that irreversibly binds to the protein of bacterial ribosomes. **Therapeutic Effect:** Interferes with protein synthesis of susceptible microorganisms. Bactericidal.

PHARMACOKINETICS

Rapid, complete absorption after IM administration. Protein binding: less than 30%. Widely distributed (doesn't cross the blood-brain barrier, low concentrations in CSF). Excreted unchanged in urine. Removed by hemodialysis. ***Half-life:*** 2–4 hr (increased in impaired renal function and neonates; decreased in

INDICATIO…

▸ **Acute pelvic, abdominal, joint, … burn wound, postope… skin or skin-structure i… complicated UTIs; septice… meningitis**

IV, IM

Adults, Elderly. Usual dosage, 3–6 mg/kg/day in divided doses q8h or 4–6.6 mg/kg once a day.

Children 5–12 yr. Usual dosage 2–2.5 mg/kg/dose q8h.

Children younger than 5 yr. Usual dosage, 2.5 mg/kg/dose q8h.

Neonates. Usual dosage 2.5–3.5 mg/kg/dose q8–12h.

▸ **Hemodialysis**

IV, IM

Adults, Elderly. 0.5–0.7 mg/kg/dose after dialysis.

Children. 1.25–1.75 mg/kg/dose after dialysis.

Intrathecal

Adults. 4–8 mg/day.

Children 3 mo–12 yr. 1–2 mg/day.

Neonates. 1 mg/day.

▸ **Superficial eye infections**

Ophthalmic Ointment

Adults, Elderly. Usual dosage, apply thin strip to conjunctiva 2–3 times a day.

Ophthalmic Solution

Adults, Elderly, Children. Usual dosage, 1–2 drops q2–4h up to 2 drops/hr.

therapy and when the solution is applied directly to the mucosa.

! Superinfections, particularly with fungal infections, may result from bacterial imbalance no matter which administration route is used.

! Ophthalmic application may cause paresthesia of conjunctiva or mydriasis.

NURSING CONSIDERATIONS

Baseline Assessment

• Expect to correct dehydration before beginning parenteral therapy.

• Establish the patient's baseline hearing acuity before starting therapy.

◂ALERT▸ Before giving gentamicin, determine if the patient has a history of allergies, especially to aminoglycosides, sulfites, and parabens (for topical and ophthalmic forms).

Lifespan Considerations

• Gentamicin readily crosses the placenta; it is unknown if it's distributed in breast milk.

• Use cautiously in neonates because their immature renal function increases gentamicin half-life and risk of toxicity.

• Age-related renal impairment may require a dosage adjustment in elderly patients.

Precautions

◂ALERT▸ Cumulative gentamicin effects may occur with concurrent systemic administration and topical application to large areas.

• Use cautiously in elderly and neonatal patients because of age-related renal insufficiency or immaturity.

• Use cautiously in patients with neuromuscular disorders because of the potential for respiratory depression.

• Use cautiously in patients with prior hearing loss, renal impairment, or vertigo.

Administration and Handling

◂ALERT▸ Space parenteral doses evenly around the clock. Gentamicin dosage is based on ideal body weight. As ordered, monitor peak and trough serum drug levels periodically to maintain the desired serum concentrations and to minimize the risk of toxicity. The therapeutic peak serum level is 6 to 10 mcg/ml, and the therapeutic trough level is 0.5 to 2 mcg/ml. The toxic peak serum level is greater than 10 mcg/ml and the toxic trough level is greater than 2 mcg/ml.

IV

• Store vials at room temperature.

• The solution normally appears clear or slightly yellow.

• Intermittent IV infusion or IV piggyback solution is stable for 24 hours at room temperature.

• Discard the IV solution if a precipitate forms.

• Dilute with 50 to 200 ml of D_5W or 0.9% NaCl. The amount of diluent for infants and children depends on individual needs.

• Infuse over 30 to 60 minutes for adults and older children. Infuse over 60 to 120 minutes for infants and young children.

IM

• To minimize injection site pain, administer the IM injection slowly and deep in the gluteus maximus rather than the lateral aspect of thigh.

Intrathecal

• Use only 2 mg/ml of the intrathecal preparation without preservative.

• Mix with 10% of the estimated CSF volume or NaCl.

• Use the intrathecal form immediately after preparation. Discard any unused portion.

• Give over 3 to 5 minutes.

Ophthalmic
• Place a gloved finger on the patient's lower eyelid, and pull it out until a pocket is formed between the eye and lower lid.
• Hold the dropper above the pocket and place the correct number of drops (or ¼ to ½ inch of ointment) into the pocket. Close the eye gently.
• After administering ophthalmic solution, apply digital pressure to the lacrimal sac for 1 to 2 minutes to minimize drainage into the nose and throat, thereby reducing the risk of systemic effects.
• After applying ophthalmic ointment, close the patient's eye for 1 to 2 minutes. Instruct the patient to roll the eyeball to increase the drug's contact with the eye.
• Use tissue to remove excess solution or ointment around the eye.

Intervention and Evaluation
• Monitor the patient's intake and output and urinalysis results as appropriate. Urge the patient to drink fluids to maintain adequate hydration. Monitor urinalysis results for casts, RBCs, WBCs, and decreased specific gravity.
• Be alert for ototoxic and neurotoxic side effects.
• Assess for pain and induration at the IM injection site.
• Evaluate the IV infusion site for signs and symptoms of phlebitis, such as heat, pain, and red streaking over the vein.
• Inspect the patient's skin for a rash.
• If giving ophthalmic gentamicin, monitor the patient's eye for burning, itching, redness, and tearing.
• If giving topical gentamicin, monitor the patient for itching and redness.
• Be alert for signs and symptoms of superinfection, particularly changes in the oral mucosa, diarrhea, and genital or anal pruritus.
• In patients with neuromuscular disorders, assess the respiratory response carefully.
• Monitor peak and trough serum drug levels.

Patient Teaching
• Advise the patient to notify the physician if any balance, hearing, urinary, or vision problems occur, even after gentamicin therapy is completed.
• Inform the patient that IM injection may cause discomfort.
• Inform the patient using ophthalmic gentamicin that blurred vision, iritation, redness, or tearing may occur briefly after each dose. Advise him or her to notify the physician if these symptoms persist.
• Instruct the patient using topical gentamicin to clean the affected area gently before applying the ointment and to notify the physician if itching or redness occurs.

kanamycin sulfate
kan-a-**mye**-sin
(Kantrex)

CATEGORY AND SCHEDULE
Pregnancy Risk Category: Unavailable for irrigating solution.

MECHANISM OF ACTION
An aminoglycoside antibiotic that irreversibly binds to protein on bacterial ribosomes. **Therapeutic Effect:** Interferes with protein synthesis of susceptible microorganisms.

AVAILABILITY
Injection: 1 g/3 ml.

INDICATIONS AND DOSAGES

▸ Wound and surgical site irrigation

Adults, Elderly. 0.25% solution to irrigate pleural space, ventricular or abscess cavities, wounds, or surgical sites.

CONTRAINDICATIONS

Hypersensitivity to kanamycin, other aminoglycosides (cross-sensitivity), or their components

INTERACTIONS

Drug

None significant.

Herbal

None significant.

Food

None significant.

DIAGNOSTIC TEST EFFECTS

None known.

SIDE EFFECTS

Occasional

Hypersensitivity reactions (fever, pruritus, rash, urticaria)

Rare

Headache

SERIOUS REACTIONS

! None known.

NURSING CONSIDERATIONS

Baseline Assessment

• Assess the patient for hypersensitivity to kanamycin or other aminoglycosides.

Lifespan Considerations

• There are no age-related precautions noted in children or the elderly.

neomycin sulfate

nee-oh-**mye**-sin

(Myciguent, NeoFradin, Neosulf[AUS])

CATEGORY AND SCHEDULE

Pregnancy Risk Category: C

OTC (topical ointment 0.5% only)

MECHANISM OF ACTION

An aminoglycoside antibiotic that binds to bacterial microorganisms. **Therapeutic Effect:** Interferes with bacterial protein synthesis.

AVAILABILITY

Tablets: 500 mg.

Ointment (Myciguent): 0.5%.

Oral Solution (Neo-Fradin): 125 mg/5 ml.

INDICATIONS AND DOSAGES

▸ Preoperative bowel antisepsis

PO

Adults, Elderly. 1 g/hr for 4 doses; then 1 g q4h for 5 doses or 1 g at 1 p.m., 2 p.m., and 10 p.m. (with erythromycin) on day before surgery.

Children. 90 mg/kg/day in divided doses q4h for 2 days or 25 mg/kg at 1 p.m., 2 p.m., and 10 p.m. on day before surgery.

▸ Hepatic encephalopathy

PO

Adults, Elderly. 4–12 g/day in divided doses q4–6h.

Children. 2.5–7 g/m^2/day in divided doses q4–6h.

▸ Diarrhea caused by *Escherichia coli*

PO

Adults, Elderly. 3 g/day in divided doses q6h.

Children. 50 mg/kg/day in divided doses q6h.

▸ Minor skin infections
Topical
Adults, Elderly, Children. Usual dosage, apply to affected area 1–3 times/day.

CONTRAINDICATIONS
Hypersensitivity to neomycin, other aminoglycosides (cross-sensitivity), or their components

INTERACTIONS
Drug
Nephrotoxic medications, other aminoglycosides, ototoxic medications: May increase nephrotoxicity and ototoxicity if significant systemic absorption occurs.
Herbal
None known.
Food
None known.

DIAGNOSTIC TEST EFFECTS
None known.

SIDE EFFECTS
Frequent
Systemic: Nausea, vomiting, diarrhea, irritation of mouth or rectal area
Topical: Itching, redness, swelling, rash
Rare
Systemic: Malabsorption syndrome, neuromuscular blockade (difficulty breathing, drowsiness, weakness)

SERIOUS REACTIONS
! Nephrotoxicity (as evidenced by increased BUN and serum creatinine levels and decreased creatinine clearance) may be reversible if the drug is stopped at the first sign of nephrotoxic symptoms.
! Irreversible ototoxicity (manifested as tinnitus, dizziness, and impaired hearing) and neurotoxicity (as evidenced by headache, dizziness, lethargy, tremor, and visual disturbances) occur occasionally.
! Severe respiratory depression and anaphylaxis occur rarely.
! Superinfections, particularly fungal infections, may occur.

NURSING CONSIDERATIONS
Baseline Assessment
• Expect to correct dehydration before beginning neomycin therapy.
• Establish the patient's baseline hearing acuity before beginning therapy.
Precautions
• Use neomycin cautiously in elderly patients, infants, and other patients with renal insufficiency or immaturity as well as those with neuromuscular disorders, hearing loss, or vertigo.
Intervention and Evaluation
• Assess the patient for signs and symptoms of ototoxicity and neurotoxicity.
• Evaluate the patient for signs and symptoms of a hypersensitivity reaction. With topical application, symptoms may include a rash, redness, or itching.
• Watch the patient for signs and symptoms of superinfection, particularly diarrhea, genital or anal pruritus, and stomatitis.
Patient Teaching
• Advise the patient to continue taking neomycin for the full course of treatment and to space doses evenly around the clock.
• Caution the patient to notify the physician if he or she experiences dizziness, impaired hearing, or ringing in the ears.
• Instruct the patient using topical neomycin to clean the affected area gently before applying the drug and to notify the physician if itching or redness occurs.

streptomycin sulfate
strep-toe-**mye**-sin

CATEGORY AND SCHEDULE
Pregnancy Risk Category: D

MECHANISM OF ACTION
An aminoglycoside that binds directly to the 30S ribosomal subunits causing a faulty peptide sequence to form in the protein chain. **Therapeutic Effect:** Inhibits bacterial protein synthesis.

AVAILABILITY
Injection: 1 g.

INDICATIONS AND DOSAGES
▸ **Tuberculosis**

IM

Adults. 15 mg/kg/day. Maximum: 1 g/day.
Elderly. 10 mg/kg/day. Maximum: 750 mg/day.
Children. 20–40 mg/kg/day. Maximum: 1 g/day.

▸ **Dosage in renal impairment:**

Creatinine Clearance	Dosage Interval
10–50 ml/min	q24–72h
less than 10 ml/min	q72–96h

CONTRAINDICATIONS
Pregnancy

INTERACTIONS
Drug

Amphotericin, loop diuretics: May increase the nephrotoxicity of streptomycin.
Neuromuscular blockers: May increase the effects of streptomycin.

Herbal

None known.

Food

None known.

DIAGNOSTIC TEST EFFECTS
None known.

SIDE EFFECTS
Occasional

Hypotension, drowsiness, headache, drug fever, paresthesia, rash, nausea, vomiting, anemia, arthralgia, weakness, tremor

SERIOUS REACTIONS
! Nephrotoxicity (as evidenced by increased BUN and serum creatinine levels and decreased creatinine clearance) may be reversible if the drug is stopped at the first sign of nephrotoxic symptoms.
! Irreversible ototoxicity (manifested as tinnitus, dizziness, ringing or roaring in the ears, and impaired hearing) and neurotoxicity (as evidenced by headache, dizziness, lethargy, tremor, and visual disturbances) occur occasionally. Symptoms of ototoxicity, nephrotoxicity, and neuromuscular toxicity may occur.

NURSING CONSIDERATIONS
Baseline Assessment

- Determine if the patient is hypersensitive to aminoglycosides, pregnant, or being treated for other medical conditions such as myasthenia gravis or parkinsonism.

Precautions

- Use streptomycin cautiously in patients with tinnitus, vertigo, neuromuscular disorders, or renal impairment.

Administration and Handling

IM

- Inject IM streptomycin deep into a large muscle mass.
- Be aware that for patients who are

unable to tolerate IM injections, streptomycin may be given as an IV infusion over 30 to 60 minutes.

Intervention and Evaluation

- Monitor the patient's hearing, renal function, and serum concentrations of streptomycin.

Patient Teaching

- Advise the patient to notify the physician if he or she experiences such symptoms as hearing loss, dizziness, or fullness or roaring in the ears.

tobramycin sulfate

tow-bra-**my**-sin

(AK-Tob, Apo-Tobramycin [CAN], Nebcin, PMS-Tobramycin, TOBI, Tobrex)

CATEGORY AND SCHEDULE

Pregnancy Risk Category: C (B, ophthalmic form)

MECHANISM OF ACTION

An aminoglycoside antibiotic that irreversibly binds to protein on bacterial ribosomes. **Therapeutic Effect:** Interferes with protein synthesis of susceptible microorganisms.

PHARMACOKINETICS

Rapid, complete absorption after IM administration. Protein binding: less than 30%. Widely distributed (doesn't cross the blood-brain barrier; low concentrations in CSF). Excreted unchanged in urine. Removed by hemodialysis. ***Half-life:*** 2–4 hr (increased in impaired renal function and neonates; decreased in cystic fibrosis and febrile or burn patients).

AVAILABILITY

Injection Solution (Nebcin): 10 mg/ml, 40 mg/ml.
Injection Powder for Reconstitution (Nebcin): 1.2 g.
Ophthalmic Ointment (Tobrex): 0.3%.
Ophthalmic Solution (AKTob, Tobrex): 0.3%.
Nebulization Solution (TOBI): 60 mg/ml.

INDICATIONS AND DOSAGES

▸ **Skin and skin-structure, bone, joint, respiratory tract, postoperative, intra-abdominal, and burn wound infections; complicated UTIs; septicemia; meningitis**

IV, IM

Adults, Elderly. 3–6 mg/kg/day in 3 divided doses or 4–6.6 mg/kg once a day.

▸ **Superficial eye infections, including blepharitis, conjunctivitis, keratitis, and corneal ulcers**

Ophthalmic Ointment

Adults, Elderly. Usual dosage, apply a thin strip to conjunctiva q8–12h (q3–4h for severe infections).

Ophthalmic Solution

Adults, Elderly. Usual dosage, 1–2 drops in affected eye q4h (2 drops/hr for severe infections).

▸ **Bronchopulmonary infections in patients with cystic fibrosis**

Inhalation Solution

Adults. Usual dosage, 60–80 mg twice a day for 28 days, then off for 28 days.

Children. 40–80 mg 2–3 times/day.

▸ **Dosage in renal impairment**

Dosage and frequency are modified based on the degree of renal impairment and the serum drug concentration. After a loading dose of 1–2 mg/kg, the maintenance dose and frequency are based on serum creatinine levels and creatinine clearance.

CONTRAINDICATIONS
Hypersensitivity to tobramycin, other aminoglycosides (cross-sensitivity), and their components

INTERACTIONS
Drug
Nephrotoxic medications, other aminoglycosides, ototoxic medications: May increase the risk of nephrotoxicity and ototoxicity.
Neuromuscular blockers: May increase neuromuscular blockade.
Herbal
None known.
Food
None known.

DIAGNOSTIC TEST EFFECTS
May increase serum bilirubin, BUN, serum creatinine, serum LDH, AST (SGOT), and ALT (SGPT) levels. May decrease serum calcium, magnesium, potassium, and sodium concentrations. Therapeutic peak serum level is 5–20 mcg/ml; therapeutic trough serum level is 0.5–2 mcg/ml. Toxic peak serum level is greater than 20 mcg/ml; toxic trough serum level is greater than 2 mcg/ml.

IV INCOMPATIBILITIES
Amphotericin B complex (Abelcet, AmBisome, Amphotec), heparin, hetastarch (Hespan), indomethacin (Indocin), propofol (Diprivan), sargramostim (Leukine, Prokine)

IV COMPATIBILITIES
Amiodarone (Cordarone), calcium gluconate, diltiazem (Cardizem), furosemide (Lasix), hydromorphone (Dilaudid), insulin, magnesium sulfate, midazolam (Versed), morphine, theophylline

SIDE EFFECTS
Occasional
IM: Pain, induration
IV: Phlebitis, thrombophlebitis
Topical: Hypersensitivity reaction (fever, pruritus, rash, urticaria)
Ophthalmic: Tearing, itching, redness, eyelid swelling
Rare
Hypotension, nausea, vomiting

SERIOUS REACTIONS
! Nephrotoxicity (as evidenced by increased BUN and serum creatinine levels and decreased creatinine clearance) may be reversible if the drug is stopped at the first sign of nephrotoxic symptoms.
! Irreversible ototoxicity (manifested as tinnitus, dizziness, ringing or roaring in ears, and hearing loss) and neurotoxicity (manifested as headache, dizziness, lethargy, tremor, and visual disturbances) occur occasionally. The risk of these reactions increases with higher dosages or prolonged therapy and when the solution is applied directly to the mucosa.
! Superinfections, particularly fungal infections, may result from bacterial imbalance with any administration route.
! Anaphylaxis may occur.

NURSING CONSIDERATIONS
Baseline Assessment
• Expect to correct dehydration before beginning parenteral tobramycin therapy.
◂ALERT▸ Determine the patient's history of allergies, especially to aminoglycosides, sulfites, and parabens (for topical and ophthalmic routes), before giving the drug.
• Establish the patient's baseline hearing acuity before beginning therapy.
Lifespan Considerations
• Tobramycin readily crosses the

placenta and is distributed in breast milk.

- Tobramycin may cause fetal nephrotoxicity. The ophthalmic form should not be used in breast-feeding mothers and only when specifically indicated in pregnant women.
- Immature renal function in neonates and premature infants may increase the risk of toxicity.
- Age-related renal impairment may require a dosage adjustment in elderly patients.

Precautions

- Use tobramycin cautiously in patients who also use neuromuscular blockers and in those with impaired renal function or auditory or vestibular impairment.

Administration and Handling

◀ALERT▶ Monitor peak and trough serum drug levels to ensure that the desired blood concentrations are maintained and to minimize the risk of toxicity. Be sure to carefully coordinate the drawing of peak and trough serum drug levels with administration times.

◀ALERT▶ Space parenteral doses evenly around the clock. Be aware that dosages are based on ideal body weight.

IV

- Store vials at room temperature.
- Solutions may be discolored by light or air, but discoloration doesn't affect drug potency.
- Dilute with 50 to 200 ml of D_5W or 0.9% NaCl. The amount of diluent for infant and children dosages depends on individual needs.
- Infuse over 20 to 60 minutes.

IM

- To minimize injection site discomfort, administer the IM injection slowly and deep into the gluteus maximus rather than the lateral aspect of the thigh.

Ophthalmic

- Place a gloved finger on the patient's lower eyelid, and pull it out until a pocket is formed between the eye and lower lid.
- Hold the dropper above the pocket and place the correct number of drops (or ¼ to ½ inch of ointment) into the pocket. Have patient close the eye gently.
- After administering ophthalmic solution, apply digital pressure to the lacrimal sac for 1 to 2 minutes to minimize drainage into the patient's nose and throat, thereby reducing the risk of systemic effects.
- After applying ophthalmic ointment, close the patient's eye for 1 to 2 minutes. Have the patient roll the eyeball to increase the drug's contact with the eye.
- Use a tissue to remove excess solution or ointment around the eye.

Intervention and Evaluation

- Monitor the patient's intake and output and urinalysis results, as appropriate. To maintain adequate hydration, encourage the patient to drink fluids. Monitor urinalysis results for casts, RBCs, WBCs, and decreased specific gravity.
- Expect to monitor peak and trough serum drug levels. The therapeutic peak serum level is 5 to 20 mcg/ml, and the therapeutic trough level is 0.5 to 2 mcg/ml; the toxic peak serum level is greater than 20 mcg/ml, and the toxic trough level is greater than 2 mcg/ml.

◀ALERT▶ Assess the patient for ototoxic and neurotoxic side effects.

- Evaluate the IV infusion site for signs and symptoms of phlebitis, such as heat, pain, and red streaking over the vein.
- Assess for pain and induration at the IM injection site.
- Inspect the patient's skin for a rash.
- Be alert for signs and symptoms of

superinfection, particularly changes in the oral mucosa, diarrhea, and genital or anal pruritus.

- In patients with neuromuscular disorders, assess the respiratory response frequently.
- Assess the patient using ophthalmic tobramycin for itching, redness, eyelid swelling, and tearing.

Patient Teaching

- Warn the patient to notify the physician if any balance, hearing, urinary, or vision problems develop, even after therapy is completed.
- Inform the patient using ophthalmic tobramycin that irritation, redness, blurred vision, or tearing may occur briefly after application.
- Advise him or her to notify the physician if these symptoms persist.

2 Antifungal Agents

amphotericin B
caspofungin acetate
fluconazole
griseofulvin
itraconazole
ketoconazole
nystatin
sertaconazole
terbinafine hydrochloride
voriconazole

Uses: Antifungal agents are used to treat systemic and superficial fungal infections. They're effective against opportunistic and nonopportunistic *systemic* fungal infections. Opportunistic infections, which include candidiasis, aspergillosis, and cryptococcosis, occur primarily in debilitated or immunocompromised patients. Nonopportunistic infections, which include blastomycosis, histoplasmosis, and coccidioidomycosis, are less common. Antifungal agents are especially effective against *superficial* fungal infections caused by *Candida* species and dermatophytes (ringworm). Candidiasis usually affects the mucous membranes and moist skin areas; in chronic infection, organisms may invade the scalp, skin, and nails. Dermatophytosis typically affects only the skin, hair, and nails.

Action: The three types of antifungal agents act in different ways. *Polyene antifungals,* such as amphotericin B and nystatin, bind to sterols in fungal cell walls, forming pores or channels that increase cell wall permeability and allow the leakage of small molecules. *Imidazole antifungals,* such as ketoconazole, inhibit cytochrome P-450 in fungal cells, which impairs ergosterol synthesis and fungal growth. *Allylamine antifungals,* such as terbinafine, disrupt the synthesis of DNA and RNA in fungal cells. (See the illustration *Sites and Mechanism of Action: Antifungal Agents,* page 18.)

COMBINATION PRODUCTS

MYCOLOG: nystatin/triamcinolone (a steroid) 100,000 units/0.1%.
MYCO-TRIACET: nystatin/triamcinolone (a steroid) 100,000 units/0.1%.

amphotericin B ⚑

am-foe-**ter**-i-sin bee
(Abelcet, AmBisome, Amphocin, Amphotec, Fungizone)

CATEGORY AND SCHEDULE

Pregnancy Risk Category: B

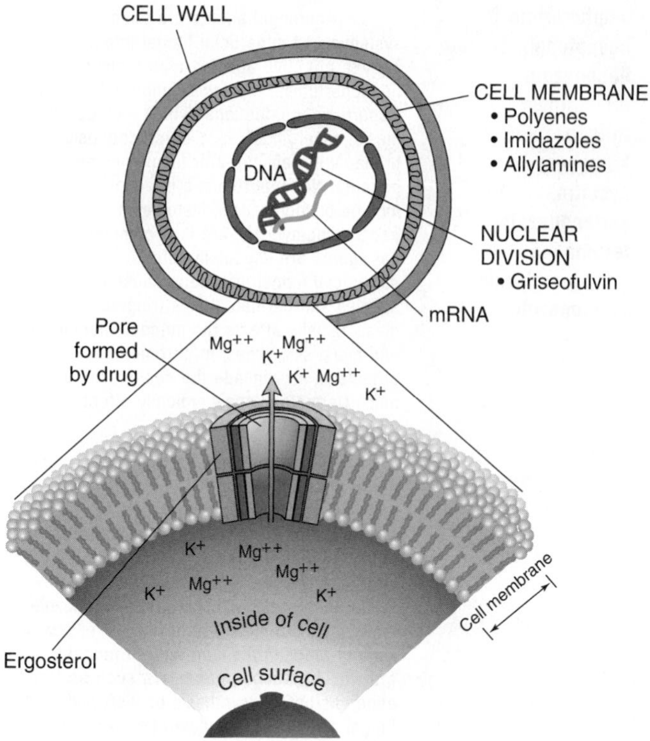

Sites and Mechanism of Action: Antifungal Agents

Antifungal agents primarily affect fungi at one of two sites: the cell membrane or the cell nucleus. Most of these agents, such as polyene, imidazole, and allylamine antifungals, act on the fungal cell membrane. Polyene antifungals, such as amphotericin B, bind to ergosterol and increase cell membrane permeability. Imidazole antifungals, such as fluconazole and ketoconazole, interfere with ergosterol synthesis by inhibiting the cytochrome P_{450} enzyme system, altering the cell membrane, and inhibiting fungal growth. Allylamine antifungals, such as terbinafine, inhibit the enzyme squaline epoxidase, which disrupts ergosterol production and cell membrane integrity. When cell membrane permeability increases, cellular components, including potassium (K^+) and magnesium (Mg^{++}), leak out. Loss of these cellular components leads to cell death.

Another antifungal agent, griseofulvin, directly affects the fungal nucleus, interfering with mitosis. By binding to structures in the mitotic spindle, it prevents cells from dividing, which eventually leads to their death.

MECHANISM OF ACTION

An antifungal and antiprotozoal that is generally fungistatic but may become fungicidal with high dosages or very susceptible microorganisms. This drug binds to sterols in the fungal cell membrane. **Therapeutic Effect:** Increases fungal cell-membrane permeability, allowing loss of potassium and other cellular components.

PHARMACOKINETICS

Protein binding: 90%. Widely distributed. Metabolic fate unknown. Cleared by nonrenal pathways. Minimal removal by hemodialysis. Amphotec and Abelcet are not dialyzable. ***Half-life:*** Fungizone, 24 hr (increased in neonates and children); Amphotec, 26–28 hr; Abelcet, 7.2 days; AmBisome, 100–153 hr.

AVAILABILITY

Cream (Fungizone): 3%.
Injection, Powder for Reconstitution (Amphotec): 50 mg, 100 mg.
Injection, Powder for Reconstitution (AmBisome, Amphocin, Fungizone): 50 mg.
Injection, Suspension (Abelcet): 5 mg/ml.

INDICATIONS AND DOSAGES

▸ **Cryptococcosis; blastomycosis; systemic candidiasis; disseminated forms of moniliasis, coccidioidomycosis, and histoplasmosis; zygomycosis; sporotrichosis; aspergillosis**

IV Infusion (Fungizone)

Adults, Elderly. Dosage based on patient tolerance and severity of infection. Initially, 1-mg test dose is given over 20–30 min. If test dose is tolerated, 5-mg dose may be given the same day. Subsequently, dosage is increased by 5 mg q12–24h until desired daily dose is reached. Alternatively, if test dose is tolerated, 0.25 mg/kg is given on same day and 0.5 mg/kg on second day; then dosage is increased until desired daily dose reached. Total daily dose: 1 mg/kg/day up to 1.5 mg/kg every other day. Maximum: 1.5 mg/kg/day.

Children. Test dose of 0.1 mg/kg/dose (maximum 1 mg) is infused over 20–60 min. If test dose is tolerated, initial dose of 0.4 mg/kg may be given on same day; dosage is then increased in 0.25–mg/kg increments as needed. Maintenance dose: 0.25–1 mg/kg/day.

Invasive fungal infections unresponsive to or intolerant of Fungizone

IV Infusion (Abelcet)

Adults, Children. 5 mg/kg at rate of 2.5 mg/kg/hr.

▸ **Empiric treatment of fungal infections in patients with febrile neutropenia; aspergillosis, candidiasis, or cryptococcosis in patients with renal impairment and those who have experienced toxicity or treatment failure with Fungizone**

IV Infusion (AmBisome)

Adults, Children. 3–5 mg/kg over 1 hr.

▸ **Invasive aspergillosis in patients with renal impairment and those who have experienced toxicity or treatment failure with Fungizone**

IV Infusion (Amphotec)

Adults, Children. 3–4 mg/kg over 2–4 hr.

▸ **Cutaneous and mucocutaneous infections caused by *Candida albicans,* such as paronychia, oral thrush, perlèche, diaper rash, and intertriginous candidiasis**

Topical

Adults, Elderly, Children. Apply liberally to affected area and rub in 2–4 times a day.

CONTRAINDICATIONS
Hypersensitivity to amphotericin B or sulfites

INTERACTIONS
Drug
Bone marrow depressants: May increase the risk of anemia.
Digoxin: May increase the risk of digoxin toxicity from hypokalemia.
Nephrotoxic medications: May increase the risk of nephrotoxicity.
Steroids: May cause severe hypokalemia.
Herbal
None known.
Food
None known.

DIAGNOSTIC TEST EFFECTS
May increase BUN, serum alkaline phosphatase, serum creatinine, serum AST (SGOT), and ALT (SGPT) levels. May decrease serum calcium, magnesium, and potassium levels.

IV INCOMPATIBILITIES
Abelcet, AmBisome, Amphotec: Don't mix with any other drug, diluent, or solution. Fungizone: Allopurinol (Aloprim), amifostine (Ethyol), aztreonam (Azactam), calcium gluconate, cefepime (Maxipime), cimetidine (Tagamet), ciprofloxacin (Cipro), docetaxel (Taxotere), dopamine (Intropin), doxorubicin (Adriamycin), enalapril (Vasotec), etoposide (VP-16), filgrastim (Neupogen), fluconazole (Diflucan), fludarabine (Fludara), foscarnet (Foscavir), gemcitabine (Gemzar), magnesium sulfate, meropenem (Merrem IV), ondansetron (Zofran), paclitaxel (Taxol), piperacillin and tazobactam (Zosyn), potassium chloride, propofol (Diprivan), vinorelbine (Navelbine)

IV COMPATIBILITIES
None known; don't mix with other medications or electrolytes.

SIDE EFFECTS
Frequent (greater than 10%)
Abelcet: Chills, fever, increased serum creatinine level, multiple organ failure
AmBisome: Hypokalemia, hypomagnesemia, hyperglycemia, hypocalcemia, edema, abdominal pain, back pain, chills, chest pain, hypotension, diarrhea, nausea, vomiting, headache, fever, rigors, insomnia, dyspnea, epistaxis, increased hepatic or renal function test results
Amphotec: Chills, fever, hypotension, tachycardia, increased serum creatinine level, hypokalemia, bilirubinemia
Fungizone: Fever, chills, headache, anemia, hypokalemia, hypomagnesemia, anorexia, malaise, generalized pain, nephrotoxicity
Topical: Local irritation, dry skin
Rare
Topical: Rash

SERIOUS REACTIONS
! Cardiovascular toxicity (as evidenced by hypotension, ventricular fibrillation, and anaphylaxis) occurs rarely.
! Altered vision and hearing, seizures, hepatic failure, coagulation defects, multiple organ failure, and sepsis may be noted.

NURSING CONSIDERATIONS
Baseline Assessment
- Determine the patient's history of allergies, especially to amphotericin B and sulfites, before giving the drug.
- Be aware that other nephrotoxic medications should be avoided, if possible.

• Obtain pre-medication orders to reduce the adverse reactions of IV therapy.

Lifespan Considerations

• Amphotericin B crosses the placenta; it is unknown if it's distributed in breast milk.

• The safety and efficacy of amphotericin B have not been established in children. Therefore, expect to use the smallest dose necessary to achieve optimal results.

• No age-related precautions have been noted for the elderly.

Precautions

• Use amphotericin B cautiously in patients with renal impairment and in those receiving antineoplastic therapy. This drug is prescribed only for progressive, potentially fatal fungal infections.

• Keep in mind that conventional amphotericin B, Fungizone, is more nephrotoxic than the amphotericin B complexes, Abelcet, AmBisome, and Amphotec.

Administration and Handling

IV (all forms)

• Obtain orders for drugs to reduce the risk or severity of adverse reactions during IV therapy, such as antiemetics, antihistamines, antipyretics, or small doses of corticosteroids.

• Observe strict aseptic technique during reconstitution because no bacteriostatic agent or preservative is present in the diluent. Be aware that the potential for thrombophlebitis may be decreased by using pediatric scalp vein needles or by adding dilute heparin solution, as prescribed.

IV (Abelcet)

• Refrigerate unreconstituted Abelcet solution. Reconstituted Abelcet solution is stable for 48 hours if refrigerated and for 6 hours at room temperature.

• Shake Abelcet 20-ml (100-mg) vial gently until contents are dissolved. Withdraw required dose using the 5-micron filter needle supplied by the manufacturer.

• Dilute each 1 ml (5 mg) of Abelcet in 4 ml of D_5W to yield a final concentration of 1 mg/ml. Reduce concentration by half (2 mg/ml) for pediatric or fluid-restricted patients.

• Infuse Abelcet over 2 hours by slow IV infusion. Shake the contents if the infusion exceeds 2 hours.

IV (AmBisome)

• Refrigerate unreconstituted AmBisome solution. Reconstituted AmBisome solution of 4 mg/ml is stable for 24 hours; reconstituted solution of 1–2 mg/ml is stable for 6 hours.

• Reconstitute each 50-mg vial of AmBisome with 12 ml sterile water for injection to provide a concentration of 4 mg/ml.

• Shake the AmBisome vial vigorously for 30 seconds. Then withdraw the required dose and empty the syringe contents through a 5-micron filter into an infusion of D_5W to provide final concentration of 1–2 mg/ml.

• Infuse AmBisome over 1–2 hours by slow IV infusion.

IV (Amphotec)

• Store unreconstituted Amphotec solution at room temperature. Reconstituted Amphotec solution is stable for 24 hours.

• Add 10 ml of sterile water for injection to each 50-mg vial of Amphotec to provide a concentration of 5 mg/ml. Shake the vial gently.

• Further dilute Amphotec only with D5W, using the specific amount recommended by the manufacturer, to provide a concentration of 0.16–0.83 mg/ml.

• Infuse Amphotec over 2–4 hours by slow IV infusion.

IV (Fungizone)

• Refrigerate unreconstituted Fungi-

zone solution. Reconstituted Fungizone solution is stable for 24 hours at room temperature or for 7 days if refrigerated. Diluted solution less than or equal to 0.1 mg/ml should be used promptly. Don't use the solution if it is cloudy or contains a precipitate.
• Rapidly inject 10 ml of sterile water for injection into each 50-mg vial of Fungizone to provide a concentration of 5 mg/ml. Immediately shake the vial until the solution is clear.
• Further dilute each 1 mg of Fungizone in at least 10 ml of D_5W to provide a concentration of 0.1 mg/ml.
• Infuse Fungizone over 2–6 hours by slow IV infusion.

Intervention and Evaluation

• Monitor BP, pulse, respirations, and temperature twice every 15 minutes, then every 30 minutes for the first 4 hours of the infusion to assess for adverse reactions. Adverse reactions include abdominal pain, anorexia, chills, fever, nausea, vomiting, and tremors. If adverse reactions occur, slow the infusion rate and give prescribed drugs to provide symptomatic relief. For patients with a severe reaction and those without orders for symptomatic relief, stop the infusion and notify the physician.
• Evaluate the IV site for signs of phlebitis (heat, pain, and red streaking over the vein).
• Monitor the patient's intake and output and renal function test results to assess for nephrotoxicity.
• Check the patient's serum potassium and magnesium levels as well as hematologic and liver function test results.
• Assess the patient's skin for burning, irritation, or pruritus.

Patient Teaching

• Explain to the patient that prolonged amphotericin B therapy over weeks or months is usually necessary to achieve the desired therapeutic effect.
• Tell the patient that the fever reaction may decrease with continued therapy.
• Inform the patient that muscle weakness may occur from drug-related loss of potassium.
• Teach the patient using topical amphotericin B to thoroughly rub in the cream or lotion.
• Inform the patient that topical amphotericin B may stain the skin or nails as well as clothing but that such stains may be removed by soap and water or dry cleaning.
• Advise the patient not to use other topical preparations or occlusive coverings without consulting the physician.
• Urge the patient to keep affected areas clean and dry, to wear light clothing, and to separate personal items that have come in direct contact with the affected area.

caspofungin acetate

cas-poe-**fun**-gin
(Cancidas)

CATEGORY AND SCHEDULE

Pregnancy Risk Category: C

MECHANISM OF ACTION

An antifungal that inhibits the synthesis of glucan, a vital component of fungal cell formation, thereby damaging the fungal cell membrane. **Therapeutic Effect:** Fungistatic.

PHARMACOKINETICS

Distributed in tissue. Extensively bound to albumin. Protein binding: 97%. Slowly metabolized in liver to active metabolite. Excreted primarily in urine and to a lesser extent in feces. Not removed by hemodialysis. ***Half-life:*** 40–50 hr.

AVAILABILITY

Powder for Injection: 50-mg, 70-mg vials.

INDICATIONS AND DOSAGES

▸ **Aspergillosis**

IV

Adults, Elderly, Children older than 12 yr. Give single 70-mg loading dose on day 1, followed by 50 mg/day thereafter. For patients with moderate hepatic insufficiency, daily dose reduced to 35 mg.

▸ **Invasive candidiasis**

IV

Adults, Elderly. Initially, 70 mg followed by 50 mg daily.

▸ **Esophageal candidiasis**

IV

Adult, Elderly. 50 mg a day.

CONTRAINDICATIONS

None known.

INTERACTIONS

Drug

Carbamazepine, cyclosporine, dexamethasone, efavirenz, nelfinavir, nevirapine, phenytoin, rifampin: May increase blood concentration of caspofungin.

Tacrolimus: May decrease the effect of tacrolimus.

Herbal

None known.

Food

None known.

DIAGNOSTIC TEST EFFECTS

May increase PT as well as serum alkaline phosphatase, serum bilirubin, serum creatinine, LDH, AST (SGOT), ALT (SGPT), serum uric acid, urine pH, urine protein, urine RBC, and urine WBC levels. May decrease Hgb, Hct, platelet count, and serum albumin, serum bicarbonate, serum protein, and serum potassium levels.

IV INCOMPATIBILITIES

Don't mix caspofungin with any other medication or use dextrose as a diluent.

SIDE EFFECTS

Frequent (26%)

Fever

Occasional (11%–4%)

Headache, nausea, phlebitis

Rare (3% or less)

Paresthesia, vomiting, diarrhea, abdominal pain, myalgia, chills, tremor, insomnia

SERIOUS REACTIONS

! Hypersensitivity reactions (characterized by rash, facial swelling, pruritus, and a sensation of warmth) may occur.

NURSING CONSIDERATIONS

Baseline Assessment

- Obtain the patient's baseline temperature, liver function test results, and history of allergies before giving caspofungin.

Lifespan Considerations

- Caspofungin crosses the placental barrier, may be embryotoxic, and is distributed in breast milk.
- The safety and efficacy of caspofungin have not been established in children.
- Age-related renal impairment may require dosage adjustment in the elderly.

Precautions

- Use caspofungin cautiously in patients with impaired hepatic function.

Administration and Handling

IV

- Refrigerate the drug but warm it to room temperature before reconstituting it.
- The reconstituted solution, may be stored at room temperature for 1 hour before infusion.
- The final infusion solution may be stored at room temperature for 24 hours.
- Discard the solution if it contains particles or is discolored.
- For a 70-mg dose, add 10.5 ml 0.9% NaCl to the 70-mg vial. Transfer 10 ml of the reconstituted solution to 250 ml 0.9% NaCl.
- For a 50-mg dose, add 10.5 ml 0.9% NaCl to the 50-mg vial. Transfer 10 ml of the reconstituted solution to 100 ml or 250 ml 0.9% NaCl.
- For 35-mg dose, add 10.5 ml 0.9% NaCl to the 50-mg vial. Transfer 7 ml of the reconstituted solution to 100 ml or 250 ml 0.9% NaCl.
- Infuse over 60 minutes.

Intervention and Evaluation

- Assess the patient for signs and symptoms of hepatic dysfunction.
- Expect to monitor liver function test results in patients with preexisting hepatic dysfunction.

Patient Teaching

- Advise the patient to notify the physician if he or she develops increased shortness of breath, itching, facial swelling, or a rash.
- Urge the patient to report pain, burning, or swelling at the IV infusion site.

fluconazole

floo-**con**-a-zole

(Apo-Fluconazole[CAN], Diflucan)

Do not confuse Diflucan with diclofenac.

CATEGORY AND SCHEDULE

Pregnancy Risk Category: C

MECHANISM OF ACTION

A fungistatic antifungal that interferes with cytochrome P-450, an enzyme necessary for ergosterol formation. **Therapeutic Effect:** Directly damages fungal membrane, altering its function.

PHARMACOKINETICS

Well absorbed from GI tract. Widely distributed, including to CSF. Protein binding: 11%. Partially metabolized in liver. Excreted unchanged primarily in urine. Partially removed by hemodialysis. ***Half-life:*** 20–30 hr (increased in impaired renal function).

AVAILABILITY

Tablets: 50 mg, 100 mg, 150 mg, 200 mg.

Powder for Oral Suspension: 10 mg/ml, 40 mg/ml.

Injection: 2 mg/ml (in 100- or 200-ml containers).

INDICATIONS AND DOSAGES

▸ **Oropharyngeal candidiasis**

PO, IV

Adults, Elderly. 200 mg once, then 100 mg/day for at least 14 days.

Children. 6 mg/kg/day once, then 3 mg/kg/day.

▸ **Esophageal candidiasis**

PO, IV

Adults, Elderly. 200 mg once, then 100 mg/day (up to 400 mg/day) for

21 days and at least 14 days following resolution of symptoms.
Children. 6 mg/kg/day once, then 3 mg/kg/day (up to 12 mg/kg/day) for 21 days at at least 14 days following resolution of symptoms.

▸ **Vaginal candidiasis**
PO
Adults. 150 mg once.

▸ **Prevention of candidiasis in patients undergoing bone marrow transplantation**
PO
Adults. 400 mg/day.

▸ **Systemic candidiasis**
PO, IV
Adults, Elderly. 400 mg once, then 200 mg/day (up to 400 mg/day) for at least 28 days and at least 14 days following resolution of symptoms.
Children. 6–12 mg/kg/day.

▸ **Cryptococcal meningitis**
PO, IV
Adults, Elderly. 400 mg once, then 200 mg/day (up to 800 mg/day) for 10–12 wk after CSF becomes negative (200 mg/day for suppression of relapse in patients with AIDS).
Children. 12 mg/kg/day once, then 6–12 mg/kg/day (6 mg/kg/day for suppression of relapse in patients with AIDS).

▸ **Onychomycosis**
PO
Adults. 150 mg/wk.

▸ **Dosage in Renal Impairment**
After a loading dose of 400 mg, the daily dosage is based on creatinine clearance:

Creatinine Clearance	% of Recommended Dose
greater than 50 ml/min	100
21–50 ml/min	50
11–20 ml/min	25
Dialysis	Dose after dialysis

OFF-LABEL USES
Treatment of coccidioidomycosis, cryptococcosis, fungal pneumonia, onychomycosis, ringworm of the hand, septicemia

CONTRAINDICATIONS
None known.

INTERACTIONS
Drug
Cyclosporine: High fluconazole doses increase cyclosporine blood concentration.
Oral antidiabetics: May increase blood concentration and effects of oral antidiabetics.
Phenytoin, warfarin: May decrease the metabolism of these drugs.
Rifampin: May increase fluconazole metabolism.
Herbal
None known.
Food
None known.

DIAGNOSTIC TEST EFFECTS
May increase serum alkaline phosphatase, serum bilirubin, AST (SGOT), and ALT (SGPT) levels.

IV INCOMPATIBILITIES
Amphotericin B (Fungizone), amphotericin B complex (Abelcet, Ambisome, Amphotec), ampicillin (Polycillin), calcium gluconate, cefotaxime (Claforan), ceftazidime (Fortaz), ceftriaxone (Rocephin), cefuroxime (Zinacef), chloramphenicol (Chloromycetin), clindamycin (Cleocin), co-trimoxazole (Bactrim), diazepam (Valium), digoxin (Lanoxin), erythromycin (Erythrocin), furosemide (Lasix), haloperidol (Haldol), hydroxyzine (Vistaril), imipenem and cilastatin (Primaxin)

IV COMPATIBILITIES
Diltiazem (Cardizem), dobutamine

(Dobutrex), dopamine (Intropin), heparin, lorazepam (Ativan), midazolam (Versed), propofol (Diprivan)

SIDE EFFECTS

Occasional (4%–1%)

Hypersensitivity reaction (including chills, fever, pruritus, and rash), dizziness, drowsiness, headache, constipation, diarrhea, nausea, vomiting, abdominal pain

SERIOUS REACTIONS

! Exfoliative skin disorders, serious hepatic effects, and blood dyscrasias (such as eosinophilia, thrombocytopenia, anemia, and leukopenia) have been reported rarely.

NURSING CONSIDERATIONS

Baseline Assessment

- Expect to obtain baseline CBC, liver function test results, and serum potassium level.

Lifespan Considerations

- It is unknown if fluconazole is excreted in breast milk.
- No age-related precautions have been noted in children.
- Age-related renal impairment may require a dosage adjustment in the elderly.

Precautions

- Use fluconazole cautiously in patients with hepatic or renal impairment, hypersensitivity to other triazoles (such as itraconazole and terconazole), or hypersensitivity to imidazoles (such as butoconazole and ketoconazole).

Administration and Handling

PO

- Give without regard to meals.
- Be aware that PO and IV therapy are equally effective and that IV therapy is for patients who can't take or tolerate the oral drug.

IV

- Store the drug at room temperature.
- Don't remove it from the outer wrap until ready to use.
- Squeeze the inner bag to check for leaks.
- Don't use the parenteral form if the seal is not intact or if the solution is cloudy or discolored or contains a precipitate.
- Don't add another medication to the solution.
- Don't exceed a flow rate of 200 mg/hour.

Intervention and Evaluation

- Assess the patient for signs and symptoms of a hypersensitivity reaction, including chills and fever.
- Expect to monitor the patient's CBC, liver and renal function test results, platelet count, and serum potassium levels.
- Advise the patient to report any itching or a rash promptly.
- Monitor the patient's temperature daily.
- Assess the patient's daily pattern of bowel activity and stool consistency.
- Evaluate the patient for dizziness and provide assistance as needed.

Patient Teaching

- Caution the patient not to drive or use machinery until his or her response to the drug is established.
- Warn the patient to notify the physician if he or she develops dark urine, pale stool, rash with or without itching, or yellow skin or eyes.
- Teach the patient with an oropharyngeal infection about good oral hygiene.
- Advise the patient to consult the physician before taking any other medications.

griseofulvin

griz-ee-oh-**full**-vin
(Fulvicin P/G, Fulvicin U/F, Grifulvin V, Gris-PEG, Grisovin[AUS])

CATEGORY AND SCHEDULE

Pregnancy Risk Category: C

MECHANISM OF ACTION

An antifungal that inhibits fungal cell mitosis by disrupting mitotic spindle structure. **Therapeutic Effect:** Fungistatic.

AVAILABILITY

Oral Suspension (Grifulvin V): 125 mg/5 ml.
Tablets (Microsize [Fulvicin-U/F]): 250 mg, 500 mg.
Tablets (Ultramicrosize [Fulvicin P/G]): 125 mg, 165 mg, 250 mg, 330 mg.
Tablets (Ultramicrosize [Gris-PEG]): 125 mg, 250 mg.

INDICATIONS AND DOSAGES

▸ **Tinea capitis, tinea corporis, tinea cruris, tinea pedis, tinea unguium**

Microsize Tablets, Oral Suspension
Adults. Usual dosage, 500–1,000 mg as a single dose or in divided doses.
Children 2 yr and older. Usual dosage, 10–20 mg/kg/day.
Ultramicrosize Tablets
Adults. Usual dosage, 330–750 mg/day as a single dose or in divided doses.
Children 2 yr and older. 5–10 mg/kg/day.

CONTRAINDICATIONS

Hepatocellular failure, porphyria

INTERACTIONS

Drug

Oral contraceptives, warfarin: May decrease the effects of these drugs.

Herbal

None known.

Food

None known.

DIAGNOSTIC TEST EFFECTS

None known.

SIDE EFFECTS

Occasional

Hypersensitivity reaction (including pruritus, rash, and urticaria), headache, nausea, diarrhea, excessive thirst, flatulence, oral thrush, dizziness, insomnia

Rare

Paresthesia of hands or feet, proteinuria, photosensitivity reaction

SERIOUS REACTIONS

! Granulocytopenia occurs rarely.

NURSING CONSIDERATIONS

Baseline Assessment

• Determine the patient's history of allergies, especially to griseofulvin and penicillins, before giving the drug.

Precautions

• Use griseofulvin cautiously in patients with hypersensitivity to penicillins and in those who are exposed to sun or ultraviolet light because photosensitivity may occur.

Intervention and Evaluation

◀ALERT▶ The duration of treatment depends on the site of infection.
• Evaluate the patient's skin for a rash and therapeutic response to the drug.
• Assess the patient's daily pattern of bowel activity and stool consistency.
◀ALERT▶ Monitor the patient's

granulocyte count as appropriate. If the patient develops granulocytopenia, notify the physician and expect to discontinue the drug.
- In patients experiencing headache, establish and document the headache's location, onset, and type.
- Assess the patient for dizziness.

Patient Teaching
- Explain to the patient that prolonged therapy over weeks or months is usually necessary.
- Advise the patient not to miss a dose and to continue therapy for as long as is ordered.
- Warn the patient to avoid consuming alcohol because flushing or tachycardia may occur.
- Advise the patient that griseofulvin may cause a photosensitivity reaction, so he or she should avoid exposure to sunlight.
- Urge the patient to maintain good hygiene to help prevent superinfection.
- Encourage the patient to separate personal items that come in direct contact with affected areas.
- Instruct the patient to keep affected areas dry and to wear light clothing for ventilation.
- Advise the patient to take griseofulvin with foods high in fat, such as milk or ice cream, to reduce GI upset and assist in drug absorption.

itraconazole

it-ra-**con**-a-zol
(Sporanox)
Do not confuse Sporanox with Suprax.

CATEGORY AND SCHEDULE

Pregnancy Risk Category: C

MECHANISM OF ACTION

A fungistatic antifungal that inhibits the synthesis of ergosterol, a vital component of fungal cell formation
Therapeutic Effect: Damages the fungal cell membrane, altering its function.

PHARMACOKINETICS

Moderately absorbed from the GI tract. Absorption is increased if the drug is taken with food. Protein binding: 99%. Widely distributed, primarily in the fatty tissue, liver, and kidneys. Metabolized in the liver to active metabolite. Primarily excreted in urine. Not removed by hemodialysis. ***Half-life:*** 21 hr; metabolite, 12 hr.

AVAILABILITY

Capsules: 100 mg.
Oral Solution: 10 mg/ml.
Injection: 10 mg/ml (25-ml ampule).

INDICATIONS AND DOSAGES

▸ **Blastomycosis, histoplasmosis**

PO

Adults, Elderly. Initially, 200 mg once a day. Maximum: 400 mg/day in 2 divided doses.

IV

Adults, Elderly. 200 mg twice a day for 4 doses, then 200 mg once a day.

▸ **Aspergillosis**

PO

Adults, Elderly. 600 mg/day in 3 divided doses for 3–4 days, then 200–400 mg/day in 2 divided doses.

IV

Adults, Elderly. 200 mg twice a day for 4 doses, then 200 mg once a day.

▸ **Esophageal candidiasis**

PO

Adults, Elderly. Swish 10 ml in mouth for several seconds, then swallow. Maximum: 200 mg/day.

▸ **Oropharyngeal candidiasis**
PO
Adults, Elderly. Vigorously swish 10 ml in mouth for several seconds (20 ml total daily dose) once a day.

OFF-LABEL USES
Suppression of histoplasmosis; treatment of disseminated sporotrichosis, fungal pneumonia and septicemia, or ringworm of the hand

CONTRAINDICATIONS
Hypersensitivity to itraconazole, fluconazole, ketoconazole, or miconazole

INTERACTIONS
Drug
Antacids, didanosine, H_2 antagonists: May decrease itraconazole absorption.
Buspirone, cyclosporine, digoxin, lovastatin, simvastatin: May increase blood concentration of these drugs.
Oral anticoagulants: May increase the effect of oral anticoagulants.
Phenytoin, rifampin: May decrease itraconazole blood concentration.
Herbal
None known.
Food
Grapefruit juice: May alter itraconazole absorption.

DIAGNOSTIC TEST EFFECTS
May increase serum LDH serum alkaline phosphatase, serum bilirubin, AST (SGOT), and ALT (SGPT) levels. May decrease serum potassium level.

IV INCOMPATIBILITIES
◂ **ALERT** ▸ Dilution compatibility of itraconazole with any solution other than 0.9% NaCl is unknown. Don't mix with D_5W or lactated Ringer's solution. Not for IV bolus administration. Don't administer any medication in same bag or through same IV line as itraconazole.

SIDE EFFECTS
Frequent (11%–9%)
Nausea, rash
Occasional (5%–3%)
Vomiting, headache, diarrhea, hypertension, peripheral edema, fatigue, fever
Rare (2% or less)
Abdominal pain, dizziness, anorexia, pruritus

SERIOUS REACTIONS
! Hepatitis (as evidenced by anorexia, abdominal pain, unusual fatigue or weakness, jaundice skin or sclera, and dark urine) occurs rarely.

NURSING CONSIDERATIONS
Baseline Assessment
- Obtain the patient's baseline temperature and liver function test results, as appropriate.
- Determine if the patient has a history of allergies before giving the drug.

Lifespan Considerations
- Itraconazole is distributed in breast milk.
- The safety and efficacy of itraconazole have not been established in children.
- Age-related renal impairment may require a dosage adjustment in the elderly.

Precautions
- Use itraconazole cautiously in patients with achlorhydria or hypochlorhydria, hepatitis, HIV infection, or impaired hepatic function.

Administration and Handling
◂ **ALERT** ▸ Doses larger than 200 mg should be given in 2 divided doses.

PO
- Give capsules with food to increase absorption.
- Give oral solution on an empty stomach.

IV
- Store ampule at room temperature. Don't freeze.
- Use only the components provided by the manufacturer.
- Don't dilute the drug with any other diluent.
- Add the full contents of the ampule (250 mg/10 ml) to the infusion bag provided (50 ml of 0.9% NaCl) and mix gently.
- Infuse the drug over 60 minutes using the extension line and infusion set provided.
- After administration, flush the infusion set with 15 to 20 ml of 0.9% NaCl over 30 seconds to 15 minutes, and discard the entire infusion line.

Intervention and Evaluation
- Assess the patient for signs and symptoms of hepatic dysfunction.
- Expect to monitor liver function test results in patients with pre-existing hepatic dysfunction.

Patient Teaching
- Instruct the patient to take itraconazole capsules and itraconazole oral solution with food if he or she experiences GI distress.
- Inform the patient that therapy will continue for at least 3 months and until laboratory tests and his or her overall condition indicate that the infection is controlled.
- Warn the patient to report decreased appetite, dark urine, nausea, vomiting, pale stools, unusual fatigue, or yellow skin to the physician.
- Caution the patient to avoid grapefruit and grapefruit juice because they may alter itraconazole absorption.

ketoconazole

kee-toe-**koe**-na-zole
(Apo-Ketocomazole[CAN], Nizoral, Nizoral AD, Sebizole[AUS])
Do not confuse Nizoral with Nasarel.

CATEGORY AND SCHEDULE

Pregnancy Risk Category: C
OTC (1% shampoo only)

MECHANISM OF ACTION

A fungistatic antifungal that inhibits the synthesis of ergosterol, a vital component of fungal cell formation. **Therapeutic Effect:** Damages the fungal cell membrane, altering its function.

AVAILABILITY

Tablets (Nizoral): 200 mg.
Cream (Nizoral): 2%.
Shampoo (Nizoral AD): 1%.

INDICATIONS AND DOSAGES

▸ **Histoplasmosis, blastomycosis, systemic candidiasis, chronic mucocutaneous candidiasis, coccidioidomycosis, paracoccidioidomycosis, chromomycosis, seborrheic dermatitis, tinea corporis, tinea capitis, tinea manus, tinea cruris, tinea pedis, tinea unguium (onychomycosis), oral thrush, candiduria**

PO
Adults, Elderly. 200–400 mg/day.
Children. 3.3–6.6 mg/kg/day. Maximum: 800 mg/day in 2 divided doses.

Topical
Adults, Elderly. Apply to affected area 1–2 times a day for 2–4 wk.

Shampoo
Adults, Elderly. Use twice weekly for 4 wk, allowing at least 3 days

between shampooing. Use intermittently to maintain control.

OFF-LABEL USES

Systemic: Treatment of fungal pneumonia, prostate cancer, septicemia

CONTRAINDICATIONS

None known.

INTERACTIONS

Drug

Alcohol, hepatotoxic medications: May increase hepatotoxicity of ketoconazole.
Antacids, anticholinergics, H_2 antagonists, omeprazole: May decrease ketoconazole absorption.
Cyclosporine, lovastatin, simvastatin: May increase blood concentration and risk of toxicity of these drugs.
Isoniazid, rifampin: May decrease blood concentration of ketoconazole.

Herbal

Echinacea: May have additive hepatotoxic effects.

Food

None known.

DIAGNOSTIC TEST EFFECTS

May increase serum alkaline phosphatase, serum bilirubin, AST (SGOT), and ALT (SGPT) levels. May decrease serum corticosteroid and testosterone concentrations.

SIDE EFFECTS

Occasional (10%–3%)
Nausea, vomiting
Rare (less than 2%)
Abdominal pain, diarrhea, headache, dizziness, photophobia, pruritus
Topical: itching, burning, irritation

SERIOUS REACTIONS

! Hematologic toxicity (as evidenced by thrombocytopenia, hemolytic anemia, and leukopenia) occurs occasionally.
! Hepatotoxicity may occur within 1 week to several months after starting therapy.
! Anaphylaxis occurs rarely.

NURSING CONSIDERATIONS

Baseline Assessment

- Confirm that a culture or histologic test was done to ensure an accurate diagnosis; therapy may begin before results are known.

Precautions

- Use ketoconazole cautiously in patients with hepatic impairment.

Administration and Handling

PO
- Give with food to minimize GI irritation.
- Tablets may be crushed.
- Ketoconazole requires acidity; give antacids, anticholinergics, H_2 blockers, or omeprazole at least 2 hours after administering the drug.

Topical
- Apply and rub gently into the affected and surrounding area.

Shampoo
- Apply to wet hair, massage for 1 minute, rinse thoroughly, reapply for 3 minutes, and then rinse.

Intervention and Evaluation

- Expect to monitor the patient's liver function test results. Be alert for signs and symptoms of hepatotoxicity, including dark urine, pale stools, jaundice, fatigue, and GI effects (anorexia, nausea, vomiting) that are not relieved by giving the drug with food.
- Monitor the patient's CBC for evidence of hematologic toxicity.
- Assess the patient's daily pattern of bowel activity and stool consistency.
- Assess the patient for dizziness; provide assistance as needed, and institute safety precautions.

• Evaluate the patient's skin for a rash, pruritus, and urticaria.
• If the patient is receiving topical ketoconazole, check his or her skin for localized burning, itching, and irritation.

Patient Teaching

• Explain to the patient that prolonged therapy over weeks or months is usually necessary.
• Instruct the patient not to miss a dose and to continue therapy for as long as directed.
• Advise the patient to avoid alcohol to minimize the risk of liver damage.
• Caution the patient to avoid tasks that require mental alertness or motor skills until his or her response to the drug is established.
• Encourage the patient to take antacids or antiulcer medications at least 2 hours after taking ketoconazole.
• Warn the patient to notify the physician if he or she develops dark urine, pale stools, yellow skin or eyes, increased irritation (with topical use), or other new symptoms.
• Teach the patient using topical ketoconazole to avoid drug contact with the eyes, to keep the skin clean and dry, to rub the drug well into affected areas, and to wear light clothing for ventilation.
• Encourage the patient to separate personal items that come in direct contact with the affected area.
• Instruct the patient to use ketoconazole shampoo initially twice weekly for 4 weeks and to wait at least 3 days between shampooing. Explain that further use of the shampoo will be based on his or her response to the initial treatment.

nystatin

nye-**stat**-in
(Mycostatin, Nilstat [CAN], Nyaderm, Nystop)
Do not confuse nystatin or Mycostatin with Nitrostat.

CATEGORY AND SCHEDULE

Pregnancy Risk Category: C

MECHANISM OF ACTION

A fungistatic antifungal that binds to sterols in the fungal cell membrane. **Therapeutic Effect:** Increases fungal cell-membrane permeability, allowing loss of potassium and other cellular components.

PHARMACOKINETICS

PO: Poorly absorbed from the GI tract. Eliminated unchanged in feces. Topical: Not absorbed systemically from intact skin.

AVAILABILITY

Oral Suspension (Mycostatin): 100,000 units/ml.
Tablets (Mycostatin): 500,000 units.
Vaginal Tablets: 100,000 units.
Cream (Mycostatin): 100,000 units/g.
Ointment: 100,000 units/g.
Topical Powder (Mycostatin, Nystop): 100,000 units/g.

INDICATIONS AND DOSAGES

▸ **Intestinal infections**

PO

Adults, Elderly. 500,000–1,000,000 units q8h.

▸ **Oral candidiasis**

PO

Adults, Elderly, Children. 400,000–600,000 units 4 times/day.
Infants. 200,000 units 4 times/day.

▸ **Vaginal infections**
Vaginal
Adults, Elderly, Adolescents. 1 tablet/day at bedtime for 14 days.
▸ **Cutaneous candidal infections**
Topical
Adults, Elderly, Children. Apply 2–4 times/day.

OFF-LABEL USES

Prophylaxis and treatment of oropharyngeal candidiasis, tinea barbae, tinea capitis

CONTRAINDICATIONS

None known.

INTERACTIONS

Drug

None known.

Herbal

None known.

Food

None known.

DIAGNOSTIC TEST EFFECTS

None known.

SIDE EFFECTS

Occasional

PO: None known
Topical: Skin irritation
Vaginal: Vaginal irritation

SERIOUS REACTIONS

! High dosages of oral form may produce nausea, vomiting, diarrhea, and GI distress.

NURSING CONSIDERATIONS

Baseline Assessment

• Confirm that cultures or histologic tests were done to ensure an accurate diagnosis before giving nystatin.

Lifespan Considerations

• It is unknown if nystatin is distributed in breast milk.
• During pregnancy, vaginal applicators may be replaced by manual insertion of tablets.
• Lozenges (troches) are not recommended for use in children younger than 5 years old. No age-related precautions have been noted for use of oral suspension or topical forms in children.
• No age-related precautions have been noted in the elderly.

Precautions

• None known.

Administration and Handling

PO
• Have the patient dissolve the lozenges (troches) slowly and completely in the mouth to ensure an optimal therapeutic effect. They should not be chewed or swallowed whole.
• Shake the oral suspension well before administration.

Intervention and Evaluation

• Assess the patient for increased irritation with topical application or increased vaginal discharge with vaginal application.

Patient Teaching

• Advise the patient not to miss a dose and to complete the full course of treatment.
• Instruct the patient to swish the oral suspension in the mouth for as long as possible before swallowing.
• Advise the patient to insert the vaginal form high into the vagina and to continue using the drug during menstruation. Tell her to consult the physician about douching and sexual intercourse.
• Caution the patient not to let the topical form come in contact with the eyes.
• Explain that nystatin cream or powder should be used sparingly on erythematous areas.
• Teach the patient to rub the topical form well into affected areas, to keep

affected areas clean and dry, and to wear light clothing for ventilation.

- Encourage the patient to separate personal items that come in contact with affected areas.
- Warn the patient to notify the physician if diarrhea, nausea, vomitting, or abdominal pain occurs.

sertaconazole

sir-tah-**con**-ah-zole
(Ertaczo)

CATEGORY AND SCHEDULE

Pregnancy Risk Category: C

MECHANISM OF ACTION

An imidazole derivative that inhibits synthesis of ergosterol, a vital component of fungal cell formation.
Therapeutic Effect: Damages fungal cell membrane.

AVAILABILITY

Cream: 2%.

INDICATIONS AND DOSAGES

▸ Tinea pedis

Topical

Adults, Elderly, Children 12 yr and older. Apply twice a day for 4 wks. Apply a sufficient amount to affected area between toes and immediate surrounding area of healthy skin.

CONTRAINDICATIONS

None known.

INTERACTIONS

Drug

None known.

Herbal

None known.

Food

None known.

DIAGNOSTIC TEST EFFECTS

None known.

SIDE EFFECTS

Rare (2%)

Burning sensation of skin at application site, erythema, dry skin, contact dermatitis, skin tenderness, hyperpigmentation, pruritus

SERIOUS REACTIONS

! None known.

NURSING CONSIDERATIONS

Baseline Assessment

- Assess patient's ability to understand and follow directions regarding application.

Lifespan Considerations

- Be aware that it is unknown if sertaconazole is excreted in breast milk.
- There are no age-related precautions noted in patients younger than 12 years of age or in the elderly.

Administration and Handling

Topical

- Rub gently into affected, surrounding areas. Avoid contact with eyes, nose, mouth.

Intervention and Evaluation

- Assess the patient's skin for dermatitis, dryness, erythema, and hyperpigmentation.
- Determine if the patient is experiencing a burning sensation or pruritus.

Patient Teaching

- Advise the patient to continue sertaconazole treatment for the full length of therapy.
- Instruct the patient to notify the physician he or she experiences increased skin irritation.
- Warn the patient to avoid sertaconazole contact with his or her eyes, mouth, and nose.

• Tell the patient to keep the affected area clean and dry.

terbinafine hydrochloride

ter-**been**-a-feen
(Apo-Terbinafine[CAN], Lamisil, Lamisil AT, Novo-Terbinafine [CAN])
Do not confuse terbinafine with terbutaline, or Lamisil with Lamictal.

CATEGORY AND SCHEDULE

Pregnancy Risk Category: B

MECHANISM OF ACTION

A fungicidal antifungal that inhibits the enzyme squalene epoxidase, thereby interfering with fungal biosynthesis. **Therapeutic Effect:** Results in death of fungal cells.

AVAILABILITY

Tablets (Lamisil): 250 mg.
Cream (Lamisil AT): 1%.
Topical Solution (Lamisil, Lamisil AT): 1%.

INDICATIONS AND DOSAGES

▸ **Tinea pedis**
Topical
Adults, Elderly, Children 12 yr and older. Apply twice a day until signs and symptoms significantly improve.
▸ **Tinea cruris, tinea corporis**
Topical
Adults, Elderly, Children 12 yr and older. Apply 1–2 times a day until signs and symptoms significantly improve.
▸ **Onychomycosis**
PO
Adults, Elderly, Children 12 yr and older. 250 mg/day for 6 wk (fingernails) or 12 wk (toenails).
▸ **Tinea versicolor**
Topical Solution
Adults, Elderly. Apply to the affected area twice a day for 7 days.
▸ **Systemic mycosis**
PO
Adults, Elderly. 250–500 mg/day for up to 16 mo.

CONTRAINDICATIONS

Oral: Children younger than 12 years, pre-existing hepatic or renal impairment (creatinine clearance of 50 ml/min or less)

INTERACTIONS

Drug
Alcohol, other hepatotoxic medications: May increase the risk of hepatotoxicity.
Hepatic enzyme inducers, including rifampin: May increase terbinafine clearance.
Hepatic enzyme inhibitors, including cimetidine: May decrease terbinafine clearance.
Herbal
None known.
Food
None known.

DIAGNOSTIC TEST EFFECTS

May increase AST (SGOT) and ALT (SGPT) levels.

SIDE EFFECTS

Frequent (13%)
Oral: Headache
Occasional (6%–3%)
Oral: Diarrhea, rash, dyspepsia, pruritus, taste disturbance, nausea
Rare
Oral: Abdominal pain, flatulence, urticaria, visual disturbance

Topical: Irritation, burning, pruritus, dryness

SERIOUS REACTIONS

! Hepatobiliary dysfunction (including cholestatic hepatitis), serious skin reactions, and severe neutropenia occur rarely.
! Ocular lens and retinal changes have been noted.

NURSING CONSIDERATIONS

Baseline Assessment

- As appropriate, monitor hepatic function in patients receiving treatment for longer than 6 weeks.

Intervention and Evaluation

◀ ALERT ▶ Topical terbinafine should be used for at least 1 week but no more than 4 weeks.

- Assess the patient for signs of a therapeutic response.
- Discontinue the drug and notify the physician if a local reaction (such as blistering, burning, irritation, pruritus, oozing, erythema, or edema) occurs.

Patient Teaching

- Teach the patient using topical terbinafine to rub the drug well into the affected and surrounding areas and not to cover the treated area with an occlusive dressing.
- Advise the patient to keep the affected area clean and dry and to wear light clothing to promote ventilation.
- Encourage the patient to separate personal items that come in contact with the affected area.
- Caution the patient not to let topical forms come in contact with eyes, mouth, nose, or other mucous membranes.
- Instruct the patient to notify the physician if diarrhea or skin irritation occurs.

voriconazole

vohr-ee-**con**-ah-zole
(Vfend)

CATEGORY AND SCHEDULE

Pregnancy Risk Category: D

MECHANISM OF ACTION

A triazole derivative that inhibits the synthesis of ergosterol, a vital component of fungal cell wall formation. **Therapeutic Effect:** Damages fungal cell wall membrane.

PHARMACOKINETICS

Rapidly and completely absorbed after PO administration. Widely distributed. Protein binding: 98%. Metabolized in the liver. Primarily excreted as a metabolite in urine. ***Half-life:*** 6 hr.

AVAILABILITY

Tablets: 50 mg, 200 mg.
Injection Powder for Reconstitution: 200 mg.
Powder for Oral Suspension: 200 mg/5 ml.

INDICATIONS AND DOSAGES

▶ **Invasive aspergillosis, other serious fungal infections caused by *Scedosporium apiospermum* and *Fusarium* species**

PO

Adults, Elderly weighing 40 kg and more. Initially, 400 mg q12h for 2 doses on day 1. Maintenance: 200 mg q12h (may increase to 200 mg q12h).
Adults, Elderly weighing less than 40 kg. Initially, 200 mg q12h for 2 doses on day 1. Maintenance: 100 mg q12h (may increase to 150 mg q12h).

▸ **Usual parenteral dosage**

IV

Adults, Elderly, Children. Initially, 6 mg/kg/dose q12h for 2 doses, then 4 mg/kg/dose q12h (may decrease to 3 mg/kg/dose if patient is unable to tolerate 4 mg/kg/dose).

▸ **Esophageal candidiasis**

PO

Adults, Elderly weighing 40 kg or more. 200 mg q12h for minimum of 14 days, then at least 7 days following resolution of symptoms.

Adults, Elderly weighing less than 40 kg. 100 mg q12h for minimum 14 days, then at least 7 days following resolution of symptoms.

CONTRAINDICATIONS

Concurrent administration of carbamazepine; ergot alkaloids; pimozide or quinidine (may cause prolonged QT interval or torsades de pointes); rifabutin; rifampin; or sirolimus

INTERACTIONS

Drug

Cyclosporine, omeprazole, phenytoin, rifabutin, sirolimus, tacrilimus, warfarin: May increase plasma concentrations of these drugs.

Phenytoin, rifabutin, rifampin: May decrease voriconazole plasma concentration.

Herbal

None known.

Food

None known.

DIAGNOSTIC TEST EFFECTS

May increase serum alkaline phosphatase and ALT (SGPT) levels.

IV INCOMPATIBILITIES

Don't mix voriconazole with any other medications.

SIDE EFFECTS

Frequent (20%–5%)

Abnormal vision, fever, nausea, rash, vomiting

Occasional (5%–2%)

Headache, chills, hallucinations, photophobia, tachycardia, hypertension

SERIOUS REACTIONS

! Hepatotoxicity occurs rarely.

NURSING CONSIDERATIONS

Baseline Assessment

- Expect to obtain baseline liver function and renal function test results before giving voriconazole.

Lifespan Considerations

- Voriconazole may cause fetal harm.
- The safety and efficacy of voriconazole have not been established in children younger than 12 years.
- No age-related precautions have been noted in the elderly.

Precautions

- Use voriconazole cautiously in patients with a hypersensitivity to other antifungals or impaired renal or hepatic function.

Administration and Handling

PO

- Give voriconazole 1 hour before or after a meal.

IV

- Store the powder for injection at room temperature.
- Use the reconstituted solution immediately.
- Don't use the reconstituted solution after 24 hours when refrigerated.
- Reconstitute a 200-mg vial with 19 ml of sterile water for injection to provide a concentration of 10 mg/ml. Further dilute the drug with 0.9% NaCl or D_5W to provide a concentration of 5 mg/ml or less.

• Infuse the drug over 1 to 2 hours at a concentration of 5 mg/ml or less.

Intervention and Evaluation

• Expect to monitor the patient's serum liver and renal function test results.

• Evaluate and monitor the patient's visual function, including color perception, visual acuity, and visual field, if drug therapy lasts longer than 28 days.

Patient Teaching

• Instruct the patient to take voriconazole at least 1 hour before or after a meal.

• Caution the patient to avoid driving at night because voriconazole may cause visual changes, such as blurred vision or photophobia.

• Advise the patient to avoid direct sunlight and to avoid performing hazardous tasks if visual changes occur.

• Inform the female patient that voriconazole may have detrimental effects on a fetus. Explain the importance of using effective contraception to avoid becoming pregnant while taking this drug.

3 Antiretroviral Agents

abacavir
amprenavir
atazanavir sulfate
delavirdine mesylate
didanosine
efavirenz
emtricitabine
enfuvirtide
fosamprenavir calcium
indinavir
lamivudine
lopinavir/ritonavir
nelfinavir
nevirapine
ritonavir
saquinavir
stavudine (d4T)
tenofovir
zalcitabine
zidovudine

Uses: Antiretroviral agents are used to treat human immunodeficiency virus (HIV) infection. HIV treatment aims to greatly reduce the viral load, which allows the CD4+ cell count to remain at a level that's adequate to fight infections. Antiretroviral therapy typically includes more than one antiretroviral agent, each with a different mechanism of action. By attacking the virus through different mechanisms of action, the risk of resistance is reduced.

Action: The five classes of antiretrovirals act in different ways. *Nucleoside reverse transcriptase inhibitors,* such as stavudine and zalcitabine, compete with natural substrates for formation of proviral DNA by reverse transcriptase inhibiting viral replication. *Fusion inhibitors,* such as enfuvirtide, inhibit fusion of viral and cellular membranes. *Nucleotide reverse transcriptase inhibitors,* such as tenofovir, inhibit reverse transcriptase by competing with the natural substrate deoxyadenosine triphosphate and by DNA chain termination. *Nonnucleoside reverse transcriptase inhibitors,* such as delavirdine and efavirenz, directly bind to reverse transcriptase and block RNA-dependent and DNA-dependent DNA polymerase activities by disrupting the enzyme's catalytic site. *Protease inhibitors,* such as indinavir and nelfinavir, bind to the active site of HIV-1 protease which prevents protease from processing HIV polyproteins. Because the structural proteins and enzymes of HIV are unable to function, the virus remains immature and noninfectious. (See the illustration *Mechanisms and Sites of Action: Antiretroviral Agents,* page 40.)

COMBINATION PRODUCTS

COMBIVIR: lamivudine/zidovudine 150 mg/300 mg.
EPZICOM: abacavir/lamivudine 600 mg/300 mg.
TRIZIVIR: abacavir/lamivudine/zidovudine 300 mg/150 mg/300 mg.
TRUVADA: emtricitabine/tenofovir 200 mg/300 mg.

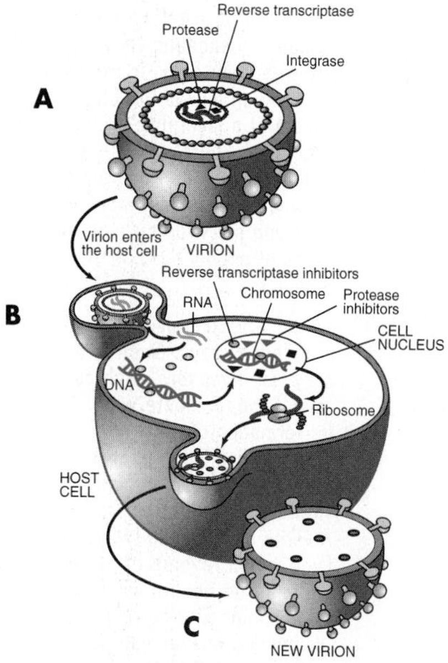

Mechanisms and Sites of Action: Antiretroviral Agents

To understand how antiretroviral agents work, you need to know how viruses reproduce. First, the infectious viral particle, or virion (A), enters the host cell. The virion attaches to the cell's surface and then inserts itself into the host cell (B). Once inside, the virion uncoats, and the enzyme reverse transcriptase makes two copies of the viral RNA: one copy is identical; the other is a mirror image. These two copies merge to form double-stranded viral DNA. This newly formed viral DNA enters the host cell's nucleus, where it inserts itself into the host cell's DNA with the help of the enzyme integrase. Then viral DNA reprograms the host cell to produce additional viral RNA, which begins the process of forming new viruses. Specifically, messenger RNA (mRNA) instructs ribosomal RNA (rRNA) to produce a new chain of proteins and enzymes that are used to form new viruses. Protease, another enzyme, cuts the chains of proteins, creating individual proteins. These individual proteins combine with new RNA to create new virions, which bud and are then released from the host cell (C).

Antiretroviral agents target specific enzymes during viral reproduction. Many of them work to inhibit reverse transcriptase. Nucleoside reverse transcriptase inhibitors, such as stavudine, interfere with the action of reverse transcriptase by mimicking naturally occurring nucleosides. Nucleotide reverse transcriptase inhibitors, such as tenofovir, block reverse transcriptase by competing with the natural substrate deoxyadenosine triphosphate and by causing DNA chain termination. Nonnucleoside reverse transcriptase inhibitors, such as delavirdine, work by directly binding to reverse transcriptase. All of these actions block the conversion of single-stranded viral RNA into double-stranded DNA. As a result, no viral DNA is available to insert itself into the host cell's DNA. Protease inhibitors, such as indinavir, bind to and interfere with the action of protease. By blocking protease, the new chain of proteins formed by rRNA can't be cut into individual proteins to make new viruses.

abacavir

ah-**bah**-cah-veer
(Ziagen)

CATEGORY AND SCHEDULE

Pregnancy Risk Category: C

MECHANISM OF ACTION

An antiretroviral that inhibits the activity of HIV-1 reverse transcriptase by competing with the natural substrate deoxyguanosine-5'-triphosphate (dGTP) and by its incorporation into viral DNA.
Therapeutic Effect: Inhibits viral DNA growth.

PHARMACOKINETICS

Rapidly and extensively absorbed after PO administration. Protein binding: 50%. Widely distributed, including to CSF and erythrocytes. Metabolized in the liver to inactive metabolites. Primarily excreted in urine. Unknown if removed by hemodialysis. ***Half-life:*** 1.5 hr.

AVAILABILITY

Tablets: 300 mg.
Oral Solution: 20 mg/ml.

INDICATIONS AND DOSAGES

▸ **HIV Infection (in combination with other antiretrovirals)**

PO

Adults. 300 mg twice a day.
Children (3 mo–16 yr). 8 mg/kg twice a day. Maximum: 300 mg twice a day.

▸ **Dosage in hepatic impairment**

Mild impairment: 200 mg 2 times/day.
Moderate to severe impairment: Not recommended.

CONTRAINDICATIONS

Hypersensitivity to abacavir or its components

INTERACTIONS

Drug

Alcohol: May increase abacavir blood concentration and half-life.

Herbal

St. John's wort: May decrease abacavir blood concentration and effect.

Food

None known.

DIAGNOSTIC TEST EFFECTS

May increase blood glucose and serum GGT, AST (SGOT), ALT (SGPT), and triglyceride levels.

SIDE EFFECTS

Adult

Frequent

Nausea (47%), nausea with vomiting (16%), diarrhea (12%), decreased appetite (11%)

Occasional

Insomnia (7%)

Children

Frequent

Nausea with vomiting (39%), fever (19%), headache, diarrhea (16%), rash (11%)

Occasional

Decreased appetite (9%)

SERIOUS REACTIONS

! A hypersensitivity reaction may be life-threatening. Signs and symptoms include fever, rash, fatigue, intractable nausea and vomiting, severe diarrhea, abdominal pain, cough, pharyngitis, and dyspnea.
! Life-threatening hypotension may occur.
! Lactic acidosis and severe hepatomegaly may occur.

NURSING CONSIDERATIONS

Baseline Assessment

- Determine if the patient is pregnant before beginning therapy.
- Expect to obtain laboratory testing, especially liver function tests, before and periodically during therapy.

Lifespan Considerations

- It is unknown whether abacavir is excreted in breast milk. However, patients taking abacavir should not breast-feed because this may increase the risk of HIV transmission and adverse effects in the infant.
- Abacavir may be used safely in children ages 3 months to 13 years.
- The safety and efficacy of abacavir have not been established in the elderly.

Precautions

- Use abacavir cautiously in patients with impaired hepatic function.

Administration and Handling

PO

- Give without regard to food.
- The oral solution may be refrigerated. Don't freeze it.

Intervention and Evaluation

- Assess the patient for nausea and vomiting.
- Determine the patient's pattern of daily bowel activity and stool consistency.
- Assess the patient's eating pattern.
- Monitor the patient for weight loss.
- Monitor laboratory values carefully, particularly liver function test results.

Patient Teaching

- Advise the patient not to take any other medications, including OTC drugs, without consulting the physician.
- Encourage the patient to eat small, frequent meals to help offset decreased appetite and nausea.
- Inform the patient that abacavir is not a cure for HIV infection, nor does it reduce the risk of transmitting HIV to others.
- Offer emotional support to the patient.

amprenavir

am-**prehn**-eh-veer
(Agenerase)
Do not confuse Agenerase with asparaginase.

CATEGORY AND SCHEDULE

Pregnancy Risk Category: C

MECHANISM OF ACTION

An antiretroviral that inhibits HIV-1 protease by binding to the enzyme's active site, thus preventing processing of viral precursors and resulting in the formation of immature, noninfectious viral particles. **Therapeutic Effect:** Impairs HIV replication and proliferation.

PHARMACOKINETICS

Rapidly absorbed after PO administration. Protein binding: 90%. Metabolized in the liver. Primarily excreted in feces. ***Half-life:*** 7.1–10.6 hr.

AVAILABILITY

Capsules: 50 mg.
Oral Solution: 15 mg/ml.

INDICATIONS AND DOSAGES

▸ **HIV-1 infection (in combination with other antiretrovirals)**

PO

Adults, Children 13–16 yr. 1,200 mg capsules twice a day.

Children 4–12 yr, and children 13–16 yr weighing less than 50 kg. 20 mg/kg twice a day or 15 mg/kg 3 times a day. Maximum: 2,400 mg/day.

Oral solution
Adults. 1,400 mg 2 times/day.
Children 4–12 yr, and children 13–16 yr weighing less than 50 kg. 22.5 mg/kg/day (1.5 ml/kg) oral solution twice a day or 17 mg/kg/day (1.1 ml/kg) 3 times a day. Maximum: 2,800 mg/day.

▸ Dosage in hepatic impairment
Dosage and frequency are modified based on the Child-Pugh score.

Child-Pugh Score	Capsules	Oral Solution
5–8	450 mg bid	513 mg bid
9–12	300 mg bid	342 mg bid

CONTRAINDICATIONS
None known.

INTERACTIONS
Drug
Amiodarone, bepridil, ergotamine, lidocaine, midazolam, oral contraceptives, quinidine, triazolam, tricyclic antidepressants: May interfere with the metabolism of these drugs.
Antacids, didanosine: May decrease amprenavir absorption.
Carbamazepine, phenobarbital, phenytoin, rifampin: May decrease amprenavir blood concentration.
Clozapine, HMG-CoA reductase inhibitors (including statins), warfarin: May increase the blood concentration of these drugs.
Herbal
St. John's wort: May decrease amprenavir blood concentration.
Food
High-fat meals: May decrease amprenavir absorption.

DIAGNOSTIC TEST EFFECTS
May increase blood cholesterol, serum glucose, and triglyceride levels.

SIDE EFFECTS
Frequent
Diarrhea or loose stools (56%), nausea (38%), oral paresthesia (30%), rash (25%), vomiting (20%)
Occasional
Peripheral paresthesia (12%), depression (4%)

SERIOUS REACTIONS
! Severe hypersensitivity reactions or Stevens-Johnson syndrome as evidenced by blisters, peeling of the skin, loosening of skin and mucous membranes, and fever may occur.

NURSING CONSIDERATIONS
Baseline Assessment
- Expect to obtain laboratory testing before and periodically during therapy.

Lifespan Considerations
- It is unknown if amprenavir crosses the placenta or is distributed in breast milk.
- The safety and efficacy of amprenavir have not established in children younger than 4 years.
- Age-related hepatic impairment may require a dosage reduction in elderly patients.

Precautions
- Use amprenavir cautiously in patients with diabetes mellitus, hemophilia, hypersensitivity to sulfa drugs, impaired hepatic function, or vitamin K deficiency from anticoagulant malabsorption.

Administration and Handling
PO
- Give amprenavir without regard to food.

Intervention and Evaluation
- Observe the patient for nausea or vomiting.
- Determine the patient's pattern of daily bowel activity and stool consistency.

• Evaluate the patient's eating pattern and monitor him or her for weight loss.
• Assess the patient for a rash and for tingling or numbness of the peripheral extremities.

Patient Teaching

• Urge the patient to avoid high-fat meals because they may decrease drug absorption.
• Encourage the patient to consume small, frequent meals to help offset decreased appetite and nausea.
• Inform the patient that amprenavir is not a cure for HIV infection, nor does it reduce the risk of transmitting HIV to others.
• Offer the patient emotional support.

atazanavir sulfate

ah-tah-**zan**-ah-veer
(Reyataz)
Do not confuse Reyataz with Retavase.

CATEGORY AND SCHEDULE

Pregnancy Risk Category: B

MECHANISM OF ACTION

An antiviral that acts as an HIV-1 protease inhibitor, selectively preventing the processing of viral precursors found in cells infected with HIV-1. **Therapeutic Effect:** Prevents the formation of mature HIV cells.

PHARMACOKINETICS

Rapidly absorbed after PO administration. Protein binding: 86%. Extensively metabolized in the liver. Excreted primarily in urine and, to a lesser extent, in feces. ***Half-life:*** 5–8 hr.

AVAILABILITY

Capsules: 100 mg, 150 mg, 200 mg.

INDICATIONS AND DOSAGES

▸ **HIV-1 infection**
PO
Adults, Elderly (antiretroviral-naive). 400 mg (2 capsules) once a day with food.
Adults, Elderly (antiretroviral-experienced). 300 mg and ritonavir (Norvir) 100 mg once a day.

▸ **HIV-1 infection (concurrent therapy with efavirenz)**
PO
Adults, Elderly. 300 mg atazanavir, 100 mg ritonavir, and 600 mg efavirenz as a single daily dose with food.

▸ **HIV-1 infection (concurrent therapy with didanosine)**
PO
Adults, Elderly. Give atazanavir with food 2 hours before or 1 hour after didanosine.

▸ **HIV-1 infection (concurrent therapy with tenofovir)**
PO
Adults, Elderly. 300 mg atazanavir and 100 mg ritonavir and 300 mg tenofovir given as a single daily dose with food.

▸ **HIV-1 infection in patients with mild to moderate hepatic impairment**
PO
Adults, Elderly. 300 mg once a day with food.

CONTRAINDICATIONS

Concurrent use with ergot derivatives, midazolam, pimozide, or triazolam; severe hepatic insufficiency

INTERACTIONS

Drug

Antacids, H_2 receptor antagonists, proton pump inhibitors, rifampin: May decrease atazanavir plasma concentrations.

Atorvastatin, calcium channel blockers, immunosuppressants, irinotecan, lovastatin, sildenafil, simvastatin, tricyclic antidepressants: May increase atazanavir plasma concentrations.

Herbal

St. John's wort: May decrease atazanavir plasma concentration.

Food

High-fat meals: May decrease atazanavir absorption.

DIAGNOSTIC TEST EFFECTS

May increase serum amylase, bilirubin, lipase, AST (SGOT), and ALT (SGPT) levels. May decrease blood Hgb level and neutrophil and platelet counts. May alter LDL and serum triglyceride levels.

SIDE EFFECTS

Frequent (16%–14%)

Nausea, headache

Occasional (9%–4%)

Rash, vomiting, depression, diarrhea, abdominal pain, fever

Rare (3% or less)

Dizziness, insomnia, cough, fatigue, back pain

SERIOUS REACTIONS

! A severe hypersensitivity reaction (marked by angioedema and chest pain) and jaundice may occur.

NURSING CONSIDERATIONS

Baseline Assessment

- Obtain laboratory testing, including CBC and liver function tests, before beginning atazanavir therapy and periodically during therapy.

Lifespan Considerations

- It is unknown if atazanavir crosses the placenta or distributed in breast milk.
- Hyperbilirubinemia, kernicterus, and lactic acidosis syndrome have been reported in pregnant and breastfeeding women.
- The safety and efficacy of atazanavir have not been established in children younger than 3 months.
- Age-related hepatic impairment may require a dosage reduction in elderly patients.

Precautions

- Use atazanavir extremely cautiously in patients with hepatic impairment.
- Also use the drug cautiously in elderly patients and patients with diabetes mellitus, impaired renal function, or pre-existing conduction system disease, including first-, second-, or third-degree AV block.

Administration and Handling

PO

- Give atazanavir with food.

Intervention and Evaluation

- Evaluate the patient's eating pattern, and assess for nausea and vomiting.
- Assess the patient's pattern of daily bowel activity and stool consistency.
- Examine the patient's skin for a rash.
- Determine if the patient experiences headache.
- Monitor the patient for the onset of depression.

Patient Teaching

- Instruct the patient to take atazanavir with food. Explain that eating small, frequent meals may offset the drug's side effects of nausea and vomiting.
- Inform the patient that atazanavir is not a cure for HIV infection, nor does it reduce the risk of transmitting HIV to others.

• Offer the patient emotional support.

delavirdine mesylate

deh-**la**-ver-deen

(Rescriptor)

Do not confuse Rescriptor with Retrovin or Ritonavir.

CATEGORY AND SCHEDULE

Pregnancy Risk Category: C

MECHANISM OF ACTION

A nonnucleoside reverse transcriptase inhibitor that binds directly to HIV-1 reverse transcriptase and blocks RNA- and DNA-dependent DNA polymerase activities. **Therapeutic Effect:** Interrupts HIV replication, slowing the progression of HIV infection.

PHARMACOKINETICS

Rapidly absorbed after PO administration. Protein binding: 98%. Primarily distributed in plasma. Metabolized in the liver. Eliminated in feces and urine. ***Half-life:*** 2–11 hr.

AVAILABILITY

Tablets: 100 mg, 200 mg.

INDICATIONS AND DOSAGES

▸ HIV infection (in combination with other antiretrovirals)

PO

Adults. 400 mg 3 times a day.

CONTRAINDICATIONS

None known.

INTERACTIONS

Drug

Benzodiazepines, calcium channel blockers: May cause life-threatening adverse reactions.

Carbamazepine, phenobarbital, phenytoin: May decrease delavirdine blood concentration.

H_2 blockers: May decrease delavirdine absorption.

Rifampin: May decrease delavirdine blood concentrations.

Herbal

None known.

Food

None known.

DIAGNOSTIC TEST EFFECTS

May increase AST (SGOT) and ALT (SGPT) levels. May decrease neutrophil count.

SIDE EFFECTS

Frequent (18%)

Rash, pruritus

Occasional (greater than 2%)

Headache, nausea, diarrhea, fatigue, anorexia

SERIOUS REACTIONS

! None known.

NURSING CONSIDERATIONS

Baseline Assessment

• Expect to obtain laboratory testing, especially liver function tests, before and periodically during delavirdine therapy.

• Offer the patient emotional support.

Lifespan Considerations

• It is unknown if delavirdine crosses the placenta or is distributed in breast milk.

• The safety and efficacy of delavirdine have not been established in children younger than 16 years and in the elderly.

Precautions

• Use delavirdine cautiously in patients with hepatic impairment.

Administration and Handling

PO

• Give delavirdine without regard to food.

• Tablets may be dispersed in water before consumption.

• Give delavirdine with orange juice or cranberry juice if the patient has achlorhydria.

Intervention and Evaluation

• Assess the patient's skin for rash.

• Determine the patient's daily pattern of bowel activity and stool consistency.

• Assess the patient's eating pattern, and monitor for nausea and weight loss.

• Expect to monitor laboratory values carefully, particularly liver function test results.

Patient Teaching

• Advise the patient not to take any other medications, including OTC drugs, without notifying the physician.

• Inform the patient that small, frequent meals may offset nausea and anorexia.

• Explain to the patient that delavirdine is not a cure for HIV infection, nor does it reduce the risk of transmitting HIV to others.

• Offer the patient emotional support.

didanosine

dye-**dan**-o-seen

(Videx, Videx-EC)

CATEGORY AND SCHEDULE

Pregnancy Risk Category: B

MECHANISM OF ACTION

A purine nucleoside analogue that is intracellularly converted into a triphosphate, which interferes with RNA-directed DNA polymerase (reverse transcriptase). **Therapeutic Effect:** Inhibits replication of retroviruses, including HIV.

PHARMACOKINETICS

Variably absorbed from the GI tract. Protein binding: less than 5%. Rapidly metabolized intracellularly to active form. Primarily excreted in urine. Partially (20%) removed by hemodialysis. ***Half-life:*** 1.5 hr; metabolite: 8–24 hr.

AVAILABILITY

Capsules (Delayed-Release): 125 mg, 200 mg, 250 mg, 400 mg.

Pediatric Powder for Oral Solution: 10 mg/ml.

Powder for Oral Solution (Single-Dose Packet): 100 mg.

Tablets (Chewable): 25 mg, 50 mg, 100 mg, 150 mg, 200 mg.

INDICATIONS AND DOSAGES

▸ **HIV infection (in combination with other antiretrovirals)**

PO (Tablets, chewable)

Adults, Children 13 yr and older weighing 60 kg or more. 200 mg q12h or 400 mg once a day.

Adults, Children 13 yr and older weighing 60 kg or less. 125 mg q12h or 250 mg once a day.

Children 3 mo to less than 13 yr. 180–300 mg/m^2/day in divided doses q12h.

Children younger than 3 mo. 50 mg/m^2/day in divided doses q12h.

PO (Delayed-Release Capsules)

Adults, Children 13 yr and older weighing 60 kg or more. 400 mg once a day.

Adults, Children 13 yr and older weighing 60 kg or less. 250 mg once a day.

PO (Oral Solution)
Adults, Children 13 yr and older weighing 60 kg or more. 250 mg q12h.
Adults, Children 13 yr and older weighing 60 kg or less. 167 mg q12h.
PO (Pediatric Powder for Oral Solution)
Children 3 mo to younger than 13 yr. 180–300 mg/m²/day in divided doses q12h.
Children younger than 3 mo. 50 mg/m²/day in divided doses q12h.

▸ Dosage in renal impairment
Patients weighing less than 60 kg:

CrCl	Tablets	Oral Solution	Delayed-Release Capsules
30–59 ml/min	75 mg twice a day	100 mg twice a day	125 mg once a day
10–29 ml/min	100 mg once a day	100 mg once a day	125 mg once a day
less than 10 ml/min	75 mg once a day	100 mg once a day	N/A

CrCl = creatinine clearance

Patients weighing 60 kg or more:

CrCl	Tablets	Oral Solution	Delayed-Release Capsules
30–59 ml/min	100 mg twice a day	100 mg twice a day	200 mg once a day
10–29 ml/min	150 mg once a day	167 mg once a day	125 mg once a day
less than 10 ml/min	100 mg once a day	100 mg once a day	125 mg once a day

CrCl = creatinine clearance

CONTRAINDICATIONS
Hypersensitivity to didanosine or any of its components

INTERACTIONS
Drug
Dapsone, flouroquinolones, itraconazole, ketoconazole, tetracyclines: May decrease absorption of these drugs.
Medications producing pancreatitis or peripheral neuropathy: May increase the risk of pancreatitis or peripheral neuropathy.
Stavudine: May increase the risk of fatal lactic acidosis in pregnancy.
Herbal
None known.
Food
All foods: Decreases absorption of didanosine.

DIAGNOSTIC TEST EFFECTS
May increase serum alkaline phosphatase, amylase, bilirubin, lipase, triglyceride, AST (SGOT), ALT (SGPT), and uric acid levels. May decrease serum potassium levels.

SIDE EFFECTS
Frequent
Adults (greater than 10%)
Diarrhea, neuropathy, chills and fever
Children (greater than 25%)
Chills, fever, decreased appetite, pain, malaise, nausea, vomiting, diarrhea, abdominal pain, headache, nervousness, cough, rhinitis, dyspnea, asthenia, rash, pruritus
Occasional
Adults (9%–2%)
Rash, pruritus, headache, abdominal pain, nausea, vomiting, pneumonia, myopathy, decreased appetite, dry mouth, dyspnea
Children (25%–10%)
Failure to thrive, weight loss, stomatitis, oral thrush, ecchymosis, arthri-

tis, myalgia, insomnia, epistaxis, pharyngitis

SERIOUS REACTIONS

! Pneumonia and opportunistic infections occur occasionally.

! Peripheral neuropathy, potentially fatal pancreatitis, retinal changes, and optic neuritis are the major toxic effects.

NURSING CONSIDERATIONS

Baseline Assessment

- Expect to obtain the patient's baseline CBC, serum renal and liver function test results, vital signs, and weight.

Lifespan Considerations

- Didanosine should be used during pregnancy only if clearly needed. Breast-feeding should be discontinued during didanosine therapy.
- Didanosine is well tolerated in children older than 3 months.
- Age-related renal impairment may require a dosage adjustment in elderly patients.

Precautions

- Use didanosine cautiously in patients with alcoholism, elevated serum triglyceride levels, renal or hepatic dysfunction, or T-cell counts less than 100 cells/mm^3.
- Use with extreme caution in patients with a history of pancreatitis.
- Use cautiously in patients with phenylketonuria and those on sodium-restricted diets because didanosine contains phenylalanine and sodium.

Administration and Handling

PO

- Store at room temperature.
- Tablets dispersed in water are stable for 1 hour at room temperature; after reconstitution of buffered powder, oral solution is stable for 4 hours at room temperature.
- After reconstitution as directed, pediatric powder for oral solution is stable for 30 days refrigerated.
- Give the drug 1 hour before or 2 hours after a meal because food decreases the rate and extent of absorption.
- Thoroughly crush and disperse the chewable tablets in at least 30 ml of water. Stir the mixture well (2 to 3 minutes), and have the patient swallow it immediately.
- Reconstitute the buffered powder for oral solution by pouring the contents of the packet into 4 oz of water; stir the mixture until completely dissolved (2 to 3 minutes). Don't mix the powder with fruit juice or any other acidic liquid because didanosine is unstable in an acidic pH.
- Add 100 to 200 ml of water to 2 g or 4 g of the unbuffered pediatric powder, respectively, to provide a concentration of 20 mg/ml. Immediately mix with an equal amount of an antacid to provide a concentration of 10 mg/ml. Shake thoroughly before administering each dose.
- Have the patient swallow the enteric-coated capsules whole on an empty stomach.

Intervention and Evaluation

◀ALERT▶ Contact the physician if the patient experiences abdominal pain, elevated serum amylase or triglyceride levels, nausea, and vomiting before taking didanosine because these symptoms may indicate pancreatitis.

- Assess the patient for signs and symptoms of peripheral neuropathy, including burning feet, restless leg syndrome (inability to find a comfortable position for legs and feet), and lack of coordination.
- Monitor the patient's pattern of

daily bowel activity and stool consistency.
- Check the patient's skin for eruptions and a rash.
- As appropriate, monitor the patient's blood chemistry values and CBC.
- Assess the patient for signs and symptoms of opportunistic infections, including cough or other respiratory symptoms, fever, and oral mucosa changes.
- Check the patient's weight at least twice a week.
- Assess the patient for visual or auditory difficulty, and provide protection from light if photophobia occurs.

Patient Teaching
- Teach the patient to shake the oral suspension well before using it, to keep it refrigerated, and to discard the solution after 30 days and obtain a new supply.
- Advise the patient to avoid consuming alcohol.
- Instruct the patient to notify the physician if he or she experiences nausea or vomiting, numbness, or persistent, severe abdominal pain.
- Explain to the patient that didanosine is not a cure for HIV infection, nor does it reduce the risk of transmitting HIV to others.
- Offer the patient emotional support.

efavirenz

e-**fahv**-er-ins
(Stocrin[AUS], Sustiva)
Do not confuse Sustiva with Survanta.

CATEGORY AND SCHEDULE
Pregnancy Risk Category: C

MECHANISM OF ACTION
A nonnucleoside reverse transcriptase inhibitor that inhibits the activity of HIV reverse transcriptase of HIV-1 and the transcription of HIV-1 RNa to DNA. **Therapeutic Effect:** Interrupts HIV replication, slowing the progression of HIV infection.

PHARMACOKINETICS
Rapidly absorbed after PO administration. Protein binding: 99%. Metabolized to major isoenzymes in the liver. Eliminated in urine and feces. ***Half-life:*** 40–55 hr.

AVAILABILITY
Capsules: 50 mg, 100 mg, 200 mg.
Tablets: 600 mg.

INDICATIONS AND DOSAGES
▸ HIV infection (in combination with other antiretrovirals)
PO
Adults, Elderly, Children 3 yr and older weighing 40 kg or more. 600 mg once a day at bedtime.
Children 3 yr and older weighing 32.5 kg–less than 40 kg. 400 mg once a day.
Children 3 yr and older weighing 25 kg–less than 32.5 kg. 350 mg once a day.
Children 3 yr and older weighing 20 kg–less than 25 kg. 300 mg once a day.
Children 3 yr and older weighing 15 kg–less than 20 kg. 250 mg once a day.
Children 3 yr and older weighing 10 kg–less than 15 kg. 200 mg once a day.

CONTRAINDICATIONS
Concurrent use with ergot derivatives, midazolam, or triazolam; efavirenz as monotherapy; hypersensitivity to efavirenz

INTERACTIONS

Drug

Alcohol, psychoactive drugs: May produce additive CNS effects.
Clarithromycin: Decreases clarithromycin plasma levels.
Ergot derivatives, midazolam, triazolam: May cause serious or life-threatening reactions, such as arrhythmias, prolonged sedation, or respiratory depression.
Indinavir, saquinavir: Decreases the plasma concentrations of these drugs.
Nelfinavir, ritonavir: Increases the plasma concentrations of these drugs.
Phenobarbital, rifabutin, rifampin: Lowers efavirenz plasma concentration.
Warfarin: Alters warfarin plasma concentration.

Herbal

None known.

Food

High-fat meals: May increase drug absorption.

DIAGNOSTIC TEST EFFECTS

May produce false-positive urine test results for cannabinoid and increase total cholesterol, AST (SGOT), ALT (SGPT), and serum triglyceride levels.

SIDE EFFECTS

Frequent (52%)

Mild to severe: Dizziness, vivid dreams, insomnia, confusion, impaired concentration, amnesia, agitation, depersonalization, hallucinations, euphoria, somnolence (mild symptoms don't interfere with daily activities; severe symptoms interrupt daily activities)

Occasional

Mild to moderate: Maculopapular rash (27%); nausea, fatigue, headache, diarrhea, fever, cough (less than 26%) (moderate symptoms may interfere with daily activities)

SERIOUS REACTIONS

! None known.

NURSING CONSIDERATIONS

Baseline Assessment

- Expect to obtain baseline AST (SGOT) and ALT (SGPT) levels in patients with a history of hepatitis B or C before giving efavirenz.
- Expect to obtain the patient's serum cholesterol and triglyceride levels before and regularly during therapy.
- Obtain the patient's medication history (including all prescription and OTC drugs) before giving the drug because efavirenz interacts with several drugs.

Lifespan Considerations

- Breast-feeding is not recommended for patients taking efavirenz.
- The safety and efficacy of efavirenz have not been established in children younger than 3 years.
- Children may be at increased risk for a rash.
- No age-related precautions have been noted in the elderly.

Precautions

- Use efavirenz cautiously in patients with a history of hepatic impairment, mental illness, or substance abuse.

Administration and Handling

PO

- Give efavirenz without regard to meals.
- High-fat meals may increase drug absorption and should be avoided.
- For adult and elderly patients, administer the drug at bedtime during the first 2 to 4 weeks because of the increased risk of temporary CNS side effects.

Intervention and Evaluation

- Monitor the patient for adverse

CNS and psychological effects, such as abnormal dreams, dizziness, impaired concentration, insomnia, severe acute depression (including suicidal ideation or attempts), and somnolence. Be aware that insomnia may begin during the first or second day of therapy and generally resolves in 2 to 4 weeks.

- Assess the patient for a rash, a common side effect.
- As appropriate, monitor the patient's liver function test results for abnormalities.
- Assess the patient for diarrhea, headache, and nausea.

Patient Teaching

- Advise the patient to take efavirenz every day as prescribed and not to stop taking it or change the dose without first notifying the physician.
- Advise the patient to avoid high-fat meals during therapy.
- Instruct the patient to notify the physician immediately if a rash appears.
- Explain to the patient that CNS and psychological side effects, such as delusions, depression, dizziness, and impaired concentration, occur in more than half of patients taking this drug. Advise the patient to notify the physician if these symptoms continue or become problematic.
- Caution the patient to avoid tasks that require mental alertness or motor skills until his or her response to the drug is established.
- Explain that efavirenz is not a cure for HIV infection, nor does it reduce the risk of transmitting HIV to others.
- Offer emotional support to the patient and family.

emtricitabine

em-trih-**sit**-ah-bean
(Emtriva)

CATEGORY AND SCHEDULE

Pregnancy Risk Category: B

MECHANISM OF ACTION

An antiretroviral that inhibits HIV-1 reverse transcriptase by incorporating itself into viral DNA, resulting in chain termination. **Therapeutic Effect:** Interrupts HIV replication, slowing the progression of HIV infection.

PHARMACOKINETICS

Rapidly and extensively absorbed from the GI tract. Excreted primarily in urine (86%) and, to a lesser extent, in feces (14%); 30% removed by hemodialysis. Unknown if removed by peritoneal dialysis. ***Half-life:*** 10 hr.

AVAILABILITY

Capsules: 200 mg.

INDICATIONS AND DOSAGES

▸ **HIV infection (in combination with other antiretrovirals)**

PO

Adults, Elderly. 200 mg once a day.

▸ **Dosage in renal impairment**

Dosage and frequency are modified based on creatinine clearance.

Creatinine Clearance	Dosage
30–49 ml/min	200 mg q48h
15–29 ml/min	200 mg q72h
less than 15 ml/min, hemodialysis patients	200 mg q96h

CONTRAINDICATIONS

None known.

INTERACTIONS

Drug

None known.

Herbal

None known.

Food

None known.

DIAGNOSTIC TEST EFFECTS

May elevate serum amylase, lipase, ALT (SGPT), AST (SGOT), and triglyceride levels. May alter blood glucose levels.

SIDE EFFECTS

Frequent (23%–13%)

Headache, rhinitis, rash, diarrhea, nausea

Occasional (14%–4%)

Cough, vomiting, abdominal pain, insomnia, depression, paresthesia, dizziness, peripheral neuropathy, dyspepsia, myalgia

Rare (3%–2%)

Arthralgia, abnormal dreams

SERIOUS REACTIONS

! Lactic acidosis and hepatomegaly with steatosis occur rarely and may be severe.

NURSING CONSIDERATIONS

Baseline Assessment

- Expect to obtain laboratory testing, especially liver function tests and serum triglyceride levels, before and periodically during emtricitabine therapy.

Lifespan Considerations

- Breast-feeding is not recommended for patients taking emtricitabine.
- The safety and efficacy of this drug have not been established in children.
- Age-related renal impairment may require a dosage adjustment in the elderly.

Precautions

- Use emtricitabine cautiously in patients with impaired hepatic or renal function.

Administration and Handling

PO

- Give emtricitabine without regard to food.

Intervention and Evaluation

- Assess the patient's daily pattern of bowel activity and stool consistency.
- Evaluate the patient for nausea and pruritus.
- Examine the patient's skin for a rash and urticaria.
- Monitor the patient's serum chemistry tests for marked abnormalities.

Patient Teaching

- Explain to the patient that emtricitabine use may cause a redistribution of body fat.
- Advise the patient to continue taking emtricitabine for the full course of treatment.
- Inform the patient that emtricitabine is not a cure for HIV infection, nor does it reduce the risk of transmitting HIV to others. Explain that he or she may continue to develop illnesses associated with advanced HIV infection.
- Offer the patient emotional support.

enfuvirtide

en-**few**-vir-tide

(Fuzeon)

Do not confuse Fuzeon with Furoxone.

CATEGORY AND SCHEDULE

Pregnancy Risk Category: B

MECHANISM OF ACTION

A fusion inhibitor that interferes with the entry of HIV-1 into CD4+ cells by inhibiting the fusion of viral and cellular membranes. **Therapeutic Effect:** Impairs HIV replication, slowing the progression of HIV infection.

PHARMACOKINETICS

Comparable absorption when injected into subcutaneous tissue of abdomen, arm, or thigh. Protein binding: 92%. Undergoes catabolism to amino acids. ***Half-life:*** 3.8 hr.

AVAILABILITY

Powder for Injection: 108-mg (approximately 90 mg/ml when reconstituted) vials.

INDICATIONS AND DOSAGES

▸ HIV infection (in combination with other antiretrovirals)

Subcutaneous

Adults, Elderly. 90 mg (1 ml) twice a day.

Children 6–16 yr. 2 mg/kg twice a day. Maximum 90 mg twice a day.

Pediatric dosing guidelines

Weight: kg (lb)	Dose: mg (ml)
11–15.5 (24–34)	27 (0.3)
15.6–20 (35–44)	36 (0.4)
20.1–24.5 (45–54)	45 (0.5)
24.6–29 (55–64)	54 (0.6)
29.1–33.5 (65–74)	63 (0.7)
33.6–38 (75–84)	72 (0.8)
38.1–42.5 (85–94)	81 (0.9)
greater than 42.5 (greater than 94)	90 (1)

CONTRAINDICATIONS

None known.

INTERACTIONS

Drug

None known.

Herbal

None known.

Food

None known.

DIAGNOSTIC TEST EFFECTS

May elevate blood glucose and serum amylase, CK, lipase, triglyceride, AST (SGOT), and ALT (SGPT) levels. May decrease blood hemoglobin levels and WBC count.

SIDE EFFECTS

Expected (98%)

Local injection site reactions (pain, discomfort, induration, erythema, nodules, cysts, pruritus, ecchymosis)

Frequent (26%–16%)

Diarrhea, nausea, fatigue

Occasional (11%–4%)

Insomnia, peripheral neuropathy, depression, cough, decreased appetite or weight loss, sinusitis, anxiety, asthenia, myalgia, cold sores

Rare (3%–2%)

Constipation, influenza, upper abdominal pain, anorexia, conjunctivitis

SERIOUS REACTIONS

! Enfuvirtide use may potentiate bacterial pneumonia.

! Hypersensitivity (rash, fever, chills, rigors, hypotension), thrombocytopenia, neutropenia, and renal insufficiency or failure may occur rarely.

NURSING CONSIDERATIONS

Baseline Assessment

- Expect to obtain laboratory testing, especially liver function tests and serum triglyceride levels, before and periodically during enfuvirtide therapy.

Lifespan Considerations

- Breast-feeding is not recommended for patients taking enfuvirtide because of the risk of transmitting HIV to the infant.

• The safety and efficacy of enfuvirtide have not been established in children 6 years and younger.
• No age-related precautions have been noted in the elderly.

Administration and Handling

• Store the drug at room temperature. Refrigerate the reconstituted solution and use it within 24 hours.
• Bring the reconstituted solution to room temperature before injection.
• Reconstitute the drug with 1.1 ml of sterile water for injection. Visually inspect the vial for particulate matter. The solution normally appears clear and colorless. Discard the unused portion.
• Administer the drug subcutaneously into the upper abdomen, anterior thigh, or arm. Rotate injection sites.

Intervention and Evaluation

• Assess the patient's skin for a hypersensitivity reaction and local injection site reactions.
• Observe the patient for evidence of fatigue or nausea.
• Evaluate the patient's sleep patterns and monitor for insomnia.
• Monitor the patient for signs and symptoms of depression.
• Monitor the patient's blood chemistry test results for marked abnormalities.

Patient Teaching

• Advise the patient to continue taking enfuvirtide for the full course of treatment.
• Warn the patient that this drug may cause bacterial pneumonia; instruct him or her to seek medical attention if cough with fever and rapid difficult breathing occurs.
• Inform the patient that enfuvirtide is not a cure for HIV infection, nor does it reduce the risk of transmitting HIV to others. Explain the need to continue practices to prevent transmission of HIV.
• Offer the patient emotional support.

fosamprenavir calcium

foss-am-**pren**-ah-vur
(Lexiva)

CATEGORY AND SCHEDULE

Pregnancy Risk Category: C

MECHANISM OF ACTION

An antiretroviral that is rapidly converted to amprenavir, which inhibits HIV-1 protease by binding to the enzyme's active site, thus preventing the processing of viral precursors and resulting in the formation of immature, noninfectious viral particles. **Therapeutic Effect:** Impairs HIV replication and proliferation.

PHARMACOKINETICS

Rapidly absorbed after PO administration. Protein binding: 90%. Metabolized in the liver. Excreted in urine and feces. ***Half-life:*** 7.7 hr.

AVAILABILITY

Tablets: 700 mg (equivalent to 600 mg amprenavir)

INDICATIONS AND DOSAGES

▸ HIV infection in patients who have not had previous protease inhibitor therapy

PO

Adults, Elderly. 1,400 mg twice daily without ritonavir; or 1,400 mg twice daily plus ritonavir 200 mg once daily; or 700 mg twice daily plus ritonavir 100 mg twice daily.

▸ **HIV infection in patients who have had previous protease inhibitor therapy**
PO
Adults, Elderly. 700 mg twice daily plus ritonavir 100 mg twice daily.
▸ **Concurrent therapy with efavirenz**
PO
Adults, Elderly. In patients receiving fosamprenavir plus once-daily ritonavir in combination with efavirenz, an additional 100 mg/day ritonavir (300 mg total/day) should be given.

CONTRAINDICATIONS

Concurrent use of amprenavir, dihydroergotamine, ergonovine, ergotamine, methylergonovine, pimozide, midazolam, or triazolam. If fosamprenavir is given concurrently with ritonavir, flecainide and propafenone are also contraindicated

INTERACTIONS

Drug

Amiodarone, bepridil, ergotamine, lidocaine, midazolam, oral contraceptives, quinidine, triazolam, tricyclic antidepressants: May interfere with the metabolism of the these drugs.
Antacids, didanosine: May decrease the absorption of fosamprenavir.
Carbamazepine, phenobarbital, phenytoin, rifampin: May decrease the fosamprenavir blood concentration.
Clozapine, HMG-CoA reductase inhibitors (statins), warfarin: May increase the blood concentrations of these drugs.

Herbal

St. John's wort: May decrease the fosamprenavir blood concentration.

Food

None known.

DIAGNOSTIC TEST EFFECTS

May increase serum lipase, triglyceride, AST (SGOT), and ALT (SGPT) levels.

SIDE EFFECTS

Frequent (39%–35%)
Nausea, rash, diarrhea
Occasional (19%–8%)
Headache, vomiting, fatigue, depression
Rare (7%–2%)
Pruritus, abdominal pain, perioral paresthesia

SERIOUS REACTIONS

! Severe and possibly life-threatening dermatologic reactions occur rarely.

NURSING CONSIDERATIONS

Baseline Assessment

• Obtain laboratory tests, especially liver function tests, before and periodically during therapy.

Lifespan Considerations

• It is unknown if fosamprenavir crosses the placenta or is distributed in breast milk.
• The safety and efficacy of fosamprenavir have not established in children younger than 4 years.
• Age-related hepatic impairment may require a dosage reduction in elderly patients.

Precautions

• Use fosamprenavir extremely cautiously in patients with hepatic impairment.
• Use fosamprenavir cautiously in elderly patients and those with diabetes mellitus, renal impairment, or a known allergy to sulfonamides.

Administration and Handling

PO
• Give fosamprenavir without regard to food.

- Don't crush or break film-coated tablets.

Intervention and Evaluation

- Closely monitor the patient for GI discomfort.
- Determine the patient's pattern of daily bowel activity and stool consistency.
- Examine the patient's skin for a rash.
- Monitor laboratory test results, especially liver function tests, for marked abnormalities.

Patient Teaching

- Instruct the patient to space doses evenly and to continue taking fosamprenavir for the full course of treatment.
- Encourage the patient to consume small, frequent meals to help offset nausea and vomiting. Suggest using OTC antidiarrheals if diarrhea occurs.
- Inform the patient that fosamprenavir is not a cure for HIV infection, nor does it reduce the risk of transmitting HIV to others.
- Offer the patient emotional support.

indinavir

in-**din**-ah-veer
(Crixivan)
Do not confuse indinavir with Denavir.

CATEGORY AND SCHEDULE

Pregnancy Risk Category: C

MECHANISM OF ACTION

A protease inhibitor that suppresses HIV protease, an enzyme necessary for splitting viral polyprotein precursors into mature and infectious viral particles. **Therapeutic Effect:** Interrupts HIV replication, slowing the progression of HIV infection.

PHARMACOKINETICS

Rapidly absorbed after PO administration. Protein binding: 60%. Metabolized in the liver. Primarily excreted in urine. Unknown if removed by hemodialysis. ***Half-life:*** 1.8 hr (increased in impaired hepatic function).

AVAILABILITY

Capsules: 100 mg, 200 mg, 333 mg, 400 mg.

INDICATIONS AND DOSAGES

▸ **HIV infection (in combination with other antiretrovirals)**

PO

Adults. 800 mg (two 400-mg capsules) q8h.

▸ **HIV infection in patients with hepatic insufficiency**

PO

Adults. 600 mg q8h.

OFF-LABEL USES

Prophylaxis following occupational exposure to HIV

CONTRAINDICATIONS

Hypersensitivity to indinavir; nephrolithiasis

INTERACTIONS

Drug

Midazolam, triazolam: Increases the risk of arrhythmias and prolonged sedation.

Herbal

St. John's wort: May decrease indinavir blood concentration and effect.

Food

Grapefruit: May decrease indinavir blood concentration and effect.

High-fat, high-calorie, and high-protein meals: May decrease indinavir blood concentration.

DIAGNOSTIC TEST EFFECTS

May increase serum bilirubin (in 10% of patients), AST (SGOT), and ALT (SGPT) levels.

SIDE EFFECTS

Frequent

Nausea (12%), abdominal pain (9%), headache (6%), diarrhea (5%)

Occasional

Vomiting, asthenia, fatigue (4%); insomnia; accumulation of fat in waist, abdomen, or back of neck

Rare

Abnormal taste sensation, heartburn, symptomatic urinary tract disease, transient renal dysfunction

SERIOUS REACTIONS

! Nephrolithiasis (flank pain with or without hematuria) occurs in 4% of patients.

NURSING CONSIDERATIONS

Baseline Assessment

- Establish the patient's baseline laboratory values.
- Monitor the patient's renal function before and during therapy, especially the results of serum creatinine and urinalysis tests.

Lifespan Considerations

- It is unknown if indinavir is excreted in breast milk. However, breast-feeding is not recommended for patients taking indinavir because of the possibility of transmitting HIV to the infant.
- The safety and efficacy of this drug have not been established in children.
- The effects of this drug on the elderly are unknown.

Precautions

- Use indinavir cautiously in patients with renal or hepatic impairment.

Administration and Handling

PO

- Store indinavir at room temperature, in the original bottle, and protect it from moisture. Keep in mind that indinavir capsules are sensitive to moisture.
- For optimal drug absorption, give indinavir with water only 1 hour before or 2 hours after a meal. However, the drug may also be given with coffee, juice, skim milk, tea, or water and with a light meal (such as dry toast with jelly).
- Don't give indinavir with meals that are high in fat, calories, or protein.
- If indinavir and didanosine are given concurrently, give the drugs at least 1 hour apart on an empty stomach.

Intervention and Evaluation

- To maintain adequate hydration, have the patient drink 48 oz (1.5 L) of liquid every day during therapy.

◀ALERT▶ Monitor the patient for signs and symptoms of nephrolithiasis (flank pain and hematuria), and notify the physician if symptoms occur. If nephrolithiasis occurs, expect therapy to be interrupted for 1 to 3 days.

- Assess the patient's pattern of daily bowel activity and stool consistency.
- Evaluate the patient for abdominal discomfort or headache.
- Expect to monitor the patient's serum amylase, bilirubin, cholesterol, lipase, and triglyceride levels; blood glucose level; CBC; CD4+ cell count; and liver function test results.

Patient Teaching

- If the patient misses a dose, instruct him or her to take the next dose at the regularly scheduled time, not to double the dose.

• Instruct the patient to take indinavir with water only 1 hour before or 2 hours after a meal for optimal drug absorption. However, explain that indinavir may also be taken with coffee, juice, skim milk, tea, or water or with a light carbohydrate meal, but should not be taken with meals high in fat, calories, or protein.
• Urge the patient to avoid St. John's wort and grapefruit or grapefruit juice during treatment because they will lower indinavir levels.
• Inform the patient that indinavir is not a cure for HIV infection, nor does it reduce the risk of transmitting HIV to others.
• Offer emotional support to the patient.

lamivudine

la-**miv**-yoo-deen
(Epivir, Epivir-HBV, Heptovir[CAN], Zeffix[AUS])
Do not confuse lamivudine with lamotrigine.

CATEGORY AND SCHEDULE

Pregnancy Risk Category: C

MECHANISM OF ACTION

An antiviral that inhibits HIV reverse transcriptase by viral DNA chain termination. Also inhibits RNA- and DNA-dependent DNA polymerase, an enzyme necessary for HIV replication. **Therapeutic Effect:** Interrupts HIV replication, slowing the progression of HIV infection.

PHARMACOKINETICS

Rapidly and completely absorbed from the GI tract. Protein binding: less than 36%. Widely distributed (crosses the blood-brain barrier). Primarily excreted unchanged in urine. Not removed by hemodialysis or peritoneal dialysis. ***Half-life:*** 11–15 hr (intracellular), 2–11 hr (serum, adults), 1.7–2 hr (serum, children). (increased in impaired renal function).

AVAILABILITY

Oral Solution (Epivir): 10 mg/ml.
Oral Solution (Epivir-HBV): 5 mg/ml.
Tablets (Epivir): 150 mg, 300 mg.
Tablets (Epivir-HBV): 100 mg.

INDICATIONS AND DOSAGES

▸ **HIV infection (in combination with other antiretrovirals)**

PO

Adults, Children 12–16 yr weighing 50 kg (100 lb) or more. 150 mg twice a day or 300 mg once a day.
Adults weighing less than 50 kg. 2 mg/kg twice a day.
Children 3 mo–11 yr. 4 mg/kg twice a day (up to 150 mg/dose).

▸ **Chronic hepatitis B**

PO

Adults, Children 17 yr and older. 100 mg/day.
Children younger than 17 yr. 3 mg/kg/day. Maximum: 100 mg/day.

▸ **Dosage in renal impairment**

Dosage and frequency are modified based on creatinine clearance.

Creatinine Clearance (ml/min)	Dosage
50 ml/min or higher	150 mg twice a day
30–49 ml/min	150 mg once a day
15–29 ml/min	150 mg first dose, then 100 mg once a day
5–14 ml/min	150 mg first dose, then 50 mg once a day
less than 5 ml/min	50 mg first dose, then 25 mg once a day

OFF-LABEL USES

Prophylaxis in health care workers at risk of acquiring HIV after occupational exposure

CONTRAINDICATIONS

None known.

INTERACTIONS

Drug

Co-trimoxazole: Increases lamivudine blood concentration.

Herbal

St. John's wort: May decrease lamivudine blood concentration and effect.

Food

None known.

DIAGNOSTIC TEST EFFECTS

May increase blood Hgb values, neutrophil count, and serum amylase, AST (SGOT), and ALT (SGPT) levels.

SIDE EFFECTS

Frequent

Headache (35%), nausea (33%), malaise and fatigue (27%), nasal disturbances (20%), diarrhea, cough (18%), musculoskeletal pain, neuropathy (12%), insomnia (11%), anorexia, dizziness, fever or chills (10%)

Occasional

Depression (9%); myalgia (8%); abdominal cramps (6%); dyspepsia, arthralgia (5%)

SERIOUS REACTIONS

! Pancreatitis occurs in 13% of pediatric patients.

! Anemia, neutropenia, and thrombocytopenia occur rarely.

NURSING CONSIDERATIONS

Baseline Assessment

• Before starting lamivudine therapy, check the patient's baseline laboratory values, especially renal function test results.

Lifespan Considerations

• Lamivudine crosses the placenta. It is unknown if lamivudine is distributed in breast milk; however, breast-feeding is not recommended for patients taking this drug because of the possibility of transmitting HIV to the infant.

• The safety and efficacy of this drug have not been established in children younger than 3 months.

• Age-related renal impairment may require a dosage adjustment in the elderly.

Precautions

• Use lamivudine cautiously in patients with impaired renal function or a history of pancreatitis or peripheral neuropathy.

• Use the drug cautiously in young children.

Administration and Handling

PO

• Give lamivudine without regard to meals.

Intervention and Evaluation

• Expect to monitor the patient's serum amylase, BUN, and serum creatinine levels.

• Evaluate the patient for altered sleep patterns, cough, dizziness, headache, and nausea.

• Assess the patient's pattern of daily bowel activity and stool consistency, and modify the patient's diet accordingly.

• If pancreatitis occurs in a pediatric patient, help the patient to sit up or flex at the waist to relieve abdominal pain aggravated by movement.

Patient Teaching

• Advise the patient to space lamivudine doses evenly around the clock and to continue taking the drug for the full course of treatment.

• Advise the parents of a pediatric

patient to closely monitor the child for symptoms of pancreatitis, such as clammy skin, hypotension, nausea, severe and steady abdominal pain that often radiates to the back, and vomiting accompanied by abdominal pain.
• Warn the patient to avoid performing tasks that require mental alertness or motor skills until his or her response to the drug has been established.
• Inform the patient that lamivudine is not a cure for HIV, nor does it reduce the risk of transmitting HIV to others. Explain that he or she may continue to experience illnesses associated with advanced HIV infection, including opportunistic infections.
• Offer the patient and family emotional support.

lopinavir/ritonavir

lop-**in**-a-veer/rit-**on**-a-veer
(Kaletra)
Do not confuse Kaletra with Keppra.

CATEGORY AND SCHEDULE

Pregnancy Risk Category: C

MECHANISM OF ACTION

A protease inhibitor combination drug in which lopinavir inhibits the activity of the enzyme protease late in the HIV replication process and ritonavir increases plasma levels of lopinavir. **Therapeutic Effect:** Formation of immature, noninfectious viral particles.

PHARMACOKINETICS

Readily absorbed after PO administration (absorption increased when taken with food). Protein binding: 98%–99%. Metabolized in the liver. Eliminated primarily in feces. Not removed by hemodialysis. ***Half-life:*** 5–6 hr.

AVAILABILITY

Capsules: 133.3 mg lopinavir/33.3 mg ritonavir.
Oral Solution: 80 mg/ml lopinavir/20 mg/ml ritonavir.

INDICATIONS AND DOSAGES

▸ HIV infection

PO

Adults. 3 capsules (400 mg lopinavir/100 mg ritonavir) or 5 ml twice a day. Increase to 4 capsules (533 mg lopinavir/133 mg ritonavir) or 6.5 ml when taken with efavirenz or nevirapine.
Children weighing 15–40 kg who are not taking efavirenz or nevirapine. 10 mg/kg twice a day.
Children weighing 7–14 kg who are not taking Alprenavir, efavirenz, nelfinavir, nevirapine. 12 mg/kg twice a day.
Children weighing 15–40 kg who are taking efavirenz or nevirapine. 11 mg/kg twice a day.
Children weighing 7–14 kg who are taking efavirenz or nevirapine. 13 mg/kg twice a day.

CONTRAINDICATIONS

Concomitant use of ergot derivatives (causes peripheral ischemia of extremities and vasospasm), flecainide, midazolam, pimozide, propafenone (increases the risk of serious cardiac arrhythmias), or triazolam (increases sedation or respiratory depression); hypersensitivity to lopinavir or ritonavir

INTERACTIONS

Drug

Atorvastatin: May increase lopi-

navir and ritonavir blood concentration and risk of myopathy.
Atovaquone, methadone, oral contraceptives: May decrease blood concentration and effects of these drugs.
Carbamazepine, corticosteroids, efavirenz, nevirapine, phenobarbital, phenytoin, rifampin: May decrease blood concentration and effects of lopinavir and ritonavir.
Clarithromycin, felodipine, immunosuppressants, nicardipine, nifedipine, rifabutin: May increase blood concentration and effects of these drugs.
Itraconzole, ketoconazole: May increase blood concentration of these drugs.
Metronidazole: May produce a disulfiram-like reaction.
Sildenafil, tadalafil, vardenafil: May increase the adverse effects of these drugs.

Herbal

St. John's wort: May decrease blood concentration and effects of lopinavir and ritonavir.

Food

None known.

DIAGNOSTIC TEST EFFECTS

May increase blood glucose, GGT, total cholesterol, and serum uric acid, AST (SGOT), ALT (SGPT), and triglyceride levels.

SIDE EFFECTS

Frequent (14%)
Mild to moderate diarrhea
Occasional (6%–2%)
Nausea, asthenia, abdominal pain, headache, vomiting
Rare (less than 2%)
Insomnia, rash

SERIOUS REACTIONS

! Anemia, leukopenia, lymphadenopathy, deep vein thrombosis, Cushing's syndrome, pancreatitis, and hemorrhagic colitis occur rarely.

NURSING CONSIDERATIONS

Baseline Assessment

• Expect to establish the patient's baseline weight, CBC, and renal and liver function test results.

Lifespan Considerations

• It is unknown if lopinavir and ritonavir is excreted in breast milk. However, breast-feeding is not recommended for patients taking this drug because of the possibility of transmitting HIV to the infant.
• The safety and efficacy of lopinavir and ritonavir have not been established in children younger than 6 months.
• In the elderly, age-related cardiac function, renal, or hepatic impairment requires caution.

Precautions

• Use lopinavir and ritonavir cautiously in patients with hepatitis B or C or impaired hepatic function.
◀ **ALERT** ▶ High-doses of itraconazole or ketoconazole are not recommended in patients taking lopinavir and rotinavir. The oral solution of lopinavir and ritonavir contains alcohol and should not be given to patients receiving metronidazole because this combination may cause a disulfiram-type reaction.

Administration and Handling

PO
• Refrigerate the drug until you dispense it, and avoid exposure to excessive heat.
• If the drug is stored at room temperature, use it within 2 months.
• Give this drug with food.

Intervention and Evaluation

• Assess the patient's pattern of daily bowel activity and stool consistency.

• Evaluate the patient for nausea and vomiting.
• Assess for signs and symptoms of opportunistic infections, such as fever, oral mucosa changes, and a cough or other respiratory symptoms.
• Check the patient's weight at least twice a week.
• Monitor the patient for signs and symptoms of pancreatitis, such as abdominal pain, nausea, and vomiting.
• Monitor the patient's CBC with differential, CD4+ cell count, HIV RNA level (viral load), liver function test results, and serum electrolyte and blood glucose levels.

Patient Teaching

• Teach the patient how to properly take lopinavir and ritonavir.
• Encourage the patient to eat small, frequent meals to offset nausea or vomiting.
• Explain to the patient that this drug is not a cure for HIV infection, nor does it reduce the risk of transmitting HIV to others.
• Offer the patient emotional support.

nelfinavir

nel-**fin**-eh-veer
(Viracept)

CATEGORY AND SCHEDULE

Pregnancy Risk Category: B

MECHANISM OF ACTION

Inhibits the activity of HIV-1 protease, the enzyme necessary for the formation of infectious HIV. **Therapeutic Effect:** Formation of immature noninfectious viral particles rather than HIV replication.

PHARMACOKINETICS

Well absorbed after PO administration (absorption increased with food). Protein binding: 98%. Metabolized in the liver. Highly bound to plasma proteins. Eliminated primarily in feces. Unknown if removed by hemodialysis. ***Half-life:*** 3.5–5 hr.

AVAILABILITY

Powder for Oral Suspension: 50 mg/g.
Tablets: 250 mg, 625 mg.

INDICATIONS AND DOSAGES

▸ **HIV infection**

PO

Adults. 750 mg (three 250-mg tablets) 3 times a day or 1,250 mg twice a day in combination with nucleoside analogues (enhances antiviral activity).
Children 2–13 yr. 20–30 mg/kg/dose 3 times a day. Maximum: 750 mg q8h.

CONTRAINDICATIONS

Concurrent administration with midazolam, rifampin, or triazolam

INTERACTIONS

Drug

Alcohol, psychoactive drugs: May produce additive CNS effects.
Anticonvulsants, rifabutin, rifampin: Decrease nelfinavir plasma concentration.
Indinavir, saquinavir: Increases plasma concentration of these drugs.
Oral contraceptives: Decreases the effects of these drugs.
Ritonavir: Increases nelfinavir plasma concentration.

Herbal

St. John's wort: May decrease plasma concentration and effects of nelfinavir.

Food

All foods: Increase nelfinavir plasma concentration.

DIAGNOSTIC TEST EFFECTS

May decrease Hgb values and neutrophil and WBC counts. May increase serum CK, AST (SGOT), and ALT (SGPT) levels.

SIDE EFFECTS

Frequent (20%)
Diarrhea
Occasional (7%–3%)
Nausea, rash
Rare (2%–1%)
Flatulence, asthenia

SERIOUS REACTIONS

! None known.

NURSING CONSIDERATIONS

Baseline Assessment

• Expect to check the patient's baseline hematologic and hepatic function test results before beginning drug therapy.

Lifespan Considerations

• It is unknown if nelfinavir is distributed in breast milk.
• No age-related precautions have been noted in children older than 2 years.
• The effects of this drug on the elderly are unknown.

Precautions

• Use nelfinavir cautiously in patients with hepatic impairment.

Administration and Handling

PO
• Give the drug with a light meal, or snack.
• Mix the oral powder with a small amount of water, milk, formula, soy formula, soy milk, or dietary supplement.
• Don't mix the powder with acidic foods or juices, such as orange juice, apple juice, or applesauce, or with water in the powder's original oral powder container.
• Be aware that the entire contents must be consumed in order to obtain the full dose.

Intervention and Evaluation

• Assess the patient's pattern of daily bowel activity and stool consistency.
• Monitor the patient's hepatic function test results for abnormalities.
◀ALERT▶ Monitor the patient for signs and symptoms of opportunistic infections, such as chills, cough, fever, and myalgia.

Patient Teaching

• Instruct the patient to take nelfinavir with food to optimize the drug's absorption.
• Advise the patient to space drug doses evenly around the clock and to take the drug every day as prescribed.
• Caution the patient not to alter the dose or discontinue the drug without first notifying the physician.
• Inform the patient that nelfinavir is not a cure for HIV infection, nor does it reduce the risk of transmitting HIV to others. Explain that he or she may continue to experience illnesses associated with advanced HIV infection, including opportunistic infections.
• Offer the patient emotional support.

nevirapine

neh-**veer**-a-peen
(Viramune)

CATEGORY AND SCHEDULE

Pregnancy Risk Category: C

MECHANISM OF ACTION
A nonnucleoside reverse transcriptase inhibitor that binds directly to HIV-1 reverse transcriptase, thus changing the shape of this enzyme and blocking RNA- and DNA-dependent polymerase activity.
Therapeutic Effect: Interferes with HIV replication, slowing the progression of HIV infection.

PHARMACOKINETICS
Readily absorbed after PO administration. Protein binding: 60%. Widely distributed. Extensively metabolized in the liver. Excreted primarily in urine. ***Half-life:*** 45 hr (single dose), 25–30 hr (multiple doses).

AVAILABILITY
Tablets: 200 mg.
Oral Suspension: 50 mg/5 ml.

INDICATIONS AND DOSAGES
▸ HIV infection
PO
Adults. 200 mg once a day for 14 days (to reduce the risk of rash). Maintenance: 200 mg twice a day in combination with nucleoside analogues.
Children older than 8 yr. 4 mg/kg once a day for 14 days; then 4 mg/kg twice a day. Maximum: 400 mg/day.
Children 2 mo–8 yr. 4 mg/kg once a day for 14 days; then 7 mg/kg twice a day.

OFF-LABEL USES
To reduce the risk of transmitting HIV from infected mother to newborn

CONTRAINDICATIONS
None known.

INTERACTIONS
Drug
Ketoconazole, oral contraceptives, protease inhibitors: May decrease the plasma concentrations of these drugs.
Rifabutin, rifampin: May decrease nevirapine blood concentration.
Herbal
St. John's wort: May decrease blood concentration and effects of nevirapine.
Food
None known.

DIAGNOSTIC TEST EFFECTS
May significantly increase serum bilirubin, GGT, AST (SGOT), and ALT (SGPT) levels. May significantly decrease Hgb level and neutrophil and platelet counts.

SIDE EFFECTS
Frequent (8%–3%)
Rash, fever, headache, nausea, granulocytopenia (more common in children)
Occasional (3%–1%)
Stomatitis (burning, erythema, or ulceration of the oral mucosa; dysphagia)
Rare (less than 1%)
Paresthesia, myalgia, abdominal pain

SERIOUS REACTIONS
! Hepatitis and rash may become severe and life-threatening.

NURSING CONSIDERATIONS
Baseline Assessment
- Check the patient's diagnostic test results and laboratory values, especially hepatic function tests, before and periodically during nevirapine therapy.
- Obtain the patient's medication history, especially regarding the use of oral contraceptives.

Lifespan Considerations
• Nevirapine crosses the placenta and is distributed in breast milk. Breast-feeding is not recommended for patients taking this drug because of the possibility of transmitting HIV to the infant.
• Granulocytopenia occurs more frequently in children.
• The effects of this drug on the elderly are unknown.

Precautions
• Use nevirapine cautiously in patients with elevated AST (SGOT) or ALT (SGPT) levels, a history of chronic hepatitis B or C, or renal or hepatic dysfunction.

Administration and Handling
◀ **ALERT** ▶ Be aware that nevirapine is always prescribed in combination with at least one additional antiretroviral because a drug-resistant virus appears rapidly when nevirapine is given as monotherapy.
PO
• Give the drug without regard to meals.

Intervention and Evaluation
• Closely monitor the patient for evidence of rash, which usually appears on the extremities, face, or trunk within the first 6 weeks of drug therapy.
• Evaluate the patient for a rash accompanied by blistering, conjunctivitis, fever, general malaise, muscle or joint aches, oral lesions, and edema, which may indicate a severe, life-threatening skin or hypersensitivity reaction.

Patient Teaching
• Advise the patient to space drug doses evenly around the clock and to continue nevirapine therapy for the full course of treatment.
• If the patient fails to take nevirapine for longer than 7 days, instruct him or her to restart therapy by taking one 200-mg tablet each day for the first 14 days, and then one 200-mg tablet twice a day.
• Warn the patient to stop therapy and notify the physician if a rash occurs.
• Explain to the patient that nevirapine is not a cure for HIV infection, nor does it reduce the risk of transmitting HIV to others.
• Offer the patient emotional support.

ritonavir
ri-**tone**-a-veer
(Norvir, Norvisec[CAN])
Do not confuse ritonavir with Retrovir.

CATEGORY AND SCHEDULE
Pregnancy Risk Category: B

MECHANISM OF ACTION
Inhibits HIV-1 and HIV-2 proteases, rendering these enzymes incapable of processing the polypeptide precursors; this results in the production of noninfectious, immature HIV particles. **Therapeutic Effect:** Impedes HIV replication, slowing the progression of HIV infection.

PHARMACOKINETICS
Well absorbed after PO administration (absorption increased with food). Protein binding: 98%–99%. Extensively metabolized in the liver to active metabolite. Primarily eliminated in feces. Unknown if removed by hemodialysis. ***Half-life:*** 2.7–5 hr.

AVAILABILITY
Oral Solution: 80 mg/ml.
Soft Gelatin Capsules: 100 mg.

INDICATIONS AND DOSAGES

▸ HIV infection

PO

Adults, Children 12 yr and older. 600 mg twice a day. If nausea occurs at this dosage, give 300 mg twice a day for 1 day, 400 mg twice a day for 2 days, 500 mg twice a day for 1 day, then 600 mg twice a day thereafter.

Children younger than 12 yr. Initially, 250 mg/m^2/dose twice a day. Increase by 50 mg/m^2/dose up to 400 mg/m^2/dose. Maximum: 600 mg/dose twice a day.

CONTRAINDICATIONS

Concurrent use of amiodarone, astemizole, bepridil, bupropion, cisapride, clozapine, encainide, flecainide, meperidine, piroxicam, propafenone, propoxyphene, quinidine, rifabutin, or terfenadine (increased risk of serious or life-threatening drug interactions, such as arrhythmias, hematologic abnormalities, and seizures); concurrent use of alprazolam, clorazepate, diazepam, estazolam, flurazepam, midazolam, triazolam, or zolpidem (may produce extreme sedation and respiratory depression)

INTERACTIONS

Drug

Desipramine, fluoxetine, other antidepressants: May increase the blood concentration of these drugs.

Disulfiram, drugs causing disulfiram-like reaction (such as metronidazole): May produce a disulfiram-like reaction.

Enzyme inducers (including carbamazepine, dexamethasone, nevirapine, phenobarbital, phenytoin, rifabutin, rifampin): May increase the metabolism and decrease the efficacy of ritonavir.

Oral contraceptives, theophylline: May decrease the effectiveness of these drugs.

Herbal

St. John's wort: May decrease the blood concentration and effect of ritonavir.

Food

None known.

DIAGNOSTIC TEST EFFECTS

May alter serum CK, GGT, triglyceride, uric acid, AST (SGOT), and ALT (SGPT) levels as well as creatinine clearance.

SIDE EFFECTS

Frequent

GI disturbances (abdominal pain, anorexia, diarrhea, nausea, vomiting), circumoral and peripheral paresthesias, altered taste, headache, dizziness, fatigue, asthenia

Occasional

Allergic reaction, flu-like symptoms, hypotension

Rare

Diabetes mellitus, hyperglycemia

SERIOUS REACTIONS

! None known.

NURSING CONSIDERATIONS

Baseline Assessment

- Check the patient's laboratory test results, if ordered, especially serum hepatic enzyme and triglyceride levels, before and periodically during ritonavir therapy.

Lifespan Considerations

- Breast-feeding is not recommended for patients taking this drug because of the possibility of transmitting HIV to the infant.
- No age-related precautions have been noted in children older than 2 years.

- The effects of this drug on the elderly are unknown.

Precautions
- Use ritonavir cautiously in patients with impaired hepatic function.

Administration and Handling
PO
- Store capsules in the refrigerator, and protect them from light.
- Refrigerate the oral solution unless it is used within 30 days and stored below 77°F.
- Give ritonavir with food if possible.
- To improve the taste of the oral solution, mix it with Advera, chocolate milk, or Ensure within 1 hour of administration.
- Patients beginning combination therapy with ritonavir and nucleoside analogues may improve GI tolerance by first taking ritonavir as monotherapy for 2 weeks and then adding the nucleosides.

Intervention and Evaluation
- Closely monitor the patient for signs and symptoms of GI or neurologic disturbances, particularly paresthesias.
- Monitor the patient's blood glucose level, CD4+ cell count, liver function test results, and plasma levels of HIV RNA.

Patient Teaching
- Advise the patient to space ritonavir doses evenly around the clock and to continue taking the drug for the full course of treatment.
- Instruct the patient to take ritonavir with food if possible.
- Suggest that the patient mix the oral solution with Advera, chocolate milk, or Ensure to improve its taste.
- Warn the patient to notify the physician if he or she experiences abdominal pain, frequent urination, increased thirst, nausea, or vomiting.
- Inform the patient that ritonavir is not a cure for HIV infection, nor does it reduce the risk of transmitting HIV to others. Explain that he or she may continue to develop illnesses associated with advanced HIV infection.
- Offer the patient and family emotional support.

saquinavir

sa-**kwin**-a-veer
(Fortovase, Invirase)
Do not confuse saquinavir with Sinequan.

CATEGORY AND SCHEDULE
Pregnancy Risk Category: B

MECHANISM OF ACTION
Inhibits HIV protease, rendering the enzyme incapable of processing the polyprotein precursors needed to generate functional proteins in HIV-infected cells. **Therapeutic Effect:** Intereferes with HIV replication, slowing the progression of HIV infection.

PHARMACOKINETICS
Poorly absorbed after PO administration (absorption increased with high-calorie and high-fat meals). Protein binding: 99%. Metabolized in the liver to inactive metabolite. Primarily eliminated in feces. Unknown if removed by hemodialysis. ***Half-life:*** 13 hr.

AVAILABILITY
Capsules (Invirase): 200 mg.
Capsules, Gelatin (Fortovase): 200 mg.
Tablets: 500 mg.

INDICATIONS AND DOSAGES

▸ HIV infection in combination with other antiretrovirals

PO

Adults, Elderly. 1,200 mg Fortovase 3 times a day or 600 mg Invirase 3 times a day within 2 hr after a full meal.

Dosage adjustments when given in combination therapy:

Delavirdine: Fortovase 800 mg 3 times/day.

Lopinavir/ritonavir: Fortovase 800 mg 2 times/day.

Nelfinavir: Fortovase 800 mg 3 times/day or 1200 mg 2 times/day.

Ritonavir: Fortovase or Invirase 1000 mg 2 times/day.

CONTRAINDICATIONS

Clinically significant hypersensitivity to saquinavir; concurrent use with ergot medications, lovastatin, midazolam, simvastatin, or triazolam

INTERACTIONS

Drug

Calcium channel blockers, clindamycin, dapsone, quinidine, triazolam: May increase the plasma concentrations of these drugs.

Carbamazepine, dexamethasone, phenobarbital, phenytoin, rifampin: May reduce saquinavir plasma concentration.

Ketoconazole: Increases saquinavir plasma concentration.

Herbal

Garlic, St. John's wort: May decrease the plasma concentration and effect of saquinavir.

Food

Grapefruit juice: May increase saquinavir plasma concentration.

DIAGNOSTIC TEST EFFECTS

May alter serum CK levels, elevate liver function test results, and lower blood glucose levels.

SIDE EFFECTS

Occasional

Diarrhea, abdominal discomfort and pain, nausea, photosensitivity, stomatitis

Rare

Confusion, ataxia, asthenia, headache, rash

SERIOUS REACTIONS

! Ketoacidosis occurs rarely.

NURSING CONSIDERATIONS

Baseline Assessment

- Check the patient's laboratory and diagnostic test results, especially liver function test results, if ordered, before and periodically during saquinavir therapy.
- Expect to obtain the patient's medication history.

Lifespan Considerations

- Breast-feeding is not recommended for patients taking saquinavir because of the possibility of transmitting HIV to the infant.
- The safety and efficacy of saquinavir have not been established in children.
- The effects of this drug on the elderly are unknown.

Precautions

- Use saquinavir cautiously in patients with diabetes mellitus or hepatic impairment.

Administration and Handling

PO

- Give saquinavir within 2 hours after a full meal because the drug may not produce antiviral activity taken on an empty stomach.
- Don't give less than 600 mg/day because the drug won't produce antiviral activity at a lower dosage. Be aware that recommended daily doses of other antiretroviral agents are zalcitabine (ddC) 0.75 mg 3

times a day or zidovudine (AZT) 200 mg 3 times a day.

Intervention and Evaluation

- Monitor the patient's blood chemistry and serum hepatic enzyme levels, CD4+ cell count and blood glucose, HIV RNA, and serum triglyceride levels.
- Closely monitor the patient for signs and symptoms of GI discomfort.
- Assess the patient's pattern of daily bowel activity and stool consistency.
- Inspect the patient's mouth for signs of mucosal ulceration.
- If the patient experience severe toxicities, such as ketoacidosis, withhold the drug and notify the physician.

Patient Teaching

- Instruct the patient to take saquinavir within 2 hours after a full meal.
- Advise the patient to space drug doses evenly around the clock and to continue taking the drug for the full course of treatment.
- Advise the patient to notify the physician if he or she experiences nausea or vomiting or persistent abdominal pain.
- Instruct the patient to avoid grapefruit products while taking saquinavir.
- Encourage the patient to avoid exposure to artificial light sources and sunlight.
- Inform the patient that saquinavir is not a cure for HIV infection, nor does it reduce the risk of transmitting HIV to others. Explain that he or she may continue to develop illnesses associated with advanced HIV infection.
- Offer emotional support to the patient.

stavudine (d4T)

stav-yoo-deen
(Zerit)

CATEGORY AND SCHEDULE

Pregnancy Risk Category: C

MECHANISM OF ACTION

Inhibits HIV reverse transcriptase by terminating the viral DNA chain. Also inhibits RNA- and DNA-dependent DNA polymerase, an enzyme necessary for HIV replication. **Therapeutic Effect:** Impedes HIV replication, slowing the progression of HIV infection.

PHARMACOKINETICS

Rapidly and completely absorbed after PO administration. Undergoes minimal metabolism. Excreted in urine. ***Half-life:*** 1.5 hr (increased in renal impairment).

AVAILABILITY

Capsules: 15 mg, 20 mg, 30 mg, 40 mg.
Oral Solution: 1 mg/ml.

INDICATIONS AND DOSAGES

▸ **HIV infection (in combination with other antiretrovirals)**

PO

Adults weighing 60 kg or more. 40 mg twice a day.
Adults weighing less than 60 kg. 30 mg twice a day.
Children weighing 30 kg or more. 20 mg twice a day.
Children weighing less than 30 kg. 2 mg/kg/day.

▸ **HIV infection in patients with a recent history and complete resolution of peripheral neuropathy or elevated liver function test results**

Adults weighing 60 kg or more. 20 mg twice a day.

Adults weighing less than 60 kg. 15 mg twice a day.

Dosage in renal impairment

Dosage and frequency are modified based on creatinine clearance and patient weight.

Creatinine Clearance	Weight 60 kg or more	Weight less than 60 kg
greater than 50 ml/min	40 mg q12h	30 mg q12h
26–50 ml/min	20 mg q12h	15 mg q12h
10–25 ml/min	20 mg q24h	15 mg q24h

CONTRAINDICATIONS

None known.

INTERACTIONS

Drug

Didanosine, ethambutol, isoniazid, lithium, phenytoin, zalcitabine: May increase the risk of peripheral neuropathy development.

Didanosine, hydroxyurea: May increase the ris of hepatotoxicity.

Zidovudine: May have antagonistic antiviral effect.

Herbal

None known.

Food

None known.

DIAGNOSTIC TEST EFFECTS

Commonly increases AST (SGOT) and ALT (SGPT) levels. May decrease neutrophil count.

SIDE EFFECTS

Frequent

Headache (55%), diarrhea (50%), chills and fever (38%), nausea and vomiting, myalgia (35%), rash (33%), asthenia (28%), insomnia, abdominal pain (26%), anxiety (22%), arthralgia (18%), back pain (20%), diaphoresis (19%), malaise (17%), depression (14%)

Occasional

Anorexia, weight loss, nervousness, dizziness, conjunctivitis, dyspepsia, dyspnea

Rare

Constipation, vasodilation, confusion, migraine, urticaria, abnormal vision

SERIOUS REACTIONS

! Peripheral neuropathy, (numbness, tingling, or pain in the hands and feet) occurs in 15% to 21% of patients.

! Ulcerative stomatitis (erythema or ulcers of oral mucosa, glossitis, gingivitis), pneumonia, and benign skin neoplasms occur occasionally.

! Pancreatitis and lactic acidosis occur rarely.

NURSING CONSIDERATIONS

Baseline Assessment

- Check the patient's laboratory test results, if ordered, especially liver function test results, before and periodically during stavudine therapy.
- Determine if the patient has a history of peripheral neuropathy.

Lifespan Considerations

- Breast-feeding is not recommended for patients taking stavudine because of the possibility of transmitting HIV to the infant.
- No age-related precautions have been noted in children.
- The effects of this drug on the elderly are unknown.

Precautions

- Use stavudine cautiously in patients with a history of peripheral neuropathy or hepatic or renal impairment.

Administration and Handling

PO

- Give stavudine without regard to meals.

Intervention and Evaluation

• Monitor the patient for signs and symptoms of peripheral neuropathy, such as numbness, pain, or tingling in the feet or hands. Be aware that these symptoms usually resolve promptly if stavudine therapy is discontinued, but they may worsen temporarily after the drug is withdrawn. If symptoms resolve completely, expect to resume drug therapy at a reduced dosage.
• Assess the patient for dizziness, headache, arthralgia, myalgia, chills, fever, a change in sleep pattern, and nausea or vomiting.
• Monitor the patient for evidence of a rash.
• Determine the patient's pattern of daily bowel activity and stool consistency.
• Assess the patient's eating pattern and check for weight loss.
• Examine the patient's eyes for signs of conjunctivitis.
• Monitor the patient's CD4+ cell count, CBC, Hgb and HIV RNA levels, and renal and liver function test results.

Patient Teaching

• Advise the patient to space doses evenly around the clock and to continue taking the drug for the full course of treatment.
• Caution the patient not to take any other medications, OTC drugs, without first notifying the physician.
• Instruct the patient to notify the physician of abdominal discomfort, shortness of breath, fatigue, nausea or vomiting, weakness, and numbness, pain, or tingling of the hands or feet.
• Inform the patient that stavudine is not a cure for HIV infection, nor does it reduce the risk of transmitting HIV to others. Explain that he or she may continue to develop illnesses associated with HIV infection, including opportunistic infections.
• Offer the patient emotional support.

tenofovir

ten-**oh**-foh-veer
(Viread)

CATEGORY AND SCHEDULE

Pregnancy Risk Category: B

MECHANISM OF ACTION

A nucleotide analogue that inhibits HIV reverse transcriptase by being incorporated into viral DNA, resulting in DNA chain termination. **Therapeutic Effect:** Slows HIV replication and reduces HIV RNA levels (viral load).

AVAILABILITY

Tablets: 300 mg.

INDICATIONS AND DOSAGES

▸ **HIV infection (in combination with other antiretrovirals)**

PO

Adults, Elderly, Children 18 yr and older. 300 mg once a day.

CONTRAINDICATIONS

None known.

INTERACTIONS

Drug

Didanosine: May increase didanosine blood concentration.
Indinavir, lamivudine, lopinavir, ritonavir: May decrease the blood concentrations of these drugs.

Herbal

None known.

Food

High-fat food: Increases tenofovir bioavailability.

DIAGNOSTIC TEST EFFECTS
May elevate liver function test results. May alter serum CK, GGT, uric acid, AST (SGOT), ALT (SGPT), and triglyceride levels as well as creatinine clearance.

SIDE EFFECTS
Occasional

GI disturbances (diarrhea, flatulence, nausea, vomiting)

SERIOUS REACTIONS
! Lactic acidosis and hepatomegaly with steatosis occur rarely, but may be severe.

NURSING CONSIDERATIONS
Baseline Assessment

- Check the patient's laboratory test results, if ordered, especially liver function test results and serum triglyceride levels, before and periodically during tenofovir therapy.

Precautions

- Use tenofovir cautiously in patients with impaired hepatic or renal function.

Administration and Handling

PO

- Give tenofovir with food.

Intervention and Evaluation

- Closely monitor the patient for signs and symptoms of GI discomfort.
- Assess the patient's pattern of daily bowel activity and stool consistency.
- Monitor the patient's CD4+ cell count, CBC, Hgb and HIV RNA plasma levels, liver function test results, and reticulocyte count.

Patient Teaching

- Instruct the patient to take tenofovir with a meal to increase the drug's absorption.
- Advise the patient to continue drug therapy for the full course of treatment.
- Advise the patient to notify the physician of nausea, vomiting, or persistent abdominal pain.
- Inform the patient that tenofovir is not a cure for HIV infection, nor does it reduce the risk of transmitting HIV to others. Explain that he or she may continue to develop illnesses associated with advanced HIV infection.
- Offer the patient and family emotional support.

zalcitabine
zal-**site**-a-been
(Hivid)

CATEGORY AND SCHEDULE
Pregnancy Risk Category: C

MECHANISM OF ACTION
A nucleoside reverse transcriptase inhibitor that inhibits viral DNA synthesis. **Therapeutic Effect:** Prevents replication of HIV-1.

PHARMACOKINETICS
Readily absorbed from the GI tract (absorption decreased by food). Protein binding: less than 4%. Undergoes phosphorylation intracellularly to the active metabolite. Primarily excreted in urine. Removed by hemodialysis. ***Half-life:*** 1–3 hr; metabolite, 2.6–10 hr (increased in impaired renal function).

AVAILABILITY
Tablets: 0.375 mg, 0.75 mg.

INDICATIONS AND DOSAGES
▸ **HIV infection (in combination with other antiretrovirals)**

PO

Adults, Children 13 yr and older. 0.75 mg q8h.

Children younger than 13 yr. 0.01 mg/kg q8h. Range: 0.005–0.01 mg/kg q8h.

▸ **Dosage in renal impairment**

Dosage and frequency are modified based on creatinine clearance.

Creatinine Clearance	Dose
10–40 ml/min	0.75 mg q12h
less than 10 ml/min	0.75 mg q24h

CONTRAINDICATIONS

Moderate or severe peripheral neuropathy

INTERACTIONS

Drug

Medications associated with peripheral neuropathy (including cisplatin, disulfiram, phenytoin, vincristine): May increase the risk of neuropathy.

Medications causing pancreatitis (including IV pentamidine): May increase the risk of pancreatitis.

Herbal

None known.

Food

None known.

DIAGNOSTIC TEST EFFECTS

May increase serum alkaline phosphatase, amylase, bilirubin, lipase, AST (SGOT), ALT (SGPT), and triglyceride levels. May decrease serum calcium, magnesium, and phosphate levels. May alter blood glucose and sodium levels.

SIDE EFFECTS

Frequent (28%–11%)

Peripheral neuropathy, fever, fatigue, headache, rash

Occasional (10%–5%)

Diarrhea, abdominal pain, oral ulcers, cough, pruritus, myalgia, weight loss, nausea, vomiting

Rare (4%–1%)

Nasal discharge, dysphagia, depression, night sweats, confusion

SERIOUS REACTIONS

! Peripheral neuropathy (characterized by numbness, tingling, burning, and pain in the lower extremities) occurs in 17% to 31% of patients. These symptoms may be followed by sharp, shooting pain and progress to a severe, continuous, burning pain that may be irreversible if the drug is not discontinued in time.

! Pancreatitis, leukopenia, neutropenia, eosinophilia, and thrombocytopenia occur rarely.

NURSING CONSIDERATIONS

Baseline Assessment

- Expect to monitor the patient's CBC, serum amylase, and serum triglyceride levels before and during therapy.

Lifespan Considerations

- It is unknown if zalcitabine crosses the placenta or is distributed in breast milk. However, breast-feeding is not recommended for patients taking this drug because of the possibility of transmitting HIV to the infant.
- No age-related precautions have been noted in children younger than 6 months.
- Children's dosages have not been established.
- Age-related renal impairment may require a dosage adjustment in the elderly.

Precautions

◂ **ALERT** ▸ Use zalcitabine with extreme caution in patients with preexisting mild peripheral neuropathy and a low CD4+ cell count because they're at increased risk for developing peripheral neuropathy. Avoid use

in patients with moderate to severe peripheral neuropathy.
• Use the drug cautiously in patients with a history of alcohol abuse, diabetes mellitus, hepatic or renal impairment, or weight loss.

Administration and Handling

PO
• Zalcitabine is best taken on an empty stomach because food decreases its absorption. However, the drug may be given with food to decrease GI distress.
• Space doses evenly around the clock.

Intervention and Evaluation

• Withhold the drug and notify the physician immediately if signs and symptoms of peripheral neuropathy develop, including burning, numbness, tingling, or shooting pains in the extremities and loss of the ankle reflex or vibratory sense.

◀ **ALERT** ▶ Assess the patient for evidence of potentially fatal pancreatitis, including abdominal pain, nausea and vomiting, and increasing serum amylase and triglyceride levels. If the patient develops any of these signs or symptoms, particularly abdominal pain, withhold the drug and notify the physician immediately.
• Assess the patient for signs and symptoms of a therapeutic response to drug therapy, including decreased fatigue, increased energy, and weight gain.
• Evaluate the patient's CBC for evidence of blood dyscrasias.

Patient Teaching

• Warn the patient to notify the physician if he or she experiences any signs or symptoms of pancreatitis or peripheral neuropathy.
• Caution the female patient of childbearing age to avoid pregnancy during therapy, and teach her about contraception use.
• Explain to the patient that zalcitabine is not a cure for HIV, nor does it reduce the risk of transmitting HIV to others. Explain that he or she may continue to develop opportunistic illnesses associated with advanced HIV infection.
• Offer emotional support to the patient.

zidovudine

zyde-**o**-vue-deen
(Apo-Zidovudine[CAN], AZT, Novo-AZT[CAN], Retrovir)
Do not confuse Retrovir with ritonavir.

CATEGORY AND SCHEDULE

Pregnancy Risk Category: C

MECHANISM OF ACTION

A nucleoside reverse transcriptase inhibitor that interferes with viral RNA-dependent DNA polymerase, an enzyme necessary for viral HIV replication. **Therapeutic Effect:** Interferes with HIV replication, slowing the progression of HIV infection.

PHARMACOKINETICS

Rapidly and completely absorbed from the GI tract. Protein binding: 25%–38%. Undergoes first-pass metabolism in the liver. Crosses the blood-brain barrier and is widely distributed, including to CSF. Primarily excreted in urine. Minimal removal by hemodialysis. ***Half-life:*** 0.8–1.2 hr (increased in impaired renal function).

AVAILABILITY

Capsules: 100 mg.
Syrup: 50 mg/5 ml.
Tablets: 300 mg.
Injection: 10 mg/ml.

INDICATIONS AND DOSAGES

▸ HIV infection

PO

Adults, Elderly, Children older than 12 yr. 200 mg q8h or 300 mg q12h.
Children 12 yr and younger. 160 mg/m²/dose q8h. Range: 90–180 mg/m²/dose q6–8h.
Neonates. 2 mg/kg/dose q6h.

IV

Adults, Elderly, Children older than 12 yr. 1–2 mg/kg/dose q4h.
Children 12 yr and younger. 120 mg/m²/dose q6h.
Neonates. 1.5 mg/kg/dose q6h.

OFF-LABEL USES

Prophylaxis in health care workers at risk of acquiring HIV after occupational exposure

CONTRAINDICATIONS

Life-threatening allergic reactions to zidovudine or its components

INTERACTIONS

Drug

Bone marrow depressants, ganciclovir: May increase myelosuppression.
Clarithromycin: May decrease zidovudine blood concentration.
Probenecid: May increase zidovudine blood concentrations and the risk of zidovudine toxicity.

Herbal

None known.

Food

None known.

DIAGNOSTIC TEST EFFECTS

May increase mean corpuscular volume.

IV INCOMPATIBILITIES

None known.

IV COMPATIBILITIES

Dexamethasone (Decadron), dobutamine (Dobutrex), dopamine (Intropin), heparin, lorazepam (Ativan), morphine, potassium chloride

SIDE EFFECTS

Expected (46%–42%)
Nausea, headache
Frequent (20%–16%)
Abdominal pain, asthenia, rash, fever, acne
Occasional (12%–8%)
Diarrhea, anorexia, malaise, myalgia, somnolence
Rare (6%–5%)
Dizziness, paresthesia, vomiting, insomnia, dyspnea, altered taste

SERIOUS REACTIONS

! Serious reactions include anemia, which occurs most commonly after 4–6 weeks of therapy, and granulocytopenia; both effects are more likely to occur in patients who have a low Hgb level or granulocyte count before beginning therapy.
! Neurotoxicity (as evidenced by ataxia, fatigue, lethargy, nystagmus, and seizures) may occur.

NURSING CONSIDERATIONS

Baseline Assessment

- Expect to obtain specimens for viral diagnostic tests before starting zidovudine therapy. Therapy may begin before results are obtained.
- Check the patient's hematology reports to establish an accurate baseline.
- Be aware that the patient should not receive drugs that are cytotoxic, myelosuppressive, or nephrotoxic because they may increase the risk of zidovudine toxicity.

Lifespan Considerations

- It is unknown if zidovudine crosses

the placenta or is distributed in breast milk.

- It is unknown if this drug causes fetal harm or affects fertility.
- No age-related precautions have been noted in children.
- The effects of this drug on the elderly are unknown.

Precautions

- Use zidovudine cautiously in patients with bone marrow depression or renal or hepatic dysfunction.

Administration and Handling

PO

- Keep capsules in a cool, dry place, and protect them from light.
- Give zidovudine without regard to food.
- Space doses evenly around the clock.
- Keep the patient in an upright position when giving the drug to prevent esophageal ulceration.

IV

- After dilution, the IV solution remains stable for 24 hours at room temperature or 48 hours if refrigerated.
- Use the solution within 8 hours if stored at room temperature or within 24 hours if refrigerated.
- Don't use the solution if it contains particulate matter or becomes discolored.
- Zidovudine must be diluted before administration. Remove a calculated dose from the vial and add it to D_5W to provide a concentration no greater than 4 mg/ml.
- Infuse the drug over 1 hour.

Intervention and Evaluation

- Monitor the patient's CD4+ cell count, CBC, Hgb and HIV RNA plasma levels, mean corpuscular volume, and reticulocyte count.
- Check the patient for bleeding, dizziness, headache, and insomnia.
- Assess the patient's pattern of daily bowel activity and stool consistency.
- Evaluate the patient's skin for acne or a rash.
- Assess the patient for signs and symptoms of opportunistic infections, such as chills, cough, fever, and myalgia.
- Monitor the patient's intake and output, as well as serum renal and liver function test results.

Patient Teaching

- Instruct the patient to space zidovudine doses evenly around the clock.
- Explain that blood tests are an essential part of therapy because of the bleeding potential.
- Warn the patient to report bleeding from the gums, nose, or rectum to the physician immediately.
- Suggest that the patient have dental work done before therapy or postpone it until blood counts return to normal, which may be weeks after therapy has stopped.
- Caution the patient not to take any other medications without the physician's prior approval.
- Warn the patient to notify the physician if he or she experiences difficulty breathing, headache, inability to sleep, muscle weakness, a rash, signs of infection, or unusual bleeding.
- Explain to the patient that zidovudine does not cure HIV infection or AIDS, but acts to reduce symptoms and slow or arrest disease progression.
- Advise the patient that zidovudine does not reduce the risk of transmitting HIV or AIDS to others.
- Offer emotional support to the patient.

4 Antitubercular Agents

ethambutol
isoniazid
pyrazinamide
rifabutin
rifampin
rifapentine

Uses: Antitubercular agents are used to treat tuberculosis, an infectious disease usually caused by *Mycobacterium tuberculosis* or *Mycobacterium bovis*. Treatment, which aims to eliminate symptoms and prevent relapse, typically consists of combination drug therapy to minimize the risk of drug resistance. Treatment may require three or more drugs and may continue for 6 to 24 months.

Action: First-line agents act in different ways, combining the greatest efficacy with an acceptable degree of toxicity. For example, *ethambutol* blocks enzymes in mycobacteria, preventing cell wall synthesis. *Isoniazid* inhibits the synthesis of mycolic acids, which are important to mycobacterial cell walls. *Pyrazinamide* affects enzymes involved in mycolic acid synthesis. *Rifabutin, rifampin,* and *rifapentine* inhibit DNA-dependent RNA polymerase in mycobacteria. (See the illustration *Sites and Mechanisms of Action: Anti-infective Agents,* page 2.)

COMBINATION PRODUCTS

RIFAMATE: isoniazid/rifampin 150 mg/300 mg.
ISONIAZID/PYRAZINRIFATER: amide/ rifampin 50 mg/300 mg/120 mg.

ethambutol

e-**tham**-byoo-tole
(Etibi[CAN], Myambutol)
Do not confuse ethambutol or Myambutol with Nembutal.

CATEGORY AND SCHEDULE

Pregnancy Risk Category: B

MECHANISM OF ACTION

An isonicotinic acid derivative that interferes with RNA synthesis. **Therapeutic Effect:** Suppresses the multiplication of mycobacteria.

PHARMACOKINETICS

Rapidly and well absorbed from the GI tract. Protein binding: 20%–30%. Widely distributed. Metabolized in the liver. Primarily excreted in urine. Removed by hemodialysis. ***Half-life:*** 3–4 hr (increased in impaired renal function).

AVAILABILITY

Tablets: 100 mg, 400 mg.

INDICATIONS AND DOSAGES

▸ **Tuberculosis**

PO

Adults, Elderly, Children. 15–25 mg/kg/day as a single dose or 50 mg/kg 2 times/wk. Maximum: 2.5 g/dose.

▸ **Atypical mycobacterial infections**
PO
Adults, Elderly, Children. 15 mg/kg/day. Maximum: 1 g/day.

▸ **Dosage in renal impairment**
Dosage interval is modified based on creatinine clearance.

Creatinine Clearance	Dosage Interval
10–50 ml/min	q24–36h
less than 10 ml/min	q48h

OFF-LABEL USES
Treatment of atypical mycobacterial infections

CONTRAINDICATIONS
Optic neuritis

INTERACTIONS
Drug
Neurotoxic medications: May increase the risk of neurotoxicity.
Herbal
None known.
Food
None known.

DIAGNOSTIC TEST EFFECTS
May increase serum uric acid levels.

SIDE EFFECTS
Occasional
Acute gouty arthritis (chills, pain, swelling of joints with hot skin), confusion, abdominal pain, nausea, vomiting, anorexia, headache
Rare
Rash, fever, blurred vision, eye pain, red-green color blindness

SERIOUS REACTIONS
! Optic neuritis (more common with high-dosage or long-term ethambutol therapy), peripheral neuritis, thrombocytopenia, and an anaphylactoid reaction occur rarely.

NURSING CONSIDERATIONS
Baseline Assessment
- Evaluate the patient's CBC and renal and liver function test results.

Lifespan Considerations
- Ethambutol crosses the placenta and is excreted in breast milk.
- The safety and efficacy of ethambutol have not been established in children younger than 13 years.
- Age-related renal impairment may require a dosage adjustment in the elderly.

Precautions
- Use ethambutol cautiously in patients with cataracts, diabetic retinopathy, recurrent ocular inflammatory conditions, gout, or renal dysfunction.
- Ethambutol use is not recommended for children 13 years and younger.

Administration and Handling
PO
- Give ethambutol with food to decrease GI upset.

Intervention and Evaluation
- Assess the patient for the first signs of vision changes, including altered color perception and decreased visual acuity. If vision changes occur, discontinue the drug and notify the physician immediately.
- Monitor the patient's serum uric acid levels. Also, assess the patient for signs and symptoms of gout, including hot, painful, or swollen joints, especially in the ankle, big toe, or knee.
- Assess the patient for signs and symptoms of peripheral neuritis, as evidenced by burning, numbness, or tingling of the extremities. Notify the physician if peripheral neuritis occurs.

Patient Teaching
- Advise the patient not to skip drug doses and to take ethambutol for the

full course of therapy, which may be months or years.

- Warn the patient to notify the physician immediately of any visual problems. Explain that visual effects are generally reversible after ethambutol is discontinued, but that in rare cases they may take up to a year to resolve or may become permanent.
- Advise the patient to promptly report burning, numbness, or tingling of the feet or hands, as well as pain and swelling of joints.

isoniazid

eye-soe-**nye**-a-zid
(INH, Isotamine[CAN], Nydrazid, PMS Isoniazid[CAN])

CATEGORY AND SCHEDULE

Pregnancy Risk Category: C

MECHANISM OF ACTION

An isonicotinic acid derivative that inhibits mycolic acid synthesis and causes disruption of the bacterial cell wall and loss of acid-fast properties in susceptible mycobacteria. Active only during bacterial cell division.
Therapeutic Effect: Bactericidal against actively growing intracellular and extracellular susceptible mycobacteria.

PHARMACOKINETICS

Readily absorbed from the GI tract. Protein binding: 10%–15%. Widely distributed (including to CSF). Metabolized in the liver. Primarily excreted in urine. Removed by hemodialysis. ***Half-life:*** 0.5–5 hr.

AVAILABILITY

Tablets: 100 mg, 300 mg.
Syrup: 50 mg/5 ml.
Injection: 100 mg/ml.

INDICATIONS AND DOSAGES

▸ **Tuberculosis (in combination with one or more antituberculars)**
PO, IM
Adults, Elderly. 5 mg/kg/day as a single dose. Maximum 300 mg/day.
Children. 10–15 mg/kg/day as a single dose. Maximum 300 mg/day.

▸ **Prevention of tuberculosis**
PO, IM
Adults, Elderly. 300 mg/day as a single dose.
Children. 10 mg/kg/day as a single dose. Maximum 300 mg/day.

CONTRAINDICATIONS

Acute hepatic disease, history of hypersensitivity reactions or hepatic injury with previous isoniazid therapy

INTERACTIONS

Drug
Alcohol: May increase isoniazid metabolism and the risk of hepatotoxicity.
Carbamazepine, phenytoin: May increase the toxicity of these drugs.
Disulfiram: May increase CNS effects.
Hepatotoxic medications: May increase the risk of hepatotoxicity.
Ketoconazole: May decrease ketoconazole blood concentration.

Herbal
None known.

Food
Tyramine-containing foods: May cause a hypertensive crisis.

DIAGNOSTIC TEST EFFECTS

May increase serum bilirubin, AST (SGOT), and ALT (SGPT) levels.

SIDE EFFECTS

Frequent
Nausea, vomiting, diarrhea, abdominal pain

Rare
Pain at injection site, hypersensitivity reaction

SERIOUS REACTIONS

! Rare reactions include neurotoxicity (as evidenced by ataxia and paraesthesia), optic neuritis, and hepatotoxicity.

NURSING CONSIDERATIONS

Baseline Assessment

◀ALERT▶ Determine if the patient has a history of hypersensitivity reactions or hepatic injury from isoniazid or a sensitivity to nicotinic acid or chemically related medications before starting drug therapy.
- Make sure that appropriate specimens are obtained for culture and sensitivity testing before beginning therapy.
- Evaluate the patient's initial liver function test results.

Lifespan Considerations

- Prophylactic use of isoniazid in pregnant women is usually postponed until after childbirth.
- Isoniazid crosses the placenta and is distributed in breast milk.
- No age-related precautions have been noted in children.
- The elderly are more susceptible to developing hepatitis.

Precautions

- Use isoniazid cautiously in alcoholic patients, those with chronic hepatic disease or severe renal impairment, and patients with hypersensitivity to nicotinic acid or other chemically related medications because of the risk of cross-sensitivity.

Administration and Handling

PO
- Give isoniazid 1 hour before or 2 hours after a meal. The drug may be given with food to decrease GI upset, but this will delay its absorption.
- Administer the drug at least 1 hour before antacids, especially those containing aluminum.

Intervention and Evaluation

◀ALERT▶ Monitor the patient's liver function test results. Also, assess the patient for signs and symptoms of hepatitis, such as anorexia, dark urine, fatigue, jaundice, nausea, vomiting, and weakness. If you suspect hepatitis, withhold the drug and notify the physician promptly.
- Assess the patient for burning, numbness, and tingling of the extremities. Be aware that patients at risk for neuropathy, such as alcoholics, those with chronic hepatic disease, diabetics, the elderly, and malnourished individuals, may receive pyridoxine prophylactically.
- Be alert for signs and symptoms of a hypersensitivity reaction, including fever and skin eruptions.

Patient Teaching

- Instruct the patient to take isoniazid 1 hour before or 2 hours after a meal. However, explain that he or she may take the drug with food if GI upset occurs.
- Advise the patient not to skip doses and to continue taking isoniazid for the full course of therapy (6 to 24 months).
- Urge the patient to avoid consuming alcohol during treatment.
- Caution the patient not to take any other drugs, including antacids, without first notifying the physician. Explain that he or she must take isoniazid at least 1 hour before taking an antacid.
- Warn the patient to avoid foods containing tyramine, including aged cheeses, sauerkraut, smoked fish, and tuna, because these foods may cause headache, a hot or clammy feeling, light-headedness, pounding heart-

beat, and red or itching skin. Advise the patient to notify the physician if any of these reactions occur. Also, provide the patient with a list of tyramine-containing foods.
- Caution the patient to notify the physician immediately of any new symptoms, such as dark urine, fatigue, nausea or vomiting, visual problems, numbness or tingling of the feet or hands, and yellowing of the skin or eyes.

pyrazinamide

pye-ra-**zin**-a-mide
(Pyrazinamide, Tebrazid[CAN], Zinamide[AUS])

CATEGORY AND SCHEDULE

Pregnancy Risk Category: C

MECHANISM OF ACTION

An antitubercular whose exact mechanism of action is unknown. **Therapeutic Effect:** Either bacteriostatic or bactericidal, depending on the drug's concentration at the infection site and the susceptibility of infecting bacteria.

AVAILABILITY

Tablets: 500 mg.

INDICATIONS AND DOSAGES

▸ Tuberculosis (in combination with other antituberculars)
PO
Adults. 15–30 mg/kg/day in 1–4 doses. Maximum: 3 g/day.
Children. 20–40 mg/kg/day in 1 or 2 doses. Maximum: 2 g/day.

CONTRAINDICATIONS

Severe hepatic dysfunction

INTERACTIONS

Drug
Allopurinol, colchicine, probenecid, sulfinpyrazone: May decrease the effects of these drugs.
Herbal
None known.
Food
None known.

DIAGNOSTIC TEST EFFECTS

May increase AST (SGOT), ALT (SGPT), and serum uric acid concentrations.

SIDE EFFECTS

Frequent
Arthralgia, myalgia (usually mild and self-limiting)
Rare
Hypersensitivity reaction (rash, pruritus, urticaria), photosensitivity, gouty arthritis

SERIOUS REACTIONS

! Hepatotoxicity, gouty arthritis, thrombocytopenia, and anemia occur rarely.

NURSING CONSIDERATIONS

Baseline Assessment
- Determine if the patient has a hypersensitivity to pyrazinamide, ethionamide, isoniazid, or niacin before beginning pyrazinamide therapy.
- Ensure that specimens for culture and sensitivity tests have been obtained before beginning drug therapy.
- Evaluate the patient's initial CBC, liver function test results, and serum uric acid levels.

Lifespan Considerations
- The safety and efficacy of pyrazinamide have not been established in children.

Precautions

• Use pyrazinamide cautiously in patients with diabetes mellitus, renal impairment, or a history of gout.
• Use the drug cautiously in patients with a hypersensitivity to ethionamide, isoniazid, or niacin.

Intervention and Evaluation

• Monitor the patient's liver function test results and be alert for hepatic reactions, such as anorexia, fever, jaundice, liver tenderness, malaise, nausea, and vomiting. If such reactions occur, stop the drug and notify the physician promptly.
• Check the patient's serum uric acid levels and assess for signs and symptoms of gout, such as hot, painful, swollen joints (especially the ankle, big toe, or knee).
• Evaluate the patient's blood glucose levels, especially in patients with diabetes mellitus, because pyrazinamide administration may make diabetes management difficult.
• Assess the patient's skin for a rash or skin eruptions.
• Monitor the patient's CBC for anemia and thrombocytopenia.

Patient Teaching

• Instruct the patient to take pyrazinamide with food to reduce GI upset.
• Advise the patient not to skip drug doses and to complete the full course of therapy, which may take months or years.
• Explain to the patient that follow-up physician office visits and laboratory tests are essential parts of treatment.
• Encourage the patient to avoid overexposure to the sun or ultraviolet light to prevent photosensitivity reactions.
• Warn the patient to immediately notify the physician of any new symptoms, especially fever; hot, painful, or swollen joints; unusual fatigue; or jaundice.

rifabutin

rif-a-byoo-ten
(Mycobutin)
Do not confuse rifabutin with rifampin.

CATEGORY AND SCHEDULE

Pregnancy Risk Category: B

MECHANISM OF ACTION

An antitubercular that inhibits DNA-dependent RNA polymerase, an enzyme in susceptible strains of *Escherichia coli* and *Bacillus subtilis*. Rifabutin has a broad spectrum of antimicrobial activity, including against mycobacteria such as *Mycobacterium avium* complex (MAC). **Therapeutic Effect:** Prevents MAC disease.

PHARMACOKINETICS

Readily absorbed from the GI tract (high-fat meals delay absorption). Protein binding: 85%. Widely distributed. Crosses the blood-brain barrier. Extensive intracellular tissue uptake. Metabolized in the liver to active metabolite. Excreted in urine; eliminated in feces. Unknown if removed by hemodialysis. ***Half-life:*** 16–69 hr.

AVAILABILITY

Capsules: 150 mg.

INDICATIONS AND DOSAGES

▸ **Prevention of MAC disease (first episode)**

PO

Adults, Elderly. 300 mg as a single dose or in 2 divided doses if GI upset occurs.

▸ **Prevention of recurrent MAC disease**
PO
Adults, Elderly. 300 mg/day (in combination)
▸ **Dosage in renal impairment**
Dosage is modified based on creatinine clearance. If creatinine clearance is less than 30 ml/min, reduce dosage by 50%.

CONTRAINDICATIONS
Active tuberculosis; hypersensitivity to other rifamycins, including rifampin

INTERACTIONS
Drug
Oral contraceptives: May decrease contraceptive effectiveness.
Zidovudine: May decrease blood concentration of zidovudine, but does not affect the drug's inhibition of HIV.
Herbal
None known.
Food
None known.

DIAGNOSTIC TEST EFFECTS
May increase serum alkaline phosphatase, AST (SGOT), and ALT (SGPT) levels.

SIDE EFFECTS
Frequent (30%)
Red-orange or red-brown discoloration of urine, feces, saliva, skin, sputum, sweat, or tears
Occasional (11%–3%)
Rash, nausea, abdominal pain, diarrhea, dyspepsia, belching, headache, altered taste, uveitis, corneal deposits
Rare (less than 2%)
Anorexia, flatulence, fever, myalgia, vomiting, insomnia

SERIOUS REACTIONS
! Hepatitis and thrombocytopenia occur rarely. Anemia and neutropenia may also occur.

NURSING CONSIDERATIONS
Baseline Assessment
• Expect the patient to undergo a biopsy of suspicious nodes, if present. Also, expect to obtain blood or sputum cultures and a chest x-ray to rule out active tuberculosis.
• If ordered, obtain the patient's baseline CBC and liver function test results.
Lifespan Considerations
• It is unknown if rifabutin crosses the placenta or is excreted in breast milk.
• No age-related precautions have been noted in children or the elderly.
Precautions
• Use rifabutin cautiously in patients with hepatic or renal impairment.
• The safety of this drug for children has not been established.
Administration and Handling
PO
• Give rifabutin with food if GI irritation occurs.
• Mix the drug with applesauce if the patient can't swallow the capsules whole.
Intervention and Evaluation
• Monitor the patient's CBC and platelet counts, Hgb level, Hct, and hepatic function test results.
• Avoid giving the patient IM injections, taking rectal temperature, and any other traumatic procedures that may induce bleeding.
• Check the patient's body temperature and notify the physician of flu-like symptoms, GI intolerance, or a rash.
Patient Teaching
• Inform the patient that urine, feces, perspiration, saliva, skin, sputum, and tears may become reddish brown or reddish orange during drug ther-

apy and that soft contact lenses may become permanently discolored.
• Caution female patients who use oral contraceptives that rifabutin may decrease the contraceptives' effectiveness. Teach such patients alternative methods of contraception.
• Advise the patient to avoid crowds and those with known infection.
• Warn the patient to notify the physician promptly if he or she experiences dark urine, flu-like symptoms, nausea or vomiting, unusual bleeding or bruising, or any visual disturbances.

rifampin

rye-fam-pin
(Rifadin, Rimactane, Rimycin[AUS], Rofact[CAN])
Do not confuse rifampin with rifabutin, Rifamate, rifapentine, or Ritalin.

CATEGORY AND SCHEDULE
Pregnancy Risk Category: C

MECHANISM OF ACTION
An antitubercular that interferes with bacterial RNA synthesis by binding to DNA-dependent RNA polymerase, thus preventing its attachment to DNA and blocking RNA transcription. **Therapeutic Effect:** Bactericidal in susceptible microorganisms.

PHARMACOKINETICS
Well absorbed from the GI tract (food delays absorption). Protein binding: 80%. Widely distributed. Metabolized in the liver to active metabolite. Primarily eliminated by the biliary system. Not removed by hemodialysis. ***Half-life:*** 3–5 hr (increased in hepatic impairment).

AVAILABILITY
Capsules (Rifadin): 150 mg, 300 mg.
Capsules (Rimactane): 300 mg.
Injection, Powder for Reconstitution (Rifadin): 600 mg.

INDICATIONS AND DOSAGES
▸ Tuberculosis
PO, IV
Adults, Elderly. 10 mg/kg/day. Maximum: 600 mg/day.
Children. 10–20 mg/kg/day in divided doses q12–24h.
▸ Prevention of meningococcal infections
PO, IV
Adults, Elderly. 600 mg q12h for 2 days.
Children 1 month and older. 20 mg/kg/day in divided doses q12–24h. Maximum: 600 mg/dose.
Infants younger than 1 mo. 10 mg/kg/day in divided doses q12h for 2 days.
▸ Staphylococcal infections
PO, IV
Adults, Elderly. 600 mg once a day.
Children. 15 mg/kg/day in divided doses q12h.
▸ *Staphylococcus aureus* infections (in combination with other anti-infectives)
PO
Adults, Elderly. 300–600 mg twice a day.
Neonates. 5–20 mg/kg/day in divided doses q12h.
▸ Prevention of *Haemophilus influenzae* infection
PO
Adults, Elderly. 600 mg/day for 4 days.
Children 1 mo and older. 20 mg/kg/day in divided doses q12h for 5–10 days.
Children younger than 1 mo. 10 mg/kg/day in divided doses q12h for 2 days.

OFF-LABEL USES
Prophylaxis of *H. influenzae* type b infection; treatment of atypical mycobacterial infection and serious infections caused by *Staphylococcus* species

CONTRAINDICATIONS
Concomitant therapy with amprenavir, hypersensitivity to rifampin or any other rifamycins

INTERACTIONS
Drug
Alcohol, hepatotoxic medications, ritonavir, saquinavir: May increase the risk of hepatotoxicity.
Aminophylline, theophylline: May increase clearance of these drugs.
Chloramphenicol, digoxin, disopyramide, fluconazole, methadone, mexiletine, oral anticoagulants, oral antidiabetics, phenytoin, quinidine, tocainide, verapamil: May decrease the effects of these drugs.
Oral contraceptives: May decrease oral contraceptive effectiveness.
Herbal
None known.
Food
None known.

DIAGNOSTIC TEST EFFECTS
May increase serum alkaline phosphatase, bilirubin, uric acid, AST (SGOT), and ALT (SGPT) levels.

IV INCOMPATIBILITIES
Diltiazem (Cardizem)

SIDE EFFECTS
Expected
Red-orange or red-brown discoloration of urine, feces, saliva, skin, sputum, sweat, or tears
Occasional (5%–2%)
Hypersensitivity reaction (such as flushing, pruritus, or rash)
Rare (2%–1%)
Diarrhea, dyspepsia, nausea, candida as evidenced by sore mouth or tongue

SERIOUS REACTIONS
! Rare reactions include hepatotoxicity (risk is increased when rifampin is taken with isoniazid), hepatitis, blood dyscrasias, Stevens-Johnson syndrome, and antibiotic-associated colitis.

NURSING CONSIDERATIONS
Baseline Assessment
- Determine if the patient has a hypersensitivity to rifampin or other rifamycins before beginning drug therapy.
- Make sure specimens for culture and sensitivity tests have been collected before beginning drug therapy.
- Evaluate the patient's initial CBC and serum hepatic enzyme levels.

Precautions
- Use rifampin cautiously in patients with active alcoholism, a history of alcohol abuse, or hepatic dysfunction.

Lifespan Considerations
- Rifampin crosses the placenta and is distributed in breast milk.
- No age-related precautions have been noted in children or the elderly.

Administration and Handling
PO
- If possible, give rifampin with 8 oz of water 1 hour before or 2 hours after a meal. Rifampin may be given with food to decrease GI upset, but this will delay its absorption.
- Mix the capsule's contents with applesauce or jelly if the patient can't swallow the capsules whole.
- Give rifampin at least 1 hour

before administering antacids, especially antacids containing aluminum.

IV

◀ALERT▶ Administer rifampin by IV infusion only. Avoid IM and subcutaneous administration.

- The reconstituted vial is stable for 24 hours.
- Once the reconstituted vial is further diluted, it is stable for 4 hours in D_5W or 24 hours in 0.9% NaCl.
- Reconstitute each 600-mg vial with 10 ml of sterile water for injection to provide a concentration of 60 mg/ml.
- Withdraw the desired dose and further dilute with 500 ml of D_5W.
- Infuse the solution over 3 hours (or over 30 minutes if diluted with 100 ml of D_5W).

Intervention and Evaluation

- Assess the IV site at least hourly during the infusion for extravasation, as evidenced by local inflammation and irritation. At the first sign of extravasation, restart the IV line at another site.
- Monitor the patient's liver function test results and assess the patient for signs and symptoms of hepatitis, such as anorexia, fatigue, nausea and vomiting, jaundice, and weakness. If such signs or symptoms occur, withhold rifampin and inform the physician immediately.
- Report hypersensitivity reactions, such as flu-like symptoms and skin eruptions, promptly.
- Assess the patient's pattern of daily bowel activity and stool consistency.
- Monitor the CBC for blood dyscrasias, and observe the patient for bleeding, ecchymosis, infection (manifested as a fever or sore throat), and unusual fatigue and weakness.

Patient Teaching

- Instruct the patient to take rifampin with 8 oz of water 1 hour before or 2 hours after a meal. If GI upset occurs, tell the patient that he or she can take rifampin with food.
- Warn the patient to avoid consuming alcohol while taking this drug.
- Instruct the patient not to take any other medications, including antacids, while taking rifampin without first consulting the physician. Advise the patient to take rifampin at least 1 hour before taking an antacid.
- Inform the patient that urine, feces, sputum, sweat, and tears may become reddish orange or reddish brown during therapy and that soft contact lenses may become permanently stained.
- Warn the patient to notify the physician immediately if he or she experiences fatigue, fever, flu-like symptoms, nausea, vomiting, unusual bleeding or bruising, weakness, yellow eyes and skin, or any other new symptoms.
- Caution female patients taking oral contraceptives to check with the physician because rifampin may decrease the effectiveness of oral contraceptives. Teach such patients alternative methods of contraception.

rifapentine

rif-a-**pen**-teen

(Priftin)

Do not confuse rifapentine with rifampin.

CATEGORY AND SCHEDULE

Pregnancy Risk Category: C

MECHANISM OF ACTION

An antitubercular that inhibits bacterial RNA synthesis by binding to DNA-dependent RNA polymerase in *Mycobacterium tuberculosis*. This action prevents the enzyme from attaching to DNA, thereby blocking

RNA transcription. **Therapeutic Effect:** Bactericidal.

AVAILABILITY

Tablets: 150 mg.

INDICATIONS AND DOSAGES

▸ Tuberculosis

PO

Adults, Elderly. Intensive phase: 600 mg twice weekly for 2 mo (interval between doses no less than 3 days). Continuation phase: 600 mg weekly for 4 mo.

CONTRAINDICATIONS

None known.

INTERACTIONS

Drug

Alcohol: May increase risk of hepatotoxicity.

Oral contraceptives, warfarin: May decrease the effects of these drugs.

Herbal

None known.

Food

None known.

DIAGNOSTIC TEST EFFECTS

May increase serum AST (SGOT), ALT (SGPT), and bilirubin levels.

SIDE EFFECTS

Rare (less than 4%)

Red-orange or red-brown discoloration of urine, feces, saliva, skin, sputum, sweat, or tears; arthralgia, pain, nausea, vomiting, headache, dyspepsia, hypertension, dizziness, diarrhea

SERIOUS REACTIONS

! Hyperuricemia, neutropenia, proteinuria, hematuria, and hepatitis occur rarely.

NURSING CONSIDERATIONS

Baseline Assessment

- Evaluate the patient's initial CBC and serum hepatic enzyme levels.

Precautions

- Use rifapentine cautiously in alcoholic patients and patients with hepatic impairment.

Administration and Handling

◂ALERT▸ Be aware that rifapentine is used only in combination with another antitubercular.

Intervention and Evaluation

- Monitor the patient's serum hepatic enzyme levels.
- Assess the patient's pattern of daily bowel activity and stool consistency.
- Evaluate the patient for diarrhea, GI upset, nausea, or vomiting.

Patient Teaching

- Inform the patient that urine, feces, sputum, sweat, and tears may become red-orange or red-brown during therapy and that soft contact lenses may become permanently stained.
- Warn the patient to notify the physician if he or she experiences dark urine, decreased appetite, fever, nausea or vomiting, or pain or swelling of the joints.
- Caution female patients taking oral contraceptives to check with the physician because rifapentine may decrease the effectiveness of oral contraceptives. Teach such patients alternative methods of contraception.

5 Antiviral Agents

acyclovir
adefovir dipivoxil
amantadine hydrochloride
cidofovir
famciclovir
fomivirsen
foscarnet sodium
ganciclovir sodium
oseltamivir
ribavirin
rimantadine hydrochloride
valacyclovir
valganciclovir hydrochloride
zanamivir

Uses: Antiviral agents are used to treat cytomegalovirus (CMV) retinitis in patients with AIDS, acute herpes zoster infection (shingles), recurrent genital herpes infection, chickenpox, influenza A viral illness, and mucosal and cutaneous infections with herpes simplex virus.

Action: To be effective, antivirals must inhibit virus-specific nucleic acid and protein synthesis. They may act by interfering with viral DNA synthesis and viral replication, inactivating viral DNA polymerases, incorporating into and halting the growth of viral DNA chains, preventing the release of viral nucleic acid into host cells, or blocking viral penetration into cells. (See the illustration *Sites and Mechanisms of Action: Anti-infective Agents,* page 2.)

COMBINATION PRODUCTS

REBETRON: ribavirin/interferon alfa-2b (an immunologic agent) Packaged as ribavirin (Rebetol) 200 mg capsules together with recombinant interferon alfa-2b (Intron A) injection as 3 million international units per 0.5 ml or 3 million international units per 0.2 ml.

acyclovir

ay-sye-kloe-ver
(Aciclovir-BC IV[AUS], Acihexal[AUS], Acyclo-V[AUS], Avirax[CAN], Lovir[AUS], Zovirax, Zyclir[AUS])
Do not confuse Zovirax with Zostrix or Zyvox.

CATEGORY AND SCHEDULE

Pregnancy Risk Category: B

MECHANISM OF ACTION

A synthetic nucleoside that converts to acyclovir triphosphate, becoming part of the DNA chain. **Therapeutic Effect:** Interferes with DNA synthesis and viral replication. Virustatic.

PHARMACOKINETICS

Poorly absorbed from the GI tract; minimal absorption following topical application. Protein binding: 9%–36%. Widely distributed. Partially metabolized in liver. Excreted primarily in urine. Removed by hemodialysis. ***Half-life:*** 2.5 hr (increased in impaired renal function).

AVAILABILITY

Capsules: 200 mg.
Tablets: 400 mg, 800 mg.
Injection, solution: 50 mg/ml.
Oral Suspension: 200 mg/5 ml.

Powder for Injection: 500 mg, 1,000 mg.
Ointment: 5%/50 mg.

INDICATIONS AND DOSAGES

▸ Genital herpes (initial episode)
PO
Adults, Elderly, Children 12 yr and older. 200 mg q4h 5 times a day.
IV
Adults, Elderly, Children 12 yr and older. 5 mg/kg q8h for 5 days.

▸ Genital herpes (recurrent)
Less than 6 episodes per year:
PO
Adults, Elderly, Children 12 yr and older. 200 mg q4h 5 times a day for 5 days.
6 episodes or more per year:
PO
Adults, Elderly, Children 12 yr and older. 400 mg 2 times a day or 200 mg 3–5 times a day for up to 12 months.

▸ Herpes simplex mucocutaneous
IV
Adults, Elderly, Children 12 yr and older. 5 mg/kg/dose q8h for 7 days.
Children younger than 12 yr. 10 mg/kg q8h for 7 days.

▸ Herpes simplex neonatal
IV
Children younger than 4 mo. 10 mg/kg q8h for 10 days.

▸ Herpes simplex encephalitis
IV
Adults, Elderly, Children 12 yr and older. 10 mg/kg q8h for 10 days.
Children 3 mo–younger than 12 yr. 20 mg/kg q8h for 10 days.

▸ Herpes zoster (caused by varicella)
IV
Adults, Elderly, Children 12 yr and older. 10 mg/kg q8h for 7 days.
Children younger than 12 yr. 20 mg/kg q8h for 7 days.

▸ Herpes zoster (shingles)
PO
Adults, Elderly, Children 12 yr and older. 800 mg q4h 5 times a day for 7–10 days.
Topical
Adults, Elderly. Apply to affected area 3–6 times a day for 7 days.

▸ Varicella (chickenpox)
PO
Adults, Elderly, Children older than 12 yr or children 2–12 yr weighing 40 kg or more. 800 mg 4 times a day for 5 days.
Children 2–12 yr weighing less than 40 kg. 20 mg/kg 4 times a day for 5 days. Maximum: 800 mg/dose.
Children younger than 2 yr. 80 mg/kg/day.

▸ Dosage in renal impairment
Dosage and frequency are modified based on severity of infection and degree of renal impairment.
PO
For creatinine clearance of 10 ml/min or less, dosage is 200 mg q12h.
IV

Creatinine Clearance	Dosage Percent	Dosage Interval
greater than 50 ml/min	100	8 hr
25–50 ml/min	100	12 hr
10–25 ml/min	100	24 hr
less than 10 ml/min	50	24 hr

OFF-LABEL USES

Treatment of herpes simplex ocular infections, infectious mononucleosis

CONTRAINDICATIONS

Use in neonates when acyclovir is reconstituted with bacteriostatic water containing benzyl alcohol

INTERACTIONS

Drug

Nephrotoxic medications (such as aminoglycosides): May increase the nephrotoxicity of acyclovir.
Probenecid: May increase acyclovir half-life.

Herbal

None known.

Food

None known.

DIAGNOSTIC TEST EFFECTS

May increase BUN and serum creatinine concentrations.

IV INCOMPATIBILITIES

Aztreonam (Azactam), cefepime (Maxipime), diltiazem (Cardizem), dobutamine (Dobutrex), dopamine (Intropin), levofloxacin (Levaquin), meropenem (Merrem IV), ondansetron (Zofran), piperacillin and tazobactam (Zosyn)

IV COMPATIBILITIES

Allopurinol (Alloprim), amikacin (Amikin), ampicillin, cefazolin (Ancef), cefotaxime (Claforan), ceftazidime (Fortaz), ceftriaxone (Rocephin), cimetidine (Tagamet), clindamycin (Cleocin), famotidine (Pepcid), fluconazole (Diflucan), gentamicin, heparin, hydromorphone (Dilaudid), imipenem (Primaxin), lorazepam (Ativan), magnesium sulfate, methylprednisolone (SoluMedrol), metoclopramide (Reglan), metronidazole (Flagyl), morphine, multivitamins, potassium chloride, propofol (Diprivan), ranitidine (Zantac), vancomycin

SIDE EFFECTS

Frequent

Parenteral (9%–7%): Phlebitis or inflammation at IV site, nausea, vomiting
Topical (28%): Burning, stinging

Occasional

Parenteral (3%): Pruritus, rash, urticaria
Oral (12%–6%): Malaise, nausea
Topical (4%): Pruritus

Rare

Oral (3%–1%): Vomiting, rash, diarrhea, headache
Parenteral (2%–1%): Confusion, hallucinations, seizures, tremors
Topical (less than 1%): Rash

SERIOUS REACTIONS

! Rapid parenteral administration, excessively high doses, or fluid and electrolyte imbalance may produce renal failure exhibited by such signs and symptoms as abdominal pain, decreased urination, decreased appetite, increased thirst, nausea, and vomiting.
! Toxicity has not been reported with oral or topical use.

NURSING CONSIDERATIONS

Baseline Assessment

- Determine if the patient has a history of allergies, particularly to acyclovir.
- Assess herpes simplex lesions before treatment to compare baseline lesions with those after treatment.

Lifespan Considerations

- Acyclovir crosses the placenta and is distributed in breast milk.
- The safety and efficacy of acyclovir have not been established in children less than 2 years (less than 1 year for IV use).
- Age-related renal impairment may require a dosage adjustment in the elderly.

Precautions

- Use acyclovir cautiously in patients with dehydration, fluid and electrolyte imbalances, neurologic abnormalities, or renal or hepatic impairment and in those using nephrotoxic agents concurrently.

Administration and Handling

PO

- Give acyclovir without regard to food.
- Don't crush or break capsules.
- Store capsules at room temperature.

IV

- Store vials at room temperature. Solutions of 50 mg/ml will remain stable for 12 hours at room temperature; they may form precipitate when refrigerated. Potency is not affected by precipitate or redissolution.
- IV infusion (piggyback) will remain stable for 24 hours at room temperature. Yellow discoloration does not affect potency.
- Add 10 ml of sterile water for injection to each 500-mg vial (50 mg/ml). Don't use bacteriostatic water for injection containing benzyl alcohol or parabens because this will cause a precipitate to form.
- Shake well until the solution is clear.
- Further dilute with at least 100 ml of D_5W or 0.9% NaCl. The final concentration should be less than or equal to 7 mg/ml.
- Infuse the drug over at least 1 hour because renal tubular damage may occur with too-rapid administration.
- Maintain adequate hydration during the infusion and for 2 hours afterward.

Topical

- Avoid eye contact with the ointment or cream.
- Use a finger cot or rubber glove to prevent autoinoculation.

Intervention and Evaluation

- Assess the IV site for signs and symptoms of phlebitis, including heat, pain, and red streaking over the vein.
- Evaluate cutaneous lesions for signs of effective drug treatment.
- Ensure adequate ventilation.
- Be sure to maintain appropriate isolation precautions in patients with chickenpox and disseminated herpes zoster.
- Provide analgesics and comfort measures, especially to the elderly.

Patient Teaching

- Encourage the patient to drink adequate fluids during therapy.
- Advise the patient not to touch lesions to prevent spreading the infection to new sites.
- Urge the genital herpes patient to space doses evenly around the clock and to continue taking acyclovir for the full course of treatment.
- Instruct the patient to use a finger cot or rubber glove when applying the ointment.
- Caution the patient with genital herpes to avoid sexual intercourse while lesions are visible to prevent infecting his or her partner.
- Inform the patient that acyclovir does not cure genital herpes.
- Encourage the female patient to have a Pap smear at least annually because of the increased risk of cervical cancer in women with genital herpes.

adefovir dipivoxil

ah-**deh**-foh-veer

(Hepsera)

CATEGORY AND SCHEDULE

Pregnancy Risk Category: C

MECHANISM OF ACTION

An antiviral that inhibits the enzyme DNA polymerase, causing DNA chain termination after its incorporation into viral DNA. **Therapeutic Effect:** Prevents cell replication of viral DNA.

PHARMACOKINETICS

Binds to proteins after PO administration. Excreted in urine. ***Half-life:*** 7 hr (increased in impaired renal function).

AVAILABILITY

Tablets: 10 mg.

INDICATIONS AND DOSAGES

▸ Chronic hepatitis B in patients with normal renal function

PO

Adults, Elderly. 10 mg once a day.

▸ Chronic hepatitis B in patients with impaired renal function

Adults, Elderly with creatinine clearance 20–49 ml/min. 10 mg q48h.

Adults, Elderly with creatinine clearance 10–19 ml/min. 10 mg q72h.

Adults, Elderly on hemodialysis. 10 mg every 7 days following dialysis.

CONTRAINDICATIONS

None known.

INTERACTIONS

Drug

Ibuprofen: Increases adefovir plasma concentration.

Herbal

None known.

Food

None known.

DIAGNOSTIC TEST EFFECTS

May increase serum amylase, creatinine, AST (SGOT) and ALT (SGPT) levels.

SIDE EFFECTS

Frequent (13%)

Asthenia

Occasional (9%–4%)

Headache, abdominal pain, nausea, flatulence

Rare (3%)

Diarrhea, dyspepsia

SERIOUS REACTIONS

! Nephrotoxicity (characterized by increased serum creatinine and decreased serum phosphorus levels) is a treatment-limiting toxicity of adefovir therapy.

! Lactic acidosis and severe hepatomegaly occur rarely, particularly in female patients.

NURSING CONSIDERATIONS

Baseline Assessment

- As ordered, obtain renal function laboratory values before therapy begins and routinely thereafter.
- Expect to adjust adefovir dosage in patients with pre-existing renal insufficiency.
- Expect to obtain a blood sample for HIV antibody testing before therapy begins because unrecognized or untreated HIV infection may result in the emergence of HIV resistance.

Precautions

- Use adefovir cautiously in patients with impaired renal function and known risk factors for hepatic disease.
- Use the drug cautiously in elderly patients.

Administration and Handling

PO

- Give adefovir without regard to food.

Intervention and Evaluation

- Monitor the patient's intake and output and serum creatinine levels.
- Closely monitor for serious reactions, especially in patients taking other drugs that are excreted by the kidneys or are known to affect renal function.

Patient Teaching

• Encourage the patient to comply with follow-up laboratory testing. Explain that these tests will help monitor the patient's kidney and liver function and hepatitis B virus levels.

◀ **ALERT** ▶ Warn the patient to immediately notify the physician if he or she experiences unusual muscle pain, abdominal pain with nausea and vomiting, a cold feeling in arms and legs, and dizziness. Explain that these signs and symptoms may signal the onset of lactic acidosis.

◀ **ALERT** ▶ Warn the patient to continue to take adefovir as prescribed because a very serious form of hepatitis may develop if the drug is stopped.

• Advise the patient to immediately notify the physician of yellow skin color or whites of the eyes or other unusual signs or symptoms. Explain that these may indicate serious liver problems.

• Instruct the patient to use reliable methods of contraception during therapy.

amantadine hydrochloride

a-**man**-ta-deen
(Endantadine[CAN], PMS-Amantadine[CAN], Symmetrel)

CATEGORY AND SCHEDULE

Pregnancy Risk Category: C

MECHANISM OF ACTION

A dopaminergic agonist that blocks the uncoating of influenza A virus, preventing penetration into the host and inhibiting M2 protein in the assembly of progeny virions. Amantadine also blocks the reuptake of dopamine into presynaptic neurons and causes direct stimulation of postsynaptic receptors. **Therapeutic Effect:** Antiviral and antiparkinsonian activity.

PHARMACOKINETICS

Rapidly and completely absorbed from the GI tract. Protein binding: 67%. Widely distributed. Primarily excreted in urine. Minimally removed by hemodialysis. ***Half-life:*** 11–15 hr (increased in the elderly, decreased in impaired renal function).

AVAILABILITY

Capsule: 100 mg.
Syrup: 50 mg/5 ml.
Tablets: 100 mg.

INDICATIONS AND DOSAGES

▸ **Prevention and symptomatic treatment of respiratory illness due to influenza A virus**

PO

Adults older than 64 yr. 100 mg/day.
Adults 13–64 yr. 200 mg/day.
Children 10–12 yr. 5 mg/kg/day up to 200 mg/day.
Children 1–9 yr. 5 mg/kg/day (up to 150 mg/day).

▸ **Parkinson's disease, extrapyramidal symptoms**

PO

Adults, Elderly. 100 mg twice a day. May increase up to 300 mg/day in divided doses.

▸ **Dosage in renal impairment**

Dose and frequency are modified based on creatinine clearance.

Creatinine Clearance	Dosage
30–50 ml/min	200 mg first day; 100 mg/day thereafter
15–29 ml/min	200 mg first day; 100 mg on alternate days
less than 15 ml/min	200 mg every 7 days

OFF-LABEL USES

Treatment of ADHD. Fatigue associated with multiple sclerosis

CONTRAINDICATIONS

None known.

INTERACTIONS

Drug

Alcohol: May increase CNS effects, including dizziness, confusion, light-headedness, and orthostatic hypotension.
Anticholinergics, antihistamines, phenothiazine, tricyclic antidepressants: May increase anticholinergic effects of amantadine.
Hydrochlorothiazide, triamterene: May increase amantadine blood concentration and risk for toxicity.

Herbal

None known.

Food

None known.

DIAGNOSTIC TEST EFFECTS

None known.

SIDE EFFECTS

Frequent (10%–5%)

Nausea, dizziness, poor concentration, insomnia, nervousness

Occasional (5%–1%)

Orthostatic hypotension, anorexia, headache, livedo reticularis (reddish blue, netlike blotching of skin), blurred vision, urine retention, dry mouth or nose

Rare

Vomiting, depression, irritation or swelling of eyes, rash

SERIOUS REACTIONS

! CHF, leukopenia, and neutropenia occur rarely.
! Hyperexcitability, seizures, and ventricular arrhythmias may occur.

NURSING CONSIDERATIONS

Baseline Assessment

• When treating infections caused by influenza A virus, expect to obtain specimens for viral diagnostic tests before giving the first dose. Therapy may begin before test results are known.

Lifespan Considerations

• It is unknown if amantadine crosses the placenta or is distributed in breast milk.
• No age-related precautions have been noted in children older than 1 year.
• The elderly may exhibit increased sensitivity to amantadine's anticholinergic effects.
• They also may require a dosage adjustment because of age-related renal impairment.

Precautions

• Use amantadine cautiously in patients with cerebrovascular disease, CHF, a history of seizures, hepatic or renal dysfunction, orthostatic hypotension, peripheral edema, or recurrent eczematoid dermatitis, and in those receiving CNS stimulants.

Administration and Handling

PO

◀ **ALERT** ▶ Give amantadine as a single dose or in 2 divided doses and without regard to food.
• Administer the nighttime dose several hours before bedtime to prevent insomnia.

Intervention and Evaluation

- Expect to monitor the patient's intake and output and renal function test results, if ordered.
- Check for peripheral edema and for skin blotching or a rash.
- Evaluate the patient's food tolerance and assess for nausea or vomiting.
- Assess the patient for dizziness.
- For patients with Parkinson's disease, assess for clinical reversal of symptoms as evidenced by an improvement of the masklike facial expression, muscle rigidity, shuffling gait, and tremor of the head and hands at rest.

Patient Teaching

- Advise the patient to space amantadine doses evenly around the clock and to continue taking the drug for the full course of treatment.
- Tell the patient to take the nighttime dose several hours before bedtime to prevent insomnia.
- Instruct the patient not to take any other medications, including OTC drugs, without first consulting the physician.
- Warn the patient to avoid alcoholic beverages.
- Caution the patient not to drive, use machinery, or engage in other activities that require alertness if he or she is experiencing dizziness or blurred vision.
- Advise the patient to get up slowly from a sitting or lying position.
- Instruct the patient to notify the physician of any new symptoms, especially blurred vision, dizziness, nausea or vomiting, and skin blotching or a rash.

cidofovir

ci-**dah**-fo-veer
(Vistide)

CATEGORY AND SCHEDULE

Pregnancy Risk Category: C

MECHANISM OF ACTION

An anti-infective that inhibits viral DNA synthesis by incorporating itself into the growing viral DNA chain. **Therapeutic Effect:** Suppresses replication of cytomegalovirus (CMV).

PHARMACOKINETICS

Protein binding: less than 6%. Excreted primarily unchanged in urine. Effect of hemodialysis unknown. ***Elimination half-life:*** 1.4–3.8 hr.

AVAILABILITY

Injection: 75 mg/ml (5-ml ampule).

INDICATIONS AND DOSAGES

▸ **CMV retinitis in patients with AIDS (in combination with probenecid)**

IV infusion

Adults. Induction: Usual dosage, 5 mg/kg at constant rate over 1 hr once weekly for 2 consecutive wk. Give 2 g of PO probenecid 3 hr before cidofovir dose, and then give 1 g 2 hr and 8 hr after completion of the 1-hr cidofovir infusion (total of 4 g). In addition, give 1 L of 0.9% NaCl over 1–2 hr immediately before the cidofovir infusion. If tolerated, a second liter may be infused over 1–3 hr at the start of the infusion or immediately afterward. Maintenance: 5 mg/kg cidofovir at constant rate over 1 hr once every 2 wk.

▸ **Dosage in renal impairment**

Dosages are modified based on creatinine clearance.

Creatinine Clearance	Induction Dose	Maintenance Dose
41–55 ml/min	2 mg/kg	2 mg/kg
30–40 ml/min	1.5 mg/kg	1.5 mg/kg
20–29 ml/min	1 mg/kg	1 mg/kg
19 ml/min or less	0.5 mg/kg	0.5 mg/kg

OFF-LABEL USES
Treatment of ganciclovir-resistant CMV, foscarnet-resistant CMV, adenovirus, and acyclovir-resistant herpes simplex virus or varicella-zoster virus

CONTRAINDICATIONS
Direct intraocular injection, history of clinically severe hypersensitivity to probenecid or other sulfa-containing drugs, hypersensitivity to cidofovir, renal function impairment (serum creatinine level greater than 1.5 mg/dl, creatinine clearance of 55 ml/min or less, or urine protein level greater than 100 mg/dl)

INTERACTIONS
Drug
Nephrotoxic medications (such as aminoglycosides, amphotericin B, foscarnet, IV pentamidine): Increase the risk of nephrotoxicity.
Herbal
None known.
Food
None known.

DIAGNOSTIC TEST EFFECTS
May decrease neutrophil count and serum bicarbonate, phosphate, and uric acid levels. May elevate serum creatinine levels.

IV INCOMPATIBILITIES
No information available for Y-site administration.

SIDE EFFECTS
Frequent
Nausea, vomiting (65%), fever (57%), asthenia (46%), rash (30%), diarrhea (27%), headache (27%), alopecia (25%), chills (24%), anorexia (22%), dyspnea (22%), abdominal pain (17%)

SERIOUS REACTIONS
! Serious adverse reactions may include proteinuria (80%), nephrotoxicity (53%), neutropenia (31%), elevated serum creatinine levels (29%), infection (24%), anemia (20%), ocular hypotony (a decrease in intraocular pressure, 12%), and pneumonia (9%).
Concurrent use of probenecid may produce a hypersensitivity reaction characterized by a rash, fever, chills, and anaphylaxis.
! Acute renal failure occurs rarely.

NURSING CONSIDERATIONS
Baseline Assessment
- For patients who also take zidovudine (AZT), expect to temporarily discontinue zidovudine administration or decrease the zidovudine dose by 50% on days of cidofovir infusion. Be aware that concurrent probenecid use reduces the metabolic clearance of zidovudine.
- Closely monitor the patient's renal function during therapy through serum creatinine levels and urinalysis results.

Lifespan Considerations
- Cidofovir is embryotoxic and results in reduced fetal body weight in animals.
- It is unknown if cidofovir is excreted in breast milk. Breast-feeding is not recommended for patients taking this drug because of the possibility of transmitting HIV to the infant.

• The safety and efficacy of cidofovir have not been established in children.
• Age-related renal impairment may require a dosage adjustment in the elderly.

Precautions

• Use cidofovir cautiously in patients with pre-existing diabetes mellitus. Patients using cidofovir should avoid concurrent use of nephrotoxic drugs, such as aminoglycosides, amphotericin B, foscarnet, and IV pentamidine.

Administration and Handling

IV

◀ALERT▶ Don't exceed the recommended dosage, frequency, or infusion rate.
• Store cidofovir at a controlled room temperature (68° to 77°F).
• Refrigerate admixtures for no more than 24 hours. Allow refrigerated admixtures to warm to room temperature before use.
• Dilute the drug in 100 ml of 0.9% NaCl and infuse over 1 hour.
• Prepare to administer IV hydration with 0.9% NaCl and probenecid with each cidofovir infusion to minimize the risk of nephrotoxicity.
• Have the patient eat before each dose of probenecid to help reduce nausea and vomiting. As prescribed, administer an antiemetic to reduce the risk of nausea.

Intervention and Evaluation

• Monitor the patient's serum creatinine and urine protein levels, and WBC count before giving each dose.
• Monitor the patient for signs and symptoms of proteinuria, which may be an early indicator of dose-dependent nephrotoxicity.
• Periodically evaluate the patient's visual acuity and check for ocular symptoms.
• Obtain an order for an antiemetic and administer it to the patient as needed.

Patient Teaching

• Explain to the patient that he or she must complete the full course of probenecid with each dose of cidofovir.
• Caution female patients of childbearing age to use effective contraception during and for 1 month after cidofovir treatment. Explain the need to avoid pregnancy because cidofovir is harmful to the embryo.
• Warn male patients to practice barrier contraceptive methods during and for 3 months after treatment.
• Instruct the patient not to breast-feed while taking cidofovir.
• Explain the importance of having regular follow-up ophthalmologic exams.

famciclovir

fam-**si**-klo-veer
(Famvir)
Do not confuse Famvir with Femhrt.

CATEGORY AND SCHEDULE

Pregnancy Risk Category: B

MECHANISM OF ACTION

A synthetic nucleoside that inhibits viral DNA synthesis. **Therapeutic Effect:** Suppresses replication of herpes simplex virus and varicella-zoster virus.

PHARMACOKINETICS

Rapidly and extensively absorbed after PO administration. Protein binding: 20%–25%. Rapidly metabolized to penciclovir by enzymes in the GI wall, liver, and plasma. Eliminated unchanged in urine. Removed by hemodialysis. ***Half-life:*** 2 hr.

AVAILABILITY

Tablets: 125 mg, 250 mg, 500 mg.

INDICATIONS AND DOSAGES

▸ Herpes zoster

PO

Adults. 500 mg q8h for 7 days.

▸ Recurrent genital herpes

PO

Adults. 125 mg twice a day for 5 days.

▸ Suppression of recurrent genital herpes

PO

Adults. 250 mg twice a day for up to 1 yr.

▸ Recurrent herpes simplex

PO

Adults. 500 mg twice a day for 7 days.

▸ Dosage in renal impairment

Dosage and frequency are modified based on creatinine clearance.

Creatinine Clearance	Herpes Zoster	Genital Herpes
40–59 ml/min	500 mg q12h	125 mg q12h
20–39 ml/min	500 mg q24h	125 mg q24h
less than 20 ml/min	250 mg q24h	125 mg q24h

▸ Dosage in hemodialysis patients

For adults with herpes zoster, give 250 mg after each dialysis treatment; for adults with genital herpes, give 125 mg after each dialysis treatment.

CONTRAINDICATIONS

None known.

INTERACTIONS

Drug

None known.

Herbal

None known.

Food

None known.

DIAGNOSTIC TEST EFFECTS

None known.

SIDE EFFECTS

Frequent

Headache (23%), nausea (12%)

Occasional (10%–2%)

Dizziness, somnolence, numbness of feet, diarrhea, vomiting, constipation, decreased appetite, fatigue, fever, pharyngitis, sinusitis, pruritus

Rare (less than 2%)

Insomnia, abdominal pain, dyspepsia, flatulence, back pain, arthralgia

SERIOUS REACTIONS

! None known.

NURSING CONSIDERATIONS

Baseline Assessment

- Determine if the patient has a history of renal impairment.
- Obtain the results of baseline diagnostic tests, which may include renal function studies.

Lifespan Considerations

- Be aware that famciclovir causes an increase in mammary adenocarcinoma in animals.
- It is unknown if famciclovir is excreted in breast milk.
- The safety and efficacy of famciclovir have not been established in children.
- Age-related renal impairment may require a dosage adjustment in the elderly.

Precautions

- Use famciclovir cautiously in patients with hepatic or renal impairment.

Administration and Handling

PO

- Give famciclovir without regard to food.

Intervention and Evaluation

- Evaluate the patient for cutaneous lesions.

• Assess the patient for signs and symptoms of neurologic effects, including dizziness and headache.
• Provide the patient with analgesics, if ordered, and comfort measures. Be aware that famciclovir administration is especially exhausting to elderly patients.

Patient Teaching

• Encourage the patient to drink adequate fluids.
• Teach the patient to keep his or her fingernails short and hands clean.
• Caution the patient not to touch the lesions for the duration of an outbreak to prevent cross-contamination and spreading the infection to new sites.
• Advise the patient with genital herpes to space doses evenly around the clock and to take famciclovir for the full course of treatment.
• Advise the patient to notify the physician if the lesions fail to improve or if they recur.

fomivirsen

foh-mih-**ver**-sen
(Vitravene)

CATEGORY AND SCHEDULE

Pregnancy Risk Category: C

MECHANISM OF ACTION

An antiviral that binds to messenger RNA, inhibiting the synthesis of viral proteins. **Therapeutic Effect:** Blocks replication of cytomegalovirus (CMV).

AVAILABILITY

Intravitreal Injection: 6.6 mg/ml.

INDICATIONS AND DOSAGES

▸ **CMV retinitis**

Intravitreal injection

Adults. 330 mcg (0.05 ml) every other week for 2 doses, then 330 mcg every 4 weeks.

CONTRAINDICATIONS

None significant.

INTERACTIONS

Drug

None significant.

Herbal

None significant.

Food

None significant.

DIAGNOSTIC TEST EFFECTS

May alter liver function test results and serum alkaline phosphatase level. May decrease blood Hgb levels and neutrophil and platelet counts.

SIDE EFFECTS

Frequent (10%–5%)

Fever, headache, nausea, diarrhea, vomiting, abdominal pain, anemia, uveitis, abnormal vision

Occasional (5%–2%)

Chest pain, confusion, dizziness, depression, neuropathy, anorexia, weight loss, pancreatitis, dyspnea, cough

SERIOUS REACTIONS

! Thrombocytopenia may occur.

NURSING CONSIDERATIONS

Precautions

• Be aware that fomivirsen use should be avoided in patients who have received cidofovir within 2 to 4 weeks of fomivirsen therapy.
• Use this drug cautiously in patients with increased intraocular pressure.

Intervention and Evaluation

• After fomivirsen injection, expect the physician to evaluate the patient's light perception, optic nerve head perfusion, and intraocular pressure.

• Monitor the patient for signs and symptoms of extraocular CMV infection, including pneumonitis and colitis. Also, assess for signs and symptoms of CMV infection in the untreated eye if only one eye is undergoing treatment.

Patient Teaching

• Inform the patient that fomivirsen treats but does not cure CMV retinitis. Explain that regular eye exams and follow-up care will be required.

foscarnet sodium

foss-**car**-net
(Foscavir)

CATEGORY AND SCHEDULE

Pregnancy Risk Category: C

MECHANISM OF ACTION

An antiviral that selectively inhibits binding sites on virus-specific DNA polymerase and reverse transcriptase. **Therapeutic Effect:** Inhibits replication of herpes virus.

PHARMACOKINETICS

Sequestered into bone and cartilage. Protein binding: 14%–17%. Primarily excreted unchanged in urine. Removed by hemodialysis. ***Half-life:*** 3.3–6.8 hr (increased in impaired renal function).

AVAILABILITY

Injection: 24 mg/ml.

INDICATIONS AND DOSAGES

▸ **Cytomegalovirus (CMV) retinitis**

IV

Adults, Elderly. Initially, 60 mg/kg q8h or 100 mg/kg q12h for 2–3 wk. Maintenance: 90–120 mg/kg/day as a single IV infusion.

▸ **Herpes infection**

IV

Adults. 40 mg/kg q8–12h for 2–3 wk or until healed.

▸ **Dosage in renal impairment**

Dosages are individualized based on creatinine clearance. Refer to the dosing guide provided by the manufacturer.

CONTRAINDICATIONS

None known.

INTERACTIONS

Drug

Nephrotoxic medications: May increase the risk of nephrotoxicity.
Pentamidine (IV): May cause reversible hypocalcemia, hypomagnesemia, and nephrotoxicity.
Zidovudine (AZT): May increase the risk of anemia.

Herbal

None known.

Food

None known.

DIAGNOSTIC TEST EFFECTS

May increase serum alkaline phosphatase, bilirubin, creatinine, AST (SGOT), and ALT (SGPT) levels. May decrease serum magnesium and potassium levels. May alter serum calcium and phosphate concentrations.

IV INCOMPATIBILITIES

Acyclovir (Zovirax), amphotericin B (Fungizone), co-trimoxazole (Bactrim), diazepam (Valium), digoxin (Lanoxin), diphenhydramine (Benadryl), dobutamine (Dobutrex), droperidol (Inapsine), ganciclovir (Cytovene), haloperidol (Haldol), leucovorin, midazolam (Versed), pentamidine (Pentam IV), prochlorperazine (Compazine), vancomycin (Vancocin)

IV COMPATIBILITIES

Dopamine (Intropin), heparin, hydromorphone (Dilaudid), lorazepam (Ativan), morphine, potassium chloride

SIDE EFFECTS

Frequent

Fever (65%); nausea (47%); vomiting, diarrhea (30%)

Occasional (5% or greater)

Anorexia, pain and inflammation at injection site, fever, rigors, malaise, headache, paresthesia, dizziness, rash, diaphoresis, abdominal pain

Rare (5%–1%)

Back or chest pain, edema, flushing, pruritus, constipation, dry mouth

SERIOUS REACTIONS

! Nephrotoxicity occurs to some extent in most patients.

! Seizures and serum mineral or electrolyte imbalances may be life-threatening.

NURSING CONSIDERATIONS

Baseline Assessment

• Expect to obtain the patient's baseline CBC, serum mineral and electrolyte levels, renal function test results, and vital signs.

Lifespan Considerations

• It is unknown if foscarnet is distributed in breast milk.

• The safety and efficacy of foscarnet have not been established in children.

• Age-related renal impairment may require a dosage adjustment in the elderly.

Precautions

• Use foscarnet cautiously in patients with altered serum calcium or other serum electrolyte levels, a history of renal impairment, or cardiac or neurologic abnormalities.

Administration and Handling

IV

• Store vials at room temperature.

• After dilution, foscarnet is stable for 24 hours at room temperature.

• Don't use the solution it it is discolored or contains particulate material.

• If you're giving the drug through a peripheral vein catheter, dilute the 24-mg/ml solution to 12 mg/ml, using only D_5W or 0.9% NaCl solution for injection. If you're using a central venous catheter for the infusion, the 24-mg/ml solution need not be diluted.

• Because foscarnet dosage is calculated based on body weight, remove the unneeded quantity before starting the infusion to avoid an overdose.

• Use an IV infusion pump to prevent an accidental overdose.

• Using aseptic technique, administer the solution within 24 hours of the first opening the sealed bottle.

◀ **ALERT** ▶ Don't give foscarnet by IV injection or rapid infusion because these routes increase the drug's toxicity. Administer foscarnet by IV infusion at a rate not faster than 1 hour for doses up to 60 mg/kg and 2 hours for doses greater than 60 mg/kg.

• To minimize the risk of phlebitis and toxicity, use central venous lines or veins with an adequate blood flow to permit rapid dilution and dissemination of foscarnet.

Intervention and Evaluation

• Monitor the patient's blood Hct and Hgb levels, renal function test results, and serum calcium, creatinine, magnesium, phosphorus, and potassium levels.

• Obtain periodic ophthalmic exams and monitor the results.

• Assess the patient for signs and symptoms of serum electrolyte imbalances, especially hypocalcemia (numbness or tingling in the extremities or around the mouth) and hypokalemia (irritability, muscle cramps, numbness or tingling of the extremities, and weakness).
• Provide sufficient fluids before and during the infusion to promote diuresis and reduce the risk of renal impairment.
• Evaluate the patient for signs and symptoms of anemia, bleeding, superinfections, and tremors. Institute safety measures for potential seizures.

Patient Teaching

• Instruct the patient to report numbness or tingling in the extremities or around the mouth during or after the infusion because this may indicate electrolyte abnormalities.
• Advise the patient to report tremors promptly because the drug may cause seizures.

ganciclovir sodium

gan-sy-clo-ver
(Cymevene[AUS], Cytovene, Vitrasert)
Do not confuse Cytovene with Cytosar.

CATEGORY AND SCHEDULE

Pregnancy Risk Category: C

MECHANISM OF ACTION

This synthetic nucleoside competes with viral DNA polymerase and is incorporated into growing viral DNA chains. **Therapeutic Effect:** Interferes with synthesis and replication of viral DNA.

PHARMACOKINETICS

Widely distributed. Protein binding: 1%–2%. Undergoes minimal metabolism. Excreted unchanged primarily in urine. Removed by hemodialysis. ***Half-life:*** 2.5–3.6 hr (increased in impaired renal function).

AVAILABILITY

Capsules (Cytovene): 250 mg, 500 mg.
Powder for Injection (Cytovene): 500 mg.
Implant (Vitrasert): 4.5 mg.

INDICATIONS AND DOSAGES

▸ Cytomegalovirus (CMV) retinitis

IV

Adults, Children 3 mo and older. 10 mg/kg/day in divided doses q12h for 14–21 days, then 5 mg/kg/day as a single daily dose.

▸ Prevention of CMV disease in transplant patients

IV

Adults, Children. 10 mg/kg/day in divided doses q12h for 7–14 days, then 5 mg/kg/day as a single daily dose.

▸ Other CMV infections

IV

Adults. Initially, 10 mg/kg/day in divided doses q12h for 14–21 days, then 5 mg/kg/day as a single daily dose. Maintenance: 1,000 mg 3 times a day or 500 mg q3h (6 times a day).
Children. Initially, 10 mg/kg/day in divided doses q12h for 14–21 days, then 5 mg/kg/day as a single daily dose. Maintenance: 30 mg/kg/dose q8h.

Intravitreal Implant

Adults. 1 implant q6–9mo plus oral ganciclovir.
Children 9 yr and older. 1 implant q6–9mo plus oral ganciclovir (30 mg/dose q8h).

▸ Adult dosage in renal impairment
Dosage and frequency are modified based on CrCl.

CrCl	Induction Dosage	Maintenance Dosage	Oral
50–69 ml/min	2.5 mg/kg q12h	2.5 mg/kg q24h	1,500 mg/day
25–49 ml/min	2.5 mg/kg q24h	1.25 mg/kg q24h	1,000 mg/day
10–24 ml/min	1.25 mg/kg q24h	0.625 mg/kg q24h	500 mg/day
less than 10 ml/min	1.25 mg/kg 3 times/wk	0.625 mg/kg 3 times/wk	500 mg 3 times/wk

CrCl = creatinine clearance

OFF-LABEL USES
Treatment of other CMV infections, such as gastroenteritis, hepatitis, and pneumonitis

CONTRAINDICATIONS
Absolute neutrophil count less than 500/mm^3, platelet count less than 25,000/mm^3, hypersensitivity to acyclovir or ganciclovir, immunocompetent patients, patients with congenital or neonatal CMV disease

INTERACTIONS
Drug
Bone marrow depressants: May increase bone marrow depression.
Imipenem and cilastatin: May increase the risk of seizures.
Zidovudine (AZT): May increase the risk of hepatotoxicity.
Herbal
None known.
Food
None known.

DIAGNOSTIC TEST EFFECTS
May increase serum alkaline phosphatase, bilirubin, AST (SGOT), and ALT (SGPT) levels.

IV INCOMPATIBILITIES
Aldesleukin (Proleukin), amifostine (Ethyol), aztreonam (Azactam), cefepime (Maxipime), cytarabine (ARA-C), doxorubicin (Adriamycin), fludarabine (Fludara), foscarnet (Foscavir), gemcitabine (Gemzar), ondansetron (Zofran), piperacillin and tazobactam (Zosyn), sargramostim (Leukine), vinorelbine (Navelbine)

IV COMPATIBILITIES
Amphotericin B, enalapril (Vasotec), filgrastim (Neupogen), fluconazole (Diflucan), propofol (Diprivan)

SIDE EFFECTS
Frequent
Diarrhea (41%), fever (40%), nausea (25%), abdominal pain (17%), vomiting (13%)
Occasional (11%–6%)
Diaphoresis, infection, paresthesia, flatulence, pruritus
Rare (4%–2%)
Headache, stomatitis, dyspepsia, phlebitis

SERIOUS REACTIONS
! Hematologic toxicity occurs commonly: leukopenia in 41%–29% of patients and anemia in 25%–19%.
! Intraocular insertion occasionally results in visual acuity loss, vitreous hemorrhage, and retinal detachment.
! GI hemorrhage occurs rarely.

NURSING CONSIDERATIONS
Baseline Assessment
• Evaluate the patient's baseline hematologic studies.
• Obtain specimens (blood, feces,

throat culture, urine) for culture and sensitivity testing, as ordered, before giving ganciclovir. Keep in mind that test results are needed to support the differential diagnosis and rule out retinal infection as the result of hematogenous dissemination.

Lifespan Considerations

• Ganciclovir should not be used during pregnancy. Breast-feeding should be discontinued during therapy but may be resumed no sooner than 72 hours after the last dose of ganciclovir.
• The safety and efficacy of ganciclovir have not been established in children younger than 12 years.
• Age-related renal impairment may require a dosage adjustment in the elderly.

Precautions

• Use ganciclovir cautiously in pediatric patients. The long-term safety of this drug has not been determined because of its potential for causing adverse reproductive and carcinogenic effects.
• Use this drug cautiously in patients with impaired renal function, neutropenia, or thrombocytopenia.

Administration and Handling

PO

• Give ganciclovir with food.

IV

• Store vials at room temperature. Do not refrigerate.
• The reconstituted solution in the vial remains stable for 12 hours at room temperature.
• After dilution, refrigerate the solution and use it within 24 hours.
• Discard the solution if precipitate forms or discoloration occurs.
• Avoid inhaling the solution. Also avoid exposing the solution to the eyes, mucous membranes, or skin. Use latex gloves and safety glasses during preparation and handling of ganciclovir solution. If the solution comes in contact with mucous membranes or the skin, wash the affected area thoroughly with soap and water; if it comes in contact with the eyes, rinse the eyes thoroughly with plain water.
• Reconstitute the 500-mg vial with 10 ml of sterile water for injection to provide a concentration of 50 mg/ml; do not use bacteriostatic water because it contains parabens, which is incompatible with ganciclovir.
• Further dilute with 100 ml of D_5W, 0.9% NaCl, lactated Ringer's, or any combination of these to provide a concentration of 5 mg/ml.

◀ALERT▶ Do not give ganciclovir by IV push or rapid IV infusion because these routes increase the risk of ganciclovir toxicity. Administer it only by IV infusion over 1 hour.

• Protect the patient from infiltration because the high pH of this drug causes severe tissue irritation.
• Use large veins to permit rapid dilution and dissemination of ganciclovir and to minimize the risk of phlebitis. Keep in mind that central venous ports tunneled under subcutaneous tissue may reduce catheter-associated infection.

Intervention and Evaluation

• Monitor the patient's intake and output, and provde adequate hydration (at least 1,500 ml/24 hours).
• Diligently evaluate the patient's hematology reports for a decreased platelet count, neutropenia, and thrombocytopenia.
• Evaluate the patient for complications and therapeutic improvement.
• Assess the patient for signs and symptoms of infiltration, phlebitis, pruritus, and a rash.
• Evaluate for altered vision in the patient receiving an intravitreal implant.

Patient Teaching

• Explain that frequent blood tests

and eye exams are necessary during therapy because of the drug's toxic nature.
• Stress the need to promptly report any new symptom to the physician.
• Inform male patients that ganciclovir may temporarily or permanently inhibit sperm production.
• Tell female patients that ganciclovir use may suppress fertility.
• Advise female patients to use effective contraception during therapy.
• Urge male patients to use barrier contraception during ganciclovir therapy and for 90 days afterward because of the drug's mutagenic potential.
• Inform the patient that ganciclovir suppresses but does not cure CMV retinitis.

oseltamivir

ah-suhl-**tahm**-ah-veer
(Tamiflu)

CATEGORY AND SCHEDULE

Pregnancy Risk Category: C

MECHANISM OF ACTION

A selective inhibitor of influenza virus neuraminidase, an enzyme essential for viral replication. Acts against both influenza A and B viruses. **Therapeutic Effect:** Suppresses the spread of infection within the respiratory system and reduces the duration of clinical symptoms.

PHARMACOKINETICS

Readily absorbed. Protein binding: 3%. Extensively converted to active drug in the liver. Primarily excreted in urine. ***Half-life:*** 6–10 hr.

AVAILABILITY

Capsules: 75 mg.
Oral Suspension: 12 mg/ml.

INDICATIONS AND DOSAGES

▸ **Influenza**

PO

Adults, Elderly. 75 mg 2 times a day for 5 days.
Children weighing more than 40 kg. 75 mg twice a day.
Children weighing 24–40 kg. 60 mg twice a day.
Children weighing 15–23 kg. 45 mg twice a day.
Children weighing less than 15 kg. 30 mg twice a day.

▸ **Prevention of influenza**

PO

Adults, Elderly. 75 mg once a day.

▸ **Dosage in renal impairment**

PO

For adult and elderly patients, dosage is decreased to 75 mg once a day for at least 7 days and possibly up to 6 wk.

CONTRAINDICATIONS

None known.

INTERACTIONS

Drug

None known.

Herbal

None known.

Food

None known.

DIAGNOSTIC TEST EFFECTS

None known.

SIDE EFFECTS

Frequent (5%)

Nausea, vomiting, diarrhea

Occasional (4%–1%)

Abdominal pain, bronchitis, dizziness, headache, cough, insomnia, fatigue, vertigo

SERIOUS REACTIONS

! Colitis, pneumonia, and pyrexia occur rarely.

NURSING CONSIDERATIONS

Lifespan Considerations

• It is unknown if oseltamivir is excreted in breast milk.
• The safety and efficacy of this drug have not been established in children younger than 1 year.
• No age-related precautions have been noted in the elderly.

Precautions

• Use oseltamivir cautiously in patients with renal impairment.

Administration and Handling

PO

• Give oseltamivir without regard to food.

Intervention and Evaluation

• Monitor the patient's renal function.
• Monitor the blood glucose levels of diabetic patients.

Patient Teaching

• Instruct the patient to begin taking oseltamivir as soon as flu symptoms appear.
• Warn the patient to avoid contact with those who are at high risk for influenza.

ribavirin

rye-ba-**vye**-rin
(Copegus, Rebetol, Virazole)
Do not confuse ribavirin with riboflavin.

CATEGORY AND SCHEDULE

Pregnancy Risk Category: X

MECHANISM OF ACTION

A synthetic nucleoside that inhibits influenza virus RNA polymerase activity and interferes with expression of messenger RNA. **Therapeutic Effect:** Inhibits viral protein synthesis and replication of viral RNA and DNA.

AVAILABILITY

Capsules (Rebetol): 200 mg.
Tablets (Cepegus): 200 mg.
Powder for Reconstitution (Aerosol [Virazole]): 6 g.
Oral Solution (Rebetol): 40 mg/ml.

INDICATIONS AND DOSAGES

▸ Chronic hepatitis C

PO (capsule or oral solution in combination with interferon alfa-2b)
Adults, Elderly. 1,000–1,200 mg/day in 2 divided doses.
Children weighing more than 60 kg. Use adult dosage. *(51–60 kg):* 400 mg 2 times/day. *(37–50 kg):* 200 mg in morning, 400 mg in evening. *(24–36 kg):* 200 mg 2 times/day.
PO (capsules in combination with peginterferon alfa-2b)
Adults, Elderly. 800 mg/day in 2 divided doses.
PO (tablets in combination with peginterferon alfa-2b)
Adults, Elderly. 800–1,200 mg/day in 2 divided doses.

▸ Severe lower respiratory tract infection caused by respiratory syncytial virus (RSV)

Inhalation
Children, Infants. Use with Viratek small-particle aerosol generator at a concentration of 20 mg/ml (6 g reconstituted with 300 ml sterile water) over 12–18 hr/day for 3–7 days.

OFF-LABEL USES

Treatment of influenza A or B and west Nile virus

CONTRAINDICATIONS

Pregnancy, women of childbearing

age who won't use contraception reliably

INTERACTIONS

Drug

Didanosine: May increase the risk of pancreatitis and peripheral neuropathy and decrease the effects of didanosine.

Nucleoside analogues (including adefovir, didanosine, lamivudine, stavudine, zalcitabine, zidovudine): May increase the risk of lactic acidosis.

Herbal

None known.

Food

None known.

DIAGNOSTIC TEST EFFECTS

None known.

SIDE EFFECTS

Frequent (greater than 10%)

Dizziness, headache, fatigue, fever, insomnia, irritability, depression, emotional lability, impaired concentration, alopecia, rash, pruritus, nausea, anorexia, dyspepsia, vomiting, decreased hemoglobin, hemolysis, arthralgia, musculoskeletal pain, dyspnea, sinusitis, flu-like symptoms

Occasional (1%–10%)

Nervousness, altered taste, weakness

SERIOUS REACTIONS

! Cardiac arrest, apnea and ventilator dependence, bacterial pneumonia, pneumonia, and pneumothorax occur rarely.

! Anemia may occur if ribavirin therapy exceeds 7 days.

NURSING CONSIDERATIONS

Baseline Assessment

- Expect to obtain sputum specimens for diagnostic testing before giving the first dose of ribavirin or during the first 24 hours of therapy.
- Establish the patient's baseline respiratory status.
- For patients taking oral ribavirin, expect to obtain a CBC with differential and to test the female patient of childbearing age monthly for pregnancy.

Precautions

- Use oral ribavirin cautiously in elderly patients, patients with cardiac or pulmonary disease, and patients with a history of psychiatric disorders.
- Use inhaled ribavirin cautiously in patients with asthma or COPD and in patients requiring mechanical ventilation.

Administration and Handling

PO

- Give capsules without regard to food.
- Give tablets with food.

Inhalation

◂ **ALERT** ▸ Ribavirin may be given by nasal or oral inhalation.

- The solution normally appears clear and colorless and is stable for 24 hours at room temperature. Discard the solution for nebulization after 24 hours. Also discard the solution if it becomes discolored or cloudy.
- Add 50 to 100 ml of sterile water for injection or inhalation to each 6-g vial.
- Transfer the solution to the flask that serves as the reservoir for the Viratek aerosol generator.
- Further dilute to a final volume of 300 ml and a concentration of 20 mg/ml.
- Use only the Viratek aerosol generator available from the drug manufacturer.
- Don't give ribavirin concurrently with other drugs administered by nebulization.

• Discard the reservoir solution when fluid levels are low and at least every 24 hours.

◀ **ALERT** ▶ Be aware that there is controversy over the safety of administering ribavirin to ventilator-dependent patients; only experienced personnel should administer the drug.

Intervention and Evaluation

• Monitor the patient's intake and output and fluid balance carefully.
• Check the patient's hematology reports for anemia due to reticulocytosis when therapy exceeds 7 days.
• For ventilator-assisted patients, watch for "rainout" (accumulation of fluid in the ventilator tubing), and empty the tubing frequently.
• Be alert for impaired ventilation and gas exchange resulting from drug precipitate.
• Periodically assess breath sounds and check the skin for a rash.
• Monitor the patient's blood pressure and respirations.

Patient Teaching

• Instruct the patient to immediately report difficulty breathing or itching, redness, or swelling of the eyes.
• Educate female patients about the need to prevent pregnancy and undergo regular pregnancy testing during ribavirin therapy.
• Teach male patients about the need to protect female partners from pregnancy.

rimantadine hydrochloride

ri-**man**-ti-deen
(Flumadine)
Do not confuse rimantadine with ranitidine, or Flumadine with flunisolide or flutamide.

CATEGORY AND SCHEDULE

Pregnancy Risk Category: C

MECHANISM OF ACTION

An antiviral that appears to exert an inhibitory effect early in the viral replication cycle. May inhibit uncoating of the virus. **Therapeutic Effect:** Prevents replication of influenza A virus.

AVAILABILITY

Syrup: 50 mg/5 ml.
Tablets: 100 mg.

INDICATIONS AND DOSAGES

▸ **Influenza A virus**

PO

Adults, Elderly. 100 mg twice a day for 7 days.

Elderly nursing home patients, patients with severe hepatic or renal impairment. 100 mg once a day for 7 days.

▸ **Prevention of influenza A virus**

PO

Adults, Elderly, Children 10 yr and older. 100 mg twice a day for at least 10 days after known exposure (usually for 6–8 wk).

Children younger than 10 yr. 5 mg/kg once a day. Maximum: 150 mg.

Elderly nursing home patients, patients with severe hepatic or renal impairment. 100 mg once a day.

CONTRAINDICATIONS
Hypersensitivity to amantadine or rimantadine

INTERACTIONS
Drug
Acetaminophen, aspirin: May decrease rimantadine blood concentration.
Anticholinergics, CNS stimulants: May increase side effects of rimantadine.
Cimetidine: May increase rimantadine blood concentration.
Herbal
None known.
Food
None known.

DIAGNOSTIC TEST EFFECTS
None known.

SIDE EFFECTS
Occasional (3%–2%)
Insomnia, nausea, nervousness, impaired concentration, dizziness
Rare (less than 2%)
Vomiting, anorexia, dry mouth, abdominal pain, asthenia, fatigue

SERIOUS REACTIONS
! None known.

NURSING CONSIDERATIONS
Precautions
• Use rimantadine cautiously in patients with a history of recurrent eczematoid dermatitis, renal or hepatic impairment, seizures, or uncontrolled psychosis.
• Use the drug cautiously in patients who also take CNS stimulants.
Administration and Handling
PO
• Give rimantadine without regard to food.
Intervention and Evaluation
• Assess the patient for anxiety, nervousness, and insomnia.
• Provide assistance if the patient experiences dizziness.
Patient Teaching
• Urge the patient to avoid contact with people who are at high risk for developing influenza A because a rimantadine-resistant virus may be shed during therapy.
• Warn the patient not to perform tasks that require mental alertness or motor skills until his or her response to the drug has been established.
• Caution the patient against taking acetaminophen, aspirin, or compounds containing these drugs.
• Inform the patient that rimantadine may cause dry mouth.

valacyclovir
val-a-**sye**-kloe-ver
(Valtrex)

CATEGORY AND SCHEDULE
Pregnancy Risk Category: B

MECHANISM OF ACTION
A virustatic antiviral that is converted to acyclovir triphosphate, becoming part of the viral DNA chain. **Therapeutic Effect:** Interferes with DNA synthesis and replication of herpes simplex virus and varicella-zoster virus.

PHARMACOKINETICS
Rapidly absorbed after PO administration. Protein binding: 13%–18%. Rapidly converted by hydrolysis to the active compound acyclovir. Widely distributed to tissues and body fluids (including CSF). Primarily eliminated in urine. Removed by hemodialysis. ***Half-life:*** 2.5–3.3 hr

(increased in impaired renal function).

AVAILABILITY
Caplets: 500 mg, 1,000 mg.

INDICATIONS AND DOSAGES
▸ Herpes zoster (shingles)
PO
Adults, Elderly. 1 g 3 times a day for 7 days.
▸ Herpes simplex (cold sores)
PO
Adults, Elderly. 2 g twice a day for 1 day.
▸ Initial episode of genital herpes
PO
Adults, Elderly. 1 g twice a day for 10 days.
▸ Recurrent episodes of genital herpes
PO
Adults, Elderly. 500 mg twice a day for 3 days.
▸ Prevention of genital herpes
PO
Adults, Elderly. 500–1,000 mg/day.
▸ Dosage in renal impairment
Dosage and frequency are modified based on creatinine clearance.

Creatinine Clearance	Herpes Zoster	Genital Herpes
50 ml/min or higher	1 g q8h	500 mg q12h
30–49 ml/min	1 g q12h	500 mg q12h
10–29 ml/min	1 g q24h	500 mg q24h
less than 10 ml/min	500 mg q24h	500 mg q24h

OFF-LABEL USES
To reduce the risk of heterosexual transmission of genital herpes

CONTRAINDICATIONS
Hypersensitivity to or intolerance of acyclovir, valacyclovir, or their components

INTERACTIONS
Drug
Cimetidine, probenecid: May increase acyclovir blood concentration.
Herbal
None known.
Food
None known.

DIAGNOSTIC TEST EFFECTS
None known.

SIDE EFFECTS
Frequent
Herpes zoster (17%–10%): Nausea, headache
Genital herpes (17%): Headache
Occasional
Herpes zoster (7%–3%): Vomiting, diarrhea, constipation (50 yr or older), asthenia, dizziness (50 yr or older)
Genital herpes (8%–3%): Nausea, diarrhea, dizziness
Rare
Herpes zoster (3%–1%): Abdominal pain, anorexia
Genital herpes (3%–1%): Asthenia, abdominal pain

SERIOUS REACTIONS
! None known.

NURSING CONSIDERATIONS
Baseline Assessment
- Determine if the patient has a history of allergies, particularly to acyclovir or valacyclovir, before beginning drug therapy.
- Expect to obtain tissue cultures from herpes simplex and herpes zoster patients before giving the first dose of valacyclovir. Therapy may proceed before test results are known.
- Assess the patient's medical history, especially in those with ad-

vanced HIV infection or hepatic or renal impairment and in those who have had a bone marrow or kidney transplant.

Lifespan Considerations

• Valacyclovir may cross the placenta and be distributed in breast milk.
• The safety and efficacy of this drug have not been established in children.
• Age-related renal impairment may require a dosage adjustment in the elderly.

Precautions

• Use valacyclovir cautiously in patients with advanced HIV infection, fluid or electrolyte imbalances, neurologic abnormalities, or renal or hepatic impairment; in dehydrated patients; in those who have had a bone marrow or kidney transplant; and in those using nephrotoxic agents concurrently.

Administration and Handling

◀ **ALERT** ▶ Be aware that valacyclovir therapy for shingles is most effective when started within 48 hours of the onset of the herpes zoster rash.

PO

• Give valacyclovir without regard to food.
• Don't crush or break caplets.

Intervention and Evaluation

• Evaluate the patient for cutaneous lesions.
• Monitor the patient's CBC, liver and renal function test results, and urinalysis results.
• Keep herpes zoster patients in strict isolation, according to your institution's policies and procedures.
• Provide analgesics, if ordered, and comfort measures for herpes zoster patients. Know that herpes zoster is especially exhausting for the elderly.
• Provide the patient with adequate fluids.
• Keep the patient's fingernails short and hands clean.

Patient Teaching

• Encourage the patient to drink adequate fluids.
• Teach the patient to start valacyclovir treatment at the first sign of a recurrent episode of genital herpes or herpes zoster. Explain that treatment is most effective when started within 48 hours after symptoms first appear.
• Caution the patient not to touch lesions to avoid spreading the infection to new sites.
• Advise the genital herpes patient to space doses evenly around the clock and to continue taking the drug for the full course of treatment.
• Warn the genital herpes patient to avoid sexual intercourse while lesions are present to prevent infecting his or her partner.
• Advise the patient to notify the physician if lesions don't improve or if they recur.
• Urge the female patient with genital herpes to have a Pap test at least annually because of the increased risk of cervical cancer associated with genital herpes.
• Inform the patient that valacyclovir treats but does not cure genital herpes.

valganciclovir hydrochloride

val-gan-**sye**-kloh-veer
(Valcyte)

CATEGORY AND SCHEDULE

Pregnancy Risk Category: C

MECHANISM OF ACTION

A synthetic nucleoside that competes with viral DNA esterases and is incorporated directly into growing viral DNA chains. **Therapeutic Effect:** Interferes with DNA synthesis and viral replication.

PHARMACOKINETICS

Well absorbed and rapidly converted to ganciclovir by intestinal and hepatic enzymes. Widely distributed. Slowly metabolized intracellularly. Primarily excreted unchanged in urine. Removed by hemodialysis. ***Half-life:*** 18 hr (increased in impaired renal function).

AVAILABILITY

Tablets: 450 mg.

INDICATIONS AND DOSAGES

▸ Cytomegalovirus (CMV) retinitis in patients with normal renal function

PO

Adults. Initially, 900 mg (two 450-mg tablets) twice a day for 21 days. Maintenance: 900 mg once a day.

▸ Prevention of CMV after transplant

PO

Adults, Elderly. 900 mg once a day beginning within 10 days of transplant and continuing until 100 days post-transplant.

▸ Dosage in renal impairment

Dosage and frequency are modified based on creatinine clearance.

Creatinine Clearance	Induction Dosage	Maintenance Dosage
60 ml/min or more	900 mg twice/day	900 mg once/day
40–59 ml/min	450 mg twice/day	450 mg once/day
25–39 ml/min	450 mg once/day	450 mg q2 days
10–24 ml/min	450 mg q2 days	450 mg twice/week

CONTRAINDICATIONS

Hypersensitivity to acyclovir or ganciclovir

INTERACTIONS

Drug

Amphotericin B, cyclosporine: May increase the risk of nephrotoxicity.

Bone marrow depressants: May increase bone marrow depression.

Imipenem and cilastatin: May increase the risk of seizures.

Probenecid: Decreases renal clearance of valganciclovir.

Zidovudine (AZT): May increase the risk of hematologic toxicity.

Herbal

None known.

Food

All foods: Maximize drug bioavailability.

DIAGNOSTIC TEST EFFECTS

May decrease blood Hct and Hgb levels, serum creatinine level, platelet count, and WBC count.

SIDE EFFECTS

Frequent (16%–9%)

Diarrhea, neutropenia, headache

Occasional (8%–3%)

Nausea, anemia, thrombocytopenia

Rare (less than 3%)

Insomnia, paraesthesia, vomiting, abdominal pain, fever

SERIOUS REACTIONS

! Hematologic toxicity, including severe neutropenia (most common), anemia, and thrombocytopenia, may occur.

! Retinal detachment occurs rarely.

! An overdose may result in renal toxicity.

! Valganciclovir may decrease sperm production and fertility.

NURSING CONSIDERATIONS

Baseline Assessment

• Evaluate the patient's baseline serum creatinine level as well as blood chemistry and hematologic test results.

Lifespan Considerations

• Valganciclovir should not be used during pregnancy because of the drug's mutagenic potential.
• Female patients should avoid breast-feeding until at least 72 hours after the last dose of valganciclovir.
• The safety and efficacy of this drug have not been established in children younger than 12 years.
• Age-related renal impairment may require a dosage adjustment in the elderly.

Precautions

• Use valganciclovir with extreme caution in children because of the drug's long-term carcinogenicity and risk of reproductive toxicity.
• Use the drug cautiously in patients with pre-existing cytopenias, a history of cytopenic reactions to other drugs, or renal impairment and in elderly patients, who have a greater risk of renal impairment.

Administration and Handling

PO
• Don't break or crush tablets (potentially carcinogenic).
• Avoid contact with skin. Wash skin with soap and water if contact occurs.
• Give valganciclovir with food.

Intervention and Evaluation

• Monitor the patient's intake and output, and ensure adequate hydration (at least 1,500 ml/24 hours).
• Carefully evaluate the CBC for decreased platelet count, WBC count, and blood Hct and Hgb levels.
• Evaluate the patient's complications, therapeutic improvement, and vision.

Patient Teaching

• Stress the need for frequent blood tests during therapy because of the drug's toxic nature.
• Instruct the patient to have an ophthalmologic exam every 4 to 6 weeks, as advised by the physician, during treatment.
• Warn the patient to report any new symptoms promptly to the physician.
• Explain to the male patient that valganciclovir may temporarily or permanently inhibit sperm production. Explain to the female patient that valganciclovir may temporarily or permanently suppress fertility.
• Advise female patients to use effective contraception during valganciclovir therapy.
• Teach male patients to use barrier contraception during and for 90 days after therapy because of the drug's mutagenic potential.
• Inform the patient that valganciclovir treats but does not cure CMV retinitis.

zanamivir

za-**na**-mi-veer
(Relenza)

CATEGORY AND SCHEDULE

Pregnancy Risk Category: B

MECHANISM OF ACTION

An antiviral that appears to inhibit the influenza virus enzyme neuraminidase, which is essential for viral replication. **Therapeutic Effect:** Prevents viral release from infected cells.

AVAILABILITY

Powder for inhalation: 5 mg/blister.

INDICATIONS AND DOSAGES

▸ Influenza virus

Inhalation

Adults, Elderly, Children 7 yr and older. 2 inhalations (one 5-mg blister per inhalation for a total dose of 10 mg) twice a day (approximately 12 hr apart) for 5 days.

▸ Prevention of influenza virus

Inhalation

Adults, Elderly. 2 inhalations once a day for the duration of the exposure period.

CONTRAINDICATIONS

None known.

INTERACTIONS

Drug

None known.

Herbal

None known.

Food

None known.

DIAGNOSTIC TEST EFFECTS

May increase serum CK level and liver function test results.

SIDE EFFECTS

Occasional (3%–2%)

Diarrhea, sinusitis, nausea, bronchitis, cough, dizziness, headache

Rare (less than 1.5%)

Malaise, fatigue, fever, abdominal pain, myalgia, arthralgia, urticaria

SERIOUS REACTIONS

! Neutropenia may occur.

! Bronchospasm may occur in those with a history of COPD or bronchial asthma.

NURSING CONSIDERATIONS

Baseline Assessment

• Patients requiring an inhaled bronchodilator at the same time as zanamivir should receive the bronchodilator before zanamivir.

Precautions

• Use zanamivir cautiously in patients with asthma or COPD.

Administration and Handling

Inhalation

• Using the Diskhaler device provided, instruct the patient to exhale completely; then, holding the mouthpiece 1 inch away from the patient's lips, instruct the patient to inhale and hold his or her breath for as long as possible before exhaling.

• Have the patient rinse his or her mouth with water immediately after inhalation to prevent mouth and throat dryness.

• Store the drug at room temperature.

Intervention and Evaluation

• Provide assistance if the patient experiences dizziness.

• Assess the patient's pattern of daily bowel activity and stool consistency.

Patient Teaching

• Teach the patient how to use the delivery device.

• Advise the patient to space doses evenly around the clock and to continue treatment for the full 5-day course.

• Urge the patient to avoid contact with those who are at high risk for influenza.

• Encourage the patient with respiratory disease to always have an inhaled bronchodilator readily available.

6 Carbapenems

ertapenem
imipenem-cilastatin sodium
meropenem

Uses: Carbapenems are used to treat a wide variety of infections caused by aerobic and anaerobic organisms, including *streptococci, enterococci, staphylococci, Pseudomonas* species, *Acinetobacter* species, and *Bacteroides fragilis.* They have a broader spectrum of activity than most other beta-lactam antibiotics.

Action: Carbapenems bind to penicillin-binding proteins, disrupting bacterial cell wall synthesis. Through this action, they're bactericidal. (See the illustration *Sites and Mechanisms of Action: Anti-infective Agents,* page 2.)

ertapenem

er-ta-**pen**-em
(Invanz)

CATEGORY AND SCHEDULE

Pregnancy Risk Category: B

MECHANISM OF ACTION

A carbapenem that penetrates the bacterial cell wall of microorganisms and binds to penicillin-binding proteins, inhibiting cell wall synthesis. **Therapeutic Effect:** Produces bacterial cell death.

PHARMACOKINETICS

Almost completely absorbed after IM administration. Protein binding: 85%–95%. Widely distributed. Primarily excreted in urine with smaller amount eliminated in feces. Removed by hemodialysis. ***Half-life:*** 4 hr.

AVAILABILITY

Injection Powder for Reconstitution: 1-g.

INDICATIONS AND DOSAGES

▸ **Intra-abdominal infection**

IM, IV

Adults, Elderly. 1 g/day for 5–14 days.

▸ **Skin and skin structure infection**

IM, IV

Adults, Elderly. 1 g/day for 7–14 days.

▸ **Pneumonia, urinary tract infection (UTI)**

IM, IV

Adults, Elderly. 1 g/day for 10–14 days.

▸ **Pelvic infection**

IM, IV

Adults, Elderly. 1 g/day for 3–10 days.

▸ **Dosage in renal impairment**

For adults and elderly patients with creatinine clearance less than 30 ml/min. Dosage is 500 mg once a day.

CONTRAINDICATIONS

History of hypersensitivity to beta-lactams (imipenem and cilastin, meropenem), hypersensitivity to amide-type local anesthetics (IM)

INTERACTIONS

Drug

Probenecid: Reduces renal excretion of ertapenem.

Herbal

None known.

Food

None known.

DIAGNOSTIC TEST EFFECTS

May increase serum alkaline phosphatase, AST (SGOT) and ALT (SGPT) levels. May decrease platelet count, blood Hct and Hgb levels, and serum potassium level.

IV INCOMPATIBILITIES

Do not mix or infuse ertapenem with any other medications. Do not use diluents or IV solutions containing dextrose.

IV COMPATIBILITIES

Sterile water for injection, 0.9% NaCl

SIDE EFFECTS

Frequent (10%–6%)

Diarrhea, nausea, headache

Occasional (5%–2%)

Altered mental status, insomnia, rash, abdominal pain, constipation, vomiting, edema, fever

Rare (less than 2%)

Dizziness, cough, oral candidiasis, anxiety, tachycardia, phlebitis at IV site

SERIOUS REACTIONS

! Antibiotic-associated colitis and other superinfections may occur.

! Anaphylactic reactions have been reported.

! Seizures may occur in those with CNS disorders (including patients with brain lesions or a history of seizures), bacterial meningitis, or severe renal impairment.

NURSING CONSIDERATIONS

Baseline Assessment

◀ALERT▶ Determine if the patient has a history of allergies, particularly to beta-lactams, cephalosporins, or penicillins before beginning ertapenem therapy.

- Determine if the patient has a history of seizures.

Lifespan Considerations

- Ertapenem is distributed in breast milk.
- The safety and efficacy of ertapenem have not been established in children younger than18 years.
- Advanced or end-stage renal insufficiency may require a dosage adjustment in the elderly.

Precautions

- Use ertapenem cautiously in patients with CNS disorders (particularly brain lesions or a history of seizures), impaired renal function, or a hypersensitivity to cephalosporins, penicillins, or other allergens.
- Probenecid use should be avoided in a patient receiving ertapenem.

Administration and Handling

IV

- The solution normally appears colorless to yellow; variations in color don't affect potency.
- Discard the solution if it contains a precipitate.
- The reconstituted solution is stable for 6 hours at room temperature and 24 hours if refrigerated.
- Dilute the 1-g vial with 10 ml of 0.9% NaCl or bacteriostatic water for injection.
- Shake well to dissolve.
- Further dilute with 50 ml of 0.9% NaCl.
- Give by intermittent IV infusion (piggyback), not by IV push. Infuse over 20 to 30 minutes.

IM

- Reconstitute the lyophilized pow-

der with 3.2 ml of 1% lidocaine injection without epinephrine.
- Shake the vial thoroughly.
- To minimize patient discomfort, slowly inject the drug deep into the gluteus maximus rather than the lateral aspect of the thigh.
- Administer the suspension within 1 hour after preparation.

Intervention and Evaluation
- Assess the patient's pattern of daily bowel activity and stool consistency.
- Evaluate the patient's hydration status, and check for nausea and vomiting.
- Check the IV injection site for inflammation.
- Inspect the patient's skin for a rash.
- Evaluate the patient's mental status, and watch for seizures and tremors.
- Assess the patient's sleep pattern for evidence of insomnia.

Patient Teaching
- Advise the patient to notify the physician if he or she experiences diarrhea, a rash, seizures, tremors, or any other new symptoms.

imipenem-cilastatin sodium

i-me-**pen**-em
(Primaxin)

CATEGORY AND SCHEDULE

Pregnancy Risk Category: C

MECHANISM OF ACTION

A fixed-combination carbapenem. Imipenem penetrates the bacterial cell membrane and binds to penicillin-binding proteins, inhibiting cell wall synthesis. Cilastatin competitively inhibits the enzyme dehydropeptidase, preventing renal metabolism of imipenem. **Therapeutic Effect:** Produces bacterial cell death.

PHARMACOKINETICS

Readily absorbed after IM administration. Protein binding: 13%–21%. Widely distributed. Metabolized in the kidneys. Primarily excreted in urine. Removed by hemodialysis. ***Half-life:*** 1 hr (increased in impaired renal function).

AVAILABILITY

IV Injection: 250 mg, 500 mg.
IM Injection: 500 mg, 750 mg.

INDICATIONS AND DOSAGES

▸ **Serious respiratory tract, skin and skin-structure, gynecologic, bone, joint, intra-abdominal, nosocomial, and polymicrobic infections; UTIs; endocarditis; septicemia**

IV

Adults, Elderly. 2–4 g/day in divided doses q6h.

▸ **Mild to moderate respiratory tract, skin and skin-structure, gynecologic, bone, joint, intra-abdominal, and polymicrobic infections; UTIs; endocarditis; septicemia**

IV

Adults, Elderly. 1–2 g/day in divided doses q6–8h.
Children older than 3 mo–12 yr. 60–100 mg/kg/day in divided doses q6h. Maximum: 4 g/day.
Children 1–3 mo. 100 mg/kg/day in divided doses q6h.
Children younger than 1 mo. 20–25 mg/kg/dose q8–24h.

IM

Adults, Elderly. 500–750 mg q12h.

▸ **Dosage in renal impairment**

Dosage and frequency are modified based on creatinine clearance and the severity of the infection.

Creatinine Clearance	Dosage (IV)
31–70 ml/min	500 mg q8h
21–30 ml/min	500 mg q12h
5–20 ml/min	250 mg q12h

CONTRAINDICATIONS
None known.

INTERACTIONS
Drug
None known.
Herbal
None known.
Food
None known.

DIAGNOSTIC TEST EFFECTS
May increase BUN level and serum alkaline phosphatase, bilirubin, creatinine, LDH, AST (SGOT) and ALT (SGPT) levels. May decrease blood Hct and Hgb levels.

IV INCOMPATIBILITIES
Allopurinol (Aloprim), amphotericin B complex (Abelcet, AmBisome, Amphotec), fluconazole (Diflucan)

IV COMPATIBILITIES
Diltiazem (Cardizem), insulin, propofol (Diprivan)

SIDE EFFECTS
Occasional (3%–2%)
Diarrhea, nausea, vomiting
Rare (2%–1%)
Rash

SERIOUS REACTIONS
! Antibiotic-associated colitis and other superinfections may occur.
! Anaphylactic reactions have been reported.

NURSING CONSIDERATIONS
Baseline Assessment
◀ALERT▶ Determine if the patient has a history of allergies, particularly to beta-lactams, cephalosporins, or penicillins, before beginning drug therapy.
- Determine if the patient has a history of seizures.

Lifespan Considerations
- Imipenem crosses the placenta and is distributed in amniotic fluid, breast milk, and cord blood.
- This drug may be used safely in children.
- Age-related renal impairment may require a dosage adjustment in the elderly.

Precautions
- Use imipenem and cilastatin cautiously in patients with a history of seizures, renal impairment, or sensitivity to penicillins.

Administration and Handling
IV
- The solution normally appears colorless to yellow; discard it if it turns brown or contains a precipitate.
- Dilute each 250- or 500-mg vial with 100 ml D_5W or 0.9% NaCl.
- Give by intermittent IV infusion (piggyback), not by IV push.
- The reconstituted solution is stable for 4 hours at room temperature and 24 hours if refrigerated.
- Infuse the drug over 20 to 30 minutes (over 40 to 60 minutes for the 1-g dose).
- Observe the patient during the initial 30 minutes of a first-time infusion for possible hypersensitivity reaction.

IM
- Reconstitute the 500-mg vial with 2 ml of 1% lidocaine HCl injection without epinephrine, and the 750-mg vial with 3 ml of 1% lidocaine, as prescribed.
- Administer the suspension within 1 hour of preparation.
- Don't mix the suspension with any other medications.

• To minimize patient discomfort, slowly inject the drug deep into a large muscle, such as the gluteus maximus rather than the lateral aspect of the thigh.

Intervention and Evaluation

• Monitor the patient's hematologic and liver and renal function test results.
• Evaluate the patient for injection site pain or phlebitis, as evidenced by heat, pain, and red streaking over the vein.
• Assess the patient for nausea and vomiting.
• Assess the patient's pattern of daily bowel activity and stool consistency.
• Inspect the patient's skin for a rash.
• Observe the patient for seizures and tremors.

Patient Teaching

• Advise the patient to immediately notify the physician if he or she experiences severe diarrhea and to avoid taking antidiarrheals until directed to do so.
• Instruct the patient to notify the physician of troublesome or serious adverse reactions, including infusion site pain, redness, or swelling; nausea or vomiting, or a rash or itching.

meropenem

murr-oh-**peh**-nem
(Merrem IV)

CATEGORY AND SCHEDULE

Pregnancy Risk Category: B

MECHANISM OF ACTION

A carbapenem that binds to penicillin-binding proteins and inhibits bacterial cell wall synthesis. **Therapeutic Effect:** Produces bacterial cell death.

PHARMACOKINETICS

After IV administration, widely distributed into tissues and body fluids, including CSF. Protein binding: 2%. Primarily excreted unchanged in urine. Removed by hemodialysis. ***Half-life:*** 1 hr.

AVAILABILITY

Powder for Injection: 500 mg, 1 g.

INDICATIONS AND DOSAGES

▸ **Mild to moderate infections**

IV

Adults, Elderly. 0.5–1 g q8h.
Children 3 mo and older. 20 mg/kg/dose q8h.
Children younger than 3 mo. 20 mg/kg/dose q8–12h.

▸ **Meningitis**

IV

Adults, Elderly, Children weighing 50 kg or more. 2 g q8h.
Children 3 mo and older weighing less than 50 kg. 40 mg/kg q8h.
Maximum: 2 g/dose.

▸ **Dosage in renal impairment**

Dosage and frequency are modified based on creatinine clearance.

Creatinine Clearance	Dosage	Interval
26–49 ml/min	Recommended dose (1,000 mg)	q12h
10–25 ml/min	½ of recommended dose	q12h
less than 10 ml/min	½ of recommended dose	q24h

OFF-LABEL USES

Lower respiratory tract infections, febrile neutropenia, gynecologic and obstetric infections, sepsis

CONTRAINDICATIONS

None known.

INTERACTIONS

Drug

Probenecid: Reduces renal excretion of meropenem.

Herbal

None known.

Food

None known.

DIAGNOSTIC TEST EFFECTS

May increase BUN level and serum alkaline phosphatase, bilirubin, creatinine, LDH, AST (SGOT), and ALT (SGPT) levels. May decrease blood Hct and Hgb levels and serum potassium levels.

IV INCOMPATIBILITIES

Acyclovir (Zovirax), amphotericin B (Fungizone), diazepam (Valium), doxycycline (Vibramycin), metronidazole (Flagyl), ondansetron (Zofran)

IV COMPATIBILITIES

Dobutamine (Dobutrex), dopamine (Intropin), heparin, magnesium

SIDE EFFECTS

Frequent (5%–3%)

Diarrhea, nausea, vomiting, headache, inflammation at injection site

Occasional (2%)

Oral candidiasis, rash, pruritus

Rare (less than 2%)

Constipation, glossitis

SERIOUS REACTIONS

! Antibiotic-associated colitis and other superinfections may occur.

! Anaphylactic reactions have been reported.

! Seizures may occur in those with CNS disorders (including brain lesions and a history of seizures), bacterial meningitis, or impaired renal function.

NURSING CONSIDERATIONS

Baseline Assessment

- Determine if the patient has a history of seizures.

Lifespan Considerations

- It is unknown if meropenem is distributed in breast milk.
- The safety and efficacy of meropenem have not been established in children younger than 3 months.
- Age-related renal impairment may require a dosage adjustment in the elderly.

Precautions

- Probenecid use should be avoided in a patient receiving meropenem.
- Use meropenem cautiously in patients with CNS disorders (particularly a history of seizures), renal impairment, or a hypersensitivity to cephalosporins, penicillins, or other allergens.

Administration and Handling

◀ ALERT ▶

IV

- Space drug doses evenly around the clock.
- Store vials at room temperature.
- Reconstitute each 500-mg vial with 10 ml of sterile water for injection to provide a concentration of 50 mg/ml. Shake to dissolve until clear.
- The solution may be further diluted with 100 ml of 0.9% NaCl or D_5W.
- After dilution with 0.9% NaCl, the solution is stable for 2 hours at room temperature and 18 hours if refrigerated; after dilution with D_5W, it's stable for 1 hour at room temperature and 8 hours if refrigerated.
- Give IV push (5 to 20 ml) over 3 to 5 minutes and IV intermittent infusion (piggyback) over 15 to 30 minutes.

Intervention and Evaluation

- Assess the patient's pattern of daily bowel activity and stool consistency.
- Evaluate the patient's hydration

status, and check for nausea and vomiting.

• Check the IV injection site for inflammation.
• Inspect the patient's skin for a rash.
• Monitor the patient's electrolyte levels (especially potassium), intake and output, and renal function test results.
• Observe the patient's mental status, and be alert for seizures or tremors.
• Assess the patient's BP and temperature at least twice a day.

Patient Teaching

• Caution the patient to immediately notify the physician if he or she experiences severe diarrhea and to avoid taking antidiarrheals until directed to do.
• Advise the patient to notify the physician of troublesome or serious adverse reactions, including infusion site pain, redness, or swelling; nausea or vomiting; or a rash or itching.

7 Cephalosporins

cefaclor
cefadroxil
cefazolin sodium
cefdinir
cefditoren
cefepime
cefixime
cefotaxime sodium
cefotetan disodium
cefoxitin sodium
cefpodoxime proxetil
cefprozil
ceftazidime
ceftibuten
ceftizoxime sodium
ceftriaxone sodium
cefuroxime axetil, cefuroxime sodium
cephalexin
loracarbef

Uses: Cephalosporins are used to treat a number of infections, including respiratory infections, skin and soft tissue infections, bone and joint infections, and GU infections. These broad-spectrum antibiotics also are used prophylactically in some surgical procedures. First-generation cephalosporins have good activity against gram-positive organisms and moderate activity against gram-negative organisms, including *Escherichia coli, Klebsiella pneumoniae,* and *Proteus mirabilis.* Second-generation cephalosporins have increased activity against gram-negative organisms. Third-generation cephalosporins are less active against gram-positive organisms, more active against the Enterobacteriaceae and somewhat active against *Pseudomonas aeruginosa.* The fourth-generation cephalosporin cefepime is active against gram-positive organisms, such as *Staphylococcus aureus,* and gram-negative organisms, such as *P. aeruginosa.*

Action: Cephalosporins inhibit bacterial cell wall synthesis or activate enzymes that disrupt the cell wall, causing a weakening in the cell wall, cell lysis, and cell death. (See the illustration *Sites and Mechanisms of Action: Anti-infective Agents,* page 2.) Cephalosporins may be bacteriostatic or bactericidal and are most effective against rapidly dividing cells.

cefaclor

sef-a-klor
(Apo-Cefaclor[CAN], Ceclor, Ceclor CD, Cefkor[AUS], Cefkor CD[AUS], Keflor[AUS])

CATEGORY AND SCHEDULE

Pregnancy Risk Category: B

MECHANISM OF ACTION

A second-generation cephalosporin that binds to bacterial cell membranes and inhibits cell wall synthesis. **Therapeutic Effect:** Bactericidal.

PHARMACOKINETICS

Well absorbed from the GI tract. Protein binding: 25%. Widely distributed. Primarily excreted unchanged in urine. Moderately removed by hemodialysis. ***Half-life:*** 0.6–0.9 hr (increased in impaired renal function).

AVAILABILITY

Capsules (Ceclor): 250 mg, 500 mg.
Oral Suspension (Ceclor): 125 mg/5 ml, 187 mg/5 ml, 250 mg/5 ml, 375 mg/5 ml.
Tablets (Extended-Release [Ceclor CD]): 375 mg, 500 mg.
Tablets (Chewable [Raniclor]): 125 mg, 187 mg, 250 mg, 375 mg.

INDICATIONS AND DOSAGES

▸ Bronchitis
PO (Extended-Release)
Adults, Elderly. 500 mg q12h for 7 days.
▸ Lower respiratory tract infections
PO
Adults, Elderly. 250–500 mg q8h.
▸ Otitis media
PO
Children. 20–40 mg/kg/day in 2–3 divided doses. Maximum: 1 g/day.
▸ Pharyngitis, skin/skin structure infections, tonsillitis
PO (Extended-Release)
Adults, Elderly. 375 mg q12h.
PO (Regular-Release)
Adults, Elderly. 250–500 mg q8h.
Children. 20–40 mg/kg/day in 2–3 divided doses. Maxiumum: 1 g/day.
▸ Urinary tract infections
PO
Adults, Elderly. 250–500 mg q8h.
Children. 20–40 mg/kg/day in 2–3 divided doses q8h. Maximum: 1 g/day.
PO (Extended-Release)
Adults, Children older than 16 yr. 375–500 mg q12h.
▸ Otitis media
PO
Children older than 1 mo. 40 mg/kg/day in divided doses q8h. Maximum: 1 g/day.
▸ Dosage in renal impairment
Decreased dosage may be necessary in patients with creatinine clearance less than 40 ml/min.

CONTRAINDICATIONS

History of anaphylactic reaction to penicillins or hypersensitivity to cephalosporins

INTERACTIONS

Drug
Probenecid: May increase cefaclor blood concentration.
Herbal
None known.
Food
None known.

DIAGNOSTIC TEST EFFECTS

May increase BUN level and serum alkaline phosphatase, bilirubin, creatinine, LDH, AST (SGOT), and ALT (SGPT) levels. May cause a positive direct or indirect Coombs' test.

SIDE EFFECTS

Frequent
Oral candidiasis, mild diarrhea, mild abdominal cramping, vaginal candidiasis
Occasional
Nausea, serum sickness-like reaction (marked by fever and joint pain; usually occurs after the second course of therapy and resolves after the drug is discontinued)
Rare
Allergic reaction (pruritus, rash, and urticaria)

SERIOUS REACTIONS

! Antibiotic-associated colitis and other superinfections may result from altered bacterial balance.
! Nephrotoxicity may occur, especially in patients with preexisting renal disease.
! Patients with a history of allergies, especially to penicillin, are at increased risk for developing a severe hypersensitivity reaction, marked by severe pruritus,

angioedema, bronchospasm, and anaphylaxis.

NURSING CONSIDERATIONS

Baseline Assessment

◀ **ALERT** ▶ Determine if the patient has a history of allergies, particularly to cefaclor, other cephalosporins, or penicillins, before beginning drug therapy.

Lifespan Considerations

- Cefaclor readily crosses the placenta and is distributed in breast milk.
- No age-related precautions have been noted in children older than 1 month.
- Age-related renal impairment may require a dosage adjustment in the elderly.

Precautions

- Use cefaclor cautiously in patients with renal impairment or a history of GI disease (especially antibiotic-associated or ulcerative colitis).
- Use the drug cautiously in patients using nephrotoxic drugs concurrently.

Administration and Handling

PO

- After reconstitution, the oral solution is stable for 14 days if refrigerated.
- Shake the oral suspension well before using.
- Give cefaclor without regard to food; however, if GI upset occurs, give it with food or milk.
- Don't cut, crush, or chew extended-release tablets.

Intervention and Evaluation

- Assess the patient's mouth for white patches on the mucous membranes and tongue.
- Assess the patient's pattern of daily bowel activity and stool consistency. Although mild GI effects may be tolerable, severe symptoms may indicate the onset of antibiotic-associated colitis.
- Monitor the patient's intake and output and renal function test results to assess for nephrotoxicity.
- Be alert for signs and symptoms of superinfection, including abdominal pain or cramping, moderate to severe diarrhea, severe anal or genital pruritus or discharge, and severe mouth or tongue soreness.

Patient Teaching

- Advise the patient to space doses evenly around the clock and to continue taking cefaclor for the full course of treatment.
- Inform the patient that cefaclor may cause GI upset; suggest that he or she take the drug with food or milk if GI upset occurs.
- Instruct the patient to refrigerate cefaclor oral suspension.

cefadroxil

sef-a-**drox**-ill
(Duricef)

CATEGORY AND SCHEDULE

Pregnancy Risk Category: B

MECHANISM OF ACTION

A first-generation cephalosporin that binds to bacterial cell membranes and inhibits cell wall synthesis. **Therapeutic Effect:** Bactericidal.

PHARMACOKINETICS

Well absorbed from the GI tract. Protein binding: 15%–20%. Widely distributed. Primarily excreted unchanged in urine. Removed by hemodialysis. ***Half-life:*** 1.2–1.5 hr (increased in impaired renal function).

AVAILABILITY

Capsules: 500 mg.
Oral Suspension: 250 mg/5 ml, 500 mg/5 ml.
Tablets: 1,000 mg.

INDICATIONS AND DOSAGES

▸ **UTIs**

PO

Adults, Elderly. 1–2 g/day as a single dose or in 2 divided doses.
Children. 30 mg/kg/day in 2 divided doses. Maximum: 2 g/day.

▸ **Skin and skin-structure infections, group A beta-hemolytic streptococcal pharyngitis, tonsillitis**

PO

Adults, Elderly. 1–2 g in 2 divided doses.
Children. 30 mg/kg/day in 2 divided doses. Maximum: 2 g/day.

▸ **Impetigo**

PO

Children. 30 mg/kg/day as a single dose or in 2 divided doses. Maximum: 2 g/day.

▸ **Dosage in renal impairment**

After an initial 1-g dose, dosage and frequency are modified based on creatinine clearance and the severity of the infection.

Creatinine Clearance	Dosage Interval
25–50 ml/min	500 mg q12h
10–25 ml/min	500 mg q24h
0–10 ml/min	500 mg q36h

CONTRAINDICATIONS

History of anaphylactic reaction to penicillins or hypersensitivity to cephalosporins

INTERACTIONS

Drug

Probenecid: Increases cefadroxil blood concentration.

Herbal

None known.

Food

None known.

DIAGNOSTIC TEST EFFECTS

May increase BUN level and serum alkaline phosphatase, bilirubin, creatinine, LDH, AST (SGOT), and ALT (SGPT) levels. May cause a positive direct or indirect Coombs' test.

SIDE EFFECTS

Frequent

Oral candidiasis, mild diarrhea, mild abdominal cramping, vaginal candidiasis

Occasional

Nausea, unusual bruising or bleeding, serum sickness-like reaction (marked by fever and joint pain; usually occurs after the second course of therapy and resolves after the drug is discontinued)

Rare

Allergic reaction (rash, pruritus, urticaria), thrombophlebitis (pain, redness, swelling at injection site)

SERIOUS REACTIONS

! Antibiotic-associated colitis and other superinfections may result from altered bacterial balance.
! Nephrotoxicity may occur, especially in patients with preexisting renal disease.
! Patients with a history of allergies, especially to penicillin, are at increased risk for developing a severe hypersensitivity reaction, marked by severe pruritus, angioedema, bronchospasm, and anaphylaxis.

NURSING CONSIDERATIONS

Baseline Assessment

◀ **ALERT** ▶ Determine if the patient

has a history of allergies, particularly to cefadroxil, other cephalosporins, or penicillins, before beginning drug therapy.

Lifespan Considerations

• Cefadroxil readily crosses the placenta and is distributed in breast milk.
• No age-related precautions have been noted in children.
• Age-related renal impairment may require a dosage adjustment in the elderly.

Precautions

• Use cefadroxil cautiously in patients with renal impairment or a history of drug allergies or GI disease (especially antibiotic-associated or ulcerative colitis).
• Use the drug cautiously in patients using nephrotoxic drugs concurrently.

Administration and Handling

PO

• After reconstitution, the oral solution is stable for 14 days if refrigerated.
• Shake the oral suspension well before using.
• Give cefadroxil without regard to food; however, if GI upset occurs, give it with food or milk.

Intervention and Evaluation

• Assess the patient's mouth for white patches on the mucous membranes and tongue.
• Assess the patient's pattern of daily bowel activity and stool consistency. Although mild GI effects may be tolerable, severe effects may indicate the onset of antibiotic-associated colitis.
• Monitor the patient's intake and output and renal function test results to assess for nephrotoxicity.
• Be alert for signs and symptoms of superinfection, such as abdominal pain or cramping, anal or genital pruritus or discharge, moderate to severe diarrhea, and severe mouth or tongue soreness.

Patient Teaching

• Advise the patient to space doses evenly around the clock and to continue taking cefadroxil for the full course of treatment.
• Explain that cefadroxil may cause GI upset; suggest taking the drug with food or milk if GI upset occurs.
• Advise the patient to refrigerate cefadroxil oral suspension.

cefazolin sodium

sef-**a**-zoe-lin
(Ancef, Kefzol)
Do not confuse cefazolin with cefprozil or Cefzil.

CATEGORY AND SCHEDULE

Pregnancy Risk Category: B

MECHANISM OF ACTION

A first-generation cephalosporin that binds to bacterial cell membranes and inhibits cell wall synthesis. **Therapeutic Effect:** Bactericidal.

PHARMACOKINETICS

Widely distributed. Protein binding: 85%. Primarily excreted unchanged in urine. Moderately removed by hemodialysis. ***Half-life:*** 1.4–1.8 hr (increased in impaired renal function).

AVAILABILITY

Injection: 500 mg, 1 g.
Ready-to-Hang Infusion: 1 g/50 ml, 2 g/100 ml.

INDICATIONS AND DOSAGES

▸ **Uncomplicated UTIs**

IV, IM

Adults, Elderly. 1 g q12h.

Mild to moderate infections
IV, IM
Adults, Elderly. 250–500 mg q8–12h.
Severe infections
IV, IM
Adults, Elderly. 0.5–1 g q6–8h.
Life-threatening infections
IV, IM
Adults, Elderly. 1–1.5 g q6h. Maximum: 12 g/day.
Perioperative prophylaxis
IV, IM
Adults, Elderly. 1 g 30–60 min before surgery, 0.5–1 g during surgery, and q6–8h for up to 24 hr postoperatively.
Usual pediatric dosage
Children. 50–100 mg/kg/day in divided doses q8h. Maximum: 6 g/day.
Neonates older than 7 days. 40–60 mg/kg/day in divided doses q8–12h.
Neonates 7 days and younger. 40 mg/kg/day in divided doses q12h.
Dosage in renal impairment
Dosing frequency is modified based on creatinine clearance.

Creatinine Clearance	Dosage Interval
10–30 ml/min	Usual dose q12h
less than 10 ml/min	Usual dose q24h

CONTRAINDICATIONS
History of anaphylactic reaction to penicillins or hypersensitivity to cephalosporins

INTERACTIONS
Drug
Probenecid: Increases cefazolin blood concentration.
Herbal
None known.
Food
None known.

DIAGNOSTIC TEST EFFECTS
May increase BUN level and serum alkaline phosphatase, bilirubin, creatinine, LDH, AST (SGOT), and ALT (SGPT) levels. May cause a positive direct or indirect Coombs' test

IV INCOMPATIBILITIES
Amikacin (Amikin), amiodarone (Cordarone), hydromorphone (Dilaudid)

IV COMPATIBILITIES
Calcium gluconate, diltiazem (Cardizem), famotidine (Pepcid), heparin, insulin (regular), lidocaine, magnesium sulfate, midazolam (Versed), morphine, multivitamins, potassium chloride, propofol (Diprivan), vecuronium (Norcuron)

SIDE EFFECTS
Frequent
Discomfort with IM administration, oral candidiasis, mild diarrhea, mild abdominal cramping, vaginal candidiasis
Occasional
Nausea, serum sickness-like reaction (marked by fever and joint pain; usually occurs after the second course of therapy and resolves after the drug is discontinued)
Rare
Allergic reaction (rash, pruritus, urticaria), thrombophlebitis (pain, redness, swelling at injection site)

SERIOUS REACTIONS
! Antibiotic-associated colitis and other superinfections may result from altered bacterial balance.
! Nephrotoxicity may occur, especially in patients with preexisting renal disease.
! Patients with a history of allergies, especially to penicillin, are at increased risk for developing a

severe hypersensitivity reaction, marked by severe pruritus, angioedema, bronchospasm, and anaphylaxis.

NURSING CONSIDERATIONS

Baseline Assessment

◀ALERT▶ Determine if the patient has a history of allergies, particularly to cefazoloin, other cephalosporins, or penicillins, before beginning drug therapy.

Lifespan Considerations

- Cefazolin readily crosses the placenta and is distributed in breast milk.
- No age-related precautions have been noted in children.
- Age-related renal impairment may require a dosage adjustment in the elderly.

Precautions

- Use cefazolin cautiously in patients with renal impairment or a history of GI disease (especially antibiotic-associated or ulcerative colitis).
- Use the drug cautiously in patients using nephrotoxic drugs concurrently.

Administration and Handling

IV

- The solution normally appears light yellow to yellow.
- The IV infusion (piggyback) is stable for 24 hours at room temperature and 96 hours if refrigerated.
- Discard the solution if a precipitate forms.
- Reconstitute each 1-g vial with at least 10 ml of sterile water for injection.
- The solution may be further diluted in 50 to 100 ml D_5W or 0.9% NaCl to decrease the incidence of thrombophlebitis.
- Administer the IV push over 3 to 5 minutes.
- Infuse the intermittent IV infusion (piggyback) over 20 to 30 minutes.

IM

- Reconstitute each 500-mg vial with 2 ml of sterile water for injection and each 1-g vial with 2.5 ml of sterile water for injection.
- To minimize patient discomfort, slowly inject the drug deep into the gluteus maximus rather than the lateral aspect of the thigh.

Intervention and Evaluation

- Evaluate the IM injection site for induration and tenderness.
- Assess the patient's mouth for white patches on the mucous membranes or tongue.
- Assess the patient's pattern of daily bowel activity and stool consistency. Although mild GI effects may be tolerable, severe symptoms may indicate the onset of antibiotic-associated colitis.
- Monitor the patient's intake and output and renal function test results to assess for nephrotoxicity.
- Be alert for signs and symptoms of superinfection, including abdominal pain or cramping, moderate to severe diarrhea, severe anal or genital pruritus or discharge, and severe mouth or tongue soreness.

Patient Teaching

- Inform the patient that IM injections may cause discomfort.

cefdinir

sef-di-neer

(Omnicef)

CATEGORY AND SCHEDULE

Pregnancy Risk Category: B

MECHANISM OF ACTION

A third-generation cephalosporin that binds to bacterial cell membranes and inhibits cell wall synthesis. **Therapeutic Effect:** Bactericidal.

PHARMACOKINETICS

Moderately absorbed from the GI tract. Protein binding: 60%–70%. Widely distributed. Not appreciably metabolized. Primarily excreted unchanged in urine. Minimally removed by hemodialysis. ***Half-life:*** 1–2 hr (increased in impaired renal function).

AVAILABILITY

Capsules: 300 mg.
Oral Suspension: 125 mg/5 ml, 250 mg/5 ml.

INDICATIONS AND DOSAGES

▸ Community-acquired pneumonia
PO
Adults, Elderly, Children 13 yr and older. 300 mg q12h for 10 days.

▸ Acute exacerbation of chronic bronchitis
PO
Adults, Elderly. 300 mg q12h for 5–10 days.

▸ Acute maxillary sinusitis
PO
Adults, Elderly, Children 13 yr and older. 300 mg q12h or 600 mg q24h for 10 days.
Children 6 mo–12 yr. 7 mg/kg q12h or 14 mg/kg q24h for 10 days.

▸ Pharyngitis or tonsillitis
PO
Adults, Elderly, Children 13 yr and older. 300 mg q12h for 5–10 days or 600 mg q24h for 10 days.
Children 6 mo–12 yr. 7 mg/kg q12h for 5–10 days or 14 mg/kg q24h for 10 days.

▸ Uncomplicated skin or skin-structure infections
PO
Adults, Elderly, Children 13 yr and older. 300 mg q12h for 10 days.
Children 6 mo–12 yr. 7 mg/kg q12h for 10 days.

▸ Acute bacterial otitis media
PO (Capsules)
Children 6 mo–12 yr. 7 mg/kg q12h or 14 mg/kg q24h for 10 days.

▸ Usual pediatric dosage for oral suspension
Children weighing 81–95 lb (37–43 kg). 12.5 ml (2.5 tsp) q12h or 25 ml (5 tsp) q24h.
Children weighing 61–80 lb (28–36 kg). 10 ml (2 tsp) q12h or 20 ml (4 tsp) q24h.
Children weighing 41–60 lb (19–27 kg). 7.5 ml (1 tsp) q12h or 15 ml (3 tsp) q24h.
Children weighing 20–40 lb (9–18 kg). 5 ml (1 tsp) q12h or 10 ml (2 tsp) q24h.
Infants weighing less than 20 lb (9 kg). 2.5 ml (½ tsp) q12h or 5 ml (1 tsp) q24h.

▸ Dosage in renal impairment
For patients with creatinine clearance less than 30 ml/min, dosage is 300 mg/day as single daily dose. For hemodialysis patients, dosage is 300 mg or 7 mg/kg/dose every other day.

CONTRAINDICATIONS

History of anaphylactic reaction to penicillins or hypersensitivity to cephalosporins

INTERACTIONS

Drug

Antacids: Decrease cefdinir blood concentration.
Probenecid: Increases cefdinir blood concentration.

Herbal

None known.

Food

None known.

DIAGNOSTIC TEST EFFECTS

May increase serum alkaline phosphatase, bilirubin, LDH, AST

(SGPT), and ALT (SGOT) levels. May produce a false-positive reaction for ketones in urine.

SIDE EFFECTS

Frequent

Oral candidiasis, mild diarrhea, mild abdominal cramping, vaginal candidiasis

Occasional

Nausea, serum sickness-like reaction (marked by fever and joint pain; usually occurs after the second course of therapy and resolves after the drug is discontinued)

Rare

Allergic reaction (rash, pruritus, urticaria)

SERIOUS REACTIONS

! Antibiotic-associated colitis and other superinfections may result from altered bacterial balance.

! Nephrotoxicity may occur, especially in patients with preexisting renal disease.

! Patients with a history of allergies, especially to penicillin, are at increased risk for developing a severe hypersensitivity reaction, marked by severe pruritus, angioedema, bronchospasm, and anaphylaxis.

NURSING CONSIDERATIONS

Baseline Assessment

◀ALERT▶ Determine the patient's history of allergies, especially to cefdinir, other cephalosporins, or penicillins, before beginning drug therapy.

Lifespan Considerations

• Cefdinir crosses the placenta but is not distributed in breast milk.
• Infants and newborns may have lower renal clearance of cefdinir.
• Age-related renal impairment may require decreased dosage or increased dosing interval in the elderly.

Precautions

• Use cefdinir cautiously in patients with renal or hepatic impairment or a history of GI disease (especially antibiotic-associated or ulcerative colitis).

Administration and Handling

PO

• Give cefdinir without regard to food.
• To reconstitute the oral suspension, add 39 ml of water to the 60-ml bottle or 65 ml of water to the 120-ml bottle.
• Shake the oral suspension well before administering.
• Store the mixed suspension at room temperature. Discard any unused portion after 10 days.

Intervention and Evaluation

• Assess the patient's pattern of daily bowel activity and stool consistency. Although mild GI effects may be tolerable, severe symptoms may indicate the onset of antibiotic-associated colitis.
• Be alert for signs and symptoms of superinfection including abdominal pain or cramping, anal or genital pruritus or discharge, moderate to severe diarrhea, severe mouth or tongue soreness, and new or increased fever.
• Monitor the patient's hematology reports.

Patient Teaching

• Advise the patient to space doses evenly around the clock and to continue taking cefdinir for the full course of treatment.
• Caution the patient to notify the nurse or physician of persistent diarrhea.
• Instruct the patient to take antacids 2 hours before or after taking cefdinir.

cefditoren

seff-di-**tore**-en
(Spectracef)

CATEGORY AND SCHEDULE

Pregnancy Risk Category: B

MECHANISM OF ACTION

A third-generation cephalosporin that binds to bacterial cell membranes and inhibits cell wall synthesis. **Therapeutic Effect:** Bactericidal.

PHARMACOKINETICS

Moderately absorbed from the gastrointestinal (GI) tract. Protein binding: 88%. Not metabolized. Excreted in the urine. Minimally removed by hemodialysis. ***Half-life:*** 1.6 hr (half-life increased with impaired renal function).

AVAILABILITY

Tablets: 200 mg.

INDICATIONS AND DOSAGES

▸ **Pharyngitis, tonsillitis, skin infections**

PO

Adults, Elderly, Children older than 12 yr. 200 mg twice a day for 10 days.

▸ **Acute exacerbation of chronic bronchitis**

PO

Adults, Elderly, Children older than 12 yr. 400 mg twice a day for 10 days.

▸ **Community-acquired pneumonia**

PO

Adults, Elderly, Children older than 12 yr. 400 mg twice a day for 14 days.

▸ **Dosage in renal impairment**

Dosage and frequency are modified based on creatinine clearance.

Creatinine Clearance	Dosage
50–80 ml/min	No adjustment necessary.
30–49 ml/min	200 mg twice a day
less than 30 ml/min	200 mg once a day

CONTRAINDICATIONS

Carnitive deficiency, inborn errors of metabolism, known allergy to cephalosporins, hypersensitivity to milk protein

INTERACTIONS

Drug

Antacids containing magnesium or aluminum, H_2 receptor antagonists: May decrese the absorption of cefditoren.
Probenecid: May increase the absorption of cefditoren.

Herbal

None known.

Food

High-fat meals. Increase the cefditoren plasma concentration.

DIAGNOSTIC TEST EFFECTS

May cause a positive direct or indirect Coombs' test and a false-positive reaction to glycosuria.

SIDE EFFECTS

Occasional (11%)
Diarrhea
Rare (4%–1%)
Nausea, headache, abdominal pain, vaginal candidiasis, dyspepsia, vomiting

SERIOUS REACTIONS

! Antibiotic-associated colitis and other superinfections may occur.
! Patients with a history of allergies, especially to penicillin, are at increased risk for developing a severe hypersensitivity reaction, marked by severe pruritus,

angioedema, bronchospasm, and anaphylaxis.

NURSING CONSIDERATIONS

Baseline Assessment

◀ALERT▶ Determine if the patient has a history of allergies to other cephalosporins or penicillins, before beginning therapy.

Lifespan Considerations

- It is unknown if cefditoren is distributed in breast milk.
- The safety and efficacy of cefditoren have not been established in children younger than 12 years.
- Age-related renal impairment may require a dosage adjustment in the elderly.

Precautions

- Use cefditoren cautiously in patients with allergies, renal impairment, a history of GI disease, or a hypersensitivity to penicillins or other drugs.

Administration and Handling

PO

- Give cefditoren with meals to enhance drug absorption.

Intervention and Evaluation

- Be alert for signs and symptoms of superinfection, including abdominal pain, moderate to severe diarrhea, severe anal or genital pruritus, and stomatitis.
- Assess the patient's pattern of daily bowel activity and stool consistency. Severe GI effects may indicate the onset of antibiotic-associated colitis.
- Monitor the patient for carnitine deficiency, as evidenced by confusion, fatigue, hypoglycemia, and muscle damage.

Patient Teaching

- Advise the patient to space doses evenly around the clock, not to skip doses, and to continue taking cefditoren for the full course of treatment.
- Encourage the patient to take cefditoren with food if he or she experiences GI upset.

cefepime

sef-e-peem

(Maxipime)

Do not confuse cefepime with ceftidine.

CATEGORY AND SCHEDULE

Pregnancy Risk Category: B

MECHANISM OF ACTION

A fourth-generation cephalosporin that binds to bacterial cell membranes and inhibits cell wall synthesis. **Therapeutic Effect:** Bactericidal.

PHARMACOKINETICS

Well absorbed after IM administration. Protein binding: 20%. Widely distributed. Primarily excreted unchanged in urine. Removed by hemodialysis. ***Half-life:*** 2–2.3 hr (increased in impaired renal function, and in the elderly).

AVAILABILITY

Powder for Injection: 500 mg, 1 g, 2 g.

INDICATIONS AND DOSAGES

▸ **Pneumonia**

IV

Adults, Elderly. 1–2 g q12h for 7–10 days.

Children 2 mo and older. 50 mg/kg q12h. Maximum: 2 g/dose.

▸ **Intra-abdominal infections**

IV

Adults, Elderly. 2 g q12h for 10 days.

▸ **Skin and skin structure infections**

IV

Adults, Elderly. 2 g q12h for 10 days.

Children 2 mo and older. 50 mg/kg q12h. Maximum: 2 g/dose.

▸ **UTIs**

IV

Adults, Elderly. 0.5–2 g q12h for 7–10 days.

Children 2 mo and older. 50 mg/kg q12h. Maximum: 2 g/dose.

▸ **Febrile neutropenia**

IV

Adults, Elderly. 2 g q8h.

Children 2 mo and older. 50 mg/kg q8h. Maximum: 2 g/dose.

▸ **Dosage in renal impairment**

Dosage and frequency are modified based on creatinine clearance and the severity of the infection.

Creatinine Clearance	Dose
30–60 ml/min	0.5–2 g q24h
11–29 ml/min	0.5–1 g q24h
10 ml/min or less	0.25–0.5 g q24h

CONTRAINDICATIONS

History of anaphylactic reaction to penicillins or hypersensitivity to cephalosporins

INTERACTIONS

Drug

Probenecid: May increase cefepime blood concentration.

Herbal

None known.

Food

None known.

DIAGNOSTIC TEST EFFECTS

May increase serum alkaline phosphatase, bilirubin, LDH, AST (SGOT), and ALT (SGPT) levels. May cause a positive direct or indirect Coombs' test.

IV INCOMPATIBILITIES

Acyclovir (Zovirax), amphotericin (Fungizone), cimetidine (Tagamet), ciprofloxacin (Cipro), cisplatin (Platinol), dacarbazine (DTIC), daunorubicin (Cerubidine), diazepam (Valium), diphenhydramine (Benadryl), dobutamine (Dobutrex), dopamine (Intropin), doxorubicin (Adriamycin), droperidol (Inapsine), famotidine (Pepcid), ganciclovir (Cytovene), haloperidol (Haldol), magnesium, magnesium sulfate, mannitol, meperidine (Demerol), metoclopramide (Reglan), morphine, ofloxacin (Floxin), ondansetron (Zofran), vancomycin (Vancocin)

IV COMPATIBILITIES

Bumetanide (Bumex), calcium gluconate, furosemide (Lasix), hydromorphone (Dilaudid), lorazepam (Ativan), propofol (Diprivan)

SIDE EFFECTS

Frequent

Discomfort with IM administration, oral candidiasis, mild diarrhea, mild abdominal cramping, vaginal candidiasis

Occasional

Nausea, serum sickness-like reaction (marked by fever and joint pain; usually occurs after the second course of therapy and resolves after the drug is discontinued)

Rare

Allergic reaction (rash, pruritus, urticaria), thrombophlebitis (pain, redness, swelling at injection site)

SERIOUS REACTIONS

! Antibiotic-associated colitis manifested and other superinfections may result from altered bacterial balance.

! Nephrotoxicity may occur, especially in patients with preexisting renal disease.

! Patients with a history of allergies, especially to penicillin, are at increased risk for developing a severe hypersensitivity reaction, marked by severe pruritus, angioedema, bronchospasm, and anaphylaxis.

NURSING CONSIDERATIONS

Baseline Assessment

◀ALERT▶ Determine if the patient has a history of allergies, particularly to cefepime, other cephalosporins, or penicillins, before beginning drug therapy.

Lifespan Considerations

- It is unknown if cefepime is distributed in breast milk.
- No age-related precautions have been noted in children older than 2 months.
- Age-related renal impairment may require decreased dosage or increased dosing interval in the elderly.

Precautions

- Use cefepime cautiously in patients with renal impairment.

Administration and Handling

IV

- The solution is stable for 24 hours at room temperature or 7 days if refrigerated.
- Add 5 ml of diluent recommended by manufacturer to each 500-mg vial (10 ml to each 1-g or 2-g vial).
- Further dilute the resulting solution with 50 to 100 ml 0.9% NaCl or D_5W.
- Administer the IV push over 3 to 5 minutes.
- Administer the intermittent IV infusion (piggyback) over 30 minutes.

IM

- Add 1.3 ml of sterile water for injection, 0.9% NaCl, or D_5W to 500-mg vial (or 2.4 ml to each 1-g and 2-g vial).
- To minimize patient discomfort, slowly inject the drug deep into a large muscle mass, such as the upper gluteus maximus, rather than the lateral aspect of the thigh.

Intervention and Evaluation

- Evaluate the IM injection site for induration and tenderness.
- Check the patient's mouth for white patches on the mucous membranes and tongue.
- Assess the patient's pattern of daily bowel activity and stool consistency. Although mild GI effects may be tolerable, severe symptoms may indicate the onset of antibiotic-associated colitis.
- Monitor the patient's intake and output and renal function test results to assess for nephrotoxicity.
- Be alert for signs and symptoms of superinfection, including abdominal pain or cramping, moderate to severe diarrhea, severe anal or genital pruritus or discharge, and severe mouth or tongue soreness.

Patient Teaching

- Inform the patient that IM injections may cause discomfort.

cefixime

sef-**ix**-ime
(Suprax)
Do not confuse Suprax with Sporanox, Surbex, or Surfak.

CATEGORY AND SCHEDULE

Pregnancy Risk Category: B

MECHANISM OF ACTION

A third-generation cephalosporin that binds to bacterial cell membranes and inhibits cell wall synthesis. **Therapeutic Effect:** Bactericidal.

PHARMACOKINETICS

Moderately absorbed from the GI tract. Protein binding: 65%–70%.

Widely distributed. Primarily excreted unchanged in urine. Minimally removed by hemodialysis. ***Half-life:*** 3–4 hr (increased in renal impairment).

AVAILABILITY

Oral Suspension: 100 mg/5 ml.
Tablets: 200 mg, 400 mg.

INDICATIONS AND DOSAGES

▸ **Otitis media, acute bronchitis, acute exacerbations of chronic bronchitis, pharyngitis, tonsillitis, and uncomplicated UTIs**

PO

Adults, Elderly, Children weighing more than 50 kg. 400 mg/day as a single dose or in 2 divided doses.
Children 6 mo–12 yr weighing less than 50 kg. 8 mg/kg/day as a single dose or in 2 divided doses.
Maximum: 400 mg.

▸ **Uncomplicated gonorrhea**

PO

Adults. 400 mg as a single dose.

▸ **Dosage in renal impairment**

Dosage is modified based on creatinine clearance.

Creatinine Clearance	% of Usual Dose
21–60 ml/min	75%
20 ml/min or less	50%

CONTRAINDICATIONS

History of anaphylactic reaction to penicillins, hypersensitivity to cephalosporins

INTERACTIONS

Drug

Probenecid: Increases serum concentration of cefixime.

Herbal

None known.

Food

None known.

DIAGNOSTIC TEST EFFECTS

May increase BUN and serum alkaline phosphatase, bilirubin, creatinine, AST (SGOT), and ALT (SGPT) levels. May increase LDH level. May cause a positive direct or indirect Coombs' test.

SIDE EFFECTS

Frequent

Oral candidiasis, mild diarrhea, mild abdominal cramping, vaginal candidiasis

Occasional

Nausea, serum sickness–like reaction (marked by arthralgia and fever; usually occurs after second course of therapy and resolves after drug is discontinued)

Rare

Allergic reaction (rash, pruritus, urticaria)

SERIOUS REACTIONS

! Antibiotic-associated colitis and other superinfections may result from altered bacterial balance.
! Nephrotoxicity may occur, especially in patients with preexisting renal disease.
! Patients with a history of allergies, especially to penicillin, are at increased risk for developing a severe hypersensitivity reaction, marked by severe pruritus, angioedema, bronchospasm, and anaphylaxis.

NURSING CONSIDERATIONS

Baseline Assessment

◂ **ALERT** ▸ Determine if the patient has a history of allergies, particularly to cephalosporins or penicillins, before beginning drug therapy.

Lifespan Considerations

- Cefixime is not recommended for use during labor and delivery.

• It is unknown if cefixime is distributed in breast milk.
• The safety and efficacy of cefixime have not been established in children younger than 6 months.
• Age-related renal impairment may require a dosage adjustment in the elderly.

Precautions

• Use cefixime cautiously in patients with a history of GI disease, hypersensitivity to penicillins or other drugs, or renal impairment.

Administration and Handling

◀ALERT▶ Use cefixime oral suspension to treat otitis media because the suspension achieves a higher peak serum level of the drug.

PO

• Give cefixime without regard to food.
• After reconstitution, the oral suspension is stable for 14 days at room temperature. Do not refrigerate.
• Shake the oral suspension well before administering it.

Intervention and Evaluation

• Check for white patches on the oral mucous membranes and tongue, which may be signs of oral candidiasis.
• Assess the patient's pattern of daily bowel activity and stool consistency. Severe GI effects may indicate the onset of antibiotic-associated colitis.
• Monitor the patient's intake and output and renal function test results for nephrotoxicity.
• Be alert for signs and symptoms of superinfection, including abdominal pain, moderate to severe diarrhea, severe anal or genital pruritus, and severe stomatitis.

Patient Teaching

• Advise the patient to space doses evenly around the clock and to complete the full course of treatment.
• Instruct the patient to take the drug with food or milk if GI upset occurs.

cefotaxime sodium

sef-oh-**taks**-eem
(Claforan)
Do not confuse cefotaxime with cefoxitin, ceftizoxime, or cefuroxime; or Claforan with Claritin.

CATEGORY AND SCHEDULE

Pregnancy Risk Category: B

MECHANISM OF ACTION

A third-generation cephalosporin that binds to bacterial cell membranes and inhibits cell wall synthesis. **Therapeutic Effect:** Bactericidal.

PHARMACOKINETICS

Widely distributed, including to CSF. Protein binding: 30%–50%. Partially metabolized in the liver to active metabolite. Primarily excreted in urine. Moderately removed by hemodialysis. ***Half-life:*** 1 hr (increased in impaired renal function).

AVAILABILITY

Powder for Injection: 500 mg, 1 g, 2 g.

INDICATIONS AND DOSAGES

▸ **Uncomplicated infections**

IV, IM

Adults, Elderly. 1 g q12h.

▸ **Mild to moderate infections**

IV, IM

Adults, Elderly. 1–2 g q8h.

▸ **Severe infections**

IV, IM

Adults, Elderly. 2 g q6–8h.

▸ **Life-threatening infections**

IV, IM

Adults, Elderly. 2 g q4h.

Children: 2 g q4h. Maximum: 12 g/day.

▸ **Gonorrhea**
IM
Adults. (Male): 1 g as a single dose. (Female): 0.5 g as a single dose.

▸ **Perioperative prophylaxis**
IV, IM
Adults, Elderly. 1 g 30–90 min before surgery.

▸ **Cesarean section**
IV
Adults. 1 g as soon as umbilical cord is clamped, then 1 g 6 and 12 hr after first dose.

▸ **Usual pediatric dosage**
Children weighing 50 kg or more. 1–2 g q6–8h.
Children 1 mo–12 yr weighing less than 50 kg. 100–200 mg/kg/day in divided doses q6–8h.

▸ **Dosage in renal impairment**
For patients with creatinine clearance less than 20 ml/min give half of dose at usual dosing intervals.

OFF-LABEL USES
Treatment of Lyme disease

CONTRAINDICATIONS
History of anaphylactic reaction to penicillins or hypersensitivity to cephalosporins

INTERACTIONS
Drug
Probenecid: May increase cefotaxime blood concentration.
Herbal
None known.
Food
None known.

DIAGNOSTIC TEST EFFECTS
May increase liver function test results and produce a positive direct or indirect Coombs' test

IV INCOMPATIBILITIES
Allopurinol (Aloprim), filgrastim (Neupogen), fluconazole (Diflucan), hetastarch (Hespan), pentamidine (Pentam IV), vancomycin (Vancocin)

IV COMPATIBILITIES
Diltiazem (Cardizem), famotidine (Pepcid), hydromorphone (Dilaudid), lorazepam (Ativan), magnesium sulfate, midazolam (Versed), morphine, propofol (Diprivan)

SIDE EFFECTS
Frequent
Discomfort with IM administration, oral candidiasis, mild diarrhea, mild abdominal cramping, vaginal candidiasis
Occasional
Nausea, serum sickness-like reaction (marked by fever and joint pain; usually occurs after the second course of therapy and resolves after the drug is discontinued)
Rare
Allergic reaction (rash, pruritus, urticaria), thrombophlebitis (pain, redness, swelling at injection site)

SERIOUS REACTIONS
! Antibiotic-associated colitis and other superinfections may result from altered bacterial balance.
! Nephrotoxicity may occur, especially in patients with preexisting renal disease.
! Patients with a history of allergies, especially to penicillin, are at increased risk for developing a severe hypersensitivity reaction, marked by severe pruritus, angioedema, bronchospasm, and anaphylaxis.

NURSING CONSIDERATIONS
Baseline Assessment
◂ **ALERT** ▸ Determine if the patient has a history of allergies, particularly to cefotaxime, other cephalosporins,

or penicillins, before beginning drug therapy.

Lifespan Considerations

• Cefotaxime readily crosses the placenta and is distributed in breast milk.
• No age-related precautions have been noted in children.
• Age-related renal impairment may require a dosage adjustment in the elderly.

Precautions

• Use cefotaxime cautiously in patients with renal impairment or a history of GI disease (especially antibiotic-associated or ulcerative colitis).
• Use cefotaxime cautiously in patients using nephrotoxic drugs concurrently.

Administration and Handling

IV

• The solution normally appears light yellow to amber. The IV infusion (piggyback) may become darker, but this doesn't affect potency.
• The IV infusion (piggyback) is stable for 24 hours at room temperature, and 5 days if refrigerated.
• Discard the solution if a precipitate forms.
• Add 10 ml of sterile water for injection to each 500-mg, 1-g, or 2-g vial to provide a concentration of 50, 95, or 180 mg/ml, respectively.
• The resulting solution may be further diluted with 50 to 100 ml of 0.9% NaCl or D_5W.
• Administer the IV push over 3 to 5 minutes.
• Administer the intermittent IV infusion (piggyback) over 20 to 30 minutes.

IM

• Reconstitute the drug with sterile water for injection or bacteriostatic water for injection.
• Add 2, 3, or 5 ml to each 500-mg, 1-g, or 2-g vial, respectively, to yield a concentration of 230, 300, or 330 mg/ml, respectively.
• To minimize patient discomfort, slowly inject the drug deep into the gluteus maximus rather than the lateral aspect of the thigh.
• Administer a 2-g IM dose at two separate sites.

Intervention and Evaluation

• Evaluate the IM injection site for induration and tenderness.
• Assess the patient's mouth for white patches on the mucous membranes and tongue.
• Assess the patient's pattern of daily bowel activity and stool consistency. Although mild GI effects may be tolerable, severe symptoms may indicate the onset of antibiotic-associated colitis.
• Monitor the patient's intake and output and renal function test results to assess for nephrotoxicity.
• Be alert for signs and symptoms of superinfection, including abdominal pain or cramping, moderate to severe diarrhea, severe anal or genital pruritus or discharge, and severe mouth or tongue soreness.

Patient Teaching

• Inform the patient that IM injections may cause discomfort.

cefotetan disodium

sef-oh-tee-tan

(Apatef [AUS], Cefotan)

Do not confuse cefotetan with cefoxitin or Ceftin.

CATEGORY AND SCHEDULE

Pregnancy Risk Category: B

MECHANISM OF ACTION

A second-generation cephalosporin that binds to bacterial cell membranes and inhibits cell wall synthesis. **Therapeutic Effect:** Bactericidal.

PHARMACOKINETICS
Protein binding: 78%–91%. Primarily excreted unchanged in urine. Minimally removed by hemodialysis. ***Half-life:*** 3–4.6 hr (increased in impaired renal function).

AVAILABILITY
Powder for Injection: 1 g, 2 g.

INDICATIONS AND DOSAGES
▸ **UTIs**
IV, IM
Adults, Elderly. 1–2 g in divided doses q12–24h.
▸ **Mild to moderate infections**
IV, IM
Adults, Elderly. 1–2 g q12h.
▸ **Severe infections**
IV, IM
Adults, Elderly. 2 g q12h.
▸ **Life-threatening infections**
IV, IM
Adults, Elderly. 3 g q12h.
▸ **Perioperative prophylaxis**
IV
Adults, Elderly. 1–2 g 30–60 min before surgery.
▸ **Cesarean section**
IV
Adults. 1–2 g as soon as umbilical cord is clamped.
▸ **Usual pediatric dosage**
Children. 40–80 mg/kg/day in divided doses q12h. Maximum: 6 g/day.
▸ **Dosage in renal impairment**
Dosing frequency is modified based on creatinine clearance and the severity of the infection.

Creatinine Clearance	Dosage Interval
10–30 ml/min	Usual dose q24h
less than 10 ml/min	Usual dose q48h

CONTRAINDICATIONS
History of anaphylactic reaction to penicillins or hypersensitivity to cephalosporins

INTERACTIONS
Drug
Alcohol: May produce a disulfiram-like reaction (facial flushing, headache, nausea, pruritus, tachycardia).
Heparin, other anticoagulants: May increase the risk of bleeding.
Herbal
None known.
Food
None known.

DIAGNOSTIC TEST EFFECTS
May increase BUN level and serum alkaline phosphatase, creatinine, AST (SGOT), and ALT (SGPT) levels. May prolong prothrombin time and produce a positive direct or indirect Coombs' test. Interferes with crossmatching procedures and hematologic tests.

IV INCOMPATIBILITIES
Vancomycin (Vancocin)

IV COMPATIBILITIES
Diltiazem (Cardizem), famotidine (Pepcid), heparin, insulin (regular), morphine, propofol (Diprivan)

SIDE EFFECTS
Frequent
Discomfort with IM administration, oral candidiasis, mild diarrhea, mild abdominal cramping, vaginal candidiasis
Occasional
Nausea, unusual bleeding or bruis-

ing, serum sickness-like reaction (marked by fever and joint pain; usually occurs after the second course of therapy and resolves after the drug is discontinued)

Rare

Allergic reaction (rash, pruritus, urticaria), thrombophlebitis (pain, redness, swelling at injection site)

SERIOUS REACTIONS

! Antibiotic-associated colitis and other superinfections may result from altered bacterial balance.

! Nephrotoxicity may occur, especially in patients with preexisting renal disease.

! Patients with a history of allergies, especially to penicillin, are at increased risk for developing a severe hypersensitivity reaction, marked by severe pruritus, angioedema, bronchospasm, and anaphylaxis.

NURSING CONSIDERATIONS

Baseline Assessment

◀ALERT▶ Determine if the patient has a history of allergies, particularly to cephalosporins or penicillins, before beginning drug therapy.

Lifespan Considerations

- Cefotetan readily crosses the placenta and is distributed in breast milk.
- The safety and efficacy of this drug have not been established in children.
- Age-related renal impairment may require a dosage adjustment in the elderly.

Precautions

- Use cefotetan cautiously in patients with renal impairment or a history GI disease (especially antibiotic-associated or ulcerative colitis).
- Use the drug cautiously in patients using nephrotoxic drugs concurrently.

Administration and Handling

◀ALERT▶ Give by IM injection, IV push, or intermittent IV infusion (piggyback) only.

IV

- The solution normally appears colorless to light yellow. A deeper yellow does not indicate loss of potency.
- The IV infusion (piggyback) is stable for 24 hours at room temperature and 96 hours if refrigerated.
- Discard the solution if a precipitate forms.
- Reconstitute each 1-g vial with 10 ml of sterile water for injection to provide a concentration of 95 mg/ml.
- The resulting solution may be further diluted with 50 to 100 ml of 0.9% NaCl or D_5W.
- Administer IV push over 3 to 5 minutes.
- Administer intermittent IV infusion (piggyback) over 20 to 30 minutes.

IM

- Add 2 ml of sterile water for injection or other appropriate diluent to each 1-g vial, or 3 ml to each 2-g vial, to provide a concentration of 400 mg/ml or 500 mg/ml, respectively.
- To minimize patient discomfort, slowly inject the drug deep into the gluteus maximus rather than the lateral aspect of the thigh.

Intervention and Evaluation

- Evaluate the IV site for signs and symptoms of phlebitis, as evidenced by heat, pain, and red streaking over the vein.
- Evaluate the IM injection site for induration and tenderness.
- Assess the patient's mouth for white patches on the mucous membranes and tongue.
- Assess the patient's pattern of daily bowel activity and stool consistency.

Although mild GI effects may be tolerable, severe symptoms may indicate the onset of antibiotic-associated colitis.

- Monitor the patient's intake and output and renal function test results to assess for nephrotoxicity.
- Be alert for signs and symptoms of superinfection, including abdominal pain or cramping, moderate to severe diarrhea, severe anal or genital pruritus or discharge, and severe mouth or tongue soreness.

Patient Teaching

- Inform the patient that IM injections may cause discomfort.
- Warn the patient to avoid consuming alcohol and alcohol-containing preparations (such as cough syrup) during treatment and for 72 hours after the last dose of cefotetan.

cefoxitin sodium

se-**fox**-i-tin

(Mefoxin)

Do not confuse cefoxitin with cefotaxime, cefotetan, or Cytoxan.

CATEGORY AND SCHEDULE

Pregnancy Risk Category: B

MECHANISM OF ACTION

A second-generation cephalosporin that binds to bacterial cell membranes and inhibits cell wall synthesis. **Therapeutic Effect:** Bactericidal.

AVAILABILITY

Powder for Injection: 1 g, 2 g.

INDICATIONS AND DOSAGES

▸ Mild to moderate infections

IV, IM

Adults, Elderly. 1–2 g q6–8h.

▸ Severe infections

IV, IM

Adults, Elderly. 1 g q4h or 2 g q6–8h up to 2 g q4h.

▸ Uncomplicated gonorrhea

IM

Adults. 2 g one time with 1 g probenecid.

▸ Perioperative prophylaxis

IV, IM

Adults, Elderly. 2 g 30–60 min before surgery, then q6h for up to 24 hr after surgery.

Children older than 3 mo. 30–40 mg/kg 30–60 min before surgery, then q6h for up to 24 hr after surgery.

▸ Cesarean section

IV

Adults. 2 g as soon as umbilical cord is clamped, then 2 g 4 and 8 hr after first dose, then q6h for up to 24 hr.

▸ Usual pediatric dosage

Children older than 3 mo. 80–160 mg/kg/day in 4–6 divided doses. Maximum: 12 g/day.

Neonates. 90–100 mg/kg/day in divided doses q6–8h.

▸ Dosage in renal impairment

After a loading dose of 1–2 g, dosage and frequency are modified based on creatinine clearance and the severity of the infection.

Creatinine Clearance	Dosage
30–50 ml/min	1–2 g q8–12h
10–29 ml/min	1–2 g q12–24h
5–9 ml/min	500 mg–1 g q12–24h
less than 5 ml/min	500 mg–1 g q24–48h

CONTRAINDICATIONS

History of anaphylactic reaction to penicillins or hypersensitivity to cephalosporins

INTERACTIONS

Drug

Probenecid: Increases serum concentration of cefoxitin.

Herbal

None known.

Food

None known.

DIAGNOSTIC TEST EFFECTS

May increase BUN level and serum alkaline phosphatase, creatinine, AST (SGOT), and ALT (SGPT) levels. May produce a positive direct or indirect Coombs' test. Interferes with crossmatching procedures and hematologic tests.

IV INCOMPATIBILITIES

Filgrastim (Neupogen), pentamidine (Pentam IV), vancomycin (Vancocin)

IV COMPATIBILITIES

Diltiazem (Cardizem), famotidine (Pepcid), heparin, hydromorphone (Dilaudid), magnesium sulfate, morphine, multivitamins, propofol (Diprivan)

SIDE EFFECTS

Frequent

Discomfort with IM administration, oral candidiasis, mild diarrhea, mild abdominal cramping, vaginal candidiasis

Occasional

Nausea, serum sickness-like reaction (marked by fever and joint pain; usually occurs after the second course of therapy and resolves after the drug is discontinued).

Rare

Allergic reaction (pruritus, rash, urticaria), thrombophlebitis (pain, redness, swelling at injection site)

SERIOUS REACTIONS

! Antibiotic-associated colitis and other superinfections may result from altered bacterial balance.

! Nephrotoxicity may occur, especially in patients with preexisting renal disease.

! Patients with a history of allergies, especially to penicillin, are at increased risk for developing a severe hypersensitivity reaction, marked by severe pruritus, angioedema, bronchospasm, and anaphylaxis.

NURSING CONSIDERATIONS

Baseline Assessment

◀ALERT▶ Determine if the patient has a history of allergies, particularly to cefoxitin, other cephalosporins, or penicillins, before beginning drug therapy.

Precautions

• Use cefoxitin cautiously in patients with renal impairment or a history of GI disease (especially antibiotic-associated or ulcerative colitis).

• Use the drug cautiously in patients using nephrotoxic drugs concurrently.

Administration and Handling

◀ALERT▶ Give by IM injection, intermittent IV infusion (piggyback), or IV push.

◀ALERT▶ Space doses evenly around the clock.

IM

• Reconstitute each 1-g vial with 2 ml of sterile water for injection or lidocaine to provide a concentration of 400 mg/ml.

• To minimize patient discomfort, slowly inject the drug deep into the gluteus maximus rather than the lateral aspect of the thigh.

IV

• The solution normally appears colorless to light amber; a darker color does not indicate loss of potency.

• The IV infusion (piggyback) is stable for 24 hours at room temperature and 48 hours if refrigerated.
• Discard the solution if a precipitate forms.
• Reconstitute each 1-g vial with 10 ml of sterile water for injection to provide a concentration of 95 mg/ml.
• The resulting solution may be further diluted with 50 to 100 ml of sterile water for injection, 0.9% NaCl, or D_5W.
• Administer IV push over 3 to 5 minutes.
• Administer intermittent IV infusion (piggyback) over 15 to 30 minutes.

Intervention and Evaluation

• Evaluate the IV site for phlebitis, as evidenced by heat, pain, and red streaking over the vein.
• Assess the IM injection site for induration and tenderness.
• Assess the patient's mouth for white patches on the mucous membranes and tongue.
• Assess the patient's pattern of daily bowel activity and stool consistency. Mild GI effects may be tolerable, but severe symptoms may indicate the onset of antibiotic-associated colitis.
• Monitor the patient's intake and output and renal function test results to assess for signs of nephrotoxicity.
• Be alert for signs and symptoms of superinfection, including abdominal pain or cramping, moderate to severe diarrhea, severe anal or genital pruritus or discharge, and severe mouth or tongue soreness.

Patient Teaching

• Inform the patient that IM injections may cause discomfort.

cefpodoxime proxetil

sef-**pod**-ox-ime
(Vantin)
Do not confuse Vantin with Ventolin.

CATEGORY AND SCHEDULE

Pregnancy Risk Category: B

MECHANISM OF ACTION

A third-generation cephalosporin that binds to bacterial cell membranes and inhibits cell wall synthesis. **Therapeutic Effect:** Bactericidal.

PHARMACOKINETICS

Well absorbed from the GI tract (food increases absorption). Protein binding: 21%–40%. Widely distributed. Primarily excreted unchanged in urine. Partially removed by hemodialysis. ***Half-life:*** 2.3 hr (increased in impaired renal function and elderly patients).

AVAILABILITY

Oral Suspension: 50 mg/5 ml, 100 mg/5 ml.
Tablets: 100 mg, 200 mg.

INDICATIONS AND DOSAGES

▸ **Chronic bronchitis, pneumonia**
PO
Adults, Elderly, Children older than 13 yr. 200 mg q12h for 10–14 days.

▸ **Gonorrhea, rectal gonococcal infection (female patients only)**
PO
Adults, Children older than 13 yr. 200 mg as a single dose.

▸ **Skin and skin-structure infections**
PO
Adults, Elderly, Children older than 13 yr. 400 mg q12h for 7–14 days.

▸ **Pharyngitis, tonsillitis**
PO
Adults, Elderly, Children older than 13 yr. 100 mg q12h for 5–10 days.
Children 6 mo–13 yr. 5 mg/kg q12h for 5–10 days. Maximum: 100 mg/dose.
▸ **Acute maxillary sinusitis**
PO
Adults, Children older than 13 yr. 200 mg twice a day for 10 days.
Children 2 mo–13 yr. 5 mg/kg q12h for 10 days. Maximum: 400 mg/day.
▸ **UTIs**
PO
Adults, Elderly, Children older than 13 yr. 100 mg q12h for 7 days.
▸ **Acute otitis media**
PO
Children 6 mo–13 yr. 5 mg/kg q12h for 5 days. Maximum: 400 mg/dose.
▸ **Dosage in renal impairment**
For patients with creatinine clearance less than 30 ml/min, usual dose is given q24h. For patients on hemodialysis, usual dose is given 3 times/wk after dialysis.

CONTRAINDICATIONS
History of anaphylactic reaction to penicillins or hypersensitivity to cephalosporins

INTERACTIONS
Drug
Antacids, H_2 antagonists: May decrease cefpodoxime absorption.
Probenecid: May increase cefpodoxime blood concentration.
Herbal
None known.
Food
None known.

DIAGNOSTIC TEST EFFECTS
May increase BUN level and serum alkaline phosphatase, bilirubin, creatinine, LDH, AST (SGOT), and ALT (SGPT) levels. May produce a positive direct or indirect Coombs' test.

SIDE EFFECTS
Frequent
Oral candidiasis, mild diarrhea, mild abdominal cramping, vaginal candidiasis
Occasional
Nausea, serum sickness-like reaction (marked by fever and joint pain; usually occurs after the second course of therapy and resolves after the drug is discontinued)
Rare
Allergic reaction (pruritus, rash, urticaria)

SERIOUS REACTIONS
! Antibiotic-associated colitis and other superinfections may result from altered bacterial balance.
! Nephrotoxicity may occur, especially in patients with preexisting renal disease.
! Patients with a history of allergies, especially to penicillin, are at increased risk for developing a severe hypersensitivity reaction, marked by severe pruritus, angioedema, bronchospasm, and anaphylaxis.

NURSING CONSIDERATIONS
Baseline Assessment
◂ALERT▸ Determine if the patient has a history of allergies, particularly to cephalosporins or penicillins, before beginning drug therapy.
Lifespan Considerations
- Cefpodoxime readily crosses the placenta and is distributed in breast milk.
- The safety and efficacy of cefpodixime have not been established in children younger than 6 months.
- Age-related renal impairment may

require a dosage adjustment in the elderly.

Precautions

- Use cefpodoxime cautiously in patients with renal impairment, a history GI disease (especially antibiotic-associated ulcerative colitis), or allergies to other drugs.
- Use the drug cautiously in patients using nephrotoxic drugs concurrently.

Administration and Handling

PO

- Administer cefpodoxime with food to enhance drug absorption.
- After reconstitution, the oral suspension is stable for 14 days if refrigerated.

Intervention and Evaluation

- Assess the patient's mouth for white patches on the mucous membranes and tongue.
- Assess the patient's pattern of daily bowel activity and stool consistency. Mild GI effects may be tolerable, but severe symptoms may indicate the onset of antibiotic-associated colitis.
- Monitor the patient's intake and output and renal function test results to assess for nephrotoxicity.
- Be alert for signs and symptoms of superinfection including abdominal pain or cramping, moderate to severe diarrhea, severe anal or genital pruritus or discharge, and severe mouth or tongue soreness.

Patient Teaching

- Advise the patient to space doses evenly around the clock and to continue cefpodoxime therapy for the full course of treatment.
- Instruct the patient using the oral suspension to refrigerate it, shake it well before using, and take it with food.

cefprozil

sef-**pro**-zil

(Cefzil)

Do not confuse cefprozil with Cefazolin; or Cefzil with Cefol, Ceftin, or Kefzol.

CATEGORY AND SCHEDULE

Pregnancy Risk Category: B

MECHANISM OF ACTION

A second-generation cephalosporin that binds to bacterial cell membranes and inhibits cell wall synthesis. **Therapeutic Effect:** Bactericidal.

PHARMACOKINETICS

Well absorbed from the GI tract. Protein binding: 36%–45%. Widely distributed. Primarily excreted unchanged in urine. Moderately removed by hemodialysis. ***Half-life:*** 1.3 hr (increased in impaired renal function).

AVAILABILITY

Oral Suspension: 125 mg/5 ml, 250 mg/5 ml.

Tablets: 250 mg, 500 mg.

INDICATIONS AND DOSAGES

▸ Pharyngitis, tonsillitis

PO

Adults, Elderly. 500 mg q24h for 10 days.

Children 2–12 yr. 7.5 mg/kg q12h for 10 days.

▸ Acute bacterial exacerbation of chronic bronchitis, secondary bacterial infection of acute bronchitis

PO

Adults, Elderly. 500 mg q12h for 10 days.

▸ **Skin and skin-structure infections**
PO
Adults, Elderly. 250–500 mg q12h for 10 days.
Children. 20 mg/kg q24h for 10 days.

▸ **Acute sinusitis**
PO
Adults, Elderly. 250–500 mg q12h for 10 days.
Children 6 mo–12 yr. 7.5–15 mg/kg q12h for 10 days.

▸ **Otitis media**
PO
Children 6 mo–12 yr. 15 mg/kg q12h for 10 days. Maximum: 1 g/day.

▸ **Dosage in renal impairment**
Patients with creatinine clearance less than 30 ml/min receive 50% of usual dose at usual interval.

CONTRAINDICATIONS
History of anaphylactic reaction to penicillins or hypersensitivity to cephalosporins

INTERACTIONS
Drug
Probenecid: Increases serum concentration of cefprozil.
Herbal
None known.
Food
None known.

DIAGNOSTIC TEST EFFECTS
May increase liver function test results. May produce a positive direct or indirect Coombs' test. Interferes with crossmatching procedures and hematologic tests.

SIDE EFFECTS
Frequent
Oral candidiasis, mild diarrhea, mild abdominal cramping, vaginal candidiasis
Occasional
Nausea, serum sickness reaction (marked by fever and joint pain; usually occurs after the second course of therapy and resolves after the drug is discontinued)
Rare
Allergic reaction (pruritus, rash, urticaria)

SERIOUS REACTIONS
! Antibiotic-associated colitis and other superinfections may result from altered bacterial balance.
! Nephrotoxicity may occur, especially in patients with preexisting renal disease.
! Patients with a history of allergies, especially to penicillin, are at increased risk for developing a severe hypersensitivity reaction, marked by severe pruritus, angioedema, bronchospasm, and anaphylaxis.

NURSING CONSIDERATIONS
Baseline Assessment
◂ **ALERT** ▸ Determine if the patient has a history of allergies, particularly to cefprozil, other cephalosporins, or penicillins, before beginning drug therapy.
Lifespan Considerations
- Cefprozil readily crosses the placenta and is distributed in breast milk.
- The safety and efficacy of cefprozil have not been established in children younger than 6 months.
- Age-related renal impairment may require a dosage adjustment in the elderly.
Precautions
- Use cefprozil cautiously in patients with a history of GI disease, especially antibiotic-associated or ulcerative colitis, and in those with renal impairment.

• Use the drug cautiously in patients using nephrotoxic drugs concurrently.

Administration and Handling

PO

• After reconstitution, the oral suspension is stable for 14 days if refrigerated.

• Shake the oral suspension well before using.

• Give cefprozil without regard to meals; however, if GI upset occurs, give it with food or milk.

Intervention and Evaluation

• Assess the patient's oral cavity for evidence of stomatitis.

• Assess the patient's pattern of daily bowel activity and stool consistency. Mild GI effects may be tolerable, but severe symptoms may indicate the onset of antibiotic-associated colitis.

• Monitor the patient's intake and output and renal function test results to assess for nephrotoxicity.

• Be alert for signs and symptoms of superinfection, including abdominal pain or cramping, moderate to severe diarrhea, severe anal or genital pruritus or discharge, and severe mouth or tongue soreness.

Patient Teaching

• Advise the patient to space drug doses evenly around the clock and to continue cefprozil therapy for the full course of treatment.

• Instruct the patient to take cefprozil with food or milk if GI upset occurs.

ceftazidime

sef-**taz**-i-deem

(Ceptaz, Fortaz, Fortum[AUS], Tazicef, Tazidime)

Do not confuse ceftazidime with ceftizoxime.

CATEGORY AND SCHEDULE

Pregnancy Risk Category: B

MECHANISM OF ACTION

A third-generation cephalosporin that binds to bacterial cell membranes and inhibits cell wall synthesis. **Therapeutic Effect:** Bactericidal.

PHARMACOKINETICS

Widely distributed (including to CSF). Protein binding: 5%–17%. Primarily excreted unchanged in urine. Removed by hemodialysis. ***Half-life:*** 2 hr (increased in impaired renal function).

AVAILABILITY

Powder for Injection (Fortaz, Tazicef, Tazidime): 500 mg, 1 g, 2 g.

INDICATIONS AND DOSAGES

▸ **UTIs**

IV, IM

Adults. 250–500 mg q8–12h.

▸ **Mild to moderate infections**

IV, IM

Adults. 1 g q8–12h.

▸ **Uncomplicated pneumonia, skin and skin-structure infections**

IV, IM

Adults. 0.5–1 g q8h.

▸ **Bone and joint infections**

IV, IM

Adults. 2 g q12h.

▸ **Meningitis, serious gynecologic and intra-abdominal infections**

IV, IM

Adults. 2 g q8h.

▸ **Pseudomonal pulmonary infections in patients with cystic fibrosis**
IV
Adults. 30–50 mg/kg q8h. Maximum: 6 g/day.

▸ **Usual elderly dosage**
Elderly (normal renal function). 500 mg–1 g q12h.

▸ **Usual pediatric dosage**
Children 1 mo–12 yr. 100–150 mg/kg/day in divided doses q8h. Maximum: 6 g/day.
Neonates 0–4 wk. 100–150 mg/kg/day in divided doses q8–12h.

▸ **Dosage in renal impairment**
After an initial 1-g dose, dosage and frequency are modified based on creatinine clearance and the severity of the infection.

Creatinine Clearance	Dosage
31–50 ml/min	1 g q12h
16–30 ml/min	1 g q24h
6–15 ml/min	500 mg q24h
less than 5 ml/min	500 mg q48h

CONTRAINDICATIONS
History of anaphylactic reaction to penicillins or hypersensitivity to cephalosporins

INTERACTIONS
Drug
None known.
Herbal
None known.
Food
None known.

DIAGNOSTIC TEST EFFECTS
May increase BUN level and serum alkaline phosphatase, creatinine, LDH, AST (SGOT), and ALT (SGPT) levels. May produce a positive direct or indirect Coombs' test. Interferes with crossmatching procedures and hematologic tests.

IV INCOMPATIBILITIES
Amphotericin B complex (AmBisome, Amphotec, Abelcet), doxorubicin liposomal (Doxil), fluconazole (Diflucan), idarubicin (Idamycin), midazolam (Versed), pentamidine (Pentam IV), vancomycin (Vancocin)

IV COMPATIBILITIES
Diltiazem (Cardizem), famotidine (Pepcid), heparin, hydromorphone (Dilaudid), morphine, propofol (Diprivan)

SIDE EFFECTS
Frequent
Discomfort with IM administration, oral candidiasis, mild diarrhea, mild abdominal cramping, vaginal candidiasis
Occasional
Nausea, serum sickness-like reaction (marked by fever and joint pain; usually occurs after the second course of therapy and resolves after the drug is discontunued)
Rare
Allergic reaction (pruritus, rash, urticaria), thrombophlebitis (pain, redness, swelling at injection site)

SERIOUS REACTIONS
! Antibiotic-associated colitis and other superinfections may result from altered bacterial balance.
! Nephrotoxicity may occur, especially in patients with preexisting renal disease.
! Patients with a history of allergies, especially to penicillin, are at increased risk for developing a severe hypersensitivity reaction, marked by severe pruritus, angioedema, bronchospasm, and anaphylaxis.

NURSING CONSIDERATIONS

Baseline Assessment

◀ALERT▶ Determine if the patient has a history of allergies, particularly to cephalosporins or penicillins, before beginning drug therapy.

Lifespan Considerations

- Ceftazidime readily crosses the placenta and is distributed in breast milk.
- No age-related precautions have been noted in children.
- Age-related renal impairment may require a dosage adjustment in the elderly.

Precautions

- Use ceftazidime cautiously in patients with a history of GI disease, especially antibiotic-associated or ulcerative colitis, and those with renal impairment.
- Use the drug cautiously in patients using nephrotoxic drugs concurrently.

Administration and Handling

◀ALERT▶ Give ceftazidime by IM injection, direct IV injection, or intermittent IV infusion (piggyback).

IV

- The solution normally appears light yellow to amber, but tends to darken; color change does not indicate loss of potency.
- The IV infusion (piggyback) is stable for 18 hours at room temperature and 7 days if refrigerated.
- Discard the solution if a precipitate forms.
- Add 10 ml of sterile water for injection to each 1-g vial to provide a concentration of 90 mg/ml.
- The resulting solution may be further diluted with 50 to 100 ml of 0.9% NaCl, D_5W, or another compatible diluent.
- Administer IV push over 3 to 5 minutes.
- Administer intermittent IV infusion (piggyback) over 15 to 30 minutes.

IM

- To reconstitute, add 1.5 ml of sterile water for injection or lidocaine 1% to 500-mg vial, if prescribed, or 3 ml to 1-g vial to provide a concentration of 280 mg/ml.
- To minimize patient discomfort, slowly inject the drug deep into the gluteus maximus rather than the lateral aspect of the thigh.

Intervention and Evaluation

- Evaluate the IV site for phlebitis, as evidenced by heat, pain, and red streaking over the vein.
- Assess the IM injection site for induration and tenderness.
- Assess the patient's mouth for white patches on the mucous membranes or tongue.
- Assess the patient's pattern of daily bowel activity and stool consistency. Mild GI effects may be tolerable, but severe symptoms may indicate the onset of antibiotic-associated colitis.
- Monitor the patient's intake and output and renal function test results to assess for nephrotoxicity.
- Be alert for signs and symptoms of superinfection including abdominal pain or cramping, moderate to severe diarrhea, severe anal or genital pruritus or discharge, and severe mouth or tongue soreness.

Patient Teaching

- Inform the patient that IM injections may cause discomfort.

ceftibuten

cef-te-bute-in

(Cedax)

CATEGORY AND SCHEDULE

Pregnancy Risk Category: B

MECHANISM OF ACTION
A third-generation cephalosporin that binds to bacterial cell membranes and inhibits cell wall synthesis. **Therapeutic Effect:** Bactericidal.

PHARMACOKINETICS
Rapidly absorbed from the gastrointestinal tract. Excreted primarily in urine. ***Half-life:*** 2–3hr.

AVAILABILITY
Capsules: 400 mg.
Oral Suspension: 90 mg/5 ml.

INDICATIONS AND DOSAGES
▸ **Chronic bronchitis**
PO
Adults, Elderly. 400 mg/day once a day for 10 days.
▸ **Pharyngitis, tonsillitis**
PO
Adults, Elderly. 400 mg once a day for 10 days.
Children older than 6 mo. 9 mg/kg once a day for 10 days. Maximum: 400 mg/day.
▸ **Otitis media**
PO
Children older than 6 mo. 9 mg/kg once a day for 10 days. Maximum: 400 mg/day.
▸ **Dosage in renal impairment**
Dosage is modified based on creatinine clearance.

Creatinine Clearance	Dosage
50 ml/min and higher	400 mg or 9 mg/kg q24h
30–49 ml/min	200 mg or 4.5 mg/kg q24h
less than 30 ml/min	100 mg or 2.25 mg/kg q24h

CONTRAINDICATIONS
History of anaphylactic reaction to penicillins or hypersensitivity to cephalosporins

INTERACTIONS
Drug
Aminoglycosides: Increased risk of nephrotoxicity.
Probenecid: Increases serum ceftibuten level.
Herbal
None known.
Food
None known.

DIAGNOSTIC TEST EFFECTS
May increase BUN level and serum alkaline phosphatase, bilirubin, creatinine, LDH, AST (SGOT), and ALT (SGPT) levels. May produce a positive direct or indirect Coombs' test.

SIDE EFFECTS
Frequent
Oral candidiasis, mild diarrhea (discharge, itching)
Occasional
Nausea, serum sickness-like reaction (marked by fever and joint pain; usually occurs after the second course of therapy and resolves after the drug is discontinued)
Rare
Allergic reaction (rash, pruritus, urticaria)

SERIOUS REACTIONS
! Antibiotic-associated colitis and other superinfections may result from altered bacterial balance.
! Nephrotoxicity may occur, especially in patients with preexisting renal disease.
! Patients with a history of allergies, especially to penicillin, are at increased risk for developing a severe hypersensitivity reaction, marked by severe pruritus,

angioedema, bronchospasm, and anaphylaxis.

NURSING CONSIDERATIONS

Baseline Assessment

◀ALERT▶ Determine if the patient has a history of allergies, particularly to ceftibuten, other cephalosporins, or penicillins, before beginning drug therapy.

Precautions

- Use ceftibuten cautiously in patients with renal impairment, a history of GI disease (especially antibiotic-associated or ulcerative colitis), or allergies to penicillins or other drugs.

Administration and Handling

◀ALERT▶ Use the oral suspension when treating otitis media to achieve higher peak blood levels.

Intervention and Evaluation

- Assess the patient's mouth for white patches on the mucous membranes and tongue.
- Assess the patient's pattern of daily bowel activity and stool consistency. Mild GI effects may be tolerable, but severe symptoms may indicate the onset of antibiotic-associated colitis.
- Monitor the patient's intake and output and renal function test results to assess for nephrotoxicity.
- Be alert for signs and symptoms of superinfection, including abdominal pain or cramping, moderate to severe diarrhea, severe anal or genital pruritus or discharge, and severe mouth or tongue soreness.

Patient Teaching

- Advise the patient to space drug doses evenly around the clock and to continue taking ceftibuten for the full course of treatment.
- Instruct the patient to take the drug with food or milk if GI upset occurs.

ceftizoxime sodium

sef-ti-**zox**-eem

(Cefizox)

Do not confuse ceftizoxime with cefotaxime or ceftazidime.

CATEGORY AND SCHEDULE

Pregnancy Risk Category: B

MECHANISM OF ACTION

A third-generation cephalosporin that binds to bacterial cell membranes and inhibits cell wall synthesis. **Therapeutic Effect:** Bactericidal.

PHARMACOKINETICS

Widely distributed (including to CSF). Protein binding: 30%. Primarily excreted unchanged in urine. Moderately removed by hemodialysis. ***Half-life:*** 1.7 hr (increased in impaired renal function).

AVAILABILITY

Powder for Injection: 500 mg, 1 g, 2 g.

INDICATIONS AND DOSAGES

▸ **Uncomplicated UTIs**

IV, IM

Adults, Elderly. 500 mg q12h.

▸ **Mild, moderate, or severe infections of the biliary, respiratory, and GU tracts; skin, bone, and intra-abdominal infections; meningitis; and septicemia**

IV, IM

Adults, Elderly. 1–2 g q8–12h.

▸ **Life-threatening infections of the biliary, respiratory, and GU tracts; skin, bone and intra-abdominal infections; meningitis; and septicemia**

IV

Adults, Elderly. 3–4 g q8h, up to 2 g q4h.

▸ **Pelvic inflammatory disease (PID)**
IV
Adults. 2 g q4–8h.
▸ **Uncomplicated gonorrhea**
IM
Adults. 1 g one time.
▸ **Usual pediatric dosage**
Children older than 6 mo. 50 mg/kg q6–8h. Maximum: 12 g/day.
▸ **Dosage in renal impairment**
After a loading dose of 0.5–1 g, dosage and frequency are modified based creatinine clearance and the severity of the infection.

Creatinine Clearance	Dosage
50–79 ml/min	0.5 g–1.5 g q8h
5–49 ml/min	0.25 g–1 g q12h
less than 5 ml/min	0.25–0.5 g q24h or 0.5 g–1 g q48h

CONTRAINDICATIONS
History of anaphylactic reaction to penicillins or hypersensitivity to cephalosporins

INTERACTIONS
Drug
Probenecid: Increases serum concentration of ceftizoxime.
Herbal
None known.
Food
None known.

DIAGNOSTIC TEST EFFECTS
May increase BUN level and serum alkaline serum phosphatase, creatinine, AST (SGOT), and ALT (SGPT) levels. May produce a positive direct or indirect Coombs' test.

IV INCOMPATIBILITIES
Filgrastim (Neupogen)

IV COMPATIBILITIES
Hydromorphone (Dilaudid), morphine, propofol (Diprivan)

SIDE EFFECTS
Frequent
Discomfort with IM administration, oral candidiasis, mild diarrhea, mild abdominal cramping, vaginal candidiasis
Occasional
Nausea, serum sickness-like reaction (fever, joint pain; usually occurs after the second course of therapy and resolves after the drug is discontinued)
Rare
Allergic reaction (rash, pruritus, urticaria), thrombophlebitis (pain, redness, swelling at injection site)

SERIOUS REACTIONS
! Antibiotic-associated colitis manifested and other superinfections may result from altered bacterial balance.
! Nephrotoxicity may occur, especially in patients with preexisting renal disease.
! Patients with a history of allergies, especially to penicillin, are at increased risk for developing a severe hypersensitivity reaction, marked by severe pruritus, angioedema, bronchospasm, and anaphylaxis.

NURSING CONSIDERATIONS
Baseline Assessment
◂ALERT▸ Determine if the patient has a history of allergies, particularly to ceftizoxime, other cephalosporins, or penicillins, before beginning drug therapy.
Lifespan Considerations
• Ceftizoxime readily crosses the placenta and is distributed in breast milk.

• Ceftizoxime use in children is associated with transient elevations of blood eosinophil count and serum CK, AST (SGOT), and ALT (SGPT) levels.
• Age-related renal impairment may require a dosage adjustment in the elderly.

Precautions

• Use ceftizoxime cautiously in patients with hepatic or renal impairment or a history of GI disease (especially antibiotic-associated or ulcerative colitis).

Administration and Handling

IV

• The solution normally appears clear to pale yellow. A change from yellow to amber does not indicate loss of potency.
• The IV infusion (piggyback) is stable for 24 hours at room temperature and 96 hours if refrigerated.
• Discard the solution if a precipitate forms.
• To reconstitute, add 5 ml of sterile water for injection to each 0.5-g vial to provide a concentration of 95 mg/ml.
• The resulting solution may be further diluted with 50 to 100 ml of 0.9% NaCl, D_5W, or another compatible fluid.
• Administer IV push over 3 to 5 minutes.
• Infuse intermittent IV infusion (piggyback) over 15 to 30 minutes.

IM

• Add 1.5 ml of sterile water for injection to each 0.5-g vial to provide a concentration of 270 mg/ml.
• Give deep IM injections slowly to minimize patient discomfort.
• When giving a 2-g dose, divide the dose and give in different large muscle masses.

Intervention and Evaluation

• Assess the patient's mouth for white patches on the mucous membranes and tongue.
• Assess the patient's pattern of daily bowel activity and stool consistency. Mild GI effects may be tolerable, but severe symptoms may indicate the onset of antibiotic-associated colitis.
• Monitor the patient's intake and output and renal function test results to assess for nephrotoxicity.
• Be alert for signs and symptoms of superinfection, including abdominal pain or cramping, moderate to severe diarrhea, severe anal or genital pruritus or discharge, and severe mouth or tongue soreness.

Patient Teaching

• Inform the patient that IM injections may cause discomfort.

ceftriaxone sodium

sef-try-**ax**-one
(Rocephin)

CATEGORY AND SCHEDULE

Pregnancy Risk Category: B

MECHANISM OF ACTION

A third-generation cephalosporin that binds to bacterial cell membranes and inhibits cell wall synthesis. **Therapeutic Effect:** Bactericidal.

PHARMACOKINETICS

Widely distributed (including to CSF). Protein binding: 83%–96%. Primarily excreted unchanged in urine. Not removed by hemodialysis. ***Half-life:*** 4.3–4.6 hr IV; 5.8–8.7 hr IM (increased in impaired renal function).

AVAILABILITY

Powder for Injection: 250 mg, 500 mg, 1 g, 2 g.

INDICATIONS AND DOSAGES

▸ **Mild to moderate infections**
IV, IM
Adults, Elderly. 1–2 g as a single dose or in 2 divided doses.

▸ **Serious infections**
IV, IM
Adults, Elderly. Up to 4 g/day in 2 divided doses.
Children. 50–75 mg/kg/day in divided doses q12h. Maximum: 2 g/day.

▸ **Skin and skin-structure infections**
IV, IM
Children. 50–75 mg/kg/day as a single dose or in 2 divided doses. Maximum: 2 g/day.

▸ **Meningitis**
IV
Children. Initially, 75 mg/kg, then 100 mg/kg/day as a single dose or in divided doses q12h. Maximum: 4 g/day.

▸ **Lyme disease**
IV
Adults, Elderly. 2–4 g a day for 10–14 days.

▸ **Acute bacterial otitis media**
IM
Children. 50 mg/kg once a day for 3 days. Maximum: 1 g/day.

▸ **Perioperative prophylaxis**
IV, IM
Adults, Elderly. 1 g 0.5–2 hrs before surgery.

▸ **Uncomplicated gonorrhea**
IM
Adults. 250 mg plus doxycycline one time.

▸ **Dosage in renal impairment**
Dosage modification is usually unnecessary but liver and renal function test results should be monitored in those with both renal and liver impairment or severe renal impairment.

CONTRAINDICATIONS

History of anaphylactic reaction to penicillins or hypersensitivity to cephalosporins

INTERACTIONS

Drug
None known.
Herbal
None known.
Food
None known.

DIAGNOSTIC TEST EFFECTS

May increase BUN level and serum alkaline phosphatase, bilirubin, creatinine, AST (SGOT), and ALT (SGPT) levels. May produce a positive direct or indirect Coombs' test. Interferes with crossmatching procedures and hematologic tests.

IV INCOMPATIBILITIES

Aminophylline, amphotericin B complex (AmBisome, Amphotec, Abelcet), filgrastim (Neupogen), fluconazole (Diflucan), labetalol (Normodyne), pentamidine (Pentam IV), vancomycin (Vancocin)

IV COMPATIBILITIES

Diltiazem (Cardizem), heparin, lidocaine, morphine, propofol (Diprivan)

SIDE EFFECTS

Frequent
Discomfort with IM administration, oral candidiasis, mild diarrhea, mild abdominal cramping, vaginal candidiasis
Occasional
Nausea, serum sickness-like reaction (marked by fever and joint pain; usually occurs after the second course of therapy and resolves after the drug is discontinued)
Rare
Allergic reaction (rash, pruritus, urticaria), thrombophlebitis (pain, redness, swelling at injection site)

SERIOUS REACTIONS

! Antibiotic-associated colitis and other superinfections may result from altered bacterial balance.

! Nephrotoxicity may occur, especially in patients with pre-existing renal disease.

! Patients with a history of allergies, especially to penicillin, are at increased risk for developing a severe hypersensitivity reaction, marked by severe pruritus, angioedema, bronchospasm, and anaphylaxis.

NURSING CONSIDERATIONS

Baseline Assessment

◀ALERT▶ Determine if the patient has a history of allergies, particularly to ceftriaxone, other cephalosporins, or penicillins, before beginning drug therapy.

Lifespan Considerations

- Ceftriaxone readily crosses the placenta and is distributed in breast milk.
- Ceftriaxone use in children may displace serum bilirubin from serum albumin.
- Use ceftriaxone cautiously in neonates, who may become hyperbilirubinemic.
- Age-related renal impairment may require a dosage adjustment in the elderly.

Precautions

- Use ceftriaxone cautiously in patients with hepatic or renal impairmen, a history of allergies, or a history of GI disease (especially antibiotic-associated or ulcerative colitis).
- Use the drug cautiously in patients using nephrotoxic drugs concurrently.

Administration and Handling

IV

- The solution normally appears light yellow to amber.
- The IV infusion (piggyback) is stable for 3 days at room temperature and 10 days if refrigerated.
- Discard the solution if a precipitate forms.
- Add 2.4 ml of sterile water for injection to each 250-mg vial, 4.8 ml to each 500-mg vial, 9.6 ml to each 1-g vial, and 19.2 ml to each 2-g vial to provide a concentration of 100 mg/ml.
- The resulting solution may be further diluted with 50 to 100 ml of 0.9% NaCl or D_5W.
- Infuse the intermittent IV infusion (piggyback) over 15 to 30 minutes for adults and over 10 to 30 minutes for children or neonates.
- Alternate IV sites and use large veins to reduce the risk of phlebitis.

IM

- Add 0.9 ml of sterile water for injection, 0.9% NaCl, D_5W, bacteriostatic water and 0.9% benzyl alcohol, or lidocaine to each 250-mg vial, 1.8 ml to each 500-mg vial, 3.6 ml to each 1-g vial, and 7.2 ml to each 2-g vial to provide a concentration of 250 mg/ml.
- To minimize patient discomfort, slowly inject the drug deep into the gluteus maximus rather than the lateral aspect of the thigh.

Intervention and Evaluation

- Assess the patient's mouth for white patches on the mucous membranes and tongue.
- Assess the patient's pattern of daily bowel activity and stool consistency. Mild GI effects may be tolerable, but severe symptoms may indicate the onset of antibiotic-associated colitis.
- Monitor the patient's intake and output and renal function test results to assess for nephrotoxicity.

• Be alert for signs and symptoms of superinfection including abdominal pain or cramping, moderate to severe diarrhea, severe anal or genital pruritus or discharge, and severe mouth or tongue soreness.

Patient Teaching

• Inform the patient that IM injections may cause discomfort.

cefuroxime axetil

sef-yur-**ox**-ime

(Ceftin, Zinnat[AUS])

Do not confuse cefuroxime with cefotaxime or deferoxamine, or Ceftin with Cefzil.

cefuroxime sodium

(Kefurox, Zinacef)

CATEGORY AND SCHEDULE

Pregnancy Risk Category: B

MECHANISM OF ACTION

A second-generation cephalosporin that binds to bacterial cell membranes and inhibits cell wall synthesis. **Therapeutic Effect:** Bactericidal.

PHARMACOKINETICS

Rapidly absorbed from the GI tract. Protein binding: 33%–50%. Widely distributed (including to CSF). Primarily excreted unchanged in urine. Moderately removed by hemodialysis. ***Half-life:*** 1.3 hr (increased in impaired renal function).

AVAILABILITY

Oral Suspension: 125 mg/5 ml, 250 mg/5 ml.
Tablets: 250 mg, 500 mg.
Powder for Injection: 750 mg, 1.5 g.

INDICATIONS AND DOSAGES

▸ Ampicillin-resistant influenza; bacterial meningitis; early Lyme disease; GU tract, gynecologic, skin, and bone infections; septicemia; gonorrhea, and other gonococcal infections

IV, IM
Adults, Elderly. 750 mg–1.5 g q8h.
Children. 75–100 mg/kg/day divided q8h. Maximum: 8 g/day.
Neonates. 50–100 mg/kg/day divided q12h.
PO
Adults, Elderly. 125–500 mg twice a day, depending on the infection.

▸ Pharyngitis, tonsillitis

PO
Children 3 mo–12 yr. 125 mg (tablets) q12h or 20 mg/kg/day (suspension) in 2 divided doses.

▸ Acute otitis media, acute bacterial maxillary sinusitis, impetigo

PO
Children 3 mo–12 yr. 250 mg (tablets) q12h or 30 mg/kg/day (suspension) in 2 divided doses.

▸ Bacterial meningitis

IV
Children 3 mo–12 yr. 200–240 mg/kg/day in divided doses q6–8h.

▸ Perioperative prophylaxis

IV
Adults, Elderly. 1.5 g 30–60 min before surgery and 750 mg q8h after surgery.

▸ Usual neonatal dosage

IV, IM
Neonates. 20–100 mg/kg/day in divided doses q12h.

▸ Dosage in renal impairment

Adult dosage and frequency are modified based on creatinine clearance and the severity of the infection.

Creatinine Clearance	Dosage
greater than 20 ml/min	750 mg–1 g q8h
10–20 ml/min	750 mg q12h
less than 10 ml/min	750 mg q24h

CONTRAINDICATIONS
History of anaphylactic reaction to penicillins or hypersensitivity to cephalosporins

INTERACTIONS
Drug
Probenecid: Increases serum concentration of cefuroxime.
Herbal
None known.
Food
None known.

DIAGNOSTIC TEST EFFECTS
May increase serum alkaline phosphatase, bilirubin, LDH, AST (SGOT), and ALT (SGPT) levels. May produce a positive direct or indirect Coombs' test. Interferes with crossmatching procedures, hematologic tests.

IV INCOMPATIBILITIES
Filgrastim (Neupogen), fluconazole (Diflucan), midazolam (Versed), vancomycin (Vancocin)

IV COMPATIBILITIES
Diltiazem (Cardizem), hydromorphone (Dilaudid), morphine, propofol (Diprivan)

SIDE EFFECTS
Frequent
Discomfort with IM administration, oral candidiasis, mild diarrhea, mild abdominal cramping, vaginal candidiasis
Occasional
Nausea, serum sickness-like reaction (marked by fever and joint pain; usually occurs after the second course of therapy and resolves after the drug is discontinued)
Rare
Allergic reaction (rash, pruritus, urticaria), thrombophlebitis (pain, redness, swelling at injection site)

SERIOUS REACTIONS
! Antibiotic-associated colitis and other superinfections may result from altered bacterial balance.
! Nephrotoxicity may occur, especially in patients with preexisting renal disease.
! Patients with a history of allergies, especially to penicillin, are at increased risk for developing a severe hypersensitivity reaction, marked by severe pruritus, angioedema, bronchospasm, and anaphylaxis.

NURSING CONSIDERATIONS
Baseline Assessment
◀ALERT▶ Determine if the patient has a history of allergies, particularly to cefuroxime, other cephalosporins, or penicillins, before beginning drug therapy.
Lifespan Considerations
• Cefuroxime readily crosses the placenta and is distributed in breast milk.
• No age-related precautions have been noted in children.
• Age-related renal impairment may require a dosage adjustment in the elderly.
Precautions
• Use cefuroxime cautiously in patients with renal impairment or a history of GI disease, especially antibiotic-associated or ulcerative colitis.
• Use the drug cautiously in patients using nephrotoxic drugs concurrently.

Administration and Handling

PO

• Give cefuroxime tablets without regard to food. However, if GI upset occurs, give with food or milk.

• Avoid crushing tablets because they have a bitter taste.

• Give the oral suspension with food.

IV

• The solution normally appears light yellow to amber; a darker color does not indicate loss of potency.

• The IV infusion (piggyback) is stable for 24 hours at room temperature and 7 days if refrigerated.

• Discard the solution if a precipitate forms.

• To reconstitute, add 8 ml of sterile water for injection to each 750-mg vial, or 14 ml to each 1.5-g vial to provide a concentration of 100 mg/ml.

• For intermittent IV infusion (piggyback), further dilute with 50 to 100 ml of 0.9% NaCl or D_5W.

• Administer the IV push over 3 to 5 minutes.

• Infuse the intermittent IV infusion (piggyback) over 15 to 60 minutes.

IM

• To minimize patient discomfort, slowly inject the drug deep into the gluteus maximus rather than the lateral aspect of the thigh.

Intervention and Evaluation

• Assess the patient's mouth for white patches on the mucous membranes and tongue.

• Assess the patient's pattern of daily bowel activity and stool consistency. Mild GI effects may be tolerable, but severe symptoms may indicate the onset of antibiotic-associated colitis.

• Monitor the patient's intake and output and renal function test results to assess for nephrotoxicity.

• Be alert for signs and symptoms of superinfection, including abdominal pain or cramping, moderate to severe diarrhea, severe anal or genital pruritus or discharge, and severe mouth or tongue soreness.

Patient Teaching

• Advise the patient taking oral cefuroxime to space doses evenly around the clock and to continue therapy for the full course of treatment.

• Instruct the patient to take the drug with food or milk if GI upset occurs.

• Inform the patient that IM injections may cause discomfort.

cephalexin

sef-a-**lex**-in

(Apo-Cephalex[CAN], Biocef, Ceporex[AUS], Ibilex[AUS], Keflex, Keftab, Novolexin[CAN])

CATEGORY AND SCHEDULE

Pregnancy Risk Category: B

MECHANISM OF ACTION

A first-generation cephalosporin that binds to bacterial cell membranes and inhibits cell wall synthesis. **Therapeutic Effect:** Bactericidal.

PHARMACOKINETICS

Rapidly absorbed from the GI tract. Protein binding: 10%–15%. Widely distributed. Primarily excreted unchanged in urine. Moderately removed by hemodialysis. ***Half-life:*** 0.9–1.2 hr (increased in impaired renal function).

AVAILABILITY

Capsules (Biocef): 500 mg.
Capsules (Keflex): 250 mg, 500 mg.
Powder for Oral Suspension (Biocef): 125 mg/5 ml, 250 mg/5 ml.
Tablets: 250 mg, 500 mg.
Tablets (Keftab): 500 mg.

INDICATIONS AND DOSAGES

▸ **Bone infections, prophylaxis of rheumatic fever, follow-up to parenteral therapy**

PO

Adults, Elderly. 250–500 mg q6h up to 4 g/day.

▸ **Streptococcal pharyngitis, skin and skin-structure infections, uncomplicated cystitis**

PO

Adults, Elderly. 500 mg q12h.

▸ **Usual pediatric dosage**

Children. 25–100 mg/kg/day in 2–4 divided doses.

▸ **Otitis media**

PO

Children. 75–100 mg/kg/day in 4 divided doses.

▸ **Dosage in renal impairment**

After usual initial dose, dosing frequency is modified based on creatinine clearance and the severity of the infection.

Creatinine Clearance	Dosage Interval
10–40 ml/min	Usual dose q8–12h
less than 10 ml/min	Usual dose q12–24h

CONTRAINDICATIONS

History of anaphylactic reaction to penicillins or hypersensitivity to cephalosporins

INTERACTIONS

Drug

Probenecid: Increases serum concentration of cephalexin.

Herbal

None known.

Food

None known.

DIAGNOSTIC TEST EFFECTS

May increase serum alkaline phosphatase, AST (SGOT), and ALT (SGPT) levels. May produce a positive direct or indirect Coombs' test. Interferes with crossmatching procedures and hematologic tests.

SIDE EFFECTS

Frequent

Oral candidiasis, mild diarrhea, mild abdominal cramping, vaginal candidiasis

Occasional

Nausea, serum sickness-like reaction (marked by fever and joint pain; ususally occurs after the second course of therapy and resolves after the drug is discontinued)

Rare

Allergic reaction (rash, pruritus, urticaria)

SERIOUS REACTIONS

! Antibiotic-associated colitis and other superinfections may result from altered bacterial balance.

! Nephrotoxicity may occur, especially in patients with preexisting renal disease.

! Patients with a history of allergies, especially to penicillin, are at increased risk for developing a severe hypersensitivity reaction, marked by severe pruritus, angioedema, bronchospasm, and anaphylaxis.

NURSING CONSIDERATIONS

Baseline Assessment

◂ALERT▸ Determine if the patient has a history of allergies, particularly to cephalexin, other cephalosporins, or penicillins, before beginning drug therapy.

Lifespan Considerations

• Cephalexin readily crosses the placenta and is distributed in breast milk.

• No age-related precautions have been noted in children.

• Age-related renal impairment may

require a dosage adjustment in the elderly.

Precautions

• Use cephalexin cautiously in patients with renal impairment or a history of GI disease, especially antibiotic-associated or ulcerative colitis.

• Use the drug cautiously in patients using nephrotoxic drugs concurrently.

Administration and Handling

◀ **ALERT** ▶ Space drug doses evenly around the clock.

PO

• After reconstitution, the oral suspension is stable for 14 days if refrigerated.

• Shake the oral suspension well before using.

• Give oral cephalexin without regard to meals. However, if GI upset occurs, give with food or milk.

Intervention and Evaluation

• Assess the patient's mouth for white patches on the mucous membranes and tongue.

• Assess the patient's pattern of daily bowel activity and stool consistency. Mild GI effects may be tolerable, but severe symptoms may indicate the onset of antibiotic-associated colitis.

• Monitor the patient's intake and output and renal function test results to assess for nephrotoxicity.

• Be alert for signs and symptoms of superinfection, including abdominal pain or cramping, moderate to severe diarrhea, severe anal or genital pruritus or discharge, and severe mouth or tongue soreness.

Patient Teaching

• Advise the patient taking oral cephalexin to space doses evenly around the clock and to continue therapy for the full course of treatment.

• Instruct the patient to take the drug with food or milk if GI upset occurs.

• Teach the patient to refrigerate the oral suspension.

loracarbef

lor-a-**kar**-bef

(Lorabid)

Do not confuse loracarbef or Lorabid with Lortab.

CATEGORY AND SCHEDULE

Pregnancy Risk Category: B

MECHANISM OF ACTION

A second-generation cephalosporin that binds to bacterial cell membranes and inhibits cell wall synthesis. **Therapeutic Effect:** Bactericidal.

AVAILABILITY

Capsules: 200 mg, 400 mg.
Powder for Oral Suspension: 100 mg/5 ml, 200 mg/5 ml.

INDICATIONS AND DOSAGES

▸ **Bronchitis**

PO

Adults, Elderly, Children 12 yr and older. 200–400 mg q12h for 7 days.

▸ **Pharyngitis**

PO

Adults, Elderly, Children 12 yr and older. 200 mg q12h for 10 days.
Children 6 mo–11 yr. 7.5 mg/kg q12h for 10 days.

▸ **Pneumonia**

PO

Adults, Elderly, Children 12 yr and older. 400 mg q12h for 14 days.

▸ **Sinusitis**

PO

Adults, Elderly, Children 12 yr and older. 400 mg q12h for 10 days.
Children 6 mo–11 yr. 15 mg/kg q12h for 10 days.

▸ **Skin and soft-tissue infections**
PO
Adults, Elderly, Children 12 yr and older. 200 mg q12h for 7 days.
Children 6 mo–11 yr. 7.5 mg/kg q12h for 7 days.
▸ **UTIs**
PO
Adults, Elderly, Children 6 mo–12 yr. 200–400 mg q12h for 7–14 days.
▸ **Otitis media**
PO
Children 6 mo–12 yr. 15 mg/kg q12h for 10 days.

CONTRAINDICATIONS

History of anaphylactic reaction to penicillins or hypersensitivity to cephalosporins

INTERACTIONS

Drug

Probenecid: Increases serum concentration and half-life of loracarbef.

Herbal

None known.

Food

None known.

DIAGNOSTIC TEST EFFECTS

May increase BUN level and serum alkaline phosphatase, creatinine, AST (SGOT), and ALT (SGPT) levels. May decrease blood leukocyte and platelet counts.

SIDE EFFECTS

Frequent

Abdominal pain, anorexia, nausea, vomiting, diarrhea

Occasional

Rash, pruritus

Rare

Dizziness, headache, vaginitis

SERIOUS REACTIONS

! Antibiotic-associated colitis and other superinfections may result from altered bacterial balance.
! Hypersensitivity reactions (ranging from rash, urticaria, and fever to anaphylaxis) occur in fewer than 5% of patients—most commonly in patients with a history of drug allergies, especially to penicillins.

NURSING CONSIDERATIONS

Baseline Assessment

◂ **ALERT** ▸ Determine if the patient has a history of allergies, particularly to laracarbef, other cephalosporins, or penicillins, before beginning drug therapy.

Precautions

• Use loracarbef cautiously in patients with a history of colitis or renal impairment.

Administration and Handling

PO
• Give loracarbef 1 hour before or 2 hours after meals.
• After reconstitution, the oral suspension may be kept at room temperature for 14 days.
• Discard any unused portion after 14 days.
• Shake the oral suspension well before using.

Intervention and Evaluation

• Assess the patient for nausea or vomiting.
• Assess the patient's pattern of daily bowel activity and stool consistency.
• Evaluate the patient's skin for a rash, especially in the diaper area in infants and toddlers.
• Monitor the patient's intake and output, renal function reports, and urinalysis results for signs of nephrotoxicity.

• Be alert for signs and symptoms of superinfection, including abdominal pain or cramping, anal or genital pruritus or discharge, moderate to severe diarrhea, and severe mouth or tongue soreness.

Patient Teaching

• Advise the patient to take loracarbef 1 hour before or 2 hours after a meal, to space doses evenly around the clock, and to continue taking the drug for the full course of treatment.

8 Macrolides

azithromycin
clarithromycin
dirithromycin
erythromycin

Uses: Macrolides are used to treat pharyngitis, tonsillitis, sinusitis, chronic bronchitis, pneumonia, and uncomplicated skin and skin structure infections.

Action: Macrolides, which can be bacteriostatic or bactericidal, act primarily against gram-positive microorganisms and gram-negative cocci by reversibly binding to the P site of the 50S ribosomal subunit of susceptible organisms. This action inhibits RNA-dependent protein synthesis and causes bacterial cell death. (See the illustration *Sites and Mechanisms of Action: Anti-infective Agents,* page 2.) Azithromycin and clarithromycin appear to be more potent than erythromycin.

COMBINATION PRODUCTS

ERYZOLE: erythromycin/sulfisoxazole (a sulfonamide) 200 mg/600 mg per 5 ml.
PEDIAZOLE: erythromycin/sulfisoxazole (a sulfonamide) 200 mg/600 mg per 5 ml.

azithromycin

ay-zi-thro-**mye**-sin
(Zithromax, Zithromax TRI-PAK, Zithromax Z-PAK)
Do not confuse azithromycin with erythromycin.

CATEGORY AND SCHEDULE

Pregnancy Risk Category: B

MECHANISM OF ACTION

A macrolide antibiotic that binds to ribosomal receptor sites of susceptible organisms, inhibiting RNA-dependent protein synthesis.
Therapeutic Effect: Bacteriostatic or bactericidal, depending on the drug dosage.

PHARMACOKINETICS

Rapidly absorbed from the GI tract. Protein binding: 7%–50%. Widely distributed. Eliminated primarily unchanged by biliary excretion. ***Half-life:*** 68 hr.

AVAILABILITY

Oral Suspension: 100 mg/5 ml, 200 mg/5 ml.
Tablets: 250 mg, 500 mg, 600 mg. Tri-Pak: 3 × 500 mg. Z-Pak: 6 × 250 mg.
Injection: 500 mg.

INDICATIONS AND DOSAGES

▸ **Respiratory tract, skin, and skin-structure infections**

PO

Adults, Elderly. 500 mg once, then 250 mg/day for 4 days.
Children 6 mo and older. 10 mg/kg once (maximum 500 mg) then 5 mg/kg/day for 4 days (maximum 250 mg).

▸ **Acute bacterial exacerbations of COPD**

PO

Adults. 500 mg/day for 3 days.

▸ Otitis media
PO
Children 6 mo and older. 10 mg/kg once (maximum 500 mg) then 5 mg/kg/day for 4 days (maximum 250 mg). Single dose: 30 mg/kg. Maximum: 1,500 mg. Three-day regimen: 10 mg/kg/day as single daily dose. Maximum: 500 mg/day.

▸ Pharyngitis, tonsillitis
PO
Children older than 2 yr. 12 mg/kg/day (maximum 500 mg) for 5 days.

▸ Chancroid
PO
Adults, Elderly: 1 g as single dose.
Children: 20 mg/kg as single dose. Maximum: 1 g.

▸ Treatment of *Mycobacterium avium* complex (MAC)
PO
Adults, Elderly. 500 mg/day in combination.
Children. 5 mg/kg/day (maximum 250 mg) in combination.

▸ Prevention of MAC
PO
Adults, Elderly. 1,200 mg/wk alone or with rifabutin.
Children. 5 mg/kg/day (maximum 250 mg) or 20 mg/kg/wk (maximum 1,200 mg) alone or with rifabutin.

▸ Nongonococcal urethritis and cervicitis due to *Chlamydia trachomatis*
PO
Adults. 1 g as a single dose.

▸ Usual pediatric dosage
PO
Children older than 6 mo. 10 mg/kg once (maximum: 500 mg) then 5 mg/kg/day for 4 days (maximum 250 mg).

▸ Usual parenteral dosage (Community Acquired Pneumonia, PID)
IV
Adults. 500 mg/day, followed by oral therapy.

OFF-LABEL USES
Chlamydial infections, gonococcal pharyngitis, uncomplicated gonococcal infections of the cervix, urethra, and rectum

CONTRAINDICATIONS
Hypersensitivity to azithromycin or other macrolide antibiotics

INTERACTIONS
Drug
Aluminum- or magnesium-containing antacids: May decrease azithromycin blood concentration.
Carbamazepine, cyclosporine, theophylline, warfarin: May increase the serum concentrations of these drugs.
Herbal
None known.
Food
None known.

DIAGNOSTIC TEST EFFECTS
May increase serum CK, AST (SGOT), and ALT (SGPT) levels.

IV INCOMPATIBILITIES
Information is not available.

IV COMPATIBILITIES
None known; don't mix with other medications.

SIDE EFFECTS
Occasional
Nausea, vomiting, diarrhea, abdominal pain
Rare
Headache, dizziness, allergic reaction

SERIOUS REACTIONS
! Antibiotic-associated colitis and other superinfections may result from altered bacterial balance.
! Acute interstitial nephritis and hepatotoxicity occur rarely.

NURSING CONSIDERATIONS

Baseline Assessment

- Determine if the patient has a history of hepatitis or allergies to azithromycin or other macrolides before beginning therapy.

Lifespan Considerations

- It is unknown if azithromycin is distributed in breast milk.
- The safety and efficacy of azithromycin have not been established in children younger than 16 years for IV use and younger than 6 months for oral use.
- No age-related precautions have been noted in elderly patients with normal renal function.

Precautions

- Use azithromycin cautiously in patients with hepatic or renal dysfunction.

Administration and Handling

PO

- Give tablets without regard to food.
- Store the oral suspension at room temperature. The suspension is stable for 10 days after reconstitution.
- Don't administer the oral suspension with food. Give it at least 1 hour before or 2 hours after a meal. Give azithromycin 1 hour before or 2 hours after antacids.

IV

- Store vials at room temperature.
- After reconstitution, the solution is stable for 24 hours at room temperature or 7 days if refrigerated.
- Reconstitute each 500-mg vial with 4.8 ml sterile water for injection to provide a concentration of 100 mg/ml.
- Shake well to ensure dissolution.
- Further dilute the solution with 250 or 500 ml 0.9% NaCl or D_5W to provide a final concentration of 2 mg/ml or 1 mg/ml, respectively.
- Infuse the drug over 60 minutes.

Intervention and Evaluation

- Assess the patient for GI discomfort, nausea, or vomiting.
- Assess the patient's pattern of daily bowel activity and stool consistency.
- Monitor the patient's liver function test results.
- Assess the patient for signs and symptoms of hepatotoxicity, such as abdominal pain, fever, GI disturbances, and malaise.
- Evaluate the patient for signs and symptoms of superinfection, including genital or anal pruritus, sore mouth or tongue, and moderate to severe diarrhea.

Patient Teaching

- Instruct the patient to take the oral suspension with 8 oz of water at least 1 hour before or 2 hours after consuming any food or beverages.
- Advise the patient to space doses evenly around the clock and to continue taking azithromycin for the full course of treatment.
- If the patient must take an antacid containing aluminum or magnesium, tell him or her to take the drug 1 hour before or 2 hours after the antacid.

clarithromycin

clare-i-thro-**mye**-sin

(Biaxin, Biaxin XL, Klacid[AUS])

CATEGORY AND SCHEDULE

Pregnancy Risk Category: C

MECHANISM OF ACTION

A macrolide that binds to ribosomal receptor sites of susceptible organisms, inhibiting protein synthesis of the bacterial cell wall. **Therapeutic Effect:** Bacteriostatic; may be bactericidal with high dosages or very susceptible microorganisms.

PHARMACOKINETICS

Well absorbed from the GI tract. Protein binding: 65%–75%. Widely distributed. Metabolized in the liver to active metabolite. Primarily excreted in urine. Not removed by hemodialysis. ***Half-life:*** 3–7 hr; metabolite 5–7 hr (increased in impaired renal function).

AVAILABILITY

Oral Suspension: 125 mg/5 ml, 250 mg/5 ml.
Tablets: 250 mg, 500 mg.
Tablets (Extended-Release): 500 mg.

INDICATIONS AND DOSAGES

▸ Bronchitis
PO
Adults, Elderly. 500 mg q12h for 7–14 days.

▸ Skin, soft tissue infections
PO
Adults, Elderly. 250 mg q12h for 7–14 days.
Children. 7.5 mg/kg q12h for 10 days.

▸ MAC prophylaxis
PO
Adults, Elderly. 500 mg 2 times/day.
Children. 7.5 mg/kg q12h. Maximum: 500 mg 2 times/day.

▸ MAC treatment
PO
Adults, Elderly. 500 mg 2 times/day in combination.
Children. 7.5 mg/kg q12h in combination. Maximum: 500 mg 2 times/day.

▸ Pharyngitis, tonsillitis
PO
Adults, Elderly. 250 mg q12h for 10 days.
Children. 7.5 mg/kg q12h for 10 days.

▸ Pneumonia
PO
Adults, Elderly. 250 mg q12h for 7–14 days.
Children. 7.5 mg/kg q12h.

▸ Maxillary sinusitis
PO
Adults, Elderly. 500 mg q12h for 14 days.
Children. 7.5 mg/kg q12h. Maximum: 500 mg 2 times/day.

▸ *H. pylori*
PO
Adults, Elderly. 500 mg q12h for 10–14 days in combination.

▸ Acute otitis media
PO
Children. 7.5 mg/kg q12h for 10 days.

▸ Dosage in renal impairment
For patients with creatinine clearance less than 30 ml/min, reduce dose by 50% and administer once or twice a day.

CONTRAINDICATIONS

Hypersensitivity to clarithromycin or other macrolide antibiotics

INTERACTIONS

Drug

Carbamazepine, digoxin, theophylline: May increase blood concentration and toxicity of these drugs.
Rifampin: May decrease clarithromycin blood concentration.
Warfarin: May increase warfarin effects.
Zidovudine: May decrease blood concentration of zidovudine.

Herbal

None known.

Food

None known.

DIAGNOSTIC TEST EFFECTS

May (rarely) increase BUN, AST (SGOT), and ALT (SGPT) levels.

SIDE EFFECTS

Occasional (6%–3%)
Diarrhea, nausea, altered taste, abdominal pain
Rare (2%–1%)
Headache, dyspepsia

SERIOUS REACTIONS

! Antibiotic-associated colitis and other superinfections may result from altered bacterial balance.
! Hepatotoxicity and thrombocytopenia occur rarely.

NURSING CONSIDERATIONS

Baseline Assessment

◀ALERT▶ Determine if the patient has a history of hepatitis or allergies to clarithromycin or other macrolides before beginning drug therapy.

Lifespan Considerations

- It is unknown if clarithromycin is distributed in breast milk.
- The safety and efficacy of this drug have not been established in children younger than 6 months.
- Age-related renal impairment may require a dosage adjustment in the elderly.

Precautions

- Use clarithromycin cautiously in patients with hepatic or renal dysfunction and in elderly patients with severe renal impairment.

Administration and Handling

PO

- Give clarithromycin without regard to food.
- Don't crush or break tablets.

Intervention and Evaluation

- Assess the patient's pattern of daily bowel activity and stool consistency. Mild GI effects may be tolerable, but severe symptoms may indicate the onset of antibiotic-associated colitis.
- Be alert for signs and symptoms of superinfection, including abdominal pain, anal or genital pruritus, moderate to severe diarrhea, and mouth soreness.

Patient Teaching

- Instruct the patient to take clarithromycin tablets with 8 oz of water. Inform the patient that the tablets and oral suspension may be taken with or without food.
- Advise the patient to space doses evenly around the clock and to continue taking clarithromycin for the full course of treatment.

dirithromycin

die-rith-ro-**my**-sin
(Dynabac)
Do not confuse Dynabac with Dynacin or DynaCirc.

CATEGORY AND SCHEDULE

Pregnancy Risk Category: C

MECHANISM OF ACTION

A macrolide that binds to ribosomal receptor sites of susceptible organisms, inhibiting bacterial protein synthesis. **Therapeutic Effect:** Bactericidal or bacteriostatic, depending on drug dosage.

PHARMACOKINETICS

Rapidly absorbed from the GI tract. Protein binding: 15%–30%.Widely distributed into tissues and within cells. Eliminated primarily unchanged by biliary excretion. Not removed by hemodialysis. ***Half-life:*** 30–44 hr.

AVAILABILITY

Tablets (Enteric-Coated): 250 mg.

INDICATIONS AND DOSAGES

▸ Pharyngitis, tonsillitis

PO

Adults, Elderly, Children 12 yr and older. 500 mg once a day for 10 days.

▸ Acute or chronic bronchitis, skin and skin-structure infections

PO

Adults, Elderly, Children 12 yr and older. 500 mg once a day for 7 days.

▸ Community-acquired pneumonia

PO

Adults, Elderly, Children 12 yr and older. 500 mg once a day for 14 days.

CONTRAINDICATIONS

Hypersensitivity to dirithromycin or other macrolide antibiotics

INTERACTIONS

Drug

Aluminum- and magnesium-containing antacids: May decrease dirithromycin blood concentration.

H_2 antagonists: Increase dirithromycin absorption.

Herbal

None known.

Food

None known.

DIAGNOSTIC TEST EFFECTS

May increase serum CK and potassium levels as well as blood eosinophil, neutrophil and platelet counts.

SIDE EFFECTS

Frequent (10%–8%)

Abdominal pain, headache, nausea, diarrhea

Occasional (3%–2%)

Vomiting, dyspepsia, dizziness, nonspecific pain, asthenia

Rare (less than 2%)

Increased cough, flatulence, rash, dyspnea, pruritus and urticaria, insomnia

SERIOUS REACTIONS

! Antibiotic-associated colitis and other superinfections may result from altered bacterial balance.

NURSING CONSIDERATIONS

Baseline Assessment

◂ALERT▸ Determine if the patient has a history of allergies to dirithromycin or other macrolides before beginning drug therapy.

Lifespan Considerations

- It is unknown if dirithromycin is distributed in breast milk.
- The safety and efficacy of dirithromycin have not been established in children younger than 12 years.
- No age-related precautions have been noted in the elderly.

Precautions

- Use dirithromycin cautiously in patients with hepatic or renal dysfunction.

Administration and Handling

PO

- Administer dirithromycin with food or within 1 hour after a meal because food increases absorption.
- Have the patient swallow the tablets whole, not chew them. Don't crush or cut the tablets.

Intervention and Evaluation

- Monitor the patient's WBC count to determine if the infection is improving.
- Evaluate the patient for diarrhea, GI discomfort, headache, and nausea.
- Assess the patient's pattern of daily bowel activity and stool consistency.
- Evaluate the patient for signs and symptoms of superinfection, including anal or genital pruritus, moderate to severe diarrhea, abdominal cramps, fever, and sore mouth or tongue.

Patient Teaching

- Instruct the patient to take dirithro-

mycin with food or within 1 hour after a meal.
• Advise the patient to continue dirithromycin therapy for the full course of treatment.
• If the patient must take an antacid containing aluminum or magnesium, tell him or her to take the drug 1 hour before or 2 hours after the antacid.

erythromycin

er-ith-roe-**mye**-sin
(A/T/S, Akne-Mycin, Apo-Erythro Base[CAN], EES, Emgel, Eryacne[AUS], Erybid[CAN], Eryc, Eryc LD[AUS], EryDerm, Erygel, EryPed, Ery-Tab, Erythra-Derm, Erythrocin, Erythromid[CAN], PCE)
Do not confuse erythromycin with azithromycin or Ethmozine, or Eryc with Emct.

CATEGORY AND SCHEDULE

Pregnancy Risk Category: B

MECHANISM OF ACTION

A macrolide that reversibly binds to bacterial ribosomes, inhibiting bacterial protein synthesis. **Therapeutic Effect:** Bacteriostatic.

PHARMACOKINETICS

Variably absorbed from the GI tract (depending on dosage form used). Protein binding: 70%–90%. Widely distributed. Metabolized in the liver. Primarily eliminated in feces by bile. Not removed by hemodialysis. ***Half-life:*** 1.4–2 hr (increased in impaired renal function).

AVAILABILITY

Topical Gel (A/T/S, Emgel, Erygel): 2%.
Injection Powder for Reconstitution (Erythrocin): 500 mg, 1 g.
Ophthalmic Ointment: 5 mg/g.
Topical Ointment (Akne-Mycin): 2%.
Oral Suspension (EryPed, EES): 200 mg/5 ml, 400 mg/5 ml.
Topical Solution (Staticin): 1.5%.
Topical Solution (A/T/S, EryDerm, Erythra-Derm): 2%.
Tablet (Chewable [Ery-Ped]): 200 mg.
Tablets (Ery-Tab): 250 mg, 333 mg, 500 mg.
Tablets (EES): 400 mg.
Tablets (Erythrocin): 250 mg, 500 mg.
Tablets (PCE): 333 mg, 500 mg.

INDICATIONS AND DOSAGES

▸ **Mild to moderate infections of the upper and lower respiratory tract, pharyngitis, skin infections**
PO
Adults, Elderly. 250 mg q6h, 500 mg q12h, or 333 mg q8h. Maximum: 4 g/day.
Children. 30–50 mg/kg/day in divided doses up to 60–100 mg/kg/day for severe infections.
Neonates. 20–40 mg/kg/day in divided doses q6–12h.
IV
Adults, Elderly, Children. 15–20 mg/kg/day in divided doses. Maximum: 4 g/day.

▸ **Preoperative intestinal antisepsis**
PO
Adults, Elderly. 1 g at 1 pm, 2 pm, and 11 pm on day before surgery (with neomycin).
Children. 20 mg/kg at 1pm, 2pm, and 11 pm on day before surgery (with neomycin).

▸ **Acne vulgaris**
Topical
Adults. Apply thin layer to affected area twice a day.

▸ **Gonococcal ophthalmia neonatorum**
Ophthalmic
Neonates. 0.5–2 cm no later than 1 hr after delivery.

OFF-LABEL USES

Systemic: Treatment of acne vulgaris, chancroid, *Campylobacter* enteritis, gastroparesis, Lyme disease
Topical: Treatment of minor bacterial skin infections
Ophthalmic: Treatment of blepharitis, conjunctivitis, keratitis, chlamydial trachoma

CONTRAINDICATIONS

Administration of fixed-combination product, Pediazole, to infants younger than 2 months; history of hepatitis due to macrolides; hypersensitivity to macrolides; pre-existing hepatic disease

INTERACTIONS

Drug

Buspirone, cyclosporine, felodipine, lovastatin, simvastatin: May increase the blood concentration and toxicity of these drugs.
Carbamazepine: May inhibit the metabolism of carbamazepine.
Chloramphenicol, clindamycin: May decrease the effects of these drugs.
Hepatotoxic medications: May increase the risk of hepatotoxicity.
Theophylline: May increase the risk of theophylline toxicity.
Warfarin: May increase warfarin's effects.

Herbal

None known.

Food

None known.

DIAGNOSTIC TEST EFFECTS

May increase serum alkaline phosphatase, bilirubin, AST (SGOT), and ALT (SGPT) levels.

IV INCOMPATIBILITIES

Fluconazole (Diflucan)

IV COMPATIBILITIES

Aminophylline, amiodarone (Cordarone), diltiazem (Cardizem), heparin, hydromorphone (Dilaudid), lidocaine, lorazepam (Ativan), magnesium sulfate, midazolam (Versed), morphine, multivitamins, potassium chloride

SIDE EFFECTS

Frequent

IV: Abdominal cramping or discomfort, phlebitis or thrombophlebitis
Topical: Dry skin (50%)

Occasional

Nausea, vomiting, diarrhea, rash, urticaria

Rare

Ophthalmic: Sensitivity reaction with increased irritation, burning, itching, and inflammation
Topical: Urticaria

SERIOUS REACTIONS

! Antibiotic-associated colitis and other superinfections may occur.
! High dosages in patients with renal impairment may lead to reversible hearing loss.
! Anaphylaxis and hepatotoxicity occur rarely.
! Ventricular arrhythmias and prolonged QT interval occur rarely with the IV drug form.

NURSING CONSIDERATIONS

Baseline Assessment

◂ALERT▸ Determine if the patient has a history of hepatitis or allergies to erythromycin or other macrolides before beginning drug therapy.

Lifespan Considerations

- Erythromycin crosses the placenta and is distributed in breast milk.
- Erythromycin estolate may increase liver function test results in pregnant women.
- No age-related precautions have been noted in children or the elderly.

Precautions

- Use erythromycin cautiously in patients with hepatic dysfunction.
- Use the combination drug Pediazole (erythromycin and sulfisoxazole) cautiously in patients with impaired renal or hepatic function, severe allergies, bronchial asthma, or glucose-6-phosphate dehydrogenase deficiency.

Administration and Handling

PO

- Store capsules and tablets at room temperature.
- The oral suspension is stable for 14 days at room temperature.
- Administer erythromycin base or stearate 1 hour before or 2 hours after a meal. Erythromycin estolate and ethylsuccinate may be given without regard to food, but are absorbed better when given on an empty stomach.
- Give tablets or capsules with 8 oz of water.
- If the patient has difficulty swallowing, sprinkle the capsule contents in a teaspoonful of applesauce and follow with water.
- Make sure the patient doesn't swallow chewable tablets whole.

IV

- Store the parenteral form at room temperature.
- The initial reconstituted solution in vial is stable for 24 hours at room temperature and 2 weeks if refrigerated.
- Diluted IV solutions are stable for 8 hours at room temperature and 24 hours if refrigerated.
- Discard the solution if a precipitate forms.
- Reconstitute each 500-mg vial with 10 ml or each 1-g vial with 20 ml sterile water for injection without a preservative to provide a concentration of 50 mg/ml.
- Further dilute with 100 to 250 ml D_5W or 0.9% NaCl.
- Administer intermittent IV infusion (piggyback) over 20 to 60 minutes.
- Administer continuous infusion over 6 to 24 hours.

Ophthalmic

- Place a gloved finger on the patient's lower eyelid, and pull it out until a pocket is formed between the eye and the lower lid. Place ¼–½ inch of ointment into the pocket.
- Have the patient close the eye for 1 to 2 minutes and roll the eyeball gently to increase the drug's distribution.
- Remove excess ointment around the eye with tissue.

Intervention and Evaluation

- Assess the patient's pattern of daily bowel activity and stool consistency.
- Examine the patient's skin for a rash.
- Evaluate the patient for signs and symptoms of hepatotoxicity, including abdominal pain, fever, GI disturbances, and malaise.
- Evaluate the patient for signs and symptoms of superinfection, such as genital and anal pruritus, sore mouth or tongue, abdominal cramps, and moderate to severe diarrhea.
- Check the patient's injection site for signs and symptoms of phlebitis, such as heat, pain, and red streaking over the vein.
- Monitor the patient for signs of hearing loss because high dosages can cause hearing loss in patients with hepatic or renal dysfunction.

Patient Teaching

- Instruct the patient to take the oral

form of erythromycin with 8 oz of water 1 hour before or 2 hours after food or beverage. Teach the patient not to swallow chewable tablets whole.

• Advise the patient to space doses evenly around the clock and to continue erythromycin therapy for the full course of treatment.

• Caution the patient using the ophthalmic form of erythromycin to notify the physician if burning, inflammation, or itching occurs.

• Advise the patient using the topical form of erythromycin to notify the physician if burning, excessive dryness, or itching occurs.

• Inform the patient being treated for acne that maximum improvement may take 3 months and that erythromycin therapy may need to be continued for months or years.

• Advise the patient being treated for acne to wait at least 1 hour before using other topical acne preparations containing abrasive or peeling agents, such as medicated soaps, and cosmetics or aftershave containing alcohol.

9 Penicillins

amoxicillin
amoxicillin/clavulanate potassium
ampicillin sodium
ampicillin/sulbactam sodium
oxacillin
penicillin G benzathine
penicillin G potassium
penicillin V potassium
piperacillin sodium/tazobactam sodium
ticarcillin disodium/clavulanate potassium

Uses: Penicillins may be used to treat a large number of infections, including pneumonia and other respiratory infections, UTIs, septicemia, meningitis, intra-abdominal infections, gonorrhea, syphilis, and bone and joint infections. These agents are classified by their antimicrobial spectrum of activity. *Natural penicillins,* such as penicillin G benzathine and penicillin V potassium, are very active against gram-positive cocci but are ineffective against most strains of *Staphylococcus aureus* because the drugs are inactivated by the enzyme penicillinase, which is produced by these organisms.

Penicillinase-resistant penicillins, such as oxacillin, are effective against penicillinase-producing *S. aureus* but are less effective against gram-positive cocci than the natural penicillins. *Broad-spectrum penicillins,* such as amoxicillin and ampicillin sodium, are effective against gram-positive cocci and some gram-negative bacteria, such as *Haemophilus influenzae, Escherichia coli,* and *Proteus mirabilis. Extended-spectrum penicillins,* such as piperacillin sodium and tazobactam sodium and ticarcillin disodium and clavulanate potassium, are effective against *Pseudomonas aeruginosa, Enterobacter* species, *Proteus* species, *Klebsiella* species, and some other gram-negative organisms.

Action: Penicillins inhibit cell wall synthesis by binding to and inactivating penicillin-binding proteins, which are enzymes responsible for bacterial cell wall development. By inactivating these enzymes, penicillins disrupt and weaken bacterial cell walls resulting in cell lysis and death. They may be bacteriostatic or bactericidal and are most effective against bacteria undergoing active growth and division. (See the illustration *Mechanisms of Action: Penicillins,* page 175.)

COMBINATION PRODUCTS

BICILLIN CR: penicillin G benzathine/penicillin procaine 600,000 units/600,000 units.

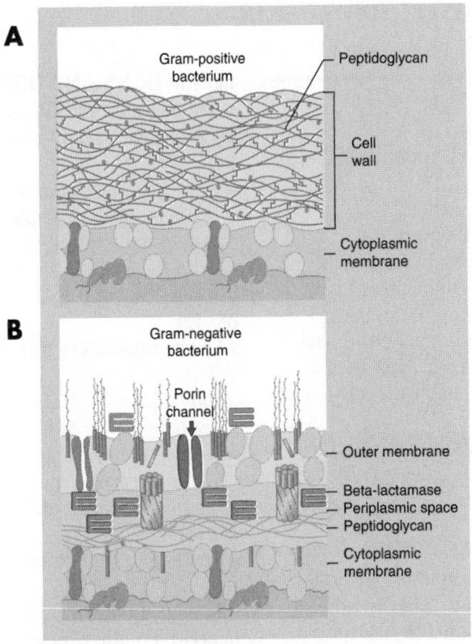

Mechanisms of Action: Penicillins

Penicillins generally act by weakening the normally rigid cell walls of bacteria. A weakened wall causes the cell to absorb excess water, leading to cellular swelling and rupture. However, penicillins' effectiveness is determined by the structure of the bacterial cell wall, which differs in gram-positive and gram-negative bacteria.

Gram-positive bacteria (A) have a rigid cell wall composed of long strands of peptidoglycan. This peptidoglycan is held together by cross-bridges, which are formed by transpeptidase and give the cell wall its strength. Autolysins (bacterial enzymes that adhere to cellular bonds in the wall) are also present in the cell wall. Bacteria use these enzymes to break down portions of the cell wall to permit growth and cell division. Penicillins inhibit transpeptidases, thereby interfering with the creation of cross-bridges and weakening the cell wall. They also activate autolysins, which leads to cell wall breakdown and cell destruction.

Gram-negative bacteria (B) have a different cell wall structure. Unlike gram-positive bacteria, which have two layers (a cell wall and a cytoplasmic membrane), gram-negative bacteria have three layers (an outer membrane, a thin cell wall, and a cytoplasmic membrane). Although penicillins can penetrate the cell wall, they must first penetrate the outer membrane. Only a few penicillins are small enough to pass through the tiny openings (porin channels) in the outer membrane to be effective against gram-negative bacteria.

In addition, gram-positive and gram-negative bacteria produce enzymes called beta-lactamases, which can render penicillins ineffective. Beta-lactamases that act specifically on penicillins are known as penicillinases. Gram-positive bacteria produce large amount of penicillinases but release them into the environment around the cell. In contrast, gram-negative bacteria produce smaller amounts of these enzymes but release them into the periplasmic space. So even if a penicillin can pass through the porin channel, it must also be resistant to penicillinase to achieve its therapeutic effect.

amoxicillin

a-**mox**-i-sill-in

(Alphamox[AUS], Amohexal[AUS], Amoxil, Amoxil Duo[AUS], Apo-Amoxi[CAN], Cilamox[AUS], Clamoxyl[AUS], DisperMox, Fisamox[AUS], Maxamox[AUS], Moxacin[AUS], Novamoxin[CAN], Polymox, Trimox, Wymox)

Do not confuse amoxicillin with amoxapine, DisperMox with Diamox, or Trimox with Tylox.

CATEGORY AND SCHEDULE

Pregnancy Risk Category: B

MECHANISM OF ACTION

A penicillin that inhibits bacterial cell wall synthesis. **Therapeutic Effect:** Bactericidal in susceptible microorganisms.

PHARMACOKINETICS

Well absorbed from the GI tract. Protein binding: 20%. Partially metabolized in the liver. Primarily excreted in urine. Removed by hemodialysis. ***Half-life:*** 1–1.3 hr (increased in impaired renal function).

AVAILABILITY

Capsules (Amoxil, Moxillin, Trimox): 250 mg, 500 mg.
Oral drops (Amoxil): 125 mg/5 ml, 200 mg/5 ml, 250 mg/5 ml, 400 mg/5 ml.
Tablets (Amoxil): 500 mg, 875 mg.
Tablets (Chewable [Amoxil]): 200 mg, 250 mg, 400 mg.
Tablets for Oral Suspension (DisperMox): 200 mg, 400 mg.

INDICATIONS AND DOSAGES

▸ **Ear, nose, throat, GU, skin, and skin-structure infections**
PO
Adults, Elderly, Children weighing more than 20 kg. 250–500 mg q8h or 500–875 mg (tablets) twice a day
Children weighing less than 20 kg. 20–40 mg/kg/day in divided doses q8–12h.

▸ **Lower respiratory tract infections**
PO
Adults, Elderly, Children weighing more than 20 kg. 500 mg q8h or 875 mg (tablets) twice a day.
Children weighing less than 20 kg. 40 mg/kg/day in divided doses q8–12h.

▸ **Acute, uncomplicated gonorrhea**
PO
Adults. 3 g one time with 1 g probenecid. Follow with tetracycline or erythromycin therapy.
Children 2 yr and older. 50 mg/kg plus probenecid 25 mg/kg as a single dose.

▸ **Acute otitis media**
PO
Children. 80–90 mg/kg/day in divided doses q12h.

▸ ***Helicobacter pylori*** **infection**
PO
Adults, Elderly. 1 g twice a day for 10 days (in combination with other antibiotics).

▸ **Prevention of endocarditis**
PO
Adults, Elderly. 2 g 1 hr before procedure.
Children. 50 mg/kg 1 hr before procedure.

▸ **Usual pediatric dosage**
Neonates, Children younger than 3 mo. 20–30 mg/kg/day in divided doses q12h.

▸ **Dosage in renal impairment**
Dosage interval is modified based on creatinine clearance.

Creatinine clearance 10–30 ml/min. Usual dose q12h.
Creatinine clearance less than 10 ml/min. Usual dose q24h.

OFF-LABEL USES

Treatment of Lyme disease and typhoid fever

CONTRAINDICATIONS

Hypersensitivity to any penicillin, infectious mononucleosis

INTERACTIONS

Drug

Allopurinol: May increase incidence of rash.
Oral contraceptives: May decrease effectiveness of oral contraceptives.
Probenecid: May increase amoxicillin blood concentration and risk of toxicity.

Herbal

None known.

Food

None known.

DIAGNOSTIC TEST EFFECTS

May increase BUN and serum LDH, bilirubin, creatinine, AST (SGOT), and ALT (SGPT) levels. May cause a positive Coombs' test.

SIDE EFFECTS

Frequent

GI disturbances (mild diarrhea, nausea, or vomiting), headache, oral or vaginal candidiasis

Occasional

Generalized rash, urticaria

SERIOUS REACTIONS

! Antibiotic-associated colitis and other superinfections may result from altered bacterial balance.
! Severe hypersensitivity reactions, including anaphylaxis and acute interstitial nephritis occur rarely.

NURSING CONSIDERATIONS

Baseline Assessment

- Determine if the patient has a history of allergies, especially to cephalosporins or penicillins, before giving the drug.

Lifespan Consideration

- Amoxicillin crosses the placenta, appears in cord blood and amniotic fluid, and is distributed in breast milk in low concentrations.
- Amoxicillin administration may lead to allergic sensitization, candidiasis, diarrhea, and skin rash in infants.
- Immature renal function in neonates and young infants may delay renal excretion of amoxicillin.
- Age-related renal impairment may require dosage adjustment in the elderly.

Precautions

- Use amoxicillin cautiously in patients with antibiotic-associated colitis or a history of allergies, especially to cephalosporins.

Administration and Handling

PO

- Store capsules or tablets at room temperature.
- Instruct the patient to chew or crush chewable tablets thoroughly before swallowing.
- After reconstitution, the oral solution is stable for 14 days either at room temperature or refrigerated.
- Give amoxicillin without regard to food.

Intervention and Evaluation

- Withhold amoxicillin and promptly notify the physician if the patient experiences a rash or diarrhea. Severe diarrhea with abdominal pain, blood or mucus in stool, and fever may indicate antibiotic-associated colitis.
- Monitor the patient for signs and symptoms of superinfection, includ-

ing anal or genital pruritus, black hairy tongue, diarrhea, increased fever, sore throat, ulceration or changes of oral mucosa, and vomiting.

Patient Teaching

- Urge the patient to space doses evenly around the clock and to continue taking amoxicillin for the full course of treatment.
- Instruct the patient to take amoxicillin with meals if GI upset occurs.
- Advise the patient to thoroughly chew or crush the chewable tablets before swallowing.
- Warn the patient to notify the physician if diarrhea, a rash, or other new symptoms occur.

amoxicillin/ clavulanate potassium

a-**mox**-i-sill-in/clav-u-**lan**-ate (Augmentin, Augmentin ES 600, Augmentin XR, Ausclay[AUS], Ausclay Duo Forte[AUS], Ausclay Duo 400[AUS], Clamoxyl[AUS], Clamoxyl Duo 400 [AUS], Clamoxyl Duo Forte[AUS], Clavulin[CAN], Clavulin Duo Forte[AUS])

Do not confuse amoxicillin with amoxapine.

CATEGORY AND SCHEDULE

Pregnancy Risk Category: B

MECHANISM OF ACTION

Amoxicillin inhibits bacterial cell wall synthesis, while clavulanate inhibits bacterial beta-lactamase. **Therapeutic Effect:** Amoxicillin is bactericidal in susceptible microorganisms. Clavulanate protects amoxicillin from enzymatic degradation.

PHARMACOKINETICS

Well absorbed from the GI tract. Protein binding: 20%. Partially metabolized in the liver. Primarily excreted in urine. Removed by hemodialysis. ***Half-life***: 1–1.3 hr (increased in impaired renal function).

AVAILABILITY

Powder for Oral Suspension: 125 mg/5 ml, 200 mg/5 ml, 250 mg/5 ml, 400 mg/5 ml, 600 mg/5 ml.
Tablets: 250 mg, 500 mg, 875 mg.
Tablets (Extended-Release): 1,000 mg.
Tablets (Chewable): 125 mg, 200 mg, 250 mg, 400 mg.

INDICATIONS AND DOSAGES

▸ **Mild to moderate infections**

PO

Adults, Elderly, Children weighing more than 40 kg. 250 mg q8h or 500 mg q12h.
Children weighing less than 40 kg. 20 mg/kg/day in divided doses q8h.

▸ **Respiratory tract and other severe infections**

PO

Adults, Elderly, Children weighing more than 40 kg. 500 mg q8h or 875 mg q12h.
Children weighing less than 40 kg. 40 mg/kg/day in divided doses q8h.

▸ **Otitis media**

PO

Children. 90 mg/kg/day in divided doses q12h for 10 days.

▸ **Sinusitis, lower respiratory tract infections**

PO

Children. 40 mg/kg/day in divided doses q8h or 45 mg/kg/day in divided doses q12h.

▸ Usual neonate dosage
PO
Neonates, Children younger than 3 mo. 30 mg/kg/day in divided doses q12h.
▸ Dosage in renal impairment
Dosage and frequency are modified based on creatinine clearance.
Creatinine clearance 10–30 ml/min. 250–500 mg q12h.
Creatinine clearance less than 10 ml/min. 250–500 mg q24h.

OFF-LABEL USES
Treatment of bronchitis and chancroid

CONTRAINDICATIONS
Hypersensitivity to any penicillins, infectious mononucleosis

INTERACTIONS
Drug
Allopurinol: May increase incidence of rash.
Oral contraceptives: May decrease effects of oral contraceptives.
Probenecid: May increase amoxicillin and clavulanate blood concentration and risk of toxicity.
Herbal
None known.
Food
None known.

DIAGNOSTIC TEST EFFECTS
May increase serum AST (SGOT) and ALT (SGPT) levels. May cause a positive Coombs' test.

SIDE EFFECTS
Frequent
GI disturbances (mild diarrhea, nausea, vomiting), headache, oral or vaginal candidiasis
Occasional
Generalized rash, urticaria

SERIOUS REACTIONS
! Antibiotic-associated colitis and other superinfections may result from altered bacterial balance.
! Severe hypersensitivity reactions, including anaphylaxis and acute interstitial nephritis occur rarely.

NURSING CONSIDERATIONS
Baseline Assessment
◂ALERT▸ Determine if the patient has a history of allergies, especially to cephalosporins or penicillins, before starting therapy.
Lifespan Considerations
- Amoxicillin and clavulanate crosses the placenta, appears in cord blood and amniotic fluid, and is distributed in breast milk in low concentrations.
- Amoxicillin and clavulanate may lead to allergic sensitization, candidiasis, diarrhea, and skin rash in infants.
- Immature renal function in neonates and young infants may delay renal excretion of amoxicillin and clavulanate.
- Age-related renal impairment may require a dosage adjustment in the elderly.

Precautions
- Use amoxicillin and clavulanate cautiously in patients with antibiotic-associated colitis or a history of allergies, especially to cephalosporins.

Administration and Handling
◂ALERT▸ Drug dosage is expressed in terms of amoxicillin. Be aware that an alternative dosage is 500 to 875 mg twice a day for adults and 200 to 400 mg twice a day for children.
PO
- Store tablets at room temperature.
- After reconstitution, the oral solu-

tion is stable for 14 days either at room temperature or refrigerated.
• Give the drug without regard to meals.
• Instruct the patient to chew or crush chewable tablets thoroughly before swallowing.

Intervention and Evaluation

• Withhold amoxicillin and promptly notify the physician if the patient experiences a rash or diarrhea. Although a rash is a common side effect of amoxicillin, it may also indicate hypersensitivity. Severe diarrhea with abdominal pain, blood or mucus in stools, and fever may indicate antibiotic-associated colitis.
• Be alert for signs and symptoms of superinfection, including anal or genital pruritus, black hairy tongue, diarrhea, increased fever, sore throat, ulceration or changes of oral mucosa, and vomiting.

Patient Teaching

• Advise the patient to space doses evenly around the clock and to continue taking amoxicillin and clavulanate for the full course of treatment.
• Instruct the patient to take the drug with meals if GI upset occurs.
• Instruct the patient to thoroughly chew or crush the chewable tablets before swallowing.
• Warn the patient to notify the physician if diarrhea, rash, or other new symptoms occur.

ampicillin sodium

am-pi-**sill**-in **soe**-dee-um
(Alphacin[AUS], Apo-Ampi[CAN], Novo-Ampicillin[CAN], Nu-Ampi[CAN], Polycillin, Principen)
Do not confuse ampicillin with aminophylline, Imipenem, or Unipen.

CATEGORY AND SCHEDULE

Pregnancy Risk Category: B

MECHANISM OF ACTION

A penicillin that inhibits cell wall synthesis in susceptible microorganisms. **Therapeutic Effect:** Bactericidal.

PHARMACOKINETICS

Moderately absorbed from the GI tract. Protein binding: 28%. Widely distributed. Partially metabolized in the liver. Primarily excreted in urine. Removed by hemodialysis. ***Half-life:*** 1–1.5 hr (increased in impaired renal function).

AVAILABILITY

Capsules: 250 mg, 500 mg.
Powder for Oral Suspension: 125 mg/5 ml, 250 mg/5 ml, 500 mg/5 ml.
Powder for Injection: 125 mg, 250 mg, 500 mg, 1 g, 2 g.

INDICATIONS AND DOSAGES

▸ **Respiratory tract, skin and skin-structure infections**

PO

Adults, Elderly. 250–500 mg q6h.
Children. 50–100 mg/kg/day in divided doses q6h. Maxiumum: 3 g/day.

IV, IM

Adults, Elderly. 500 mg to 3 g q6h. Maxiumum: 14 g/day.

Children. 100–200 mg/kg/day in divided doses q6h.
Neonates. 50–100 mg/kg/day in divided doses q6–12h.

▸ **Meningitis**

IV

Children. 200–400 mg/kg/day in divided doses q6h. Maxiumum: 12 g/day
Neonates. 100–200 mg/kg/day in divided doses q6–12h.

▸ **Gonococcal infections**

PO

Adults. 3.5 g one time with 1 g probenecid.

▸ **Perioperative prophylaxis**

IV, IM

Adults, Elderly. 2 g 30 min before procedure. May repeat in 8 hr.
Children. 50 mg/kg 30 min before procedure. May repeat in 8 hr.

▸ **Dosage in renal impairment**

Creatinine Clearance	% of Normal Dosage
10–30 ml/min	give q6–12h
less than 10 ml/min	give q12h

CONTRAINDICATIONS

Hypersensitivity to any penicillin, infectious mononucleosis

INTERACTIONS

Drug

Allopurinol: May increase incidence of rash.
Oral contraceptives: May decrease effectiveness of oral contraceptives.
Probenecid: May increase ampicillin blood concentration and risk of ampicillin toxicity.

Herbal

None known.

Food

None known.

DIAGNOSTIC TEST EFFECTS

May increase AST (SGOT) and ALT (SGPT) levels. May cause a positive Coombs' test.

IV INCOMPATIBILITIES

Amikacin (Amikin), diltiazem (Cardizem), gentamicin, midazolam (Versed)

IV COMPATIBILITIES

Calcium gluconate, cefepime (Maxipime), dopamine (Intropin), famotidine (Pepcid), furosemide (Lasix), heparin, hydromorphone (Dilaudid), insulin (regular), levofloxacin (Levaquin), magnesium sulfate, morphine, multivitamins, potassium chloride, propofol (Diprivan)

SIDE EFFECTS

Frequent

Pain at IM injection site, GI disturbances (mild diarrhea, nausea, vomiting), oral or vaginal candidiasis

Occasional

Generalized rash, urticaria, phlebitis or thrombophlebitis (with IV administration), headache

Rare

Dizziness, seizures (especially with IV therapy)

SERIOUS REACTIONS

! Antibiotic-associated colitis and other superinfections may result from altered bacterial balance.
! Severe hypersensitivity reactions, including anaphylaxis and acute interstitial nephritis, occur rarely.

NURSING CONSIDERATIONS

Baseline Assessment

◂**ALERT**▸ Determine if the patient has a history of allergies, especially to cephalosporins or penicillins, before starting drug therapy.

Lifespan Considerations

- Ampicillin readily crosses the placenta, appears in cord blood and

amniotic fluid, and is distributed in breast milk in low concentrations.
- Ampicillin may lead to allergic sensitization, candidiasis, diarrhea, and a rash in infants.
- Immature renal function in neonates and young infants may delay renal excretion of ampicillin.

◀ALERT▶ Keep in mind that higher dosages may be needed for neonatal meningitis.
- Age-related renal impairment may require a dosage adjustment in the elderly.

Precautions
- Use ampicillin cautiously in patients with antibiotic-associated colitis or a history of allergies, particularly to cephalosporins.

Administration and Handling

PO
- Store capsules at room temperature.
- After reconstitution, the oral suspension is stable for 7 days at room temperature and 14 days if refrigerated
- Give oral forms 1 hour before or 2 hours after meals for maximum absorption.

IV
- An IV solution diluted with 0.9% NaCl is stable for 2 to 8 hours at room temperature or 3 days if refrigerated.
- An IV solution diluted with D_5W is stable for 2 hours at room temperature or 3 hours if refrigerated.
- Discard the IV solution if a precipitate forms.
- For IV injection, dilute each 125-, 250-, or 500-mg vial with 5 ml sterile water for injection and each 1- or 2-g vial with 10 ml.
- For intermittent IV infusion (piggyback), further dilute with 50 to 100 ml 0.9% NaCl or D_5W.
- Administer each 125-, 250-, or 500-mg dose over 3 to 5 minutes and each 1- to 2-g dose over 10 to 15 minutes.
- Infuse intermittent IV infusion (piggyback) over 20 to 30 minutes.
- Because of the potential for hypersensitivity and anaphylaxis, start the initial dose at a few drops per minute, increase the dosage slowly to the prescribed rate, and stay with the patient for the first 10 to 15 minutes. Then assess the patient every 10 minutes during the infusion for signs and symptoms of hypersensitivity or anaphylaxis.
- Expect to switch to the oral route as soon as possible.

IM
- Reconstitute each vial with sterile water for injection or bacteriostatic water for injection. Consult individual ampicillin vials or package insert for specific volumes of diluent.
- The reconstituted solution is stable for 1 hour. Inject the drug deep into a large muscle mass.

Intervention and Evaluation
- Withhold ampicillin and promptly notify the physician if the patient experiences a rash or diarrhea. Although a rash is a common side effect of ampicillin, it also may indicate hypersensitivity. Severe diarrhea with abdominal pain, blood or mucus in stools, and fever may indicate antibiotic-associated colitis.
- Evaluate the IV site for signs of phlebitis, such as heat, pain, and red streaking over the vein.
- Check the IM injection site for pain and swelling.
- Monitor the patient's intake and output, renal function tests, and urinalysis results.
- Assess the patient for signs and symptoms of superinfection, such as anal or genital pruritus, black hairy tongue, oral ulceration or pain, diarrhea, increased fever, sore throat, and vomiting.

Patient Teaching

- Inform the patient that ampicillin is more effective if taken 1 hour before or 2 hours after consuming food or a beverage.
- Advise the patient to space doses evenly around the clock and to take ampicillin for the full course of treatment.
- Inform the patient that IM injections may cause discomfort.
- Warn the patient to notify the physician if diarrhea, rash, or other new symptoms occur.

ampicillin/sulbactam sodium

am-pi-sill-in/sul-**bac**-tam
(Unasyn)

CATEGORY AND SCHEDULE

Pregnancy Risk Category: B

MECHANISM OF ACTION

Ampicillin inhibits bacterial cell wall synthesis, while sulbactam inhibits bacterial beta-lactamase. **Therapeutic Effect:** Ampicillin is bactericidal in susceptible microorganisms. Sulbactam protects ampicillin from enzymatic degradation

PHARMACOKINETICS

Protein binding: 28%–38%. Widely distributed. Partially metabolized in the liver. Primarily excreted in urine. Removed by hemodialysis. ***Half-life:*** 1 hr (increased in impaired renal function).

AVAILABILITY

Powder for Injection: 1.5 g (ampicillin 1 g/sublactam 500 g), 3 g (ampicillin 2 g/sublactam 1 g).

INDICATIONS AND DOSAGES

▸ **Skin/skin-structure, intra-abdominal, and gynecologic infections**

IV, IM

Adults, Elderly. 1.5 g (1 g ampicillin/500 mg sulbactam) to 3 g (2 g ampicillin/1 g sulbactam) q6h.

▸ **Skin and skin-structure infections**

IV

Children 1–12 yr. 150–300 mg/kg/day in divided doses q6h.

▸ **Dosage in renal impairment**

Dosage and frequency are modified based on creatinine clearance and the severity of the infection.

Creatinine Clearance	Dosage
greater than 30 ml/min	0.5–3 g q6–8h
15–29 ml/min	1.5–3 g q12h
5–14 ml/min	1.5–3 g q24h
less than 5 ml/min	Not recommended

CONTRAINDICATIONS

Hypersensitivity to any penicillin, infectious mononucleosis

INTERACTIONS

Drug

Allopurinol: May increase incidence of rash.

Oral contraceptives: May decrease effectiveness of oral contraceptives.

Probenecid: May increase ampicillin blood concentration and risk of ampicillin toxicity.

Herbal

None known.

Food

None known.

DIAGNOSTIC TEST EFFECTS

May increase serum LDH, alkaline phosphatase, creatinine, AST (SGOT), and ALT (SGPT) levels. May cause a positive Coombs' test.

IV INCOMPATIBILITIES

Diltiazem (Cardizem), idarubicin (Idamycin), ondansetron (Zofran), sargramostim (Leukine)

IV COMPATIBILITIES

Famotidine (Pepcid), heparin, insulin (regular), morphine

SIDE EFFECTS

Frequent

Diarrhea and rash (most common), urticaria, pain at IM injection site, thrombophlebitis with IV administration, oral or vaginal candidiasis

Occasional

Nausea, vomiting, headache, malaise, urine retention

SERIOUS REACTIONS

! Severe hypersensitivity reactions, including anaphylaxis, acute interstitial nephritis, and blood dyscrasias may occur.

! Antibiotic-associated colitis and other superinfections may result from altered bacterial balance.

! Overdose may produce seizures.

NURSING CONSIDERATIONS

Baseline Assessment

◀ALERT▶ Determine if the patient has a history of allergies, especially to cephalosporins or penicillins, before giving the drug.

Lifespan Considerations

- Ampicillin readily crosses the placenta, appears in cord blood and amniotic fluid, and is distributed in breast milk in low concentrations.
- Ampicillin may lead to allergic sensitization, candidiasis, diarrhea, and a rash in infants.
- The safety and efficacy of ampicillin and sulbactam have not been established in children younger than 1 year.
- Age-related renal impairment may require a dosage adjustment in the elderly. Elderly, age-related renal impairment may require dosage adjustment.

Precautions

- Use ampicillin and sulbactam cautiously in patients with antibiotic-associated colitis or a history of allergies, particularly to cephalosporins.

Administration and Handling

IV

- When reconstituted with 0.9% NaCl, the IV solution is stable for 8 hours at room temperature or 48 hours if refrigerated. Stability may differ with other diluents.
- Discard the IV solution if a precipitate forms.
- For IV injection, dilute with 10 to 20 ml sterile water for injection.
- For intermittent IV infusion (piggyback), further dilute with 50 to 100 ml D_5W or 0.9% NaCl.
- Administer IV injection slowly, over 10 to 15 minutes.
- Administer intermittent IV infusion (piggyback) over 15 to 30 minutes.
- Because of the potential for hypersensitivity and anaphylaxis, start the initial dose at a few drops per minute, and then increase the dose slowly to the ordered rate. Stay with the patient for the first 10 to 15 minutes; then check the patient every 10 minutes during the infusion for signs and symptoms of hypersensitivity or anaphylaxis.
- Expect to switch to an oral antibiotic as soon as possible.

IM

- Reconstitute each 1.5-g vial with 3.2 ml or each 3-g vial with 6.4 ml of sterile water for injection to provide a concentration of 250 mg ampicillin/125 mg sulbactam per milliliter.
- Administer the injection deep into

a large muscle mass within 1 hour of preparation.

Intervention and Evaluation

- Withhold ampicillin and promptly notify the physician if the patient experiences a rash or diarrhea. Although a rash is a common side effect of ampicillin, it may also indicate hypersensitivity. Severe diarrhea with abdominal pain, blood or mucus in stools, and fever may indicate antibiotic-associated colitis.
- Evaluate the IV site for signs of phlebitis, such as heat, pain, and red streaking over vein.
- Check the IM injection site for pain and swelling.
- Monitor the patient's intake and output, renal function test results, and urinalysis results.
- Assess the patient for signs and symptoms of superinfection, such as anal or genital pruritus, black hairy tongue, changes in oral mucosa, diarrhea, increased fever, sore throat, and vomiting.

Patient Teaching

- Advise the patient to space doses evenly around the clock and to take ampicillin for the full course of treatment.
- Inform the patient that IM injections may cause discomfort.
- Warn the patient to notify the physician if diarrhea, rash, or other new symptoms occur.

oxacillin

ox-a-**sill**-in

CATEGORY AND SCHEDULE

Pregnancy Risk Category: B

MECHANISM OF ACTION

A penicillin that binds to bacterial membranes. **Therapeutic Effect:** Bactericidal.

AVAILABILITY

Powder for Injection: 1-g vials, 2-g vials.

INDICATIONS AND DOSAGES

▸ Upper respiratory tract, skin, and skin-structure infections

IV, IM

Adults, Elderly, Children weighing 40 kg or more. 250–500 mg q4–6h.

Children weighing less than 40 kg. 50 mg/kg/day in divided doses q6h. Maximum: 12 g/day.

▸ Lower respiratory tract and other serious infections

IV, IM

Adults, Elderly, Children weighing 40 kg or more. 1 g q4–6h. Maximum: 12 g/day.

Children weighing less than 40 kg. 100 mg/kg/day in divided doses q4–6h.

CONTRAINDICATIONS

Hypersensitivity to any penicillin

INTERACTIONS

Drug

Probenecid: May increase oxacillin blood concentration and risk of toxicity.

Herbal

None known.

Food

None known.

DIAGNOSTIC TEST EFFECTS

May increase AST (SGOT) levels. May cause a positive Coombs' test.

SIDE EFFECTS

Frequent

Mild hypersensitivity reaction (fever, rash, pruritus), GI effects (nausea, vomiting, diarrhea)

Occasional
Phlebitis, thrombophlebitis (more common in elderly), hepatotoxicity (with high IV dosage)

SERIOUS REACTIONS

! Antibiotic-associated colitis and other superinfections may result from altered bacterial balance.
! A mild to severe hypersensitivity reaction may occur in those allergic to penicillins.

NURSING CONSIDERATIONS

Baseline Assessment
• Determine if the patient has a history of allergies, especially to cephalosporins or penicillin, before starting oxacillin therapy.
Precautions
• Use oxacillin cautiously in patients with impaired renal function or a history of allergies, especially to cephalosporins.
Administration and Handling
IV
• Store vials at room temperature.
• Once reconstituted, the solution remains stable for 3 days at room temperature or 7 days refrigerated. When further diluted with D_5W or 0.9% NaCl, the solution is stable for 24 hours.
• Add 10 ml sterile water for injection to each 1-g vial to provide a concentration of 100 mg/ml.
• For piggyback administration, further dilute with 50 to 100 mg D_5W or 0.9% NaCl.
• Administer IV push over 10 minutes and IV piggyback over 30 minutes.
Intervention and Evaluation
• Withhold oxacillin as prescribed, and promptly notify the physician if the patient experiences a rash or diarrhea with abdominal pain, blood or mucus in stools, fever.
• Evaluate the patient's IV site frequently for signs of phlebitis, such as heat, pain, and red streaking over the vein.
• Monitor the patient's intake and output, renal function test results, and urinalysis results.
• Assess the patient for signs and symptoms of superinfection, such as anal or genital pruritus, black hairy tongue, oral ulceration or pain, diarrhea, increased fever, sore throat, and vomiting.
Patient Teaching
• Tell the patient to immediately report burning or pain at the IV site.
• Instruct the patient to immediately report signs of an allergic reaction, such as shortness of breath, chest tightness, or hives.
• Encourage the patient to practice good oral hygiene.

penicillin G benzathine

pen-ih-**sil**-lin G **benz**-ah-thene
(Bicillin LA, Permapen)
Do not confuse penicillin G benzathine with penicillin G potassium or penicillin G procaine.

CATEGORY AND SCHEDULE

Pregnancy Risk Category: B

MECHANISM OF ACTION

A penicillin that inhibits bacterial cell wall synthesis by binding to one or more of the penicillin-binding proteins of bacteria. **Therapeutic Effect:** Bactericidal.

AVAILABILITY

Injection (Prefilled Syringe [Bicillin LA, Permapen]): 600,000 units/ml.

INDICATIONS AND DOSAGES

▸ Group A streptococcal infections

IM

Adults, Elderly. 1.2 million units as a single dose.

Children. 25,000–50,000 units/kg as a single dose.

▸ Prevention of rheumatic fever

IM

Adults, Elderly. 1.2 million units every 3–4wk or 600,000 units twice monthly.

Children. 25,000–50,000 units/kg every 3–4wk.

▸ Early syphilis

IM

Adults, Elderly. 2.4 million units divided and administered in two separate injection sites.

▸ Congenital syphilis

IM

Children. 50,000 units/kg weekly for 3 wk.

▸ Syphilis of more than 1 year's duration

IM

Adults, Elderly. 2.4 million units divided and administered in two separate injection sites weekly for 3 wk.

Children. 50,000 units/kg weekly for 3 wk.

CONTRAINDICATIONS

Hypersensitivity to any penicillin

INTERACTIONS

Drug

Erythromycin: May antagonize effects of penicillin.

Probenecid: Increases serum concentration of penicillin.

Herbal

None known.

Food

None known.

DIAGNOSTIC TEST EFFECTS

May cause a positive Coombs' test.

SIDE EFFECTS

Occasional

Lethargy, fever, dizziness, rash, pain at injection site

Rare

Seizures, interstitial nephritis

SERIOUS REACTIONS

! Hypersensitivity reactions, ranging from chills, fever, and rash to anaphylaxis, may occur.

NURSING CONSIDERATIONS

Baseline Assessment

- Determine if the patient has a history of allergies, particularly to cephalosporins or penicillins, before beginning drug therapy.

Precautions

- Use penicillin G benzathine cautiously in patients with a hypersensitivity to cephalosporins, impaired cardiac or renal function, or seizure disorders.

Administration and Handling

IM

- Store prefilled syringes in the refrigerator. Do not freeze them.
- Administer the drug undiluted by deep IM injection.

◂ALERT▸ Do not administer penicillin G benzathine IV, intra-arterially, or subcutaneously because doing so may cause heart attack, severe neurovascular damage, thrombosis, and death.

Intervention and Evaluation

- Monitor the patient's CBC, renal function test results, and urinalysis results.

Patient Teaching

- Inform the patient that he or she may experience temporary pain at the injection site.
- Warn the patient to immediately report chills, fever, rash, or any other unusual signs or symptoms.

penicillin G potassium

pen-ih-**sil**-lin G
(Megacillin[CAN], Novepen-G[CAN], Pfizerpen)
Do not confuse penicillin G potassium with penicillin G benzathine or penicillin G procaine.

CATEGORY AND SCHEDULE

Pregnancy Risk Category: B

MECHANISM OF ACTION

A penicillin that inhibits bacterial cell wall synthesis by binding to one or more of the penicillin-binding proteins of bacteria. **Therapeutic Effect:** Bactericidal.

AVAILABILITY

Injection: 5 million units.
Premixed Dextrose Solution: 1 million units, 2 million units, 3 million units.

INDICATIONS AND DOSAGES

▸ **Sepsis, meningitis, pericarditis, endocarditis, pneumonia due to susceptible gram-positive organisms (not *Staphylococcus aureus*) and some gram-negative organisms**
IV, IM
Adults, Elderly. 2–24 million units/day in divided doses q4–6h.
Children. 100,000–400,000 units/kg/day in divided doses q4–6h.
▸ **Dosage in renal impairment**
Dosage interval is modified based on creatinine clearance.

Creatinine Clearance	Dosage Interval
10–30 ml/min	Usual dose q8–12h
less than 10 ml/min	Usual dose q12–18h

CONTRAINDICATIONS

Hypersensitivity to any penicillin

INTERACTIONS

Drug
Erythromycin: May antagonize effects of penicillin.
Probenecid: Increases serum concentration of penicillin.
Herbal
None known.
Food
Food, milk: Decrease penicillin absorption.

DIAGNOSTIC TEST EFFECTS

May cause a positive Coombs' test.

IV INCOMPATIBILITIES

Amikacin (Amikin), aminophylline, amphotericin B, dopamine (Intropin)

IV COMPATIBILITIES

Amiodarone (Cordarone), calcium gluconate, diltiazem (Cardizem), diphenhydramine (Benadryl), furosemide (Lasix), heparin, hydromorphone (Dilaudid), lidocaine, magnesium sulfate, methylprednisolone (Solu-Medrol), morphine, potassium chloride

SIDE EFFECTS

Occasional
Lethargy, fever, dizziness, rash, electrolyte imbalance, diarrhea, thrombophlebitis
Rare
Seizures, interstitial nephritis

SERIOUS REACTIONS

! Hypersensitivity reactions ranging from rash, fever, and chills to anaphylaxis may occur.

NURSING CONSIDERATIONS

Baseline Assessment
◂ALERT▸ Determine if the patient

has a history of allergies, particularly to cephalosporins or penicillins, before beginning drug therapy.

Precautions

- Use penicillin G potassium cautiously in patients with a hypersensitivity to cephalosporins, impaired hepatic or renal function, or seizure disorders.

Administration and Handling

IV

- The reconstituted solution is stable for 7 days if refrigerated.
- Follow the manufacturer's guidelines for dilution.
- After reconstitution, further dilute with 50 to 100 ml D_5W or 0.9% NaCl to yield a final concentration of 100,000 to 500,000 units/ml (50,000 units/ml for infants and neonates).
- Infuse the solution over 15 to 60 minutes.

Intervention and Evaluation

- Monitor the patient's CBC, electrolyte levels, renal function test results, and urinalysis results.

Patient Teaching

- Advise the patient to space doses evenly and to continue taking the drug for the full course of treatment.
- Warn the patient to immediately notify the physician if he or she experiences diarrhea, a rash, fever or chills, or any other unusual signs or symptoms.

penicillin V potassium

pen-ih-**sil**-lin V

(Abbocillin VK[AUS], Apo-Pen-VK[CAN], Cilicaine VK[AUS], L.P.V.[AUS], Novo-Pen-VK[CAN], Veetids)

CATEGORY AND SCHEDULE

Pregnancy Risk Category: B

MECHANISM OF ACTION

A penicillin that inhibits cell wall synthesis by binding to bacterial cell membranes. **Therapeutic Effect:** Bactericidal.

PHARMACOKINETICS

Moderately absorbed from the GI tract. Protein binding: 80%. Widely distributed. Metabolized in the liver. Primarily excreted in urine. ***Half-life:*** 1 hr (increased in impaired renal function).

AVAILABILITY

Tablets: 250 mg, 500 mg.
Powder for Oral Solution: 125 mg/5 ml, 250 mg/5 ml.

INDICATIONS AND DOSAGES

▸ **Mild to moderate respiratory tract or skin or skin-structure infections, otitis media, necrotizing ulcerative gingivitis**

PO

Adults, Elderly, Children 12 yr and older. 125–500 mg q6–8h.
Children younger than 12 yr. 25–50 mg/kg/day in divided doses q6–8h. Maximum: 3 g/day.

▸ **Primary prevention of rheumatic fever**

PO

Adults, Elderly. 500 mg 2–3 times/day for 10 days.
Children. 250 mg 2–3 times/day for 10 days.

▸ **Primary prevention of rheumatic fever**

PO

Adults, Elderly, Children. 250 mg twice a day.

CONTRAINDICATIONS

Hypersensitivity to any penicillin

INTERACTIONS

Drug

Probenecid: May increase penicillin blood concentration and risk of toxicity.

Herbal
None known.

Food
None known.

DIAGNOSTIC TEST EFFECTS
May cause positive a Coombs' test.

SIDE EFFECTS
Frequent
Mild hypersensitivity reaction (chills, fever, rash), nausea, vomiting, diarrhea
Rare
Bleeding, allergic reaction

SERIOUS REACTIONS
! Severe hypersensitivity reactions, including anaphylaxis, may occur.
! Nephrotoxicity, antibiotic-associated colitis, and other superinfections may result from high dosages or prolonged therapy.

NURSING CONSIDERATIONS

Baseline Assessment
◀ALERT▶ Determine if the patient has a history of allergies, particularly to aspirin, cephalosporins, or penicillins, before beginning drug therapy.

Lifespan Considerations
- Penicillin V potassium readily crosses the placenta, appears in amniotic fluid and cord blood, and is distributed in breast milk in low concentrations.
- Use of penicillin V potassium may lead to allergic sensitization, candidiasis, diarrhea, and a rash in infants.
- Use caution when giving penicillin V to neonates and young infants because their immature renal function may delay renal excretion of the drug.
- Age-related renal impairment may require a dosage adjustment in the elderly.

Precautions
- Use penicillin V potassium cautiously in patients with renal impairment, a history of seizures, or a history of allergies, particularly to cephalosporins.

Administration and Handling
PO
- Store tablets at room temperature.
- After reconstitution, the oral solution is stable for 14 days if refrigerated.
- Space drug doses evenly around the clock.
- Give the drug without regard to food.

Intervention and Evaluation
- Withhold penicillin V potassium and promptly notify the physician if the patient experiences diarrhea or a rash. Severe diarrhea with abdominal pain, fever, and mucus or blood in stools may indicate antibiotic-associated colitis; a rash may indicate a hypersensitivity reaction.
- Monitor the patient's intake and output, renal function test results, and urinalysis results for signs of nephrotoxicity.
- Be alert for signs and symptoms of superinfection, including anal or genital pruritus, vaginal discharge, diarrhea, increased fever, nausea and vomiting, sore throat, and stomatitis.
- Review the patient's blood Hgb levels.
- Check the patient for signs of bleeding, including ecchymosis, overt bleeding, and swelling of tissue.

Patient Teaching
- Advise the patient to space doses evenly around the clock and to continue taking penicillin V potassium for the full course of treatment.
- Warn the patient to immediately notify the physician if he or she

experiences bleeding, bruising, diarrhea, a rash, or any other new symptoms.

piperacillin sodium/ tazobactam sodium

pip-ur-ah-**sill**-in/tay-zoe-**back**-tam
(Tazocin[CAN], Zosyn)
Do not confuse Zosyn with Zofran or Zyvox.

CATEGORY AND SCHEDULE

Pregnancy Risk Category: B

MECHANISM OF ACTION

Piperacillin inhibits cell wall synthesis by binding to bacterial cell membranes. Tazobactam inactivates bacterial beta-lactamase. **Therapeutic Effect:** Piperacillin is bactericidal in susceptible organisms. Tazobactam protects piperacillin from enzymatic degradation, extends its spectrum of activity, and prevents bacterial overgrowth.

PHARMACOKINETICS

Protein binding: 16%–30%. Widely distributed. Primarily excreted unchanged in urine. Removed by hemodialysis. ***Half-life:*** 0.7–1.2 hr (increased in hepatic cirrhosis and impaired renal function).

AVAILABILITY

◀ALERT▶ Piperacillin/tazobactam is a combination product in an 8:1 ratio of piperacillin to tazobactam.
Powder for Injection: 2.25 g, 3.375 g, 4.5 g.
Premix Ready to Use: 2.25 g, 3.375 g, 4.5 g.

INDICATIONS AND DOSAGES

▸ **Severe infections**
IV
Adults, Elderly, Children 12 yr and older. 4 g/0.5 g q8h or 3 g/0.375 g q6h. Maximum: 18 g/2.25 g daily.

▸ **Moderate infections**
IV
Adults, Elderly, Children 12 yr and older. 2 g/0.225g q6–8h.

▸ **Dosage in renal impairment**
Dosage and frequency are modified based on creatinine clearance.

Creatinine Clearance	Dosage
20–40 ml/min	8 g/1 g/day (2.25 g q6h)
less than 20 ml/min	6 g/0.75 g/day (2.25 g q8h)

▸ **Dosage in hemodialysis patients**
IV
Adults, Elderly. 2.25 g q8h with additional dose of 0.75 g after each dialysis session.

CONTRAINDICATIONS

Hypersensitivity to any penicillin

INTERACTIONS

Drug

Hepatotoxic medications: May increase the risk of hepatotoxicity.
Probenecid: May increase piperacillin blood concentration and risk of toxicity.

Herbal

None known.

Food

None known.

DIAGNOSTIC TEST EFFECTS

May increase serum sodium, alkaline phosphatase, bilirubin, LDH, AST (SGOT), and ALT (SGPT) levels. May decrease serum potassium level. May cause a positive Coombs' test.

IV INCOMPATIBILITIES

Amphotericin B (Fungizone), amphotericin B complex (Abelcet, AmBisome, Amphotec), chlorpromazine (Thorazine), dacarbazine (DTIC), daunorubicin (Cerubidine), dobutamine (Dobutrex), doxorubicin (Adriamycin), doxorubicin liposomal (Doxil), droperidol (Inapsine), famotidine (Pepcid), haloperidol (Haldol), hydroxyzine (Vistaril), idarubicin (Idamycin), minocycline (Minocin), nalbuphine (Nubain), prochlorperazine (Compazine), promethazine (Phenergan), vancomycin (Vancocin)

IV COMPATIBILITIES

Aminophylline, bumetanide (Bumex), calcium gluconate, diphenhydramine (Benadryl), dopamine (Intropin), enalapril (Vasotec), furosemide (Lasix), granisetron (Kytril), heparin, hydrocortisone (Solu-Cortef), hydromorphone (Dilaudid), lorazepam (Ativan), magnesium sulfate, methylprednisolone (Solu-Medrol), metoclopramide (Reglan), morphine, ondansetron (Zofran), potassium chloride

SIDE EFFECTS

Frequent

Diarrhea, headache, constipation, nausea, insomnia, rash

Occasional

Vomiting, dyspepsia, pruritus, fever, agitation, candidiasis, dizziness, abdominal pain, edema, anxiety, dyspnea, rhinitis

SERIOUS REACTIONS

! Antibiotic-associated colitis and other superinfections may result from altered bacterial balance.

! Seizures and other neurologic reactions are more likely to occur in patients with renal impairment and those who have received an overdose.

! Severe hypersensitivity reactions, including anaphylaxis, occur rarely.

NURSING CONSIDERATIONS

Baseline Assessment

◀ALERT▶ Determine if the patient has a history of allergies, especially to cephalosporins or penicillins, before beginning drug therapy.

Lifespan Considerations

- Piperacillin readily crosses the placenta, appears in amniotic fluid and cord blood, and is distributed in breast milk in low concentrations.
- Piperacillin use in infants may lead to allergic sensitization, candidiasis, diarrhea, and a rash.
- Piperacillin dosage has not been established for children younger than 12 years.
- Age-related renal impairment may require a dosage adjustment in the elderly.

Precautions

- Use piperacillin and tazobactam cautiously in patients with a history of allergies, especially to cephalosporins, a pre-existing seizure disorder, or renal impairment.

Administration and Handling

IV

- Reconstitute each 1-g vial with 5 ml D_5W or 0.9% NaCl. Shake vigorously to dissolve.
- The reconstituted vial is stable for 24 hours at room temperature and 48 hours if refrigerated.
- Further dilute with at least 50 ml D_5W, 0.9% NaCl, dextrose 5% in 0.9% NaCl, or lactated Ringer's solution.
- After further dilution, the solution is stable for 24 hours at room temperature and 7 days if refrigerated.
- Infuse the drug over 30 minutes.

Intervention and Evaluation

- Assess the patient's pattern of daily bowel activity and stool consistency. Mild GI effects may be tolerable, but severe symptoms may indicate the onset of antibiotic-associated colitis.
- Be alert for signs and symptoms of superinfection, including abdominal pain, moderate to severe diarrhea, severe anal or genital pruritus, and stomatitis.
- Monitor the patient's electrolyte levels (especially potassium), intake and output, renal function test results, and urinalysis results.

Patient Teaching

- Advise the patient to immediately notify the physician if he or she experiences severe diarrhea and to avoid taking antidiarrheals until directed to do so.
- Instruct the patient to notify the physician if pain, redness, or swelling occurs at the infusion site.
- Because piperacillin contains sodium, advise the patient to consult the physician about possibly reducing salt intake.

ticarcillin disodium/ clavulanate potassium

tie-car-**sill**-in/klah-view-**lan**-ate
(Timentin)

CATEGORY AND SCHEDULE

Pregnancy Risk Category: B

MECHANISM OF ACTION

Ticarcillin binds to bacterial cell walls, inhibiting cell wall synthesis. Clavulanate inhibits the action of bacterial beta-lactamase. **Therapeutic Effect:** Ticarcillin is bactericidal in susceptible organisms. Clavulanate protects ticarcillin from enzymatic degradation.

PHARMACOKINETICS

Widely distributed. Protein binding: ticarcillin 45%–60%, clavulanate 9%–30%. Minimally metabolized in the liver. Primarily excreted unchanged in urine. Removed by hemodialysis. ***Half-life:*** 1–1.2 hr (increased in impaired renal function).

AVAILABILITY

Powder for Injection: 3.1 g.
Premixed Solution for Infusion: 3.1 g/100 ml.

INDICATIONS AND DOSAGES

▸ Skin and skin-structure, bone, joint, and lower respiratory tract infections; septicemia; endometriosis

IV

Adults, Elderly. 3.1 g (3 g ticarcillin) q4–6h. Maximum: 18–24 g/day.
Children 3 mo and older. 200–300 mg (as ticarcillin) q4–6h.

▸ UTIs

IV

Adults, Elderly. 3.1 g q6–8h.

▸ Dosage in renal impairment

Dosage interval is modified based on creatinine clearance.

Creatinine Clearance	Dosage Interval
10–30 ml/min	Usual dose q8h
less than 10 ml/min	Usual dose q12h

CONTRAINDICATIONS

Hypersensitivity to any penicillin

INTERACTIONS

Drug

Anticoagulants, heparin, NSAIDs, thrombolytics: May increase the

risk of hemorrhage with high dosages of ticarcillin.
Probenecid: May increase ticarcillin blood concentration and risk of toxicity.

Herbal

None known.

Food

None known.

DIAGNOSTIC TEST EFFECTS

May increase bleeding time and serum alkaline phosphatase, bilirubin, creatinine, LDH, AST (SGOT), and ALT (SGPT) levels. May decrease serum potassium, sodium, and uric acid levels. May cause a positive Coombs' test.

IV INCOMPATIBILITIES

Amphotericin B complex (Abelcet, AmBisome, Amphotec), vancomycin (Vancocin)

IV COMPATIBILITIES

Diltiazem (Cardizem), heparin, insulin, morphine, propofol (Diprivan)

SIDE EFFECTS

Frequent

Phlebitis or thrombophlebitis (with IV dose), rash, urticaria, pruritus, altered smell or taste

Occasional

Nausea, diarrhea, vomiting

Rare

Headache, fatigue, hallucinations, bleeding or ecchymosis

SERIOUS REACTIONS

! Overdosage may produce seizures and other neurologic reactions.
! Antibiotic-associated colitis and other superinfections may result from bacterial imbalance.
! Severe hypersensitivity reactions, including anaphylaxis, occur rarely.

NURSING CONSIDERATIONS

Baseline Assessment

◀ALERT▶ Determine if the patient has a history of allergies, especially to cephalosporins or penicillins, before beginning drug therapy.

Lifespan Considerations

- Ticarcillin readily crosses the placenta, appears in amniotic fluid and cord blood, and is distributed in breast milk in low concentrations.
- Ticarcillin use in infants may lead to allergic sensitization, candidiasis, diarrhea, and a rash.
- The safety and efficacy of this drug have not been established in children younger than 3 months.
- Age-related renal impairment may require a dosage adjustment in the elderly.

Precautions

- Use ticarcillin and clavulanate cautiously in patients with renal impairment or a history of allergies, especially to cephalosporins.

Administration and Handling

IV

- The solution normally appears colorless to pale yellow; a darker color indicates a loss of potency.
- The reconstituted IV infusion (piggyback) is stable for 24 hours at room temperature and 3 days if refrigerated.
- Discard the solution if a precipitate forms.
- This drug is available in ready-to-use containers.
- For IV infusion (piggyback), reconstitute each 3.1-g vial with 13 ml sterile water for injection or 0.9% NaCl to provide a concentration of 200 mg ticarcillin and 6.7 mg clavulanic acid per milliliter.
- Shake the vial to assist reconstitution.
- Further dilute with 50 to 100 ml D_5W or 0.9% NaCl.

- Infuse the drug over 30 minutes.
- Because of the potential for hypersensitivity reactions such as anaphylaxis, start the initial dose at a few drops per minute, and then increase it slowly to the ordered rate. Stay with the patient for the first 10 to 15 minutes during the initial dose; then check the patient every 10 minutes during the infusion for signs and symptoms of hypersensitivity or anaphylaxis.

Intervention and Evaluation

- Withhold the drug and promptly notify the physician of the patient experiences diarrhea or a rash. Severe diarrhea with fever, abdominal pain, and mucus or blood in stools may indicate antibiotic-associated colitis; a rash may be a sign of hypersensitivity.
- Assess the patient's food tolerance.
- Provide the patient with mouth care and sugarless gum or hard candy to offset the drug's bad taste and smell.
- Evaluate the IV site for signs and symptoms of phlebitis, such as heat, pain, and red streaking over the vein.
- Monitor the patient's intake and output, renal function test results, and urinalysis results.
- Assess the patient for ecchymosis, overt bleeding, and tissue swelling.
- Monitor the patient's hematology reports and serum electrolyte levels, particularly potassium.
- Be alert for signs and symptoms of superinfection, including anal or genital pruritus, diarrhea, increased fever, sore throat, vomiting, and pain or stomatitis.

Patient Teaching

- Advise the patient to immediately notify the physician if he or she experiences pain, redness, or swelling at the infusion site.
- Warn the patient to immediately notify the physician if he or she experiences severe diarrhea, a rash, itching, or any other unusual signs or symptoms.

10 Quinolones

ciprofloxacin hydrochloride
gatifloxacin
gemifloxacin mesylate
levofloxacin
lomefloxacin hydrochloride
moxifloxacin hydrochloride
norfloxacin
ofloxacin

Uses: Quinolones are used primarily to treat lower respiratory infections, skin and skin-structure infections, UTIs, and sexually transmitted diseases.

Action: Quinolones are bactericidal and act against a wide range of gram-negative and gram-positive organisms. In susceptible microorganisms, they inhibit DNA gyrase, the enzyme responsible for unwinding and supercoiling DNA before it replicates. By inhibiting DNA gyrase, quinolones interfere with bacterial cell replication and repair and cause cell death. (See the illustration *Sites and Mechanisms of Action: Anti-infective Agents,* page 2.)

COMBINATION PRODUCTS

CIPRODEX OTIC: ciprofloxacin/dexamethasone (a steroid) 0.3%/0.1%.
CIPRO HC OTIC: ciprofloxacin/hydrocortisone (a steroid) 0.2%/1%.

ciprofloxacin hydrochloride

sip-ro-**floks**-a-sin
(C-Flox[AUS], Ciloquin[AUS], Ciloxan, Cipro, Ciproxin[AUS])
Do not confuse ciprofloxacin or Ciloxan with cinoxacin or Cytoxan.

CATEGORY AND SCHEDULE

Pregnancy Risk Category: C

MECHANISM OF ACTION

A fluoroquinolone that inhibits the enzyme DNA gyrase in susceptible bacteria, interfering with bacterial cell replication. **Therapeutic Effect:** Bactericidal.

PHARMACOKINETICS

Well absorbed from the GI tract (food delays absorption). Protein binding: 20%–40%. Widely distributed (including to CSF). Metabolized in the liver to active metabolite. Primarily excreted in urine. Minimal removal by hemodialysis. ***Half-life:*** 4–6 hr (increased in impaired renal function and the elderly).

AVAILABILITY

Tablets (Cipro): 100 mg, 250 mg, 500 mg, 750 mg.
Tablets (Extended-Release [Cipro XR]): 500 mg, 1000 mg.
Infusion: 200 mg/100 ml, 400 mg/200 ml.
Ophthalmic Ointment (Ciloxan): 0.3%.
Ophthalmic Suspension (Ciloxan): 0.3%.

INDICATIONS AND DOSAGES

▸ **Mild to moderate UTIs**
PO
Adults, Elderly. 250 mg q12h.
IV
Adults, Elderly. 200 mg q12h.

▸ Complicated UTIs, mild to moderate respiratory tract, bone, joint, skin and skin-structure infections; infectious diarrhea
PO
Adults, Elderly. 500 mg q12h.
IV
Adults, Elderly. 400 mg q12h.
▸ Severe, complicated infections
PO
Adults, Elderly. 750 mg q12h.
IV
Adults, Elderly. 400 mg q12h.
▸ Prostatitis
PO
Adults, Elderly. 500 mg q12h for 28 days.
▸ Uncomplicated bladder infection
PO
Adults. 100 mg twice a day for 3 days.
▸ Acute sinusitis
PO
Adults. 500 mg q12h.
▸ Uncomplicated gonorrhea
PO
Adults. 250 mg as a single dose.
▸ Cystic fibrosis
IV
Children. 30 mg/kg/day in 2–3 divided doses. Maximum: 1.2 g/day.
PO
Children. 40 mg/kg/day. Maximum: 2 g/day.
▸ Corneal ulcer
Ophthalmic
Adults, Elderly. 2 drops q15min for 6 hr, then 2 drops q30min for the remainder of first day, 2 drops q1h on second day, and 2 drops q4h on days 3–14.
▸ Conjunctivitis
Ophthalmic
Adults, Elderly. 1–2 drops q2h for 2 days, then 2 drops q4h for next 5 days.
▸ Dosage in renal impairment
Dosage and frequency are modified based on creatinine clearance and the severity of the infection.

Creatinine Clearance	Dosage Interval
less than 30 ml/min	Usual dose q18–24h

▸ Hemodialysis
Adults, Elderly. 250–500 mg q24h (after dialysis).
▸ Peritoneal Dialysis
Adults, Elderly. 250–500 mg q24h (after dialysis).

OFF-LABEL USES
Treatment of chancroid

CONTRAINDICATIONS
Hypersensitivity to ciprofloxacin or other quinolones; for ophthalmic administration: vaccinia, varicella, epithelial herpes simplex, keratitis, mycobacterial infection, fungal disease of ocular structure, use after uncomplicated removal of a foreign body

INTERACTIONS
Drug
Antacids, iron preparations, sucralfate: May decrease ciprofloxacin absorption.
Caffeine, oral anticoagulants: May increase the effects of these drugs.
Theophylline: Decreases clearance and may increase blood concentration and risk of toxicity of theophylline.
Herbal
None known.
Food
None known.

DIAGNOSTIC TEST EFFECTS
May increase BUN and serum alkaline phosphatase, bilirubin, creatinine, LDH, AST (SGOT), and ALT (SGPT) levels.

IV INCOMPATIBILITIES
Aminophylline, ampicillin and

sulbactam (Unasyn), cefepime (Maxipime), dexamethasone (Decadron), furosemide (Lasix), heparin, hydrocortisone (Solu-Cortef), methylprednisolone (Solu-Medrol), phenytoin (Dilantin), sodium bicarbonate

IV COMPATIBILITIES

Calcium gluconate, diltiazem (Cardizem), dobutamine (Dobutrex), dopamine (Intropin), lidocaine, lorazepam (Ativan), magnesium, midazolam (Versed), potassium chloride

SIDE EFFECTS

Frequent (5%–2%)
Nausea, diarrhea, dyspepsia, vomiting, constipation, flatulence, confusion, crystalluria
Ophthalmic: Burning, crusting in corner of eye

Occasional (less than 2%)
Abdominal pain or discomfort, headache, rash
Ophthalmic: Bad taste, sensation of something in eye, eyelid redness or itching

Rare (less than 1%)
Dizziness, confusion, tremors, hallucinations, hypersensitivity reaction, insomnia, dry mouth, paresthesia

SERIOUS REACTIONS

! Superinfection (especially enterococcal or fungal), nephropathy, cardiopulmonary arrest, chest pain, and cerebral thrombosis may occur.
! Hypersensitivity reactions, including photosensitivity (as evidenced by rash, pruritus, blisters, edema, and burning skin), have occurred in patients receiving fluoroquinolones.
! Arthropathy may occur if the drug is given to children younger than 18 years.
! Sensitization to the ophthalmic form of the drug may contraindicate later systemic use of ciprofloxacin.

NURSING CONSIDERATIONS

Baseline Assessment
◀ **ALERT** ▶ Determine if the patient has a history of hypersensitivity to ciprofloxacinor other quinolones before beginning drug therapy.

Lifespan Considerations
- It is unknown if ciprofloxacin is distributed in breast milk. If possible, pregnant or breast-feeding women should avoid taking the drug because of the risk of arthropathy in the fetus or infant.
- The safety and efficacy of ciprofloxacin have not been established in children younger than 18 years.
- Age-related renal impairment may require a dosage adjustment in the elderly.

Precautions
- Use ciprofloxacin cautiously in patients with CNS disorders, renal impairment, or seizures and those taking caffeine or theophylline.
- Don't administer the oral suspension by NG tube.

Administration and Handling
PO
- Ciprofloxacin may be given without regard to food, but the preferred administration time is 2 hours after a meal.
- Don't administer antacids containing aluminum or magnesium within 2 hours of ciprofloxacin.
- Provide the patient with sufficient amounts of citrus fruits and cranberry juice to acidify urine.
- The oral suspension may be stored for 14 days at room temperature.

IV
- Store the injection form at room temperature.
- The solution normally appears clear and colorless or slightly yellow.

• After withdrawing the drug from a 200-mg or 400-mg vial, further dilute it with D_5W or 0.9% NaCl for injection to a final concentration of 1 to 2 mg/ml.
• Infuse the drug over 60 minutes.
• IV ciprofloxacin is also available prediluted in ready-to-use infusion containers.

Ophthalmic
• Tilt the patient's head back, and place the solution in the conjunctival sac of the affected eye.
• Close the patient's eye and then press gently on the lacrimal sac for 1 minute.
• Don't use ophthalmic solutions for injection.
• Unless the infection is very superficial, systemic administration generally accompanies ophthalmic use.

Intervention and Evaluation
• Evaluate the patient's food tolerance.
• Assess the patient's pattern of daily bowel activity and stool consistency.
• Evaluate the patient for dizziness, headache, tremors, and visual problems.
• Assess the patient for chest and joint pain.
• Observe patients receiving the ophthalmic form for a therapeutic response.

Patient Teaching
• Advise the patient not to skip drug doses and to take ciprofloxacin for the full course of therapy.
• Instruct the patient to take ciprofloxacin during meals with 8 oz of water and to drink several glasses of water between meals.
• Teach the patient to shake the oral suspension well before taking it and not to chew the microcapsules in the suspension.
• Encourage the patient to consume foods and juices that are high in ascorbic acid (such as citrus fruits and cranberry juice) to prevent crystalluria.
• Caution the patient not to take antacids within 2 hours of ciprofloxacin because they may reduce or destroy ciprofloxacin's effectiveness.
• Inform the patient that sugarless gum or hard candy may relieve ciprofloxacin's bad taste.
• Explain to patients receiving the ophthalmic form of ciprofloxacin that a crystal precipitate may form but usually resolves in 1 to 7 days.

gatifloxacin

gah-tee-**floks**-a-sin
(Tequin, Zymar)

CATEGORY AND SCHEDULE

Pregnancy Risk Category: C

MECHANISM OF ACTION

A fluoroquinolone that inhibits two enzymes, topoisomerase II and IV, in susceptible microorganisms. **Therapeutic Effect:** Interferes with bacterial DNA replication. Prevents or delays resistance emergence. Bactericidal.

PHARMACOKINETICS

Well absorbed from the gastrointestinal (GI) tract after PO administration. Protein binding: 20%. Widely distributed. Metabolized in liver. Primarily excreted in urine. ***Half-life:*** 7–14 hr.

AVAILABILITY

Tablets (Tequin): 200 mg, 400 mg.
Injection (Tequin): 200-mg, 400-mg vials.
Ophthalmic Solution (Zymar): 0.3%.

INDICATIONS AND DOSAGES

▸ **Chronic bronchitis, complicated urinary tract infections, pyelonephritis, skin infections**
PO/IV
Adults, Elderly. 400 mg/day for 7–10 days (5 days for chronic bronchitis).

▸ **Sinusitis**
PO, IV
Adults, Elderly. 400 mg/day for 10 days.

▸ **Pneumonia**
PO, IV
Adults, Elderly. 400 mg/day for 7–14 days.

▸ **Cystitis**
PO, IV
Adults, Elderly. 400 mg as a single dose or 200 mg/day for 3 days.

▸ **Urethral gonorrhea in men and women, endocervical and rectal gonorrhea in women**
PO, IV
Adults, Elderly. 400 mg as a single dose.

▸ **Topical treatment of bacterial conjunctivitis due to susceptible strains of bacteria**
Ophthalmic
Adults, Elderly, Children 1 yr and older. 1 drop q2h while awake for 2 days, then 1 drop up to 4 times/day for days 3–7.

▸ **Dosage in renal impairment**

Creatinine Clearance	Dosage
40 ml/min	400 mg/day
less than 40 ml/min	Initially, 400 mg/day then 200 mg/day
Hemodialysis	Initially, 400 mg/day then 200 mg/day
Peritoneal dialysis	Initially, 400 mg/day then 200 mg/day

CONTRAINDICATIONS

Hypersensitivity to quinolones

INTERACTIONS

Drug

Antacids, digoxin, iron preparations: May decrease gatifloxacin plasma concentration and half-life.
Probenecid: May increase gatifloxacin plasma concentration and half-life.

Herbal

None known.

Food

None known.

DIAGNOSTIC TEST EFFECTS

None known.

IV INCOMPATIBILITIES

Amphotericin (Fungizone), potassium phosphate

IV COMPATIBILITIES

Aminophylline, calcium gluconate, hydromorphone (Dilaudid), lidocaine, lorazepam (Ativan), magnesium sulfate, methylprednisolone (Solu-Medrol), metoclopramide (Reglan), midazolam (Versed), morphine, nitroglycerin, potassium chloride, sodium phosphate

SIDE EFFECTS

Occasional (8%–3%)
Nausea, vaginitis, diarrhea, headache, dizziness
Ophthalmic: conjunctival irritation, increased tearing, corneal inflammation

Rare (3%–0.1%)
Abdominal pain, constipation, dyspepsia, stomatitis, edema, insomnia, abnormal dreams, diaphoresis, altered taste, rash
Ophthalmic: corneal swelling, dry eye, eye pain, eyelid swelling, headache, red eye, reduced visual acuity, altered taste

SERIOUS REACTIONS

! Pseudomembranous colitis as evidenced by severe abdominal pain and cramps, severe watery diarrhea, and fever may occur.

! Superinfection manifested as genital or anal pruritus, ulceration or changes in oral mucosa, and moderate to severe diarrhea may occur.

NURSING CONSIDERATIONS

Baseline Assessment

◀ALERT▶ Determine the patient's history of hypersensitivity to gatifloxacin and quinolones before beginning drug therapy

Lifespan Considerations

- Be aware that it is unknown if gatifloxacin is distributed in breast milk.
- The safety and efficacy of gatifloxacin have not been established in children.
- In the elderly, age-related renal impairment may require dosage adjustment.

Precautions

- Use cautiously in patients with cerebral atherosclerosis, central nervous system (CNS) disorders, liver or renal impairment, seizures, and those with a prolonged QT interval.
- Use cautiously in patients taking other medications known to prolong the QT interval (e.g., erythromycin, tricyclic antidepressants).
- Use cautiously in patients with uncorrected hypokalemia and those receiving amiodarone, quinidine, procainamide, and sotalol.

Administration and Handling

PO

- Give without regard to meals.
- Administer oral gatifloxacin 4 hours before giving antacids, buffered tablets or solutions, ferrous sulfate, or multivitamins.

Ophthalmic

- Tilt the patient's head backward and have the patient look up.
- Gently pull the patient's lower eyelid down until a pocket is formed.
- Hold the dropper above the pocket, and without touching the eyelid or conjunctival sac, place drops into the center of the pocket.
- Close the patient's eye, then apply gentle digital pressure to the lacrimal sac at the inner canthus.
- Remove excess solution around the patient's eye with a tissue.

IV

- Know that the drug is available prediluted and ready for use and that it's also available in 20- and 40-ml vials, which must be diluted in 100–200 ml D_5W, 0.9% NaCl.
- Infuse over 60 minutes.
- Do not give by rapid or bolus IV.

Intervention and Evaluation

- Assess the patient's pattern of daily bowel activity and stool consistency.
- Assist the patient with ambulation if he or she experiences dizziness.
- Evaluate the patient for headache, nausea, signs of infection, and vaginitis.
- Monitor the patient's mental status and white blood cell (WBC) count.

Patient Teaching

- Advise the patient not to skip a drug dose and to take gatifloxacin for the full course of therapy.
- Instruct the patient to take gatifloxacin with 8 oz water and to drink several glasses of water between meals.
- Warn the patient not to take antacids within 4 hours of taking the medication as antacids would reduce or destroy gatifloxacin's effectiveness.
- Urge the patient to avoid exposure

to direct sunlight during therapy and for several days after treatment.
• Warn the patient not to perform tasks that require mental alertness or motor skills until his or her response to the drug has been established.

gemifloxacin mesylate

gem-ih-**flocks**-ah-sin
(Factive)

CATEGORY AND SCHEDULE

Pregnancy Risk Category: C

MECHANISM OF ACTION

A fluoroquinolone that inhibits the enzyme DNA gyrase in susceptible microorganisms, interfering with bacterial cell replication and repair.
Therapeutic Effect: Bactericidal.

PHARMACOKINETICS

Rapidly and well absorbed from the GI tract. Protein binding: 70%. Widely distributed. Penetrates well into lung tissue and fluid. Undergoes limited metabolism in the liver. Primarily excreted in feces; lesser amount eliminated in urine. Partially removed by hemodialysis. ***Half-life:*** 4–12 hr.

AVAILABILITY

Tablets: 320 mg.

INDICATIONS AND DOSAGES

▸ Acute bacterial exacerbation of chronic bronchitis
PO
Adults, Elderly. 320 mg once a day for 5 days.
▸ Community-acquired pneumonia
PO
Adults, Elderly. 320 mg once a day for 7 days.
▸ Dosage in renal impairment
Dosage and frequency are modified based on creatinine clearance.

Creatinine Clearance	Dosage
greater than 40 ml/min	320 mg once a day
40 ml/min or less	160 mg once a day

CONTRAINDICATIONS

Concurrent use of amiodarone, quinidine, procainamide, or sotalol; history of prolonged QTc interval; hypersensitivity to fluoroquinolones; uncorrected electrolyte disorders (such as hypokalemia and hypomagnesemia)

INTERACTIONS

Drug
Aluminum and magnesium-containing antacids, bismuth subsalicylate, didanosine, iron preparations and other metals, sucralfate, zinc preparations: May decrease the absorption of gemifloxacin.
Antipsychotics, class 1A and class III antiarrhythmics, erythromycin, tricyclic antidepressants: May increase the risk of prolonged QTc interval and life-threatening arrhythmias.
Cyclosporine: Increases the risk of nephrotoxicity.
Probenecid: Increases gemifloxacin serum concentration.
Herbal
None known.
Food
None known.

DIAGNOSTIC TEST EFFECTS

May increase BUN and serum alkaline phosphatase, bilirubin, LDH, creatinine, AST (SGOT), and ALT (SGPT) levels.

SIDE EFFECTS

Occasional (4%–2%)
Diarrhea, rash, nausea
Rare (1% or less)
Headache, abdominal pain, dizziness

SERIOUS REACTIONS

! Antibiotic-associated colitis may result from altered bacterial balance. Hypersensitivity reactions, including photosensitivity (as evidenced by rash, pruritus, blisters, edema, and burning skin), have occurred in patients receiving fluoroquinolones.

NURSING CONSIDERATIONS

Baseline Assessment

◀ **ALERT** ▶ Determine if the patient has a history of hypersensitivity to fluoroquinolones.

- Measure the patient's baseline QT interval, and calculate the QTc interval.
- Plan to obtain baseline laboratory tests, especially serum electrolyte levels. Expect to administer supplements, as needed, for low electrolyte levels.

Lifespan Considerations

- Gemifloxacin may be teratogenic. Substitute formula feedings for breast-feeding.
- The safety and efficacy of gemifloxacin have not been established in children 18 years of age and younger.
- Age-related renal impairment may require a dosage adjustment in the elderly.

Precautions

- Use gemifloxacin cautiously in patients with acute myocardial ischemia, clinically significant bradycardia, or impaired hepatic or renal function.

Administration and Handling

PO

- Give gemifloxacin without regard to food.
- Don't crush or break tablets.
- Don't administer antacids within 2 hours of gemifloxacin.

Intervention and Evaluation

- Monitor the patient's liver function test results and WBC count.
- Monitor the patient for signs and symptoms of infection.
- Assess the patient's daily pattern of daily bowel activity and stool consistency.
- Examine the patient's skin for a rash.
- Be alert for signs and symptoms of superinfection, including genital pruritus and oral candidiasis.
- Calculate the QT and QTc intervals to check for prolongation.

Patient Teaching

- Instruct the patient to complete the full course of gemifloxacin therapy.
- Advise the patient to take each drug dose with 8 oz of water. Explain that gemifloxacin may be taken with or without food.
- Encourage the patient to drink several glasses of water between meals.
- Warn the patient not to take antacids within 2 hours of a gemifloxacin because they may destroy or reduce the drug's effectiveness.

levofloxacin

levo-**flox**-a-sin
(Iquix, Levaquin, Quixin)

CATEGORY AND SCHEDULE

Pregnancy Risk Category: C

MECHANISM OF ACTION

A fluoroquinolone that inhibits the

DNA enzyme gyrase in susceptible microorganisms, interfering with bacterial cell replication and repair. **Therapeutic Effect:** Bactericidal.

PHARMACOKINETICS

Well absorbed after both PO and IV administration. Protein binding: 8%–24%. Penetrates rapidly and extensively into leukocytes, epithelial cells, and macrophages. Lung concentrations are 2-5 times higher than those of plasma. Eliminated unchanged in the urine. Partially removed by hemodialysis. ***Half-life:*** 8 hr.

AVAILABILITY

Oral Solution: 25 mg/ml.
Tablets (Levaquin): 250 mg, 500 mg, 750 mg.
Injection (Levaquin): 500-mg/20-ml vials.
Premixed Solution (Levaquin): 250 mg/50 ml, 500 mg/100 ml, 750 mg/150 ml.
Ophthalmic Solution (Quixin): 1.5%
Ophthalmic Solution (Iquix): 0.5%.

INDICATIONS AND DOSAGES

▸ **Bronchitis**
PO, IV
Adults, Elderly. 500 mg q24h for 7 days.

▸ **Community-acquired pneumonia**
PO
Adults, Elderly. 750 mg/day for 5 days.

▸ **Pneumonia**
PO, IV
Adults, Elderly. 500 mg q24h for 7–14 days.

▸ **Acute maxillary sinusitis**
PO, IV
Adults, Elderly. 500 mg q24h for 10–14 days.

▸ **Skin and skin-structure infections**
PO, IV
Adults, Elderly. 500 mg q24h for 7–10 days.

▸ **UTIs, acute pyelonephritis**
PO, IV
Adults, Elderly. 250 mg q24h for 10 days.

▸ **Bacterial conjunctivitis**
Ophthalmic
Adults, Elderly, Children 1 yr and older. 1–2 drops q2h for 2 days (up to 8 times a day), then 1–2 drops q4h for 5 days.

▸ **Corneal ulcer**
Ophthalmic
Adults, Elderly, Children older than 5 yr. Days 1–3: Instill 1–2 drops q30min to 2 hours while awake and 4–6 hours after retiring. Days 4 through completion: 1–2 drops q1–4h while awake.

▸ **Dosage in renal impairment**
For bronchitis, pneumonia, sinusitis, and skin and skin-structure infections, dosage and frequency are modified based on creatinine clearance.

Creatinine Clearance	Dosage
50–80 ml/min	No change
20–49 ml/min	500 mg initially, then 250 mg q24h
10–19 ml/min	500 mg initially, then 250 mg q48h

Dialysis 500 mg initially, then 250 mg q48h
For UTIs and pyelonephritis, dosage and frequency are modified based on creatinine clearance.

Creatinine Clearance	Dosage
20 ml/min	No change
10–19 ml/min	250 mg initially, then 250 mg q48h

CONTRAINDICATIONS

Hypersensitivity to levofloaxcin, other fluoroquinolones, or nalidixic acid

INTERACTIONS

Drug

Antacids, iron preparations, sucralfate, zinc: Decrease levofloxacin absorption.
NSAIDs: May increase the risk of CNS stimulation or seizures.

Herbal

None known.

Food

None known.

DIAGNOSTIC TEST EFFECTS

May alter blood glucose levels.

IV INCOMPATIBILITIES

Furosemide (Lasix), heparin, insulin, nitroglycerin, propofol (Diprivan)

IV COMPATIBILITIES

Aminophylline, dobutamine (Dobutrex), dopamine (Intron), fentanyl (Sublimaze), lidocaine, lorazepam (Ativan), morphine

SIDE EFFECTS

Occasional (3%–1%)

Diarrhea, nausea, abdominal pain, dizziness, drowsiness, headache, light-headedness
Ophthalmic: Local burning or discomfort, margin crusting, crystals or scales, foreign body sensation, ocular itching, altered taste

Rare (less than 1%)

Flatulence; altered taste; pain; inflammation or swelling in calves, hands, or shoulder; chest pain; difficulty breathing; palpitations; edema; tendon pain
Ophthalmic: Corneal staining, keratitis, allergic reaction, eyelid swelling, tearing, reduced visual acuity

SERIOUS REACTIONS

! Antibiotic-associated colitis and other superinfections may occur from altered bacterial balance.
Hypersensitivity reactions, including photosensitivity (as evidenced by rash, pruritus, blisters, edema, and burning skin), have occurred in patients receiving fluoroquinolones.

NURSING CONSIDERATIONS

Baseline Assessment

◀ALERT▶ Determine if the patient has a history of hypersensitivity to levofloxacin or other fluoroquinolones before beginning drug therapy.

Lifespan Considerations

- Levofloxacin is excreted in breast milk and should be avoided during pregnancy and breast-feeding.
- The safety and efficacy of levofloxacin have not been established in children younger than 18 years.
- Age-related renal impairment may require a dosage adjustment in the elderly.

Precautions

- Use levofloxacin cautiously in patients with bradycardia, cardiomyopathy, hypokalemia, hypomagnesemia, impaired renal function, seizure disorder, or suspected CNS disorder.

Administration and Handling

PO

- Give levofloxacin without regard to food.
- Don't administer antacids (containing aluminum or magnesium), sucralfate, iron preparations, or multivitamins containing zinc within 2 hours of levofloxacin because these drugs significantly reduce levofloxacin absorption.
- Provide the patient with citrus fruits and cranberry juice to acidify urine.

IV

- Levofloxacin is available in single-dose 20-ml (500-mg) vials and as a premixed (with D_5W), ready-to-infuse solution.
- For infusion using the single-dose vial, withdraw the desired amount (10 ml for 250 mg, 20 ml for 500 mg). Dilute each 10 ml (250 mg) with at least 40 ml 0.9% NaCl or D_5W.
- Administer the drug slowly, over not less than 60 minutes.

Ophthalmic

- Place a gloved finger on the patient's lower eyelid, and pull it out until a pocket is formed between the eye and lower lid.
- Hold the dropper above the pocket, and place the correct number of drops into the pocket.
- Close the patient's eye gently. Apply digital pressure to the lacrimal sac for 1 to 2 minutes to minimize drainage of the medication into the patient's nose and throat, reducing the risk of systemic effects.

Intervention and Evaluation

- Monitor the patient's blood glucose levels and liver and renal function test results.
- Promptly report any hypersensitivity reactions, including photosensitivity, pruritus, skin rash, and urticaria to the physician.
- Be alert for signs and symptoms of superinfection, such as anal or genital pruritus, moderate to severe diarrhea, new or increased fever, and ulceration or changes in the oral mucosa.
- Provide symptomatic relief for nausea.
- Evaluate the patient's food tolerance and change in taste sensation.

Patient Teaching

- Encourage the patient to drink 6 to 8 glasses of fluid a day, including citrus and cranberry juices to acidify urine.
- Advise the patient to avoid tasks that require mental alertness or motor skills until his or her response to the drug is established.
- Warn the patient to notify the physician if he or she experiences chest pain, difficulty breathing, palpitations, persistent diarrhea, edema, or tendon pain.

lomefloxacin hydrochloride

low-meh-**flocks**-ah-sin
(Maxaquin)

CATEGORY AND SCHEDULE

Pregnancy Risk Category: C

MECHANISM OF ACTION

A quinolone that inhibits the enzyme DNA gyrase in susceptible microorganisms, interfering with bacterial cell replication and repair. **Therapeutic Effect:** Bactericidal.

PHARMACOKINETICS

Well absorbed from the GI tract. Protein binding: 10%. Widely distributed. Metabolized in the liver. Primarily excreted in urine. Not removed by hemodialysis. ***Half-life:*** 4–6 hr (increased with impaired renal function and in the elderly).

AVAILABILITY

Tablets: 400 mg.

INDICATIONS AND DOSAGES

▸ Complicated UTIs

PO

Adults, Elderly. 400 mg/day for 10–14 days.

▸ **Uncomplicated UTIs**
PO
Adults (females). 400 mg/day for 3 days.
▸ **Lower respiratory tract infections**
PO
Adults, Elderly. 400 mg/day for 10 days.
▸ **Surgical prophylaxis**
PO
Adults, Elderly. 400 mg 2–6 hr before surgery.
▸ **Dosage in renal impairment**
Dosage and frequency are modified based on creatinine clearance.

Creatinine Clearance	Dosage
41 ml/min and higher	No change
10–40 ml/min	400 mg initially, then 200 mg/day for 10–14 days

CONTRAINDICATIONS
Hypersensitivity to quinolones

INTERACTIONS
Drug
Antacids, iron preparations, sucralfate: May decrease lomefloxacin absorption.
Caffeine, oral anticoagulants: May increase the effects of these drugs.
Theophylline: Decreases clearance and may increase blood concentration and risk of toxicity of theophylline.
Herbal
None known.
Food
None known.

DIAGNOSTIC TEST EFFECTS
May increase BUN and serum alkaline phosphatase, bilirubin, creatinine, LDH, AST (SGOT), and ALT (SGPT) levels.

SIDE EFFECTS
Occasional (3%–2%)
Nausea, headache, photosensitivity, dizziness
Rare (1%)
Diarrhea

SERIOUS REACTIONS
! Antibiotic-associated colitis and other superinfections may result from altered bacterial balance.
! Hypersensitivity reactions, including photosensitivity (as evidenced by rash, pruritus, blisters, edema, and burning skin), have occurred in patients receiving fluoroquinolones.
! Arthropathy may occur if the drug is given to children younger than 18 years.

NURSING CONSIDERATIONS
Baseline Assessment
◂ **ALERT** ▸ Determine if the patient has a history of hypersensitivity to lomefloxacin or other quinolones before beginning drug therapy.
Lifespan Considerations
• It is unknown if lomefloxacin is distributed in breast milk. If possible, pregnant or breast-feeding women should avoid taking the drug because of the risk of arthropathy in the fetus or infant.
• The safety and efficacy of lomefloxacin have not been established in children.
• Age-related renal impairment may require a dosage adjustment in the elderly.
Precautions
• Use lomefloxacin cautiously in patients with CNS disorders, renal impairment, or seizures, and those taking caffeine or theophylline.
Administration and Handling
PO
• Lomefloxacin may be given with-

out regard to food, but the preferred administration time is 2 hours after a meal.
• Don't administer antacids containing aluminum or magnesium within 2 hours of lomefloxacin.
• Provide the patient with citrus fruits and cranberry juice to acidify urine.

Intervention and Evaluation
• Monitor the patient for dizziness, headache, and signs and symptoms of infection.
• Monitor the patient's mental status and WBC count.
• Be alert for signs and symptoms of superinfection, such as anal or genital pruritus, fever, oral candidiasis, and vaginitis.

Patient Teaching
• Advise the patient not to skip drug doses and to continue taking lomefloxacin for the full course of therapy.
• Warn the patient not to take antacids while on lomefloxacin because antacids may reduce or destroy lomefloxacin's effectiveness.
• Urge the patient to avoid exposure to sunlight and ultraviolet light and to wear sunscreen and protective clothing if photosensitivity develops.

moxifloxacin hydrochloride

moks-i-**floks**-a-sin
(Avelox, Avelox IV, Vigamox)
Do not confuse Avelox with Avonex.

CATEGORY AND SCHEDULE
Pregnancy Risk Category: C

MECHANISM OF ACTION
A fluoroquinolone that inhibits two enzymes, topoisomerase II and IV, in susceptible microorganisms. **Therapeutic Effect:** Interferes with bacterial DNA replication. Prevents or delays emergence of resistant organisms. Bactericidal.

PHARMACOKINETICS
Well absorbed from the gastrointestinal (GI) tract after PO administration. Protein binding: 50%. Widely distributed throughout body with tissue concentration often exceeding plasma concentration. Metabolized in liver. Primarily excreted in urine with a lesser amount in feces. ***Half-life:*** 10.7–13.3 hr.

AVAILABILITY
Tablets (Avelox): 400 mg.
Injection (Avelox IV): 400 mg.
Ophthalmic Solution (Vigamox): 0.5%.

INDICATIONS AND DOSAGES
▸ **Acute bacterial sinusitis, community-acquired pneumonia**
IV, PO
Adults, Elderly. 400 mg q24h for 10 days.
▸ **Acute bacterial exacerbation of chronic bronchitis**
IV, PO
Adults, Elderly. 400 mg q24h for 5 days.
▸ **Skin and skin-structure infection**
IV, PO
Adults, Elderly. 400 mg once a day for 7 days.
▸ **Topical treatment of bacterial conjunctivitis due to susceptible strains of bacteria**
Ophthalmic
Adults, Elderly, Children older than 1 yr. 1 drop 3 times/day for 7 days.

CONTRAINDICATIONS
Hypersensitivity to quinolones

INTERACTIONS

Drug

Antacids, didanosine chewable, buffered tablets or pediatric powder for oral solution, iron preparations, sucralfate: May decrease moxifloxacin absorption.

Herbal

None known.

Food

None known.

DIAGNOSTIC TEST EFFECTS

None known.

IV INCOMPATIBILITIES

Do not add or infuse other drugs simultaneously through the same IV line. Flush line before and after use if same IV line is used with other medications.

SIDE EFFECTS

Frequent (8%–6%)

Nausea, diarrhea

Occasional (3%–2%)

Dizziness, headache, abdominal pain, vomiting

Ophthalmic (6%–1%): conjunctival irritation, reduced visual acuity, dry eye, keratitis, eye pain, ocular itching, swelling of tissue around cornea, eye discharge, fever, cough, pharyngitis, rash, rhinitis

Rare (1%)

Change in sense of taste, dyspepsia (heartburn, indigestion), photosensitivity

SERIOUS REACTIONS

! Pseudomembranous colitis as evidenced by fever, severe abdominal cramps or pain, and severe watery diarrhea may occur.

! Superinfection manifested as anal or genital pruritus, moderate to severe diarrhea, and stomatitis may occur.

NURSING CONSIDERATIONS

Baseline Assessment

◀ALERT▶ Determine the patient's history of hypersensitivity to moxifloxacin and quinolones before beginning drug therapy.

Lifespan Considerations

- Be aware that moxifloxacin may be distributed in breast milk and may produce teratogenic effects.
- Be aware that the safety and efficacy of moxifloxacin have not been established in children.
- There are no age-related precautions noted in the elderly.

Precautions

- Use cautiously in patients with cerebral arthrosclerosis, CNS disorders, liver or renal impairment; seizures, those with a prolonged QT interval, and uncorrected hypokalemia.
- Use cautiously in patients receiving amiodarone, procainamide, quinidine, and sotalol.

Administration and Handling

◀ALERT▶ Infuse IV over 60 minutes or more.

PO

- Give without regard to meals.
- Administer oral moxifloxacin 4 hours before or 8 hours after antacids, didanosine chewable, buffered tablets or pediatric powder for oral solution, iron preparations, multivitamins, or sucralfate.

Ophthalmic

- Tilt the patient's head back and instruct the patient to look up.
- With a gloved finger, gently pull the patient's lower eyelid down until a pocket is formed.
- Hold the dropper above the pocket and, without touching the eyelid or conjunctival sac, place drops into the center of the pocket.
- Close the patient's eye gently and

apply gentle digital pressure to the lacrimal sac at the inner canthus.
- Remove excess solution around the patient's eye with a tissue.

IV
- Store at room temperature.
- Do not refrigerate.
- Available in ready-to-use containers.
- Give by IV infusion only.
- Avoid rapid or bolus IV infusion.
- Infuse over 60 minutes or more.

Intervention and Evaluation
- Assess the patient's pattern of daily bowel activity and stool consistency.
- Assist the patient with ambulation if he or she experiences dizziness.
- Evaluate the patient for abdominal pain, altered sense of taste, dyspepsia (heartburn, indigestion), headache, and vomiting.
- Monitor the patient for signs of infection.
- Monitor the patient's white blood cell (WBC) count.

Patient Teaching
- Explain to the patient that moxifloxacin may be taken without regard to food.
- Encourage the patient to drink plenty of fluids.
- Urge the patient to avoid exposure to direct sunlight as this may cause a photosensitivity reaction.
- Instruct the patient not to take antacids 4 hours before or 8 hours after moxifloxacin dose.
- Advise the patient to take moxifloxacin for the full course of therapy.

norfloxacin
nor-**flox**-a-sin
(Apo-Norflox[CAN], Insensye [AUS], Norfloxacine[CAN], Noroxin, Novo-Norfloxacin[CAN], PMS-Norfloxacin[CAN], Roxin [AUS])

CATEGORY AND SCHEDULE
Pregnancy Risk Category: C

MECHANISM OF ACTION
A quinolone that inhibits DNA gyrase in susceptible microorganisms, interfering with bacterial cell replication and repair. **Therapeutic Effect:** Bactericidal.

AVAILABILITY
Tablets: 400 mg.

INDICATIONS AND DOSAGES
▸ **Urinary tract infections (UTIs)**
PO
Adults, Elderly. 400 mg twice a day for 7-21 days.

▸ **Prostatitis**
PO
Adults. 400 mg twice a day for 28 days.

▸ **Uncomplicated gonococcal infections**
PO
Adults. 800 mg as a single dose.

▸ **Dosage in renal impairment**
Dosage and frequency are modified based on creatinine clearance.

Creatinine Clearance	Dosage
30 ml/min or higher	400 mg twice a day
less than 30 ml/min	400 mg once a day

CONTRAINDICATIONS
Children younger than 18 years because of risk arthropathy; hyper-

sensitivity to norfloxacin, other quinolones, or their components

INTERACTIONS

Drug

Antacids, sucralfate: May decrease norfloxacin absorption.
Oral anticoagulants: May increase effects of oral anticoagulants.
Theophylline: Decreases clearance and may increase blood concentration and risk of toxicity of theophylline.

Herbal

None known.

Food

None known.

DIAGNOSTIC TEST EFFECTS

May increase BUN level and serum alkaline phosphatase, bilirubin, creatinine, LDH, AST (SGOT), and ALT (SGPT) levels.

SIDE EFFECTS

Frequent
Nausea, headache, dizziness
Rare
Vomiting, diarrhea, dry mouth, bitter taste, nervousness, drowsiness, insomnia, photosensitivity, tinnitus, crystalluria, rash, fever, seizures

SERIOUS REACTIONS

! Superinfection, anaphylaxis, Stevens-Johnson syndrome, and arthropathy occur rarely.
! Hypersensitivity reactions, including photosensitivity (as evidenced by rash, pruritus, blisters, edema, and burning skin), have occurred in patients receiving fluoroquinolones.

NURSING CONSIDERATIONS

Baseline Assessment

◀ALERT▶ Determine if the patient has a history of hypersensitivity to norfloxacin or other quinolones before beginning drug therapy.

Precautions

- Use norfloxacin cautiously in patients with impaired renal function and a predisposition to seizures.

Administration and Handling

PO

- Give norfloxacin with 8 oz of water 1 hour before or 2 hours after a meal.
- Provide the patient with several glasses of water between meals as well as citrus fruits and cranberry juice to acidify urine.
- Don't administer antacids within 2 hours of norfloxacin.

Intervention and Evaluation

- Assess the patient for chest pain, dizziness, headache, joint pain, and nausea.
- Evaluate the patient's food tolerance.

Patient Teaching

- Instruct the patient to take norfloxacin with 8 oz of water 1 hour before or 2 hours after a meal.
- Advise the patient to complete the full course of norfloxacin therapy.
- Encourage the patient to drink several glasses of water between meals.
- Inform the patient that norfloxacin may cause dizziness or drowsiness.
- Instruct the patient not to take antacids within 2 hours of norfloxacin because they may reduce or destroy norfloxacin's effectiveness.

ofloxacin

o-**flox**-a-sin

(Apo-Oflox[CAN], Floxin, Floxin Otic, Ocuflox)

Do not confuse Floxin with Flexeril or Flexon, or Ocuflox with Ocufen.

CATEGORY AND SCHEDULE

Pregnancy Risk Category: C

MECHANISM OF ACTION

A fluoroquinolone antibiotic that inhibits DNA gyrase in susceptible microorganisms, interfering with bacterial cell replication and repair. **Therapeutic Effect:** Bactericidal.

PHARMACOKINETICS

Rapidly and well absorbed from the GI tract. Protein binding: 20%–25%. Widely distributed (including to CSF). Metabolized in the liver. Primarily excreted in urine. Removed by hemodialysis. ***Half-life:*** 4.7–7 hr (increased in impaired renal function, cirrhosis, and the elderly).

AVAILABILITY

Tablets (Floxin): 200 mg, 300 mg, 400 mg.
Injection Solution (Floxin): 40 mg/ml.
Premixed Infusion Solution (Floxin): 200 mg/50 ml, 400 mg/100 ml.
Ophthalmic Solution (Ocuflox): 0.3%.
Otic Solution (Floxin): 0.3%.

INDICATIONS AND DOSAGES

▸ UTIs

PO, IV

Adults. 200 mg q12h.

▸ Pelvic inflammatory disease (PID)

PO

Adults. 400 mg q12h for 10-14 days.

▸ Lower respiratory tract, skin and skin-structure infections

PO, IV

Adults. 400 mg q12h for 10 days.

▸ Prostatitis, sexually transmitted diseases (cervicitis, urethritis)

PO

Adults. 300 mg q12h.

▸ Prostatitis

IV

Adults. 300 mg q12h.

▸ Sexually transmitted diseases

IV

Adults. 400 mg as a single dose.

▸ Acute, uncomplicated gonorrhea

PO

Adults. 400 mg 1 time.

▸ Usual elderly dosage

PO

Elderly. 200–400 mg q12–24h for 7 days up to 6 wk.

▸ Bacterial conjunctivitis

Ophthalmic

Adults, Elderly. 1–2 drops q2–4h for 2 days, then 4 times a day for 5 days.

▸ Corneal ulcers

Ophthalmic

Adults. 1–2 drops q30min while awake for 2 days, then q60min while awake for 5–7 days, then 4 times a day.

▸ Acute otitis media

Otic

Children 1–12 yr. 5 drops into the affected ear 2 times/day for 10 days.

▸ Otitis externa

Otic

Adults, Elderly, Children 12 yr and older. 10 drops into the affected ear once a day for 7 days.

Children 6 mo–11 yr. 5 drops into the affected ear once a day for 7 days.

▸ Dosage in renal impairment

After a normal initial dose, dosage and frequency are based on creatinine clearance.

Creatinine Clearance	Adjusted Dose	Dosage Interval
greater than 50 ml/min	None	q12h
10–50 ml/min	None	q24h
less than 10 ml/min		q24h

CONTRAINDICATIONS
Children younger than 18 years, hypersensitivity to any quinolones

INTERACTIONS
Drug
Antacids, sucralfate: May decrease absorption and effects of ofloxacin.
Caffeine: May increase the effects of caffeine.
Theophylline: May increase theophylline blood concentration and risk of toxicity.
Herbal
None known.
Food
None known.

DIAGNOSTIC TEST EFFECTS
None known.

IV INCOMPATIBILITIES
Amphotericin B complex (Abelcet, AmBisome, Amphotec), cefepime (Maxipime), doxorubicin liposomal (Doxil)

IV COMPATIBILITIES
Propofol (Diprivan)

SIDE EFFECTS
Frequent (10%–7%)
Nausea, headache, insomnia
Occasional (5%–3%)
Abdominal pain, diarrhea, vomiting, dry mouth, flatulence, dizziness, fatigue, drowsiness, rash, pruritus, fever
Rare (less than 1%)
Constipation, paraesthesia

SERIOUS REACTIONS
! Antibiotic-associated colitis and other superinfections may occur from altered bacterial balance.
! Hypersensitivity reactions, including photosensitivity (as evidenced by rash, pruritus, blisters, edema, and burning skin), have occurred in patients receiving fluoroquinolones.
! Arthropathy (swelling, pain, and clubbing of fingers and toes, degeneration of stress-bearing portion of a joint) may occur if the drug is given to children.

NURSING CONSIDERATIONS
Baseline Assessment
◀ALERT▶ Determine if the patient has a history of hypersensitivity to ofloxacin or other quinolones before beginning drug therapy.
Lifespan Considerations
- Ciprofloxacin is distributed in breast milk. If possible, pregnant or breast-feeding women should avoid taking the drug because of the risk of arthropathy in the fetus or infant.
- The safety and efficacy of ofloxacin have not been established in children younger than 1 year for otic form.
- Age-related renal impairment may require a dosage adjustment for oral and parenteral forms in the elderly.
- No age-related precautions for the otic form have been noted in the elderly.
Precautions
- Use ofloxacin cautiously in patients with CNS disorders, renal impairment, or seizures and those taking caffeine or theophylline.
- Use the drug cautiously in patients with syphilis because ofloxacin may mask or delay symptoms of syphilis; serologic test for syphilis should be

done at diagnosis and 3 months after treatment.

Administration and Handling

PO

- Don't give ofloxacin with food. The preferred dosing time is 1 hour before or 2 hours after a meal.
- Give the drug with 8 oz of water and provide additional liquids between meals.
- Provide the patient with citrus fruits and cranberry juice to acidify urine.
- Administer antacids containing aluminum or magnesium or products containing iron or zinc within 2 hours before or after taking ofloxacin.

IV

- Store single-use vial at room temperature.
- Know that ofloxacin is also available in premixed, ready-to-hang solutions.
- Dilute each 200-mg vial with 50 ml D_5W or 0.9% NaCl (each 400-mg vial with 100 ml) to provide a concentration of 4 mg/ml.
- After dilution, the IV solution may be stored for 72 hours at room temperature and 14 days if refrigerated.
- Give by IV infusion only over at least 60 minutes; avoid rapid or bolus IV administration.
- Discard unused portions.
- Don't infuse other medications simultaneously through the same IV line.

Ophthalmic

- Tilt the patient's head back and place the solution in the conjunctival sac.
- Close the patient's eye; then press gently on the lacrimal sac for 1 minute.
- Don't use ophthalmic solutions for injection.
- Unless the infection is very superficial, expect to also administer systemic drug therapy.

Otic

- Instruct the patient to lie down with the head turned so that the affected ear is upright.
- Instill drops toward the canal wall, not directly on the eardrum.
- Pull the auricle down and back in children and up and back in adults.

Intervention and Evaluation

- Monitor the patient for signs and symptoms of infection.
- Monitor the patient's mental status and WBC count.
- Examine the patient's skin for a rash. Withhold the drug and promptly notify the physician at the first sign of a rash or another allergic reaction.
- Assess the patient's pattern of daily bowel activity and stool consistency.
- Observe the patient for insomnia.
- Evaluate the patient for dizziness, headache, tremors, and visual difficulties.
- Provide assistance with ambulation as needed.
- Be alert for signs of superinfection, such as anal or genital pruritus, fever, stomatitis, and vaginitis.

Patient Teaching

- Teach the patient that ofloxacin is best taken 1 hour before or 2 hours after a meal.
- Instruct the patient not to take antacids within 2 hours before or after taking ofloxacin.
- Inform the patient that ofloxacin may cause dizziness, drowsiness, headache, and insomnia.
- Advise the patient to avoid tasks requiring mental alertness or motor skills until his or her response to ofloxacin is established.

11 Tetracyclines

demeclocycline hydrochloride
doxycycline
minocycline hydrochloride
tetracycline hydrochloride

Uses: Tetracyclines are used to treat rickettsial diseases (such as typhus fever and Q fever), *Chlamydia trachomatis* infections, brucellosis, cholera, pneumonia caused by *Mycoplasma pneumoniae,* Lyme disease, *Helicobacter pylori* gastric infections (in combination therapy), and periodontal disease. Topical formulations are used to treat acne.

Action: Tetracyclines are bacteriostatic. They inhibit bacterial protein synthesis by binding to the 30S ribosomal subunit and preventing the binding of transfer RNA to messenger RNA. (See the illustration *Mechanism of Action: Tetracyclines,* page 216.)

demeclocycline hydrochloride

dem-e-kloe-**sye**-kleen
(Declomycin, Ledermycin[AUS])

CATEGORY AND SCHEDULE

Pregnancy Risk Category: D

MECHANISM OF ACTION

A tetracycline antibiotic that inhibits bacterial protein synthesis by binding to ribosomal receptor sites; also inhibits ADH-induced water reabsorption. **Therapeutic Effect:** Bacteriostatic; also produces water diuresis.

AVAILABILITY

Tablets: 150 mg, 300 mg.

INDICATIONS AND DOSAGES

▸ **Mild to moderate infections, including acne, pertussis, chronic bronchitis, and UTIs**

PO

Adults, Elderly. 150 mg 4 times a day or 300 mg 2 times a day.
Children older than 8 yr. 8–12 mg/kg/day in 2–4 divided doses.

▸ **Uncomplicated gonorrhea**

PO

Adults. Initially, 600 mg, then 300 mg q12h for 4 days for total of 3 g.

▸ **Syndrome of inappropriate ADH secretion (SIADH)**

PO

Adults, Elderly. Initially, 900–1,200 mg/day in 3–4 divided doses, then decrease dose to 600–900 mg/day in divided doses.

CONTRAINDICATIONS

Children 8 years and younger, last half of pregnancy

INTERACTIONS

Drug

Antacids containing aluminum, calcium, or magnesium; laxatives containing magnesium; oral iron preparations: Impair the absorption of demeclocycline.
Cholestyramine, colestipol: May decrease demeclocycline absorption.
Oral contraceptives: May decrease the effects of oral contraceptives.

Herbal

None known.

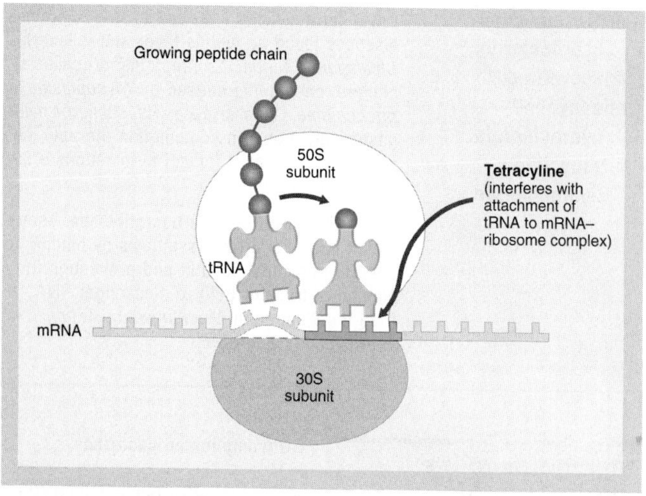

Mechanism of Action: Tetracyclines

Like certain other anti-infectives, tetracyclines work by interfering with bacterial protein synthesis. Protein synthesis normally occurs when the ribosomal subunits 50S and 30S bind to messenger RNA (mRNA), which arranges amino acids into peptide chains that form proteins. Then transfer RNA (tRNA) helps carry out genetic instructions from mRNA to arrange certain amino acids in a specific sequence to form a growing peptide chain. Once the peptide chain is complete, mRNA detaches from the ribosomal subunits, and the new protein is created.

Tetracyclines inhibit bacterial protein synthesis by attaching to the 30S ribosomal subunit. As a result, tRNA can't bind with the mRNA-ribosome complex, and no new amino acids can be synthesized or added to the growing peptide chain.

Food

Dairy products: May decrease demeclocycline absorption.

DIAGNOSTIC TEST EFFECTS

May increase BUN and serum alkaline phosphatase, amylase, bilirubin, AST (SGOT), and ALT (SGPT) levels.

SIDE EFFECTS

Frequent

Anorexia, nausea, vomiting, diarrhea, dysphagia, possibly severe photosensitivity (with moderate to high demeclocycline dosage).

Occasional

Urticaria, rash; diabetes insipidus syndrome, marked by polydipsia, polyuria, and weakness (with long-term therapy).

SERIOUS REACTIONS

! Superinfection (especially fungal), anaphylaxis, and benign intracranial hypertension occur rarely.

! Bulging fontanelles occur rarely in infants.

NURSING CONSIDERATIONS

Baseline Assessment

◀ALERT▶ Determine if the patient has a history of allergies, especially to tetracyclines, before beginning drug therapy.

Precautions

- Use demeclocycline cautiously in patients with renal impairment, and in those who can't avoid sun or ultraviolet exposure, because such exposure may produce a severe photosensitivity reaction.

Administration and Handling

PO

- Give antacids containing aluminum, calcium, or magnesium; laxatives containing magnesium; or oral iron preparations 1 to 2 hours before or after demeclocycline because they may impair the drug's absorption.

Intervention and Evaluation

- Assess the patient's pattern of daily bowel activity and stool consistency.
- Evaluate the patient's food intake and tolerance.
- Monitor the patient's intake and output and renal function test results.
- Examine the patient's skin for a rash.
- Be alert for signs and symptoms of superinfection, such as anal or genital pruritus, diarrhea, and ulceration or changes of the oral mucosa or tongue.
- Monitor the patient's BP and LOC because of the potential for increased intracranial pressure.

Patient Teaching

- Instruct the patient to take demeclocycline doses on an empty stomach with a full glass of water.
- Advise the patient to space drug doses evenly around the clock and to continue taking demeclocycline for the full course of treatment.
- Encourage the patient to avoid overexposure to sun or ultraviolet light to prevent photosensitivity reactions.

doxycycline

dox-i-**sye**-kleen

(Adoxa, Apo-Doxy[CAN], Doryx, Doxsig[AUS], Doxy-100, Doxycin[CAN], Doxyhexal[AUS], Doxylin[AUS], Monodox, Periostat, Vibramycin, Vibra-Tabs)

Do not confuse doxycycline with Dicyclomine or doxylamine, or Monodox with Monopril.

CATEGORY AND SCHEDULE

Pregnancy Risk Category: D

MECHANISM OF ACTION

A tetracycline antibiotic that inhibits bacterial protein synthesis by binding to ribosomes. **Therapeutic Effect:** Bacteriostatic.

AVAILABILITY

Capsules (Doryx): 75 mg, 100 mg.
Capsules (Monodox): 50 mg, 100 mg.
Capsules (Vibramycin): 100 mg.
Oral Suspension (Vibramycin): 25 mg/5 ml.
Syrup (Vibramycin): 50 mg/5 ml.
Tablets (Adoxa): 50 mg, 75 mg, 100 mg.
Tablets (Periostat): 20 mg.
Tablets (Vibra-Tabs): 100 mg.
Injection, Powder for Reconstitution (Doxy-100): 100 mg.

INDICATIONS AND DOSAGES

▸ Respiratory, skin, and soft-tissue infections; UTIs; pelvic inflammatory disease (PID); brucellosis; trachoma; Rocky Mountain spotted fever; typhus; Q fever; rickettsia; severe acne (Adoxa); smallpox; psittacosis; ornithosis; granuloma inguinale; lymphogranuloma venereum; intestinal amebiasis (adjunctive treatment); prevention of rheumatic fever

PO

Adults, Elderly. Initially, 100 mg q12h, then 100 mg/day as single dose or 50 mg q12h for severe infections.

Children 8 yr and older and weighing more than 45 kg. 2–4 mg/kg/day divided q12–24h. Maximum: 200 mg/day.

IV

Adults, Elderly. Initially, 200 mg as 1–2 infusions; then 100–200 mg/day in 1–2 divided doses.

Children 8 yr and older. 2–4 mg/kg/day divided q12–24h. Maximum: 200 mg/day.

▸ Acute gonococcal infections

PO

Adults. Initially, 200 mg, then 100 mg at bedtime on first day; then 100 mg twice a day for 14 days.

▸ Syphilis

PO, IV

Adults. 200 mg/day in divided doses for 14–28 days.

▸ Traveler's diarrhea

PO

Adults, Elderly. 100 mg/day during a period of risk (up to 14 days) and for 2 days after returning home.

▸ Periodontitis

PO

Adults. 20 mg twice a day.

OFF-LABEL USES

Treatment of atypical mycobacterial infections, rheumatoid arthritis, gonorrhea, and malaria; prevention of Lyme disease; prevention or treatment of traveler's diarrhea

CONTRAINDICATIONS

Children 8 years and younger, hypersensitivity to tetracyclines or sulfites, last half of pregnancy, severe hepatic dysfunction

INTERACTIONS

Drug

Antacids containing aluminum, calcium, or magnesium; laxatives containing magnesium: Decrease doxycycline absorption.
Barbiturates, carbamazepine, phenytoin: May decrease doxycycline blood concentrations.
Cholestyramine, colestipol: May decrease doxycycline absorption.
Oral contraceptives: May decrease the effects of oral contraceptives.
Oral iron preparations: Impair absorption of doxycycline.

Herbal

None known.

Food

None known.

DIAGNOSTIC TEST EFFECTS

May increase serum alkaline phosphatase, amylase, bilirubin, AST (SGOT), and ALT (SGPT) levels. May alter CBC.

IV INCOMPATIBILITIES

Allopurinol (Aloprim), heparin, piperacillin and tazobactam (Zosyn)

IV COMPATIBILITIES

Amiodarone (Cordarone), diltiazem (Cardizem), hydromorphone (Dilaudid), magnesium sulfate, morphine, propofol (Diprivan)

SIDE EFFECTS

Frequent

Anorexia, nausea, vomiting, diarrhea, dysphagia, possibly severe photosensitivity

Occasional

Rash, urticaria

SERIOUS REACTIONS

! Superinfection (especially fungal) and benign intracranial hypertension (headache, visual changes) may occur.

! Hepatoxicity, fatty degeneration of the liver, and pancreatitis occur rarely.

NURSING CONSIDERATIONS

Baseline Assessment

◀ **ALERT** ▶ Determine if the patient has a history of allergies, especially to tetracyclines or sulfites before beginning drug therapy.

Precautions

- Use doxycycline cautiously in patients who can't avoid sun or ultraviolet light exposure because such exposure may produce a severe photosensitivity reaction.

Administration and Handling

PO

- Store capsules and tablets at room temperature.
- Store oral suspension for up to 2 weeks at room temperature.
- Give doxycycline with a full glass of fluid. It may also be given with food or milk.
- Give oral doxycycline 1 to 2 hours before or after antacids that contain aluminum, calcium, or magnesium; laxatives that contain magnesium; or oral iron preparations because these drugs may impair doxycycline absorption.

IV

◀ **ALERT** ▶ Don't administer doxycycline IM or subcutaneously. Space doses evenly around clock.

- After reconstitution, the IV piggyback infusion may be stored for up to 12 hours at room temperature or up to 72 hours if refrigerated.
- Protect the drug from direct sunlight. Discard it if a precipitate forms.
- Reconstitute each 100-mg vial with 10 ml of sterile water for injection to yield a concentration of mg/ml.
- Further dilute each 100 mg with at least 100 ml of D_5W, 0.9% NaCl, or lactated Ringer's solution.
- Give the intermittent IV (piggyback) infusion over 1 to 4 hours.

Intervention and Evaluation

- Assess the patient's pattern of daily bowel activity and stool consistency.
- Examine the patient's skin for a rash.
- Monitor the patient's LOC because of the potential for benign intracranial hypertension.
- Be alert for signs and symptoms of superinfection, such as anal or genital pruritus, diarrhea, and ulceration or changes of the oral mucosa.

Patient Teaching

- Advise the patient to continue taking doxycycline for the full course of therapy.
- Instruct the patient not to take doxycycline with antacids or iron products because they decrease the drug's absorption.
- Encourage the patient to avoid overexposure to sun or ultraviolet light to prevent photosensitivity reactions.

minocycline hydrochloride

mi-noe-**sye**-kleen
(Akamin[AUS], Dynacin, Minocin, Minomycin[AUS], Myrac, Novo Minocycline[CAN])
Do not confuse Dynacin with Dynabac, or Minocin with Mithracin or niacin.

CATEGORY AND SCHEDULE

Pregnancy Risk Category: D

MECHANISM OF ACTION

A tetracycline antibiotic that inhibits bacterial protein synthesis by binding to ribosomes. **Therapeutic Effect:** Bacteriostatic.

AVAILABILITY

Capsules (Dynacin, Minocin): 50 mg, 75 mg, 100 mg.
Capsules (Pellet-Filled [Minocin]): 50 mg, 100 mg.
Tablets (Minocin, Myrac): 50 mg, 75 mg, 100 mg.
Powder for Injection (Minocin, Myrac): 100 mg.

INDICATIONS AND DOSAGES

▸ **Mild, moderate, or severe prostate, urinary tract, and CNS infections (excluding meningitis); uncomplicated gonorrhea; inflammatory acne; brucellosis; skin granulomas; cholera; trachoma; nocardiasis; yaws; and syphilis when penicillins are contraindicated**
PO
Adults, Elderly. Initially, 100–200 mg, then 100 mg q12h or 50 mg q6h.
IV
Adults, Elderly. Initially, 200 mg, then 100 mg q12h up to 400 mg/day.
PO, IV
Children older than 8 yr. Initially, 4 mg/kg, then 2 mg/kg q12h.

OFF-LABEL USES

Treatment of atypical mycobacterial infections, rheumatoid arthritis, scleroderma

CONTRAINDICATIONS

Children younger than 8 years, hypersensitivity to tetracyclines, last half of pregnancy

INTERACTIONS

Drug

Carbamazepine, phenytoin: May decrease minocycline blood concentration.
Cholestyramine, colestipol: May decrease minocycline absorption.
Oral contraceptives: May decrease the effects of oral contraceptives.

Herbal

St. John's wort: May increase the risk of photosensitivity.

Food

None known.

DIAGNOSTIC TEST EFFECTS

May increase serum alkaline phosphatase, amylase, bilirubin, AST (SGOT), and ALT (SGPT) levels.

IV INCOMPATIBILITIES

Piperacillin and tazobactam (Zosyn)

IV COMPATIBILITIES

Heparin, magnesium, potassium

SIDE EFFECTS

Frequent

Dizziness, light-headedness, diarrhea, nausea, vomiting, abdominal cramps, possibly severe photosensitivity, drowsiness, vertigo

Occasional

Altered pigmentation of skin or mucous membranes, rectal or genital pruritus, stomatitis

SERIOUS REACTIONS

! Superinfection (especially fungal),

anaphylaxis, and benign intracranial hypertension may occur.
! Bulging fontanelles occur rarely in infants.

NURSING CONSIDERATIONS

Baseline Assessment

◀ALERT▶ Determine if the patient has a history of allergies, especially to tetracyclines or sulfites, before beginning drug therapy.

Precautions

- Use minocycline cautiously in patients with renal impairment and in those who can't avoid sun or ultraviolet exposure because such exposure may produce a severe photosensitivity reaction.

Administration and Handling

◀ALERT▶ Space drug doses evenly around the clock.

PO

- Store the oral drug at room temperature.
- Give capsules and tablets with a full glass of water.

IV

- The IV solution may be stored for up to 24 hours at room temperature.
- Discard the solution if a precipitate forms.
- For intermittent IV (piggyback) infusion, reconstitute each 100-mg vial with 5 to 10 ml of sterile water for injection to provide a concentration of 20 or 10 mg/ml, respectively.
- Further dilute with 500 to 1,000 ml D_5W or 0.9% NaCl.
- Administer the piggyback IV infusion immediately after reconstitution. Infuse it over 6 hours.

Intervention and Evaluation

- Assess the patient's ability to ambulate because minocycline may cause dizziness, drowsiness, or vertigo.
- Assess the patient's pattern of daily bowel activity and stool consistency.
- Examine the patient's skin for a rash.
- Check the patient's BP and LOC because of the potential for benign intracranial hypertension.
- Be alert for signs and symptoms of superinfection, such as anal or genital pruritus, diarrhea, and stomatitis.

Patient Teaching

- Instuct the patient to drink a full glass of water with minocycline capsules or tablets and to avoid bedtime doses.
- Advise the patient to space drug doses evenly around the clock and to continue taking minocycline for the full course of treatment.
- Warn the patient to avoid tasks that require mental alertness or motor skills until his or her response to the drug is established.
- Instruct the patient to notify the physician if diarrhea, rash, or other new symptoms occur.
- Encourage the patient to avoid overexposure to the sun or ultraviolet light.

tetracycline hydrochloride

tet-ra-**sye**-kleen
(Achromycin, Apo-Tetra[CAN], Latycin[AUS], Mysteclin[AUS], Novotetra[CAN], Sumycin, Tetrex[AUS])

CATEGORY AND SCHEDULE

Pregnancy Risk Category: D
(B with topical form)

MECHANISM OF ACTION

A tetracycline antibiotic that inhibits bacterial protein synthesis by binding to ribosomes. **Therapeutic Effect:** Bacteriostatic.

PHARMACOKINETICS

Readily absorbed from the GI tract. Protein binding: 30%–60%. Widely distributed. Excreted in urine; eliminated in feces through biliary system. Not removed by hemodialysis. **Half-life:** 6–11 hr (increased in impaired renal function).

AVAILABILITY

Capsules: 250 mg, 500 mg.
Oral Suspension: 125 mg/5 ml.
Tablets: 250 mg, 500 mg.
Topical Solution: 2.2 mg/ml.
Topical Ointment: 3%.

INDICATIONS AND DOSAGES

▸ **Inflammatory acne vulgaris, Lyme disease, mycoplasmal disease, *Legionella* infections, Rocky Mountain spotted fever, chlamydial infections in patients with gonorrhea**
PO
Adults, Elderly. 250–500 mg q6–12h.
Children older than 8 yr. 25–50 mg/kg/day in 4 divided doses. Maximum: 3 g/day.

▸ ***Helicobacter pylori* infections**
PO
Adults, Elderly. 500 mg 2–4 times a day (in combination).
Topical
Adults, Elderly. Apply twice a day (once in the morning, once in the evening).

▸ **Dosage in renal impairment**
Dosage interval is modified based on creatinine clearance.

Creatinine Clearance	Dosage Interval
50–80 ml/min	Usual dose q8–12h
10–50 ml/min	Usual dose q12–24h
less than 10 ml/min	Usual dose q24h

CONTRAINDICATIONS

Children 8 years and younger, hypersensitivity to tetracyclines or sulfites

INTERACTIONS

Drug

Carbamazepine, phenytoin: May decrease tetracycline blood concentration.
Cholestyramine, colestipol: May decrease tetracycline absorption.
Oral contraceptives: May decrease the effects of oral contraceptives.

Herbal

St. John's wort: May increase the risk of photosensitivity.

Food

Dairy products: Inhibit tetracycline absorption.

DIAGNOSTIC TEST EFFECTS

May increase BUN and serum alkaline phosphatase, amylase, bilirubin, AST (SGOT), and ALT (SGPT) levels.

SIDE EFFECTS

Frequent

Dizziness, light-headedness, diarrhea, nausea, vomiting, abdominal cramps, possibly severe photosensitivity
Topical: Dry, scaly skin; stinging or burning sensation

Occasional

Pigmentation of skin or mucous membranes, rectal or genital pruritus, sore mouth or tongue
Topical: Pain, redness, swelling, or other skin irritation.

SERIOUS REACTIONS

! Superinfection (especially fungal), anaphylaxis, and benign intracranial hypertension may occur.
! Bulging fontanelles occur rarely in infants.

NURSING CONSIDERATIONS

Baseline Assessment

◀ALERT▶ Determine if the patient has a history of allergies, especially to tetracyclines or sulfites, before beginning drug therapy.

Lifespan Considerations

- Tetracycline readily crosses the placenta and is distributed in breast milk.
- Women in the last half of pregnancy should avoid using tetracycline because it may inhibit skeletal growth of the fetus.
- Tetracycline use is not recommended for children 8 years and younger because it may cause permanent discoloration of teeth or enamel hypoplasia and may inhibit skeletal growth.
- No age-related precautions have been noted in the elderly.

Precautions

- Use tetracycline cautiously in patients who can't avoid sun or ultraviolet light exposure because such exposure may produce a severe photosensitivity reaction.

Administration and Handling

PO

◀ALERT▶ Space drug doses evenly around the clock.

- Give capsules and tablets with a full glass of water 1 hour before or 2 hours after a meal.

Topical

- Cleanse the area gently before application.
- Because of the drug's potential for staining skin, wear gloves during application and apply the drug only to the affected area.

Intervention and Evaluation

- Assess the patient's pattern of daily bowel activity and stool consistency.
- Monitor the patient's food intake and tolerance.
- Examine the patient's skin for a rash.
- Be alert for signs and symptoms of superinfection, such as anal or genital pruritus, diarrhea, and ulceration or changes of the oral mucosa.
- Monitor the patient's BP and LOC because of the potential for benign intracranial hypertension.

Patient Teaching

- Instruct the patient to take oral tetracycline on an empty stomach 1 hour before or 2 hours after consuming beverages or food.
- Teach the patient to drink a full glass of water with tetracycline capsules and to avoid bedtime tetracycline doses.
- Advise the patient to space drug doses evenly around the clock and to continue taking tetracycline for the full course of treatment.
- Warn the patient to notify the physician if diarrhea, rash, or any other new symptoms occur.
- Encourage the patient to avoid overexposure to the sun or ultraviolet light to prevent photosensitivity reactions.
- Instruct the patient not to take any other medications, including OTC drugs, without consulting the physician.
- Inform the patient that topical tetracycline may turn his or her skin yellow but that washing removes the solution. Also explain that fabrics may be stained by heavy topical application.
- Warn the patient not to apply topical tetracycline to deep or open wounds.

12 Miscellaneous Anti-infective Agents

atovaquone
aztreonam
bacitracin
chloramphenicol
clindamycin
clofazimine
co-trimoxazole (sulfamethoxazole and trimethoprim)
dapsone
daptomycin
drotrecogin alfa
fosfomycin tromethamine
hydroxychloroquine sulfate
linezolid
metronidazole hydrochloride
nitrofurantoin sodium
pentamidine isethionate
quinupristin-dalfopristin
rifaximin
sulfasalazine
telithromycin
tinidazole
trimethoprim
vancomycin hydrochloride

Uses: Miscellaneous anti-infective agents have a wide variety of uses because they belong to many different subclasses. Some agents, such as atovaquone, chloramphenicol, and linezolid, are used for serious infections when other, less toxic agents have failed or aren't appropriate. Others are prescribed to treat uncommon infections, such as malaria (hydroxychloroquine), leprosy (dapsone), and trichomoniasis and amebiasis (metronidazole). Several, including aztreonam, clindamycin, and quinupristin-dalfopristin, combat a broad range of systemic infections, whereas others are used for just one indication, such as fosfomycin and nitrofurantoin, which are used solely to treat UTIs. In addition to treatment, some miscellaneous anti-infectives are used prophylactically, such as vancomycin (to prevent bacterial endocarditis) and co-trimoxazole and pentamidine (to prevent *Pneumocystis carinii* pneumonia).

Action: Miscellaneous anti-infective agents may be bacteriostatic or bactericidal and work in many different ways. (See the illustration *Sites and Mechanisms of Action: Anti-infective Agents,* page 2.) For details, see the specific drug entries.

COMBINATION PRODUCTS

BACTRIM: trimethoprim/sulfamethoxazole (a sulfonamide) 16 mg/80 mg/ml (injection), 40 mg/200 mg/5 ml (suspension), 80 mg/400 mg or 160 mg/800 mg (tablets).
HELIDAC: metronidazole/bismuth (an antisecretory)/tetracycline (an anti-infective) 250 mg/262 mg/500 mg.
MYCITRACIN: bacitracin/polymyxin B (an anti-infective)/neomycin (an aminoglycoside). 400 units/5,000 units/3.5 mg per/g, 500 units/5,000 units/3.5 mg/g.

NEOSPORIN OINTMENT, TRIPLE ANTIBIOTIC: bacitracin/neomycin (an aminoglycoside)/polymyxin B (an anti-infective) 400 units/3.5 mg/5,000 units, 400 units/3.5 mg/10,000 units.
POLYSPORIN: bacitracin/polymyxin B (an anti-infective) 500 units/10,000 units/g.
SEPTRA: trimethoprim/sulfamethoxazole (a sulfonamide) 16 mg/80 mg/ml (injection), 40 mg/200 mg/5 ml (suspension), 80 mg/400 mg or 160 mg/800 mg (tablets).
ZOTRIM: trimethoprim/sulfamethoxazole (a sulfonamide)/phenazopyridine (a urinary analgesic) 160 mg/800 mg/200 mg.

atovaquone

a-**toe**-va-kwone
(Mepron, Wellvone[AUS])

CATEGORY AND SCHEDULE

Pregnancy Risk Category: C

MECHANISM OF ACTION

A systemic anti-infective that inhibits the mitochondrial electron-transport system at the cytochrome bc1 complex (Complex III), which interrupts nucleic acid and adenosine triphosphate synthesis. **Therapeutic Effect:** Antiprotozoal and antipneumocystic activity.

PHARMACOKINETICS

Absorption increased with a high-fat meal. Protein binding: greater than 99%. Metabolized in liver. Primarily excreted in feces. ***Half-life:*** 2–3 days.

AVAILABILITY

Oral Suspension: 750 mg/5 ml.

INDICATIONS AND DOSAGES

▸ ***Pneumocystis carinii*** **pneumonia (PCP)**
PO
Adults. 750 mg twice a day with food for 21 days.
Children. 40 mg/kg/day in 2 divided doses. Maximum: 1,500 mg/day.

▸ **Prevention of PCP**
PO
Adults. 1,500 mg once a day with food.
Children 4–24 mo. 45 mg/kg/day as single dose. Maximum: 1,500 mg/day.
Children 1–3 mo and older than 24 mos. 30 mg/kg/day as single dose. Maximum: 1,500 mg/day.

▸ **Usual pediatric dosage**
PO
Children. 40 mg/kg/day with food.

CONTRAINDICATIONS

Development or history of potentially life-threatening allergic reaction to the drug

INTERACTIONS

Drug
Rifampin: May decrease atovaquone blood concentration and increase rifampin blood concentration.
Herbal
None known.
Food
None known.

DIAGNOSTIC TEST EFFECTS

May increase serum alkaline phosphatase, amylase, AST (SGOT), and ALT (SGPT) levels. May decrease serum sodium levels.

SIDE EFFECTS

Frequent (greater than 10%)
Rash, nausea, diarrhea, headache, vomiting, fever, insomnia, cough

Occasional (less than 10%)
Abdominal discomfort, thrush, asthenia, anemia, neutropenia

SERIOUS REACTIONS

! None known.

NURSING CONSIDERATIONS

Baseline Assessment

• Determine the patient's history of allergies to atovaquone before beginning drug therapy.
• Evaluate the patient's history for medical problems that may interfere with the drug's absorption, such as GI disorders.

Lifespan Considerations

• It is unknown if atovaquone is distributed in breast milk.
• The safety and efficacy of atovaquone have not been established in children.
• No age-related precautions have been noted in the elderly.

Precautions

• Use atovaquone cautiously in elderly patients and in patients with chronic diarrhea, malabsorption syndromes, or severe PCP.

Intervention and Evaluation

• Assess the patient for GI discomfort, nausea, and vomiting.
• Assess the patient's pattern of daily bowel activity and stool consistency.
• Examine the patient's skin for a rash.
• Monitor the patient's Hgb levels, intake and output, and renal function test results.
• Monitor elderly patients closely because of age-related cardiac, hepatic, and renal impairment.

Patient Teaching

• Advise the patient to continue taking atovaquone for the full course of treatment.
• Instruct the patient not to take any other medications without first notifying the physician.
• Urge the patient to notify his or her physician if diarrhea, rash, or other new symptoms occur.

aztreonam

az-**tree**-oo-nam
(Azactam)

CATEGORY AND SCHEDULE

Pregnancy Risk Category: B

MECHANISM OF ACTION

A monobactam antibiotic that inhibits bacterial cell wall synthesis.
Therapeutic Effect: Bactericidal.

PHARMACOKINETICS

Completely absorbed after IM administration. Protein binding: 56%–60%. Partially metabolized by hydrolysis. Primarily excreted unchanged in urine. Removed by hemodialysis. ***Half-life:*** 1.4–2.2 hr (increased in impaired renal or hepatic function).

AVAILABILITY

Injection Powder for Reconstitution: 500 mg, 1 g, 2 g.

INDICATIONS AND DOSAGES

▸ **UTIs**
IV, IM
Adults, Elderly. 500 mg–1 g q8–12h.

▸ **Moderate to severe systemic infections**
IV, IM
Adults, Elderly. 1–2 g q8–12h.

▸ **Severe or life-threatening infections**
IV
Adults, Elderly. 2 g q6–8h.

▸ **Cystic fibrosis**
IV
Children. 50 mg/kg/dose q6–8h up to 200 mg/kg/day. Maximum: 8 g/d.
▸ **Mild to severe infections in children**
IV
Children. 30 mg/kg q6–8h. Maximum: 120 mg/kg/day.
Neonates. 60–120 mg/kg/day q6–12h.
▸ **Dosage in renal impairment**
Dosage and frequency are modified based on creatinine clearance and the severity of the infection:

Creatinine Clearance	Dosage
10–30 ml/min	1–2 g initially, then ½ usual dose at usual intervals
less than 10 ml/min	1–2 g initially; then ¼ usual dose at usual intervals

OFF-LABEL USES
Treatment of bone and joint infections

CONTRAINDICATIONS
None known.

INTERACTIONS
Drug
None known.
Herbal
None known.
Food
None known.

DIAGNOSTIC TEST EFFECTS
May increase serum alkaline phosphatase, creatinine, LDH, AST (SGOT), and ALT (SGPT) levels. Produces a positive Coombs' test.

IV INCOMPATIBILITIES
Acyclovir (Zovirax), amphotericin (Fungizone), daunorubicin (Cerubidine), ganciclovir (Cytovene), lorazepam (Ativan), metronidazole (Flagyl), vancomycin (Vancocin)

IV COMPATIBILITIES
Aminophylline, bumetanide (Bumex), calcium gluconate, cimetidine (Tagamet), diltiazem (Cardizem), dobutamine (Dobutrex), dopamine (Intropin), famotidine (Pepcid), furosemide (Lasix), heparin, hydromorphone (Dilaudid), insulin (regular), magnesium sulfate, morphine, potassium chloride, propofol (Diprivan)

SIDE EFFECTS
Occasional (less than 3%)
Discomfort and swelling at IM injection site, nausea, vomiting, diarrhea, rash
Rare (less than 1%)
Phlebitis or thrombophlebitis at IV injection site, abdominal cramps, headache, hypotension

SERIOUS REACTIONS
! Antibiotic-associated colitis and other superinfections may result from altered bacterial balance.
! Severe hypersensitivity reactions, including anaphylaxis, occur rarely.

NURSING CONSIDERATIONS

Baseline Assessment
◂ **ALERT** ▸ Determine if the patient has a history of allergies, especially to antibiotics, before giving aztreonam.
Lifespan Considerations
- Aztreonam crosses the placenta, and is distributed in amniotic fluid and in low concentrations in breast milk.
- The safety and efficacy of aztreonam have not been established in children less than 9 months old.

- Age-related renal impairment may require a dosage adjustment in the elderly.

Precautions

- Use aztreonam cautiously in patients with hepatic or renal impairment or a history of allergies, especially to antibiotics.

Administration and Handling

IV

- Store vials at room temperature.
- The solution normally appears colorless to light yellow.
- After reconstitution, the solution is stable for 48 hours at room temperature and 7 days if refrigerated.
- Discard the solution if a precipitate forms. Discard unused portions of solution.
- For IV push, dilute each gram with 6–10 ml of sterile water for injection.
- For intermittent IV infusion, further dilute with 50 to 100 ml of D_5W or 0.9% NaCl.
- Administer IV push, over 3 to 5 minutes.
- Administer IV infusion, over 20 to 60 minutes.

IM

- Shake the vial immediately and vigorously after adding the diluent.
- Inject the drug deep into a large muscle mass.
- After reconstitution for IM injection, the solution is stable for 48 hours at room temperature and 7 days if refrigerated.

Intervention and Evaluation

- Evaluate the patient for signs and symptoms of phlebitis, such as heat, pain, and red streaking over the vein and pain at the IM injection site.
- Observe the patient for GI discomfort, nausea, or vomiting.
- Assess the patient's pattern of daily bowel activity and stool consistency.
- Examine the patient's skin for a rash.
- Be alert for signs and symptoms of superinfection, including anal or genital pruritus, black hairy tongue, vomiting, diarrhea, fever, sore throat, and ulceration or changes of oral mucosa.

Patient Teaching

- Urge the patient to report any diarrhea, nausea, rash, or vomiting he or she experiences.

bacitracin

bass-i-**tray**-sin

(Baciguent, Baci-IM, Bacitracin)

Do not confuse bacitracin with Bactrim or Bactroban.

CATEGORY AND SCHEDULE

Pregnancy Risk Category: C

OTC

MECHANISM OF ACTION

An antibiotic that interferes with plasma membrane permeability and inhibits bacterial cell wall synthesis in susceptible bacteria. **Therapeutic Effect:** Bacteriostatic.

AVAILABILITY

Powder for Irrigation: 50,000 units.
Ophthalmic Ointment: 500 units/g.
Topical Ointment: 500 units/g.

INDICATIONS AND DOSAGES

▸ **Superficial ocular infections**

Ophthalmic

Adults. ½-inch ribbon in conjunctival sac q3–4h.

▸ **Skin abrasions, superficial skin infections**

Topical

Adults, Children. Apply to affected area 1–5 times a day.

▸ **Surgical treatment and prophylaxis**

Irrigation

Adults, Elderly. 50,000–150,000 units, as needed.

CONTRAINDICATIONS
None known.

INTERACTIONS
Drug
None known.
Herbal
None known.
Food
None known.

DIAGNOSTIC TEST EFFECTS
None known.

SIDE EFFECTS
Rare
Ophthalmic: Burning, itching, redness, swelling, pain
Topical: Hypersensitivity reaction (allergic contact dermatitis, burning, inflammation, pruritus)

SERIOUS REACTIONS
! Severe hypersensitivity reactions, including apnea and hypotension, occur rarely.

NURSING CONSIDERATIONS
Baseline Assessment
Determine the patient's history of allergies to bacitracin before beginning drug therapy.
Precautions
◀ALERT▶ When administering a fixed-combination product containing bacitracin, familiarize yourself with the side effects of each of the product's drug components.
Administration and Handling
Ophthalmic
- Place a gloved finger on the patient's lower eyelid and pull it out until a pocket is formed between the eye and lower lid. Place ¼ to ½ inch of the ointment in the pocket.
- Have the patient close the eye gently for 1 to 2 minutes and roll the eyeball to increase the drug's contact with the eye.
- Remove excess ointment around the eye with a tissue.
Intervention and Evaluation
Topical
- If the patient is using the ophthalmic ointment, assess his or her eye for a therapeutic response or a hypersensitivity reaction (increased burning, pruritus, redness, and swelling).
- If the patient is using the topical ointment, be alert for signs and symptoms of hypersensitivity, such as burning, inflammation, and pruritus.
- When using preparations containing corticosteroids, closely monitor the patient for any unusual signs or symptoms because corticosteroids may mask clinical signs.
Patient Teaching
- Advise the patient to space drug doses evenly around the clock and to continue using bacitracin for the full course of treatment.
- Urge the patient to report burning, itching, increased irritation, or rash.

chloramphenicol
klor-am-**fen**-i-kole
(Chloromycetin, Chloroptic, Chlorsig[AUS], Poenfenicol[AUS])
Do not confuse chloramphenicol with chlorambucil.

CATEGORY AND SCHEDULE
Pregnancy Risk Category: C

MECHANISM OF ACTION
A dichloroacetic acid derivative that inhibits bacterial protein synthesis by binding to bacterial ribosomal receptor sites. **Therapeutic Effect:** Bacteriostatic (may be bactericidal in high concentrations).

AVAILABILITY

Powder for Injection: 100 mg/ml.
Ophthalmic Ointment: 10 mg/g.
Ophthalmic Solution: 5 mg/ml.

INDICATIONS AND DOSAGES

▸ Mild to moderate infections caused by organisms resistant to other less toxic antibiotics

IV

Adults, Elderly. 50–100 mg/kg/day in divided doses q6h. Maximum: 4 g/day.

Children older than 1 mo. 50–75 mg/kg/day in divided doses q6h. Maximum: 4 g/day

▸ Meningitis

IV

Children older than 1 mo. 50–100 mg/kg/day in divided doses q6h.

▸ Usual ophthalmic dosage

Adults, Elderly, Children. 1–2 drops 4–6 times/day.

CONTRAINDICATIONS

Hypersensitivity to chloramphenicol

INTERACTIONS

Drug

Anticonvulsants, bone marrow depressants: May increase myelosuppression.

Clindamycin, erythromycin: May antagonize the effects of these drugs.

Oral antidiabetics: May increase the effects of these drugs.

Phenobarbital, phenytoin, warfarin: May increase blood concentrations of these drugs.

Vitamin B_{12}: May decrease the effects of vitamin B_{12} in patients with pernicious anemia.

Herbal

None known.

Food

None known.

DIAGNOSTIC TEST EFFECTS

Therapeutic blood level: 10–20 mcg/ml; toxic blood level: greater than 25 mcg/ml. When administered with iron salts, may increase serum iron levels.

SIDE EFFECTS

Occasional

Systemic: Nausea, vomiting, diarrhea

Ophthalmic: Blurred vision, burning, stinging, hypersensitivity reaction

Otic: Hypersensitivity reaction

Rare

"Gray baby" syndrome in neonates (abdominal distention, blue-gray skin color, cardiovascular collapse, unresponsiveness), rash, shortness of breath, confusion, headache, optic neuritis (blurred vision, eye pain), peripheral neuritis (numbness and weakness in feet and hands)

SERIOUS REACTIONS

! Superinfection due to bacterial or fungal overgrowth may occur.

! There is a narrow margin between effective therapy and toxic levels producing blood dyscrasias.

! Myelosuppression, with resulting aplastic anemia, hypoplastic anemia, and pancytopenia, may occur weeks or months later.

NURSING CONSIDERATIONS

Baseline Assessment

- Determine if the patient is also receiving other drugs that cause myelosuppression because chloramphenicol should not be given concurrently with these drugs, if possible.
- Expect to obtain baseline blood studies before beginning chloramphenicol therapy.

Precautions

- Use chloramphenicol cautiously in patients with myelosuppression, or renal or hepatic impairment, and in those who have previously under-

gone cytotoxic drug therapy or radiation therapy.
• Use chloramphenicol cautiously in children younger than 2 years.

Intervention and Evaluation

• Assess the patient for nausea and vomiting.
• Assess the patient's pattern of daily bowel activity and stool consistency.
• Evaluate the patient's mental status.
• Determine if the patient is experiencing visual disturbances.
• Examine the patient's skin for a rash.
• Be alert for signs and symptoms of superinfection, such as anal or genital pruritus, a change in the oral mucosa, diarrhea, and increased fever.
• Monitor the patient's drug blood levels (therapeutic blood level is 10 to 20 mcg/ml; toxic blood level is greater than 25 mcg/ml).

Patient Teaching

• Advise the patient to space drug doses evenly around the clock and to continue taking chloramphenicol for the full course of treatment.
• Instruct the patient using the ophthalmic form to continue treatment for at least 48 hours after the eye returns to normal appearance.

clindamycin

klin-da-**mye**-sin
(Cleocin, Cleocin HCl[AUS], Clindesse, Dalacin[CAN], Dalacin C[AUS])

CATEGORY AND SCHEDULE

Pregnancy Risk Category: B

MECHANISM OF ACTION

A lincosamide antibiotic that inhibits protein synthesis of the bacterial cell wall by binding to bacterial ribosomal receptor sites. Topically, it decreases fatty acid concentration on the skin. **Therapeutic Effect:** Bacteriostatic. Prevents outbreaks of acne vulgaris.

PHARMACOKINETICS

Rapidly absorbed from the GI tract. Protein binding: 92%–94%. Widely distributed. Metabolized in the liver to some active metabolites. Primarily excreted in urine. Not removed by hemodialysis. ***Half-life:*** 2.4–3 hr (increased in impaired renal function and premature infants).

AVAILABILITY

Capsules: 75 mg, 150 mg, 300 mg.
Oral Solution: 75 mg/5 ml.
Injection: 150 mg/ml.
Topical Gel: 1%.
Topical Solution: 1%.
Vaginal Cream (Clindesse): 2%.
Vaginal Suppository: 100 mg.

INDICATIONS AND DOSAGES

▸ **Chronic bone and joint, respiratory tract, skin and soft-tissue, intra-abdominal, and female GU infections; endocarditis; septicemia**

PO

Adults, Elderly. 150–450 mg/dose q6–8h.
Children. 10–30 mg/kg/day in 3–4 divided doses. Maximum: 1.8 g/day.

IV, IM

Adults, Elderly. 1.2–1.8 g/day in 2–4 divided doses.
Children. 25–40 mg/kg/day in 3–4 divided doses. Maximum: 4.8 g/day.

▸ **Bacterial vaginosis**

PO

Adults, Elderly. 300 mg twice a day for 7 days.

Intravaginal

Adults. One applicatorful at bedtime for 3–7 days or 1 suppository at bedtime for 3 days.

▸ **Acne vulgaris**
Topical
Adults. Apply thin layer to affected area twice a day.

OFF-LABEL USES
Treatment of malaria, otitis media, *Pneumocystis carinii* pneumonia, toxoplasmosis

CONTRAINDICATIONS
History of antibiotic-associated colitis, regional enteritis, or ulcerative colitis; hypersensitivity to clindamycin or lincomycin; known allergy to tartrazine dye

INTERACTIONS
Drug
Adsorbent antidiarrheals: May delay absorption of clindamycin.
Chloramphenicol, erythromycin: May antagonize the effects of clindamycin.
Neuromuscular blockers: May increase the effects of these drugs.
Herbal
None known.
Food
None known.

DIAGNOSTIC TEST EFFECTS
May increase serum alkaline phosphatase, AST (SGOT), and ALT (SGPT) levels.

IV INCOMPATIBILITIES
Allopurinol (Aloprim), filgrastim (Neupogen), fluconazole (Diflucan), idarubicin (Idamycin)

IV COMPATIBILITIES
Amiodarone (Cordarone), diltiazem (Cardizem), heparin, hydromorphone (Dilaudid), magnesium sulfate, midazolam (Versed), morphine, multivitamins, propofol (Diprivan)

SIDE EFFECTS
Frequent
Systemic: Abdominal pain, nausea, vomiting, diarrhea
Topical: Dry scaly skin
Vaginal: Vaginitis, pruritus
Occasional
Systemic: Phlebitis or thrombophlebitis with IV administration, pain and induration at IM injection site, allergic reaction, urticaria, pruritus
Topical: Contact dermatitis, abdominal pain, mild diarrhea, burning or stinging
Vaginal: Headache, dizziness, nausea, vomiting, abdominal pain
Rare
Vaginal: Hypersensitivity reaction

SERIOUS REACTIONS
! Antibiotic-associated colitis and other superinfections may occur during and several weeks after clindamycin therapy (including the topical form).
! Blood dyscrasias (leukopenia, thrombocytopenia) and nephrotoxicity (proteinuria, azotemia, oliguria) occur rarely.

NURSING CONSIDERATIONS
Baseline Assessment
◂ALERT▸ Determine if the patient has a history of allergies, particularly to aspirin, clindamycin, or lincomycin, before beginning drug therapy.
- Determine if the patient is also receiving neuromuscular blockers; avoid concurrent use, if possible.

Lifespan Considerations
- Systemic clindamycin readily crosses the placenta and is distributed in breast milk.
- It is unknown if the topical and vaginal forms of clindamycin are distributed in breast milk.
- Use clindamycin cautiously in children less than 1 month old.

• No age-related precautions have been noted in the elderly.

Precautions

• Use clindamycin cautiously in patients with severe renal or hepatic dysfunction and in patients using neuromuscular blockers concurrently.

• Don't apply topical preparations to abraded areas or near the eyes.

Administration and Handling

PO

• Store capsules at room temperature.

• Give capsules with 8 oz of water and without regard to food.

• After reconstitution, the oral solution is stable for 2 weeks at room temperature.

• Don't refrigerate the oral solution to avoid thickening it.

IV

• The IV infusion (piggyback) is stable at room temperature for up to 16 days.

• Dilute 300 to 600 mg with 50 ml D_5W or 0.9% NaCl (900 to 1,200 mg with 100 ml). Never exceed a concentration of 18 mg/ml.

• Infuse 50-ml (300- to 600-mg) piggyback solution over 10 to 20 minutes; infuse 100-ml (900-mg to 1.2-g) piggyback solution over 30 to 40 minutes. Be aware that severe hypotension or cardiac arrest can occur with too-rapid administration.

• Don't administer more than 1.2 g in a single infusion.

IM

• Don't exceed 600 mg/dose.

• Give by deep IM injection.

Intervention and Evaluation

• Assess the patient's pattern of daily bowel activity and stool consistency. Report diarrhea promptly to the physician because of the potential for developing serious colitis (even with topical or vaginal clindamycin).

• Assess the patient's skin for dryness, irritation, and rash with topical application.

• Be alert for signs and symptoms of superinfection, such as anal or genital pruritus, a change in oral mucosa, increased fever, and severe diarrhea.

Patient Teaching

• Instruct the patient to take oral doses with 8 oz water.

• Advise the patient to space drug doses evenly around the clock and to continue taking clindamycin for the full course of treatment.

• Warn the patient to use caution when applying topical clindamycin concurrently with abrasive, peeling acne agents, soaps, or alcohol-containing cosmetics to avoid a cumulative effect.

• Instruct the patient not to apply topical preparations near the eyes or on abraded areas.

• Direct the patient to rinse her eyes with copious amounts of cool tap water if the vaginal form of clindamycin accidentally comes in contact with her eyes.

• Advise the patient not to engage in sexual intercourse during treatment with the vaginal form of clindamycin.

clofazimine

kloe-**faz**-i-meen

(Lamprene)

CATEGORY AND SCHEDULE

Pregnancy Risk Category: C

MECHANISM OF ACTION

An antibiotic that binds to mycobacterial DNA. **Therapeutic Effect:** Inhibits mycobacterial growth and produces anti-inflammatory action.

AVAILABILITY

Capsules: 50 mg.

INDICATIONS AND DOSAGES

▸ Leprosy

PO

Adults, Elderly. 100 mg/day in combination with dapsone and rifampin for 3 yr then 100 mg/day as monotherapy.

Children. 1 mg/kg/day in combination with dapsone and rifampin.

▸ Erythema nodosum

PO

Adults, Elderly. 100–200 mg/day for up to 3 mo, then 100 mg/day.

CONTRAINDICATIONS

None significant.

INTERACTIONS

Drug

Dapsone: May decrease the effects of clofazimine.

Herbal

None significant.

Food

All foods: May increase the absorption of clofazimine.

DIAGNOSTIC TEST EFFECTS

May increase blood glucose levels.

SIDE EFFECTS

Frequent (greater than 10%)

Dry skin, abdominal pain, nausea, vomiting, diarrhea, skin discoloration (pink to brownish-black)

Occasional (10%–1%)

Rash; pruritus; eye irritation; discoloration of sputum, sweat, and urine

SERIOUS REACTIONS

! None significant.

NURSING CONSIDERATIONS

Baseline Assessment

- Assess the patient for sensitivity to clofazimine.

Precautions

- Use clofazimine cautiously in patients with GI problems, including abdominal pain and diarrhea.

Administration and Handling

PO

- Clofazimine may be given with food.

Intervention and Evaluation

- Monitor the patient's GI signs and symptoms.
- Notify the physician if the patient complains of crampy or colicky abdominal pain.

Patient Teaching

- Instruct the patient to take clofazimine with meals to decrease GI discomfort.
- Inform the patient that clofazimine may cause skin discoloration.

co-trimoxazole (sulfamethoxazole and trimethoprim)

koe-trye-**mox**-a-zole

(Apo-Sulfatrim[CAN], Bactrim, Bactrim DS, Cosig Forte[AUS], Novotrimel[CAN], Resprim[AUS], Resprim Forte[AUS], Septra, Septra DS, Septrin[AUS], Septrin Forte[AUS], Sulfatrim Pediatric)

Do not confuse Bactrim with bacitracin, co-trimoxazole with clotrimazole, or Septra with Sectral or Septa.

CATEGORY AND SCHEDULE

Pregnancy Risk Category: C

MECHANISM OF ACTION

A sulfonamide and folate antagonist that blocks bacterial synthesis of essential nucleic acids. **Therapeutic Effect:** Bactericidal in susceptible microorganisms.

PHARMACOKINETICS

Rapidly and well absorbed from the GI tract. Protein binding: 45%–60%. Widely distributed. Metabolized in the liver. Excreted in urine. Minimally removed by hemodialysis. ***Half-life:*** sulfamethoxazole 6–12 hr, trimethoprim 8–10 hr (increased in impaired renal function).

AVAILABILITY

◀ **ALERT** ▶ All dosage forms have same 5:1 ratio of sulfamethoxazole (SMX) to trimethoprim (TMP).
Oral Suspension (Septra, Sulfatrim Pediatric): SMX 200 mg and TMP 40 mg per 5 ml.
Tablets (Bactrim, Septra): SMX 400 mg and TMP 80 mg.
Tablets (Double Strength [Bactrim DS, Septra DS]): SMX 800 mg and TMP 160 mg.
Injection (Septra): SMX 80 mg and TMP 16 mg per ml.

INDICATIONS AND DOSAGES

▸ **Mild to moderate infections**
PO, IV
Adults, Elderly, Children older than 2 mo. 6–12 mg/kg/day in divided doses q12h.
▸ **Serious infections, *Pneumocystis Carinii* pneumonia (PCP)**
PO, IV
Adults, Elderly, Children older than 2 mo. 15–20 mg/kg/day in divided doses q6–8 h.
▸ **Prevention of PCP**
PO
Adults. One double-strength tablet each day.
Children. 150 mg/m^2/day on 3 consecutive days/wk.
▸ **Traveler's diarrhea**
PO
Adults, Elderly. One double-strength tablet q12h for 5 days.
▸ **Acute exacerbation of chronic bronchitis**
PO
Adults, Elderly. One double-strength tablet q12h for 14 days.
▸ **Prevention of UTIs**
PO
Adults, Elderly, children older than 2 mo. 2 mg/kg/dose once a day.
▸ **Dosage in renal impairment**
Dosage and frequency are modified based on creatinine clearance, the severity of the infection and the serum concentration of the drug. For those with creatinine clearance of 15–30 ml/min, a 50% dosage reduction is recommended.

OFF-LABEL USES

Treatment of bacterial endocarditis; gonorrhea; meningitis; septicemia; sinusitis; and biliary tract, bone, joint, chancroid, chlamydial, intra-abdominal, skin, and soft-tissue infections

CONTRAINDICATIONS

Hypersensitivity to trimethoprim or any sulfonamides, infants younger than 2 months old, megaloblastic anemia due to folate deficiency

INTERACTIONS

Drug

Hemolytics: May increase the risk of toxicity.
Hepatotoxic medications: May increase the risk of hepatotoxicity.
Hydantoin anticonvulsants, oral antidiabetics, warfarin: May increase or prolong the effects of these drugs and increase their risk of toxicity.
Methenamine: May form a precipitate.

Methotrexate: May increase the effects of methotrexate.

Herbal

None known.

Food

None known.

DIAGNOSTIC TEST EFFECTS

May increase BUN and serum alkaline phosphatase, creatinine, potassium, AST (SGOT), and ALT (SGPT) levels.

IV INCOMPATIBILITIES

Fluconazole (Diflucan), foscarnet (Foscavir), midazolam (Versed), vinorelbine (Navelbine)

IV COMPATIBILITIES

Diltiazem (Cardizem), heparin, hydromorphone (Dilaudid), lorazepam (Ativan), magnesium sulfate, morphine

SIDE EFFECTS

Frequent

Anorexia, nausea, vomiting, rash (generally 7–14 days after therapy begins), urticaria

Occasional

Diarrhea, abdominal pain, pain or irritation at the IV infusion site

Rare

Headache, vertigo, insomnia, seizures, hallucinations, depression

SERIOUS REACTIONS

! Rash, fever, sore throat, pallor, purpura, cough, and shortness of breath may be early signs of serious adverse reactions.

! Fatalities have occasionally occurred after Stevens-Johnson syndrome, toxic epidermal necrolysis, fulminant hepatic necrosis, agranulocytosis, aplastic anemia, and other blood dyscrasias in patients taking sulfonamides.

! Myelosuppression, decreased platelet count and severe dermatologic reactions may occur, especially in the elderly.

NURSING CONSIDERATIONS

Baseline Assessment

◀ALERT▶ Determine if the patient has a history of bronchial asthma, hypersensitivity to trimethoprim or any sulfonamide, or sulfite sensitivity before beginning drug therapy.

- Expect to establish the patient's hematologic, hepatic, and renal baselines.

Lifespan Considerations

- Co-trimoxazole use is contraindicated during pregnancy at term and during breast-feeding.
- Co-trimoxazole readily crosses the placenta and is distributed in breast milk.
- Co-trimoxazole use is contraindicated in children younger than 2 months old; if given to newborns, it may produce kernicterus.
- Elderly patients have an increased risk of developing myelosuppression, decreased platelet count, and severe skin reactions.

Precautions

- Use co-trimoxazole cautiously in patients with impaired renal or hepatic function or glucose-6-phosphate dehydrogenase deficiency.

Administration and Handling

◀ALERT▶ Be aware that drug potency is expressed in terms of trimethoprim content.

PO

- Store tablets and oral suspension at room temperature.
- Give the oral form with 8 oz water on an empty stomach. Have the patient drink several additional glasses of water each day.

IV

- For piggyback IV infusion, dilute each 5-ml vial with 75 to 125 ml D_5W.

• Discard the solution if it is cloudy or contains a precipitate.
• Don't mix co-trimoxazole with other drugs or solutions.
• Be aware that the piggyback IV infusion solution is stable for 2 to 6 hours. Use the solution immediately.
• Infuse the solution over 60 to 90 minutes. Avoid bolus or rapid infusion and IM injection.
• Ensure that the patient is adequately hydrated.

Intervention and Evaluation

• Monitor the patient's intake and output.
• Assess the patient's pattern of daily bowel activity and stool consistency.
• Examine the patient's skin for pallor, purpura, and rash.
• Check the patient's IV site and flow rate.
• Monitor the patient's hematology studies and renal and liver function test reports.
• Evaluate the patient for CNS symptoms, such as hallucinations, headache, insomnia, and vertigo.
• Monitor the patient's vital signs at least twice a day.
• Evaluate the patient for cough or shortness of breath.
• Assess the patient for ecchymosis, overt bleeding, or edema.

Patient Teaching

• Instruct the patient to take oral co-trimoxazole doses with 8 oz of water and to drink several extra glasses of water each day.
• Advise the patient to space drug doses evenly around the clock and to continue taking co-trimoxazole for the full course of treatment.
• Warn the patient to notify the physician immediately if he or she experiences any new symptoms, especially bleeding, bruising, fever, sore throat, and a rash or other skin changes.

dapsone

dap-sone
(Dapsone)

CATEGORY AND SCHEDULE

Pregnancy Risk Category: C

MECHANISM OF ACTION

An antibiotic that is a competitive antagonist of para-aminobenzoic acid (PABA); it prevents normal bacterial utilization of PABA for synthesis of folic acid. **Therapeutic Effect:** Inhibits bacterial growth.

AVAILABILITY

Tablets: 25 mg, 100 mg.

INDICATIONS AND DOSAGES

▸ **Leprosy**

PO

Adults, Elderly. 50–100 mg/day for 3–10 yr.
Children. 1–2 mg/kg/24 hr. Maximum: 100 mg/day.

▸ **Dermatitis herpetiformis**

PO

Adults, Elderly. Initially, 50 mg/day. May increase up to 300 mg/day.

▸ ***Pneumocystis carinii* pneumonia (PCP)**

PO

Adults, Elderly. 100 mg/day in combination with trimethoprim for 21 days.

▸ **Prevention of PCP**

PO

Adults, Elderly. 100 mg/day.
Children older than 1 mo. 2 mg/kg/day. Maximum: 100 mg/day.

OFF-LABEL USES

Treatment of inflammatory bowel disorders, malaria

CONTRAINDICATIONS

None significant.

INTERACTIONS

Drug

Methotrexate: May increase hematologic reactions.
Probenecid: May decrease the excretion of dapsone.
Protease inhibitors (including ritonavir): May increase dapsone blood concentration.
Rifampin: May decrease rifampin blood concentration.
Trimethoprim: May increase the risk of toxic effects.

Herbal

St. John's wort: May decrease dapsone blood concentration.

Food

None significant.

DIAGNOSTIC TEST EFFECTS

None significant.

SIDE EFFECTS

Frequent (greater than 10%)
Hemolytic anemia, methemoglobinemia, rash
Occasional (10%–1%)
Hemolysis, photosensitivity reaction

SERIOUS REACTIONS

! Agranulocytosis and blood dyscrasias may occur.

NURSING CONSIDERATIONS

Baseline Assessment

- Obtain the patient's baseline CBC as ordered.
- Determine if the patient has a hypersensitivity to dapsone or its derivatives, such as sulfoxone sodium.

Precautions

- Use dapsone cautiously in patients with agranulocytosis, severe anemia, aplastic anemia, glucose-6-phosphate dehydrogenase deficiency, or a hypersensitivity to dapsone or its derivatives (such as sulfoxone sodium).

Administration and Handling

PO
- Give dapsone without regard to food.

Intervention and Evaluation

- Assess the patient's skin for a dermatologic reaction.
- Monitor the patient for signs and symptoms of hemolysis, such as jaundice.
- Monitor the patient's CBC.

Patient Teaching

- Explain to the patient that frequent blood tests are necessary, especially during early dapsone therapy.
- Instruct the patient to notify the physician and discontinue dapsone if a rash occurs.
- Advise the patient to report persistent fatigue, fever, or sore throat.
- Encourage the patient to avoid overexposure to sun or ultraviolet light.

daptomycin

dap-toe-my-sin
(Cubicin)

CATEGORY AND SCHEDULE

Pregnancy Risk Category: B

MECHANISM OF ACTION

A lipopeptide antibacterial agent that binds to bacterial membranes and causes a rapid depolarization of the membrane potential. The loss of membrane potential leads to inhibition of protein, DNA, and RNA synthesis. **Therapeutic Effect:** Bactericidal.

PHARMACOKINETICS

Widely distributed. Protein binding: 90%. Primarily excreted unchanged in urine. Moderately removed by hemodialysis. ***Half-life:*** 7–8 hr (increased in impaired renal function).

AVAILABILITY
Powder for Injection: 250 mg/vial, 500 mg/vial.

INDICATIONS AND DOSAGES
▸ **Complicated skin and skin-structure infections**
IV
Adults, Elderly. 4 mg/kg every 24 hr for 7–14 days.
▸ **Dosage in renal impairment**
For patients with creatinine clearance of less than 30 ml/min, dosage is 4 mg/kg q48h for 7–14 days.

CONTRAINDICATIONS
None known.

INTERACTIONS
Drug
HMG-CoA reductase inhibitors: May cause myopathy.
Tobramycin: Increases the serum concentration of daptomycin.
Herbal
None known.
Food
None known.

DIAGNOSTIC TEST EFFECTS
May increase serum CPK levels. May alter liver function test results.

IV INCOMPATIBILITIES
Diluents containing dextrose. If the same IV line is used to administer different drugs, the line should be flushed with 0.9% NaCl.

SIDE EFFECTS
Frequent (6%–5%)
Constipation, nausea, peripheral injection site reactions, headache, diarrhea
Occasional (4%–3%)
Insomnia, rash, vomiting
Rare (less than 3%)
Pruritus, dizziness, hypotension

SERIOUS REACTIONS
! Skeletal muscle myopathy, characterized by muscle pain and weakness, particularly of the distal extremities, occurs rarely.
! Antibiotic-associated colitis and other superinfections may result from altered bacterial balance.

NURSING CONSIDERATIONS
Baseline Assessment
• Obtain culture and sensitivity tests, as ordered, before giving the first dose of daptomycin. Therapy may begin before the test results are known.
Lifespan Considerations
• It is unknown if daptomycin is distributed in breast milk.
• The safety and efficacy of this drug have not been established in children younger than 18 years of age.
• No age-related precautions have been noted in the elderly.
Precautions
• Use daptomycin cautiously in pregnant patients and patients with a history of or current musculoskeletal disorders or renal impairment.
• Avoid concurrent use of HMG-CoA reductase inhibitors because they may cause myopathy.
Administration and Handling
IV
• Store the drug in the refrigerator.
• The drug normally appears as a pale yellow to light brown lyophilized cake.
• Discard the solution if it contains particulate matter.
• Reconstitute the 250-mg vial with 5 ml 0.9% NaCl and the 500 mg vial with 10 ml 0.9% NaCl.
• Further dilute in 50 ml 0.9% NaCl.
• The reconstituted solution is stable for 12 hours at room temperature and up to 48 hours if refrigerated.

• Infuse the intermittent IV (piggyback) infusion over 30 minutes.

Intervention and Evaluation

• Check for white patches on the patient's mucous membranes and tongue.
• Assess the patient's pattern of daily bowel activity and stool consistency. Mild GI effects may be tolerable, but severe symptoms may indicate the onset of antibiotic-associated colitis.
• Be alert for signs and symptoms of superinfection, including abdominal pain, moderate to severe diarrhea, severe anal or genital pruritus, and severe mouth soreness.
• Monitor the patient for dizziness and institute appropriate safety measures.

Patient Teaching

• Instruct the patient to notify the physician if he or she experiences headache, nausea, rash, severe diarrhea, new muscle weakness, or any other new symptoms.

drotrecogin alfa

droh-tree-**koh**-gen
(Xigris)

CATEGORY AND SCHEDULE

Pregnancy Risk Category: C

MECHANISM OF ACTION

A recombinant form of human-activated protein C that exerts an antithrombotic effect by inhibiting Factors Va and VIIIa and may exert an indirect profibrinolytic effect by inhibiting plasminogen activator inhibitor-1 and limiting the generation of activated thrombin-activatable-fibrinolysis-inhibitor. The drug may also exert an anti-inflammatory effect by inhibiting tumor necrosis factor production by monocytes, by blocking leukocyte adhesion to selectins, and by limiting thrombin-induced inflammatory responses. **Therapeutic Effect:** Produces anti-inflammatory, antithrombotic, and profibrinolytic effects.

PHARMACOKINETICS

Inactivated by endogenous plasma protease inhibitors. Clearance occurs within 2 hr of initiating infusion. ***Half-life:*** 1.6 hr.

AVAILABILITY

Powder for Infusion: 5 mg, 20 mg.

INDICATIONS AND DOSAGES

▸ **Severe sepsis**

IV Infusion

Adults, Elderly. 24 mcg/kg/hr for 96 hr.

CONTRAINDICATIONS

Active internal bleeding, evidence of cerebral herniation, intracranial neoplasm or mass lesion, presence of an epidural catheter, recent (within the past 3 mo) hemorrhagic stroke, recent (within the past 2 mo) intracranial or intraspinal surgery or severe head trauma, trauma with an increased risk of life-threatening bleeding

INTERACTIONS

Drug

None known.

Herbal

None known.

Food

None known.

DIAGNOSTIC TEST EFFECTS

May prolong aPTT.

IV INCOMPATIBILITIES

Don't mix drotrecogin alfa with other medications.

IV COMPATIBILITIES

Lactated Ringer's solution, 0.9% NaCl, and dextrose are the only solutions that can be administered through the same line.

SIDE EFFECTS

None known.

SERIOUS REACTIONS

! Bleeding (intrathoracic, retroperitoneal, GI, GU, intra-abdominal, intracranial) occurs in about 2% of patients.

NURSING CONSIDERATIONS

Baseline Assessment

- The following criteria must be met before initiating drotrecogin alfa therapy: age of at least 18 years; weight less than 135 kg; no pregnancy or breast-feeding; 3 or more systemic inflammatory response criteria (fever, heart rate greater than 90 beats/minute, respiratory rate greater than 20 breaths/minute, increased WBC count); and at least one sepsis-induced organ or system failure (cardiovascular, hepatic, renal, respiratory, or unexplained metabolic acidosis).

Lifespan Considerations

- It is unknown if drotrecogin alfa causes fetal harm or is excreted in breast milk.
- The safety and efficacy of drotrecogin alfa have not been established in children or the elderly.

Precautions

- Use drotrecogin alfa cautiously in patients with chronic, severe hepatic disease, intracranial aneurysm, platelet count less than 30,000/mm^3, or prolonged prothrombin time and in those who have had GI bleeding within the past 6 weeks.
- Use the drug cautiously in patients who are using heparin concurrently and in those who have had thrombolytic therapy within the past 3 days or anticoagulant or aspirin therapy within the past 7 days.
- Use caution when administering other drugs that affect hemostasis.

Administration and Handling

IV

- Store unreconstituted vials at room temperature.
- Reconstitute the 5-mg and 20-mg vials by slowly adding 2.5 ml or 10 ml of sterile water for injection, respectively, to yield a concentration of 2 mg/ml.
- Swirl the vial gently to mix; don't shake or invert it.
- Add the reconstituted drug to an infusion bag containing 0.9% NaCl, and dilute to a final concentration of 100 to 200 mcg/ml. Direct the stream to the side of the bag to minimize agitation.
- Invert the infusion bag to mix the solution.
- Start the infusion within 3 hours after reconstitution.
- Administer the drug through a dedicated IV line or a dedicated lumen of a multilumen central venous catheter at a rate of 24 mcg/kg/hr for 96 hours.
- If the infusion is interrupted, restart it at 24 mcg/kg/hr, as prescribed.

Intervention and Evaluation

- Monitor the patient closely for hemorrhagic complications.

Patient Teaching

- Inform the patient that bleeding may occur for up to 28 days after treatment. Warn the patient to immediately notify the physician if signs or symptoms of unusual bleeding occur.

fosfomycin tromethamine

foss-fo-**mye**-sin
(Monurol)
Do not confuse Monurol with Monopril.

CATEGORY AND SCHEDULE

Pregnancy Risk Category: B

MECHANISM OF ACTION

An antibiotic that prevents bacterial cell wall formation by inhibiting the synthesis of peptidoglycan. **Therapeutic Effect:** Bactericidal.

AVAILABILITY

Powder for Oral Solution: 3 g.

INDICATIONS AND DOSAGES

▸ **Uncomplicated UTIs**

PO

Females. 3 g mixed in 4 oz water as a single dose.
Males. 3 g/day for 2–3 days.

CONTRAINDICATIONS

None known.

INTERACTIONS

Drug

Metoclopramide: Lowers serum concentration and urinary excretion of fosfomycin.

Herbal

None known.

Food

None known.

DIAGNOSTIC TEST EFFECTS

May increase blood eosinophil count and serum alkaline phosphatase, bilirubin, AST (SGOT), and ALT (SGPT) levels. May alter platelet and WBC counts. May decrease blood Hct and Hgb levels.

SIDE EFFECTS

Occasional (9%–3%)
Diarrhea, nausea, headache, back pain
Rare (less than 2%)
Dysmenorrhea, pharyngitis, abdominal pain, rash

SERIOUS REACTIONS

! None known.

NURSING CONSIDERATIONS

Administration and Handling

• Give fosfomycin without regard to food.

Patient Teaching

• Instruct the patient to always mix fosfomycin with water before consuming.
• Inform the patient that symptoms should improve 2 to 3 days after the initial dose of fosfomycin.

hydroxychloroquine sulfate

hye-drox-ee-**klor**-oh-kwin
(Apo-Hydroxyquine [CAN], Plaquenil)
Do not confuse hydroxychloroquine with hydrocortisone or hydroxyzine.

CATEGORY AND SCHEDULE

Pregnancy Risk Category: C

MECHANISM OF ACTION

An antimalarial and antirheumatic that concentrates in parasite acid vesicles, increasing the pH of the vesicles and interfering with parasite protein synthesis. Antirheumatic action may involve suppressing formation of antigens responsible for hypersensitivity reactions. **Therapeutic Effect:** Inhibits parasite growth.

AVAILABILITY

Tablets: 200 mg (155 mg base).

INDICATIONS AND DOSAGES

▸ **Treatment of acute attack of malaria (dosage in mg base)**

PO

Dose	Times	Adults	Children
Initial	Day 1	620 mg	10 mg/kg
Second	6 hr later	310 mg	5 mg/kg
Third	Day 2	310 mg	5 mg/kg
Fourth	Day 3	310 mg	5 mg/kg

▸ **Suppression of malaria**

PO

Adults. 310 mg base weekly on same day each week, beginning 2 wk before entering an endemic area and continuing for 4–6 wk after leaving the area.

Children. 5 mg base/kg/wk, beginning 2 wk before entering an endemic area and continuing for 4–6 wk after leaving the area. If therapy is not begun before exposure, administer a loading dose of 10 mg base/kg in 2 equally divided doses 6 hr apart, followed by the ususal dosage regimen.

▸ **Rheumatoid arthritis**

PO

Adults. Initially, 400–600 mg (310–465 mg base) daily for 5–10 days, gradually increased to optimum response level. Maintenance (usually within 4–12 wk): Dosage decreased by 50% and then continued at maintenance dose of 200–400 mg/day. Maximum effect may not be seen for several months.

▸ **Lupus erythematosus**

PO

Adults. Initially, 400 mg once or twice a day for several weeks or months. Maintenance: 200–400 mg/day.

OFF-LABEL USES

Treatment of juvenile arthritis, sarcoid-associated hypercalcemia

CONTRAINDICATIONS

Long-term therapy for children, porphyria, psoriasis, retinal or visual field changes

INTERACTIONS

Drug

Penicillamine: May increase blood penicillamine concentration and the risk of hematologic, renal, or severe skin reactions.

Herbal

None known.

Food

None known.

DIAGNOSTIC TEST EFFECTS

None known.

SIDE EFFECTS

Frequent

Mild, transient headache; anorexia; nausea; vomiting

Occasional

Visual disturbances, nervousness, fatigue, pruritus (especially of palms, soles, and scalp), irritability, personality changes, diarrhea

Rare

Stomatitis, dermatitis, impaired hearing

SERIOUS REACTIONS

! Ocular toxicity, especially retinopathy, may occur and may progress even after drug is discontinued.

! Prolonged therapy may result in peripheral neuritis, neuromyopathy, hypotension, EKG changes, agranulocytosis, aplastic anemia, thrombocytopenia, seizures, and psychosis.

! Overdosage may result in headache, vomiting, visual disturbances, drowsiness, seizures, and hypokalemia followed by cardiovascular collapse and death.

NURSING CONSIDERATIONS

Baseline Assessment

• Evaluate the patient's CBC and liver function test results.

Precautions

• Use hydroxychloroquine cautiously in patients with glucose-6-phosphate dehydrogenase deficiency, hepatic disease, alcoholism, or a history of alcohol abuse.

• Be aware that children are especially susceptible to hydroxychloroquine's fatal effects.

Administration and Handling

◀ALERT▶ Be aware that 200 mg hydroxychloroquine equals 155 mg base.

• Give the drug dose with food for treatment of malaria.

Intervention and Evaluation

• Monitor the patient for visual disturbances and impaired hearing, and promptly report them to the physician.

• Evaluate the patient for GI distress.

• Monitor the patient's liver function test results.

• Assess the patient's buccal mucosa and skin, and check for pruritus.

Patient Teaching

• Advise the patient to continue taking hydroxychloroquine for the full course of treatment.

• Inform the patient that a therapeutic response may not be evident for up to 6 months.

• Warn the patient to immediately notify the physician of any new symptoms, such as decreased hearing, tinnitus, muscle weakness, and visual difficulties.

linezolid

li-**nee**-zoh-lid

(Zyvox, Zyvoxam)

Do not confuse Zyvox with Zoverax or Vioxx.

CATEGORY AND SCHEDULE

Pregnancy Risk Category: C

MECHANISM OF ACTION

An oxalodinone anti-infective that binds to a site on bacterial 23S ribosomal RNA, preventing the formation of a complex that is essential for bacterial translation. **Therapeutic Effect:** Bacteriostatic against enterococci and staphylococci; bactericidal against streptococci.

PHARMACOKINETICS

Rapidly and extensively absorbed after PO administration. Protein binding: 31%. Metabolized in the liver by oxidation. Excreted in urine. ***Half-life:*** 4–5.4 hr.

AVAILABILITY

Powder for Oral Suspension: 100 mg/5 ml.
Tablets: 400 mg, 600 mg.
Injection: 2 mg/ml in 100-ml, 200-ml, 300-ml bags.

INDICATIONS AND DOSAGES

▸ **Vancomycin-resistant infections**

PO, IV

Adults, Elderly, Children older than 11 yr. 600 mg q12h for 14–28 days.

▸ **Pneumonia, complicated skin and skin structure infections**

PO, IV

Adults, Elderly, Children older than 11 yr. 600 mg q12h for 10–14 days.

▸ **Uncomplicated skin and skin structure infections**
PO
Adults, Elderly. 400 mg q12h for 10–14 days.
Children older than 11 yr. 600 mg q12h for 10–14 days.
Children 5–11 yr. 10 mg/kg/dose q12h for 10–14 days.
▸ **Usual neonate dosage**
PO, IV
Neonates. 10 mg/kg/dose q8–12h.

CONTRAINDICATIONS
None known.

INTERACTIONS
Drug
Adrenergic agents (sympathomimetics): Increase the effects of linezolid.
MAOIs: Decrease the effects of MAOIs.
Herbal
None known.
Food
Tyramine-containing foods and beverages: Excessive amounts may cause significant hypertension.

DIAGNOSTIC TEST EFFECTS
May decrease blood Hgb, platelet count, WBC count, and ALT (SGPT) levels.

IV INCOMPATIBILITIES
Amphotericin B complex (Abelcet, AmBisome, Amphotec), chlorpromazine (Thorazine), co-trimoxazole (Bactrim), diazepam (Valium), erythromycin (Erythrocin), pentamidine (Pentam IV), phenytoin (Dilantin)

SIDE EFFECTS
Occasional (5%–2%)
Diarrhea, nausea, headache
Rare (less than 2%)
Altered taste, vaginal candidiasis, fungal infection, dizziness, tongue discoloration

SERIOUS REACTIONS
! Thrombocytopenia and myelosuppression occur rarely.
! Antibiotic-associated colitis and other superinfections may result from altered bacterial balance.

NURSING CONSIDERATIONS
Lifespan Considerations
• It is unknown if linezolid is distributed in breast milk.
• The safety and efficacy of linezolid have not been established in children.
• No age-related precautions have been noted in the elderly.
Precautions
• Use linezolid cautiously in patients with carcinoid syndrome, pheochromocytoma, severe renal or hepatic impairment, uncontrolled hypertension, or untreated hyperthyroidism.
Administration and Handling
PO
• Give linezolid without regard to food.
• Use the oral suspension within 21 days of reconstitution.
IV
◂ **ALERT** ▸ Don't mix linezolid with other medications. If the same line is used to administer another drug, flush it with a compatible fluid (D_5W, 0.9% NaCl, lactated Ringer's).
• Store the drug at room temperature and protect it from light. A yellow color does not affect potency.
• Infuse the drug over 30 to 120 minutes.
Intervention and Evaluation
• Assess the patient's pattern of daily bowel activity and stool consistency. Mild GI effects may be tolerable, but severe symptoms may indicate the onset of antibiotic-associated colitis.

• Be alert for signs and symptoms of superinfection, such as abdominal pain, moderate to severe diarrhea, severe anal or genital pruritus, and severe mouth soreness.
• Monitor the patient's CBC weekly.

Patient Teaching

• Advise the patient to space drug doses evenly around the clock and to continue linezolid therapy for the full course of treatment.
• Tell the patient that he or she may take linezolid with food or milk if GI upset occurs.
• Advise the patient to avoid excessive amounts of tyramine-containing foods (such as aged cheese and red wine) as these foods may cause severe reactions including diaphoresis, neck stiffness, palpitations, and severe headache. Give the patient a list of these foods.

metronidazole hydrochloride

me-troe-**ni**-da-zole
(Apo-Metronidazole[CAN], Flagyl, Flagyl ER, MetroCream, MetroGel, Metrogyl[AUS], MetroLotion, Metronidazole IV [AUS], Metronide[AUS], NidaGel[CAN], Noritate, Novonidazol[CAN], Rozex[AUS])

CATEGORY AND SCHEDULE

Pregnancy Risk Category: B

MECHANISM OF ACTION

A nitroimidazole derivative that disrupts bacterial and protozoal DNA, inhibiting nucleic acid synthesis.
Therapeutic Effect: Produces bactericidal, antiprotozoal, amebicidal, and trichomonacidal effects. Produces anti-inflammatory and immunosuppressive effects when applied topically.

PHARMACOKINETICS

Well absorbed from the GI tract; minimally absorbed after topical application. Protein binding: less than 20%. Widely distributed; crosses blood-brain barrier. Metabolized in the liver to active metabolite. Primarily excreted in urine; partially eliminated in feces. Removed by hemodialysis. ***Half-life:*** 8 hr (increased in alcoholic hepatic disease and in neonates).

AVAILABILITY

Capsules (Flagyl): 375 mg.
Tablets (Flagyl): 250 mg, 500 mg.
Tablets (Extended-Release [Flagyl ER]): 750 mg.
Injection (Infusion): 500 mg/100 ml.
Lotion: 0.75%.
Topical Gel (MetroGel): 0.75%.
Topical Cream (MetroCream): 0.75%.
Topical Cream (Noritate): 1%.
Vaginal Gel (MetroGel-Vaginal): 0.75%.

INDICATIONS AND DOSAGES

▸ **Amebiasis**

PO

Adults, Elderly. 500–750 mg q8h.
Children. 35–50 mg/kg/day in divided doses q8h.

▸ **Trichomoniasis**

PO

Adults, Elderly. 250 mg q8h or 2 g as a single dose.
Children. 15–30 mg/kg/day in divided doses q8h.

▸ **Anaerobic skin and skin-structure, CNS, lower respiratory tract, bone, joint, intra-abdominal, and gynecologic infections; endocarditis; septicemia**

PO, IV

Adults, Elderly, Children. 30 mg/kg/day in divided doses q6h. Maximum: 4 g/day.

▸ **Antibiotic-associated pseudomembranous colitis**
PO
Adults, Elderly. 250–500 mg 3–4 times a day for 10–14 days.
Children. 30 mg/kg/day in divided doses q6h for 7–10 days.
▸ ***Helicobacter pylori* infections**
PO
Adults, Elderly. 250–500 mg 3 times a day (in combination).
Children. 15–20 mg/kg/day in 2 divided doses.
▸ ***Bacterial vaginosis***
PO
Adults. 750 mg at bedtime for 7 days.
▸ **Intravaginal**
Adults. One applicatorful twice a day or once a day at bedtime for 5 days.
▸ **Rosacea**
Topical
Adults. Apply thin layer of lotion to affected area twice a day or cream once a day.

OFF-LABEL USES
Treatment of bacterial vaginosis, grade III-IV decubitus ulcers with anaerobic infection, *H. pylori*–associated gastritis and duodenal ulcer, inflammatory bowel disease; topical treatment of acne rosacea

CONTRAINDICATIONS
Hypersensitivity to metronidazole or other nitroimidazole derivatives (also parabens with topical application)

INTERACTIONS
Drug
Alcohol: May cause a disulfiram-type reaction.
Disulfiram: May increase the risk of toxicity.
Oral anticoagulants: May increase the effects of these drugs.

Herbal
None known.
Food
None known.

DIAGNOSTIC TEST EFFECTS
May increase serum LDH, AST (SGOT), and ALT (SGPT) levels.

IV INCOMPATIBILITIES
Amphotericin B complex (Abelcet, AmBisome, Amphotec), filgrastim (Neupogen)

IV COMPATIBILITIES
Diltiazem (Cardizem), dopamine (Intropin), heparin, hydromorphone (Dilaudid), lorazepam (Ativan), magnesium sulfate, midazolam (Versed), morphine

SIDE EFFECTS
Frequent
Systemic: Anorexia, nausea, dry mouth, metallic taste
Vaginal: Symptomatic cervicitis and vaginitis, abdominal cramps, uterine pain
Occasional
Systemic: Diarrhea or constipation, vomiting, dizziness, erythematous rash, urticaria, reddish brown urine
Topical: Transient erythema, mild dryness, burning, irritation, stinging, tearing when applied too close to eyes
Vaginal: Vaginal, perineal, or vulvar itching; vulvar swelling
Rare
Mild, transient leukopenia; thrombophlebitis with IV therapy

SERIOUS REACTIONS
! Oral therapy may result in furry tongue, glossitis, cystitis, dysuria, pancreatitis, and flattening of T waves on EKG readings.
! Peripheral neuropathy, manifested as numbness and tingling in hands or

feet, is usually reversible if treatment is stopped immediately after neurologic symptoms appear.
! Seizures occur occasionally.

NURSING CONSIDERATIONS

Baseline Assessment

• Determine if the patient has a history of hypersensitivity to metronidazole or other nitroimidazole derivatives (and parabens with topical form) before beginning therapy.
• Obtain patient specimens for diagnostic tests and cultures before giving the first dose of metronidazole. Therapy may begin before the test results are known.

Lifespan Considerations

• Metronidazole readily crosses the placenta and is distributed in breast milk.
• Metronidazole use is contraindicated during the first trimester of pregnancy in women with trichomoniasis. Topical use during pregnancy or breast-feeding is discouraged.
• No age-related precautions have been noted in children; however, the safety and efficacy of topical administration in those younger than 21 years have not been established.
• Age-related hepatic impairment may require a dosage adjustment in the elderly.

Precautions

• Use metronidazole cautiously in patients with blood dyscrasias, CNS disorders, severe hepatic dysfunction, or a predisposition to edema.
• Use the drug cautiously in patients receiving corticosteroid therapy concurrently.

Administration and Handling

PO
• Give metronidazole without regard to food. However, give it with food if GI upset occurs.

IV
• Store ready-to-use infusion bags at room temperature.
• Infuse the drug IV over 30 to 60 minutes. Don't give as an IV bolus injection.

Intervention and Evaluation

• Avoid prolonged use of indwelling catheters.
• Assess the patient's pattern of daily bowel activity and stool consistency. Document the number and characteristics of stools in amebiasis patients.
• Monitor the patient's intake and output and assess the patient for urinary problems.
• Be alert for neurologic symptoms, such as dizziness and paresthesia.
• Examine the patient for rash and urticaria.
• Be alert for signs and symptoms of superinfection, such as anal or genital pruritus, furry tongue, ulceration or change of oral mucosa, and vaginal discharge.

Patient Teaching

• Explain to the patient that his or her urine may become reddish brown during metronidazole therapy.
• Urge the patient to avoid alcohol and alcohol-containing preparations (such as cough syrups and elixirs) while taking metronidazole.
• Warn the patient to avoid tasks requiring mental alertness or motor skills until his or her response to the drug is established.
• Instruct the patient taking metronidazole for trichomoniasis to refrain from sexual intercourse until the full treatment is completed.
• Caution patients using topical metronidazole to avoid drug contact with eyes. Explain that cosmetics may be applied after the drug is applied.
• Inform the patient that metronidazole acts on papules, pustules, and erythema, but has no effect on ocular

problems (conjunctivitis, keratitis, blepharitis), rhinophyma (hypertrophy of nose), or telangiectasia.
• Urge rosacea patients to avoid alcohol, excessive sunlight, exposure to very hot and cold temperatures, and hot and spicy foods.

nitrofurantoin sodium

nye-troe-**fyoor**-an-toyn
(Apo-Nitrofurantoin[CAN], Furadantin, Macrobid, Macrodantin, Novo-Furan[CAN], Ralodantin[AUS])

CATEGORY AND SCHEDULE
Pregnancy Risk Category: B

MECHANISM OF ACTION
An antibacterial UTI agent that inhibits the synthesis of bacterial DNA, RNA, proteins, and cell walls by altering or inactivating ribosomal proteins. **Therapeutic Effect:** Bacteriostatic (bactericidal at high concentrations).

PHARMACOKINETICS
Microcrystalline form rapidly and completely absorbed; macrocrystalline form more slowly absorbed. Food increases absorption. Protein binding: 40%. Primarily concentrated in urine and kidneys. Metabolized in most body tissues. Primarily excreted in urine. Removed by hemodialysis. ***Half-life:*** 20–60 min.

AVAILABILITY
Capsules (Macrobid [macrocrystalline]): 100 mg.
Capsules (Macrodantin [macrocrystalline]): 25 mg, 50 mg, 100 mg
Oral Suspension (Furadantin [microcrystalline]): 25 mg/5 ml.

INDICATIONS AND DOSAGES
▸ **Urinary tract infections (UTIs)**
PO (Furadantin, Macrodantin)
Adults, Elderly. 50–100 mg q6h. Maximum: 400 mg/day.
Children. 5–7 mg/kg/day in divided doses q6h. Maximum: 400 mg/day.
PO (Macrobid)
Adults, Elderly. 100 mg twice a day. Maximum: 400 mg/day.
▸ **Long-term prevention of UTIs**
PO
Adults, Elderly. 50–100 mg at bedtime.
Children. 1–2 mg/kg/day as a single dose. Maximum: 100 mg/day.

OFF-LABEL USES
Prevention of bacterial UTIs

CONTRAINDICATIONS
Anuria, oliguria, substantial renal impairment (creatinine clearance less than 40 ml/min); infants younger than 1 mo old because of the risk of hemolytic anemia

INTERACTIONS
Drug
Hemolytics: May increase the risk of nitrofurantoin toxicity.
Neurotoxic medications: May increase the risk of neurotoxicity.
Probenecid: May increase blood concentration and toxicity of nitrofurantoin.
Herbal
None known.
Food
None known.

DIAGNOSTIC TEST EFFECTS
None known.

SIDE EFFECTS
Frequent
Anorexia, nausea, vomiting, dark urine

Occasional
Abdominal pain, diarrhea, rash, pruritus, urticaria, hypertension, headache, dizziness, drowsiness
Rare
Photosensitivity, transient alopecia, asthmatic exacerbation in those with history of asthma

SERIOUS REACTIONS

! Superinfection, hepatotoxicity, peripheral neuropathy (may be irreversible), Stevens-Johnson syndrome, permanent pulmonary function impairment, and anaphylaxis occur rarely.

NURSING CONSIDERATIONS

Baseline Assessment

- Determine if the patient has a history of asthma.
- Evaluate the patient's baseline renal and liver function test results.

Lifespan Considerations

- Nitrofurantoin readily crosses the placenta and is distributed in breast milk.
- Nitrofurantoin use is contraindicated at term and during breast-feeding if the infant is suspected of having glucose-6-phosphate dehydrogenase (G6PD) deficiency.
- No age-related precautions have been noted in children older than 1 month.
- Elderly patients are more likely to develop acute pneumonitis and peripheral neuropathy and may require a dosage adjustment because of age-related renal impairment.

Precautions

- Use nitrofurantoin cautiously in debilitated patients (greater risk of peripheral neuropathy) and in patients with anemia, diabetes mellitus, electrolyte imbalance, G6PD deficiency (greater risk of hemolytic anemia), renal impairment, or vitamin B deficiency.

Administration and Handling

PO

- Give nitrofurantoin with food or milk to enhance absorption and reduce GI upset.

Intervention and Evaluation

- Monitor the patient's intake and output and renal function test results.
- Assess the patient's pattern of daily bowel activity and stool consistency.
- Examine the patient's skin for a rash and urticaria.
- Be alert for signs and symptoms of peripheral neuropathy, such as numbness or tingling, especially in the lower extremities.
- Observe the patient for signs and symptoms of hepatotoxicity, such as arthralgia, fever, hepatomegaly, and rash.
- Perform a respiratory assessment by auscultating the patient's lungs and checking for chest pain, cough, and difficulty breathing.

Patient Teaching

- Instruct the patient to take nitrofurantoin with food or milk for best results and to reduce GI upset.
- Advise the patient to continue taking nitrofurantoin for the full course of therapy.
- Inform the patient that urine may become dark yellow or brown with nitrofurantoin use.
- Urge the patient to avoid exposure to the sun and ultraviolet light and to use sunscreen and wear protective clothing when outdoors.
- Warn the patient to notify the physician if chest pain, cough, difficult breathing, fever, or numbness and tingling of fingers or toes occurs.
- Explain to the patient that hair loss may occur but is only temporary.

pentamidine isethionate

pen-**tam**-i-deen
(NebuPent, Pentacarinat[CAN], Pentam-300)

CATEGORY AND SCHEDULE

Pregnancy Risk Category: C

MECHANISM OF ACTION

An anti-infective, that interferes with nuclear metabolism and incorporation of nucleotides, inhibiting DNA, RNA, phospholipid, and protein synthesis. **Therapeutic Effect:** Produces antibacterial and antiprotozoal effects.

PHARMACOKINETICS

Well absorbed after IM administration; minimally absorbed after inhalation.Widely distributed. Primarily excreted in urine. Minimally removed by hemodialysis. ***Half-life:*** 6.5 hr (increased in impaired renal function).

AVAILABILITY

Injection (Pentam-300): 300 mg.
Powder for Nebulization (Nebupent): 300 mg.

INDICATIONS AND DOSAGES

▸ ***Pneumocystis carinii*** **pneumonia (PCP)**

IV, IM

Adults, Elderly. 4 mg/kg/day once a day for 14–21 days.
Children. 4 mg/kg/day once a day for 10–14 days.

▸ **Prevention of PCP**

Inhalation

Adults, Elderly. 300 mg once q4wk.
Children 5 yr and older. 300 mg q3–4wk.
Children younger than 5 yr. 8 mg/kg/dose once q3–4wk.

OFF-LABEL USES

Treatment of African trypanosomiasis, cutaneous or visceral leishmaniasis

CONTRAINDICATIONS

Concurrent use with didanosine

INTERACTIONS

Drug

Blood dyscrasia-producing medications, bone marrow depressants: May increase the abnormal hematologic effects of pentamidine.
Didanosine: May increase the risk of pancreatitis.
Foscarnet: May increase the risk of hypocalcemia, hypomagnesemia, and nephrotoxicity of pentamidine.
Nephrotoxic medications: May increase the risk of nephrotoxicity.

Herbal

None known.

Food

None known.

DIAGNOSTIC TEST EFFECTS

May increase BUN and serum alkaline phosphatase, bilirubin, creatinine, AST (SGOT), and ALT (SGPT) levels. May decrease serum calcium and magnesium levels. May alter blood glucose levels.

IV INCOMPATIBILITIES

Cefazolin (Ancef), cefotaxime (Claforan), ceftazidime (Fortaz), ceftriaxone (Rocephin), fluconazole (Diflucan), foscarnet (Foscavir), interleukin (Proleukin)

IV COMPATIBILITIES

Diltiazem (Cardizem), zidovudine (Retrovir)

SIDE EFFECTS

Frequent

Injection (greater than 10%): Abscess, pain at injection site

Inhalation (greater than 5%): Fatigue, metallic taste, shortness of breath, decreased appetite, dizziness, rash, cough, nausea, vomiting, chills

Occasional

Injection (10%–1%): Nausea, decreased appetite, hypotension, fever, rash, altered taste, confusion

Inhalation (5%–1%): Diarrhea, headache, anemia, muscle pain

Rare

Injection (less than 1%): Neuralgia, thrombocytopenia, phlebitis, dizziness

SERIOUS REACTIONS

! Rare reactions include life-threatening or fatal hypotension, arrhythmias, hypoglycemia, leukopenia, nephrotoxicity or renal failure, anaphylactic shock, Stevens-Johnson syndrome, and toxic epidural necrolysis.

! Hyperglycemia and insulin-dependent diabetes mellitus (often permanent) may occur even months after therapy has stopped.

NURSING CONSIDERATIONS

Baseline Assessment

• Establish the patient's baseline blood glucose level and BP.

• Obtain specimens for diagnostic tests before giving the first dose of pentamidine.

• Determine if patient is receiving nephrotoxic drugs and avoid concurrent use.

Lifespan Considerations

• It is unknown if pentamidine crosses the placenta or is distributed in breast milk.

• No age-related precautions have been noted in children.

• No information is available regarding pentamidine use in the elderly.

Precautions

• Use pentamidine cautiously in patients with diabetes mellitus, hypertension, hypotension, or renal or hepatic impairment.

Administration and Handling

◀ **ALERT** ▶ Make sure the patient is in the supine position during administration and has frequent BP checks until he or she is stable because of the risk of a life-threatening hypotensive reaction. Have resuscitative equipment readily available.

IV

• Store vials at room temperature.

• For intermittent IV infusion (piggyback), reconstitute each vial with 3 to 5 ml D_5W or sterile water for injection.

• Withdraw the desired dose and further dilute with 50 to 250 ml D_5W.

• After reconstitution, the IV solution is stable at room temperature for 48 hours.

• Infuse the drug over 60 minutes. Discard any unused portion.

• Don't give the drug by IV injection or rapid IV infusion because this increases the risk of severe hypotension.

IM

• Reconstitute each 300-mg vial with 3 ml sterile water for injection to provide a concentration of 100 mg/ml.

Aerosol (Nebulizer)

• Store the aerosol at room temperature for 48 hours.

• Reconstitute each 300-mg vial with 6 ml sterile water for injection. Avoid using 0.9% NaCl because it may cause a precipitate to form.

• Don't mix pentamidine with other medications in the nebulizer reservoir.

Intervention and Evaluation

- Monitor the patient's BP and keep him or her supine until stable during both IM and IV pentamidine administration.

◀ **ALERT** ▶ Check the patient's blood glucose levels and assess for signs and symptoms of hypoglycemia (diaphoresis, double vision, headache, incoordination, lightheadedness, nervousness, numbness of lips, palpitations, tachycardia, and tremor) and hyperglycemia (abdominal pain, headache, malaise, nausea, polydipsia, polyphagia, polyuria, visual changes, and vomiting).

- Evaluate the patient's IM sites for induration, pain, and redness.
- Evaluate the patient's IV sites for evidence of phlebitis, such as heat, pain, and red streaking over the vein.
- Monitor the patient's hematology, liver, and renal function test results.
- Examine the patient's skin for a rash.
- Be alert for respiratory difficulty when administering pentamidine by inhalation.

Patient Teaching

- Teach the patient to remain flat in bed during pentamidine administration and to get up slowly and with assistance only when his or her BP becomes stable.
- Warn the patient to notify the nurse immediately if he or she experiences light-headedness, palpitations, shakiness, or sweating.
- Warn the patient to notify the physician if cough, fever, or shortness of breath occurs.
- Inform the patient that drowsiness, decreased appetite, and increased thirst and urination may develop in the months following therapy.
- Instruct the patient to drink plenty of water to maintain adequate hydration.
- Urge the patient to avoid consuming alcohol during therapy.

quinupristin-dalfopristin

kwin-**yoo**-pris-tin/**dal**-foh-pris-tin
(Synercid)

CATEGORY AND SCHEDULE

Pregnancy Risk Category: B

MECHANISM OF ACTION

Two chemically distinct compounds that, when given together, bind to different sites on bacterial ribosomes, inhibiting protein synthesis. **Therapeutic Effect:** Bactericidal.

PHARMACOKINETICS

After IV administration, both are extensively metabolized in the liver, with dalfopristin to active metabolite. Protein binding: quinupristin, 23%–32%; dalfopristin, 50%–56%. Primarily eliminated in feces. ***Half-life:*** quinupristin, 0.85 hr; dalfopristin, 0.7 hr.

AVAILABILITY

Injection: 500-mg vial (150 mg quinupristin/350 mg dalfopristin).

INDICATIONS AND DOSAGES

▶ **Infections due to vancomycin-resistant *Enterococcus faecium***

IV

Adults, Elderly. 7.5 mg/kg/dose q8h.

▶ **Skin and skin-structure infections**

IV

Adults, Elderly. 7.5 mg/kg/dose q12h.

CONTRAINDICATIONS

None known.

INTERACTIONS

Drug

None known.

Herbal

None known.

Food

None known.

DIAGNOSTIC TEST EFFECTS

May increase serum bilirubin, creatinine, LDH, AST (SGOT), and ALT (SGPT) levels.

IV INCOMPATIBILITIES

Heparin, sodium chloride

IV COMPATIBILITIES

Aztreonam (Azactam), ciprofloxacin (Cipro), fluconazole (Diflucan), haloperidol (Haldol), metoclopramide (Reglan), morphine, potassium chloride

SIDE EFFECTS

Frequent

Mild erythema, pruritus, pain, or burning at infusion site (with doses greater than 7 mg/kg)

Occasional

Headache, diarrhea

Rare

Vomiting, arthralgia, myalgia

SERIOUS REACTIONS

! Antibiotic-associated colitis and other superinfections may result from bacterial imbalance.

! Hepatic function abnormalities and severe venous pain and inflammation may occur.

NURSING CONSIDERATIONS

Baseline Assessment

- Assess the patient's BP, body temperature, pulse, and respiratory rate.
- Expect to obtain the patient's baseline BUN level, CBC, hepatic function test results, and urinalysis results.

Lifespan Considerations

- It is unknown if quinupristin and dalfopristin crosses the placenta or is distributed in breast milk.
- The safety and efficacy of quinupristin and dalfopristin have not been established in children.
- No age-related precautions have been noted in the elderly.

Precautions

- Use quinupristin and dalfopristin cautiously in patients with renal or hepatic dysfunction.

Administration and Handling

IV

- Refrigerate unopened vials.
- To reconstitute, slowly add 5 ml D_5W or sterile water for injection to each vial to yield a concentration of 100 mg/ml. Gently swirl the vial contents to minimize foaming.
- Further dilute with D_5W to a final concentration of 2 mg/ml (5 mg/ml if using a central line).
- Reconstituted vials are stable for 1 hour at room temperature. Diluted infusion bags are stable for 6 hours at room temperature or 54 hours if refrigerated.
- Infuse the solution over 60 minutes.
- After the infusion, flush the line with D_5W to minimize vein irritation. Don't flush with 0.9% NaCl because it's incompatible with the drug.

Intervention and Evaluation

- Monitor the patient's CBC and hepatic function test results.
- Withhold the drug and promptly inform the physician if diarrhea occurs. Diarrhea with abdominal pain, fever, and mucus or blood in stools may indicate antibiotic-associated colitis.
- Evaluate the IV site for redness,

vein irritation, burning, pruritus, mild erythema, and pain.

• Be alert for signs and symptoms of superinfection, such as anal or genital pruritus, diarrhea, increased fever, nausea and vomiting, sore throat, and stomatitis.

Patient Teaching

• Advise the patient to immediately notify the physician if he or she experiences pain, redness, or swelling at the infusion site.

• Warn the patient to immediately notify the physician if he or she experiences severe diarrhea and to avoid taking antidiarrheals until instructed to do so.

rifaximin

rye-**fax**-ih-min

(Xifaxan)

CATEGORY AND SCHEDULE

Pregnancy Risk Category: C

MECHANISM OF ACTION

An anti-infective that binds subunit of bacterial DNA-dependent RNA polymerase. **Therapeutic Effect:** Inhibits bacterial RNA synthesis.

PHARMACOKINETICS

Less than 0.4% absorbed following oral administration. ***Half-life:*** 5.85 hr.

AVAILABILITY

Tablets: 200 mg.

INDICATIONS AND DOSAGES

▸ Traveler's diarrhea

PO

Adults, Elderly, Children 12 yr and older. 200 mg three times a day for 3 days.

▸ Hepatic encephalopathy

PO

Adults, Elderly. 1,200 mg/day for 15–21 days.

OFF-LABEL USES

Treatment of hepatic encephalopathy

CONTRAINDICATIONS

Hypersensitivity to rifaximin antimicrobial agents

INTERACTIONS

Drug

None known.

Herbal

None known.

Food

None known.

DIAGNOSTIC TEST EFFECTS

None known.

SIDE EFFECTS

Occasional (11%–5%)

Flatulence, headache, abdominal discomfort, rectal tenesmus, defecation urgency, nausea

Rare (4%–2%)

Constipation, pyrexia, vomiting

SERIOUS REACTIONS

! Hypersensitivity reaction, including dermatitis, angioneurotic edema, pruritus, rash, and urticaria may occur.

! Superinfection occurs rarely.

NURSING CONSIDERATIONS

Baseline Assessment

• Check the patient's baseline hydration status by assessing mucous membranes for dryness, skin turgor, and urinary status.

Lifespan Considerations

• Be aware that it is unknown if rifaximin is excreted in breast milk.

• Be aware that the safety and effi-

cacy of rifaximin have not been established in children younger than 12 years of age.
• In the elderly, there are no age-related precautions noted.

Administration and Handling

PO
• Store at room temperature.
• Do not break or crush film-coated tablets.
• Give without regard to food.

Intervention and Evaluation

• Encourage the patient to drink adequate fluids.
• Assess the patient's bowel sounds for peristalsis.
• Monitor the patient's pattern of daily bowel activity and stool consistency.
• Assess the patient for GI disturbances.

Patient Teaching

• Warn the patient to notify the physician if his or her diarrhea worsens, if blood in the stool appears within 48 hours, or if he or she develops a fever.

sulfasalazine

sul-fa-**sal**-a-zeen
(Alti-Sulfasalazine[CAN], Azulfidine, Azulfidine EN-tabs, Pyralin EN[AUS], Salazopyrin[CAN], Salazopyrin EN[AUS], Salazopyrin EN-Tabs[CAN])

Do not confuse Azulfidine with azathioprine, or sulfasalazine with sulfadiazine or sulfisoxazole.

CATEGORY AND SCHEDULE

Pregnancy Risk Category: B (D if given near term)

MECHANISM OF ACTION

A sulfonamide that inhibits prostaglandin synthesis, acting locally in the colon. **Therapeutic Effect:** Decreases inflammatory response, interferes with GI secretion.

PHARMACOKINETICS

Poorly absorbed from the GI tract. Cleaved in colon by intestinal bacteria, forming sulfapyridine and mesalamine (5-ASA). Absorbed in colon. Widely distributed. Metabolized in the liver. Primarily excreted in urine. ***Half-life:*** sulfapyridine, 6–14 hr; 5-ASA, 0.6–1.4 hr.

AVAILABILITY

Tablets (Azulfidine): 500 mg.
Tablets (Delayed-Release [Azulfidine EN-Tabs]): 500 mg.

INDICATIONS AND DOSAGES

▸ Ulcerative colitis

PO
Adults, Elderly. 1 g 3–4 times a day in divided doses q4–6h. Maintenance: 2 g/day in divided doses q6–12h. Maximum: 6 g/day.
Children. 40–75 mg/kg/day in divided doses q4–6h. Maximum: 6 g/day. Maintenance: 30–50 mg/kg/day in divided doses q4–8h. Maximum: 2 g/day.

▸ Rheumatoid arthritis

PO
Adults, Elderly. Initially, 0.5–1 g/day for 1 wk. Increase by 0.5 g/wk, up to 3 g/day.

▸ Juvenile rheumatoid arthritis

PO
Children. Initially, 10 mg/kg/day. May increase by 10 mg/kg/day at weekly intervals. Range: 30–50 mg/kg/day. Maximum: 2 g/day.

OFF-LABEL USES

Treatment of ankylosing spondylitis

CONTRAINDICATIONS

Children younger than 2 years;

hypersensitivity to carbonic anhydrase inhibitors, local anesthetics, salicylates, sulfonamides, sulfonylureas, sunscreens containing PABA, or thiazide or loop diuretics; intestinal or urinary tract obstruction; porphyria; pregnancy at term; severe hepatic or renal dysfunction

INTERACTIONS

Drug

Anticonvulsants, methotrexate, oral anticoagulants, oral antidiabetics: May increase the effects of these drugs.
Hemolytics: May increase the toxicity of sulfasalazine.
Hepatotoxic medications: May increase the risk of hepatotoxicity.

Herbal

None known.

Food

None known.

DIAGNOSTIC TEST EFFECTS

None known.

SIDE EFFECTS

Frequent (33%)
Anorexia, nausea, vomiting, headache, oligospermia (generally reversed by withdrawal of drug)
Occasional (3%)
Hypersensitivity reaction (rash, urticaria, pruritus, fever, anemia)
Rare (less than 1%)
Tinnitus, hypoglycemia, diuresis, photosensitivity

SERIOUS REACTIONS

! Anaphylaxis, Stevens-Johnson syndrome, hematologic toxicity (leukopenia, agranulocytosis), hepatotoxicity, and nephrotoxicity occur rarely.

NURSING CONSIDERATIONS

Baseline Assessment

◀ALERT▶ Determine the patient's hypersensitivity to medications, including carbonic anhydrase inhibitors, local anesthetics, salicylates, sulfonamides, sulfonylureas, thiazide or loop diuretics, and sunscreens containing PABA, before beginning drug therapy.
- Check the patient's initial CBC, liver and renal function test results, and urinalysis test results.

Lifespan Considerations

- Sulfasalazine may produce infertility and oligospermia in men.
- Sulfasalazine readily crosses the placenta and is excreted in breast milk. Lactating patients should not breast-feed premature infants or those with hyperbilirubinemia or glucose-6-phosphate dehydrogenase (G6PD) deficiency.
- If given near term, sulfasalazine may produce hemolytic anemia, jaundice, and kernicterus in the newborn.
- No age-related precautions have been noted in children older than 2 years or the elderly.

Precautions

- Use sulfasalazine cautiously in patients with bronchial asthma, G6PD deficiency, impaired hepatic or renal function, or severe allergies.

Administration and Handling

PO
- Space drug doses evenly, at intervals not to exceed 8 hours.
- Administer sulfasalazine after meals, if possible, to prolong intestinal passage.
- Have the patient swallow delayed-release tablets whole without chewing or crushing them.
- Give the drug with 8 oz of water.

Intervention and Evaluation

- Monitor the patient's intake and

output and renal function and urinalysis test results.
• Ensure that the patient drinks plenty of water to maintain adequate hydration (minimum output 1,500 ml/24 hr) and prevent nephrotoxicity.
• Examine the patient's skin for a rash. Withhold the drug and notify the physician at the first sign of a rash.
• Assess the patient's pattern of daily bowel activity and stool consistency. The drug dosage may need to be increased if diarrhea continues or recurs.
• Closely monitor the patient's CBC.
• Check for hematologic effects, such as bleeding, ecchymosis, fever, jaundice, pallor, purpura, pharyngitis, and weakness. If they occur, notify the physician immediately.

Patient Teaching

• Instruct the patient to take sulfasalazine after food with 8 oz of water and to drink several glasses of water between meals.
• Advise the patient to space drug doses around the clock and to continue sulfasalazine therapy for the full course of treatment. Explain that the drug therapy may need to continue even after symptoms are relieved.
• Stress the importance of complying with follow-up and laboratory tests.
• Tell the patient to inform the dentist or surgeon of sulfasalazine therapy if he or she will have a dental or other surgical procedures.
• Urge the patient to avoid exposure to sun and ultraviolet light until his or her photosensitivity is determined. Explain that photosensitivity may last for months after the last dose of sulfasalazine.

telithromycin

teh-**lith**-row-my-sin
(Ketek)

CATEGORY AND SCHEDULE

Pregnancy Risk Category: C

MECHANISM OF ACTION

A ketolide that blocks protein synthesis by binding to ribosomal receptor sites of bacterial cell wall. **Therapeutic Effect:** Produces bacterial cell lysis, death.

PHARMACOKINETICS

Partially metabolized by the liver. Concentration in white blood cells (WBCs) exceeds the concentration in plasma and is eliminated more slowly from WBCs than from plasma. Minimally excreted in the feces and urine. Protein binding: 60%–70%. ***Half-life:*** 10 hr.

AVAILABILITY

Tablets: 400 mg.

INDICATIONS AND DOSAGES

▸ **Chronic bronchitis, sinusitis**

PO

Adults, Elderly. 800 mg once a day for 5 days.

▸ **Community-acquired pneumonia**

PO

Adults, Elderly. 800 mg once a day for 7–10 days.

CONTRAINDICATIONS

Hypersensitivity to macrolide antibiotics, concurrent use with cisapride or pimozide

INTERACTIONS

Drug

Atorvastatin, digoxin, lovastatin, metoprolol, pimozide, simvastatin, theophylline: May increase blood

concentration and toxicity of these drugs.
Carbamazepine, Phenobarbital, phenytoin, rifampin: May decrease telithromycin blood concentration.
Cisapride: Increases blood concentration of this drug, resulting in significant increase in QT interval.
Itraconazole, ketoconazole: May increase the blood concentration of telithromycin.
Sotalol: Decreases blood concentration of this drug.

Herbal

None known.

Food

None known.

DIAGNOSTIC TEST EFFECTS

May increase platelet count, transaminase, AST (SGOT), and ALT (SGPT) levels.

SIDE EFFECTS

Occasional (11%–4%)
Diarrhea, nausea, headache, dizziness

Rare (3%–2%)
Vomiting, loose stools, dysgeusia, dry mouth, flatulence, visual disturbances

SERIOUS REACTIONS

! Hepatic dysfunction, severe hypersensitivity reaction, and atrial arrhythmias occur rarely.

! Superinfections, especially antibiotic-associated colitis manifested as abdominal cramps, diarrhea, fever, and watery severe diarrhea, may result from altered bacterial balance.

NURSING CONSIDERATIONS

Baseline Assessment

- Determine if the patient is currently taking cisapride or pimozide. These drugs contraindicate the use of telithromycin.

Lifespan Considerations

- Be aware that it is unknown if telithromycin crosses the placenta.
- Be aware that telithromycin may be distributed in breast milk.
- Be aware that the safety and efficacy of telithromycin in children has not been established.
- There are no age-related precautions noted in the elderly.

Precautions

- Use cautiously in patients with impaired renal or hepatic function.

Administration and Handling

PO

- Store at room temperature.
- Do not break or crush film-coated tablets.
- Give without regard to food.

Intervention and Evaluation

- Assess the patient's pattern of daily bowel activity and stool consistency.
- Give telithromycin with food if the patient experiences nausea.
- Assess the patient's hepatic function panel for hepatotoxicity.

Patient and Teaching

- Instruct the patient to avoid quickly looking at objects close and then far from him or her.
- Explain to the patient that telithromycin may produce temporary difficulty in focusing that may last several hours after the first or second dose.
- Warn the patient to avoid tasks that require mental alertness or motor skills until his or her response to the drug has been established.

tinidazole

tin-**nid**-ah-zole
(Tindamax)

CATEGORY AND SCHEDULE

Pregnancy Risk Category: C

MECHANISM OF ACTION

A nitroimidazole derivative that is converted to the active metabolite by reduction of cell extracts of *Trichomonas.* The active metabolite causes DNA damage in pathogens.
Therapeutic Effect: Produces antiprotozoal effect.

PHARMACOKINETICS

Rapidly and completely absorbed. Protein binding: 12%. Distributed in all body tissues and fluids; crosses blood-brain barrier. Significantly metabolized. Primarily excreted in urine; partially eliminated in feces. ***Half-life:*** 12–14 hr.

AVAILABILITY

Tablets: 250 mg, 500 mg.

INDICATIONS AND DOSAGES

▸ Intestinal amebiasis

PO

Adults, Elderly. 2 g/day for 3 days.
Children 3 yr and older. 50 mg/kg/day (up to 2 g) for 3 days.

▸ Amebic hepatic abscess

PO

Adults, Elderly. 2 g/day for 3 to 5 days.
Children 3 yr and older. 50 mg/kg/day (up to 2 g) for 3 to 5 days.

▸ Giardiasis

PO

Adults, Elderly. 2 g single dose.
Children 3 yr and older. 50 mg/kg (up to 2 g) single dose.

▸ Trichomoniasis

PO

Adults, Elderly. 2 g single dose.

CONTRAINDICATIONS

Hypersensitivity to nitroimidazole derivatives, first trimester of pregnancy

INTERACTIONS

Drug

Alcohol: May cause a disulfiram-type reaction.
Cholestyramine, oxytetracycline: May decrease effectiveness of tinidazole; separate dosage times.
Cimetidine, fosphenytoin, ketoconazole, phenobarbital, rifampin: Reduces the metabolism of tinidazole.
Cyclosporine, fluorouracil, IV phenytoin, lithium, tacrolimus: May increase blood levels of these drugs.
Disulfiram: May increase the risk of psychotic reactions (separate doses by 2 weeks).
Oral anticoagulants: Increase the risk of bleeding.

Herbal

None known.

Food

None known.

DIAGNOSTIC TEST EFFECTS

May increase AST (SGOT), ALT (SGPT), LDH, and triglyceride levels.

SIDE EFFECTS

Occasional (4%–2%)

Metallic or bitter taste, nausea, weakness or fatigue or malaise

Rare (less than 2%)

Epigastric distress, anorexia, vomiting, headache, dizziness

SERIOUS REACTIONS

! Peripheral neuropathy characterized by numbness and paresthesia is

usually reversible if tinidazole treatment is stopped immediately upon appearance of neurologic symptoms.
! Superinfection, hypersensitivity, and seizures occur rarely.

NURSING CONSIDERATIONS

Baseline Assessment
- Determine the patient's history of hypersensitivity to metronidazole or other nitroimidazole derivatives.
- Obtain patient specimens for diagnostic tests before giving first dose. Tinidazole therapy may begin before test results are known.

Lifespan Considerations
- Be aware that tinidazole is mutagenic and spermatogenic.
- Be aware that tinidazole readily crosses the placenta and is distributed in breast milk.
- Tinidazole use is contraindicated during the first trimester of pregnancy.
- Be aware that the safety and efficacy of tinidazole have not been established in children younger than 3 years of age.
- In the elderly, age-related hepatic impairment may require dosage adjustment.

Precautions
- Use cautiously in patients with central nervous system (CNS) diseases, hepatic function impairment, and a history of blood abnormalities.

Administration and Handling
PO
- Store tinidazole at room temperature.
- Scored tinidazole tablets may be crushed.
- Give tinidazole with food to minimize epigastric distress.

Intervention and Evaluation
- Be alert to neurologic symptoms including dizziness, numbness, and tingling or paresthesia of extremities.
- Assess the patient for nausea and vomiting and initiate appropriate measures.
- Observe the patient for the onset of superinfection characterized by anal or genital pruritus, furry tongue, stomatitis, and vaginal discharge.

Patient Teaching
- Instruct the patient to take tinidazole with food.
- Explain to the patient that tinidazole use may turn his or her urine red-brown or darken it.
- Urge the patient to avoid alcoholic beverages and alocohol-containing preparations such as cough syrups during therapy and for 3 days after completion of treatment.
- Warn the patient to avoid performing tasks that require mental alertness or motor skills if he or she experiences dizziness as a side effect of tinidazole use.

trimethoprim
trye-**meth**-oh-prim
(Apo-Tremethoprim [CAN], Primsol, Proloprim)

CATEGORY AND SCHEDULE
Pregnancy Risk Category: C

MECHANISM OF ACTION
A folate antagonist that blocks bacterial biosynthesis of nucleic acids and proteins by interfering with the metabolism of folinic acid. **Therapeutic Effect:** Bacteriostatic.

PHARMACOKINETICS
Rapidly and completely absorbed from the GI tract. Protein binding: 42%–46%. Widely distributed, including to CSF. Metabolized in the liver. Primarily excreted in urine. Moderately removed by hemodialy-

sis. ***Half-life:*** 8–10 hr (increased in impaired renal function and newborns; decreased in children).

AVAILABILITY

Oral Solution (Primsol): 50 mg/5 ml.
Tablets (Proloprim): 100 mg, 200 mg.

INDICATIONS AND DOSAGES

▸ **Acute, uncomplicated UTI**

PO

Adults, Elderly, Children 12 yr and older. 100 mg q12h or 200 mg once a day for 10 days.
Children younger than 12 yr. 4–6 mg/kg/day in 2 divided doses for 10 days.

▸ **Dosage in renal impairment**

Dosage and frequency are modified based on creatinine clearance.

Creatinine Clearance	Dosage Interval
greater than 30 ml/min	No change
15–29 ml/min	50 mg q12h

OFF-LABEL USES

Prevention of bacterial UTIs, treatment of pneumonia caused by *Pneumocystis carinii*

CONTRAINDICATIONS

Infants younger than 2 months, megaloblastic anemia due to folic acid deficiency

INTERACTIONS

Drug

Folate antagonists (including methotrexate): May increase the risk of megaloblastic anemia.

Herbal

None known.

Food

None known.

DIAGNOSTIC TEST EFFECTS

May increase BUN and serum bilirubin, creatinine, AST (SGOT), and ALT (SGPT) levels.

SIDE EFFECTS

Occasional

Nausea, vomiting, diarrhea, decreased appetite, abdominal cramps, headache

Rare

Hypersensitivity reaction (pruritus, rash), methemoglobinemia (bluish fingernails, lips, or skin; fever; pale skin; sore throat; unusual tiredness), photosensitivity

SERIOUS REACTIONS

! Stevens-Johnson syndrome, erythema multiforme, exfoliative dermatitis, and anaphylaxis occur rarely.

! Hematologic toxicity (thrombocytopenia, neutropenia, leukopenia, megaloblastic anemia) is more likely to occur in elderly, debilitated, or alcoholic patients; in patients with impaired renal function; and in those receiving prolonged high dosage.

NURSING CONSIDERATIONS

Baseline Assessment

- Assess the patient's baseline hematology and serum renal function test reports.

Lifespan Considerations

- Trimethoprim readily crosses the placenta and is distributed in breast milk.
- The safety and efficacy of trimethoprim have not been established in children.
- No age-related precautions have been noted in the elderly, but they may have an increased incidence of thrombocytopenia.

Precautions

• Use trimethoprim cautiously in patients with impaired hepatic or renal function or folic acid deficiency.

Administration and Handling

PO

• Space doses evenly around the clock to maintain a constant drug level in urine.

• Give trimethoprim without regard to food (or with food if stomach upset occurs).

Intervention and Evaluation

• Examine the patient's skin for a rash.

• Evaluate the patient's food tolerance.

• Monitor the patient's serum hematology reports and liver or renal function test results.

• Observe the patient for signs and symptoms of hematologic toxicity, such as bleeding, ecchymosis, fever, malaise, pallor, and sore throat.

Patient Teaching

• Instruct the patient to space drug doses evenly around the clock and to complete the full course of trimethoprim therapy, which usually lasts 10–14 days.

• Advise the patient to take trimethoprim with food if stomach upset occurs.

• Urge the patient to avoid sun and ultraviolet light and to use sunscreen and wear protective clothing when outdoors.

• Warn the patient to immediately report bleeding, bruising, skin discoloration, fever, pallor, rash, sore throat, and tiredness.

vancomycin hydrochloride

van-koe-**mye**-sin
(Vancocin, Vancocin CP[AUS], Vancocin HCl Pulvules[AUS])

CATEGORY AND SCHEDULE

Pregnancy Risk Category: B

MECHANISM OF ACTION

A tricyclic glycopeptide antibiotic that binds to bacterial cell walls, altering cell membrane permeability and inhibiting RNA synthesis. **Therapeutic Effect:** Bactericidal.

PHARMACOKINETICS

PO: Poorly absorbed from the GI tract. Primarily eliminated in feces. Parenteral: Widely distributed. Protein binding: 55%. Primarily excreted unchanged in urine. Not removed by hemodialysis. ***Half-life:*** 4–11 hr (increased in impaired renal function).

AVAILABILITY

Capsules: 125 mg, 250 mg.
Powder for Oral Suspension (Vancocin): 1 g (provides 250 mg/5 ml after mixing).
Powder for Injection: 500 mg, 1 g.
Infusion (Premix): 500 mg/100 ml, 1 g/200 ml.

INDICATIONS AND DOSAGES

▸ **Treatment of bone, respiratory tract, skin and soft-tissue infections, endocarditis, peritonitis, and septicemia; prevention of bacterial endocarditis in those at risk (if penicillin is contraindicated) when undergoing biliary, dental, GI, GU, or respiratory surgery or invasive procedures**

IV

Adults, Elderly. 500 mg q6h or 1 g q12h.

Children older than 1 mo. 40 mg/kg/day in divided doses q6–8h. Maximum: 3–4 g/day.
Neonates. Initially, 15 mg/kg, then 10 mg/kg q8–12h.

▸ **Staphylococcal enterocolitis, antibiotic-associated pseudomembranous colitis caused by *Clostridium difficile***

PO

Adults, Elderly. 0.5–2 g/day in 3–4 divided doses for 7–10 days.
Children. 40 mg/kg/day in 3–4 divided doses for 7–10 days. Maximum: 2 g/day.

▸ **Dosage in renal impairment**

After a loading dose, subsequent dosages and frequency are modified based on creatinine clearance, the severity of the infection, and the serum concentration of the drug.

OFF-LABEL USES

Treatment of brain abscess, perioperative infections, staphylococcal or streptococcal meningitis

CONTRAINDICATIONS

None known.

INTERACTIONS

Drug

Aminoglycosides, amphotericin B, aspirin, bumetanide, carmustine, cisplatin, cyclosporine, ethacrynic acid, furosemide, streptozocin: May increase the risk of ototoxicity and nephrotoxicity of parenteral vancomycin.
Cholestyramine, colestipol: May decrease the effects of oral vancomycin.

Herbal

None known.

Food

None known.

DIAGNOSTIC TEST EFFECTS

May increase BUN level. Therapeutic peak serum level is 20–40 mcg/ml; therapeutic trough serum level is 5–15 mcg/ml. Toxic peak serum level is greater than 40 mcg/ml; toxic trough serum level is greater than 15 mcg/ml.

IV INCOMPATIBILITIES

Albumin, amphotericin B complex (Abelcet, AmBisome, Amphotec), aztreonam (Azactam), cefazolin (Ancef), cefepime (Maxipime), cefotaxime (Claforan), cefotetan (Cefotan), cefoxitin (Mefoxin), ceftazidime (Fortaz), ceftriaxone (Rocephin), cefuroxime (Zinacef), foscarnet (Foscavir), heparin, idarubicin (Idamycin), nafcillin (Nafcil), piperacillin and tazobactam (Zosyn), ticarcillin and clavulanate (Timentin)

IV COMPATIBILITIES

Amiodarone (Cordarone), calcium gluconate, diltiazem (Cardizem), hydromorphone (Dilaudid), insulin, lorazepam (Ativan), magnesium sulfate, midazolam (Versed), morphine, potassium chloride, propofol (Diprivan)

SIDE EFFECTS

Frequent

PO: Bitter or unpleasant taste, nausea, vomiting, mouth irritation (with oral solution)

Rare

Parenteral: Phlebitis, thrombophlebitis, or pain at peripheral IV site; dizziness; vertigo; tinnitus; chills; fever; rash; necrosis with extravasation
PO: Rash.

SERIOUS REACTIONS

! Nephrotoxicity and ototoxicity may occur.

! "Red-neck" syndrome (redness on face, neck, arms, and back; chills; fever; tachycardia; nausea or vomiting; pruritus; rash; unpleasant taste) may result from too-rapid injection.

NURSING CONSIDERATIONS

Baseline Assessment

• If possible, don't administer vancomycin concurrently with other ototoxic and nephrotoxic medications. If concurrent use is necessary, administer the drugs cautiously.
• Obtain culture and sensitivity tests before giving the first dose of vancomycin. Therapy may begin before test results are known.

Lifespan Considerations

• Vancomycin crosses the placenta; it is unknown if it's distributed in breast milk.
• Close monitoring of serum drug levels is recommended in premature neonates and young infants.
• Age-related renal impairment may increase the risk of ototoxicity and nephrotoxicity in the elderly. Dosage adjustment is recommended.

Precautions

• Use vancomycin cautiously in patients with pre-existing hearing impairment or renal dysfunction and in patients taking other ototoxic or nephrotoxic medications concurrently.

Administration and Handling

PO

• Be aware that vancomycin is usually not given for systemic infections because it's poorly absorbed from the GI tract; however, some patients with colitis may absorb the drug effectively.
• Reconstitute powder for oral solution as appropriate and administer it orally or by NG tube. Don't use powder for oral solution for IV administration.
• The refrigerated oral solution is stable for 2 weeks.

IV

◀ALERT▶ Give vancomycin by intermittent IV infusion (piggyback) or continuous IV infusion. Don't give by IV push because this may result in exaggerated hypotension.
• For intermittent IV infusion (piggyback), reconstitute each 500-mg or 1-g vial with 10 ml or 20 ml, respectively, of sterile water for injection to provide a concentration of 50 mg/ml.
• Further dilute to a final concentration of no more than 5 mg/ml.
• Discard the solution if a precipitate forms.
• After reconstitution, the IV solution may be refrigerated and should be used within 14 days.
• Administer the solution over 60 minutes or more.
• Monitor the patient's BP closely during the infusion.
• ADD-Vantage vials should not be used in neonates, infants, and children requiring less than a 500-mg dose.

Intervention and Evaluation

• Monitor the patient's intake and output and renal function test results.
• Assess the patient's skin for rash.
• Evaluate the patient's balance and hearing acuity.
• Evaluate the patient's IV site for phlebitis, as evidenced by heat, pain, and red streaking over the vein.
• Know that the vancomycin therapeutic peak serum level is 20 to 40 mcg/ml, and the trough level is 5 to 15 mcg/ml. The toxic peak serum level is greater than 40 mcg/ml, and the trough level is greater than 15 mcg/ml.

Patient Teaching

- Advise the patient to space drug doses evenly around the clock and to continue vancomycin therapy for the full course of treatment.
- Warn the patient to notify the physician if he or she experiences a rash, tinnitus, or signs and symptoms of nephrotoxicity.
- Inform the patient that laboratory tests are an important part of the therapy regimen.

13 Alkylating Agents

busulfan
carboplatin
carmustine
chlorambucil
cisplatin
cyclophosphamide
estramustine phosphate sodium
ifosfamide
lomustine
melphalan
oxaliplatin
thiotepa

Uses: Alkylating agents are used to treat many types of cancer, including acute and chronic leukemias, lymphomas, multiple myeloma, and solid tumors in the breasts, ovaries, uterus, lungs, bladder, and stomach.

Action: Alkylating agents form cross-links on DNA strands, which disturb DNA synthesis and cell division. In this way, these agents interfere with DNA integrity and function in rapidly proliferating tissues. They affect all phases of the cell cycle. (See the illustration *Sites and Mechanisms of Action: Antineoplastic Agents,* p. 268).

busulfan

bew-**sull**-fan
(Busulfex, Myleran)
Do not confuse Myleran with Alkeran, Leukeran, or Mylicon.

CATEGORY AND SCHEDULE

Pregnancy Risk Category: D

MECHANISM OF ACTION

An alkylating agent that interferes with DNA replication and RNA synthesis. Cell cycle-phase nonspecific. **Therapeutic Effect:** Disrupts nucleic acid function and causes myelosuppression.

PHARMACOKINETICS

Completely absorbed from the GI tract. Protein binding: 33%. Metabolized in the liver. Primarily excreted in urine. Minimally removed by hemodialysis. ***Half-life:*** 2.5 hr.

AVAILABILITY

Tablets (Myleran): 2 mg.
Injection (Busulfan): 60-mg ampule.

INDICATIONS AND DOSAGES

▸ **Remission induction in chronic myelogenous leukemia (CML)**
PO
Adults. 4–8 mg/day until WBC count falls below 15,000/mm^3.
Children. 0.06–0.12 mg/kg once a day.

▸ **Maintenance treatment of CML**
PO
Adults. Induction dose (4–8 mg/day) when total leukocyte count reaches 50,000/mm^3. If remission occurs in less than 3 mo, 1–3 mg/day may produce satisfactory response.
Elderly. Initially, lowest dosage for adults.

▸ **Conditioning regimen before allogeneic hematopoietic cell transplantation in patients with CML**
IV
Adults. 0.8 mg/kg q6h (as 2-hr infusion) for 16 doses.
Children. 0.06–0.12 mg/kg once a day.

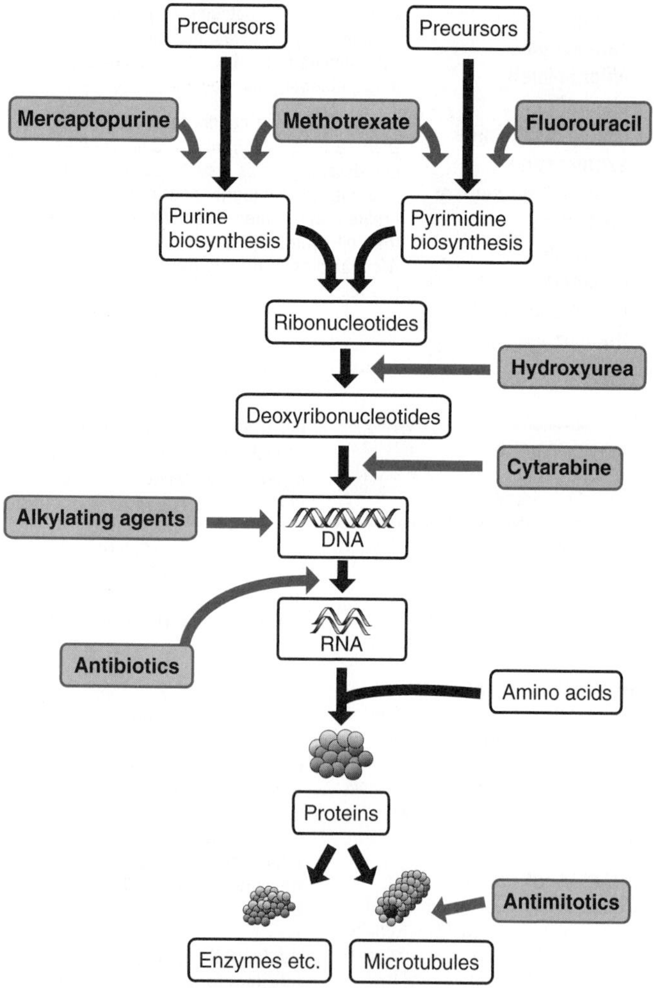

Sites and Mechanisms of Action: Antineoplastic Agents

Antineoplastic agents fight cancer by inhibiting or destroying multiplying cancer cells, Unfortunately these drugs also can damage healthy cells that rapidly divide, which accounts for the severity of adverse reactions. Most agents in some way target the cell's deoxyribonucleic acid (DNA) synthesis, which ultimately affects ribonucleic acid (RNA) and protein synthesis.

Alkalating agents, such as cyclophosphamide, work by forming bonds with nucleic acids and cross-linking DNA strands, preventing DNA replication. Ultimately, protein synthesis is hampered and cell growth stops.

Antineoplastic antibiotics, such as doxorubicin, inhibit RNA synthesis by binding with and destabilizing DNA, preventing cell growth.

Antimetabolites treat certain types of cancer by mimicking natural metabolites and blocking essential enzymes responsible for DNA synthesis and function. Methotrexate interferes with purine and pyrimidine synthesis by blocking the enzyme dihydrofolate reductase, which is responsible for converting folic acid to tetrahydrofolic acid. Mercaptopurine blocks purine synthesis by incorporating itself into the DNA and RNA. Fluorouracil inhibits thymidylate synthetase and prevents the formation of pyrimidine. Hydroxyurea inhibits ribonucleotide reductase, preventing the formation of deoxyribonucleotides needed for DNA synthesis. Cytarabine blocks DNA polymerase, and DNA formation.

Antimitotics, such as vincristine, inhibit cell division by binding to tubulin and inhibiting the microtubules needed to form mitotic spindles.

OFF-LABEL USES

Treatment of acute myelocytic leukemia

CONTRAINDICATIONS

Disease resistance to previous therapy with this drug

INTERACTIONS

Drug

Antigout medications: May decrease the effects of these drugs.
Bone marrow depressants: May increase the risk of myelosuppression.
Live-virus vaccines: May potentiate virus replication, increase vaccine side effects, and decrease the patient's antibody response to the vaccine.

Herbal

None known.

Food

None known.

DIAGNOSTIC TEST EFFECTS

May decrease serum magnesium, potassium, phosphates, and sodium levels. May increase blood glucose, BUN, and serum calcium, alkaline phosphatase, bilirubin, creatinine, and ALT (SGPT) levels.

IV INCOMPATIBILITIES

Don't mix busulfan with any other medications.

SIDE EFFECTS

Expected (98%–72%)

Nausea, stomatitis, vomiting, anorexia, insomnia, diarrhea, fever, abdominal pain, anxiety

Frequent (69%–44%)

Headache, rash, asthenia, infection, chills, tachycardia, dyspepsia

Occasional (38%–16%)

Constipation, dizziness, edema, pruritus, cough, dry mouth, depression, abdominal enlargement, pharyngitis, hiccups, back pain, alopecia, myalgia

Rare (13%–5%)

Injection site pain, arthralgia, confusion, hypotension, lethargy

SERIOUS REACTIONS

! Busulfan's major adverse effect is myelosuppression resulting in hematologic toxicity, as evidenced by anemia, severe leukopenia, and severe thrombocytopenia.

! Very high busulfan dosages may produce blurred vision, muscle twitching, and tonic-clonic seizures.

! Long-term therapy (more than 4 years) may produce pulmonary syndrome ("busulfan lung"), characterized by persistent cough, congestion, crackles, and dyspnea.

! Hyperuricemia may produce uric acid nephropathy, renal calculi, and acute renal failure.

NURSING CONSIDERATIONS

Baseline Assessment

• Expect to perform baseline and weekly hematologic studies, including blood Hct and Hgb levels, WBC count and differential, platelet count, and liver and renal function tests. Know that busulfan's dosage is based on baseline and ongoing hematologic values.

Lifespan Considerations

• Busulfan use should be avoided during pregnancy, if possible, especially in the first trimester.

• Busulfan use may cause fetal harm. It is unknown if the drug is distributed in breast milk; however, breastfeeding is not recommended for patients taking this drug.

• No age-related precautions have been noted in children or the elderly.

Precautions

• Use busulfan extremely cautiously in patients with myelosuppression.

• Use busulfan cautiously in patients with chickenpox, herpes zoster, infection, or a history of gout.

Administration and Handling

◀ALERT▶ Busulfan dosage is individualized based on the patient's clinical response and tolerance of the drug's adverse effects. When administering this drug in combination therapy, consult specific protocols for optimum dosage and sequence of drug administration.

◀ALERT▶ Because busulfan may be carcinogenic, mutagenic, or teratogenic, handle it with extreme care during preparation and administration. Use of gloves is recommended. If the drug comes in contact with skin or mucosa, wash the area thoroughly with water.

PO

• Give busulfan at the same time each day.

• Give it on an empty stomach if nausea or vomiting occurs.

IV

◀ALERT▶ Premedicate the patient with phenytoin to decrease the risk of seizures.

• Refrigerate ampules.

• Dilute bisulfan with 0.9% NaCl or D_5W only. The volume of diluent must be 10 times the volume of busulfan (for example, 9.3 ml busulfan must be diluted with 93 ml diluent).

• Use a filter to withdraw busulfan from the ampule, and add busulfan to the calculated amount of diluent. After dilution with 0.9% NaCl or D_5W, the solution is stable for 8 hours at room temperature and 12 hours if refrigerated.

• Lock the infusion pump when administering busulfan. Infuse it over 2 hours.

• Before and after the infusion, flush the catheter line with 5 ml 0.9% NaCl or D_5W.

Intervention and Evaluation

• Closely monitor the patient's laboratory values for evidence of myelosuppression.

• Examine the patient's mouth for evidence of stomatitis, such as difficulty swallowing, gum inflammation, and redness or ulceration of the oral mucosa.

• Give the patient an antiemetic to prevent nausea or vomiting.
• Assess the patient's pattern of daily bowel activity and stool consistency.

Patient Teaching

• Teach the patient to take busulfan at the same time each day.
• Instruct the patient to maintain adequate daily fluid intake to protect against renal impairment.
• Inform the patient and family about the expected side effects of busulfan treatment.
• Warn the patient to report congestion, consistent cough, difficulty breathing, easy bruising, fever, signs of local infection, sore throat, or unusual bleeding from any site.
• Urge the patient to avoid receiving vaccinations without the physician's approval and to avoid contact with anyone who has recently received a live-virus vaccine because busulfan lowers the body's resistance.
• Caution women of childbearing age to avoid pregnancy during therapy, and teach them contraception options.

carboplatin

car-**bow**-play-tin
(Paraplatin)
Do not confuse carboplatin with Cisplatin or Platinol.

CATEGORY AND SCHEDULE

Pregnancy Risk Category: D

MECHANISM OF ACTION

A platinum coordination complex that inhibits DNA synthesis by cross-linking with DNA strands, preventing cell division. Cell cycle-phase nonspecific. **Therapeutic Effect:** Interferes with DNA function.

PHARMACOKINETICS

Protein binding: Low. Hydrolyzed in solution to active form. Primarily excreted in urine. ***Half-life:*** 2.6–5.9 hr.

AVAILABILITY

Powder for Injection: 50 mg, 150 mg, 450 mg.
Injection Solution: 10 mg/ml.

INDICATIONS AND DOSAGES

▸ Ovarian carcinoma (monotherapy)

IV

Adults. 360 mg/m^2 on day 1, every 4 wk. Don't repeat dose until neutrophil and platelet counts are within acceptable levels. Adjust drug dosage in previously treated patients based on lowest post-treatment platelet or neutrophil count. Increase dosage only once to no more than 125% of starting dose.

▸ Ovarian carcinoma (combination therapy)

IV

Adults. 300 mg/m^2 (with cyclophosphamide) on day 1, every 4 wk. Don't repeat dose until neutrophil and platelet counts are within acceptable levels.

Children. 300–600 mg/m^2 every 4 wk for solid tumor, or 175 mg/m^2 every 4 wk for brain tumor.

▸ Dosage in renal impairment

Initial dosage is based on creatinine clearance; subsequent dosages are based on the patient's tolerance and degree of myelosuppression.

Creatinine Clearance	Dosage Day 1
60 ml/min or greater	360 mg/m^2
41–59 ml/min	250 mg/m^2
16–40 ml/min	200 mg/m^2

OFF-LABEL USES

Treatment of bony and soft-tissue

sarcomas; germ cell tumors; neuroblastoma; pediatric brain tumor; small-cell lung cancer; solid tumors of the bladder, cervix, and testes; squamous cell carcinoma of the esophagus

CONTRAINDICATIONS

History of severe allergic reaction to cisplatin, platinum compounds, or mannitol; severe bleeding, severe myelosuppression

INTERACTIONS

Drug

Bone marrow depressants: May increase myelosuppression.
Live-virus vaccines: May potentiate virus replication, increase vaccine side effects, and decrease the patient's antibody response to the vaccine.
Nephrotoxic, ototoxic medications: May increase the risk of nephrotoxicity.

Herbal

None known.

Food

None known.

DIAGNOSTIC TEST EFFECTS

May decrease serum electrolyte levels, including calcium, magnesium, potassium, and sodium. High dosages (more than 4 times the recommended dosage) may elevate BUN and serum alkaline phosphatase, bilirubin, creatinine, and AST (SGOT) levels.

IV INCOMPATIBILITIES

Amphotericin B complex (Abelcet, AmBisome, Amphotec)

IV COMPATIBILITIES

Etoposide (VePesid), granisetron (Kytril), ondansetron (Zofran), paclitaxel (Taxol)

SIDE EFFECTS

Frequent

Nausea (75%–80%), vomiting (65%)

Occasional

Generalized pain (17%), diarrhea or constipation (6%), peripheral neuropathy (4%)

Rare (3%–2%)

Alopecia, asthenia, hypersensitivity reaction (erythema, pruritus, rash, urticaria)

SERIOUS REACTIONS

! Myelosuppression may be severe, resulting in anemia, infection, (sepsis, pneumonia), and bleeding.
! Prolonged treatment may result in peripheral neurotoxicity.

NURSING CONSIDERATIONS

Baseline Assessment

- Be aware that treatment should not be repeated until the patient's WBC count recovers from previous therapy.

Lifespan Considerations

- Carboplatin use should be avoided during pregnancy, if possible, especially in the first trimester.
- Carboplatin use may cause fetal harm. It is unknown if carboplatin is distributed in breast milk; however, breast-feeding is not recommended for patients taking this drug.
- The safety and efficacy of carboplatin have not been established in children.
- The elderly are at increased risk for peripheral neurotoxicity and severe myelotoxicity. They also may require decreased dosage and more careful monitoring of blood counts because of age-related renal impairment.

Precautions

- Use carboplatin cautiously in patients with chickenpox, herpes zoster, infection, or renal impairment.

Administration and Handling

◀ALERT▶ Arboplatin dosage is individualized based on the patient's clinical response and tolerance of the drug's adverse effects. Also, know that platelets must be greater than 100,000 mm^3 and neutrophils greater than 2,000 mm^3 before giving any dosage.

◀ALERT▶ Know that carboplatin may be carcinogenic, mutagenic, or teratogenic. Handle with extreme care during preparation and administration.

IV

- Store vials at room temperature.
- Reconstitute the drug immediately before use.
- Don't use aluminum needles or administration sets that come in contact with drug because this may produce black precipitate and a loss of potency.
- Reconstitute each 50 mg vial with 5 ml sterile water for injection, D_5W, or 0.9% NaCl to provide a concentration of 10 mg/ml.
- Further dilute the solution with D_5W or 0.9% NaCl to provide a concentration as low as 0.5 mg/ml, if needed.
- After reconstitution, the solution is stable for 8 hours. Discard any unused portion after 8 hours.
- Infuse the solution over 15 to 60 minutes.
- Be aware that an anaphylactic reaction may occur minutes after administration. Use epinephrine and corticosteroid, as prescribed, to alleviate symptoms.

Intervention and Evaluation

- Monitor the patient's hematologic status, pulmonary function studies, and liver and renal function test results. Be aware that myelosuppression is increased in those who have received previous carboplatin therapy or have impaired renal function.
- Expect to administer transfusions to patients receiving prolonged therapy.
- Monitor the patient for signs and symptoms of hematologic toxicity, such as ecchymosis, fever, signs of local infection, sore throat, excessive fatigue or weakness, and unusual bleeding from any site.

Patient Teaching

- Inform the patient that nausea and vomiting may occur, but generally abate in less than 24 hours.
- Urge the patient to avoid receiving vaccinations without the physician's approval and to avoid contact with anyone who recently received a live-virus vaccine because carboplatin lowers the body's resistance.

carmustine

car-**muss**-teen

(BiCNU, Gliadel)

CATEGORY AND SCHEDULE

Pregnancy Risk Category: D

MECHANISM OF ACTION

An alkylating agent and nitrosourea that inhibits DNA and RNA synthesis by cross-linking with DNA and RNA strands, preventing cell division. Cell cycle-phase nonspecific. **Therapeutic Effect:** Interferes with DNA and RNA function.

AVAILABILITY

Powder for Injection (BiCNu): 100 mg.

Wafer (Gliadel): 7.7 mg.

INDICATIONS AND DOSAGES

▸ **Disseminated Hodgkin's disease, non-Hodgkin's lymphoma, multiple**

myeloma, and primary and metastatic brain tumors in previously untreated patients (monotherapy).
IV (BiCNu)
Adults, Elderly. 150–200 mg/m^2 as a single dose or 75–100 mg/m^2 on 2 successive days.
Children. 200–250 mg/m^2 every 4–6 wk as a single dose.
◀ **ALERT** ▶ Next dosage is based on clinical and hematologic response to previous dose (platelets greater than 100,000/mm^3 and leukocytes greater than 4000/mm^3).
Implantation (Gliadel)
Adults, Elderly, Children. Up to 8 wafers may be placed in resection cavity.

OFF-LABEL USES

Treatment of hepatic or GI carcinoma, malignant melanoma, mycosis fungoides

CONTRAINDICATIONS

None known.

INTERACTIONS

Drug

Bone marrow depressants, cimetidine: May enhance carmustine's myelosuppressive effect.
Hepatotoxic, nephrotoxic medications: May increase the risk of hepatotoxicity or nephrotoxicity.
Live virus vaccines: May potentiate virus replication, increase vaccine side effects, and decrease the patient's antibody response to the vaccine.

Herbal

None known.

Food

None known.

DIAGNOSTIC TEST EFFECTS

May increase BUN, and serum alkaline phosphatase, bilirubin, AST (SGOT), and ALT (SGPT) levels.

IV INCOMPATIBILITIES

Allopurinol (Aloprim)

SIDE EFFECTS

Frequent
Nausea and vomiting within minutes to 2 hr after administration (may last up to 6 hr)
Occasional
Diarrhea, esophagitis, anorexia, dysphagia
Rare
Thrombophlebitis

SERIOUS REACTIONS

! Hematologic toxicity due to myelosuppression occurs frequently. Thrombocytopenia occurs about 4 weeks after carmustine treatment begins and lasts 1 to 2 weeks.
! Leukopenia is evident 5 to 6 weeks after treatment begins and lasts 1 to 2 weeks. Anemia occurs less frequently and is less severe.
! Mild, reversible hepatotoxicity also occurs frequently.
! Prolonged high-dose carmustine therapy may produce impaired renal function and pulmonary toxicity (pulmonary infiltrate or fibrosis).

NURSING CONSIDERATIONS

Baseline Assessment

- Expect to perform liver function studies before and periodically during therapy.
- Monitor the patient's blood counts before, weekly during, and for at least 6 weeks after carmustine therapy ends.

Precautions

- Use carmustine cautiously in patients with decreased erythrocyte, leukocyte, and platelet counts.

Administration and Handling

◀ **ALERT** ▶ Carmustine dosage is individualized based on the patient's clinical response and tolerance of the drug's adverse effects. When administering this drug in combination therapy, consult specific protocols for optimum dosage and sequence of drug administration.

◀ALERT▶ Carmustine may be carcinogenic, mutagenic, or teratogenic and may cause transient burning and brown staining of the skin. Wear protective gloves during drug preparation.

IV

- Refrigerate unopened vials of dry powder.
- Reconstituted vials are stable for up to 8 hours at room temperature and up to 24 hours if refrigerated.
- Solutions further diluted to 0.2 mg/ml with D_5W or 0.9% NaCl are stable for an additional 8 hours at room temperature and for 48 hours if refrigerated.
- The solution normally appears clear and colorless to yellow. Discard the solution if the color changes, a precipitate forms, or an oily film develops on the bottom of the vial.
- Reconstitute each 100-mg vial with 3 ml sterile dehydrated (absolute) alcohol, followed by 27 ml sterile water for injection to provide a concentration of 3.3 mg/ml.
- Further dilute with 50 to 250 ml D_5W or 0.9% NaCl.
- Infuse the solution over 1 to 2 hours (shorter duration may produce intense burning pain at the injection site and intense flushing of the skin or conjunctiva).
- Flush the IV line with 5 to 10 ml 0.9% NaCl or D_5W before and after administration to prevent irritation at the injection site.

Intervention and Evaluation

- Monitor the patient's CBC; BUN level; serum alkaline phosphatase and bilirubin levels; and pulmonary, liver, and renal function test results.
- Monitor the patient for signs and symptoms of anemia (excessive fatigue and weakness) and hematologic toxicity (ecchymosis, fever, signs of local infection, sore throat, and unusual bleeding from any site.
- Evaluate the patient for signs and symptoms of pulmonary toxicity, including dyspnea and fine crackles.

Patient Teaching

- Instruct the patient to maintain adequate daily fluid intake to protect against renal impairment.
- Urge the patient to avoid receiving vaccinations without the physician's approval and to avoid contact with anyone who has recently received a live-virus vaccine because carmustine lowers the body's resistance.
- Advise the patient to contact the physician if nausea or vomiting continues at home.

chlorambucil

klor-am-bew-sill

(Leukeran)

Do not confuse Leukeran with Alkeran, Chloromycetin, Leukine, or Myleran.

CATEGORY AND SCHEDULE

Pregnancy Risk Category: D

MECHANISM OF ACTION

An alkylating agent and nitrogen mustard that inhibits DNA and RNA synthesis by cross-linking with DNA and RNA strands. Cell cycle-phase nonspecific. **Therapeutic Effect:** Interferes with nucleic acid function.

PHARMACOKINETICS

Rapidly and completely absorbed from the GI tract. Protein binding: 99%. Rapidly metabolized in the liver to active metabolite. Not removed by hemodialysis. ***Half-life:*** 1.5 hr; metabolite 2.5 hr.

AVAILABILITY

Tablets: 2 mg.

INDICATIONS AND DOSAGES

▸ **Palliative treatment of advanced Hodgkin's disease, advanced malignant (non-Hodgkin's) lymphoma (including giant follicular lymphoma and lymphosarcoma), chronic lymphocytic leukemia**

PO

Adults, Elderly, Children. For initial or short-course therapy, 0.1–0.2 mg/kg/day as a single or in divided doses for 3–6 wk (average dose, 4–10 mg/day). Alternatively, 0.4 mg/kg initially as a single daily dose every 2 wk and increased by 0.1 mg/kg every 2 wk until response and myelosuppression occur. Maintenance: 0.03–0.1 mg/kg/day (average dose, 2–4 mg/day).

OFF-LABEL USES

Treatment of hairy cell leukemia, nephrotic syndrome, ovarian or testicular carcinoma, polycythemia vera

CONTRAINDICATIONS

Previous allergic reaction or disease resistance to drug

INTERACTIONS

Drug

Antigout medications: May decrease the effect of these drugs.
Bone marrow depressants: May increase bone myelosuppression.
Live-virus vaccines: May potentiate virus replication, increase vaccine side effects and decrease the patient's antibody response to the vaccine.
Other immunosuppressants (including steroids): May increase the risk of infection or development of neoplasms.

Herbal

None known.

Food

None known.

DIAGNOSTIC TEST EFFECTS

May increase serum alkaline phosphatase, serum uric acid, and AST (SGOT) levels.

SIDE EFFECTS

Expected

GI effects such as nausea, vomiting, anorexia, diarrhea, and abdominal distress (generally mild, last less than 24 hr and occur only if single dose exceeds 20 mg).

Occasional

Rash or dermatitis, pruritus, cold sores

Rare

Alopecia, urticaria, erythema, hyperuricemia

SERIOUS REACTIONS

! Hematologic toxicity due to myelosuppression occurs frequently and may include neutropenia, leukopenia, progressive lymphopenia, anemia, and thrombocytopenia.
! After discontinuation of short-course therapy, thrombocytopenia and leukopenia usually last for 1 to 2 weeks but may persist for 3 to 4 weeks.
! The neutrophil count may continue to decrease for up to 10 days after the last dose.
! Hematologic toxicity appears to be less severe with intermittent rather than continuous drug administration.
! Overdosage may produce seizures in children.
! Excessive serum uric acid level and hepatotoxicity occur rarely.

NURSING CONSIDERATIONS

Baseline Assessment

- Expect to obtain a CBC before and each week during chlorambucil therapy.
- Expect to obtain a WBC count 3 to 4 days after each weekly CBC during the first 3 to 6 weeks of chlorambucil therapy (or 4 to 6 weeks if the patient is on an intermittent dosing schedule).

Lifespan Considerations

- Chlorambucil use should be avoided during pregnancy, if possible, especially in the first trimester.
- Breast-feeding is not recommended for patients taking this drug.
- No age-related precautions have been noted in children or the elderly.

Precautions

- Use chlorambucil extremely cautiously within 4 weeks after full-course radiation therapy or myelosuppressive drug regimen.
- Be aware that seizures may increase when chlorambucil is taken for nephrotic syndrome.

Administration and Handling

◀ALERT▶ Chlorambucil may be carcinogenic, mutagenic, or teratogenic. Handle the drug with extreme care during administration.

- Chlorambucil dosage is individualized based on the patient's clinical response and tolerance of the drug's adverse effects. When administering this drug in combination therapy, consult specific protocols for optimum dosage and sequence of drug administration.

PO

- Give chlorambucil without regard to food.

Intervention and Evaluation

- Monitor the patient for signs and symptoms of hematologic toxicity, such as ecchymosis, fever, signs of local infection, sore throat, excessive fatigue or weakness, and unusual bleeding from any site.
- Assess the patient's skin for rash, pruritus, and urticaria.

Patient Teaching

- Instruct the patient to maintain adequate daily fluid intake to protect against renal impairment.
- Warn the patient to report congestion, consistent cough, difficulty breathing, easy bruising, fever, signs of local infection, sore throat, or unusual bleeding from any site.
- Urge the patient to avoid receiving vaccinations without the physician's approval and to avoid contact with anyone who has recently received a live-virus vaccine because chlorambucil lowers the body's resistance.

cisplatin ⚑

sis-**plah**-tin

(Platinol-AQ)

Do not confuse cisplatin with carboplatin, or Platinol with Paraplatin or Patanol.

CATEGORY AND SCHEDULE

Pregnancy Risk Category: D

MECHANISM OF ACTION

A platinum coordination complex that inhibits DNA and to a lesser extent, RNA, protein synthesis by cross-linking with DNA strands, preventing cell division. Cell cycle-phase nonspecific. **Therapeutic Effect:** Interferes with DNA function.

PHARMACOKINETICS

Widely distributed. Protein binding: greater than 90%. Undergoes rapid nonenzymatic conversion to inactive metabolite. Excreted in urine. Removed by hemodialysis. ***Half-life:***

58–73 hr (increased with impaired renal function).

AVAILABILITY

Injection: 10-mg (CAN) 50-mg, 100-mg vials.

INDICATIONS AND DOSAGES

▸ **Advanced bladder carcinoma, metastatic ovarian tumors, metastatic testicular tumors**

IV

Adults, Elderly, Children. For intermittent dosage schedule, 37–75 mg/m^2 once every 2–3 wk or 50–100 mg/m^2 over 4–8 hr once every 21–28 days. For daily dosage schedule, 15–20 mg/m^2/day for 5 days every 3–4 wk.

▸ **Dosage in renal impairment**

Dosage is modified based on creatinine clearance.

Creatinine Clearance	% of Dose
10–50 ml/min	75%
less than 10 ml/min	50%

OFF-LABEL USES

Breast, cervical, endometrial, gastric, head and neck, lung, and prostate carcinomas; germ cell tumors; neuroblastoma; osteosarcoma

CONTRAINDICATIONS

Hearing impairment, myelosuppression, pregnancy

INTERACTIONS

Drug

Antigout medications: May decrease the effects of these drugs.
Bone marrow depressants: May increase myelosuppression.
Live-virus vaccines: May potentiate virus replication, increase vaccine side effects, and decrease the patient's antibody response to the vaccine.
Nephrotoxic, ototoxic medications: May increase the risk of nephrotoxicity or ototoxicity.

Herbal

None known.

Food

None known.

DIAGNOSTIC TEST EFFECTS

May increase BUN and serum creatinine, uric acid, and AST (SGOT) levels. May decrease creatinine clearance and serum calcium, magnesium, phosphate, potassium, and sodium levels. May cause a positive Coombs' test result.

IV INCOMPATIBILITIES

Amifostine (Ethyol), amphotericin B complex (Abelcet, AmBisome, Amphotec), cefepime (Maxipime), piperacillin and tazobactam (Zosyn), thiotepa

IV COMPATIBILITIES

Etoposide (VePesid), granisetron (Kytril), heparin, hydromorphone (Dilaudid), lorazepam (Ativan), magnesium sulfate, mannitol, morphine, ondansetron (Zofran)

SIDE EFFECTS

Frequent

Nausea, vomiting (generally beginning 1–4 hr after administration and lasting up to 24 hr); myelosuppression (affecting 25%–30% of patients with recovery generally occurring in 18–23 days).

Occasional

Peripheral neuropathy (with prolonged therapy [4–7 mo]).
Pain or redness at injection site, loss of taste or appetite

Rare

Hemolytic anemia, blurred vision, stomatitis

SERIOUS REACTIONS

! An anaphylactic reaction manifested as angioedema, wheezing, tachycardia, and hypotension may occur in the first few minutes of IV administration in patients previously exposed to cisplatin.

! Nephrotoxicity occurs in 28%–36% of patients treated with a single dose of cisplatin, usually during the second week of therapy.

! Ototoxicity, including tinnitus and hearing loss, occurs in 31% of patients treated with a single dose of cisplatin. It may be more severe in children and may become more frequent or severe with repeated doses.

NURSING CONSIDERATIONS

Baseline Assessment

• Keep patients well hydrated before and 24 hours after receiving cisplatin to ensure adequate urinary output and decrease the risk of nephrotoxicity.

Lifespan Considerations

• Cisplatin use should be avoided during pregnancy, if possible, especially in the first trimester.

• Breast-feeding is not recommended for patients taking this drug.

• The ototoxic effects of this drug may be more severe in children.

• Age-related renal impairment may require a dosage adjustment in the elderly.

Precautions

• Use cisplatin cautiously in patients who have previously been treated with other antineoplastics or radiation.

Administration and Handling

◀ALERT▶ Verify any cisplatin dose exceeding 120 mg/m^2 per course. Cisplatin dosage is individualized based on the patient's clinical response and tolerance of the drug's adverse effects. When administering this drug in combination therapy, consult specific protocols for optimum dosage and sequence of drug administration. Be aware that repeat courses should not be given more often than every 3 to 4 weeks. Also, the course should not be repeated unless the patient's auditory acuity is within normal limits, serum creatinine level is less than 1.5 mg/dl, BUN level is less than 25 mg/dl, and platelet and WBC counts are within acceptable levels.

◀ALERT▶ Because cisplatin may be carcinogenic, mutagenic, or teratogenic, wear protective gloves and handle the drug with extreme care during preparation and administration.

IV

• After reconstitution, the solution normally appears clear and colorless. Protect it from direct sunlight.

• The reconstituted solution is stable for up to 20 hours at room temperature. Don't refrigerate it because a precipitate may form. Discard it if a precipitate forms.

• Reconstitute the 10-mg vial with 10 ml sterile water for injection (50-mg vial with 50 ml) to provide a concentration of 1 mg/ml.

• For IV infusion, dilute the desired dose in up to 1,000 ml D_5W, 0.33% or 0.45% NaCl containing 12.5 to 50 g mannitol/L.

• Infuse the solution over 2 to 24 hours. Avoid rapid infusion because this increases the risk of nephrotoxicity and ototoxicity.

• Monitor the patient for an anaphylactic reaction during the first few minutes of the IV infusion.

Intervention and Evaluation

• Measure all of the patient's vomitus. If the patient vomits 750 ml or more over 8 hours, notify the physician immediately.

• Monitor the patient's intake and output every 1 to 2 hours, beginning with pretreatment hydration and continuing for 48 hours after cisplatin therapy. If urine output is less than 100 ml/hour, notify the physician immediately.
• Assess the patient's vital signs every 1 to 2 hours during the infusion.
• Monitor the patient's urinalysis and renal function test results for evidence of nephrotoxicity.

Patient Teaching

• Instruct the patient to report hearing loss or ringing or roaring in the ears.
• Urge the patient to avoid receiving vaccinations without the physician's approval and to avoid contact with anyone who has recently received an oral polio vaccine because cisplatin lowers the body's resistance.
• Advise the patient to contact the physician if nausea or vomiting continues at home.
• Teach the patient to recognize signs and symptoms of peripheral neuropathy.

cyclophosphamide

sye-kloe-**foss**-fa-mide
(Cycloblastin[AUS], Cytoxan, Endoxan Asta[AUS], Endoxon Asta[AUS], Neosar, Procytox[CAN])
Do not confuse Cytoxan with cefoxitin, Ciloxan, cyclosporine, or Cytotec.

CATEGORY AND SCHEDULE

Pregnancy Risk Category: D

MECHANISM OF ACTION

An alkylating agent that inhibits DNA and RNA protein synthesis by cross-linking with DNA and RNA strands, preventing cell growth. Cell cycle-phase nonspecific. **Therapeutic Effect:** Potent immunosuppressant.

PHARMACOKINETICS

Well absorbed from the GI tract. Protein binding: Low. Crosses the blood-brain barrier. Metabolized in the liver to active metabolites. Primarily excreted in urine. Removed by hemodialysis. ***Half-life:*** 3–12 hr.

AVAILABILITY

Tablets (Cytoxan): 25 mg, 50 mg.
Powder for Injection (Neosar): 100 mg, 200 mg.
Powder for Injection (Cytoxan, Neosar): 500 mg, 1 g, 2 g.

INDICATIONS AND DOSAGES

▸ Ovarian adenocarcinoma, breast carcinoma, Hodgkin's disease, non-Hodgkin's lymphoma, multiple myeloma, leukemia (acute lymphoblastic, acute myelogenous, acute monocytic, chronic granulocytic, chronic lymphocytic), mycosis fungoides, disseminated neuroblastoma, retinoblastoma

PO
Adults. 1–5 mg/kg/day.
Children. Initially, 2–8 mg/kg/day. Maintenance: 2–5 mg/kg twice a week.
IV
Adults. 40–50 mg/kg in divided doses over 2–5 days; or 10–15 mg/kg every 7–10 days or 3–5 mg/kg twice a week.
Children. 2–8 mg/kg/day for 6 days or total dose for 7 days once a week.

▸ Biopsy-proven minimal-change nephrotic syndrome

PO
Adults, Children. 2.5–3 mg/kg/day for 60–90 days.

OFF-LABEL USES

Treatment of carcinoma of bladder, cervix, endometrium, lung, prostate, or testicles; germ cell ovarian tumors; osteosarcoma; rheumatoid arthritis; systemic lupus erythematosus

CONTRAINDICATIONS

None known.

INTERACTIONS

Drug

Allopurinol, bone marrow depressants: May increase myelosuppression.
Antigout medications: May decrease the effects of these drugs.
Cytarabine: May increase the risk of cardiomyopathy.
Immunosuppressants: May increase the risk of infection and development of neoplasms.
Live-virus vaccines: May potentiate virus replication, increase vaccine side effects, and decrease the patient's antibody response to the vaccine.

Herbal

None known.

Food

None known.

DIAGNOSTIC TEST EFFECTS

May increase serum uric acid levels.

IV INCOMPATIBILITIES

Amphotericin B complex (Abelcet, AmBisome, Amphotec)

IV COMPATIBILITIES

Granisetron (Kytril), heparin, hydromorphone (Dilaudid), lorazepam (Ativan), morphine, ondansetron (Zofran), propofol (Diprivan)

SIDE EFFECTS

Expected

Marked leukopenia 8–15 days after initial therapy

Frequent

Nausea, vomiting (beginning about 6 hr after administration and lasting about 4 hr); alopecia (33%)

Occasional

Diarrhea, darkening of skin and fingernails, stomatitis, headache, diaphoresis

Rare

Pain or redness at injection site

SERIOUS REACTIONS

! Cyclophosphamide's major toxic effect is myelosuppression resulting in blood dyscrasias, such as leukopenia, anemia, thrombocytopenia, and hypoprothrombinemia.
! Expect leukopenia to resolve in 17 to 28 days. Anemia generally occurs after large doses or prolonged therapy. Thrombocytopenia may occur 10–15 days after drug initiation.
! Hemorrhagic cystitis occurs commonly in long-term therapy, especially in pediatric patients.
! Pulmonary fibrosis and cardiotoxicity have been noted with high doses.
! Amenorrhea, azoospermia, and hyperkalemia may also occur.

NURSING CONSIDERATIONS

Baseline Assessment

- Expect to obtain the patient's WBC count weekly during cyclophosphamide therapy or until the drug's maintenance dose is established and then at 2- to 3-week intervals.

Precautions

- Use cyclophosphamide cautiously in patients with severe leukopenia, thrombocytopenia, or tumor infiltration of bone marrow and in those who have previously been treated with other antineoplastics or radiation.

Lifespan Considerations

• Cyclophosphamide use should be avoided during pregnancy because of the risk of fetal malformations, such as cardiac anomalies, hernias, and limb abnormalities.
• Cyclophosphamide is distributed in breast milk, so breast-feeding is not recommended for patients taking this drug.
• No age-related precautions have been noted in children.
• Age-related renal impairment may require cautious use of this drug in the elderly.

Administration and Handling

◀ **ALERT** ▶ Cyclophosphamide dosage is individualized based on the patient's clinical response and tolerance of the drug's adverse effects. When administering this drug in combination therapy, consult specific protocols for optimum dosage and sequence of drug administration.
◀ **ALERT** ▶ Because cyclophosphamide may be carcinogenic, mutagenic, or teratogenic, handle the drug with extreme care during drug preparation and administration.

PO

• Give cyclophosphamide on an empty stomach. If GI upset occurs, give with food.

IV

• Reconstituted solution is stable for up to 24 hours at room temperature or up to 6 days if refrigerated.
• For IV push, reconstitute each 100-mg vial with 5 ml sterile water for injection or bacteriostatic water for injection to provide a concentration of 20 mg/ml.
• Shake the solution to dissolve, and allow it to stand until clear.
• Give by IV push or further dilute with 250 ml D_5W, 0.9% NaCl, 0.45% NaCl, lactated Ringer's (LR) solution or D_5LR.
• Infuse each 100 mg or fraction thereof over 15 minutes or longer.

Intervention and Evaluation

• Monitor the patient's blood chemistry results, CBC, and serum uric acid concentration.
• Monitor the patient's WBC closely during initial therapy. Be alert for diaphoresis, facial flushing, faintness, and oropharyngeal sensation with IV drug administration.
• Monitor the patient for signs and symptoms of hematologic toxicity, such as ecchymosis, fever, signs of local infection, sore throat, excessive fatigue or weakness, and unusual bleeding from any site.

Patient Teaching

• To help prevent cystitis, encourage the patient to drink plenty of fluids before, during, and after therapy and to void frequently.
• Urge the patient to avoid receiving vaccinations without the physician's approval and to avoid contact with anyone who has recently received a live-virus vaccine because cyclophosphamide lowers the body's resistance.
• Advise the patient to report easy bruising, fever, signs of local infection, sore throat, or unusual bleeding from any site.
• Explain to the patient that hair loss is reversible, but that new hair may have a different color or texture.

estramustine phosphate sodium

es-trah-**mew**-steen
(Emcyt)
Do not confuse Emcyt with Eryc.

CATEGORY AND SCHEDULE
Pregnancy Risk Category: C

MECHANISM OF ACTION
An alkylating agent, estrogen and nitrogen mustard that binds to microtubule-associated proteins, causing their disassembly. **Therapeutic Effect:** Reduces serum testosterone concentration.

PHARMACOKINETICS
Well absorbed from the GI tract. Highly localized in prostatic tissue. Rapidly dephosphorylated during absorption into peripheral circulation. Metabolized in the liver. Primarily eliminated in feces by biliary system. ***Half-life:*** 20 hr.

AVAILABILITY
Capsules: 140 mg.

INDICATIONS AND DOSAGES
▸ **Prostatic carcinoma**
PO
Adults, Elderly. 10–16 mg/kg/day or 140 mg 4 times/day.

CONTRAINDICATIONS
Active thrombophlebitis or thromboembolic disorders (unless the tumor is the cause of the thromboembolic disorder and the benefits outweigh the risk), hypersensitivity to estradiol or nitrogen mustard

INTERACTIONS
Drug
Calcium-containing antacids: May impair estramustine absorption.
Hepatotoxic medications: May increase the risk of hepatotoxicity.
Herbal
None known.
Food
Milk, dairy products, and other calcium-rich foods: May impair estramustine absorption.

DIAGNOSTIC TEST EFFECTS
May increase blood glucose level and serum bilirubin, cortisol, LDH, phospholipid, prolactin, AST (SGOT), sodium, and triglyceride levels. May decrease urine pregnanediol level and serum antithrombin III, folate, and phosphate levels. May alter thyroid function test results.

SIDE EFFECTS
Frequent
Peripheral edema of lower extremities, breast tenderness or enlargement, diarrhea, flatulence, nausea
Occasional
Increase in BP, thirst, dry skin, ecchymosis, flushing, alopecia, night sweats
Rare
Headache, rash, fatigue, insomnia, vomiting

SERIOUS REACTIONS
! Estramustine use may exacerbate CHF and increase the risk of pulmonary emboli, thrombophlebitis, and cerebrovascular accident.

NURSING CONSIDERATIONS

Lifespan Considerations
• Estramustine is not used in pregnant women or in children.

• Age-related renal impairment and peripheral vascular disease may require cautious use of this drug in the elderly.

Precautions

• Use estramustine cautiously in patients with cerebrovascular or coronary artery disease; a history of thrombophlebitis, thrombosis, or thromboembolic disorders; impaired hepatic function; or metabolic bone disease in those with hypercalcemia or renal insufficiency.

Administration and Handling

PO

• Refrigerate capsules. The drug may be stored at room temperature for 24 to 48 hours without loss of potency.
• Give estramustine with water 1 hour before or 2 hours after a meal.

Intervention and Evaluation

• Monitor the patient's BP periodically.

Patient Teaching

• Advise the patient to take estramustine with water 1 hour before or 2 hours after a meal.
• Instruct the patient not to take estramustine with calcium-containing antacids, milk, dairy products, or other calcium-rich foods.
• Encourage the patient to use contraceptive measures during estramustine therapy.
• Warn the patient to notify the physician if he or she experiences calf pain, speech or vision disturbances, dizziness, severe or migraine headache, heaviness in the chest, numbness, shortness of breath, unexplained cough, or vomiting.

ifosfamide

eye-**fos**-fah-mid
(Holoxan[AUS], Ifex)

CATEGORY AND SCHEDULE

Pregnancy Risk Category: D

MECHANISM OF ACTION

An alkylating agent that inhibits DNA and RNA protein synthesis by cross-linking with DNA and RNA strands, preventing cell growth. Cell cycle-phase nonspecific. **Therapeutic Effect:** Interferes with DNA and RNA function.

PHARMACOKINETICS

Metabolized in the liver to active metabolite. Crosses the blood-brain barrier (to a limited extent). Primarily excreted in urine. Removed by hemodialysis. ***Half-life:*** 15 hr.

AVAILABILITY

Powder for Injection: 1 g, 3 g.

INDICATIONS AND DOSAGES

▸ Germ cell testicular carcinoma

IV

Adults. 700–2,000 mg/m^2/day for 5 consecutive days. Repeat every 3wk or after recovery from hematologic toxicity. Administer with mesna.
Children. 1,200–1,800 mg/m^2/day for 5 days every 21–28 days.

OFF-LABEL USES

Treatment of Ewing's sarcoma; non-Hodgkin's lymphoma; and lung, pancreatic, and soft-tissue carcinoma

CONTRAINDICATIONS

Pregnancy, severe myelosuppression

INTERACTIONS

Drug

Bone marrow depressants: May increase myelosuppression.
Live-virus vaccines: May potentiate virus replication, increase vaccine side effects, and decrease the patient's antibody response to the vaccine.

Herbal

None known.

Food

None known.

DIAGNOSTIC TEST EFFECTS

May increase BUN and serum bilirubin, creatinine, uric acid, AST (SGOT), and ALT (SGPT) levels.

IV INCOMPATIBILITIES

Cefepime (Maxipime), methotrexate

IV COMPATIBILITIES

Granisetron (Kytril), ondansetron (Zofran)

SIDE EFFECTS

Frequent

Alopecia (83%); nausea, vomiting (58%)

Occasional (15%–5%)

Confusion, somnolence, hallucinations, infection

Rare (less than 5%)

Dizziness, seizures, disorientation, fever, malaise, stomatitis

SERIOUS REACTIONS

! Hemorrhagic cystitis with hematuria and dysuria occurs frequently if a protective agent (mesna) is not used.
! Myelosuppression, characterized by leukopenia and, to a lesser extent, thrombocytopenia occurs frequently.
! Pulmonary toxicity, hepatotoxicity, nephrotoxicity, cardiotoxicity, and CNS toxicity (manifested as confusion, hallucinations, somnolence, and coma) may require discontinuation of therapy.

NURSING CONSIDERATIONS

Baseline Assessment

- Obtain the patient's urinalysis test results, as appropriate, before each dose. If hematuria occurs, as evidenced by more than 10 RBCs per field, notify the physician because therapy will have to be withheld until resolution occurs.
- Expect to obtain the patient's blood Hgb level and WBC and platelet counts before each dose.

Precautions

- Use ifosfamide cautiously in patients with myelosuppression or impaired hepatic or renal function.

Lifespan Considerations

- Ifosfamide use should be avoided during pregnancy, if possible, especially in the first trimester because it may cause fetal harm.
- Ifosfamide is distributed in breast milk. Breast-feeding is not recommended for patients taking this drug.
- Ifosfamide is not intended for use in children.
- Age-related renal impairment may require a dosage adjustment in the elderly.

Administration and Handling

◀ALERT▶ Ifosfamide dosage is individualized based on the patient's clinical response and tolerance of the drug's adverse effects. When administering this drug in combination therapy, consult specific protocols for optimum dosage and sequence of drug administration.

◀ALERT▶ Hemorrhagic cystitis occurs if mesna is not given concurrently with ifosfamide. Mesna should always be given with ifosfamide.

IV

- Store vials at room temperature.

- After reconstitution with bacteriostatic water for injection, the solution may be stored for up to 1 week at room temperature, or up to 3 weeks if refrigerated. A solution that is further diluted may be refreigerated for up to 6 weeks.
- If the solution is prepared with other diluents, it should be used within 6 hours.
- Reconstitute each 1-g vial with 20 ml sterile water for injection or bacteriostatic water for injection to provide a concentration of 50 mg/ml. Shake to dissolve.
- Further dilute with D_5W or 0.9% NaCl to provide a concentration of 0.6 to 20 mg/ml.
- Infuse the drug over at least 30 minutes.
- Give with at least 2,000 ml PO or IV fluid to prevent bladder toxicity.
- Give with a prescribed protectant against hemorrhagic cystitis, such as mesna. Mesna should always be given with ifosfamide to prevent other adverse reactions, including chills, fever, jaundice, joint pain, sore throat, stomatitis, or unusual bleeding or bruising.

Intervention and Evaluation

- Monitor the patient's hematologic studies and urinalysis results diligently.
- Assess the patient for signs and symptoms of hematologic toxicity, such as ecchymosis, fever, signs of local infection, sore throat, excessive fatigue or weakness, and unusual bleeding from any site.

Patient Teaching

- Advise the patient that alopecia related to ifosfamide use is reversible, but that new hair growth may have a different color or texture.
- Encourage the patient to drink plenty of fluids to protect against cystitis.
- Urge the patient to avoid receiving vaccinations without the physician's approval and to avoid contact with crowds, anyone with a known infection, and anyone who has recently received a live-virus vaccine because ifosfamide lowers the body's resistance.
- Warn the patient to notify the physician if he or she experiences chills, fever, joint pain, sores in the mouth or on the lips, sore throat, yellowing of the skin or eyes, or unusual bleeding or bruising.

lomustine

low-**meuw**-steen
(CeeNU)

CATEGORY AND SCHEDULE

Pregnancy Risk Category: D

MECHANISM OF ACTION

An alkylating agent and nitrosourea that inhibits DNAand RNA protein synthesis by cross-linking with DNA and RNA strands, preventing cell division. Cell cycle-phase nonspecific. **Therapeutic Effect:** Interferes with DNA and RNA function.

AVAILABILITY

Capsules: 10 mg, 40 mg, 100 mg.

INDICATIONS AND DOSAGES

▸ Disseminated Hodgkin's disease, primary and metastatic brain tumors

PO

Adults, Elderly. 100–130 mg/m^2 as single dose. Repeat dose at intervals of at least 6 wk but not until circulating blood elements have returned to acceptable levels. Adjust dose based on hematologic response to previous dose.

Children. 75–150 mg/m^2 as a single dose every 6wk.

OFF-LABEL USES
Breast, GI, lung, or renal carcinoma; malignant melanoma; multiple myeloma

CONTRAINDICATIONS
Pregnancy

INTERACTIONS
Drug
Bone marrow depressants: May increase myelosuppression.
Live-virus vaccines: May potentiate virus replication, increase vaccine side effects, and decrease the patient's antibody response to the vaccine.
Herbal
None known.
Food
None known.

DIAGNOSTIC TEST EFFECTS
May increase liver function test results.

SIDE EFFECTS
Frequent
Nausea, vomiting (occuring 45 min-6 hr after dose and lasting 12–24 hr); anorexia (often follows for 2–3 days).
Occasional
Neurotoxicity (confusion, slurred speech), stomatitis, darkening of skin, diarrhea, rash, pruritus, alopecia

SERIOUS REACTIONS
! Myelosuppression may result in hematologic toxicity, manifested principally as leukopenia, mild anemia, and thrombocytopenia. Leukopenia occurs about 6 weeks after a dose, thrombocytopenia about 4 weeks after a dose; both persist for 1–2 weeks.
! Refractory anemia and thrombocytopenia occur commonly if lomustine therapy continues for more than 1 year.
! Hepatotoxicity occurs infrequently.
! Large cumulative doses of lomustine may result in renal damage.

NURSING CONSIDERATIONS
Baseline Assessment
• As ordered, obtain weekly blood counts as recommended by the manufacturer. Experts recommend that the first blood count be obtained 2 to 3 weeks after initial therapy and that subsequent blood counts be obtained based on prior hematologic toxicity.
• Give antiemetics, as prescribed, to reduce the duration and frequency of nausea and vomiting.
Precautions
• Use lomustine cautiously in patients with depressed erythrocyte, leukocyte, or platelet counts.
Administration and Handling
◀ **ALERT** ▶ Lomustine dosage is individualized based on the patient's clinical response and tolerance of the drug's adverse effects. When administering this drug in combination therapy, consult specific protocols for optimum dosage and sequence of drug administration.
Intervention and Evaluation
• Monitor the patient's CBC with differential; platelet count; and liver, renal, and pulmonary function test results.
• Assess the patient for signs and symptoms of stomatitis, such as burning or erythema of the oral mucosa, difficulty swallowing, and sore throat.

• Monitor the patient for signs and symptoms of hematologic toxicity, such as ecchymosis, fever, signs of local infection, sore throat, excessive fatigue or weakness, and unusual bleeding from any site.

Patient Teaching

• Inform the patient that nausea or vomiting usually abates in less than a day and that fasting before therapy can reduce the frequency and duration of GI effects.
• Teach the patient to maintain fastidious oral hygiene to prevent stomatitis.
• Urge the patient to avoid receiving vaccinations without the physician's approval and to avoid contact with crowds, anyone with a known illness, and anyone who has recently received a live-virus vaccine because lomustine lowers the body's resistance.
• Warn the patient to notify the physician if he or she experiences easy bruising, fever, yellow eyes or skin, signs of local infection, sore throat, swelling of the legs and feet, and unusual bleeding from any site.

melphalan

mel-fah-lan
(Alkeran)
Do not confuse Alkeran with Leukeran, or melphalan with Mephyton or Myleran.

CATEGORY AND SCHEDULE

Pregnancy Risk Category: D

MECHANISM OF ACTION

An alkylating agent that inhibits protein synthesis primarily by cross-linking with strands of DNA and RNA, producing cell death. Cell cycle-phase nonspecific. **Therapeutic Effect:** Disrupts nucleic acid function.

AVAILABILITY

Tablets: 2 mg.
Powder for Injection: 50 mg.

INDICATIONS AND DOSAGES

▸ Ovarian carcinoma

PO

Adults, Elderly. 0.2 mg/kg/day for 5 successive days. Repeat at 4- to 6-wk intervals.

▸ Multiple myeloma

PO

Adults. Initially, 6 mg once a day, adjusted as indicated; or 0.15 mg/kg/day for 7 days or 0.25 mg/kg/day for 4 days. Repeat at 4- to 6-wk intervals.

IV

Adults. 16 mg/m^2/dose every 2 wk for 4 doses, then repeated monthly according to protocol.

▸ Dosage in renal impairment

PO, IV

BUN level greater than 30 mg/dl. Decrease melphalan dosage by 50%.
Serum creatinine level greater than 1.5 mg/dl. Decrease the melphalan dosage by 50%.

OFF-LABEL USES

Treatment of breast carcinoma, neuroblastoma, rhabdomyosarcoma, testicular carcinoma

CONTRAINDICATIONS

Pregnancy, severe myelosuppression

INTERACTIONS

Drug

Antigout medications: May decrease the effects of these drugs.
Bone marrow depressants: May increase myelosuppression.
Live-virus vaccines: May potentiate virus replication, increase vaccine

side effects, and decrease the patient's antibody response to the vaccine.

Herbal

None known.

Food

None known.

DIAGNOSTIC TEST EFFECTS

May increase serum uric acid level and cause a positive direct Coombs' test.

IV INCOMPATIBILITIES

Don't mix melphalan with any other medications.

SIDE EFFECTS

Frequent

Nausea, vomiting (may be severe with large dose)

Occasional

Diarrhea, stomatitis, rash, pruritus, alopecia

SERIOUS REACTIONS

! Myelosuppression may cause hematologic toxicity, manifested principally as leukopenia and thrombocytopenia and to lesser extent, anemia, pancytopenia, and agranulocytosis. Leukopenia may occur as early as 5 days after drug initiation.

! WBC and platelet counts return to normal levels during the 5th week of therapy, but leukopenia and thrombocytopenia may last more than 6 weeks after the drug is discontinued.

! Hyperuricemia, marked by hematuria, crystalluria, and flank pain, may occur.

NURSING CONSIDERATIONS

Baseline Assessment

• Expect to obtain blood counts weekly. Expect dosage to be decreased or discontinued if the WBC count falls below 3,000/mm^3 or the platelet count falls below 100,000/mm^3.

• Expect to give antiemetics, if ordered, to prevent or treat nausea and vomiting.

Precautions

• Use melphalan cautiously in patients with myelosuppression, impaired renal function, and a leukocyte count less than 3,000/mm^3 or platelet count less than 100,000/mm^3.

Administration and Handling

◀ALERT▶ Because melphalan may be carcinogenic, mutagenic, or teratogenic, handle the drug with extreme care during preparation and administration. Know that melphalan dosage is individualized on the basis of the patient's clinical response and tolerance of the drug's adverse effects. When used in combination therapy, consult specific protocols for optimum dosage and sequence of drug administration. Be aware that leukocyte count is usually maintained between 3,000 to 4,000/mm^3.

IV

• Store melphalan at room temperature and protect it from light.

• Once reconstituted, the solution is stable for up to 90 minutes at room temperature. Don't refrigerate it.

• Reconstitute the 50-mg vial with diluent supplied by the manufacturer to yield a 5-mg/ml solution.

• Further dilute with 0.9% NaCl to a final concentration of no more than 2 mg/ml for a central line or 0.45 mg/ml for a peripheral line.

• Infuse the solution over 15 to 30 minutes at a rate not to exceed 10 mg/min.

Intervention and Evaluation

• Monitor the patient's blood Hgb and serum electrolyte levels, CBC with differential, and platelet count.

- Evaluate the patient for signs and symptoms of stomatitis.
- Monitor the patient for signs and symptoms of hematologic toxicity (including excessive fatigue or weakness, ecchymosis, fever, signs of local infection, sore throat, and unusual bleeding from any site), and hyperuricemia (including hematuria and flank pain).

Patient Teaching

- Instruct the patient to avoid IM injections, rectal temperatures, and other traumatic procedures that may induce bleeding.
- Encourage the patient to drink plenty of fluids to protect against hyperuricemia.
- Advise the patient to maintain fastidious oral hygiene.
- Inform the patient that hair loss is reversible but that new hair may have a different color or texture.
- Stress the importance of avoiding crowds and those with known infections.
- Warn the patient to notify the physician if bleeding, bruising, cough, fever, shortness of breath, or sore throat occurs.

oxaliplatin

ahks-al-eh-**plah**-tin
(Eloxatin)

CATEGORY AND SCHEDULE

Pregnancy Risk Category: D

MECHANISM OF ACTION

A platinum-containing complex that cross-links with DNA strands, preventing cell division. Cell cycle–phase nonspecific. **Therapeutic Effect:** Inhibits DNA replication.

PHARMACOKINETICS

Rapidly distributed. Protein binding: 90%. Undergoes rapid, extensive nonenzymatic biotransformation. Excreted in urine. ***Half-life:*** 70 hr.

AVAILABILITY

Powder for Injection: 50-mg, 100-mg vials.

INDICATIONS AND DOSAGES

▸ **Metastatic colon or rectal cancer in patients whose disease has recurred or progressed during or within 6 months of completing first-line therapy with bolus 5-fluorouracil (5-FU), leucovorin, and irinotecan**

IV

Adults. Day 1: Oxaliplatin 85 mg/m^2 in 250–500 ml D_5W and leucovorin 200 mg/m^2, both given simultaneously over more than 2 hr in separate bags using a Y-line, followed by 5-FU 400 mg/m^2 IV bolus given over 2–4 min, followed by 5-FU 600 mg/m^2 in 500 ml D_5W as a 22-hr continuous IV infusion. Day 2: Leucovorin 200 mg/m^2 IV infusion given over more than 2 hr, followed by 5-FU 400 mg/m^2 IV bolus given over 2–4 min, followed by 5-FU 600 mg/m^2 in 500 ml D_5W as a 22-hr continuous IV infusion.

▸ **Ovarian cancer**

IV

Adults. Cisplatin 100 mg/m^2 and oxaliplatin 130 mg/m^2 every 3 wk.

OFF-LABEL USES

Treatment of ovarian cancer

CONTRAINDICATIONS

History of allergy to platinum compounds

INTERACTIONS

Drug

Live-virus vaccines: May potentiate virus replication, increase vaccine side effects, and decrease the patient's antibody response to the vaccine.

Nephrotic medications: May decrease the clearance of oxaliplatin.

Herbal

None known.

Food

None known.

DIAGNOSTIC TEST EFFECTS

May alter serum bilirubin, AST (SGOT), and ALT (SGPT) levels. May decrease blood Hgb and Hct levels and platelet count.

IV INCOMPATIBILITIES

Don't infuse oxaliplatin with alkaline medications.

SIDE EFFECTS

Frequent (76%–20%)

Peripheral or sensory neuropathy (usually occurs in hands, feet, perioral area, and throat but may present as jaw spasm, abnormal tongue sensation, eye pain, chest pressure, or difficulty walking, swallowing, or writing), nausea (64%), fatigue, diarrhea, vomiting, constipation, abdominal pain, fever, anorexia

Occasional (14%–10%)

Stomatitis, earache, insomnia, cough, difficulty breathing, backache, edema

Rare (7%–3%)

Dyspepsia, dizziness, rhinitis, flushing, alopecia

SERIOUS REACTIONS

! Peripheral or sensory neuropathy can occur, sometimes precipitated or exacerbated by drinking or holding a glass of cold liquid during the IV infusion.

! Pulmonary fibrosis, characterized by a nonproductive cough, dyspnea, crackles, and radiologic pulmonary infiltrates, may require drug discontinuation.

! Hypersensitivity reaction (rash, urticaria, pruritus) occurs rarely.

NURSING CONSIDERATIONS

Baseline Assessment

- Ensure that the patient doesn't suck on ice or drink or touch a glass of cold liquid during the IV infusion because this can precipitate or exacerbate neuropathy, which may occur within hours or days of a dose and may last for up to 14 days.
- Assess the patient's baseline BUN and serum creatinine levels, platelet count, and WBC count.

Lifespan Considerations

- Oxaliplatin use should be avoided during pregnancy, if possible, especially in the first trimester because it may cause fetal harm.
- Breast-feeding is not recommended for patients taking this drug.
- The safety and efficacy of oxaliplatin have not been established in children.
- Elderly patients are at increased risk for dehydration, diarrhea, fatigue, and hypokalemia.

Precautions

- Use oxaliplatin cautiously in patients with peripheral neuropathy (past or present), impaired renal function, or infection; in pregnant or immunosuppressed patients; and in those who have previously been treated with other antineoplastics or radiation.

Administration and Handling

◀ALERT▶ Pretreat the patient with antiemetics (5-HT_3 antagonists), if ordered. Know that repeat courses should not be given more frequently than every 2 weeks.

◀ALERT▶ Because oxaliplatin may be mutagenic, teratogenic, and carcinogenic, wear protective gloves during drug preparation and administration. If the solution comes in contact with your skin, wash the skin immediately with soap and water. Don't use aluminum needles or administration sets that may come in contact with the drug because they may cause degradation of platinum compounds.
◀ALERT▶ Don't allow the patient to suck on ice or drink or touch glasses of cold liquids during the infusion because this can precipitate or exacerbate acute neuropathy.
◀ALERT▶ Never reconstitute oxaliplatin with sodium chloride or other chloride-containing solutions.

IV

- After reconstitution, the solution is stable for up to 6 hours at room temperature and up to 24 hours in the refrigerator.
- Reconstitute each 50-mg vial with 10 ml sterile water for injection or D_5W (100-mg vial with 20 ml). Further dilute with 150 to 500 ml D_5W.
- Administer the drug at the prescribed infusion rate or according to protocol.

Intervention and Evaluation

- Although myelosuppression is minimal, monitor the patient for a decrease in platelet or WBC count.
- Evaluate the patient for diarrhea and signs of GI bleeding, such as bright red or tarry stools.
- Monitor the patient's intake and output.
- Assess the patient for signs and symptoms of stomatitis, including erythema of the oral mucosa, sore throat, and ulceration of the lips or mouth.

Patient Teaching

- Warn the patient to promptly report easy bruising, fever, signs of local infection, sore throat, or unusual bleeding from any site.
- Urge the patient not to receive vaccinations during therapy and to avoid contact with anyone who has recently received an oral polio vaccine.

thiotepa

thigh-oh-**teh**-pah
(Thioplex)

CATEGORY AND SCHEDULE
Pregnancy Risk Category: D

MECHANISM OF ACTION

An alkylating agent that inhibits DNA and RNA protein synthesis by cross-linking with DNA and RNA strands, preventing cell growth. Cell cycle–phase nonspecific. **Therapeutic Effect:** Interferes with DNA and RNA function.

AVAILABILITY

Powder for Injection: 15 mg.

INDICATIONS AND DOSAGES

▸ **Adenocarcinoma of breast and ovary, Hodgkin's disease, lymphosarcoma, superficial papillary carcinoma of urinary bladder**

IV

Adults, Elderly. Initially, 0.3–0.4 mg/kg every 1–4 wk. Maintenance dose adjusted weekly based on blood counts.

Children. 25–65 mg/m^2 as a single dose every 3–4wk.

▸ **Control of pericardial, peritoneal, or pleural effusions due to metastatic tumors**

Intracavitary Injection

Adults, Elderly. 0.6–0.8 mg/kg every 1–4wk.

OFF-LABEL USES
Treatment of lung carcinoma

CONTRAINDICATIONS
Pregnancy, severe myelosuppression (leukocyte count less than 3,000/mm^3 or platelet count less than 150,000/mm^3)

INTERACTIONS
Drug
Antigout medications: May decrease the effects of these drugs.
Bone marrow depressants: May increase myelosuppression.
Live-virus vaccines: May potentiate virus replication, increase vaccine side effects, and decrease the patient's antibody response to the vaccine.
Herbal
None known.
Food
None known.

DIAGNOSTIC TEST EFFECTS
May increase serum uric acid levels.

IV INCOMPATIBILITIES
Cisplatin (Platinol-AQ), filgrastim (Neupogen)

IV COMPATIBILITIES
Allopurinol (Aloprim), bumetanide (Bumex), calcium gluconate, carboplatin (Paraplatin), cyclophosphamide (Cytoxan), dexamethasone (Decadron), diphenhydramine (Benadryl), doxorubicin (Adriamycin), etoposide (VePesid), fluorouracil, gemcitabine (Gemzar), granisetron (Kytril), heparin, hydromorphone (Dilaudid), leucovorin, lorazepam (Ativan), magnesium sulfate, morphine, ondansetron (Zofran), paclitaxel (Taxol), potassium chloride, vincristine (Oncovin), vinorelbine (Navelbine)

SIDE EFFECTS
Occasional
Pain at injection site, headache, dizziness, urticaria, rash, nausea, vomiting, anorexia, stomatitis
Rare
Alopecia, cystitis, hematuria (after intravesical dose)

SERIOUS REACTIONS
! Hematologic toxicity, manifested as leukopenia, anemia, thrombocytopenia, and pancytopenia, may occur from bone marrow depression.
! Although the WBC count falls to its lowest point 10–14 days after initial therapy, the initial effects on bone marrow may not evident for 30 days.
! Stomatitis and ulceration of intestinal mucosa may occur.

NURSING CONSIDERATIONS
Baseline Assessment
• Expect the patient to undergo hematologic testing at least weekly during therapy and for 3 weeks after therapy is discontinued.
Precautions
• Use thiotepa cautiously in patients with myelosuppressionor hepatic or renal impairment.
Administration and Handling
◀ALERT▶ Thiotepa dosage is individualized based on the patient's clinical response and tolerance of the drug's adverse effects. When administering this drug in combination therapy, consult specific protocols for optimum thiotepa dosage and sequence of drug administration.
◀ALERT▶ Because thiotepa may be carcinogenic, mutagenic, or teratogenic, handle the drug with extreme care during preparation and administration.
◀ALERT▶ Know that the drug may be given by intrapericardial, intraperito-

neal, intrapleural, intratumoral, or IV injection and by intravesical instillation.

IV
- Refrigerate unopened vials.
- Reconstituted solution normally appears clear to slightly opaque. Refrigerated solution may be stored for up to 5 days. Discard the solution if it appears grossly opaque or contains a precipitate.
- Reconstitute each 15-mg vial with 1.5 ml sterile water for injection to provide a concentration of 10 mg/ml. Shake the solution gently and let it stand to clear.
- Withdraw the reconstituted drug through a 0.22-micron filter before administering. Give IV push over 5 minutes at a concentration of 10 mg/ml. Give IV infusion at a concentration of 1 mg/ml.

Intervention and Evaluation
- Interrupt thiotepa therapy if the patient's platelet count falls below 150,000/mm^3, WBC count falls below 3,000/mm^3, or either count declines rapidly.
- Monitor the patient's hematology test results and serum uric acid levels.
- Assess the patient for signs and symptoms of stomatitis.
- Monitor the patient for signs and symptoms of symptoms of hematologic toxicity, including excessive fatigue and weakness, ecchymosis, fever, signs of local infection, sore throat, or unusual bleeding from any site.
- Examine the patient's skin for urticaria and rash.

Patient Teaching
- Teach the patient to maintain fastidious oral hygiene to guard against stomatitis.
- Urge the patient to avoid receiving vaccinations and contact with crowds, anyone with a known infection, and anyone who has recently received a live-virus vaccine.
- Warn the patient to promptly notify the physician if he or she experiences easy bruising, fever, signs of local infection, sore throat, or unusual bleeding from any site.

14 Antibiotics

bleomycin sulfate
daunorubicin
doxorubicin
epirubicin
idarubicin hydrochloride
mitomycin
valrubicin

Uses: Antineoplastic antibiotics are cytotoxic and are therefore only used to treat cancer and not infections. *Bleomycin* is prescribed for germ cell tumors of the testes and ovaries. *Daunorubicin* is effective in acute lymphocytic and acute myelogenous leukemias. *Doxorubicin* is used in acute leukemias, malignant lymphomas, and breast cancer. *Epirubicin* is used only in breast cancer. *Idarubicin* is active against acute myelogenous leukemia. *Mitomycin* may be prescribed for carcinoma of the cervix, stomach, breast, bladder, head, or neck. *Valrubicin* is a useful treatment for urinary bladder cancer.

Action: Originally isolated from cultures of *Streptomyces,* antineoplastic antibiotics act by inhibiting RNA synthesis and binding with DNA. (See the illustration *Sites and Mechanisms of Action: Antineoplastic Agents,* page 268.) These actions cause fragmentation of DNA molecules.

bleomycin sulfate

blee-oh-**my**-sin
(Blenamax[AUS], Blenoxane)

CATEGORY AND SCHEDULE
Pregnancy Risk Category: D

MECHANISM OF ACTION
A glycopeptide antibiotic whose mechanism of action is unknown. Is most effective in the G_2 phase of cell division. **Therapeutic Effect:** Appears to inhibit DNA synthesis and, to a lesser extent, RNA and protein synthesis.

AVAILABILITY
Powder for Injection: 15 units, 30 units.

INDICATIONS AND DOSAGES
▸ **As monotherapy to treat testicular carcinoma; lymphomas (including Hodgkin's disease, choriocarcinoma, reticulum cell sarcoma, and lymphosarcoma); and squamous cell carcinomas of the head and neck (including mouth, tongue, tonsil, nasopharynx, oropharynx, sinus, palate, lip, buccal mucosa, gingiva, epiglottis, and larynx).**
IV, IM, Subcutaneous
Adults, Elderly. 10–20 units/m^2 (0.25–0.5 units/kg) 1–2 times/wk.
IV (continuous)
Adults, Elderly. 15 units/m^2 over 24 hr for 4 days.
▸ **In combination therapy to treat testicular carcinoma; lymphomas (including Hodgkin's disease,**

choriocarcinoma, reticulum cell sarcoma, and lymphosarcoma); and squamous cell carcinomas of the head and neck (including mouth, tongue, tonsil, nasopharynx, oropharynx, sinus, palate, lip, buccal mucosa, gingiva, epiglottis, and larynx).
IV, IM
Adults, Elderly. 3–4 units/m^2.
As a sclerosing agent to treat malignant pleural effusions and prevent recurrent pleural effusions.
Intrapleural
Adults, Elderly. 60–240 units as a single injection.

OFF-LABEL USES
Treatment of mycosis fungoides, osteosarcoma, ovarian tumors, renal carcinoma, soft-tissue sarcoma

CONTRAINDICATIONS
Previous allergic reaction

INTERACTIONS
Drug
Cisplatin: May decrease bleomycin clearance and increase the risk of bleomycin toxicity (from cisplatin-induced renal impairment).
Live-virus vaccines: May potentiate virus replication, increase vaccine side effects, and decrease the patient's antibody response to the vaccine.
Other antineoplastics: May increase the risk of bleomycin toxicity.
Herbal
None known.
Food
None known.

DIAGNOSTIC TEST EFFECTS
None known.

IV INCOMPATIBILITIES
None known by Y-site administration.

IV COMPATIBILITIES
Cefepime (Maxipime), dacarbazine (DTIC), dexamethasone (Decadron), diphenhydramine (Benadryl), fludarabine (Fludara), gemcitabine (Gemzar), ondansetron (Zofran), paclitaxel (Taxol), piperacillin and tazobactam (Zosyn), vinblastine (Velban), vinorelbine (Navelbine)

SIDE EFFECTS
Frequent
Anorexia, weight loss, erythematous skin swelling, urticaria, rash, striae, vesiculation, hyperpigmentation (particularly at areas of pressure, skin folds, cuticles, IM injection sites, and scars), stomatitis (usually evident 1 to 3 weeks after initial therapy); may also be accompanied by decreased skin sensitivity followed by skin hypersensitivity, nausea, vomiting, alopecia, and—with parenteral form—fever or chills (typically occurring a few hours after large single dose and lasting 4–12 hr).

SERIOUS REACTIONS
! Interstitial pneumonitis occurs in 10% of patients and occasionally progresses to pulmonary fibrosis. This condition appears to be dose- or age-related, occurring more often in patients receiving a total dose greater than 400 units and those older than 70 years.
! Nephrotoxicity and hepatotoxicity occur infrequently.

NURSING CONSIDERATIONS
Baseline Assessment
• Expect the patient to have chest X-rays performed every 1 to 2 weeks during bleomycin therapy.
Precautions
• Use bleomycin cautiously in pa-

tients with severe pulmonary or renal impairment.

Administration and Handling

◀ **ALERT** ▶ Bleomycin dosage is individualized based on the patient's clinical response and tolerance of the drug's adverse effects. When administering this drug in combination therapy, consult specific protocols for optimum dosage and sequence of drug administration. Be aware that cumulative doses greater than 400 units increase the risk of developing pulmonary toxicity. For lymphoma patients, administer test doses of 2 units or less for the first 2 doses, as ordered, because they're at increased risk for an anaphylactoid reaction.

◀ **ALERT** ▶ Because bleomycin may be carcinogenic, mutagenic, or teratogenic, handle the drug with extreme care during preparation and administration.

IV

- Refrigerate the powder for injection.
- After reconstitution with 0.9% NaCl, the solution may be stored for up to 24 hours at room temperature.
- Reconstitute the 15-unit vial with at least 5 ml (30-unit vial with at least 10 ml) 0.9% NaCl to provide a concentration not greater than 3 units/ml.
- Administer the IV injection over at least 10 minutes.

IM, Subcutaneous

- Refrigerate the powder for injection.
- After reconstitution with 0.9% NaCl, the solution is stable for up to 24 hours at room temperature.
- Reconstitute the 15-unit vial with 1–5 ml (30-unit vial with 2–10 ml) sterile water for injection, 0.9% NaCl injection, or bacteriostatic water for injection to provide a concentration of 3–15 units/ml. Do not use D_5W.

Intervention and Evaluation

- Monitor the patient's breath sounds for pulmonary toxicity as evidenced by dyspnea, fine crackles, and rhonchi.
- Observe the patient for dyspnea.
- Monitor the patient's hematologic and oxygen saturation tests and liver and renal function test results, including BUN, serum bilirubin, serum creatinine, AST (SGOT), and ALT (SGPT) levels.
- Assess the patient's skin each day for signs of cutaneous toxicity.
- Monitor the patient for signs and symptoms of anemia (excessive fatigue and weakness), hematologic toxicity (easy bruising, fever, signs of local infection, sore throat, unusual bleeding), and stomatitis (burning or erythema of oral mucosa of lips, palate, and tongue).

Patient Teaching

- Inform the patient that fever and chills occur less frequently with continued bleomycin therapy.
- Explain to the patient that Hodgkin's disease and testicular tumors usually improve within 2 weeks of bleomycin treatment and squamous cell carcinoma within 3 weeks of treatment.
- Urge the patient not to receive vaccinations and to avoid contact with anyone who has recently received a live-virus vaccine.

daunorubicin

dawn-oh-**rue**-bih-sin
(Cerubidine, DaunoXome)
Do not confuse daunorubicin with dactinomycin or doxorubicin.

CATEGORY AND SCHEDULE

Pregnancy Risk Category: D

MECHANISM OF ACTION

An anthracycline antibiotic that inhibits DNA and DNA-dependent RNA synthesis by binding with DNA strands. Liposomal encapsulation increases uptake by tumors, prolongs drug action, and may decrease toxicity. **Therapeutic Effect:** Prevents cell division.

PHARMACOKINETICS

Widely distributed. Protein binding: High. Does not cross the blood-brain barrier. Metabolized in the liver to active metabolite. Excreted in urine; eliminated by biliary excretion. ***Half-life:*** 18.5 hr; metabolite: 26.7 hr.

AVAILABILITY

Powder for Injection (Cerubidine): 20 mg.
Solution for Injection (Cerubidine): 5 mg/ml.
Injection (DaunoXome): 2 mg/ml.

INDICATIONS AND DOSAGES

▸ **Acute lymphocytic leukemia**
IV
Adults. 45 mg/m² on days 1–3 of induction course.
Children. 25–45 mg/m² on days 1 and 8 of cycle.

▸ **Acute lymphocytic leukemia (ALL)**
IV
Adults, Elderly. 45 mg/m² on days 1–3 of induction course.
Children. 25–45 mg/m² on days 1 and 8 of cycle.

▸ **Acute myeloid leukemia (AML), Acute non-lympocytic leukemia (ANLL)**
IV
Adults, Elderly. 45 mg/m² on days 1–3 of first cycle and on days 1 and 2 of subsequent courses.
Children. 30–60 mg/m² on days 1–3 of cycle.

▸ **Kaposi's sarcoma**
IV (DaunoXome)
Adults. 20–40 mg/m² over 1 hr repeated q2wk; or 100 mg/m² q3wk.

▸ **Dosage in renal impairment**
ALL, AML, ANLL
Creatinine clearance less than 10 ml/min. 75% of normal dose.
Serum creatinine greater than 3 mg/dL. 50% of normal dose.
Kaposi's Sarcoma
Serum creatinine greater than 3 mg/dL. 50% of normal dose.

▸ **Dosage in hepatic impairment**
ALL, AML, ANLL
Bilirubin 1.2–3 mg/dL. 75% of normal dose.
Bilirubin 3.1–5 mg/dL. 50% of normal dose.
Bilirubin greater than 5 mg/dL. Daunorubicin is not recommended for use in this patient population.
Kaposi's Sarcoma
Bilirubin 1.2–3 mg/dL. 75% of normal dose.
Bilirubin greater than 3 mg/dL. 50% of normal dose.

OFF-LABEL USES

Treatment of chronic myelocytic leukemia, Ewing's sarcoma, neuroblastoma, non-Hodgkin's lymphoma, Wilms' tumor

CONTRAINDICATIONS

Arrhythmias, CHF, left ventricular

ejection fraction less than 40%, pre-existing myelosuppression

INTERACTIONS

Drug

Antigout medications: May decrease the effects of these drugs.
Bone marrow depressants: May enhance myelosuppression.
Live-virus vaccines: May potentiate virus replication, increase vaccine side effects, and decrease the patient's antibody response to the vaccine.

Herbal

None known.

Food

None known.

DIAGNOSTIC TEST EFFECTS

May increase serum alkaline phosphatase, bilirubin, uric acid, and AST (SGOT) levels.

IV INCOMPATIBILITIES

Allopurinol (Aloprim), aztreonam (Azactam), cefepime (Maxipime), fludarabine (Fludara), piperacillin and tazobactam (Zosyn)
DaunoXome: Don't mix with any other solution, especially NaCl or bacteriostatic agents (such as benzyl alcohol).

IV COMPATIBILITIES

Cytarabine (Cytosar), etoposide (VePesid), filgrastim (Neupogen), granisetron (Kytril), ondansetron (Zofran)

SIDE EFFECTS

Frequent

Complete alopecia (scalp, axillary, pubic), nausea, vomiting (beginning a few hours after administration and lasting 24–48 hours)
DaunoXome: Mild to moderate nausea, fatigue, fever

Occasional

Diarrhea, abdominal pain, esophagitis, stomatiti, transverse pigmentation of fingernails and toenails

Rare

Transient fever, chills

SERIOUS REACTIONS

! Myelosuppression may cause hematologic toxicity, manifested as severe leukopenia, anemia, and thrombocytopenia. Platelet and WBC counts typically decrease in 10–14 days and return to normal levels by the third week of daunorubicin treatment.
! The risk of cardiotoxicity (either acute, manifested as transient EKG abnormalities, or chronic, manifested as CHF) increases when the total cumulative dose exceeds 550 mg/m^2 in adults, 300 mg/m^2 in children older than 2 years, or 10 mg/kg in children younger than 2 years.

NURSING CONSIDERATIONS

Baseline Assessment

- Expect to obtain the patient's erythrocyte, platelet, and WBC counts before beginning and regularly during daunorubicin therapy.
- Obtain the patient's baseline EKG before beginning daunorubicin therapy.
- Give antiemetics, if ordered, to the patient to prevent and treat nausea.

Lifespan Considerations

- Daunorubicin use should be avoided during pregnancy, especially in the first trimester, because it may cause fetal harm. Breast-feeding is not recommended for patients taking this drug.
- The safety and efficacy of daunorubicin have not been established in children.
- Use daunorubicin cautiously in elderly patients, who are at increased

risk for cardiotoxicity and myelosuppression. They may also require a dosage adjustment because of age-related renal impairment.

Precautions

• Use daunorubicin cautiously in patients with biliary, hepatic, or renal impairment.

Administration and Handling

◀ **ALERT** ▶ Daunorubicin dosage is individualized based on the patient's clinical response and tolerance of the drug's adverse effects. When administering this drug in combination therapy, consult specific protocols for optimum dosage and sequence of drug administration.

IV

◀ **ALERT** ▶ To decrease the risk of cardiotoxicity, don't exceed a total cumulative dose of 500 mg/m^2 in adults, 450 mg/m^2 in those who have received irradiation of the cardiac region, 300 mg/m^2 in children older than 2 years, and 10 mg/kg in children younger than 2 years. Use body weight to calculate the dosage for children younger than 2 years or with a body surface area less than 0.5 m^2. Expect to reduce dosage in those with hepatic or renal impairment.

◀ **ALERT** ▶ Give daunorubicin by IV push. Although daunorubicin may be given by IV infusion, this route is not recommended because of the risk of thrombophlebitis and vein irritation. Avoid areas overlying joints and tendons, small veins, and swollen or edematous extremities. Because daunorubicin may be carcinogenic, mutagenic, or teratogenic, handle the drug with extreme care during preparation and administration.

IV

Cerubidine

• The reconstituted solution may be stored for up to 24 hours at room temperature or up to 48 hours if refrigerated.

• Discard the solution if the color changes from red to blue-purple because this indicates decomposition.

• Reconstitute each 20-mg vial with 4 ml sterile water for injection to provide a concentration of 5 mg/ml.

• Gently agitate the vial until the contents have completely dissolved.

• For IV push, withdraw the desired dose into a syringe containing 10 to 15 ml 0.9% NaCl. Inject over 2 to 3 minutes into tubing of running IV solution of D_5W or 0.9% NaCl.

• For IV infusion, further dilute with 100 ml D_5W or 0.9% NaCl. Infuse over 30 to 45 minutes.

• Know that extravasation produces immediate pain and severe local tissue damage. If extravasation occurs, stop the infusion immediately and aspirate as much infiltrated drug as possible. Then infiltrate the area with 50 to 100 mg hydrocortisone sodium succinate injection or 1 ml 5% ascorbic acid injection, as ordered and apply cold compresses.

IV

DaunoXome

• Refrigerate unopened vials.

• The reconstituted solution is stable for 6 hours if refrigerated.

• Don't use the solution if it appears opaque.

• Dilute the drug with an equal amount of D_5W to provide a concentration of 1 mg/ml. Don't use any other diluent.

• Infuse DaunoXome over 60 minutes.

Intervention and Evaluation

• Monitor the patient for signs and symptoms of stomatitis (including burning and erythema of oral mucosa), which may lead to ulceration within 2 to 3 days.

• Assess the patient's nailbeds for hyperpigmentation.

• Monitor the patient's hematologic

status, liver and renal function studies, and serum uric acid level.
- Give antiemetics, if ordered, to prevent or treat nausea.
- Assess the patient's pattern of daily bowel activity and stool consistency.
- Monitor the patient for signs and symptoms of hematologic toxicity, including excessive fatigue and weakness, ecchtmosis, fever, signs of local infection, sore throat and unusual bleeding from any site.

Patient Teaching
- Inform the patient that urine may turn a reddish color for 1 to 2 days after beginning daunorubicin therapy.
- Caution the patient to notify the physician if nausea and vomiting persist at home.
- Warn the patient to notify the physician if he or she experiences easy bruising, fever, signs of local infection, sore throat, or unusual bleeding from any site.
- Urge the patient to drink plenty of fluids to help protect against hyperuricemia.
- Advise the patient to maintain fastidious oral hygiene.
- Urge the patient not to receive vaccinations and to avoid contact with anyone who has recently received a live-virus vaccine.
- Inform the patient that hair growth will resume about 5 weeks after the last dose of doxorubicin but that new hair may have a different color and texture.

doxorubicin

dox-o-**roo**-bi-sin
(Adriamycin, Caelyx, Doxil, Rubex)
Do not confuse doxorubicin with daunorubicin, or Adriamycin with idamycin or idarubicin.

CATEGORY AND SCHEDULE
Pregnancy Risk Category: D

MECHANISM OF ACTION
An anthracycline antibiotic that inhibits DNA and DNA-dependent RNA synthesis by binding with DNA strands. Liposomal encapsulation increases uptake by tumors, prolongs drug action, and may decrease toxicity. **Therapeutic Effect:** Prevents cell division.

PHARMACOKINETICS
Widely distributed. Protein binding: 74%–76%. Does not cross the blood-brain barrier. Metabolized rapidly in the liver to active metabolite. Primarily eliminated by biliary system. Not removed by hemodialysis. ***Half-life:*** 16 hr; metabolite, 32 hr.

AVAILABILITY
Injection, Powder for Reconstitution (Adriamycin RDF): 10 mg, 20 mg, 50 mg, 150 mg.
Injection, Powder for Reconstitution (Rubex): 50 mg, 100 mg.
Injection Solution (Adriamycin PFS): 2 mg/ml.
Lipid Complex (Doxil): 2 mg/ml.

INDICATIONS AND DOSAGES

▸ **To produce regression in acute lymphoblastic and myeloblastic leukemia; breast, bronchogenic, gastric, ovarian, thyroid, and transitional cell bladder carcinomas; Hodgkin's disease; non-Hodgkin's lymphomas; neuroblastoma; primary liver cancer; soft-tissue and bone sarcomas; and Wilms' tumor**

IV

Adults. 60–75 mg/m^2 as a single dose every 21 days, 20 mg/m^2 once weekly, or 25–30 mg/m^2/day on 2–3 successive days q4wk. Because of the risk of cardiotoxicity, don't exceed a cumulative dose of 550 mg/m^2 (400–450 mg/m^2 for those previously treated with related compounds or irradiation of cardiac region).

Children. 35–75 mg/m^2 as a single dose q3wk or 20–30 mg/m^2 weekly, or 60–90 mg/m^2 as continuous infusion over 96 hr q3–4wk.

▸ **Kaposi's sarcoma**

IV (Doxil)

Adults. 20 mg/m^2 q3wk infused over 30 min.

▸ **Ovarian cancer**

IV (Doxil)

Adults. 50 mg/m^2 q4wk.

▸ **Dosage in hepatic impairment**

Dosage is modified based on serum bilirubin level.

Serum Bilirubin Concentration	% of Normal Dose
1.2–3 mg/dl	50%
greater than 3 mg/dl	25%

OFF-LABEL USES

Treatment of cervical, head or neck, endometrial, liver, pancreatic, prostatic, and testicular carcinomas; germ cell tumors; multiple myeloma

CONTRAINDICATIONS

Cardiomyopathy; pre-existing myelosuppression; previous or concomitant treatment with cyclophosphamide, idarubicin, mitoxantrone, or irradiation of the cardiac region; severe CHF

INTERACTIONS

Drug

Antigout medications: May decrease the effects of these drugs.
Bone marrow depressants: May increase myelosuppression.
Daunorubicin: May increase the risk of cardiotoxicity.
Live-virus vaccines: May potentiate virus replication, increase vaccine side effects, and decrease the patient's antibody response to the vaccine.

Herbal

None known.

Food

None known.

DIAGNOSTIC TEST EFFECTS

May cause EKG changes and increase serum uric acid level. Doxil may reduce neutrophil and RBC counts.

IV INCOMPATIBILITIES

Doxorubicin: Allopurinol (Aloprim), amphotericin B complex (Abelcet, AmBisome, Amphotec), cefepime (Maxipime), furosemide (Lasix), ganciclovir (Cytovene), heparin, piperacillin and tazobactam (Zosyn), propofol (Diprivan)
Doxil: Don't mix with any other medications.

IV COMPATIBILITIES

Dexamethasone (Decadron), diphenhydramine (Benadryl), etoposide (VePesid), granisetron (Kytril), hydromorphone (Dilaudid), lorazepam (Ativan), morphine, ondansetron (Zofran), paclitaxel (Taxol)

SIDE EFFECTS

Frequent

Complete alopecia (scalp, axillary, pubic hair), nausea, vomiting, stomatitis, esophagitis (especially if drug is given on several successive days), reddish urine

Doxil: Nausea

Occasional

Anorexia, diarrhea; hyperpigmentation of skin, nailbeds, and phalangeal and dermal creases

Rare

Fever, chills, conjunctivitis, lacrimation

SERIOUS REACTIONS

! Myelosuppression may cause hematologic toxicity (manifested principally as leukopenia and, to lesser extent, anemia and thrombocytopenia), usually within 10–15 days of starting therapy. Blood counts typically return to normal levels by the third week.

! Cardiotoxicity (either acute, manifested as transient EKG abnormalities, or chronic, manifested as CHF) may occur.

NURSING CONSIDERATIONS

Baseline Assessment

- As ordered, obtain the patient's blood Hct and Hgb levels, platelet count, and WBC count before and periodically during doxorubicin therapy.
- Obtain a baseline EKG before starting doxorubicin therapy.
- As ordered, obtain liver function studies before administering each dose.

Lifespan Considerations

- Doxorubicin use should be avoided, if possible, during pregnancy, especially in the first trimester. Breast-feeding is also not recommended for patients taking this drug.
- Patients older than 70 years and children younger than 2 years are at increased risk for cardiotoxicity.

Precautions

- Use doxorubicin cautiously in patients with impaired hepatic function.

Administration and Handling

◀ALERT▶ Doxorubicin dosage is individualized based on the patient's clinical response and tolerance of the drug's adverse effects. When administering this drug, in combination therapy, consult specific protocols for optimum dosage and sequence of drug administration.

◀ALERT▶ Because doxorubicin may be carcinogenic, mutagenic, or teratogenic, wear gloves when preparing or administering the drug. If doxorubicin powder or solution comes in contact with your skin, wash the area thoroughly. When accessing a vein for infusion, avoid areas overlying joints and tendons, small veins, and swollen or edematous extremities.

IV

- Store at room temperature.
- The reconstituted solution is stable for up to 24 hours at room temperature or up to 48 hours if refrigerated.
- Protect the reconstituted solution from prolonged exposure to sunlight; discard any unused portions.
- Reconstitute each 10-mg vial with 5 ml preservative-free 0.9% NaCl (20-mg vial with 10 ml, 50-mg vial with 25 ml) to provide a concentration of 2 mg/ml.
- Shake the vial and allow the contents to dissolve.
- Withdraw an appropriate volume of air from the vial during reconstitution to avoid excessive pressure buildup.

• Further dilute the solution with 50 ml D_5W or 0.9% NaCl, if necessary, and administer it as a continuous infusion through a central venous line.
• For IV push, administer the drug into the tubing of a free-flowing IV infusion of D_5W or 0.9% NaCl, preferably through a butterfly needle. To avoid facial flushing and erythematous streaking along the vein, administer over no less than 3 to 5 minutes.
• Test for flashback every 30 seconds to make sure that the needle remains in the vein during injection.
• Be aware that extravasation produces immediate pain and severe local tissue damage. If extravasation occurs, stop drug administration immediately; withdraw as much medication as possible, obtain an extravasation kit, and follow protocol.

IV

Doxil
• Refrigerate unopened vials.
• Dilute each dose in 250 ml D_5W. Don't use any diluent except D_5W.
• Use the solution within 24 hours of dilution.
• Infuse Doxil over more than 30 minutes.
• Don't use in-line filters.

Intervention and Evaluation
• Monitor the patient for signs and symptoms of stomatitis, including burning or erythema of oral mucosa and difficulty swallowing. Be aware that stomatitis may lead to ulceration of mucous membranes within 2 to 3 days.
• Examine the patient's nailbeds and skin for hyperpigmentation.
• Monitor the patient's hematologic status, liver and renal function test results, and serum uric acid levels.
• Assess the patient's pattern of daily bowel activity and stool consistency.
• Give antiemetics, if ordered, to prevent or treat nausea.
• Monitor the patient for signs and symptoms of hematologic toxicity, including excessive fatigue and weakness, ecchymosis, fever, signs of local infection, sore throat, and unusual bleeding from any site.

Patient Teaching
• Warn the patient to notify the physician if he or she experiences easy bruising, fever, signs of local infection, sore throat, or unusual bleeding from any site or if nausea and vomiting persist after discharge.
• Urge the patient receiving the lipid complex form of doxorubicin to avoid consuming alcohol during therapy because alcohol may cause GI irritation such as nausea.
• Caution the patient not to receive vaccinations and to avoid contact with anyone who has recently received a live-virus vaccine.
• Advise the patient to maintain fastidious oral hygiene.
• Inform the patient that hair growth will resume 2 to 3 months after the last dose of doxorubicin but new hair may have a different color and texture.

epirubicin

eh-pea-**rew**-bih-sin
(Ellence, Pharmorubicin)

CATEGORY AND SCHEDULE
Pregnancy Risk Category: D

MECHANISM OF ACTION
An anthracycline antibiotic whose exact mechanism is unknown but may include formation of a complex with DNA and subsequent inhibition of DNA, RNA, and protein synthesis. Also inhibits DNA helicase

activity, preventing enzymatic separation of double-stranded DNA and interfering with replication and transcription. **Therapeutic Effect:** Produces antiproliferative and cytotoxic activity.

PHARMACOKINETICS

Widely distributed into tissues. Protein binding: 77%. Metabolized in the liver and RBCs. Primarily eliminated through biliary excretion. Not removed by hemodialysis. ***Half-life:*** 33 hr.

AVAILABILITY

Injection: 2-mg/ml single-use vials.

INDICATIONS AND DOSAGES

▸ Breast cancer

IV

Adults. Initially, 100–120 mg/m^2 in repeated cycles of 3–4 wk, in combination with fluorouracil (5-FU) and Cytoxan. Total dose may be given on day 1 of each cycle or in equally divided doses on days 1 and 8 of each cycle.

OFF-LABEL USES

Treatment of lung or ovarian carcinoma, non-Hodgkin's lymphoma, sarcomas

CONTRAINDICATIONS

Baseline neutrophil count less than 1,500/mm^3, hypersensitivity to epirubicin, previous treatment with anthracyclines up to maximum cumulative dose, recent MI, severe hepatic impairment, severe myocardial insufficiency

INTERACTIONS

Drug

Blood dyscrasia-causing medications: May increase the patient's risk of developing leukopenia or thrombocytopenia.

Bone marrow depressants: May cause additive bone marrow suppression.

Calcium channel blockers: May increase the patient's risk of developing heart failure.

Cimetidine: May increase epirubicin serum concentration and toxicity.

Hepatotoxic medications: May increase the risk of hepatic toxicity.

Live-virus vaccines: May potentiate virus replication, increase vaccine side effects, and decrease the patient's antibody response to the vaccine.

Herbal

None known.

Food

None known.

DIAGNOSTIC TEST EFFECTS

None known.

IV INCOMPATIBILITIES

Heparin, 5-FU. Don't mix epirubicin in same syringe with other medications.

SIDE EFFECTS

Frequent (83%–70%)

Nausea, vomiting alopecia, amenorrhea

Occasional (9%–5%)

Stomatitis, diarrhea, hot flashes

Rare (2%–1%)

Rash, pruritus, fever, lethargy, conjunctivitis

SERIOUS REACTIONS

! The risk of cardiotoxicity (either acute, manifested as transient EKG abnormalities, or chronic, manifested as CHF) increases when the total cumulative dose exceeds 900 mg/m^2.

! Extravasation during administration may result in severe local tissue necrosis.

! Myelosuppression may cause hematologic toxicity, manifested principally as leukopenia and, to lesser extent, anemia and thrombocytopenia.

NURSING CONSIDERATIONS

Baseline Assessment

• As ordered, obtain the patient's blood Hct and Hgb levels, platelet count, and WBC count before and periodically during epirubicin therapy.
• Obtain a baseline EKG, if ordered, before starting epirubicin therapy.
• As ordered, obtain liver function studies before each epirubicin dose.
• Give antiemetics, if ordered, to prevent or treat nausea.

Lifespan Considerations

• Epirubicin may cause fetal harm. It is unknown if epirubicin is distributed in breast milk.
• The safety and efficacy of epirubicin have not been established in children.
• No age-related precautions have been noted in the elderly, but monitor them for toxicity.

Precautions

• Use epirubicin cautiously in patients with hepatic or renal impairment.

Administration and Handling

◀ALERT▶ Be aware that a dosage adjustment is necessary for patients with bone marrow dysfunction, hematologic toxicities, hepatic dysfunction, or severe renal impairment.
◀ALERT▶ Wear protective clothing when handling epirubicin. If the drug accidentally comes in contact with your skin or eyes, flush the area immediately with copious amounts of water. Exclude pregnant staff from working with epirubicin.

IV

◀ALERT▶ Know that venous sclerosis may result if epirubicin is infused into a small vein.
• Refrigerate unopened vials and protect them from light.
• Use the solution within 24 hours of first penetration of rubber stopper. Discard any unused portion.
• Ready-to-use vials require no reconstitution.
• Infuse the drug into the tubing of a free-flowing IV infusion of 0.9% NaCl or D_5W over 3 to 5 minutes.

Intervention and Evaluation

• Monitor the patient for signs and symptoms of stomatitis, which may lead to ulceration of mucous membranes within 2 to 3 days.
• Monitor the patient's blood Hct and Hgb levels, platelet count, and WBC count for signs of myelosuppression. Also monitor cardiac function and liver and renal function test results.
• Assess the patient's pattern of daily bowel activity and stool consistency.
• Monitor the patient for signs and symptoms of hematologic toxicity, including excessive fatigue and weakness, ecchymosis, fever, signs of local infection, sore throat, and unusual bleeding from any site.

Patient Teaching

• Warn the patient to notify the physician if he or she experiences easy bruising, fever, signs of local infection, sore throat, or unusual bleeding from any site.
• Instruct the patient to maintain fastidious oral hygiene.
• Urge the patient not to receive vaccinations and to avoid contact with anyone who has recently received a live-virus vaccine.
• Inform the patient that hair growth will resume 2 to 3 months after the last dose of epirubicin but that new hair may have a different color and texture.

idarubicin hydrochloride

eye-dah-**roo**-bi-sin
(Idamycin PFS, Zavedos)
Do not confuse idarubicin with doxorubicin, or Idamycin with Adriamycin.

CATEGORY AND SCHEDULE
Pregnancy Risk Category: D

MECHANISM OF ACTION
An anthracycline antibiotic that inhibits nucleic acid synthesis by interacting with the enzyme topoisomerase II, which promotes DNA strand supercoiling. **Therapeutic Effect:** Causes death of rapidly dividing cells.

PHARMACOKINETICS
Widely distributed. Protein binding: 97%. Rapidly metabolized in the liver to active metabolite. Primarily eliminated by biliary excretion. Not removed by hemodialysis. ***Half-life:*** 4–46 hr; metabolite: 8–92 hr.

AVAILABILITY
Injection: 1 mg/ml in 5 ml, 10 ml vials.

INDICATIONS AND DOSAGES
▸ **Acute myeloid leukemia**

IV

Adults. 8–12 mg/m^2/day for 3 days in combination with Ara-C.
Children (solid tumor). 5 mg/m^2 once a day for 3 days.
Children (leukemia). 10–12 mg/m^2 once a day for 3 days.

▸ **Dosage in hepatic or renal impairment**

Dosage is modified based on serum creatinine or bilirubin level.

Serum Level	Dose Reduction
Serum creatinine 2 mg/dl or more	25%
Serum bilirubin greater than 2.5 mg/dl	50%
Serum bilirubin greater than 5 mg/dl	Do not give

CONTRAINDICATIONS
Pre-existing arrhythmias, cardiomyopathy, myelosuppression, pregnancy, severe CHF

INTERACTIONS
Drug
Antigout medications: May decrease the effects of these drugs.
Bone marrow depressants: May increase myelosuppression.
Live-virus vaccines: May potentiate virus replication, increase vaccine side effects, and decrease the patient's antibody response to the vaccine.
Herbal
None known.
Food
None known.

DIAGNOSTIC TEST EFFECTS
May increase serum alkaline phosphatase, bilirubin, uric acid, AST (SGOT), and ALT (SGPT) levels. May cause EKG changes.

IV INCOMPATIBILITIES
Acyclovir (Zovirax), allopurinol (Aloprim), ampicillin and sulbactam (Unasyn), cefazolin (Ancef, Kefzol), cefepime (Maxipime), ceftazidime (Fortaz), clindamycin (Cleocin), dexamethasone (Decadron), furosemide (Lasix), hydrocortisone (Solu-Cortef), lorazepam (Ativan), meperidine (Demerol), methotrexate, piperacillin and tazobactam (Zosyn), sodium bicarbonate, teniposide

(Vumon), vancomycin (Vancocin), vincristine (Oncovin)

IV COMPATIBILITIES

Diphenhydramine (Benadryl), granisetron (Kytril), magnesium, potassium

SIDE EFFECTS

Frequent

Nausea, vomiting (82%); complete alopecia (scalp, axillary, pubic hair) (77%); abdominal cramping, diarrhea (73%); mucositis (50%)

Occasional

Hyperpigmentation of nailbeds, phalangeal and dermal creases (46%); fever (36%); headache (20%)

Rare

Conjunctivitis, neuropathy

SERIOUS REACTIONS

! Myelosuppression may cause hematologic toxicity (manifested principally as leukopenia and, to lesser extent, anemia and thrombocytopenia), usually within 10 to 15 days of starting therapy. Blood counts typically return to normal levels by the third week.

! Cardiotoxicity (either acute, manifested as transient EKG abnormalities, or chronic, manifested as CHF) may occur.

NURSING CONSIDERATIONS

Baseline Assessment

- Evaluate the patient's baseline CBC and liver and renal function test results.
- Obtain an EKG, as ordered, before starting idarubicin therapy.
- Give an antiemetic before and during idarubicin therapy, if ordered, to prevent or treat nausea and vomiting.

Lifespan Considerations

- Idarubicin use should be avoided during pregnancy because the drug may be embryotoxic.
- It is unknown if idarubicin is distributed in breast milk; however, the patient should stop breast-feeding before starting idarubicin therapy.
- The safety and efficacy of idarubicin have not been established in children.
- Elderly patients are at increased risk for cardiotoxicity. They may also require a dosage adjustment because of age-related renal impairment.
- Use idarubicin cautiously in elderly patients with inadequate bone marrow reserves.

Precautions

- Use idarubicin cautiously in patients receiving concurrent radiation therapy and in those with impaired hepatic or renal function.

Administration and Handling

◀ALERT▶ Idarubicin dosage is individualized based on the patient's clinical response and tolerance of the drug's adverse effects. When administering this drug in combination therapy, consult specific protocols for optimum dosage and sequence of drug administration.

◀ALERT▶ Give idarubicin by free-flowing IV infusion and never by the subcutaneous or IM route. When accessing a vein for infusion, avoid areas overlying joints and tendons, small veins, and swollen or edematous extremities. Use gloves, gowns, and eye goggles when preparing and administering this drug. If idarubicin powder or solution comes in contact with skin, wash thoroughly.

IV

- The reconstituted solution is stable for up to 3 days at room temperature or up to 7 days if refrigerated.
- Discard unused solution.
- Reconstitute each 10-mg vial with 10 ml (or each 5 mg-vial with 5 ml)

of 0.9% NaCl to provide a concentration of 1 mg/ml.

- Administer over 10 to 15 minutes into the tubing of a free-flowing IV infusion of D_5W or 0.9% NaCl, preferably through a butterfly needle.
- Monitor for signs and symptoms of extravasation, such as immediate pain and severe local tissue damage. If extravasation occurs, stop the infusion immediately. Apply cold compresses immediately, then continue every 30 minutes 4 times a day for 3 days. Keep the affected extremity elevated.

Intervention and Evaluation

- Monitor the patient's CBC with differential, EKG, platelet count, and liver and renal function test results.
- Monitor the patient for signs and symptoms of hematologic toxicity, including excessive fatigue and weakness, ecchymosis, fever, signs of local infection, sore throat, and unusual bleeding from any site.
- Avoid procedures that may precipitate bleeding, such as adminsitration of IM injections or rectal medications.
- Assess the patient for signs and symptoms of life-threatening CHF (dyspnea, edema, crackles) and arrhythmias.

Patient Teaching

- Teach the patient and family how to recognize the early signs and symptoms of bleeding and infection.
- Urge the patient to avoid crowds and those with known infections.
- Instruct the patient to notify the physician if he or she experiences easy bruising, bleeding, fever, or sore throat.
- Inform the patient that idarubicin use may turn urine pink or red.
- Teach the patient to maintain fastidious oral hygiene.
- Urge the patient to use contraceptive measures during idarubicin therapy.
- Inform the patient about the likelihood of total body hair loss. Explain that new hair growth will resume 2 to 3 months after the last dose of idarubicin but that new hair may have a different color or texture.

mitomycin

my-toe-**my**-sin
(Mutamycin, Mytomycin C-Kyowa)

CATEGORY AND SCHEDULE

Pregnancy Risk Category: Safety in pregnancy has not been established.

MECHANISM OF ACTION

An antibiotic that acts similar to an alkylating agent, cross-linking with strands of DNA. **Therapeutic Effect:** Inhibits DNA and RNA synthesis.

PHARMACOKINETICS

Widely distributed. Does not cross the blood-brain barrier. Primarily metabolized in the liver and excreted in urine. ***Half-life:*** 50 min.

AVAILABILITY

Powder for Injection: 5 mg, 20 mg, 40 mg.

INDICATIONS AND DOSAGES

▸ Disseminated adenocarcinoma of pancreas and stomach

IV

Adults, Elderly, Children. Initially, 10–20 mg/m^2 as single dose. Repeat q6–8wk. Give additional courses only after platelet and WBC counts are within acceptable levels, as shown below.

Leukocytes/ mm^3	Platelets/ mm^3	% of Prior Dose to Give
4,000	more than 100,000	100%
3,000–3,999	75,000–99,000	100%
2,000–2,999	25,000–74,999	70%
1,999 or less	less than 25,000	50%

▸ Dosage in renal impairment
Patients with creatinine clearance less than 10 ml/min should receive 75% of normal dose.

OFF-LABEL USES
Treatment of biliary, bladder, breast, cervical, colorectal, head and neck, and lung carcinomas; chronic myelocytic leukemia

CONTRAINDICATIONS
Coagulation disorders and bleeding tendencies, platelet count less than $75,000/mm^3$, serious infection, serum creatinine level greater than 1.7 mg/dl, WBC count less than $3,000/mm^3$

INTERACTIONS
Drug
Bone marrow depressants: May increase myelosuppression.
Live-virus vaccines: May potentiate virus replication, increase vaccine side effects, and decrease the patient's antibody response to the vaccine.
Herbal
None known.
Food
None known.

DIAGNOSTIC TEST EFFECTS
May increase BUN and serum creatinine levels.

IV INCOMPATIBILITIES
Aztreonam (Azactam), bleomycin (Blenoxane), cefepime (Maxipime), filgrastim (Neupogen), heparin, piperacillin/tazobactam (Zosyn), sargramostin (Leukine), vinorelbine (Navelbine)

IV COMPATIBILITIES
Cisplatin (Platinol AQ), cyclophosphamide (Cytoxan), doxorubicin (Adriamycin), 5-fluorouracil, granisetron (Kytril), leucovorin, methotrexate, ondansetron (Zofran), vinblastine (Velban), vincristine (Oncovin)

SIDE EFFECTS
Frequent (greater than 10%)
Fever, anorexia, nausea, vomiting
Occasional (10%–2%)
Stomatitis, paraesthesia, purple color bands on nails, rash, alopecia, unusual fatigue
Rare (less than 1%)
Thrombophlebitis, cellulitis, extravasation

SERIOUS REACTIONS
! Marked myelosuppression may result in hematologic toxicity (manifested as leukopenia, thrombocytopenia and to a lesser extent, anemia), usually within 2 to 4 weeks after the start of therapy.
! Renal toxicity (manifested as increased BUN and serum creatinine levels) and pulmonary toxicity (manifested as dyspnea, cough, hemoptysis, and pneumonia) may occur.
! Long-term therapy may produce hemolytic uremic syndrome, characterized by hemolytic anemia, thrombocytopenia, renal failure, and hypertension.

NURSING CONSIDERATIONS

Baseline Assessment

• If ordered, obtain the patient's bleeding time, CBC, and PT before and periodically during mitomycin therapy.
• Give antiemetics before and during mitomycin therapy, if ordered, to prevent or treat nausea and vomiting.

Lifespan Considerations

• Mitomycin use should be avoided during pregnancy, especially in the first trimester. Breast-feeding is not recommended for patients taking this drug.
• No age-related precautions have been noted in children.
• In the elderly, age-related renal impairment may require cautious use.

Precautions

• Use cautiously in patients with impaired hepatic or renal function and myelosuppression.

Administration and Handling

◀ALERT▶ Mitomycin dosage is individualized based on the patient's clinical response and tolerance of the drug's adverse effects. When administering this drug in combination therapy, consult specific protocols for optimum dosage and sequence of drug administration.

◀ALERT▶ Because mitomycin may be carcinogenic, mutagenic, or teratogenic, handle the drug with extreme care during preparation and administration.

IV

• Reconstitute a 5-mg vial with 10 ml (and a 20-mg vial with 40 ml) of sterile water for injection to provide a concentration of 0.5 mg/ml.
• Don't shake the vial to dissolve. Allow the vial to stand at room temperature until complete dissolution occurs.
• A concentration of 0.5 mg/ml is stable for up to 7 days at room temperature or up to 2 weeks if refrigerated.
• For IV infusion, further dilute with 50 to 100 ml D_5W or 0.9% NaCl.
• If further diluted with D_5W, the solution is stable for up to 3 hours at room temperature; if further diluted with 0.9% NaCl, the solution is stable for up to 24 hours at room temperature.
• Use only clear, blue-gray solutions.
• Give IV push over 5 to 10 minutes.
• Give reconstituted solution through the tubing of a functioning IV infusion.

◀ALERT▶ Be aware that mitomycin is extremely irritating to veins and may produce pain with induration, paresthesia, and thrombophlebitis during the infusion.

• Monitor for signs and symptoms of extravasation, which may produce cellulitis, tissue sloughing, and ulceration. If extravasation occurs, stop the infusion immediately and inject the ordered antidote, as appropriate. Apply ice intermittently for up to 72 hours, and keep the affected area elevated.

Intervention and Evaluation

• Assess the patient's IV site for evidence of extravasation and phlebitis.
• Monitor the patient for signs and symptoms of renal toxicity including elevated BUN and serum creatinine levels and foul-smelling urine.
• Monitor the patient for signs and symptoms of hematologic toxicity, including excessive fatigue and weakness, ecchymosis, fever, signs of local infection, sore throat, and unusual bleeding from any site.

Patient Teaching

• Warn the patient to immediately report burning or pain at the injection site.
• Urge the patient to avoid vaccina-

tions and contact with anyone who has recently received a live-virus vaccine.
• Advise the patient to notify the physician if he or she experiences painful urination, fever, nausea and vomiting, shortness of breath, sore throat, easy bruising, or unusual bleeding from any site.
• Instruct the patient to maintain fastidious oral hygiene.
• Inform the patient that hair growth will resume 2 to 3 months after the last dose of mitomycin but that new hair may have a different color and texture.

valrubicin

val-**rue**-bih-sin
(VaHaxan [CAN], Valstar)
Do not confuse valrubicin with valsartan.

CATEGORY AND SCHEDULE
Pregnancy Risk Category: C

MECHANISM OF ACTION
An anthracycline antibiotic that inhibits incorporation of nucleosides into nucleic acids after penetrating cells. **Therapeutic Effect:** Causes chromosomal damage, arresting cells in the G_2 phase of cell division, and interferes with DNA synthesis.

AVAILABILITY
Solution for Intravesical Instillation: 40 mg/ml.

INDICATIONS AND DOSAGES
▸ **Bladder cancer**
Intravesical
Adults, Elderly. 800 mg once weekly for 6 wk.

CONTRAINDICATIONS
Perforated bladder, sensitivity to valrubicin, severe irritated bladder, small bladder capacity, UTI

SIDE EFFECTS
Frequent
Local intravesical reaction (10%): Local bladder symptoms, urinary frequency or urgency, dysuria, hematuria, bladder pain, cystitis, bladder spasms
Systemic (15%–5%): Abdominal pain, nausea, UTI
Occasional
Local intravesical reaction (less than 10%): Nocturia, local burning, urethral pain, pelvic pain, gross hematuria
Systemic (5%–2%): Diarrhea, vomiting, urine retention, microscopic hematuria, asthenia, headache, malaise, back pain, chest pain, dizziness, rash, anemia, fever, vasodilation
Rare
Systemic (1%): Flatus, peripheral edema, hyperglycemia, pneumonia, myalgia

NURSING CONSIDERATIONS
Baseline Assessment
• Determine if the patient is breast-feeding, pregnant, or sensitive to valrubicin before beginning therapy.
• Assess and document the patient's medical history and medication use.
Lifespan Considerations
• Breast-feeding is not recommended for patients taking this drug.
Administration and Handling
◂ **ALERT** ▸ Valrubicin is not for IM or IV use.
• Wear gloves during drug preparation to prevent skin reactions from accidental exposure.
• If you accidentally expose your eye

to the drug, immediately and thoroughly flush the eye.
• Insert a urinary catheter to drain the bladder. Then instill valrubicin into the bladder through the catheter over several minutes by gravity flow. Remove the catheter and have the patient retain the drug for 2 hours before voiding.

Intervention and Evaluation

• Monitor the patient for disease recurrence about every 3 months through the results of cytoscopy, biopsy, or urine cytology.
• Provide the patient with adequate fluids to maintain hydration during valrubicin therapy.

Patient Teaching

• Urge the patient to use reliable contraceptive measures during valrubicin therapy.
• Inform the patient that urine may be red-tinged during the first 24 hours after drug administration. Advise the patient to notify the physician if the red color persists.

15 Antimetabolites

capecitabine
clofarabine
cytarabine
fludarabine phosphate
fluorouracil, 5-FU
gemcitabine hydrochloride
hydroxyurea
mercaptopurine
methotrexate sodium
pemetrexed

Uses: Antimetabolites produce the best response in patients with lymphomas, acute leukemias, cancer of the GI tract, or breast cancer.

Action: Structurally similar to natural metabolites, antimetabolites act by disrupting critical metabolic processes. Some agents inhibit enzymes that synthesize essential cellular components; others are incorporated into DNA, interfering with DNA replication and function. (See the illustration *Sites and Mechanisms of Action: Antineoplastic Agents,* page 268.) By altering DNA synthesis and metabolism, antimetabolites affect the S phase of the cell cycle.

capecitabine

cap-eh-**site**-ah-bean
(Xeloda)
Do not confuse Xeloda with Xenical.

CATEGORY AND SCHEDULE

Pregnancy Risk Category: D

MECHANISM OF ACTION

An antimetabolite that is enzymatically converted to 5-fluorouracil. Inhibits enzymes necessary for synthesis of essential cellular components. **Therapeutic Effect:** Interferes with DNA synthesis, RNA processing, and protein synthesis.

PHARMACOKINETICS

Readily absorbed from the GI tract. Protein binding: less than 60%. Metabolized in the liver. Primarily excreted in urine. ***Half-life:*** 45 min.

AVAILABILITY

Tablets: 150 mg, 500 mg.

INDICATIONS AND DOSAGES

▸ **Metastatic breast cancer, colon cancer**

PO

Adults, Elderly. Initially, 2,500 mg/m^2/day in 2 equally divided doses approximately q12h for 2 wk. Follow with a 1-wk rest period; given in 3-wk cycles.

CONTRAINDICATIONS

Severe renal impairment

INTERACTIONS

Drug

Warfarin: May alter the effects of warfarin.

Herbal

None known.

Food

None known.

DIAGNOSTIC TEST EFFECTS

May increase serum alkaline phosphatase, bilirubin, AST (SGOT), and ALT (SGPT) levels. May decrease blood Hct, Hgb level, and WBC count.

SIDE EFFECTS

Frequent (greater than 5%)
Diarrhea (sometimes severe), nausea, vomiting, stomatitis, hand-and-foot syndrome (painful palmar-plantar swelling with paresthesia, erythema, and blistering), fatigue, anorexia, dermatitis

Occasional (less than 5%)
Constipation, dyspepsia, nail disorder, headache, dizziness, insomnia, edema, myalgia

SERIOUS REACTIONS

! Serious reactions may include myelosuppression (evidenced by neutropenia, thrombocytopenia, and anemia), cardiovascular toxicity (marked by angina, cardiomyopathy, and deep vein thrombosis), respiratory toxicity (marked by dyspnea, epistaxis, and pneumonia), and lymphedema.

NURSING CONSIDERATIONS

Baseline Assessment

- Assess the patient's history of sensitivity to capecitabine or 5-fluorouracil.
- As ordered, obtain the patient's baseline Hct and Hgb blood levels.

Lifespan Considerations

- Capecitabine use should be avoided during pregnancy because the drug may cause fetal malformations.
- It is unknown if capecitabine is distributed in breast milk; however, breast-feeding is not recommended for patients taking this drug.
- The safety and efficacy of capecitabine in children younger than 18 years have not been established.
- The elderly may be more sensitive to capecitabine's GI side effects.

Precautions

- Use capecitabine cautiously in patients with chickenpox, preexisting myelosuppresion, herpes zoster, or hepatic or renal impairment, and in those who have previously undergone cytotoxic or radiation therapy.

Administration and Handling

- Give capecitabine 30 minutes before a meal.

Intervention and Evaluation

- Evaluate the patient for severe diarrhea. If dehydration occurs, fluid and electrolyte replacement therapy should be ordered.
- Assess the patient's hands and feet for chemotherapy-induced edema and erythema.
- Monitor the patient's CBC for evidence of myelosuppresion.
- Monitor the patient for signs and symptoms of blood dyscrasias, including excessive fatigue or weakness, echymosis, fever, signs of local infection, sore throat, and unusual bleeding from any site.

Patient Teaching

- Instruct the patient to notify the physician if he or she experiences nausea and vomiting, severe diarrhea, stomatitis, signs of hand-and-foot syndrome, easy bruising, a fever higher than 100.5° F, signs of local infection, sore throat, or unusual bleeding from any site.
- Urge the patient not to receive vaccinations and to avoid contact with anyone who has recently received a live-virus vaccine.

clofarabine

klo-**fare**-ah-been
(Clolar)

CATEGORY AND SCHEDULE

Pregnancy Risk Category: D

MECHANISM OF ACTION

An antimetabolite that is metabolized intracellularly to rhibonucleotide reductase, alters mitochondrial membrane, necessary in DNA synthesis. **Therapeutic Effect:** Decreases cell replication, affects cell repair, produces cell death.

AVAILABILITY

Injection Solution: 20 ml (20 mg) vial.

INDICATIONS AND DOSAGES

▸ Acute lymphoblastic leukemia (ALL)

IV

Children 1–21 yr. 52 mg/m^2 over 2 hours once daily for 5 consecutive days; repeat every 2–6 weeks following recovery or return to baseline organ function.

CONTRAINDICATIONS

None known.

INTERACTIONS

Drug

None known.

Herbal

None known.

Food

None known.

DIAGNOSTIC TEST EFFECTS

May increase serum bilirubin, creatinine, uric acid, AST (SGOT), and ALT (SGPT) levels. May decrease Hct, Hgb, thrombocytes, and WBC levels.

IV INCOMPATIBILITIES

Do not administer any other medications through the same IV line.

SIDE EFFECTS

Frequent (83%–20%)

Vomiting, nausea, diarrhea, pruritus, headache, fever, dermatitis, rigors, abdominal pain, fatigue, tachycardia, epistaxis, anorexia, petechiae, limb pain, hypotension, anxiety, constipation, edema

Occasional (19%–11%)

Cough, mucosal inflammation, erythema, flushing, hematuria, dizziness, gingival bleeding, myalgia, injection site pain, respiratory distress, pharyngitis, back pain, palmar-plantar erythrodysesthesia syndrome, hypertension, depression, irritability, arthralgia

Rare (10%)

Tremor, weight gain, somnolence

SERIOUS REACTIONS

! Neutropenia occurs in 57% of patients.

! Pericardial effusion occurs in 35% of patients.

! Left ventricular systolic dysfunction occurs in 27% of patients.

! Hepatomegaly and jaundice occur in 15% of patients.

! Pleural effusion, pneumonia, and bacteremia occur in 10% of patients.

! Capillary leak syndrome occurs in less than 10% of patients.

NURSING CONSIDERATIONS

Precautions

- Use clofarabine cautiously in patients with hepatic or renal impairment.

Administration and Handling

IV

- Store undiluted and diluted solution at room temperature; diluted solution must be used within 24 hours.
- Filter clofarabine through a sterile 0.2-micrometer syringe filter prior to further dilution with D_5W or 0.9% NaCl.
- Administer clofarabine over 2 hours. Continuous IV fluids are

encouraged to decrease tumor lysis syndrome and other adverse events.

cytarabine

sigh-**tar**-ah-bean
(Ara-C, Cytosar[CAN], Cytosar-U)
Do not confuse cytarabine with Cytadren, Cytovene, or vidarabine.

CATEGORY AND SCHEDULE

Pregnancy Risk Category: D

MECHANISM OF ACTION

An antimetabolite that is converted intracellularly to a nucleotide. Cell cycle-specific for S phase of cell division. **Therapeutic Effect:** May inhibit DNA synthesis. Potent immunosuppressive activity.

PHARMACOKINETICS

Widely distributed; moderate amount crosses the blood-brain barrier. Protein binding: 15%. Primarily excreted in urine. ***Half-life:*** 1–3 hr.

AVAILABILITY

Injection Powder: 100 mg, 500 mg, 1 g, 2 g.
Injection Solution: 20 mg/ml, 100 mg/ml.

INDICATIONS AND DOSAGES

▸ To induce remission in acute lymphocytic leukemia, acute and chronic myelocytic leukemia, meningeal leukemia, or non-Hodgkin's lymphoma in children

IV

Adults, Elderly, Children. 200 mg/m²/day for 5 days q2wk as monotherapy or 100–200 mg/m²/day for 5- to 10-day course of therapy every q2–4wk in combination therapy.

Intrathecal

Adults, Elderly, Children. 5–7.5 mg/m² every 2–7 days.

▸ To maintain remission in acute lymphocytic leukemia, acute and chronic myelocytic leukemia, meningeal leukemia, or non-Hodgkin's lymphoma in children

IV

Adults, Elderly, Children. 70–200 mg/m²/day for 2–5 days every month.

IM, Subcutaneous

Adults, Elderly, Children. 1–1.5 mg/m² as single dose q1–4wk.

Intrathecal

Adults, Elderly, Children. 5–7.5 mg/m² every 2–7 days.

OFF-LABEL USES

Treatment of Hodgkin's disease, myelodysplastic syndrome

CONTRAINDICATIONS

None known.

INTERACTIONS

Drug

Antigout medications: May decrease the effects of these drugs.
Bone marrow depressants: May increase myelosuppression.
Cyclophosphamide: May increase the risk of cardiomyopathy.
Live-virus vaccines: May potentiate virus replication, increase vaccine side effects, and decrease the patient's antibody response to the vaccine.

Herbal

None known.

Food

None known.

DIAGNOSTIC TEST EFFECTS

May increase serum alkaline phosphatase, bilirubin, uric acid, and AST (SGOT) levels.

IV INCOMPATIBILITIES
Amphotericin B complex (Abelcet, AmBisome, Amphotec), ganciclovir (Cytovene), heparin, insulin (regular)

IV COMPATIBILITIES
Dexamethasone (Decadron), diphenhydramine (Benadryl), filgrastim (Neupogen), granisetron (Kytril), hydromorphone (Dilaudid), lorazepam (Ativan), morphine, ondansetron (Zofran), potassium chloride, propofol (Diprivan)

SIDE EFFECTS
Frequent
IV, Subcutaneous (33%–16%): Asthenia, fever, pain, altered taste and smell, nausea, vomiting (risk greater with IV push than with continuous IV infusion)
Intrathecal (28%–11%): Headache, asthenia, altered taste and smell, confusion, somnolence, nausea, vomiting
Occasional
IV, Subcutaneous (11%–7%): Abnormal gait, somnolence, constipation, back pain, urinary incontinence, peripheral edema, headache, confusion
Intrathecal (7%–3%): Peripheral edema, back pain, constipation, abnormal gait, urinary incontinence

SERIOUS REACTIONS
! Myelosuppression may result in blood dyscrasias, such as leukopenia, anemia, thrombocytopenia, megaloblastosis, and reticulocytopenia, after a single IV dose.
! Leukopenia, anemia, and thrombocytopenia should be expected with daily or continuous IV therapy.
! Cytarabine syndrome (as evidenced by fever, myalgia, rash, conjunctivitis, malaise, and chest pain) and hyperuricemia may occur.
! High-dose cytarabine therapy may produce severe CNS, GI, and pulmonary toxicity.

NURSING CONSIDERATIONS
Baseline Assessment
- Expect the patient's leukocyte count to decrease within 24 hours after the initial cytarabine dose, continue to decrease for 7 to 9 days; show a brief rise at 12 days, decrease again at 15 to 24 days, and finally rise rapidly for the next 10 days.
- Expect the patient's platelet count to decrease 5 days after the initial cytarabine dose, reach its lowest point at 12 to 15 days, and then rise rapidly for the next 10 days.

Lifespan Considerations
- Cytarabine use should be avoided during pregnancy because the drug may cause fetal malformations.
- It is unknown if cytarabine is distributed in breast milk; however, breast-feeding is not recommended for patients taking this drug.
- There are no age-related precautions noted in children.
- In the elderly, age-related renal impairment may require dosage adjustment.

Precautions
- Use cytarabine cautiously in patients with impaired hepatic function.

Administration and Handling
◀ALERT▶ Cytarabine dosage is individualized based on the patient's clinical response and tolerance of the drug's adverse effects. When administering this drug in combination therapy, consult specific protocols for optimum dosage and sequence of drug administration. Expect to modify the dosage when serious myelosuppression occurs.
IV, Subcutaneous, Intrathecal
◀ALERT▶ Cytarabine may be given by subcutaneous injection, IV infu-

sion, IV push, or intrathecally. Because cytarabine may be carcinogenic, mutagenic, or teratogenic, handle the drug with extreme care during preparation and administration.
• Reconstituted solutions are stable for up to 48 hours at room temperature.
• IV infusion solutions at concentrations of up to 0.5 mg/ml are stable for up to 7 days at room temperature.
• Discard solution that develops a slight haze.
• Reconstitute the 100-mg vial with 5 ml (500 mg vial with 10 ml, 1-g vial with 10 ml, 2-g vial with 20 ml) bacteriostatic water for injection with benzyl alcohol to provide a concentration of 20 mg/ml, 50 mg/ml, 100 mg/ml, and 100 mg/ml, respectively.
• Further dilute the dose, if necessary, with up to 1,000 ml D_5W or 0.9% NaCl for IV infusion.
• For intrathecal use, reconstitute the vial with preservative-free 0.9% NaCl or the patient's spinal fluid. Be aware that the dose is usually administered in 5 to 15 ml of solution, after an equivalent volume of CSF is removed.
• Administer IV push, over 1 to 3 minutes. Administer IV infusion over 30 minutes to 24 hours.

Intervention and Evaluation
• Monitor the patient's CBC for signs of myelosuppression.
• Monitor the patient for signs and symptoms of blood dyscrasias, including excessive fatigue and weakness, ecchymosis, fever, signs of local infection, sore throat, and unusual bleeding from any site.
• Evaluate the patient for signs and symptoms of neuropathy, such as gait disturbances, difficulty writing, and numbness.

Patient Teaching
• Instruct the patient to drink plenty of fluids to help protect against hyperuricemia.
• Urge the patient not to receive vaccinations and to avoid contact with anyone who has recently received a live-virus vaccine.
• Warn the patient to promptly report easy bruising, fever, signs of local infection, sore throat, or unusual bleeding from any site.

fludarabine phosphate ⚑
flew-**dare**-ah-bean
(Fludara)
Do not confuse Fludara with FUDR.

CATEGORY AND SCHEDULE
Pregnancy Risk Category: D

MECHANISM OF ACTION
An antimetabolite that inhibits DNA synthesis by interfering with DNA polymerase alpha, ribonucleotide reductase, and DNA primase. **Therapeutic Effect:** Induces cell death.

PHARMACOKINETICS
Rapidly dephosphorylated in serum, then phosphorylated intracellularly to active triphosphate. Primarily excreted in urine. ***Half-life:*** 7–20 hr.

AVAILABILITY
Injection Powder for Reconstitution: 50 mg.

INDICATIONS AND DOSAGES
▸ **Chronic lymphocytic leukemia**
IV
Adults. 25 mg/m^2 daily for 5 consecutive days. Continue for up to 3 additional cycles. Begin each course of treatment every 28 days.

▸ **Non-Hodgkin's lymphoma**
IV
Adults, Elderly. Initially, 20 mg/m^2, then 30 mg/m^2/day for 48 hr.
▸ **Dosage in renal impairment**

Creatinine Clearance	Dosage
30–70 ml/min	decrease dose by 20%
less than 30 ml/min	not recommended

CONTRAINDICATIONS
Concurrent use with pentostatin

INTERACTIONS
Drug
Antigout medications: May decrease the effects of these drugs.
Bone marrow depressants: May increase the risk of myelosuppression.
Live-virus vaccines: May potentiate virus replication, increase vaccine side effects, and decrease the patient's antibody response to the vaccine.
Herbal
None known.
Food
None known.

DIAGNOSTIC TEST EFFECTS
May increase serum alkaline phosphatase, uric acid, and AST (SGOT) levels.

IV INCOMPATIBILITIES
Acyclovir (Zovirax), amphotericin B (Fungizone), hydroxyzine (Vistaril), prochlorperazine (Compazine)

IV COMPATIBILITIES
Heparin, hydromorphone (Dilaudid), lorazepam (Ativan), magnesium sulfate, morphine, multivitamins, potassium chloride

SIDE EFFECTS
Frequent
Fever (60%), nausea and vomiting (36%), chills (11%)
Occasional (20%–10%)
Fatigue, generalized pain, rash, diarrhea, cough, asthenia, stomatitis, dyspnea, peripheral edema
Rare (7%–3%)
Anorexia, sinusitis, dysuria, myalgia, paresthesia, headaches, visual disturbances

SERIOUS REACTIONS
! Pneumonia occurs frequently.
! Severe hematologic toxicity (as evidenced by anemia, thrombocytopenia, and neutropenia) and GI bleeding may occur.
! Tumor lysis syndrome may start with flank pain and hematuria and may include hypercalcemia, hyperphosphatemia, hyperuricemia and renal failure.
! High-dosage therapy may produce acute leukemia, blindness, and coma.

NURSING CONSIDERATIONS
Baseline Assessment
- Assess the patient's baseline CBC and serum creatinine level.
- Expect to discontinue fludarabine if intractable diarrhea, GI bleeding, stomatitis, or vomiting occurs.

Lifespan Considerations
- Because fludarabine may cause fetal harm, pregnant women should avoid using this drug, if possible, especially in the first trimester.
- It is unknown if fludarabine is distributed in breast milk; however, breast-feeding is not recommended for patients taking this drug.
- The safety and efficacy of fludarabine have not been established in children.
- In the elderly, age-related renal

impairment may require dosage adjustment.

Precautions

• Use fludarabine cautiously in patients with pre-existing myelosuppression, neurologic problems, or renal insufficiency.

Administration and Handling

◀ALERT▶ Fludarabine dosage is individualized based on the based on the patient's clinical response, tolerance of the drug's adverse effects, and actual weight (ideal weight in edematous or obese patients). When administering this drug in combination therapy, consult specific protocols for optimum dosage and sequence of drug administration.

IV

◀ALERT▶ Give fludarabine by IV infusion. Don't add this drug to other IV infusions.

◀ALERT▶ Because fludarabine may be carcinogenic, mutagenic, or teratogenic, handle the drug with extreme care during preparation and administration. If the drug comes in contact with skin or mucous membranes, wash the area thoroughly with soap and water; if it comes in contact with eyes, rinse the eyes carefully with plain water.

• Store the drug in the refrigerator.
• Reconstitute the 50-mg vial with 2 ml sterile water for injection to provide a concentration of 25 mg/ml.
• Further dilute with 100 to 125 ml 0.9% NaCl or D_5W.
• After reconstitution, use the drug within 8 hours; discard unused portion.
• Infuse over 30 minutes.

◀ALERT▶ When accessing a vein for infusion, avoid areas overlying joints and tendons, small veins, and swollen or edematous extremities.

• Infuse fludarabine over 30 minutes.

Intervention and Evaluation

• Assess the patient for fatigue, peripheral edema, pneumonia, and visual disturbances.
• Monitor the patient for cough, diarrhea, dyspnea, GI bleeding (including bright red or tarry stools), intractable vomiting, and rapidly falling WBC count.
• Check for signs and symptoms of stomatitis, such as difficulty swallowing, sore throat, and ulceration and erythema of the oral mucosa.
• Inspect the patient's skin for a rash.
• Be alert for signs and symptoms of tumor lysis syndrome, such as hematuria and flank pain.

Patient Teaching

• Urge the patient to avoid crowds and exposure to those with known infections.
• Warn the patient to notify the physician if he or she experiences easy bruising, fever, signs of local infection, sore throat, or unusual bleeding from any site.
• Advise the patient to contact the physician if nausea and vomiting continue at home.
• Teach the patient to maintain fastidious oral hygiene.

fluorouracil, 5-FU

phlur-oh-**your**-ah-sill
(Adrucil, Carac, Efudex, Efudix[AUS], Fluoroplex)
Do not confuse Efudex with Efidac.

CATEGORY AND SCHEDULE

Pregnancy Risk Category: D

MECHANISM OF ACTION

An antimetabolite that blocks formation of thymidylic acid. Cell cycle-specific for S phase of cell division. **Therapeutic Effect:** Inhibits DNA and RNA synthesis. Topical form destroys rapidly proliferating cells.

PHARMACOKINETICS

Widely distributed. Crosses the blood-brain barrier. Rapidly metabolized in tissues to active metabolite, which is localized intracellularly. Primarily excreted by lungs as carbon dioxide. Removed by hemodialysis. ***Half-life:*** 20 hr.

AVAILABILITY

Injection (Adrucil): 50 mg/ml.
Topical Cream (Carac, Fluoroplex): 1%.
Topical Cream (Efudex): 5%.
Topical Solution (Efudex): 2%.
Topical Solution (Fluoroplex): 1%.

INDICATIONS AND DOSAGES

▸ **Carcinoma of breast, colon, pancreas, rectum, and stomach; in combination with levamisole after surgical resection in patients with Duke's stage C colon cancer**

IV

Adults, Elderly, Children. Initially, 12 mg/kg/day for 4–5 days. Maximum: 800 mg/day. Maintenance: 6 mg/kg every other day for 4 doses repeated in 4 wk; or 15 mg/kg as a single bolus dose; or 5–15 mg/kg/wk as a single dose, not to exceed 1 g.

▸ **Multiple actinic or solar keratoses**

Topical (Efudex, Fluoroplex)

Adults, Elderly. Apply twice a day.

Topical (Carac)

Adults, Elderly. Apply once a day.

▸ **Basal cell carcinoma**

Topical (Efudex)

Adults, Elderly. Apply 2 times/day.

OFF-LABEL USES

Parenteral: Treatment of bladder, cervical, endometrial, head and neck, liver, lung, ovarian, or prostate carcinomas; pericardial, peritoneal, or pleural effusions
Topical: Treatment of actinic cheilitis, radiodermatitis

CONTRAINDICATIONS

Major surgery within previous month, myelosuppression, poor nutritional status, potentially serious infections

INTERACTIONS

Drug

Bone marrow depressants: May increase the risk of myelosuppression.
Live-virus vaccines: May potentiate virus replication, increase vaccine side effects, and decrease the patient's antibody response to the vaccine.

Herbal

None known.

Food

None known.

DIAGNOSTIC TEST EFFECTS

May decrease serum albumin level. May increase excretion of 5-hydroxyindoleacetic acid (5-HIAA) in urine. Topical form may cause eosinophilia, leukocytosis, thrombocytopenia, and toxic granulation.

IV INCOMPATIBILITIES

Amphotericin B complex (Abelcet, AmBisome, Amphotec), droperidol (Inapsine), filgrastim (Neupogen), ondansetron (Zofran), vinorelbine (Navelbine)

IV COMPATIBILITIES

Granisetron (Kytril), heparin, hydromorphone (Dilaudid), leucovorin, morphine, potassium chloride, propofol (Diprivan)

SIDE EFFECTS

Occasional

Parenteral: Anorexia, diarrhea, minimal alopecia, fever, dry skin, skin fissures, scaling, erythema
Topical: Pain, pruritus, hyperpigmentation, irritation, inflammation, and burning at application site; photosensitivity

Rare

Nausea, vomiting, anemia, esophagitis, proctitis, GI ulcer, confusion, headache, lacrimation, visual disturbances, angina, allergic reactions

SERIOUS REACTIONS

! The earliest sign of toxicity, which may occur 4–8 days after beginning therapy, is stomatitis (as evidenced by dry mouth, burning sensation, mucosal erythema, and ulceration at inner margin of lips).

! Hematologic toxicity may be manifested as leukopenia (generally within 9–14 days after drug administration, but possibly as late as the 25th day), thrombocytopenia (within 7–17 days after administration), pancytopenia, or agranulocytosis.

! The most common dermatologic toxicity is a pruritic rash on the extremities or, less frequently, the trunk.

NURSING CONSIDERATIONS

Baseline Assessment

- Monitor the patient's CBC with differential, liver and renal function test results, and platelet count.

Lifespan Considerations

- Because 5-fluorouracil may cause fetal harm, pregnant women should avoid using this drug if possible, especially in the first trimester.
- It is unknown whether 5-fluorouracil is distributed in breast milk; however, breast-feeding is not recommended for patients taking this drug.
- No age-related precautions have been noted in children.
- In the elderly, age-related renal impairment may require dosage adjustment.

Precautions

- Use 5-fluorouracil cautiously in patients with impaired hepatic or renal function, metastatic cell infiltration of bone marrow, or a history of high-dose pelvic irradiation.

Administration and Handling

◀ALERT▶ Dosage of 5-fluorouracil is individualized based on the patient's clinical response, tolerance of the drug's adverse effects, and actual weight (ideal weight in edematous or obese patients). When administering this drug in combination therapy, consult specific protocols for optimum dosage and sequence of drug administration.

IV

◀ALERT▶ Give 5-fluorouracil by IV injection or IV infusion. Don't add this drug to other IV infusions. Because 5-fluorouracil may be carcinogenic, mutagenic, or teratogenic, handle the drug with extreme care during preparation and administration.

- The solution normally appears colorless to faint yellow. Slight discoloration does not adversely affect potency or safety.
- If a precipitate forms, redissolve the solution by heating it and shaking it vigorously; then allow it to cool to body temperature.
- Administer IV push as undiluted or unreconstituted, as appropriate. Inject it through a Y-tube or 3-way stopcock of free-flowing solution.
- For IV infusion, further dilute with D_5W or 0.9% NaCl.
- Give IV push slowly over 1 to 2 minutes.

◀ **ALERT** ▶ When accessing a vein for infusion, avoid areas overlying joints and tendons, small veins, and swollen or edematous extremities.
• Administer the IV infusion over 30 minutes to 24 hours.
• Monitor the patient for signs and symptoms of extravasation, including immediate pain and severe local tissue damage. If this occurs, follow your facility's protocol.

Intervention and Evaluation
• Monitor the patient for signs of GI bleeding, including bright red or tarry stools, intractable diarrhea, and rapidly falling WBC count.
• Assess the patient for signs and symptoms of stomatitis, including difficulty swallowing, sore throat, and ulceration and erythema of the oral mucosa.
• Expect to discontinue 5-fluorouracil if intractable diarrhea, GI bleeding, or stomatitis occurs.
• Examine the patient's skin for a rash.

Patient Teaching
• Warn the patient to notify the physician if he or she experiences bleeding, easy bruising, chest pain, diarrhea, nausea, palpitations, signs and symptoms of infection, or visual changes.
• Encourage the patient to avoid overexposure to sun or ultraviolet light and to wear protective clothing, sunglasses, and sunscreen when outdoors.
• Instruct the patient using topical 5-fluorouracil to apply the drug only to the affected area and not to cover it with occlusive dressings. Advise the patient to be careful when applying the drug near the eyes, mouth, and nose and to wash hands thoroughly after application. Inform the patient that treated areas may be unsightly for several weeks after therapy.
• Teach the patient to maintain fastidious oral hygiene.

gemcitabine hydrochloride

gem-**cih**-tah-bean
(Gemzar)

CATEGORY AND SCHEDULE
Pregnancy Risk Category: D

MECHANISM OF ACTION
An antimetabolite that inhibits ribonucleotide reductase, the enzyme necessary for catalyzing DNA synthesis. **Therapeutic Effect:** Produces death in cells undergoing DNA synthesis.

PHARMACOKINETICS
Not extensively distributed after IV infusion (increased with length of infusion). Protein binding: less than 10%. Excreted primarily in urine as metabolite. ***Half-life***: 42–94 min (influenced by gender of patient and duration of infusion).

AVAILABILITY
Powder for Reconstitution: 200 mg, 1-g vials.

INDICATIONS AND DOSAGES
▶ **Non small-cell lung cancer (in combination with cisplatin)**
IV
Adults, Elderly, Children. 1,000 mg/m^2 on days 1, 8, and 15, repeated every 28 days; or 1,250 mg/m^2 on days 1 and 8. Repeat every 21 days.
▶ **Pancreatic cancer**
IV
Adults. 1,000 mg/m^2 once weekly for up to 7 wk or until toxicity necessitates decreasing dosage or withholding the dose, followed by 1 wk

of rest. Subsequent cycles should consist of once-weekly dose for 3 consecutive wk out of every 4 wk. For patients completing cycles at 1,000 mg/m^2, increase dose to 1,250 mg/m^2 as tolerated. Dose for next cycle may be increased to 1,500 mg/m^2.

▸ **Dosage reduction guidelines**

Dosage adjustments should be based on granulocyte count and platelet count, as follows:

Absolute Granulocyte Counts (cells/mm^3)	Platelet Count (cells/mm^3)	% of Full Dose
1,000 and	100,000	100
500–999	50,000–99,000	75
less than 500	less than 50,000	Hold

OFF-LABEL USES

Treatment of biliary tract carcinoma, gallbladder carcinoma, Hodgkins lymphoma, non-Hodgskin's lymphoma, ovarian carcinoma

CONTRAINDICATIONS

None known.

INTERACTIONS

Drug

Bone marrow depressants: May increase the risk of myelosuppression.

Live-virus vaccines: May potentiate virus replication, increase vaccine side effects, and decrease the patient's antibody response to the vaccine.

Herbal

None known.

Food

None known.

DIAGNOSTIC TEST EFFECTS

May increase BUN level and serum alkaline phosphatase, bilirubin, creatinine, AST (SGOT), and ALT (SGPT) levels.

IV INCOMPATIBILITIES

Acyclovir (Zovirax), amphotericin B (Fungizone), cefoperazone (Cefobid), furosemide (Lasix), ganciclovir (Cytovene), imipenem and cilastatin (Primaxin), irinotecan (Camptosar), methotrexate, methylprednisolone (Solu-Medrol), mitomycin (Mutamycin), piperacillin and tazobactam (Zosyn), prochlorperazine (Compazine)

IV COMPATIBILITIES

Bumetanide (Bumex), calcium gluconate, dexamethasone (Decadron), diphenhydramine (Benadryl), dobutamine (Dobutrex), dopamine (Intropin), granisetron (Kytril), heparin, hydrocortisone (Solu-Cortef), lorazepam (Ativan), ondansetron (Zofran), potassium

SIDE EFFECTS

Frequent

Nausea and vomiting (69%); generalized pain (48%); fever (41%); mild to moderate pruritic rash (30%); mild to moderate dyspnea, constipation (23%); peripheral edema (20%)

Occasional (19%–10%)

Diarrhea, petechiae, alopecia, stomatitis, infection, somnolence, paresthesia

Rare

Diaphoresis, rhinitis, insomnia, malaise

SERIOUS REACTIONS

! Severe myelosuppression, as evidenced by anemia, thrombocytopenia, and leukopenia, is a common reaction.

NURSING CONSIDERATIONS

Baseline Assessment

- Obtain CBC and liver and renal function test results before and periodically during gemcitabine therapy.
- Expect to stop the drug or modify the dosage if myelosuppression occurs.

Lifespan Considerations

- Because gemcitabine may cause fetal harm, pregnant women should avoid using it, if possible, expecially in the first trimester.
- It is unknown if gemcitabine is distributed in breast milk; however, breast-feeding is not recommended for patients taking this drug.
- The safety and efficacy of gemcitabine have not been established in children.
- Elderly patients are at increased risk for hematologic toxicity.

Precautions

- Use gemcitabine cautiously in patients with impaired renal function or hepatic insufficiency.

Administration and Handling

◀ **ALERT** ▶ Gemcitabine dosage is individualized based on the patient's clinical response and tolerance of the drug's adverse effects. When administering this drug in combination therapy, consult specific protocols for optimum dosage and sequence of drug administration.

◀ **ALERT** ▶ Because gemcitabine may be carcinogenic, mutagenic, or teratogenic, handle the drug with extreme care during preparation and administration.

◀ **ALERT** ▶ Increase gemcitabine dosage, as prescribed, provided that the absolute granulocyte count and platelet count nadirs exceed 1,500/mm^3 and 100,000/mm^3, respectively.

IV

- Store the unreconstituted form at room temperature because refrigeration may cause crystallization.
- The reconstituted solution is stable for up to 24 hours at room temperature.
- Reconstitute the 200-mg or 1-g vial with 5 ml or 25 ml, respectively, of 0.9% NaCl injection without preservative, to provide a concentration of 40 mg/ml.
- Shake to dissolve and give without further dilution, as appropriate.
- The solution may be further diluted with 0.9% NaCl, if necessary, to a concentration as low as 0.1 mg/ml.
- Infuse over 30 minutes.

Intervention and Evaluation

- Evaluate all of the patient's laboratory test results before giving each gemcitabine dose.
- Monitor the patient for dyspnea, fever, and pruritic rash, and dehydration due to vomiting.
- Assess the patient for signs and symptoms of stomatitis, including difficulty swallowing, sore throat, and ulceration and erythema of the oral mucosa.
- Examine the patient's skin for a rash.
- Notify the physician if the patient develops diarrhea.
- Provide antiemetics, if ordered.

Patient Teaching

- Urge the patient to avoid crowds and exposure to those with known infections.
- Warn the patient to notify the physician if he or she experiences easy bruising, fever, signs of local infection, rash, or sore throat.
- Caution the patient to notify the physician if nausea or vomiting continues at home.
- Teach the patient to maintain fastidious oral hygiene.

hydroxyurea

high-**drocks**-ee-your-e-ah
(Droxia, Hydrea, Mylocel)

CATEGORY AND SCHEDULE
Pregnancy Risk Category: D

MECHANISM OF ACTION
A synthetic urea analogue that inhibits DNA synthesis without interfering with RNA synthesis or protein. **Therapeutic Effect:** Interferes with the normal repair process of cancer cells damaged by irradiation.

AVAILABILITY
Capsules (Droxia): 200 mg, 300 mg, 400 mg.
Capsules (Hydrea): 500 mg.
Tablets (Mylocel): 1,000 mg.

INDICATIONS AND DOSAGES
▸ **Melanoma; recurrent, metastatic, or inoperable ovarian carcinoma**
PO
Adults, Elderly. 80 mg/kg every 3 days or 20–30 mg/kg/day as a single dose.
▸ **Control of primary squamous cell carcinoma of the head and neck, excluding lips (in combination with radiation therapy)**
PO
Adults, Elderly. 80 mg/kg every 3 days, beginning at least 7 days before starting radiation therapy.
▸ **Resistant chronic myelocytic leukemia**
PO
Adults, Elderly. 20–30 mg/kg once a day.
Children. 10–20 mg/kg once a day.
▸ **HIV infection**
PO
Adults, Elderly. 500 mg twice a day with didanosine.
▸ **Sickle cell anemia**
PO
Adults, Elderly, Children. Initially, 15 mg/kg once a day. May increase by 5 mg/kg/day. Maximum: 35 mg/kg/day.

OFF-LABEL USES
Treatment of cervical carcinoma, polycythemia vera; long-term suppression of HIV infection

CONTRAINDICATIONS
WBC count less than 2,500/mm^3 or platelet count less than 100,000/mm^3

INTERACTIONS
Drug
Antigout medications: May decrease the effects of these drugs.
Bone marrow depressants: May increase myelosuppression.
Live-virus vaccines: May potentiate virus replication, increase vaccine side effects, and decrease the patient's antibody response to the vaccine.
Herbal
None known.
Food
None known.

DIAGNOSTIC TEST EFFECTS
May increase BUN and serum creatinine and uric acid levels.

SIDE EFFECTS
Frequent
Nausea, vomiting, anorexia, constipation or diarrhea
Occasional
Mild, reversible rash; facial flushing; pruritus; fever; chills; malaise
Rare
Alopecia, headache, drowsiness, dizziness, disorientation

SERIOUS REACTIONS
! Myelosuppression may cause

hematologic toxicity (manifested as leukopenia and, to a lesser extent, thrombocytopenia and anemia).

NURSING CONSIDERATIONS

Baseline Assessment

• Expect the patient to undergo bone marrow studies and liver and renal function tests before and periodically during hydroxyurea therapy.
• Obtain blood Hgb and serum uric acid levels and platelet and WBC counts before and weekly during hydroxyurea therapy.

Precautions

• Use hydroxyurea cautiously in patients with impaired hepatic or renal function and in those who have had previous radiation therapy or are using other cytotoxic drugs.

Administration and Handling

◀ALERT▶ Hydroxyurea dosage is individualized based on the patient's clinical response, tolerance of the drug's adverse effects, and actual or ideal body weight, whichever is less. When administering this drug in combination therapy, consult specific protocols for optimum dosage and sequence of drug administration.
◀ALERT▶ Expect therapy to be interrupted when platelet count falls below 100,000/mm^3 or WBC count falls below 2,500/mm^3 and to resume when counts return to normal.

Intervention and Evaluation

• Assess the patient's pattern of daily bowel activity and stool consistency.
• Monitor the patient for signs and symptoms of hematologic toxicity, including excessive fatigue and weakness, ecchymosis, fever, signs of local infection, sore throat, or unusual bleeding from any site.
• Examine the patient's skin for erythema or a rash.
• Know that those patients with marked renal impairment may develop auditory or visual hallucinations and marked hematologic toxicity.
• Monitor the patient's blood Hgb level, CBC with differential (including platelet and WBC counts), liver and renal function test results, and serum uric acid levels.

Patient Teaching

• Warn the patient to notify the physician if he or she experiences easy bruising, fever, signs of local infection, sore throat, or unusual bleeding from any site.
• Urge the patient to avoid crowds and exposure to those with known infections.

mercaptopurine

mur-cap-**tow**-pure-een
(Purinethol)

CATEGORY AND SCHEDULE

Pregnancy Risk Category: D

MECHANISM OF ACTION

An antimetabolite that is incorporated into RNA and DNA, blocks purine synthesis, and inhibits DNA and RNA synthesis. **Therapeutic Effect:** Causes death of cancer cells.

AVAILABILITY

Tablets: 50 mg.

INDICATIONS AND DOSAGES

▸ **Acute lymphoblastic leukemia**
PO
Adults, Elderly, Children. 2.5–5 mg/kg once a day as induction dose. Maintenance: 1.5–2.5 mg/kg/day.
▸ **Dosage in renal impairment:**
If creatinine clearance is less than 50 ml/min. Administer usual dose q48h.

CONTRAINDICATIONS
Pregnancy, severe myelosuppression or hepatic disease

INTERACTIONS
Drug
Alcohol: May increase the risk of toxicity of mercaptopurine.
Allopurinol, doxorubicin, hepatotoxic medications: May increase the effects and risk of toxicity of mercaptopurine.
Bone marrow depressants: May increase the risk of myelosuppression.
Live-virus vaccines: May potentiate virus replication, increase vaccine side effects, and decrease the patient's antibody response to the vaccine.
Warfarin: May decrease the effects of this drug.
Herbal
None known.
Food
All foods: Decrease the bioavailability of mercaptopurine.

DIAGNOSTIC TEST EFFECTS
None known.

SIDE EFFECTS
Frequent (greater than 10%)
Myelosuppression (leading to leukopenia, thrombocytopenia, anemia), intrahepatic cholestasis, hepatic necrosis
Occasional (10%–1%)
Drug fever, hyperpigmentation, rash, hyperuricemia, nausea, vomiting, diarrhea, stomatitis, anorexia, abdominal pain, mucositis

SERIOUS REACTIONS
! Myelosuppression, hepatic necrosis, and gastroenteritis may occur.

NURSING CONSIDERATIONS
Baseline Assessment
- Determine if the patient is pregnant or breast-feeding (not recommended) and taking other medications, especially allopurinol, other bone marrow depressants, and other hepatotoxic medications, before beginning mercaptopurine therapy.
Precautions
- Use mercaptopurine cautiously in patients with infection, renal or hepatic impairment, prior myelosuppression, or a history of gout.
Administration and Handling
PO
- Don't administer mercaptopurine with meals.
Intervention and Evaluation
- Monitor the patient's hepatic and renal function tests result, platelet count, and serum uric acid level.
Patient Teaching
- Urge the patient to avoid consuming alcohol beverages during mercaptopurine therapy because alcohol may increase the risk of drug-induced toxicity.
- Urge the patient to avoid vaccinations and exposure to persons with known infections during mercaptopurine therapy.
- Warn the patient to notify the physician if he or she experiences unusual bleeding or bruising.

methotrexate sodium

meth-oh-**trex**-ate
(Apo-Methotrexate [CAN], Ledertrexate[AUS], Methoblastin[AUS], Rheumatrex, Trexall)
Do not confuse Trexall with Trexan.

CATEGORY AND SCHEDULE

Pregnancy Risk Category: D (X for patients with psoriasis or rheumatoid arthritis)

MECHANISM OF ACTION

An antimetabolite that competes with enzymes necessary to reduce folic acid to tetrahydrofolic acid, a component essential to DNA, RNA, and protein synthesis. This action inhibits DNA, RNA, and protein synthesis. **Therapeutic Effect:** Causes death of cancer cells.

PHARMACOKINETICS

Variably absorbed from the GI tract. Completely absorbed after IM administration. Protein binding: 50%–60%. Widely distributed. Metabolized intracellularly in the liver. Primarily excreted in urine. Removed by hemodialysis but not by peritoneal dialysis. ***Half-life:*** 8–12 hr (large doses, 8–15 hr).

AVAILABILITY

Tablets (Rheumatrex): 2.5 mg.
Tablets (Trexall): 5 mg, 7.5 mg, 10 mg, 15 mg.
Injection Solution: 25 mg/ml.
Injection Powder for Reconstitution: 20 mg, 1 g.

INDICATIONS AND DOSAGES

▸ Trophoblastic neoplasms
PO, IM
Adults, Elderly. 15–30 mg/day for 5 days; repeat in 7 days for 3–5 courses.

▸ Head and neck cancer
PO, IV, IM
Adults, Elderly. 25–50 mg/m^2 once weekly.

▸ Choriocarcinoma, chorioadenoma destruens, hydatidiform mole
PO, IM
Adults, Elderly. 15–30 mg/day for 5 days; repeat 3–5 times with 1–2 wk between courses.

▸ Breast cancer
IV
Adults, Elderly. 30–60 mg/m^2 days 1 and 8 q3–4wk.

▸ Acute lymphocytic leukemia
PO, IV, IM
Adults, Elderly. Induction: 3.3 mg/m^2/day in combination with other chemotherapeutic agents. Maintenance: 30 mg/m^2/wk PO or IM in divided doses or 2.5 mg/kg IV every 14 days.

▸ Burkitt's lymphoma
PO
Adults. 10–25 mg/day for 4–8 days; repeat with 7- to 10-day rest between courses.

▸ Lymphosarcoma
PO
Adults, Elderly. 0.625–2.5 mg/kg/day.

▸ Mycosis fungoides
PO
Adults, Elderly. 2.5–10 mg/day.
IM
Adults, Elderly. 50 mg/wk or 25 mg twice a week.

▸ Rheumatoid arthritis
PO
Adults, Elderly. 7.5 mg once weekly or 2.5 mg q12h for 3 doses once weekly. Maximum: 20 mg/wk.

▸ Juvenile rheumatoid arthritis
PO, IM, Subcutaneous
Children. 5–15 mg/m^2/wk as a single dose or in 3 divided doses given q12h.

▸ **Psoriasis**
PO
Adults, Elderly. 10–25 mg once weekly or 2.5–5 mg q12h for 3 doses once weekly.
IM
Adults, Elderly. 10–25 mg once weekly.

▸ **Antineoplastic dosage for children**
PO, IM
Children. 7.5–30 mg/m²/wk or q2wk.
IV
Children. 10–33,000 mg/m² bolus or continuous infusion over 6–42 hr.

▸ **Dosage in renal impairment**
Creatinine clearance 61–80 ml/min. Reduce dose by 25%.
Creatinine clearance 51–60 ml/min. Reduce dose by 33%.
Creatinine clearance 10–50 ml/min. Reduce dose by 50%–70%.

OFF-LABEL USES
Treatment of acute myelocytic leukemia; bladder, cervical, ovarian, prostatic, renal, and testicular carcinomas; psoriatic arthritis; systemic dermatomyositis

CONTRAINDICATIONS
Pre-existing myelosuppression, severe hepatic or renal impairment

INTERACTIONS
Drug
Acyclovir (parenteral): May increase the risk of neurotoxicity.
Alcohol, hepatotoxic medications: May increase the risk of hepatotoxicity.
Asparaginase: May decrease the effects of methotrexate.
Bone marrow depressants: May increase myelosuppression.
Live virus vaccines: May potentiate virus replication, increase vaccine side effects, and decrease the patient's antibody response to the vaccine.
NSAIDs: May increase the risk of methotrexate toxicity.
Probenecid, salicylates: May increase blood methotrexate concentration and risk of toxicity.
Herbal
None known.
Food
None known.

DIAGNOSTIC TEST EFFECTS
May increase serum uric acid and AST (SGOT) levels.

IV INCOMPATIBILITIES
Chlorpromazine (Thorazine), droperidol (Inapsine), gemcitabine (Gemzar), idarubicin (Idamycin), midazolam (Versed), nalbuphine (Nubain)

IV COMPATIBILITIES
Cisplatin (Platinol AQ), cyclophosphamide (Cytoxan), daunorubicin (DaunoXome), doxorubicin (Adriamycin), etoposide (VePesed), 5-fluorouracil, granisetron (Kytril), leucovorin, mitomycin (Mutamycin), ondansetron (Zofran), paclitaxel (Taxol), vinblastine (Velban), vincristine (Oncovin), vinorelbine (Navelbine)

SIDE EFFECTS
Frequent (10%–3%)
Nausea, vomiting, stomatitis; burning and erythema at psoriatic site (in patients with psoriasis)
Occasional (3%–1%)
Diarrhea, rash, dermatitis, pruritus, alopecia, dizziness, anorexia, malaise, headache, drowsiness, blurred vision

SERIOUS REACTIONS
! GI toxicity may produce gingivitis,

glossitis, pharyngitis, stomatitis, enteritis, and hematemesis.
! Hepatotoxicity is more likely to occur with frequent small doses than with large intermittent doses.
! Pulmonary toxicity may be characterized by interstitial pneumonitis.
! Hematologic toxicity, which may develop rapidly from marked myelosuppression, may be manifested as leukopenia, thrombocytopenia, anemia, and hemorrhage.
! Dermatologic toxicity may produce a rash, pruritus, urticaria, pigmentation, photosensitivity, petechiae, ecchymosis, and pustules.
! Severe nephrotoxicity may produce azotemia, hematuria, and renal failure.

NURSING CONSIDERATIONS

Baseline Assessment

- Determine if the patient with psoriasis or rheumatoid arthritis is pregnant before initiating methotrexate therapy because the drug has a pregnancy risk category of X in these patients.
- Evaluate diagnostic test results, including renal and liver function tests, Hgb and Hct levels, and platelet count, before and periodically during methotrexate therapy.
- Give antiemetics, if ordered, to prevent or treat nausea and vomiting.

Lifespan Considerations

- Because methotrexate may cause congenital anomalies and fetal death, female patients should avoid becoming pregnant during therapy and for at least one ovulatory cycle after therapy is completed, and male patients should avoid impregnating their partners during therapy and for at least 3 months after therapy is completed.
- Because methotrexate is distributed in breast milk, breast-feeding is not recommended for patients taking this drug.
- In children and the elderly, decreased hepatic and renal function requires cautious use of the drug and may require a dosage adjustment.

Precautions

- Use methotrexate cautiously in patients with ascites, myelosuppression, peptic ulcer disease, pleural effusion, or ulcerative colitis.

Administration and Handling

◀ALERT▶ Because methotrexate may be carcinogenic, mutagenic, or teratogenic, handle the drug with extreme care during preparation and administration. Wear gloves when preparing the solution. If powder or solution comes in contact with skin, wash the area immediately and thoroughly with soap and water.

- Be aware that the drug may be given IM, IV, intra-arterially, or intrathecally.

IV

- Store vials at room temperature.
- Reconstitute each 5-mg vial with 2 ml sterile water for injection or 0.9% NaCl to provide a concentration of 2.5 mg/ml up to a maximum of 25 mg/ml.
- The solution may be further diluted with D_5W or 0.9% NaCl.
- For intrathecal use, dilute with preservative-free 0.9% NaCl to provide a concentration of 1 mg/ml.
- Give IV push at 10 mg/minute.
- Give IV infusion over 30 minutes to 4 hours.

Intervention and Evaluation

- Monitor the patient's blood Hgb and Hct levels, chest x-rays, liver and renal function test results, serum uric acid level, urinalysis results, platelet count, and WBC count with differential.
- Monitor the patient for signs and

symptoms of hematologic toxicity, including excessive fatigue and weakness, ecchymosis, fever, signs of local infection, sore throat, and unusual bleeding from any site.
- Examine the patient's skin for evidence of dermatologic toxicity.
- As prescribed, administer IV fluids to keep the patient well hydrated and medication to alkalinize the urine, such as bicarbonate.
- Avoid giving IM injections, taking rectal temperatures, and performing traumatic procedures that may cause bleeding.
- Apply pressure to the IV site for 5 full minutes after administration has been completed.

Patient Teaching
- Urge the patient to avoid receiving vaccinations and contact with crowds and those with known infections.
- Urge the patient to avoid alcohol and salicylates and overexposure to sun or ultraviolet light during methotrexate therapy.
- Teach both male and female patients contraceptive methods to use during therapy and for a certain period afterward.
- Warn the patient to report easy bruising, fever, signs of local infection, sore throat, and unusual bleeding from any site.
- Teach the patient to maintain fastidious oral hygiene.
- Inform the patient that alopecia is reversible but that new hair may have a different color or texture.
- Caution the patient to notify the physician if nausea and vomiting continue at home.

pemetrexed

pem-eh-**trex**-ed
(Alimta)

CATEGORY AND SCHEDULE
Pregnancy Risk Category: D

MECHANISM OF ACTION
An antimetabolite that disrupts folate-dependent enzymes essential for cell replication. **Therapeutic Effect:** Inhibits the growth of mesothelioma cell lines.

PHARMACOKINETICS
Protein binding: 81%. Drug is not metabolized; excreted in urine. ***Half-life:*** 3.5 hr.

AVAILABILITY
Powder for Injection: 500 mg.

INDICATIONS AND DOSAGES
◀ALERT▶ Pre-treatment with dexamethasone (or equivalent) will reduce the risk and severity of a cutaneous reaction; treatment with folic acid and vitamin B_{12} beginning 1 week before treatment and continuing for 21 days after the last pemetrexed dose will reduce the risk of side effects.

▸ **Malignant pleural mesothelioma**
IV
Adults, Elderly. 600 mg/m^2 every 3 wk when used as a single agent; 500 mg/m^2 every 3 wk when used in combination with cisplatin 75 mg/m^2.

CONTRAINDICATIONS
None known.

INTERACTIONS
Drug
Nephrotoxic agents, probenecid: May delay pemetrexed clearance.

NSAIDs (particularly ibuprofen): Increase the risk of myelosuppression and GI and renal toxicity.

Herbal

None known.

Food

None known.

DIAGNOSTIC TEST EFFECTS

May decrease platelet, RBC, and WBC counts.

IV INCOMPATIBILITIES

Use only 0.9% NaCl to reconstitute; flush the line before and after the infusion. Don't add any other medications to the IV line.

SIDE EFFECTS

Frequent(12%–10%)

Fatigue, nausea, vomiting, rash or desquamation

Occasional (8%–4%)

Stomatitis, pharyngitis, diarrhea, anorexia, hypertension, chest pain

Rare (less than 3%)

Constipation, depression, dysphagia

SERIOUS REACTIONS

! Myelosuppression, manifested as neutropenia, thrombocytopenia, or anemia, may occur.

NURSING CONSIDERATIONS

Baseline Assessment

- Determine if the patient is pregnant or breast-feeding before beginning therapy.
- Obtain CBC and other blood chemistry tests before and during pemetrexed therapy.

Lifespan Considerations

- Pemetrexed use may cause fetal harm; this drug is not recommended for use during pregnancy.
- It is unknown if pemetrexed is distributed in breast milk. However, women should not breast-feed while taking pemetrexed.
- The safety and efficacy of pemetrexed have not been established in children younger than 18 years.
- Patients 65 years and older have a higher incidence of fatigue, leukopenia, neutropenia, and thrombocytopenia.

Precautions

- Use pemetrexed cautiously in patients with impaired hepatic or renal function.

Administration and Handling

IV

- Store vials at room temperature. The reconstituted solution is stable for up to 24 hours at room temperature or if refrigerated.
- Dilute the 500-mg vial with 20 ml 0.9% NaCl to provide a concentration of 25 mg/ml.
- Gently swirl each vial until the powder is completely dissolved. The solution should appear clear and colorless to yellow or green-yellow.
- Further dilute the reconstituted solution with 100 ml 0.9% NaCl.
- Infuse pemetrexed solution over 10 minutes.

Intervention and Evaluation

- Monitor the patient's Hct, Hgb level, and platelet and WBC counts.
- Assess the patient for hematologic toxicity, characterized by ecchymosis, fever, signs and symptoms of local infection, sore throat, signs of local infection, and unusual bleeding from any site, and for signs and symptoms of anemia, such as excessive fatigue and weakness.
- Examine the patient's skin for a rash or desquamation.
- Keep the patient well-hydrated to alkalinize urine.
- Monitor the patient's WBC count for nadir and recovery.

Patient Teaching

- Instruct the patient to use effective contraceptive measures during pemetrexed therapy.
- Urge the patient to promptly report fever, signs of local infection, sore throat, bruising, and unusual bleeding from any site.
- Instruct the patient to maintain fastidious oral hygiene.
- Advise the patient to avoid receiving immunizations without the physician's prior approval because pemetrexed lowers the body's resistance. Also urge the patient to avoid crowds and people with known infections.

16 Antimitotic Agents

docetaxel
paclitaxel
vinblastine sulfate
vincristine sulfate
vinorelbine

Uses: Antimitotic agents are used to treat lymphoma, lymphosarcomas, neuroblastomas, multiple myeloma, and cancer of the testes, breasts, kidneys, lungs, and ovaries.

Action: Antimitotic agents include two groups that act in different ways—vinca alkaloids and taxoids. *Vinca alkaloids,* which include vinblastine, vincristine, and vinorelbine, block mitosis during metaphase (M phase) by disrupting the assembly of microtubules (filaments that move chromosomes during cell division). This action prevents cell division. (See the illustration *Sites and Mechanisms of Action: Antineoplastic Agents,* page 268.) *Taxoids,* such as docetaxel and paclitaxel, act during the late G_2 phase to enhance the formation of stable microtubules, which prevents cell division.

docetaxel

dox-eh-**tax**-el
(Taxotere)
Do not confuse docetaxel with Taxol.

CATEGORY AND SCHEDULE

Pregnancy Risk Category: D

MECHANISM OF ACTION

An antimitotic agent belonging to the taxoid family that disrupts the microtubular cell network, which is essential for cellular function. **Therapeutic Effect:** Inhibits cellular mitosis.

PHARMACOKINETICS

Distributed into peripheral compartments. Protein binding: 94%. Extensively metabolized. Excreted primarily in feces, with lesser amount in urine. ***Half-life:*** 11.1 hr.

AVAILABILITY

Injection: 20 mg/0.5 ml with diluent, 80 mg/2 ml with diluent.

INDICATIONS AND DOSAGES

▸ **Breast carcinoma**

IV

Adults. 60–100 mg/m² given over 1 hr q3wk. If patient develops febrile neutropenia, a neutrophil count less than 500 cells/mm³ for longer than 1 wk, severe or cumulative cutaneous reactions, or severe peripheral neuropathy with initial dose of 100 mg/m², dosage should be decreased to 75 mg/m². If reaction continues, dosage should be further reduced to 55 mg/m² or therapy should be discontinued. Patients who don't experience the above symptoms at a dose of 60 mg/m² may tolerate an increased docetaxel dose.

▸ **Non–small cell lung carcinoma**

IV

Adults. 75 mg/m² q3wk. Adjust dosage if toxicity occurs.

OFF-LABEL USES

Treatment of small cell-bladder, head and neck, lung, ovarian, or prostate cancer

CONTRAINDICATIONS

History of severe hypersensitivity to docetaxel or other drugs formulated with polysorbate 80, neutrophil count less than 1,500 cells/mm^3

INTERACTIONS

Drug

Bone marrow depressants: May increase myelosuppression.
Cyclosporine, erythromycin, ketoconazole: May significantly inhibit docetaxel metabolism.
Live-virus vaccines: May potentiate replication, increase vaccine side effects, and decrease the patient's antibody response to the vaccine.

Herbal

None known.

Food

None known.

DIAGNOSTIC TEST EFFECTS

May significantly increase BUN level and serum alkaline phosphatase, bilirubin, creatinine, AST (SGOT), and ALT (SGPT) levels. Reduces blood neutrophil, thrombocyte, and WBC counts.

IV INCOMPATIBILITIES

Amphotericin B (Fungizone), doxorubicin liposomal (DaunoXome), methylprednisolone (Solu-Medrol), nalbuphine (Nubain)

IV COMPATIBILITIES

Bumetanide (Bumex), calcium gluconate, dexamethasone (Decadron), diphenhydramine (Benadryl), dobutamine (Dobutrex), dopamine (Inotropin), furosemide (Lasix), granisetron (Kytril), heparin, hydromorphone (Dilaudid), lorazepam (Ativan), magnesium sulfate, mannitol, morphine, ondansetron (Zofran), potassium chloride

SIDE EFFECTS

Frequent

Alopecia (80%), asthenia (62%), hypersensitivity reaction such as dermatitis (59%, decreases to 16% in those pretreated with oral corticosteroids), fluid retention (49%), stomatitis (43%), nausea and diarrhea (40%), fever (30%), nail changes (28%), vomiting (24%), myalgia (19%)

Occasional

Hypotension, edema, anorexia, headache, weight gain, infection (urinary tract, injection site, indwelling catheter tip), dizziness

Rare

Dry skin, sensory disorders (vision, speech, taste), arthralgia, weight loss, conjunctivitis, hematuria, proteinuria

SERIOUS REACTIONS

! In patients with normal liver function tests, neutropenia (neutrophil count less than 2,000 cells/mm^3) and leukopenia (WBC count less than 4,000 cells/mm^3) occur in 96% of patients; anemia (hemoglobin level less than 11 g/dl) occurs in 90% of patients; thrombocytopenia (platelet count less than 100,000 cells/mm^3) occurs in 8% of patients; and infection occurs in 28% of patients.

! Neurosensory and neuromotor effects, such as distal paresthesias and weakness, occur in 54% and 13% of patients, respectively.

NURSING CONSIDERATIONS

Baseline Assessment

- Give antiemetics, if ordered, to prevent or treat nausea and vomiting.
- Pretreat the patient with corticosteroids, as ordered, before initiating docetaxel therapy to reduce the severity of fluid retention and hypersensitivity reactions.

Lifespan Considerations
• Docetaxel use should be avoided during pregnancy because the drug may cause fetal harm. It is unknown if docetaxel is distributed in breast milk; however, patients receiving docetaxel should not breast-feed.
• The safety and efficacy of docetaxel have not been established in children younger than 16 years.
• No age-related precautions have been noted in the elderly.

Precautions
• Use docetaxel cautiously in patients with myelosuppression, chickenpox, herpes zoster, infection, impaired hepatic function, or preexisting pleural effusion and in those who have received chemotherapy or radiation.

Administration and Handling
IV
• Dilute the drug before administration.
• Refrigerate the vial and protect it from bright light. Know that freezing won't adversely affect the drug.
• Let the vial stand at room temperature for 5 minutes before administering. Don't store the drug in polyvinyl chloride bags.
• The reconstituted solution is stable for up to 8 hours either at room temperature or refrigerated.
• Transfer the entire contents of the diluent vial to the vial of docetaxel.
• Gently rotate the vial to ensure that the contents are thoroughly mixed; the resulting solution should have a concentration of 10 mg/ml.
• Withdraw the prescribed dose and add it to a 250-ml glass or polyolefin container of 0.9% NaCl or D_5W to provide a final concentration of 0.3–0.9 mg/ml.
• Administer the drug as a 1-hour infusion.
• Monitor the patient closely for signs and symptoms of a hypersensitivity reaction, including bronchospasm, flushing, and a localized skin reaction, which may occur within a few minutes after beginning the infusion.

Intervention and Evaluation
• Frequently monitor the patient's blood test results, particularly liver and renal function studies, neutrophil count, and serum uric acid levels. A neutrophil count of less than 1,500 cells/mm^3 requires discontinuation of docetaxel therapy.
• Observe the patient for cutaneous reactions characterized by a rash with eruptions, mainly on the feet or hands.
• Assess the patient for signs of extravascular fluid accumulation, such as dependent edema, dyspnea at rest, crackles, and pronounced abdominal distention from ascites.
• Offer emotional support to the patient and family.

Patient Teaching
• Urge the patient not to receive vaccinations and to avoid contact with anyone who has recently received a live-virus vaccine.
• Inform the patient that hair growth will resume 2 to 3 months after last dose of docetaxel but that new hair may have a different color or texture.
• Advise the patient to maintain fastidious oral hygiene.

paclitaxel

pass-leh-**tax**-ell
(Abraxane, Anzatax[AUS], Onxol, Taxol)
Do not confuse paclitaxel with Paxil, or Taxol with Taxotere.

CATEGORY AND SCHEDULE
Pregnancy Risk Category: D

MECHANISM OF ACTION

An antimitotic agent in the taxoid family that disrupts the microtubular cell network, which is essential for cellular function. Blocks cells in the late G_2 phase and M phase of the cell cycle. **Therapeutic Effect:** Inhibits cellular mitosis and replication.

PHARMACOKINETICS

Does not readily cross the blood-brain barrier. Protein binding: 89%–98%. Metabolized in the liver to active metabolites; eliminated by bile. Not removed by hemodialysis. ***Half-life:*** 1.3–8.6 hr.

AVAILABILITY

Injection (Abraxane): 100 mg vial.
Injection (Onxol, Taxol): 6 mg/ml.

INDICATIONS AND DOSAGES

▸ Ovarian cancer

IV

Adults. 135–175 mg/m²/dose over 1–24 hr q3wk.

▸ Breast carcinoma

IV

Adults, Elderly. 175 mg/m² over 3 hr q3wk.

▸ Non–small cell lung carcinoma

IV

Adults, Elderly. 135 mg/m² over 24 hr, followed by cisplatin 75 mg/m² q3wk.

▸ Kaposi's sarcoma

IV

Adults, Elderly. 135 mg/m²/dose over 3 hr q3wk or 100 mg/m²/dose over 3 hr q2wk.

▸ Dosage in hepatic impairment

Total Bilirubin	Total Dose
more than 3 mg/dl	less than 50 mg/m²
1.6–3 mg/dl	less than 75 mg/m²
1.5 mg/dl or less	less than 135 mg/m²

OFF-LABEL USES

Treatment of upper GI tract adenocarcinoma, head and neck cancer, hormone-refractory prostate cancer, non-Hodgkin's lymphoma, small-cell lung cancer, transitional cell cancer of urothelium

CONTRAINDICATIONS

Baseline neutropenia (neutrophil count 1,500 cells/mm³), hypersensitivity to drugs developed with Cremophor EL (polyoxyethylated castor oil)

INTERACTIONS

Drug

Bone marrow depressants: May increase myelosuppression.
Live-virus vaccines: May potentiate virus replication, increase vaccine side effects, and decrease the patient's antibody response to the vaccine.

Herbal

None known.

Food

None known.

DIAGNOSTIC TEST EFFECTS

May elevate serum alkaline phosphatase, bilirubin, AST (SGOT), and ALT (SGPT) levels. Decreases blood Hgb and Hct levels and platelet, RBC, and WBC counts.

IV INCOMPATIBILITIES

Amphotericin B complex (Abelcet, AmBisome, Amphotec), chlorpromazine (Thorazine), doxorubicin liposomal (Doxil), hydroxyzine (Vistaril), methylprednisolone (Solu-Medrol), mitoxantrone (Novantrone)

IV COMPATIBILITIES

Carboplatin (Paraplatin), cisplatin (Platinol AQ), cyclophosphamide (Cytoxan), cytarabine (Cytosar), dacarbazine (DTIC-Dome), dexamethasone (Decadron), diphenhydramine (Benadryl), doxorubicin (Adriamycin), etoposide (VePesid), gemcitabine (Gemzar), granisetron (Kytril), hydromorphone (Dilaudid), magnesium sulfate, mannitol, methotrexate, morphine, ondansetron (Zofran), potassium chloride, vinblastine (Velban), vincristine (Oncovin)

SIDE EFFECTS

Expected (90%–70%)
Diarrhea, alopecia, nausea, vomiting
Frequent (48%–46%)
Myalgia or arthralgia, peripheral neuropathy
Occasional (20%–13%)
Mucositis, hypotension during infusion, pain or redness at injection site
Rare (3%)
Bradycardia

SERIOUS REACTIONS

! Neutropenic nadir occurs at approximately day 11 of paclitaxel therapy.
! Anemia and leukopenia are common reactions. Thrombocytopenia occurs occasionally.
! A severe hypersensitivity reaction, including dyspnea, severe hypotension, angioedema, and generalized urticaria, occurs rarely.

NURSING CONSIDERATIONS

Baseline Assessment

- Assess the patient's blood counts, particularly neutrophil and platelet counts, before each course of paclitaxel therapy or as clinically indicated.

Lifespan Considerations

- Paclitaxel use should be avoided during pregnancy because the drug may cause fetal harm. It is unknown if paclitaxel is distributed in breast milk; however, patients receiving this drug should not breast-feed.
- The safety and efficacy of paclitaxel have not been established in children.
- No age-related precautions have been noted in the elderly.

Precautions

- Use paclitaxel cautiously in patients with hepatic impairment, peripheral neuropathy, or severe neutropenia.

Administration and Handling

◀ALERT▶ Pretreat the patient with corticosteroids, diphenhydramine, and H_2 antagonists, as prescribed.
◀ALERT▶ Because paclitaxel may be carcinogenic, mutagenic, or teratogenic, wear gloves when handling the drug. If the drug comes in contact with skin, wash the skin thoroughly with soap and water. If the drug comes in contact with mucous membranes, flush the area with water.

IV

- Refrigerate unopened vials.
- The reconstituted solution is stable at room temperature for up to 24 hours.
- Store diluted solutions in bottles or plastic bags, and administer them through polyethylene-lined administration sets. Avoid storing diluted solutions in plasticized polyvinyl chloride equipment or devices.
- Dilute with 0.9% NaCl or D_5W to a final concentration of 0.3–1.2 mg/ml.
- Administer at the ordered rate through in-line filter not greater than 0.22 micron.
- Monitor the patient's vital signs during the infusion, especially during the first hour.
- Discontinue paclitaxel administration and notify the physician if the patient experiences a severe hypersensitivity reaction.

Intervention and Evaluation
- Use strict aseptic technique during patient care, and protect the patient from infection.
- Monitor the patient's CBC, hepatic function test results, platelet count, and vital signs.
- Monitor the patient for signs and symptoms of hematologic toxicity, including excessive fatigue and weakness, ecchymosis, fever, signs of local infection, sore throat, and unusual bleeding.
- Assess the patient's response to the drug.
- Monitor the patient for and report diarrhea.
- Avoid giving the patient IM injections, taking rectal temperatures, and performing traumatic procedures that may induce bleeding.
- Apply pressure to the IV site for a full 5 minutes after administration.
- Offer emotional support to the patient and family.

Patient Teaching
- Warn the patient to immediately notify the physician if he or she experiences signs of infection, including fever and flu-like symptoms.
- Caution the patient to notify the physician if nausea and vomiting continue at home.
- Teach the patient to recognize the signs and symptoms of peripheral neuropathy.
- Urge the patient not to receive vaccinations and to avoid contact with crowds and people with known infections.
- Warn the patient to avoid pregnancy during paclitaxel therapy. Teach the patient various contraception methods.
- Inform the patient that alopecia is reversible but that new hair may have a different color or texture.

vinblastine sulfate

vin-**blass**-teen
(Oncovin[AUS], Velban, Velbe[AUS])
Do not confuse vinblastine with vincristine or vinorelbine.

CATEGORY AND SCHEDULE
Pregnancy Risk Category: D

MECHANISM OF ACTION
A vinca alkaloid that binds to microtubular protein of mitotic spindle, causing metaphase arrest. **Therapeutic Effect:** Inhibits cell division.

PHARMACOKINETICS
Does not cross the blood-brain barrier. Protein binding: 75%. Metabolized in the liver to active metabolite. Primarily eliminated in feces by biliary system. ***Half-life:*** 24.8 hr.

AVAILABILITY
Injection: 1 mg/ml.
Powder for Injection: 10 mg.

INDICATIONS AND DOSAGES
▸ Remission induction in advanced testicular carcinoma, advanced mycosis fungoides, breast carcinoma, choriocarcinoma, disseminated Hodgkin's disease, non-Hodgkin's lymphoma, Kaposi's sarcoma, or Letterer-Siwe disease
IV
Adults, Elderly. Initially, 3.7 mg/m^2 as a single dose. Increase dose by about 1.8 mg/m^2 at weekly intervals until desired therapeutic response is attained, WBC count falls below 3,000/mm^3, or maximum weekly dose of 18.5 mg/m^2 is reached.
Children. Initially, 2.5 mg/m^2 as a single dose. Increase dose by about 1.25 mg/m^2 at weekly intervals until desired therapeutic response is

attained, WBC count falls below $3,000/mm^3$, or maximum weekly dose of 7.5–12.5 mg/m^2 is reached.

▸ **Maintenance dose for treatment of advanced testicular carcinoma, advanced mycosis fungoides, breast carcinoma, choriocarcinoma, disseminated Hodgkin's disease, non-Hodgkin's lymphoma, Kaposi's sarcoma, or Letterer-Siwe disease**

IV

Adults, Elderly, Children. Administer one increment less than dose required to produce WBC count of $3,000/mm^3$. Each subsequent dose given when WBC count returns to $4,000/mm^3$ and at least 7 days have elapsed since previous dose.

OFF-LABEL USES

Treatment of bladder, head and neck, kidney, or lung carcinoma; chronic myelocytic leukemia; germ cell ovarian tumors; neuroblastoma

CONTRAINDICATIONS

Bacterial infection, severe leukopenia, significant granulocytopenia (unless it stems from disease being treated)

INTERACTIONS

Drug

Antigout medications: May decrease the effects of these drugs.
Bone marrow depressants: May increase myelosuppression.
Live-virus vaccines: May potentiate virus replication, increase vaccine side effects, and decrease the patient's antibody response to the vaccine.

Herbal

None known.

Food

None known.

DIAGNOSTIC TEST EFFECTS

May increase serum uric acid levels.

IV INCOMPATIBILITIES

Cefepime (Maxipime), furosemide (Lasix)

IV COMPATIBILITIES

Allopurinol (Aloprim), cisplatin (Platinol AQ), cyclophosphamide (Cytoxan), doxorubicin (Adriamycin), etoposide (VePesid), 5-fluorouracil, gemcitabine (Gemzar), granisetron (Kytril), heparin, leucovorin, methotrexate, ondansetron (Zofran), paclitaxel (Taxol), vinorelbine (Navelbine)

SIDE EFFECTS

Frequent

Nausea, vomiting, alopecia

Occasional

Constipation or diarrhea, rectal bleeding, headache, paraesthesia (occur 4–6 hr after administration and persist for 2–10 hr); malaise; asthenia; dizziness; pain at tumor site; jaw or face pain; depression; dry mouth

Rare

Dermatitis, stomatitis, phototoxicity, hyperuricemia

SERIOUS REACTIONS

! Hematologic toxicity is manifested as leukopenia and, less commonly, anemia. The WBC count reaches its nadir 4 to 10 days after initial therapy and recovers within 7 to 14 days (21 days with high vinblastine dosages).

! Thrombocytopenia is usually mild and transient, with recovery occurring in few days.

! Hepatic insufficiency may increase the risk of toxic drug effects.

! Acute shortness of breath or bronchospasm may occur, particularly when vinblastine is administered concurrently with mitomycin.

NURSING CONSIDERATIONS

Baseline Assessment

- Give antiemetics, if ordered, to control nausea and vomiting.
- Expect to discontinue therapy if WBC and thrombocyte counts fall abruptly. However, the physician may continue the drug if it is clearly destroying tumor cells in bone marrow.
- Expect to obtain a CBC weekly or before each vinblastine dose.

Lifespan Considerations

- Vinblastine use should be avoided during pregnancy, especially in the first trimester, because it may cause fetal harm. Breast-feeding is not recommended for patients taking this drug.
- No age-related precautions have been noted in children or the elderly.

Precautions

- Use vinblastine cautiously in patients with hepatic impairment or neurotoxicity and in those who have recently received radiation therapy or chemotherapy.

Administration and Handling

◀ALERT▶ Vinblastine dosage is individualized based on the patient's clinical response and tolerance of the drug's adverse effects. When administering this drug in combination therapy, consult specific protocols for optimum dosage and sequence of drug administration.

◀ALERT▶ Wait at least 7 days and until the WBC count is at least 4,000/mm^3 before giving repeat doses.

◀ALERT▶ Because vinblastine may be carcinogenic, mutagenic, or teratogenic, handle the drug with extreme care during preparation and administration. If the solution comes in contact with the eye, irrigate the eye with water immediately to prevent severe eye irritation and possible corneal ulceration.

IV

◀ALERT▶ Give vinblastine by IV injection. Use extreme caution in calculating the dosage and administering the drug because overdose may result in serious or fatal outcomes. Know that leakage from the IV site into surrounding tissue may produce extreme irritation.

- Refrigerate unopened vials.
- The solution normally appears clear and colorless. Discard the solution if it becomes discolored or contains a precipitate.
- After reconstitution, the solution is stable for up to 30 days if refrigerated.
- Reconstitute the 10-mg vial with 10 ml 0.9% NaCl preserved with phenol or benzyl alcohol to provide a concentration of 1 mg/ml.
- Inject the dose into the tubing of a running IV infusion or directly into a vein over 1 minute.
- Don't inject the drug into an extremity with impaired or potentially impaired circulation caused by an invading neoplasm, phlebitis, or varicosity.
- Be aware that extravasation may result in cellulitis, phlebitis, and tissue sloughing. If extravasation occurs, stop the injection immediately, notify the physician, administer hyaluronidase locally, if ordered, and apply warm compresses to the affected area.
- After completing administration directly into a vein, withdraw a minute amount of venous blood before withdrawing the needle to minimize the risk of extravasation.

Intervention and Evaluation

- Be alert for signs and symptoms of infection if the patient's WBC count falls below 2,000/mm^3.
- Assess the patient for signs and

symptoms of stomatitis, including burning or erythema of oral mucosa, difficulty swallowing, oral ulceration, and sore throat.
• Monitor the patient for signs and symptoms of hematologic toxicity, including excessive fatigue and weakness, ecchymosis, fever, signs of local infection, sore throat, and unusual bleeding from any site.
• Assess the patient's pattern of daily bowel activity and stool consistency. Take measures to prevent constipation.

Patient Teaching

• Warn the patient to immediately notify the physician if pain or burning occurs at the injection site during administration.
• Inform the patient that he or she may experience pain at the tumor site during or shortly after vinblastine injection.
• Urge the patient not to receive vaccinations and to avoid contact with crowds and those with known infections.
• Caution the patient to promptly notify the physician if he or she experiences easy bruising, fever, signs of local infection, sore throat, or unusual bleeding from any site.
• Instruct the patient to notify the physician if nausea and vomiting continue at home.
• Teach the patient measures to avoid constipation, such as increasing intake of fluids and fiber and exercising.
• Encourage the patient to maintain fastidious oral hygiene.
• Inform the patient that alopecia is reversible but that new hair may have a different color and texture.

vincristine sulfate

vin-**cris**-teen
(Oncovin, Vincasar PFS)
Do not confuse vincristine with vinblastine, or Oncovin with Ancobon.

CATEGORY AND SCHEDULE

Pregnancy Risk Category: D

MECHANISM OF ACTION

A vinca alkaloid that binds to microtubular protein of mitotic spindle, causing metaphase arrest. **Therapeutic Effect:** Inhibits cell division.

PHARMACOKINETICS

Does not cross the blood-brain barrier. Protein binding: 75%. Metabolized in the liver. Primarily eliminated in feces by biliary system. ***Half-life:*** 10–37 hr.

AVAILABILITY

Injection: 1 mg/ml.

INDICATIONS AND DOSAGES

▸ **Acute leukemia, advanced non-Hodgkin's lymphoma, disseminated Hodgkin's disease, neuroblastoma, rhabdomyosarcoma, Wilms' tumor**

IV

Adults, Elderly. 0.4–1.4 mg/m^2 once a week.
Children. 1–2 mg/m^2 once a week.
Children weighing less than 10 kg or with a body surface area less than 1 m^2. 0.05 mg/kg. Maximum: 2 mg.

▸ **Dosage in hepatic impairment**

Reduce dosage by 50% in patients with a direct serum bilirubin concentration more than 3 mg/dl.

OFF-LABEL USES

Treatment of breast, cervical, colorectal, lung, and ovarian carcinomas; chronic lymphocytic and chronic myelocytic leukemias; germ cell ovarian tumors; idiopathic thrombocytopenic purpura; malignant melanoma; multiple myeloma; mycosis fungoides

CONTRAINDICATIONS

Patients receiving radiation therapy through ports that include the liver

INTERACTIONS

Drug

Asparaginase, neurotoxic medications: May increase the risk of neurotoxicity.
Antigout medications: May decrease the effects of these drugs.
Doxorubicin: May increase the risk of myelosuppression.
Live-virus vaccines: May potentiate virus replication, increase vaccine side effects, and decrease the patient's antibody response to the vaccine.

Herbal

None known.

Food

None known.

DIAGNOSTIC TEST EFFECTS

May increase serum uric acid levels.

IV INCOMPATIBILITIES

Cefepime (Maxipime), furosemide (Lasix), idarubicin (Idamycin)

IV COMPATIBILITIES

Allopurinol (Aloprim), cisplatin (Platinol AQ), cyclophosphamide (Cytoxan), cytarabine (Ara-C, Cytosar), doxorubicin (Adriamycin), etoposide (VePesid), 5-fluorouracil, gemcitabine (Gemzar), granisetron (Kytril), leucovorin, methotrexate, ondansetron (Zofran), paclitaxel (Taxol), vinorelbine (Navelbine)

SIDE EFFECTS

Expected
Peripheral neuropathy (occurs in nearly every patient; first clinical sign is depression of Achilles tendon reflex)
Frequent
Peripheral paraesthesia, alopecia, constipation or obstipation (upper colon impaction with empty rectum), abdominal cramps, headache, jaw pain, hoarseness, diplopia, ptosis or drooping of eyelid, urinary tract disturbances
Occasional
Nausea, vomiting, diarrhea, abdominal distention, stomatitis, fever
Rare
Mild leukopenia, mild anemia, thrombocytopenia

SERIOUS REACTIONS

! Acute shortness of breath and bronchospasm may occur, especially when vincristine is administered concurrently with mitomycin.
! Prolonged or high-dose therapy may produce foot or wrist drop, difficulty walking, slapping gait, ataxia, and muscle wasting.
! Acute uric acid nephropathy may occur.

NURSING CONSIDERATIONS

Baseline Assessment

- Monitor the patient's hematologic status, liver and renal function test results, and serum uric acid levels.

Lifespan Considerations

- Vincristine use should be avoided during pregnancy, especially in the first trimester, because it may cause fetal harm. Breast-feeding is not recommended for patients taking this drug.
- No age-related precautions have been noted in children.

• The elderly are more susceptible to the drug's neurotoxic effects.

Precautions

• Use vincristine cautiously in patients with hepatic impairment, neurotoxicity, or pre-existing neuromuscular disease.

Administration and Handling

◀ **ALERT** ▶ Vincristine dosage is individualized based on the patient's clinical response and tolerance of the drug's adverse effects. When administering this drug in combination therapy, consult specific protocols for optimum dosage and sequence of drug administration.

◀ **ALERT** ▶ Because vincristine may be carcinogenic, mutagenic, or teratogenic, handle the drug with extreme care during preparation and administration.

IV

◀ **ALERT** ▶ Give vincristine by IV injection. Use extreme caution in calculating the dosage and administering the drug because overdose may result in serious or fatal outcomes.

• Refrigerate unopened vials.
• The solution normally appears clear and colorless. Discard the solution if it becomes discolored or contains a precipitate.
• Vincristine may be given undiluted.
• Inject the dose into the tubing of a running IV infusion or directly into a vein over more than 1 minute.
• Don't inject vincristine into an extremity with impaired or potentially impaired circulation caused by an invading neoplasm, phlebitis, or varicosity.
• Be aware that extravasation produces burning, edema, and stinging at the injection site. If this occurs, stop the injection immediately, notify the physician, inject hyaluronidase locally, if ordered, and apply heat to the affected area to disperse vincristine and minimize cellulitis and discomfort.

Intervention and Evaluation

• Assess the patient's Achilles tendon reflex for evidence of peripheral neuropathy.
• Assess the patient's pattern of daily bowel activity and stool consistency.
• Monitor the patient for development of diplopia or ptosis.
• Evaluate the patient's urine output for changes.

Patient Teaching

• Warn the patient to immediately notify the physician if pain or burning occurs at the injection site during administration.
• Urge the patient not to receive vaccinations and to avoid contact with crowds and those with known infections.
• Advise the patient to notify the physician if nausea and vomiting continue at home.
• Teach the patient to recognize the signs of peripheral neuropathy.
• Instruct the patient to notify the physician if he or she experiences easy bruising, fever, signs of infection, sore throat, shortness of breath, or unusual bleeding from any site.
• Inform the patient that alopecia is reversible but that new hair may have a different color and texture.

vinorelbine

vin-oh-**rell**-bean
(Navelbine)
Do not confuse vinorelbine with vinblastine.

CATEGORY AND SCHEDULE

Pregnancy Risk Category: D

MECHANISM OF ACTION
A semisynthetic vinca alkaloid that interferes with mitotic microtubule assembly. **Therapeutic Effect:** Prevents cell division.

PHARMACOKINETICS
Widely distributed after IV administration. Protein binding: 80%–90%. Metabolized in the liver. Primarily eliminated in feces by biliary system. ***Half-life:*** 28–43 hr.

AVAILABILITY
Injection: 10 mg/ml (1-ml, 5-ml vials).

INDICATIONS AND DOSAGES
▸ **Unresectable, advanced non–small cell lung cancer (as monotherapy or in combination with cisplatin)**
IV
Adults, Elderly. 30 mg/m^2 administered weekly over 6–10 min.
▸ **Dosage adjustment guidelines**
Dosage adjustments should be based on granulocyte count obtained on the day of treatment, as follows:

Granulocyte Count (cells/mm^3) on Day of Treatment	Dose
1,500 or higher	30 mg/m^2
1,000–1,499	15 mg/m^2
less than 1,000	Do not administer

▸ **Combination therapy (with cisplatin)**
IV Injection
Adults, Elderly. 25 mg/m^2 every week or 30 mg/m^2 on days 1 and 29, then q6wk.

OFF-LABEL USES
Treatment of breast cancer, cisplatin-resistant ovarian carcinoma, Hodgkin's disease

CONTRAINDICATIONS
Granulocyte count before treatment of less than 1,000 cells/mm^3

INTERACTIONS
Drug
Bone marrow depressants: May increase the risk of myelosuppression.
Cisplatin: Significantly increases the risk of granulocytopenia.
Live-virus vaccines: May potentiate virus replication, increase vaccine side effects, and decrease the patient's antibody response to the vaccine.
Mitomycin: May produce an acute pulmonary reaction.
Herbal
None known.
Food
None known.

DIAGNOSTIC TEST EFFECTS
May increase total serum bilirubin and AST (SGOT) levels and liver function test results. Decreases granulocyte, leukocyte, thrombocyte, and RBC counts.

IV INCOMPATIBILITIES
Acyclovir (Zovirax), allopurinol (Aloprim), amphotericin B (Fungizone), amphotericin B complex (Abelcet, AmBisome, Amphotec), ampicillin (Omnipen), cefazolin (Ancef), cefoperazone (Cefobid), cefotetan (Cefotan), ceftriaxone (Rocephin), cefuroxime (Zinacef), 5-fluorouracil, furosemide (Lasix), ganciclovir (Cytovene), methylprednisolone (Solu-Medrol), sodium bicarbonate

IV COMPATIBILITIES

Calcium gluconate, carboplatin (Paraplatin), cisplatin (Platinol AQ), cyclophosphamide (Cytoxan), cytarabine (ARA-C, Cytosar), dacarbazine (DTIC-Dome), daunorubicin (Cerubidine), dexamethasone (Decadron), diphenhydramine (Benadryl), doxorubicin (Adriamycin), etoposide (VePesid), gemcitabine (Gemzar), granisetron (Kytril), hydromorphone (Dilaudid), idarubicin (Idamycin), methotrexate, morphine, ondansetron (Zofran), teniposide (Vumon), vinblastine (Velban), vincristine (Oncovin)

SIDE EFFECTS

Frequent

Asthenia (35%); mild or moderate nausea (34%); constipation (29%); erythema, pain, or vein discoloration at injection site (28%); fatigue (27%); peripheral neuropathy manifested as paraesthesia and hyperesthesia (25%); diarrhea (17%); alopecia (12%)

Occasional

Phlebitis (10%), dyspnea (7%), loss of deep tendon reflexes (5%)

Rare

Chest pain, jaw pain, myalgia, arthralgia, rash

SERIOUS REACTIONS

! Bone marrow depression is manifested mainly as granulocytopenia, which may be severe. Other hematologic toxicities, including neutropenia, thrombocytopenia, leukopenia, and anemia, increase the risk of infection and bleeding.

! Acute shortness of breath and severe bronchospasm occur infrequently, particularly in patients with pre-existing pulmonary dysfunction and in those receiving mitomycin concurrently.

NURSING CONSIDERATIONS

Baseline Assessment

• Review the patient's medication history.
• Assess the patient's hematologic values, including blood Hgb level and platelet count, before giving each vinorelbine dose.
• Know that granulocyte count should be at least 1,000 cells/mm^3 before vinorelbine administration and that granulocyte nadir occurs 7–10 days after a dose.
• Be aware that hematologic growth factors should not be given within 24 hours before or after administration of chemotherapy.

Lifespan Considerations

• Vinorelbine use should be avoided during pregnancy, especially during the first trimester, because it may cause fetal harm. Breast-feeding is not recommended for patients taking this drug.
• The safety and efficacy of vinorelbine have not been established in children.
• No age-related precautions have been noted in the elderly.

Precautions

• Use vinorelbine extremely cautiously in immunocompromised patients.
• Use the drug cautiously in patients with current or recent chickenpox, herpes zoster, impaired pulmonary function, infection, leukopenia, and severe liver injury or hepatic impairment.

Administration and Handling

◀ALERT▶ Know that the patient's granulocyte count should be at least 1,000 cells/mm^3 before vinorelbine administration.

◀ALERT▶ Be careful to correctly position the IV needle or catheter before vinorelbine administration because leakage into surrounding tissue produces extreme irritation, local tissue necrosis, or thrombophlebitis. Wear gloves when preparing the solution. If the solution comes in contact with skin or mucosa, wash the affected area immediately and thoroughly with soap and water.

IV

- Refrigerate unopened vials and protect them from light.
- Unopened vials are stable at room temperature for up to 72 hours.
- Don't administer the solution if it contains particulate matter.
- Vinorelbine must be diluted and administered by syringe or IV bag.
- For administration by syringe, dilute the calculated vinorelbine dose with D_5W or 0.9% NaCl to a concentration of 1.5 to 3 mg/ml.
- For administration by IV bag, dilute the calculated vinorelbine dose with D_5W, 0.45% or 0.9% NaCl, Ringer's solution, or lactated Ringer's solution to a concentration of 0.5 to 2 mg/ml.
- Diluted vinorelbine is stable for up to 24 hours when stored in polypropylene syringes or polyvinyl chloride bags at room temperature and in normal room light.
- Administer diluted vinorelbine over 6 to 10 minutes into the side port of a free-flowing IV line closest to the IV bag; then flush the vein with 75 to 125 ml of one of the solutions.
- If extravasation occurs, stop the injection immediately notify the physician, inject hyaluronidase locally, if ordered, and apply heat to the affected area to disperse the drug and minimize cellulitis and discomfort. Also, administer the remainder of the dose in another vein.

Intervention and Evaluation

- Diligently monitor the injection site for pain, redness, and swelling.
- Frequently monitor the patient for signs and symptoms of myelosuppression both during and after vinorelbine therapy.
- Assess the patient for signs and symptoms of hematologic toxicity, including excessive fatigue and weakness, ecchymosis, fever, signs of local infection, sore throat, and unusual bleeding from any site.
- Monitor patients who develop severe granulocytopenia for evidence of infection or fever.
- Give the patient crackers, dry toast, and cola to help relieve nausea.
- Assess the patient's pattern of daily bowel activity and stool consistency.
- Determine if the patient experiences burning, numbness, or tingling of the feet and hands, which are symptoms of peripheral neuropathy, or complains of feeling like "walking on glass," which is a symptom of hyperesthesia.

Patient Teaching

- Instruct the patient to immediately report pain, redness, or swelling at the injection site.
- Warn the patient to notify the physician if he or she experiences difficulty breathing, easy bruising, fever, signs of local infection, sore throat, or unusual bleeding from any site.
- Urge the patient not to receive vaccinations and to avoid contact with crowds and those with known infections.
- Caution the patient to avoid pregnancy during vinorelbine therapy.
- Explain to the patient that alopecia is reversible but that new hair may have a different color and texture.

17 Cytoprotective Agents

amifostine
dexrazoxane
mesna

Uses: During antineoplastic therapy, specific cytoprotective agents are used to help prevent or reduce the severity of specific adverse reactions. For example, *amifostine* may be used to reduce nephrotoxicity caused by cisplatin and other alkylating agents and to minimize xerostomia caused by radiation therapy. *Dexrazoxane* reduces the risk of cardiomyopathy related to doxorubicin therapy. *Mesna* protects against hemorrhagic cystitis, which may result from cyclophosphamide or ifosfamide.

Action: Each cytoprotective agent works by a different action. *Amifostine* is converted to an active metabolite that binds with and detoxifies the reactive metabolites of cisplatin and other alkylating agents. In myocardial cell membranes, *dexrazoxane* binds with intracellular iron, preventing the generation of free radicals by the anthracycline doxorubicin. *Mesna* binds with and detoxifies the urotoxic metabolites of cyclophosphamide and ifosfamide.

amifostine

am-ih-**fos**-teen
(Ethyol)
Do not confuse Ethyol with ethanol.

CATEGORY AND SCHEDULE

Pregnancy Risk Category: C

MECHANISM OF ACTION

An antineoplastic adjunct and cytoprotective agent that is converted to an active metabolite by alkaline phosphatase in tissues. The active metabolite binds to and detoxifies metabolites of cisplatin. These actions occur more readily in normal tissues than in tumor tissue. **Therapeutic Effect:** Reduces the toxic effect of the chemotherapeutic agent cisplatin.

PHARMACOKINETICS

Rapidly cleared from plasma. Converted in tissue to active free thiol metabolite. Tissue uptake highest in bone marrow, skin, GI mucosa, salivary glands. ***Half-life:*** less than 1 minute. Less than 10% remains in plasma 6 min after drug administration.

AVAILABILITY

Powder for Injection: 500 mg in a 10-ml single-use vial.

INDICATIONS AND DOSAGES

▸ **To reduce cumulative renal toxicity from repeated administration of cisplatin in patients with advanced ovarian cancer**

IV

Adults. 910 mg/m^2 once a day as

15-min infusion, beginning 30 min before chemotherapy. A 15-min infusion is better tolerated than extended infusions. If the full dose can't be administered, dose for subsequent cycles should be 740 mg/m^2.

▸ **Treatment of postoperative radiation-induced xerostomia in patients with head and neck cancer**

IV

Adults. 200 mg/m^2 once a day as 3-min infusion, starting 15–30 min before radiation therapy.

Subcutaneous

Adults. 500 mg/day during radiation therapy.

OFF-LABEL USES

To protect lung fibroblasts from damaging effects of chemotherapeutic agent paclitaxel

CONTRAINDICATIONS

Sensitivity to aminothiol compounds or mannitol

INTERACTIONS

Drug

Antihypertensive medications or drugs that may potentiate hypotension: May increase the risk of hypotension.

Herbal

None known.

Food

None known.

DIAGNOSTIC TEST EFFECTS

May reduce serum calcium levels, especially in patients with nephrotic syndrome.

IV INCOMPATIBILITIES

Don't mix amifostine in any solution other than 0.9% NaCl.

IV COMPATIBILITIES

Mannitol, potassium chloride

SIDE EFFECTS

Frequent (62%)

Transient reduction in BP (usually starts 14 min into infusion, lasts about 6 min and returns to normal in 5–15 min); severe nausea, vomiting

Occasional (20%–10%)

Flushing or feeling of warmth or chills or feeling of coldness; dizziness, hiccups, sneezing, somnolence

Rare (less than 1%)

Clinically relevant hypocalcemia, mild rash

SERIOUS REACTIONS

! A pronounced drop in BP may require temporary cessation of amifostine and fluid resuscitation.

NURSING CONSIDERATIONS

Baseline Assessment

• Make sure the patient is adequately hydrated before beginning the infusion.

Precautions

• Use amifostine cautiously in patients with uncorrected dehydration or hpotension or pre-existing cardiovascular or cerebrovascular conditions, such as arrhythmias, CHF, ischemic heart disease, and a history of cerebrovascular accident or transient ischemic attack.

• Use the drug cautiously in patients receiving antihypertensive therapy that cannot be discontinued 24 hours before amifostine treatment begins and in patients receiving chemotherapy for potentially curable malignancies.

Administration and Handling

IV

• Don't use the solution if it is discolored or contains particulate matter.

• Reconstitute with 9.7 ml 0.9% NaCl. The reconstituted solution remains stable for 5 hours at room temperature or 24 hours if refrigerated.
• Further dilute with 0.9% NaCl for a concentration of 5 to 40 mg/ml.
• Administer amifostine over 15 minutes, beginning about 30 minutes before chemotherapy or 15 to 30 minutes before radiation therapy of the head and neck.
• Keep the patient in the supine position during the infusion.
• Monitor BP every 5 minutes during the infusion.
• Stop the infusion if systolic BP decreases significantly from baseline (for a baseline of less than 100 mm Hg, a drop of 20 mm Hg; for a baseline of 100 to 119 mm Hg, a drop of 25 mm Hg; for a baseline of 120 to 139 mm Hg, a drop of 30 mm Hg; for a baseline of 140 to 179 mm Hg, a drop of 40 mm Hg; for a baseline of more than 180 mm Hg, a drop of 50 mm Hg). If systolic BP returns to normal within 5 minutes and the patient appears asymptomatic, restart the infusion so that the full dose can be administered.

◀**ALERT**▶ If hypotension requires interruption of therapy, place the patient in the Trendelenburg position and administer a bolus infusion of normal saline solution through a separate IV line.
• Because amifostine may cause severe nausea and vomiting, administer an antiemetic, IV dexamethasone 20 mg, and a serotonin receptor antagonist before and concurrently with amifostine.

Intervention and Evaluation

• Carefully monitor the patient's fluid balance to ensure adequate hydration.
• Monitor serum calcium levels in patients at risk for hypocalcemia or nephrotic syndrome.

Patient Teaching

• Instruct the patient to remain lying down during the infusion.
• Inform the patient that BP will be monitored frequently.
• Advise the patient to immediately report chills, nausea, vomiting, a rash, or other side effects.

dexrazoxane

dex-rah-**zox**-ann
(Zinecard)

CATEGORY AND SCHEDULE
Pregnancy Risk Category: C

MECHANISM OF ACTION

An antineoplastic adjunct and cytoprotective agent that binds to intracellular iron in myocardial cell membranes preventing the generation of free radicals by anthracyclines such as doxorubicin. **Therapeutic Effect:** Protects against anthracycline-induced cardiomyopathy.

PHARMACOKINETICS

Rapidly distributed after IV administration. Not bound to plasma proteins. Primarily excreted in urine. Removed by peritoneal dialysis. ***Half-life:*** 2.1–2.5 hr.

AVAILABILITY

Powder for Injection: 250 mg (10 mg/ml reconstituted in 25-ml single-use vial), 500 mg (10 mg/ml reconstituted in 50-ml single-use vial).

INDICATIONS AND DOSAGES

▶ **Reduction of incidence and severity of cardiomyopathy associated with doxorubicin therapy in women with metastatic breast cancer**

IV

Adults, Children. Recommended dosage ratio is 10 parts dexrazoxane to 1 part doxorubicin (for example, 500 mg/m^2 dexrazoxane for every 50 mg/m^2 doxorubicin).

CONTRAINDICATIONS

Chemotherapy regimens that don't contain an anthracycline

INTERACTIONS

Drug

Concurrent FAC (5-fluorouracil, Adriamycin, cyclophosphamide) therapy: May produce severe blood dyscrasias.

Herbal

None known.

Food

None known.

DIAGNOSTIC TEST EFFECTS

Concurrent FAC therapy may produce abnormal liver or renal function test results.

IV INCOMPATIBILITIES

Don't mix dexrazoxane with other medications.

SIDE EFFECTS

Frequent

Alopecia, nausea, vomiting, fatigue, malaise, anorexia, stomatitis, fever, infection, diarrhea

Occasional

Pain at injection site, neurotoxicity, phlebitis, dysphagia, streaking or erythema at injection site

Rare

Urticaria, skin reaction

SERIOUS REACTIONS

! Patients receiving FAC therapy concurrently with dexrazoxane are at increased risk for severe leukopenia, granulocytopenia, and thrombocytopenia.

! In case of overdose, excess dexrazoxane can be removed with peritoneal dialysis or hemodialysis.

NURSING CONSIDERATIONS

Baseline Assessment

- Give antiemetics, if ordered, to prevent or treat nausea.

Lifespan Considerations

- Dexrazoxane may be embryotoxic or teratogenic. It is unknown if dexrazoxane is distributed in breast milk; however, breast-feeding is not recommended for patients taking this drug.
- The safety and efficacy of dexrazoxane have not been established in children.
- No information is available on dexrazoxane use in the elderly.

Precautions

- Use dexrazoxane cautiously in patients taking chemotherapeutic agents that increase the risk of myelosuppression or those also receiving FAC therapy.

Administration and Handling

◀ **ALERT** ▶ Dexrazoxane should be used only in patients who have received a cumulative doxorubicin dose of 300 mg/m^2 and are continuing with doxorubicin therapy.

◀ **ALERT** ▶ Don't mix dexrazoxane with other drugs. Use caution and wear gloves when handling and preparing the solution. If the powder or solution comes in contact with skin, wash immediately with soap and water.

IV

- Store vials at room temperature.
- The reconstituted solution is stable

for up to 6 hours at room temperature or if refrigerated. Discard any unused portion.
• Reconstitute with 0.167 molar (M/6) sodium lactate injection to provide a concentration of 10 mg dexrazoxane for each ml of sodium lactate.
• The solution may be further diluted with 0.9% NaCl or D_5W to a concentration of 1.3 to 5 mg/ml.
• Administer the reconstituted solution by slow IV push or IV infusion over 15 to 30 minutes.
• After the dexrazoxane infusion is completed, and within 30 minutes of starting the infusion, administer doxorubicin by IV injection.

Intervention and Evaluation

• Frequently monitor the patient's CBC with differential for evidence of blood dyscrasias.
• Monitor the patient for signs and symptoms of stomatitis, including burning or erythema of oral mucosa, difficulty swallowing, and sore throat.
• Monitor the patient's cardiac function, hematologic status, and liver and renal function studies.
• Assess the patient's pattern of daily bowel activity and stool consistency.
• Monitor the patient for signs and symptoms of hematologic toxicity, including ecchymosis, fever, signs of local infection, sore throat, and unusual bleeding from any site.

Patient Teaching

• Warn the patient to notify the physician if he or she experiences fever, signs of local infection, or sore throat or if nausea and vomiting persist at home.
• Instruct the patient to maintain fastidious oral hygiene.
• Inform the patient that hair growth will resume 2 to 3 months after the last dose of dexrazoxane but that new hair may have a different color or texture.

mesna

mess-na
(Mesnex, Uromitexan[CAN])

CATEGORY AND SCHEDULE

Pregnancy Risk Category: B

MECHANISM OF ACTION

An antineoplastic adjunct and cytoprotective agent that binds with and detoxifies urotoxic metabolites of ifosfamide and cyclophosphamide. **Therapeutic Effect:** Inhibits ifosfamide- and cyclophosphamide-induced hemorrhagic cystitis.

PHARMACOKINETICS

Rapidly metabolized after IV administration to mesna disulfide, which is reduced to mesna in kidney. Excreted in urine. ***Half-life:*** 24 min.

AVAILABILITY

Tablets: 400 mg.
Injection: 100 mg/ml.

INDICATIONS AND DOSAGES

▸ Prevention of hemorrhagic cystitis in patients receiving ifosfamide

IV

Adults, Elderly. 20% of ifosfamide dose at time of ifosfamide administration and 4 and 8 hr after each dose of ifosfamide. Total dose: 60% of ifosfamide dosage. Range: 60%–160% of the daily ifosfamide dose.

▸ Prevention of hemorrhagic cystitis in patients receiving cyclophosphamide

PO

Adults, Elderly. 40% of cyclophosphamide dose q4h for 3 doses.

IV
Adults, Elderly. 20% of cyclophosphamide dose at time of cyclophosphamide administration and q3h for 3–4 doses.

CONTRAINDICATIONS
None known.

INTERACTIONS
Drug
None known.
Herbal
None known.
Food
None known.

DIAGNOSTIC TEST EFFECTS
May produce false-positive test result for urinary ketones.

IV INCOMPATIBILITIES
Amphotericin B complex (Abelcet, AmBisome, Amphotec)

IV COMPATIBILITIES
Allopurinol (Aloprim), docetaxel (Taxotere), doxorubicin (Adriamycin), etoposide (VePesid), gemcitabine (Gemzar), granisetron (Kytril), methotrexate, ondansetron (Zofran), paclitaxel (Taxol), vinorelbine (Navelbine)

SIDE EFFECTS
Frequent (more than 17%)
Bad taste, soft stools
Large doses: Diarrhea, myalgia, headache, fatigue, nausea, hypotension, allergic reaction

SERIOUS REACTIONS
! Hematuria occurs rarely.

NURSING CONSIDERATIONS
Baseline Assessment
◀**ALERT**▶ Administer each mesna dose with ifosfamide, as prescribed.

Lifespan Considerations
- It is unknown if mesna crosses the placenta or is distributed in breast milk.
- The safety and efficacy of mesna have not been established in children.
- No information is available on mesna use in the elderly.

Administration and Handling
PO
- Dilute mesna solution in carbonated cola, fruit juices, or milk before oral administration to decrease sulfur odor, if desired.

IV
- Store parenteral form at room temperature.
- After reconstitution, the solution is stable for up to 24 hours at room temperature. Use is recommended within 6 hours. Discard unused medication.
- Dilute with D_5W or 0.9% NaCl to concentration of 1 to 20 mg/ml, as appropriate.
- Add mesna to solutions containing ifosfamide or cyclophosphamide, as appropriate.
- Administer the drug by IV infusion (piggyback) over 15 to 30 minutes or by continuous infusion.

Intervention and Evaluation
- Test the patient's morning urine specimen for hematuria. If hematuria occurs, mesna may need to be discontinued or dosage reduced.
- Assess the patient's pattern of daily bowel activity and stool consistency. Record the time of evacuation.
- Monitor the patient's BP for hypotension.

Patient Teaching
- Warn the patient to notify the physician or nurse if he or she experiences headache, myalgia, or nausea.

18 Hormones

abarelix
anastrozole
bicalutamide
exemestane
flutamide
fulvestrant
goserelin acetate
letrozole
leuprolide acetate
megestrol acetate
nilutamide
tamoxifen citrate
toremifene citrate
triptorelin pamoate

Uses: In antineoplastic therapy, hormones are used to treat cancers that are hormone dependent, including cancer of the breasts, endometrium, and prostate. Antineoplastic hormones are less toxic than other antineoplastic agents.

Action: Antineoplastic hormones may act as agonists that inhibit tumor cell growth or as antagonists that compete with endogenous hormones. These agents include *antiandrogens,* such as bicalutamide, flutamide, and nilutamide; *antiestrogens,* such as fulvestrant and tamoxifen; *aromatase inhibitors,* such as anastrozole and letrozole; *progestins,* such as megestrol; and *gonadotropin-releasing hormone analogues,* such as goserelin and leuprolide. Antiandrogens act primarily by inhibiting androgen uptake or preventing androgen from binding to androgen receptors in target tissue. Antiestrogens compete with endogenous estrogen at estrogen-receptor binding sites. Aromatase inhibitors interfere with aromatase, the enzyme that catalyzes the final step in estrogen production; this, in turn, decreases circulating estrogen levels. Progestins suppress the release of luteinizing hormone (LH) from the anterior pituitary gland. Gonadotropin-releasing hormone analogues stimulate the release of LH and follicle-stimulating hormone from the anterior pituitary gland.

abarelix

ah-**bar**-eh-lex
(Plenaxis)

CATEGORY AND SCHEDULE

Pregnancy Risk Category: X

MECHANISM OF ACTION

A luteinizing hormone-releasing hormone (LHRH) antagonist that inhibits gonadotropin and androgen production by blocking gonadotropin-releasing hormone receptors in the pituitary. **Therapeutic Effect:** Suppresses luteinizing hormone, follicle-stimulating hormone secretion, reducing the secretion of testosterone by the testes.

PHARMACOKINETICS

Slowly absorbed following intramuscular administration. Distributed extensively. Protein binding: 96%–99%. ***Half-life:*** 13.2 days.

AVAILABILITY

Powder for Injection: 113 mg kit containing 10 ml 0.9% NaCl, 18-gauge needle, 22-gauge needle.

INDICATIONS AND DOSAGES

▸ **Prostate cancer**

IM

Adults, Elderly. 100 mg on days 1, 15, 29 and every 4 weeks thereafter. Treatment failure can be detected by obtaining serum testosterone concentration prior to abarelix administration, day 19 and every 8 weeks thereafter.

CONTRAINDICATIONS

This drug should not be used in women and children

INTERACTIONS

Drug

None known.

Herbal

None known.

Food

None known.

DIAGNOSTIC TEST EFFECTS

May increase serum transaminase, serum AST (SGOT), ALT (SGPT), and serum triglyceride levels. May slightly decrease blood hemoglobin concentrations. May decrease bone mineral density.

SIDE EFFECTS

Frequent (79%–30%)

Hot flashes, sleep disturbances, breast enlargement

Occasional (20%–11%)

Breast pain, nipple tenderness, back pain, constipation, peripheral edema, dizziness, upper respiratory tract infection, diarrhea

Rare (10%)

Fatigue, nausea, dysuria, micturition frequency, urinary retention, urinary tract infection

SERIOUS REACTIONS

! Immediate-onset systemic allergic reaction characterized by hypotension, urticaria, pruritus, periorbital and/or circumoral edema, shortness of breath, wheezing, and syncope may occur.

! Prolongation of the QT interval may occur. Tightening of throat, tongue swelling, wheezing, shortness of breath, and low blood pressure occur rarely.

NURSING CONSIDERATIONS

Baseline Assessment

- Inform patient of the duration of treatment and required monitoring procedures.
- Plan to obtain serum transaminase levels prior to treatment and periodically thereafter.

Lifespan Considerations

- Be aware that this drug is not for use in women or children.
- Be aware that there are no age-related precautions noted in the elderly.

Precautions

- Use cautiously in patients with a prolonged QT interval or who weigh more than 225 lbs (103 kg).

Administration and Handling

IM

- Store at room temperature. Shake abarelix vial gently before reconstituting.
- Withdraw 2.2 ml of 0.9% NaCl using 18-gauge needle and a 3-ml syringe.
- Insert the needle into the abarelix vial and inject the diluent quickly.
- Shake immediately for 15 seconds.
- Allow vial to stand for 2 minutes.
- Tap the vial to reduce foaming and swirl the vial.
- Shake the vial again for 15 seconds and allow to stand again for 2 minutes.

• Insert 18-gauge needle, invert the vial, and draw up some of the suspension into the syringe. Without removing the needle from the vial, re-inject it at any remaining solids in the vial. Repeat this process until all solids are dispersed.
• Swirl the vial before withdrawal, then withdraw the entire contents, about 2.2 ml.
• Reconstitution will provide a concentration of 50 mg/ml and should be used within 1 hour of reconstitution.
• Exchange the 18-gauge needle with the 22-gauge needle and give entire suspension IM into the dorsogluteal or ventrogluteal region of the buttock.
• Monitor the patient for 30 minutes. The cumulative risk for allergic reaction increases with each injection.

Intervention and Evaluation

• Measure serum testosterone concentration prior to administration beginning on day 29 and every 8 weeks therafter.
• Periodically monitor the patient's serum PSA levels.

Patient Teaching

• Make sure the patient and caregiver know about preparing and injecting the drug, if the patient is to take it at home.
• Be sure to immediately notify the physician if the patient develops rash, hives, itching, tingling, or flushing. The skin reaction may occur immediately after injection or several days later.
• Tell the patient about potential side effects, including hot flashes, sleep disturbances, breast enlargement, and nipple tenderness.

anastrozole

ah-**nas**-trow-zole
(Arimidex)
Do not confuse Arimidex with Imitrex.

CATEGORY AND SCHEDULE

Pregnancy Risk Category: D

MECHANISM OF ACTION

Decreases the circulating estrogen level by inhibiting aromatase, the enzyme that catalyzes the final step in estrogen production. **Therapeutic Effect:** Inhibitis the growth of breast cancers that are stimulated by estrogens.

PHARMACOKINETICS

Well absorbed into systemic circulation (absorption not affected by food). Protein binding: 40%. Extensively metabolized in the liver. Eliminated by biliary system and, to a lesser extent, kidneys. ***Mean half-life:*** 50 hr in postmenopausal women. Steady-state plasma levels reached in about 7 days.

AVAILABILITY

Tablets: 1 mg.

INDICATIONS AND DOSAGES

▸ Breast cancer

PO

Adults, Elderly. 1 mg once a day.

CONTRAINDICATIONS

None known.

INTERACTIONS

Drug

None known.

Herbal

None known.

Food

None known.

DIAGNOSTIC TEST EFFECTS
May elevate serum GGT level in patients with liver metastasis. May increase serum LDL, serum alkaline phosphate, AST (SGOT), ALT (SGPT), and total cholesterol levels.

SIDE EFFECTS
Frequent (16%–8%)
Asthenia, nausea, headache, hot flashes, back pain, vomiting, cough, diarrhea
Occasional (6%–4%)
Constipation, abdominal pain, anorexia, bone pain, pharyngitis, dizziness, rash, dry mouth, peripheral edema, pelvic pain, depression, chest pain, paresthesia
Rare (2%–1%)
Weight gain, diaphoresis

SERIOUS REACTIONS
! Thrombophlebitis, anemia, leukopenia, and vaginal hemorrhage occur rarely.
! Vaginal hemorrhage occurs rarely (2%).

NURSING CONSIDERATIONS
Baseline Assessment
• Determine if the patient is or may be pregnant.
Lifespan Considerations
• Anastrozole is indicated only for postmenopausal women.
• Women who are or may be pregnant should not use anastrozole because the drug crosses the placenta and may cause fetal harm.
• It is unknown if anastrozole is excreted in breast milk.
• The safety and efficacy of anastrozole have not been established in children.
• No age-related precautions have been noted in the elderly.
Administration and Handling
PO
• Give anastrozole without regard to food.
Intervention and Evaluation
• Assist the patient with ambulation if weakness or dizziness occurs.
• If the patient has diarrhea, give an antidiarrheal as prescribed. If the patient is nauseous or vomiting, administer an antiemetic as prescribed.
Patient Teaching
• Instruct the patient to notify the physician if asthenia, hot flashes, and nausea become unmanageable.

bicalutamide
by-kale-**yew**-tah-myd
(Casodex, Cosudex[AUS])

CATEGORY AND SCHEDULE
Pregnancy Risk Category: X

MECHANISM OF ACTION
An antiandrogen antineoplastic agent that competitively inhibits androgen action by binding to androgen receptors in target tissue. **Therapeutic Effect:** Decreases growth of prostatic carcinoma.

PHARMACOKINETICS
Well absorbed from the GI tract. Protein binding: 96%. Metabolized in the liver to inactive metabolite. Excreted in urine and feces. Not removed by hemodialysis. ***Half-life:*** 5.8 days.

AVAILABILITY
Tablets: 50 mg.

INDICATIONS AND DOSAGES

▸ Prostatic carcinoma

PO

Adults, Elderly. 50–100 mg once a day in morning or evening, given concurrently with a luteinizing hormone-releasing hormone (LHRH) analogue or after surgical castration.

CONTRAINDICATIONS

None known.

INTERACTIONS

Drug

Warfarin: May increase warfarin's effects.

Herbal

None known.

Food

None known.

DIAGNOSTIC TEST EFFECTS

May increase BUN level and serum alkaline phosphatase, bilirubin, AST (SGOT), and ALT (SGPT) levels. May decrease blood Hgb level and WBC count.

SIDE EFFECTS

Frequent

Hot flashes (49%), breast pain (38%), muscle pain (27%), constipation (17%), diarrhea (10%), asthenia (15%), nausea (11%)

Occasional (9%–8%)

Nocturia, abdominal pain, peripheral edema

Rare (7%–3%)

Vomiting, weight loss, dizziness, insomnia, rash, impotence, gynecomastia

SERIOUS REACTIONS

! Sepsis, CHF, hypertension, and iron deficiency anemia may occur.

NURSING CONSIDERATIONS

Baseline Assessment

- Obtain liver function test results before beginning therapy.

Lifespan Considerations

- Bicalutamide may inhibit spermatogenesis; this drug is not used in women.
- The safety and efficacy of bicalutamide have not been established in children.
- No age-related precautions have been noted in the elderly.

Precautions

- Use bicalutamide cautiously in patients with moderate to severe hepatic impairment.

Administration and Handling

PO

- Give bicalutamide at the same time each day and without regard to food.

Intervention and Evaluation

- Assess the patient for diarrhea, nausea, and vomiting.

Patient Teaching

- Instruct the patient to take bicalutamide at the same time each day.
- Caution the patient against abruptly discontinuing the drug. Explain that both bicalutamide and the LHRH analogue must be continued to achieve the desired therapeutic effect.
- Inform the patient about the most common side effects.
- Advise the patient to notify the physician if nausea and vomiting persist.

exemestane

x-eh-**mess**-tane

(Aromasin)

CATEGORY AND SCHEDULE

Pregnancy Risk Category: D

MECHANISM OF ACTION

Inactivates aromatase, the principal enzyme that converts androgens to estrogens in both premenopausal and postmenopausal women, thereby lowering the circulating estrogen level. **Therapeutic Effect:** Inhibits the growth of breast cancers that are stimulated by estrogens.

PHARMACOKINETICS

Rapidly absorbed after PO administration. Protein binding: 90%. Distributed extensively into tissues. Metabolized in the liver; eliminated in urine and feces. ***Half-life:*** 24 hr.

AVAILABILITY

Tablets: 25 mg.

INDICATIONS AND DOSAGES

▸ Breast cancer

PO

Adults, Elderly. 25 mg once a day after a meal.

OFF-LABEL USES

Prevention of prostate cancer

CONTRAINDICATIONS

Hypersensitivity to exemestane

INTERACTIONS

Drug

None known.

Herbal

None known.

Food

None known.

DIAGNOSTIC TEST EFFECTS

May increase serum alkaline phosphatase, AST (SGOT), and ALT (SGPT) levels.

SIDE EFFECTS

Frequent (22%–10%)

Fatigue, nausea, depression, hot flashes, pain, insomnia, anxiety, dyspnea

Occasional (8%–5%)

Headache, dizziness, vomiting, peripheral edema, abdominal pain, anorexia, flulike symptoms, diaphoresis, constipation, hypertension

Rare (4%)

Diarrhea

SERIOUS REACTIONS

! None known.

NURSING CONSIDERATIONS

Baseline Assessment

• Document baseline vital signs, especially blood pressure, because exemestane may cause hypertension.

Lifespan Considerations

• Exemestane is indicated only for postmenopausal women.
• This drug is not used in children.
• No age-related precautions have been noted in the elderly.

Precautions

• Don't give exemestane to premenopausal women.

Administration and Handling

PO

• Give exemestane after a meal.

Intervention and Evaluation

• Monitor the patient for headache, insomnia, and signs of depression.
• Assist the patient with ambulation if dizziness occurs.
• Give antiemetics, if ordered, to prevent or treat nausea and vomiting.

Patient Teaching

• Instruct the patient to take exemestane after a meal and at the same time each day.
• Caution the patient to notify the physician if nausea or hot flashes become unmanageable.
• Advise the patient to avoid tasks that require mental alertness or motor skills until his or her response to the drug is established.

flutamide

flew-tah-myd
(Euflex[CAN], Eulexin, Flugerel[AUS], Flutamin[AUS], Fugerel[AUS], Novo-Flutamide[CAN])
Do not confuse flutamide with Flumadine.

CATEGORY AND SCHEDULE

Pregnancy Risk Category: D

MECHANISM OF ACTION

An antiandrogen hormone that inhibits androgen uptake and prevents androgen from binding to androgen receptors in target tissue. Used in conjuction with leuprolide to inhibit the stimulant effects of flutamide on serum testosterone levels. **Therapeutic Effect:** Suppresses testicular androgen production and decreases growth of prostate carcinoma.

PHARMACOKINETICS

Completely absorbed from the GI tract. Protein binding: 94%–96%. Metabolized in the liver to active metabolite. Primarily excreted in urine. Not removed by hemodialysis. ***Half-life:*** 6 hr (increased in elderly).

AVAILABILITY

Capsules: 125 mg.

INDICATIONS AND DOSAGES

▸ **Prostatic carcinoma (in combination with leuprolide)**
PO
Adults, Elderly. 250 mg q8h.

CONTRAINDICATIONS

Severe hepatic impairment

INTERACTIONS

Drug
None known.
Herbal
None known.
Food
None known.

DIAGNOSTIC TEST EFFECTS

May increase blood glucose level and serum estradiol, testosterone, bilirubin, creatinine, AST (SGOT), and ALT (SGPT) levels.

SIDE EFFECTS

Frequent
Hot flashes (50%); decreased libido, diarrhea (24%); generalized pain (23%); asthenia (17%); constipation (12%); nausea, nocturia (11%)
Occasional (8%–6%)
Dizziness, paresthesia, insomnia, impotence, peripheral edema, gynecomastia
Rare (5%–4%)
Rash, diaphoresis, hypertension, hematuria, vomiting, urinary incontinence, headache, flu-like syndromes, photosensitivity

SERIOUS REACTIONS

! Hepatoxicity, including hepatic encephalopathy, and hemolytic anemia may be noted.

NURSING CONSIDERATIONS

Baseline Assessment
• Expect to obtain liver function test results before beginning drug therapy.
Lifespan Considerations
• Flutamide is not used in pregnant women or in children.
• No age-related precautions have been noted in the elderly.

Administration and Handling

PO

- Give flutamide without regard to food.

Intervention and Evaluation

- Periodically monitor liver function test results in patients on long-term flutamide therapy.

Patient Teaching

- Caution the patient against abruptly discontinuing the drug.
- Advise the patient that urine may become amber or yellow-green during flutamide therapy.
- Encourage the patient to avoid overexposure to the sun or ultraviolet light and to wear protective clothing outdoors until his or her tolerance of ultraviolet light is determined.

fulvestrant

full-ves-trant

(Faslodex)

Do not confuse Faslodex with Fosamax.

CATEGORY AND SCHEDULE

Pregnancy Risk Category: D

MECHANISM OF ACTION

An estrogen antagonist that competes with endogenous estrogen at estrogen receptor binding sites. **Therapeutic Effect:** Inhibits tumor growth.

PHARMACOKINETICS

Extensively and rapidly distributed after IM administration. Protein binding: 99%. Metabolized in the liver. Eliminated by hepatobiliary route; excreted in feces. ***Half-life:*** 40 days in postmenopausal women. Peak serum levels occur in 7–9 days.

AVAILABILITY

Prefilled Syringe: 50 mg/ml in 2.5-ml and 5-ml syringes.

INDICATIONS AND DOSAGES

▸ **Breast cancer**

IM

Adults, Elderly. 250 mg given once monthly.

CONTRAINDICATIONS

Known or suspected pregnancy

INTERACTIONS

Drug

None known.

Herbal

None known.

Food

None known.

DIAGNOSTIC TEST EFFECTS

None known.

SIDE EFFECTS

Frequent (26%–13%)

Nausea, hot flashes, pharyngitis, asthenia, vomiting, vasodilatation, headache

Occasional (12%–5%)

Injection site pain, constipation, diarrhea, abdominal pain, anorexia, dizziness, insomnia, paresthesia, bone or back pain, depression, anxiety, peripheral edema, rash, diaphoresis, fever

Rare (2%–1%)

Vertigo, weight gain

SERIOUS REACTIONS

! UTIs, vaginitis, anemia, thromboembolic phenomena, and leukopenia occur rarely.

NURSING CONSIDERATIONS

Baseline Assessment

- Expect the patient to undergo an

estrogen receptor assay test before initiating fulvestrant therapy.
- Also expect the patient to undergo a computed tomography scan before and periodically after therapy to evaluate tumor regression.

Lifespan Considerations
- Don't administer fulvestrant to pregnant women.
- It is unknown if fulvestrant is excreted in breast milk.
- Fulvestrant is not for use in children.
- No age-related precautions have been noted in the elderly.

Precautions
- Use fulvestrant cautiously in patients receiving anticoagulant therapy and those with bleeding diathesis, estrogen receptor-negative breast cancer, hepatic disease or reduced hepatic flow, and thrombocytopenia.

Administration and Handling
IM
- Administer the drug slowly into the buttock as a single 5-ml injection or two concurrent 2.5-ml injections.

Intervention and Evaluation
- Monitor the patient's blood chemistry and plasma lipid levels.
- Evaluate the patient's level of bone pain and ensure adequate pain relief if pain increases.
- Assess the patient for edema, especially in dependent areas.
- Monitor the patient for asthenia and dizziness and provide assistance with ambulation if these symptoms occur.
- Assess the patient for headache.
- Offer the patient an antiemetic, if ordered, to prevent or treat nausea and vomiting.

Patient Teaching
- Warn the patient to notify the physician if weakness, hot flashes, or nausea become unmanageable.

goserelin acetate

gos-**er**-ah-lin
(Zoladex, Zoladex Implant[AUS], Zoladex LA)

CATEGORY AND SCHEDULE
Pregnancy Risk Category: D (advanced breast cancer), X (endometriosis, endometrial thinning)

MECHANISM OF ACTION
A gonadotropin-releasing hormone analogue and antineoplastic agent that stimulates the release of luteinizing hormone (LH) and follicle-stimulating hormone (FSH) from the anterior pituitary gland. In males, increases testosterone concentrations initially, then suppresses secretion of LH and FSH, resuting in decreased testosterone levels. **Therapeutic Effect:** In females, causes a reduction in ovarian size and function, reduction in uterine and mammary gland size, and regression of sex-hormone-responsive tumors. In males, produces pharmacologic castration and decreases the growth of abnormal prostate tissue.

AVAILABILITY
Implant: 3.6 mg, 10.8 mg.

INDICATIONS AND DOSAGES
▸ **Prostatic carcinoma**
Implant
Adults older than 18 yr, Elderly. 3.6 mg every 28 days or 10.8 mg q12wk subcutaneously into upper abdominal wall.

▸ **Breast carcinoma, endometriosis**
Implant
Adults. 3.6 mg every 28 days subcutaneously into upper abdominal wall.

▸ **Endometrial thinning**
Implant
Adults. 3.6 mg subcutaneously into upper abdominal wall as a single dose or in 2 doses 4 wk apart.

CONTRAINDICATIONS
Pregnancy

INTERACTIONS
Drug
None known.
Herbal
None known.
Food
None known.

DIAGNOSTIC TEST EFFECTS
May increase serum prostatic acid phosphatase and testosterone levels.

SIDE EFFECTS
Frequent
Headache (60%), hot flashes (55%), depression (54%), diaphoresis (45%), sexual dysfunction (21%), decreased erection (18%), lower urinary tract symptoms (13%)
Occasional (10%–5%)
Pain, lethargy, dizziness, insomnia, anorexia, nausea, rash, upper respiratory tract infection, hirsutism, abdominal pain
Rare
Pruritus

SERIOUS REACTIONS
! Arrhythmias, CHF, and hypertension occur rarely.
! Ureteral obstruction and spinal cord compression have been observed. An immediate orchiectomy may be necessary if these conditions occur.

NURSING CONSIDERATIONS
Baseline Assessment
- Determine if the patient is pregnant before beginning drug therapy.

Lifespan Considerations
- Goserelin crosses the placenta and may cause fetal harm. Women who are or may be pregnant shouldn't use this drug.
- It is unkown if goserelin is excreted in breast milk.
- The safety and efficacy of goserelin have not been established in children.
- No age-related precautions have been noted in the elderly.

Administration and Handling
Implant
- Inspect the package for damage before opening. If the package is damaged, don't use the syringe.
- Remove the sterile syringe from the package immediately before use. Examine the syringe for damage, and check that goserelin is visible in the translucent chamber.
- Clean an area of skin on the upper abdominal wall with an alcohol swab.
- Grasp the safety clip tab, pull it out and away from the needle, and discard it immediately. Then remove the needle cover.
- Using aseptic technique, stretch or pinch the patient's skin with one hand, and grip the syringe barrel. Insert the needle into the subcutaneous tissue.

◂**ALERT**▸ The goserelin syringe should not be used for aspiration. If the needle penetrates a large vessel, you'll see blood instantly in the syringe chamber. If a vessel is penetrated, withdraw the needle and use a new syringe elsewhere.
- Direct the needle so that it parallels the abdominal wall. Push the needle in until the barrel hub touches the

patient's skin. Withdraw the needle 1 cm to create a space to discharge goserelin. Fully depress the plunger to discharge the drug.
• Withdraw the needle. Then bandage the site. Confirm the discharge of goserelin by ensuring that the tip of the plunger is visible within the tip of the needle.
• Dispose of the used needle and syringe in a safe manner.

Intervention and Evaluation

• Monitor the patient for worsening signs and symptoms of prostatic cancer, especially during the first month of goserelin therapy.

Patient Teaching

• Urge the female patient to use nonhormonal contraceptive measures during goserelin therapy, and teach her about contraceptive options if needed.
• Warn the female patient to notify the physician if regular menstruation persists or she becomes pregnant. Inform her that breakthrough menstrual bleeding may occur if she misses a goserelin dose.

letrozole

leh-troe-zoll
(Femara)
Do not confuse Femara with Femhrt.

CATEGORY AND SCHEDULE

Pregnancy Risk Category: D

MECHANISM OF ACTION

Decreases the level of circulating estrogen by inhibiting aromatase, an enzyme that catalyzes the final step in estrogen production. **Therapeutic Effect:** Inhibits the growth of breast cancers that are stimulated by estrogens.

PHARMACOKINETICS

Rapidly and completely absorbed. Metabolized in the liver. Primarily eliminated by the kidneys. Unknown if removed by hemodialysis. ***Half-life:*** Approximately 2 days.

AVAILABILITY

Tablets: 2.5 mg.

INDICATIONS AND DOSAGES

▸ Breast cancer

PO

Adults, Elderly. 2.5 mg/day. Continue until tumor progression is evident.

CONTRAINDICATIONS

None known.

INTERACTIONS

Drug

None known.

Herbal

None known.

Food

None known.

DIAGNOSTIC TEST EFFECTS

May increase serum calcium, cholesterol, GGT, AST (SGOT), and ALT (SGPT) levels.

SIDE EFFECTS

Frequent (21%–9%)

Musculoskeletal pain (back, arm, leg), nausea, headache

Occasional (8%–5%)

Constipation, arthralgia, fatigue, vomiting, hot flashes, diarrhea, abdominal pain, cough, rash, anorexia, hypertension, peripheral edema

Rare (4%–1%)

Asthenia, somnolence, dyspepsia, weight gain, pruritus

SERIOUS REACTIONS

! None known.

NURSING CONSIDERATIONS

Baseline Assessment

- Determine if the patient is pregnant before beginning drug therapy.
- Document baseline vital signs, especially blood pressure, because letrozole may cause hypertension.

Lifespan Considerations

- Women who are or may be pregnant shouldn't use this drug.
- It is unknown if letrozole is distributed in breast milk.
- The safety and efficacy of letrozole have not been established in children.
- No age-related precautions have been noted in the elderly.

Precautions

- Use letrozole cautiously in patients with hepatic or renal impairment.

Administration and Handling

PO

- Give letrozole without regard to food.

Intervention and Evaluation

- Monitor the patient for asthenia and dizziness, and assist with ambulation if either condition occurs.
- Assess the patient for headache.
- Administer an antiemetic, if ordered, to prevent or treat nausea and vomiting.
- Monitor the patient's CBC, serum electrolyte levels, thyroid function, and liver and renal function test results.
- Evaluate the patient for evidence of musculoskeletal pain, and provide analgesics, if ordered.

Patient Teaching

- Advise the patient to notify the physician if weakness, hot flashes, or nausea become unmanageable.

leuprolide acetate

loo-proe-lide

(Eligard, Lucrin[AUS], Lucrin Depot Inj[AUS], Lupron, Lupron Depot, Lupron Depot Ped, Viadur)

Do not confuse leuprolide or Lupron with Lopurin or Nuprin.

CATEGORY AND SCHEDULE

Pregnancy Risk Category: X

MECHANISM OF ACTION

A gonadotropin-releasing hormone analogue and antineoplastic agent that stimulates the release of luteinizing hormone (LH) and follicle-stimulating hormone (FSH) from the anterior pituitary gland. **Therapeutic Effect:** Produces pharmacologic castration and decreases the growth of abnormal prostate tissue in males; causes endometrial tissue to become inactive and atrophic in females; and decreases the rate of pubertal development in children with central precocious puberty.

PHARMACOKINETICS

Rapidly and well absorbed after subcutaneous administration. Absorbed slowly after IM administration. Protein binding: 43%–49%. ***Half-life:*** 3–4 hr.

AVAILABILITY

Implant (Viadur): 65 mg.
Injection Depot Formulation (Eligard): 7.5 mg, 22.5 mg, 30 mg, 45 mg.
Injection Depot Formulation (Lupron Depot): 3.75 mg, 7.5 mg, 11.25 mg, 22.5 mg, 30 mg.
Injection Depot Formulation (Lupron Depot-Ped): 7.5 mg, 11.25 mg, 15 mg.

Injection solution (Lupron): 5 mg/ml.

INDICATIONS AND DOSAGES

▸ Advanced prostatic carcinoma
IM (Lupron Depot)
Adults, Elderly. 7.5 mg every month or 22.5 mg every 3 months or 30 mg every 4 months.
Subcutaneous (Eligard)
Adults, Elderly. 7.5 mg every month or 22.5 mg every 3 months or 30 mg every 4 months.
Subcutaneous (Lupron)
Adults, Elderly. 1 mg/day.
Subcutaneous (Viadur)
Adults, Elderly. 65 mg implanted q12mo.

▸ Endometriosis
IM (Lupron Depot)
Adults, Elderly. 3.75 mg/mo for up to 6 months or 11.25 mg every 3 months for up to 2 doses.

▸ Uterine leiomyomata
IM (with iron) (Lupron Depot)
Adults, Elderly. 3.75 mg/mo for up to 3 months or 11.25 mg as a single injection.

▸ Precocious puberty
IM (Lupron Depot Ped)
Children. 0.3 mg/kg/dose every 28 days. Minimum: 7.5 mg. If down regulation is not achieved, titrate upward in 3.75-mg increments q4wk.
Subcutaneous (Lupron)
Children. 20–45 mcg/kg/day. Titrate upward by 10 mcg/kg/day if down regulation is not achieved.

CONTRAINDICATIONS

Pernicious anemia, pregnancy

INTERACTIONS

Drug
None known.
Herbal
None known.
Food
None known.

DIAGNOSTIC TEST EFFECTS

May increase serum prostatic acid phosphatase (PAP) levels. Initially increases, then decreases, serum testosterone concentration.

SIDE EFFECTS

Frequent
Hot flashes (ranging from mild flushing to diaphoresis)
Females: Amenorrhea, spotting
Occasional
Arrhythmias; palpitations; blurred vision; dizziness; edema; headache; burning or itching, or swelling at injection site; nausea; insomnia; weight gain
Females: Deepening voice, hirsutism, decreased libido, increased breast tenderness, vaginitis, altered mood
Males: Constipation, decreased testicle size, gynecomastia, impotence, decreased appetite, angina
Rare
Males: Thrombophlebitis

SERIOUS REACTIONS

! Signs and symptoms of metastatic prostatic carcinoma (such as bone pain, dysuria or hematuria, and weakness or paresthesia of the lower extremities) occasionally worsen 1 to 2 weeks after the initial dose but then subside with continued therapy.
! Pulmonary embolism and MI occur rarely.

NURSING CONSIDERATIONS

Baseline Assessment
• Determine if the patient is pregnant before initiating leuprolide therapy.
• Expect to obtain serum testosterone and PAP levels periodically during leuprolide therapy. Be aware that serum testosterone and PAP levels should increase during the first week of therapy. The testosterone level

should decrease to baseline level or less within 2 weeks, and the PAP level should decrease within 4 weeks.

Lifespan Considerations

- Leuprolide use is contraindicated in pregnancy because the drug may cause spontaneous abortion.
- The long-term safety of leuprolide in children has not been established.
- No age-related precautions have been noted in the elderly.

Precautions

- Use leuprolide cautiously in children receiving long-term therapy.

Administration and Handling

◀ALERT▶ Because leuprolide may be carcinogenic, mutagenic, or teratogenic, handle it with extreme care during preparation and administration.

Subcutaneous
(Lupron)

- Refrigerate vials.
- The injection should appear clear and colorless. Discard the solution if it appears discolored or contains precipitate.
- Administer the drug undiluted into the abdomen, anterior thigh, or deltoid muscle.

IM
(Lupron Depot)

- Store at room temperature. Do not freeze. Protect from light and heat.
- Reconstitute only with the diluent provided. Follow mixing instructions provided by the manufacturer.
- Use the reconstituted solution immediately.
- Do not use needles smaller than 22 gauge; use syringes provided by the manufacturer (0.5 ml low-dose insulin syringes may be used as an alternative).

IM
(Eligard)

- Store the drug in the refrigerator.
- Allow drug to warm to room temperature before reconstitution.
- Follow mixing instructions provided by the manufacturer.
- Administer the drug within 30 minutes after reconstitution.

Intervention and Evaluation

- Monitor the patient for arrhythmias and palpitations.
- Assess the patient for peripheral edema.
- Evaluate the patient's sleep pattern.
- Monitor the patient for visual difficulties.
- Assist the patient with ambulation if dizziness occurs.
- Administer antiemetics, if ordered, to prevent or treat nausea and vomiting.

Patient Teaching

- Explain to the patient with prostate cancer that signs and symptoms of the disease may worsen temporarily during the first few weeks of leuprolide therapy.
- Urge the female patient to use nonhormonal contraceptive measures during leuprolide therapy.
- Warn the female patient to notify the physician if regular menstruation persists or she becomes pregnant.
- Inform the patient that hot flashes tend to decrease in frequency with continued leuprolide therapy.
- Warn the patient to avoid performing tasks that require mental alertness or motor skills until his or her response to the drug has been established.

megestrol acetate

me-**jess**-trole
(Apo-Megestrol[CAN], Megace, Megostat[AUS])

CATEGORY AND SCHEDULE

Pregnancy Risk Category: X (for suspension), D (for tablets)

MECHANISM OF ACTION

A hormone and antineoplastic agent that suppresses the release of luteinizing hormone from the anterior pituitary gland by inhibiting pituitary function. **Therapeutic Effect:** Shrinks tumors. Also increases appetite by an unknown mechanism.

PHARMACOKINETICS

Well absorbed from the GI tract. Metabolized in the liver; excreted in urine.

AVAILABILITY

Tablets: 20 mg, 40 mg.
Suspension: 40 mg/ml.

INDICATIONS AND DOSAGES

▸ **Palliative treatment of advanced breast cancer**
PO
Adults, Elderly. 160 mg/day in 4 equally divided doses.

▸ **Palliative treatment of advanced endometrial carcinoma**
PO
Adults, Elderly. 40–320 mg/day in divided doses. Maximum: 800 mg/day in 1–4 divided doses.

▸ **Anorexia, cachexia, weight loss**
PO
Adults, Elderly. 800 mg (20 ml)/day.

OFF-LABEL USES

Appetite stimulant, treatment of hormone-dependent or advanced prostate carcinoma

CONTRAINDICATIONS

None known.

INTERACTIONS

Drug
None known.
Herbal
None known.
Food
None known.

DIAGNOSTIC TEST EFFECTS

May increase blood glucose level.

SIDE EFFECTS

Frequent
Weight gain secondary to increased appetite
Occasional
Nausea, breakthrough bleeding, backache, headache, breast tenderness, carpal tunnel syndrome
Rare
Feeling of coldness

SERIOUS REACTIONS

! Thrombophlebitis and pulmonary embolism occur rarely.

NURSING CONSIDERATIONS

Baseline Assessment
- Determine if the patient is pregnant before initiating megestrol therapy. Inform her that megestrol has a pregnancy risk category of X in suspension form and D in tablet form.

Lifespan Considerations
- Megestrol use should be avoided during pregnancy, if possible, especially in the first 4 months.
- Breast-feeding is not recommended for patients taking this drug.
- The safety and efficacy of megestrol have not been established in children.
- No age-related precautions have been noted in the elderly.

Precautions
• Use megestrol cautiously in patients with a history of thrombophlebitis.
Intervention and Evaluation
• Monitor the patient for signs and symptoms of a therapeutic response to the drug.
• Provide support to the patient and family since this drug is palliative, not a cure.
Patient Teaching
• Caution the patient that contraception is imperative during megestrol therapy.
• Instruct the patient to notify the physician if she experiences calf pain, difficulty breathing, or vaginal bleeding.
• Advise the patient that megestrol may cause backache, breast tenderness, headache, nausea, and vomiting.

nilutamide

nih-**lute**-ah-myd
(Anandron[CAN], Nilandron)

CATEGORY AND SCHEDULE
Pregnancy Risk Category: C

MECHANISM OF ACTION
An antiandrogen hormone and antineoplastic agent that competitively inhibits androgen action by binding to androgen receptors in target tissue. **Therapeutic Effect:** Decreases growth of abnormal prostate tissue.

AVAILABILITY
Tablets: 150 mg.

INDICATIONS AND DOSAGES
▸ Prostatic carcinoma
PO
Adults, Elderly. 300 mg once a day for 30 days, then 150 mg once a day. Begin on day of, or day after, surgical castration.

CONTRAINDICATIONS
Severe hepatic impairment, severe respiratory insufficiency

INTERACTIONS
Drug
None known.
Herbal
None known.
Food
None known.

DIAGNOSTIC TEST EFFECTS
May increase serum bilirubin, creatinine, AST (SGOT), and ALT (SGPT) levels.

SIDE EFFECTS
Frequent (greater than 10%)
Hot flashes, delay in recovering vision after bright illumination (such as sun, television, bright lights), decreased libido, diminished sexual function, mild nausea, gynecomastia, alcohol intolerance
Occasional (less than 10%)
Constipation, hypertension, dizziness, dyspnea, UTIs

SERIOUS REACTIONS
! Interstitial pneumonitis occurs rarely.

NURSING CONSIDERATIONS
Baseline Assessment
• Expect to obtain a baseline chest x-ray and liver function test results before beginning nilutamide therapy.
Precautions
• Use nilutamide cautiously in patients with hepatitis or markedly increased serum hepatic function test results.

Intervention and Evaluation

- Monitor the patient's BP and liver function test results periodically during long-term nilutamide therapy.

Patient Teaching

- Warn the patient to notify the physician if he experiences any side effects at home, especially signs of hepatotoxicity, such as abdominal pain, dark urine, fatigue, and jaundice.
- Caution the patient about driving at night. Recommend tinted glasses to help decrease the visual effect of bright headlights and streetlights.

tamoxifen citrate

tam-**ox**-ih-fen

(Apo-Tamox[CAN], Genox[AUS], Istubol, Nolvadex, Nolvadex-D[CAN], Novo-Tamoxifen[CAN], Tamofen[CAN], Tamosin[AUS])

CATEGORY AND SCHEDULE

Pregnancy Risk Category: D

MECHANISM OF ACTION

A nonsteroidal antiestrogen that competes with estradiol for estrogen-receptor binding sites in the breasts, uterus, and vagina. **Therapeutic Effect:** Inhibits DNA synthesis and estrogen response.

PHARMACOKINETICS

Well absorbed from the GI tract. Metabolized in the liver. Primarily eliminated in feces by biliary system. ***Half-life:*** 7 days.

AVAILABILITY

Tablets: 10 mg, 20 mg.

INDICATIONS AND DOSAGES

▸ Adjunctive treatment of breast cancer

PO

Adults, Elderly. 20–40 mg/day. Give doses greater than 20 mg/day in divided doses.

▸ Prevention of breast cancer in high-risk women

PO

Adults, Elderly. 20 mg/day.

OFF-LABEL USES

Induction of ovulation

CONTRAINDICATIONS

None known.

INTERACTIONS

Drug

Estrogens: May decrease the effects of tamoxifen.

Herbal

None known.

Food

None known.

DIAGNOSTIC TEST EFFECTS

May increase serum cholesterol, calcium, and triglyceride levels.

SIDE EFFECTS

Frequent

Women (greater than 10%): Hot flashes, nausea, vomiting

Occasional

Women (9%–1%): Changes in menstruation, genital itching, vaginal discharge, endometrial hyperplasia or polyps

Men: Impotence, decreased libido

Men and women: Headache, nausea, vomiting, rash, bone pain, confusion, weakness, somnolence

SERIOUS REACTIONS

! Retinopathy, corneal opacity, and decreased visual acuity have been noted in patients receiving extremely high dosages (240–320 mg/day) for longer than 17 months.

NURSING CONSIDERATIONS

Baseline Assessment

• Check the results of the patient's estrogen receptor assay test, if ordered, before beginning tamoxifen therapy.

• Monitor the patient's CBC and serum calcium levels before and periodically during tamoxifen therapy.

Lifespan Considerations

• Tamoxifen use should be avoided during pregnancy, especially during the first trimester, because it may cause fetal harm. It's unknown if tamoxifen is distributed in breast milk; however, breast-feeding is not recommended for patients taking this drug.

• Tamoxifen use is safe and effective in girls aged 2 to 10 years with McCune Albright syndrome and precocious puberty.

• No age-related precautions have been noted in the elderly.

Precautions

• Use tamoxifen cautiously in patients with leukopenia or thrombocytopenia.

Administration and Handling

PO

• Give tamoxifen without regard to food.

Intervention and Evaluation

• Be alert for reports of increased bone pain and provide adequate pain relief as ordered.

• Monitor the patient's intake and output and weight.

• Examine the patient for dependent edema.

• Assess the patient for signs and symptoms of hypercalcemia, including constipation, deep bone or flank pain, excessive thirst, hypotonicity of muscles, increased urine output, nausea and vomiting, and renal calculi.

Patient Teaching

• Warn the patient to notify the physician if he or she experiences leg cramps, weakness, weight gain, or vaginal bleeding, itching, or discharge.

• Inform the patient that he or she may initially experience an increase in bone and tumor pain, which appears to indicate a good tumor response to tamoxifen.

• Caution the patient to notify the physician if nausea and vomiting continue at home.

• Urge the patient to use nonhormonal contraception during tamoxifen treatment.

toremifene citrate

tore-mih-feen
(Fareston)

CATEGORY AND SCHEDULE

Pregnancy Risk Category: D

MECHANISM OF ACTION

A nonsteroidal antiestrogen and antineoplastic agent that binds to estrogen receptors on tumors, producing a complex that decreases DNA synthesis and inhibits estrogen effects. **Therapeutic Effect:** Blocks growth-stimulating effects of estrogen in breast cancer.

PHARMACOKINETICS

Well absorbed after PO administration. Metabolized in the liver. Eliminated in feces. ***Half-life:*** Approximately 5 days.

AVAILABILITY

Tablets: 60 mg.

INDICATIONS AND DOSAGES

▸ Breast cancer

PO

Adults. 60 mg/day until disease progression is observed.

OFF-LABEL USES

Treatment of desmoid tumors, endometrial carcinoma

CONTRAINDICATIONS

History of thromboembolic disease

INTERACTIONS

Drug

Carbamazepine, phenobarbital, phenytoin: May decrease toremifene blood concentration.

Warfarin: May increase PT.

Herbal

None known.

Food

None known.

DIAGNOSTIC TEST EFFECTS

May increase serum alkaline phosphatase, bilirubin, calcium, and AST (SGOT) levels.

SIDE EFFECTS

Frequent

Hot flashes (35%); diaphoresis (20%); nausea (14%); vaginal discharge (13%); dizziness, dry eyes (9%)

Occasional (5%–2%)

Edema, vomiting, vaginal bleeding

Rare

Fatigue, depression, lethargy, anorexia

SERIOUS REACTIONS

! Ocular toxicity (cataracts, glaucoma, decreased visual acuity) and hypercalcemia may occur.

NURSING CONSIDERATIONS

Baseline Assessment

- Expect the patient to undergo an estrogen receptor assay before starting toremifene therapy.
- Monitor the patient's CBC and serum calcium levels before and periodically during toremifene therapy.

Lifespan Considerations

- Toremifene use should be avoided during pregnancy because this drug may cause fetal harm.
- It's unknown if toremifene is distributed in breast milk; however, breast-feeding is not recommended for patients taking this drug.
- Toremifene is not prescribed for children; the safety and efficacy of this drug in children have not been established.
- No age-related precautions have been noted in the elderly.

Precautions

- Use toremifene cautiously in patients with pre-existing endometrial hyperplasia, leukopenia, or thrombocytopenia.

Administration and Handling

PO

- Give toremifene without regard to food.

Intervention and Evaluation

- Assess the patient for signs and symptoms of hypercalcemia, including constipation, deep bone or flank pain, excessive thirst, hypotonicity of muscles, increased urine output, nausea and vomiting, and renal calculi.
- Monitor the patient's CBC, WBC count, liver function test results, and serum calcium levels.

Patient Teaching

- Inform the patient that she may experience an initial flare-up of symptoms, including bone pain and

hot flashes, that will subside with continued therapy.
- Warn the patient to notify the physician if she experiences leg cramps, shortness of breath, weakness, weight gain, or vaginal bleeding, discharge, or itching.
- Advise the patient to notify the physician if nausea and vomiting continue at home.
- Urge the patient to use nonhormonal methods of contraception during toremifene therapy.

triptorelin pamoate

trip-toe-**ree**-linn
(Trelstar Depot, Trelstar LA)

CATEGORY AND SCHEDULE
Pregnancy Risk Category: X

MECHANISM OF ACTION
A gonadotropin-releasing hormone (GnRH) analogue and antineoplastic agent that inhibits gonadotropin hormone secretion through a negative feedback mechanism. Circulating levels of luteinizing hormone, follicle-stimulating hormone, testosterone, and estradiol rise initially, then subside with continued therapy. **Therapeutic Effect:** Suppresses growth of abnormal prostate tissue.

AVAILABILITY
Powder for Injection (Trelstar Depot): 3.75 mg.
Powder for Injection (Trelstar LA): 11.25 mg.

INDICATIONS AND DOSAGES
▸ Prostate cancer
IM (Trelstar Depot)
Adults, Elderly. 3.75 mg once q28days.
IM (Trelstar LA)
Adults, Elderly. 11.25 mg q84days.

CONTRAINDICATIONS
Hypersensitivity to luteinizing hormone-releasing hormone (LHRH) or LHRH agonists

INTERACTIONS
Drug
Hyperprolactinemic drugs: Reduce the number of pituitary gonadotropin-releasing hormone (GnRH) receptors.
Herbal
None known.
Food
None known.

DIAGNOSTIC TEST EFFECTS
May alter serum pituitary-gonadal function test results. May cause transient increase in serum testosterone levels, usually during first week of treatment.

SIDE EFFECTS
Frequent (greater than 5%)
Hot flashes, skeletal pain, headache, impotence
Occasional (5%–2%)
Insomnia, vomiting, leg pain, fatigue
Rare (less than 2%)
Dizziness, emotional lability, diarrhea, urine retention, UTIs, anemia, pruritus

SERIOUS REACTIONS
! Bladder outlet obstruction, skeletal pain, hematuria, and spinal cord compression (with weakness or paralysis of the lower extremities) may occur.

NURSING CONSIDERATIONS
Baseline Assessment
- Determine if the patient is pregnant before beginning triptorelin therapy.

Lifespan Considerations

• Women who are or may be pregnant shouldn't use this drug.
• It is unknown if triptorelin is excreted in breast milk.
• The safety and efficacy of triptorelin have not been established in children.
• No age-related precautions have been noted in the elderly.

Intervention and Evaluation

• Expect to obtain prostatic acid phosphatase (PAP), prostate-specific antigen (PSA), and serum testosterone levels periodically during therapy. Serum testosterone and PAP levels should increase during the first week of therapy. The testosterone level should then decrease to baseline level or less within 2 weeks, and the PAP level should decrease within 4 weeks.
• Monitor the patient closely for worsening signs and symptoms of prostatic cancer, especially during the first week of therapy, due to a transient increase in testosterone level.

Patient Teaching

• Caution the patient against missing monthly injections.
• Inform the patient that he may experience blood in urine, increased skeletal pain, and urine retention initially but that these symptoms usually subside within 1 week.
• Tell the patient that he may have hot flashes during triptorelin therapy.
• Warn the patient to notify the physician if he experiences difficulty breathing, infection at the injection site, numbness of the arms or legs, breast pain or swelling, persistent nausea or vomiting, or rapid heartbeat.

19 Monoclonal Antibodies

alemtuzumab
bevacizumab
bexarotene
bortezomib
cetuximab
efalizumab
gefitinib
gemtuzumab ozogamicin
imatinib mesylate
rituximab
tositumomab and iodine ^{131}I-tositumomab
trastuzumab

Uses: Each monoclonal antibody is used to treat different types of cancer, including breast cancer, low-grade B-cell non-Hodgkin's lymphoma, and B-cell chronic lymphocytic leukemia. For details, see the specific drug entries.

Action: Although their exact mechanism of action is unknown, monoclonal antibodies may act by binding to specific cell-surface antigens. The agents' cytotoxic effects may be related to T-cell mediated recognition of the bound antibody and interference with cell proliferation.

alemtuzumab

al-lem-**two**-zoo-mab
(Campath)

CATEGORY AND SCHEDULE

Pregnancy Risk Category: C

MECHANISM OF ACTION

Binds to CD52, a cell surface glycoprotein, found on the surface of all B and T lymphocytes, most monocytes, macrophages, natural killer cells, and granulocytes. **Therapeutic Effect:** Produces cytotoxicity reducing tumor size.

PHARMACOKINETICS

Half-life: About 12 days. Peak and trough levels rise during first few weeks of therapy and approach steady state by about week 6.

AVAILABILITY

Solution for Injection: 30 mg/3 ml.

INDICATIONS AND DOSAGES

▸ **Chronic lymphocytic leukemia**

IV

Adults, Elderly. Initially, 3 mg/day as a 2-hr infusion. When the 3-mg daily dose is tolerated (with only low-grade or no infusion-related toxicities), increase daily dose to 10 mg. When the 10 mg/day dose is tolerated, maintenance dose may be initiated. Maintenance: 30 mg/day 3 times a week on alternate days (such as Monday, Wednesday, and Friday or Tuesday, Thursday, and Saturday) for up to 12 wk. The increase to 30 mg/day is usually achieved in 3–7 days.

CONTRAINDICATIONS

Active systemic infections, history of hypersensitivity or anaphylactic reaction to the drug, immunosuppression

INTERACTIONS

Drug

Live-virus vaccines: May potentiate viral replication, increase side effects, and decrease the patient's antibody response to the vaccine.

Herbal

None known.

Food

None known.

DIAGNOSTIC TEST EFFECTS

May decrease Hgb level, platelet count, and WBC count.

IV INCOMPATIBILITIES

Don't mix alemtuzumab with any other medications.

SIDE EFFECTS

Frequent

Rigors, tremors (86%), fever (85%), nausea (54%), vomiting (41%), rash (40%), fatigue (34%), hypotension (32%), urticaria (30%), pruritus, skeletal pain, headache (24%), diarrhea (22%), anorexia (20%)

Occasional (less than 10%)

Myalgia, dizziness, abdominal pain, throat irritation, vomiting, neutropenia, rhinitis, bronchospasm, urticaria

SERIOUS REACTIONS

! Neutropenia occurs in 85% of patients, anemia occurs in 80% of patients, and thrombocytopenia occurs in 72% of patients.

! A rash occurs in 40% of patients.

! Respiratory toxicity, manifested as dyspnea, cough, bronchitis, pneumonitis, and pneumonia, occurs in 26%–16% of patients.

NURSING CONSIDERATIONS

Baseline Assessment

◀ALERT▶ Expect to pretreat the patient with 650 mg acetaminophen and 50 mg diphenhydramine before each infusion to prevent infusion-related side effects.

- Expect to obtain a CBC frequently during and after therapy to assess for anemia, neutropenia, and thrombocytopenia.

Lifespan Considerations

- Alemtuzumab has the potential to cause depletion of B- and T-lymphocytes in the fetus. Advise the patient to discontinue breastfeeding during treatment and for at least 3 months after the last dose.
- The safety and efficacy of alemtuzumab have not been established in children.
- No age-related precautions have been noted in the elderly.

Administration and Handling

IV

- Refrigerate ampules before dilution. Don't freeze them.
- Use the solution within 8 hours after dilution. The diluted solution may be stored at room temperature or refrigerated.
- Discard the solution if it becomes discolored or contains particulate matter.
- Withdraw the needed amount from the ampule into a syringe. Inject it into 100-ml 0.9% NaCl or D_5W, using a low-protein binding, nonfiber-releasing 5-micron filter.
- Invert the bag to mix the contents; don't shake it.
- Give the 100-ml solution as a 2-hour IV infusion. Do not give alemtuzumab by IV push or bolus.

Intervention and Evaluation

- Monitor the patient for infusion-related reactions, including chills, fever, hypotension, and rigors, which usually occur 30 minutes to 2 hours after starting the first infusion. These reactions may resolve by slowing the drip rate.
- Monitor for signs and symptoms of hematologic toxicity, including

excessive fatigue or weakness, ecchymosis, fever, signs of local infection, sore throat or unusual bleeding from any site.

Patient Teaching

• Instruct the patient to avoid crowds and those with known infection.

• Urge the patient to avoid vaccinations and contact with anyone who has recently received a live-virus vaccine.

bevacizumab

be-vah-**ciz**-you-mab
(Avastin)

CATEGORY AND SCHEDULE

Pregnancy Risk Category: C

MECHANISM OF ACTION

An antineoplastic that binds to and inhibits vascular endothelial growth factor, a protein that plays a major role in the formation of new blood vessels to tumors. **Therapeutic Effect:** Inhibits metastatic disease progression.

PHARMACOKINETICS

Clearance varies by body weight, gender, and tumor burden. ***Half-life:*** 20 days (range, 11–50 days).

AVAILABILITY

Injection: 25-mg/ml vial.

INDICATIONS AND DOSAGES

▸ **First-line treatment of metastatic carcinoma of the colon or rectum in combination with 5-fluorouracil (5-FU)**

IV

Adults, Elderly. 5 mg/kg once every 14 days.

OFF-LABEL USES

Adjunctive therapy in breast cancer, renal cell carcinoma

CONTRAINDICATIONS

GI perforation, hypertensive crisis, nephrotic syndrome, recent hemoptysis, serious bleeding, wound dehiscence requiring medical intervention

INTERACTIONS

Drug

None known.

Herbal

None known.

Food

None known.

DIAGNOSTIC TEST EFFECTS

May decrease serum potassium, sodium, and hemoglobin levels; hematocrit; and WBC and platelet counts.

IV INCOMPATIBILITIES

Don't mix bevacizumab with dextrose solutions.

SIDE EFFECTS

Frequent (73%–25%)

Asthenia, vomiting, anorexia, hypertension, epistaxis, stomatitis, constipation, headache, dyspnea

Occasional (21%–15%)

Altered taste, dry skin, exfoliative dermatitis, dizziness, flatulence, excessive lacrimation, skin discoloration, weight loss, myalgia

Rare (8%–6%)

Nail disorder, skin ulcer, alopecia, confusion, abnormal gait, dry mouth

SERIOUS REACTIONS

! UTIs, manifested as urinary frequency or urgency and proteinuria, occur frequently.

! CHF, deep vein thrombosis, GI perforation, hypertensive crisis, nephrotic syndrome, and severe hemorrhage are the most serious reactions that occur.

! Anemia, neutropenia, and thrombocytopenia occur occasionally.

! Hypersensitivity reactions occur rarely.

NURSING CONSIDERATIONS

Baseline Assessment

• Monitor the patient's BP, CBC, and serum potassium and sodium levels before and regularly during bevacizumab treatment.

• Assess the patient's urine for proteinuria. Patients with a urine dipstick reading of 2+ or more should have a 24-hour urine collection.

Lifespan Considerations

• Bevacizumab is teratogenic and has the potential to impair fertility. Its use by pregnant women may decrease maternal and fetal body weight and increase the risk of fetal skeletal abnormalities.

• Breast-feeding women should not take bevacizumab.

• The safety and efficacy of bevacizumab have not been established in children.

• Patients older than 65 years have a higher incidence of serious adverse reactions.

Precautions

• Use bevacizumab cautiously in patients with CHF, epistaxis, hypertension, proteinuria, or renal insufficiency.

Administration and Handling

IV

◀ALERT▶ Don't give bevacizumab by IV push or IV bolus.

• Refrigerate vials.

• Withdraw the amount of bevacizumab needed for a dose of 5 mg/kg, and dilute it in 100 ml 0.9% NaCl. Discard any unused portion.

• The diluted solution may be refrigerated for up to 8 hours.

• Infuse the initial dose of bevacizumab over 90 minutes after chemotherapy.

• If the patient tolerates the first infusion well, the second infusion may be administered over 60 minutes.

• If the patient tolerates the 60-minute infusion well, all subsequent infusions may be administered over 30 minutes.

Intervention and Evaluation

• Assess the patient for asthenia (loss of energy or strength), and help the patient with ambulation if he or she experiences this side effect.

• Assess the patient for abdominal pain, chills, and fever.

• Offer the patient an antiemetic if he or she experiences nausea or vomiting.

• Assess the patient's pattern of daily bowel activity and stool consistency.

Patient Teaching

• Advise the patient not to receive immunizations without the physician's approval and to avoid contact with crowds, people with known infections, and anyone who has recently received a live-virus vaccine because bevacizumab lowers the body's resistance to infection.

• Inform the female patient of childbearing age that becoming pregnant during bevacizumab therapy may pose risks to the fetus.

bexarotene

becks-**aye**-row-teen

(Targretin)

CATEGORY AND SCHEDULE

Pregnancy Risk Category: X

MECHANISM OF ACTION

This retinoid antineoplastic agent binds to and activates retinoid X receptor subtypes, which regulate the genes that control cellular differentiation and proliferation. **Therapeutic Effect:** Inhibits growth of tumor cell lines of hematopoietic and squamous cell origin and induces tumor regression.

PHARMACOKINETICS

Moderately absorbed from the GI tract. Protein binding: greater than 99%. Metabolized in the liver. Primarily eliminated through the hepatobiliary system. ***Half-life:*** 7 hr.

AVAILABILITY

Capsules (Soft Gelatin): 75 mg.

INDICATIONS AND DOSAGES

▸ Cutaneous T-cell lymphoma refractory to at least one prior systemic therapy

PO

Adults. 300 mg/m^2/day. If no response and initial dose is well tolerated, may be increased to 400 mg/m^2/day. If not tolerated, may decrease to 200 mg/m^2/day, then to 100 mg/m^2/day.

Topical

Adults. Initially, apply once every other day. May increase at weekly intervals up to 4 times a day.

OFF-LABEL USES

Treatment of diabetes mellitus; head, neck, lung, and renal cell carcinomas; Kaposi's sarcoma

CONTRAINDICATIONS

None known.

INTERACTIONS

Drug

Antidiabetics: May enhance the effects of these drugs.

Erythromycin, itraconazole, ketoconazole: May increase bexarotene blood concentrations.

Phenytoin, rifampin: May decrease bexarotene blood concentrations.

Herbal

None known.

Food

Grapefruit juice: May increase bexarotene blood concentration and risk of toxicity.

DIAGNOSTIC TEST EFFECTS

May increase serum cholesterol, triglyceride, and total and LDL cholesterol levels. May increase CA-125 assay value in patients with ovarian cancer. May decrease serum HDL cholesterol levels. May produce abnormal liver function test results.

SIDE EFFECTS

Frequent

Hyperlipidemia (79%), headache (30%), hypothyroidism (29%), asthenia (20%)

Occasional

Rash (17%); nausea (15%); peripheral edema (13%); dry skin, abdominal pain (11%); chills, exfoliative dermatitis (10%); diarrhea (7%)

SERIOUS REACTIONS

! Pancreatitis, hepatic failure, and pneumonia occur rarely.

NURSING CONSIDERATIONS

Baseline Assessment

- Assess the patient's baseline lipid profile, liver function, thyroid function, and WBC count.
- Determine if the patient is pregnant before initiating bexarotene therapy.

Lifespan Considerations

- Bexarotene use should be avoided during pregnancy because the drug may cause fetal harm.

• It is unknown if bexarotene is distributed in breast milk; however, breast-feeding is not recommended for patients taking this drug.
• The safety and efficacy of bexarotene have not been established in children.
• No age-related precautions have been noted in the elderly.

Precautions

• Use bexarotene cautiously in patients with diabetes mellitus, lipid abnormalities, or hepatic impairment.

Administration and Handling

PO

• Give bexarotene with food.

Intervention and Evaluation

• Monitor the patient's serum cholesterol and triglyceride levels, CBC, and liver and thyroid function test results.

Patient Teaching

• Warn the female patient of child-bearing age (even if infertile) about the potential risks to the fetus if she becomes pregnant during bexarotene therapy. Instruct her to use a reliable contraceptive method during therapy and for 1 month afterward and to notify the physician if she plans to become or becomes pregnant.
• Advise the patient not to use abrasive, drying, or medicated soaps during therapy.

bortezomib

bor-**teh**-zoe-mib
(Velcade)

CATEGORY AND SCHEDULE

Pregnancy Risk Category: D

MECHANISM OF ACTION

A proteasome inhibitor, antineoplastic agent that degrades conjugated proteins required for cell-cycle progression and mitosis, disrupting cell proliferation. **Therapeutic Effect:** Produces antitumor and chemosensitizing activity and cell death.

PHARMACOKINETICS

Distributed to tissues and organs, with highest level in the GI tract and liver. Protein binding: 83%. Primarily metabolized by enzymatic action. Rapidly cleared from the circulation. Significant biliary excretion, with lesser amount excreted in the urine. ***Half-life:*** 9–15 hr.

AVAILABILITY

Powder for Injection: 3.5 mg.

INDICATIONS AND DOSAGES

▸ Multiple myeloma

IV

Adults, Elderly. Treatment cycle consists of 1.3 mg/m^2 twice weekly on days 1, 4, 8, and 11 for 2 wk followed by a 10-day rest period on days 12 to 21. Consecutive doses separated by at least 72 hr.

▸ Dosage adjustment guidelines

Therapy is withheld at onset of grade 3 nonhematological or grade 4 hematological toxicities, excluding neuropathy. When symptoms resolve, therapy is restarted at a 25% reduced dosage.

▸ Neuropathic pain, peripheral sensory neuropathy

IV

Adults, Elderly. For grade 1 with pain or grade 2 (interfering with function but not activities of daily living [ADL]), 1 mg/m^2. For grade 2 with pain or grade 3 (interfering with ADL), withhold drug until toxicity is resolved, then reinitiate with 0.7 mg/m^2. For grade 4 (permanent sensory loss that interferes with function), discontinue bortezomib.

CONTRAINDICATIONS

Hypersensitivity to boron or mannitol

INTERACTIONS

Drug

Oral antidiabetics: May alter the response of these drugs.

Food

None known.

Herbal

None known.

DIAGNOSTIC TEST EFFECTS

May significantly decrease blood Hgb and Hct levels and neutrophil, platelet, and WBC counts.

SIDE EFFECTS

Expected (65%–36%)

Fatigue, malaise, asthenia, nausea, diarrhea, anorexia, constipation, fever, vomiting

Frequent (28%–21%)

Headache, insomnia, arthralgia, limb pain, edema, paresthesia, dizziness, rash

Occasional (18%–11%)

Dehydration, cough, anxiety, bone pain, muscle cramps, myalgia, back pain, abdominal pain, taste alteration, dyspepsia, pruritus, hypotension (including orthostatic hypotension), rigors, blurred vision

SERIOUS REACTIONS

! Thrombocytopenia occurs in 40% of patients. Platelet count peaks at day 11 and returns to baseline by day 21. GI and intracerebral hemorrhage are associated with drug-induced thrombocytopenia.

! Anemia occurs in 32% of patients.

! New onset or worsening neuropathy occurs in 37% of patients. Symptoms may improve in some patients when bortezomib is discontinued.

! Pneumonia occurs occasionally.

NURSING CONSIDERATIONS

Baseline Assessment

- Keep in mind that bortezomib is used to treat patients with refractory or relapsed multiple myeloma, who have received at least two prior therapies and who have demonstrated disease progression with the last therapy.
- As ordered, obtain and monitor the patient's CBC, especially platelet count, before and throughout bortezomib treatment.
- Give antiemetics, if ordered, to prevent or treat nausea and vomiting.
- Administer antidiarrheals, if ordered, to prevent or treat diarrhea.

Lifespan Considerations

- Bortezomib may induce degenerative effects in the ovaries and testes and may affect male and female fertility. Breast-feeding is not recommended for patients receiving this drug.
- The safety and efficacy of bortezomib have not been established in children.
- Elderly patients are at increased risk for grade 3 and 4 thrombocytopenia.

Precautions

- Use bortezomib cautiously in patients with a history of syncope.
- Use the drug cautiously in patients receiving any medication that increases the risk of dehydration, hypotension, and hepatic or renal function impairment.

Administration and Handling

IV

- Store unopened vials at room temperature.
- The reconstituted solution is stable at room temperature for up to 8 hours.
- Reconstitute the vial with 3.5 ml 0.9% NaCl.

• Give bortezomib as a bolus IV injection.

Intervention and Evaluation

• Routinely assess the patient's BP. Monitor the patient for signs and symptoms of orthostatic hypotension.
• Closely monitor intake and output.
• Monitor the patient's temperature and be alert for fever.
• Assess the patient for signs and symptoms of peripheral neuropathy, including a burning sensation, hyperesthesia, neuropathic pain, and paresthesia of the extremities.
• Avoid giving the patient IM injections or rectal medications and performing other procedures that may induce trauma and bleeding.

Patient Teaching

• Caution women of childbearing age to avoid pregnancy while taking bortezomib. Teach the patient about effective forms of contraception, and stress the importance of pregnancy testing.
• Instruct the patient to drink plenty of fluids to prevent dehydration.
• Warn the patient to avoid tasks that require mental alertness or motor skills until his or her response to the drug is established.

cetuximab

ceh-**tux**-ih-mab
(Erbitux)

CATEGORY AND SCHEDULE

Pregnancy Risk Category: C

MECHANISM OF ACTION

A monoclonal antibody that binds to the epidermal growth factor receptor (EGFR), a glycoprotein on normal and tumor cells, thus inhibiting cell growth and inducing apoptosis. **Therapeutic Effect:** Inhibits the growth and survival of tumor cells that overexpress EGFR.

PHARMACOKINETICS

Reaches steady state levels by the third weekly infusion. Clearance decreases as dose increases. ***Half-life:*** 114 hr (range, 75–188 hr).

AVAILABILITY

Injection: 2 mg/ml.

INDICATIONS AND DOSAGES

▸ Metastatic colorectal carcinoma

IV

Adults, Elderly. Initially, 400 mg/m^2 as a loading dose. Maintenance: 250 mg/m^2 infused over 60 minutes weekly.

CONTRAINDICATIONS

None known.

INTERACTIONS

Drug

None known.

Herbal

None known.

Food

None known.

DIAGNOSTIC TEST EFFECTS

May decrease WBC count, hematocrit, and hemoglobin level.

IV COMPATIBILITIES

Irinotecan (Camptosar)

SIDE EFFECTS

Frequent (90%–25%)

Acneiform rash, malaise, fever, nausea, diarrhea, constipation, headache, abdominal pain, anorexia, vomiting

Occasional (16%–10%)

Nail disorder, back pain, stomatitis, peripheral edema, pruritus, cough, insomnia

Rare (9%–5%)
Weight loss, depression, dyspepsia, conjunctivitis, alopecia

SERIOUS REACTIONS

! Anemia occurs in 10% of patients.
! A severe infusion reaction, characterized by rapid onset of airway obstruction, a precipitous drop in blood pressure, and severe urticaria, occurs rarely.
! Dermatologic toxicity, pulmonary embolus, leukopenia, and renal failure occur rarely.

NURSING CONSIDERATIONS

Baseline Assessment

- Monitor the patient's hematocrit and hemoglobin level.
- Assess the patient for signs and symptoms of anemia.
- Determine if the patient is pregnant.

Lifespan Considerations

- Cetuximab crosses the placental barrier and may cause fetal harm or spontaneous abortion.
- Female patients should not breast-feed while taking cetuximab.
- The safety and efficacy of cetuximab have not been established in children.
- No age-related precautions have been noted in the elderly.

Precautions

- Use cetuximab cautiously in patients with a hypersensitivity to murine proteins.

Administration and Handling

◀ **ALERT** ▶ Premedicate the patient with 50 mg diphenhydramine IV. Cetuximab may be used as monotherapy or in combination with irinotecan.
◀ **ALERT** ▶ Do not give cetuximab by IV push or bolus.

IV
- Refrigerate vials.
- Preparations in infusion containers are stable for up to 8 hours at room temperature or 12 hours if refrigerated. Discard any unused portion.
- The solution should appear clear and colorless; it may contain a small amount of visible white particulates.
- Don't shake or dilute the vials.
- Infuse the drug using a low-protein-binding 0.22-micron in-line filter.
- Give the first dose as a 120-minute IV infusion.
- Administer maintenance infusions over 60 minutes. The maximum infusion rate is 5 ml/minute.

Intervention and Evaluation

- Diligently monitor the patient for signs and symptoms of an infusion reaction, such as rapid onset of bronchospasm, hoarseness, hypotension, stridor, and urticaria. Patients may experience their first severe infusion reaction during subsequent infusions.
- Assess the patient's skin for evidence of dermatologic toxicity, such as dry skin, exfoliative dermatitis or rash, and inflammatory sequelae.
- Instruct the patient not to receive vaccinations and to avoid contact with crowds, persons with a known infection, and anyone who has recently received a live-virus vaccine.
- Instruct the patient to limit sun exposure and wear sunscreen when outdoors during cetuximab therapy because sunlight can exacerbate skin reactions.
- Advise the patient to avoid becoming pregnant during cetuximab therapy because of the drug's potential to cause fetal harm.

efalizumab

ef-ah-**liz**-ewe-mab
(Raptiva)

CATEGORY AND SCHEDULE
Pregnancy Risk Category: C

MECHANISM OF ACTION
A monoclonal antibody that interferes with lymphocyte activation by binding to the lymphocyte antigen, inhibiting the adhesion of leukocytes to other cell types. **Therapeutic Effect:** Prevents the release of cytokines and the growth and migration of circulating total lymphocytes, predominant in psoriatic lesions.

PHARMACOKINETICS
Clearance is affected by body weight, not by gender or race, after subcutaneous injection. Serum concentration reaches steady state at 4 wk. Mean time to elimination: 25 days.

AVAILABILITY
Powder for Injection: 150 mg, designed to deliver 125 mg/1.25 ml.

INDICATIONS AND DOSAGES
▸ Psoriasis

Subcutaneous

Adults, Elderly. Initially, 0.7 mg/kg followed by weekly doses of 1 mg/kg. Maximum: 200 mg (single dose).

CONTRAINDICATIONS
Concurrent use of immunosuppressive agents

INTERACTIONS
Drug

Immunosuppressive agents: Increase the risk of infection.

Live-virus vaccines: Decrease the immune response.

Herbal

None known.

Food

None known.

DIAGNOSTIC TEST EFFECTS
May increase the lymphocyte count.

SIDE EFFECTS
Frequent (32%–10%)

Headache, chills, nausea, injection site pain

Occasional (8%–7%)

Myalgia, flu-like symptoms, fever

Rare (4%)

Back pain, acne

SERIOUS REACTIONS
! Hypersensitivity reaction, malignancies, serious infections (abscess, cellulitis, postoperative wound infection, pneumonia), thrombocytopenia, and worsening of psoriasis occur rarely.

NURSING CONSIDERATIONS

Baseline Assessment

- Obtain the patient's CBC, lymphocyte, and platelet counts before beginning therapy and periodically thereafter.
- Examine the patient's skin before beginning efalizumab therapy, and document the extent and location of psoriasis lesions.

Lifespan Considerations

- It is unknown if efalizumab is distributed in breast milk.
- Efalizumab is not indicated for use in children.
- Age-related increased incidence of infection requires cautious use in the elderly.

Precautions

- Use efalizumab cautiously in patients with asthma, chronic infections, a history of allergic reactions, or a history of malignancy.

Administration and Handling

Subcutaneous

- Refrigerate unopened vials.
- Reconstituted solution may be stored at room temperature for up to 8 hours.
- Slowly inject 1.3 ml of sterile water for injection into the efalizumab vial using the provided prefilled diluent syringe.
- Swirl the vial gently to dissolve; do not shake it because foaming will occur.
- Dissolution takes less than 5 minutes.
- Administer the injection into the abdomen, buttocks, thigh, or upper arm.

Intervention and Evaluation

- Examine the patient's skin throughout efalizumab therapy. Document improvement or worsening of psoriasis lesions.

Patient Teaching

- Teach the patient and caregiver the proper sterile technique for preparing and injecting efalizumab.
- Advise the patient that efalizumab treatment increases the risk of developing an infection.
- Inform the patient about the duration of efalizumab treatment and the required monitoring procedures.
- Caution the patient to notify the health care provider if he or she experiences bleeding from the gums, bruising or petechiae of the skin, or signs of infection.
- If the patient is diagnosed with a new malignancy, tell him or her to inform the physician about efalizumab use.
- Advise the patient not to undergo phototherapy treatments.

gefitinib

geh-**fih**-tih-nib

(Iressa)

CATEGORY AND SCHEDULE

Pregnancy Risk Category: D

MECHANISM OF ACTION

Blocks the signaling pathway that binds to the epidermal growth factor receptor (EGFR) on the surface of normal and cancer cells. EGFR activates the enzyme tyrosine kinase, which sends signals instructing the cells to grow. **Therapeutic Effect:** Inhibits the growth of cancer cells.

PHARMACOKINETICS

Slowly absorbed and extensively distributed throughout the body. Protein binding: 90%. Undergoes extensive metabolism in the liver. Excreted in the feces. ***Half-life:*** 48 hr.

AVAILABILITY

Tablets: 250 mg.

INDICATIONS AND DOSAGES

▸ Non–small cell lung cancer

PO

Adults, Elderly. 250 mg/day; may increase to 500 mg/day for patients receiving drugs that may decrease gefitinib blood concentrations, such as rifampin and phenytoin.

CONTRAINDICATIONS

None known.

INTERACTIONS

Drug

Cimetidine, phenytoin, ranitidine, rifampin, sodium bicarbonate: May decrease gefitinib blood concentration and effectiveness.

Itraconazole, ketoconazole: Increases gefitinib blood concentration.
Metoprolol: Increases the effect of metoprolol.
Warfarin: Increases the risk of bleeding.

Herbal

None known.

Food

None known.

DIAGNOSTIC TEST EFFECTS

May increase serum alkaline phosphatase, bilirubin, AST (SGOT), and ALT (SGPT) levels.

SIDE EFFECTS

Frequent (48%–25%)
Diarrhea, rash, acne
Occasional (13%–8%)
Dry skin, nausea, vomiting, pruritus
Rare (7%–2%)
Anorexia, asthenia, weight loss, peripheral edema, eye pain

SERIOUS REACTIONS

! Pancreatitis and ocular hemorrhage occur rarely.
! Hypersensitivity reaction produces angioedema and urticaria.

NURSING CONSIDERATIONS

Baseline Assessment

- Give the patient antidiarrheals and antiemetics, if ordered, to help prevent and treat diarrhea, nausea, and vomiting. For patients who can't tolerate diarrhea, expect to interrupt gefitinib therapy for up to 14 days.

Lifespan Considerations

- Gefitinib may cause fetal harm and result in termination of pregnancy. Pregnant or breast-feeding women should not receive this drug.
- The safety and efficacy of gefitinib have not been established in children.
- No age-related precautions have been noted in the elderly.

Precautions

- Use gefitinib cautiously in patients with hepatic impairement or severe renal impairment.

Administration and Handling

- Give gefitinib without regard to food. Don't crush or break film-coated tablets.

Intervention and Evaluation

- Encourage the patient to drink adequate fluids.
- Auscultate the patient's bowel sounds for hyperactivity.
- Assess the patient's pattern of daily bowel activity and stool consistency.
- Examine the patient's skin for a rash.

Patient Teaching

- Warn the patient to immediately notify the physician if he or she experiences signs and symptoms of infection, including fever and flu-like symptoms.
- Advise the patient to notify the physician if he or she experiences anorexia, nausea, vomiting, or persistent or severe diarrhea.
- Urge the patient not to receive vaccinations without the physician's approval and to avoid crowds and people with known infections.
- Caution female patients to avoid becoming pregnant during gefitinib therapy and to use contraceptive methods during treatment and for up to 12 months afterward.

gemtuzumab ozogamicin

gem-**too**-zoo-mab
(Mylotarg)

CATEGORY AND SCHEDULE

Pregnancy Risk Category: D

MECHANISM OF ACTION

Binds to an antigen on the surface of leukemic blast cells, resulting in the formation of a complex that leads to the release of the antibiotic inside the myeloid cells. The antibiotic then binds to DNA, resulting in DNA double-strand breaks and cell death. **Therapeutic Effect:** Inhibits colony formation in cultures of adult leukemic bone marrow cells.

PHARMACOKINETICS

Elimination half-life: 45 hr after first infusion; 60 hr after second infusion

AVAILABILITY

Powder for Injection: 5 mg.

INDICATIONS AND DOSAGES

▸ **CD33 positive acute myeloid leukemia**

IV

Adults 60 yr and older. 9 mg/m^2 repeated in 14 days for a total of 2 doses.

CONTRAINDICATIONS

None known.

INTERACTIONS

Drug

None known.

Herbal

None known.

Food

None known.

DIAGNOSTIC TEST EFFECTS

May increase serum bilirubin, AST (SGOT), and ALT (SGPT) levels. May decrease blood Hgb and Hct levels, platelet count, WBC count, and serum magnesium and potassium levels.

IV INCOMPATIBILITIES

Don't mix gemtuzumab with any other medications.

SIDE EFFECTS

◂**ALERT**▸ Most patients experience a postinfusion symptom complex of fever (85%), chills (73%), nausea (70%), and vomiting (63%) that resolves within 2–4 hours with supportive therapy.

Frequent (44%–31%)

Asthenia, diarrhea, abdominal pain, headache, stomatitis, dyspnea, epistaxis

Occasional (25%–15%)

Constipation, neutropenic fever, nonspecific rash, herpes simplex infection, hypertension, hypotension, petechiae, peripheral edema, dizziness, insomnia, back pain

Rare (14%–10%)

Pharyngitis, ecchymosis, dyspepsia, tachycardia, hematuria, rhinitis

SERIOUS REACTIONS

! Severe myelosuppression, characterized by neutropenia, anemia, and thrombocytopenia, occurs in 98% of all patients.

! Sepsis occurs in 25% of patients.

! Hepatotoxicity also may occur.

NURSING CONSIDERATIONS

Baseline Assessment

• Monitor the patient's baseline serum chemistry levels, CBC (to monitor for myelosuppression), and liver function test results.

Lifespan Considerations

• Pregnant women should not receive gemtuzumab because it may cause fetal harm. It is unknown if gemtuzumab is excreted in breast milk; however, women receiving this drug should not breast-feed.

• The safety and efficacy of gemtuzumab have not been established in children.

• No age-related precautions have been noted in the elderly.

Precautions

• Use gemtuzumab cautiously in patients with hepatic impairment.

Administration and Handling

◀ **ALERT** ▶ Give diphenhydramine 50 mg and acetaminophen 650 to 1,000 mg 1 hour before administering gemtuzumab, as prescribed. Follow with acetaminophen 650 to 1,000 mg every 4 hours for 2 doses, then every 4 hours as prescribed and as needed. Full recovery from hematologic toxicities is not a requirement for giving the second gemtuzumab dose.

IV

• Protect the drug from direct and indirect sunlight and unshielded fluorescent light during preparation and administration.

• Refrigerate—don't freeze—the powder for injection.

• Use strict aseptic technique in preparing the drug to protect the patient from infection.

• Prepare the drug in a biological safety hood with the fluorescent light off.

• Before reconstitution, let the vials come to room temperature.

• Using sterile syringes, reconstitute each vial with 5 ml sterile water for injection to provide a concentration of 1 mg/ml.

• Gently swirl the vial; then inspect for particulate matter or discoloration.

• After reconstitution, protect the solution from light. The solution is stable for up to 8 hours if refrigerated.

• Withdraw the desired volume from each vial and inject into an IV bag containing 100 ml 0.9% NaCl; place the IV bag into an ultraviolet protectant bag.

• Administer the solution as soon as it has been diluted in 100 ml 0.9% NaCl.

• Infuse the drug over 2 hours, using a separate peripheral or central line equipped with a low-protein-binding 1.2-micron filter.

• Don't give gemtuzumab by IV push or bolus.

Intervention and Evaluation

• Monitor the patient's blood chemistriy values, CBC, and liver function studies.

• Assess the patient for signs and symptoms of anemia (excessive fatigue and weakness) and myelosuppression (ecchymosis, fever, signs of local infection, sore throat, and unusual bleeding from any site).

• Evaluate the patient for signs and symptoms of stomatitis (burning or erythema of oral mucosa, ulceration, sore throat, difficulty swallowing).

• Monitor the patient's BP for evidence of hypertension or hypotension.

Patient Teaching

• Urge the patient not to receive vaccinations and to avoid contact with anyone who has recently received a live-virus vaccine.

• Instruct the patient to notify the physician if he or she experiences easy bruising, fever, signs of local infection, sore throat, or unusual bleeding from any site.

imatinib mesylate

im-a-tin-ib
(Gleevec, Glivec[AUS])

CATEGORY AND SCHEDULE
Pregnancy Risk Category: D

MECHANISM OF ACTION
Inhibits Bcr-Abl tyrosine kinase, an enzyme created by the Philadelphia chromosome abnormality found in patients with chronic myeloid leukemia (CML). **Therapeutic Effect:** Suppresses tumor growth during the three stages of CML; blast crisis, accelerated phase, and chronic phase.

PHARMACOKINETICS
Well absorbed after PO administration. Binds to plasma proteins, particularly albumin. Metabolized in the liver. Eliminated mainly in the feces as metabolites. ***Half-life:*** 18 hr.

AVAILABILITY
Tablets: 100 mg, 400 mg.

INDICATIONS AND DOSAGES
▸ **CML**

PO

Adults, Elderly. 400 mg/day for patients in chronic-phase CML; 600 mg/day for patients in accelerated phase or blast crisis. May increase dosage from 400 to 600 mg/day for patients in chronic phase or from 600 to 800 mg (given as 300–400 mg twice a day) for patients in accelerated phase or blast crisis in the absence of a severe drug reaction or severe neutropenia or thrombocytopenia in the following circumstances: progression of the disease, failure to achieve a satisfactory hematologic response after 3 months or more of treatment, or loss of a previously achieved hematologic response.

Children. 260 mg/m^2 a day as a single daily dose or in 2 divided doses.

CONTRAINDICATIONS
Known hypersensitivity to imatinib

INTERACTIONS
Drug

Carbamazepine, dexamethasone, phenobarbital, phenytoin, rifampicin: Decrease imatinib plasma concentration.
Clarithromycin, erythromycin, itraconazole, ketoconazole: Increase imatinib plasma concentration.
Cyclosporine, pimozide: May alter the therapeutic effects of these drugs.
Dihydropyridine calcium channel blockers, simvastatin, triazolobenzodiazepines: May increase the blood concentration of these drugs.
Live-virus vaccines: May potentiate viral replication, increase vaccine side effects, and decrease the patient's antibody response to the vaccine.
Warfarin: Reduces the effect of warfarin.

Herbal

St. John's wort: Decreases imatinib concentration.

Food

None known.

DIAGNOSTIC TEST EFFECTS
May increase serum bilirubin AST (SGOT), and ALT (SGPT) levels. May decrease platelet count, WBC count, and serum potassium level.

SIDE EFFECTS
Frequent (68%–24%)

Nausea, diarrhea, vomiting, headache, fluid retention (periorbital, lower extremities), rash, musculoskeletal pain, muscle cramps, arthralgia

Occasional (23%–10%)
Abdominal pain, cough, myalgia, fatigue, fever, anorexia, dyspepsia, constipation, night sweats, pruritus
Rare (less than 10%)
Nasopharyngitis, petechiae, asthenia, epistaxis

SERIOUS REACTIONS

! Severe fluid retention (manifested as pleural effusion, pericardial effusion, pulmonary edema, and ascites) and hepatotoxicity occur rarely.
! Neutropenia and thrombocytopenia are expected responses to the drug.
! Respiratory toxicity, manifested as dyspnea and pneumonia, may occur.

NURSING CONSIDERATIONS

Baseline Assessment

- Expect to obtain the patient's CBC weekly for the first month, biweekly for the second month, and periodically thereafter.
- Monitor the patient's liver function tests, including serum alkaline phosphatase, bilirubin, AST (SGOT), and ALT (SGPT) levels, before imatinib treatment begins and monthly thereafter.

Lifespan Considerations

- Because imatinib may cause severe teratogenic effects, female patients should avoid becoming pregnant and breast-feeding while taking this drug.
- The safety and efficacy of imatinib have not been established in children.
- Elderly patients are at increased risk for fluid retention.

Precautions

- Use imatinib cautiously in patients with hepatic or renal impairment.

Administration and Handling

PO

- Give imatinib with a meal and a large glass of water.

Intervention and Evaluation

- Assess the patient's periorbital area and lower extremities for early evidence of fluid retention.
- Weigh and monitor the patient for unexpected rapid weight gain.
- Administer antiemetics, if ordered, to control nausea and vomiting.
- Assess the patient's pattern of daily bowel activity and stool consistency.
- Monitor the patient's CBC for evidence of neutropenia and thrombocytopenia and liver function test results for evidence of hepatotoxicity. Neutropenia and thrombocytopenia usually last 2 to 4 weeks.

Patient Teaching

- Instruct the patient to take imatinib with food and a full glass of water.
- Urge the patient to avoid receiving vaccinations and coming in contact with crowds, people with known infections, and anyone who has recently received a live-virus vaccine.

rituximab

rye-**tucks**-ih-mab
(Mabthera[AUS], Rituxan)

CATEGORY AND SCHEDULE

Pregnancy Risk Category: C

MECHANISM OF ACTION

Binds to CD20, the antigen found on the surface of B lymphocytes and B-cell non-Hodgkin's lymphomas. **Therapeutic Effect:** Produces cytotoxicity, reducing tumor size.

PHARMACOKINETICS

Rapidly depletes B cells. ***Half-life:*** 59.8 hr after first infusion and 174 hr after fourth infusion.

AVAILABILITY
Injection: 10 mg/ml.

INDICATIONS AND DOSAGES
▸ Non-Hodgkin's lymphoma

IV

Adults. 375 mg/m^2 once weekly for 4–8 wk. May administer a second 4-wk course.

CONTRAINDICATIONS
Hypersensitivity to murine proteins

INTERACTIONS
Drug
None known.

Herbal
None known.

Food
None known.

DIAGNOSTIC TEST EFFECTS
None known.

IV INCOMPATIBILITIES
Don't mix rituximab with any other medications.

SIDE EFFECTS
Frequent
Fever (49%), chills (32%), asthenia (16%), headache (14%), angioedema (13%), hypotension (10%), nausea (18%), rash or pruritus (10%)

Occasional (less than 10%)
Myalgia, dizziness, abdominal pain, throat irritation, vomiting, neutropenia, rhinitis, bronchospasm, urticaria

SERIOUS REACTIONS
! A hypersensitivity reaction marked by hypotension, bronchospasm, and angioedema may occur.

! Arrhythmias may occur, particularly in those with a history of preexisting cardiac conditions.

NURSING CONSIDERATIONS
Baseline Assessment
- Expect to obtain the patient's CBC before and regularly during therapy.

Lifespan Considerations
- Be aware that rituximab may cause fetal B-cell depletion.
- Female patients with childbearing potential should use contraceptive methods during treatment and for up to 12 months afterward.
- It is unknown if rituximab is distributed in breast milk.
- The safety and efficacy of rituximab have not been established in children.
- No age-related precautions have been noted in the elderly.

Precautions
- Use rituximab cautiously in patients with a history of cardiac disease.

Administration and Handling
◀ALERT▶ Expect to pretreat the patient with acetaminophen and diphenhydramine before each infusion to help prevent infusion-related reactions.

IV

◀ALERT▶ Don't give rituximab by IV push or bolus.
- Refrigerate unopened vials.
- Withdraw the needed amount into an infusion bag, and dilute it with 0.9% NaCl or D_5W to a final concentration of 1 to 4 mg/ml.
- The diluted solution is stable for up to 24 hours if refrigerated and up to 36 hours if stored at room temperature.
- For the initial infusion, infuse the drug at 50 mg/hour. The infusion rate may be increased, as necessary, in increments of 50 mg/hour every 30 minutes to a maximum rate of 400 mg/hour.
- For subsequent infusions, the drug may be administered initially at 100

mg/hour and increased in increments of 100 mg/hour every 30 minutes to a maximum rate of 400 mg/hr.

Intervention and Evaluation

• Monitor the patient for infusion-related reactions, including chills, fever, hypotension, and rigors, which usually occur 30 minutes to 2 hours after beginning the first rituximab infusion. Slowing the infusion resolves these symptoms.

Patient Teaching

• Advise the patient to immediately report chills, fever, or shaking.

• Instruct female patients of child-bearing age to use contraceptive methods during rituximab treatment and for up to 12 months afterward.

tositumomab and iodine ^{131}I-tositumomab

toe-sit-**two**-mo-mab
(Bexxar)

CATEGORY AND SCHEDULE

Pregnancy Risk Category: X

MECHANISM OF ACTION

A monoclonal antibody composed of an antibody conjoined with a radiolabeled antitumor antibody. The antibody portion binds specifically to the CD20 antigen, which is found on pre-B and B lymphocytes and on more than 90% of B-cell non-Hodgkin lymphomas resulting in formation of a complex. **Therapeutic Effect:** Induces cytotoxicity associated with ionizing radiation from the radioisotope. Depletes circulating CD20-positive cells.

PHARMACOKINETICS

Elimination of iodine 131 (^{131}I) occurs by decay and excretion in urine. ***Half-life:*** 8 days. Patients with high tumor burden, splenomegaly, or bone marrow involvement have a faster clearance, shorter half-life, and larger volume of distribution.

AVAILABILITY

Kit (Dosimetric [Bexxar]): tositumomab 225 mg/16.1 ml (2 vials), tositumomab 35 mg/2.5 ml (1 vial), and ^{131}I-tositumomab 0.1 mg/ml (1 vial).
Kit (Therapeutic [Bexxar]): tositumomab 225 mg/16.1 ml (2 vials), tositumomab 35 mg/2.5 ml (1 vial), and ^{131}I-tositumomab 1.1 mg/ml (1 or 2 vials).

INDICATIONS AND DOSAGES

▸ Non-Hodgkin's lymphoma

IV

Adults, Elderly. Dosage contains 4 components. Day 0: tositumomab 450 mg/50 NaCl over 60 min. Then ^{131}I-tositumomab 35 mg in 30 ml NaCl over 20 min. Day 7: tositumomab 450 mg/50 NaCl over 60 min. Then, ^{131}I-tositumomab to deliver 65–75 cGy total body irradiation and tositumomab 35 mg over 20 min.

CONTRAINDICATIONS

Hypersensitivity to murine proteins

INTERACTIONS

Drug

Anticoagulants, medications that interfere with platelet function: Increase the risk of bleeding and hemorrhage.

Herbal

None known.

Food

None known.

DIAGNOSTIC TEST EFFECTS

May decrease blood Hct and Hgb levels, platelet and WBC counts, and thyroid-stimulating hormone level.

SIDE EFFECTS

Frequent (46%–18%)
Asthenia, fever, nausea, cough, chills
Occasional (17%–10%)
Rash, headache, abdominal pain, vomiting, anorexia, myalgia, diarrhea, pharyngitis, arthralgia, rhinitis, pruritus
Rare (9%–5%)
Peripheral edema, diaphoresis, constipation, dyspepsia, back pain, hypotension, vasodilation, dizziness, somnolence

SERIOUS REACTIONS

! Infusion toxicity, characterized by fever, rigors, diaphoresis, hypotension, dyspnea, and nausea, may occur during or within 48 hours of the infusion.
! Severe, prolonged myelosuppression, characterized by neutropenia, anemia, and thrombocytopenia, occurs in 71% of patients.
! Sepsis occurs in 45% of patients.
! Hemorrhage occurs in 12% of patients.
! Myelodysplastic syndrome occurs in 8% of patients.

NURSING CONSIDERATIONS

Baseline Assessment

- Obtain the patient's CBC before beginning therapy and at least weekly after administration for at least 10 weeks.

Lifespan Considerations

- The use of the ^{131}I-tositumomab component is contraindicated during pregnancy and causes severe, possibly irreversible hypothyroidism in neonates.
- Because ^{131}I-tositumomab is excreted in breast milk, patients taking this drug should not breast-feed.
- The safety and efficacy of this drug have not been established in children.
- Elderly patients (older than 65 years) have exhibited a lower overall response rate to the drug. They've also had a lower incidence, but longer duration, of severe hematologic toxicity.

Precautions

- Use this drug cautiously in patients with active systemic infection, immunosuppression, or impaired renal function.

Administration and Handling

◀ALERT▶ Pretreat by administering diphenhydramine 50 mg and acetaminophen 650–1,000 mg 1 hour before administering tositumomab; followed by acetaminophen 650–1,000 mg every 4 hours for 2 doses, then every 4 hours as needed. Full recovery from hematologic toxicities is not a requirement for giving the second dose.

◀ALERT▶ Be aware that the regimen consists of 4 components given in 2 separate steps: the dosimetric step, followed 7 to 14 days later by the therapeutic step. During the infusion, use IV tubing with an in-line 0.22-micron filter, and use the same tubing for both the dosimetric and therapeutic steps because changing the filter results in drug loss. Plan to reduce the infusion rate by 50% for mild to moderate infusion toxicity and to interrupt the infusion for severe infusion toxicity. Expect to resume therapy at 50% of the infusion rate when toxic reactions have resolved.

◀ALERT▶ Administer a thyroid protective agent such as potassium iodide, as prescribed, beginning 24 hours before administration of the ^{131}I-tositumomab dosimetric step and continuing for 2 weeks after administration of the therapeutic step.

◀ALERT▶ Remember that reconstitution amounts and rates of administration are the same for both the dosimetric and therapeutic steps.

IV

• Refrigerate tositumomab vials before dilution. Protect from strong light.

• After dilution, tositumomab solution is stable for 24 hours if refrigerated and 8 hours at room temperature. Discard any unused portion left in the vial. Do not shake.

• Use strict aseptic technique in preparing the drug to protect the patient from infection. Follow radiation safety protocols.

• Reconstitute 450 mg tositumomab in 50 ml 0.9% NaCl.

• Infuse tositumomab over 60 minutes.

• Keep ^{131}I-tositumomab frozen until thawing it before drug administration.

• Thawed ^{131}I-tositumomab doses are stable for 8 hours if refrigerated. Discard any unused portion.

• Reconstitute ^{131}I-tositumomab in 30 ml 0.9% NaCl.

• Infuse ^{131}I-tositumomab over 20 minutes.

Intervention and Evaluation

• Monitor the patient's laboratory values for evidence of severe and prolonged anemia, neutropenia, and thrombocytopenia.

• Know that time to nadir is 4 to 7 weeks and the duration of cytopenias (predominantly grade 3 and 4 thrombocytopenia and grade 3 and 4 neutropenia) is approximately 30 days.

• Monitor the patient for signs and symptoms of hematologic toxicity (including excessive fatigue and weakness, chills, fever, ecchymosis, and unusual bleeding from any site) and hypothyroidism (including fatigue, sensitivity to cold, unexplained weight gain, and constipation).

Patient Teaching

• Inform the female patient that tositumomab has a pregnancy risk category of X, which means that she must guard against becoming pregnant while receiving this drug.

• Warn the patient to notify the physician if he or she experiences easy bruising, fever, signs of local infection, sore throat, or unusual bleeding from any site.

• Urge the patient not to receive immunizations during therapy and to avoid contact with those who have recently received a live-virus vaccine.

trastuzumab

traz-**two**-zoo-mab
(Herceptin)

CATEGORY AND SCHEDULE

Pregnancy Risk Category: B

MECHANISM OF ACTION

Binds to the HER-2 protein, which is overexpressed in 25%–30% of primary breast cancers, thereby inhibiting proliferation of tumor cells. **Therapeutic Effect:** Inhibits the growth of tumor cells and mediates antibody-dependent cellular cytotoxicity.

PHARMACOKINETICS

Half-life: 5.8 days (range: 1–32 days).

AVAILABILITY

Injection, Powder for Reconstitution: 440 mg.

INDICATIONS AND DOSAGES

▸ **Breast cancer**

IV

Adults, Elderly. Initially, 4 mg/kg as a 30- to 90-min infusion, then 2 mg/kg weekly as a 30-min infusion.

CONTRAINDICATIONS

Pre-existing cardiac disease

INTERACTIONS

Drug

Cyclophosphamide, doxorubicin, epirubicin: May increase the risk of cardiac dysfunction.

Herbal

None known.

Food

None known.

DIAGNOSTIC TEST EFFECTS

None known.

IV INCOMPATIBILITIES

Don't mix trastuzumab with any other medications or with D_5W.

SIDE EFFECTS

Frequent (greater than 20%)

Pain, asthenia, fever, chills, headache, abdominal pain, back pain, infection, nausea, diarrhea, vomiting, cough, dyspnea

Occasional (15%–5%)

Tachycardia, CHF, flulike symptoms, anorexia, edema, bone pain, arthralgia, insomnia, dizziness, paresthesia, depression, rhinitis, pharyngitis, sinusitis

Rare (less than 5%)

Allergic reaction, anemia, leukopenia, neuropathy, herpes simplex

SERIOUS REACTIONS

! Cardiomyopathy, ventricular dysfunction, and CHF occur rarely.

! Pancytopenia may occur.

NURSING CONSIDERATIONS

Baseline Assessment

- Evaluate the patient's left ventricular function, and obtain a baseline EKG and multigated acquisition (MUGA) scan before starting therapy.
- Expect to obtain the patient's CBC before and periodically during therapy.

Lifespan Considerations

- It is unknown if trastuzumab is distributed in breast milk.
- The safety and efficacy of trastuzumab have not been established in children.
- Age-related cardiac dysfunction may require cautious use in the elderly.

Precautions

- Use trastuzumab cautiously in patients who have previously received cardiotoxic drug therapy or radiation therapy to the chest wall and in those with a known hypersensitivity to the drug.

Administration and Handling

◂ALERT▸ Don't give trastuzumab by IV push or IV bolus. Do not use dextrose solutions for reconstitution.

IV

- Refrigerate unopened vials.
- Reconstitute the vial with 20 ml bacteriostatic water for injection (with benzyl alcohol) to yield a concentration of 21 mg/ml. If the patient is hypersensitive to benzyl alcohol, use sterile water for injection.
- Add the calculated dose from the vial to an IV solution of 250 ml 0.9% NaCl (do not use D_5W).
- Gently mix contents in bag.
- The reconstituted IV solution normally appears colorless to pale yellow.
- After reconstitution of the vial with bacteriostatic water for injection, the

solution is stable for 28 days if refrigerated. After reconstitution of the vial with sterile water for injection without a preservative, use the solution immediately; discard unused portions.

- IV solution reconstituted in 0.9% NaCl is stable for up to 24 hours if refrigerated.
- Give loading dose (4 mg/kg) over 90 minutes. Give maintenance infusion (2 mg/kg) over 30 minutes.

Intervention and Evaluation

- Frequently monitor the patient for signs and symptoms of deteriorating cardiac function.
- Assess the patient for asthenia, and assist the patient with ambulation if needed.
- Monitor the patient for abdominal pain, back pain, chills, and fever.
- Administer antiemetics, if ordered, to treat nausea or vomiting.
- Assess the patient's pattern of daily bowel activity and stool consistency.

Patient Teaching

- Urge the patient to avoid receiving vaccinations and coming in contact with crowds, people with known infections, and anyone who has recently received an oral polio vaccine.

20 Miscellaneous Antineoplastic Agents

arsenic trioxide
asparaginase
azacitidine
BCG, intravesical
dacarbazine
erlotinib
etoposide, VP-16
interleukin-2 (aldesleukin)
irinotecan
mitotane
mitoxantrone
palifermin
pegaspargase
procarbazine hydrochloride
temozolomide
teniposide
topotecan

Uses: Miscellaneous antineoplastic agents have a wide range of specific uses. *Arsenic trioxide* is used to treat acute promyelocytic leukemia in patients who don't respond to other treatments. The enzyme *asparaginase* and its derivative *pegaspargase* are used to treat acute lymphocytic leukemia; asparaginase is also given with other drugs to treat lymphoma. *Azacitidine* is used to treat refractory anemia as well as chronic myelomonocytic leukemia. *Bacillus Calmette-Guerin (also known as BCG)* is used to treat and prevent bladder carcinoma in situ. *Dacarbazine* is used to treat metastatic malignant melanoma and, with other drugs, Hodgkin's disease. *Erlotinib* is used to treat an overactive bladder. The podophyllotoxins *etoposide* and *teniposide* are used in acute lymphocytic leukemia; etoposide is also used to treat testicular tumors, small-cell lung carcinoma, and other cancers. *Interleukin-2* is prescribed to treat metastic renal cell carcinoma and metastic melanoma. Of the DNA topoisomerase inhibitors, *irinotecan* is used for metastatic colon or rectal cancer, whereas *topotecan* is used for metastatic ovarian cancer and small-cell lung cancer. Because of its antiadrenal activity, *mitotane* is used to treat adrenocortical carcinoma as well as Cushing's syndrome. *Mitoxantrone* is helpful not only in leukemias and prostate cancer, but also in multiple sclerosis. *Palifermin* is used to treat mucositis. *Procarbazine* is used primarily to treat advanced Hodgkin's disease. *Temozolomide* is prescribed for gliomas, metastatic melanoma, and some types of anaplastic astrocytoma.

Action: Because these antineoplastic agents belong to many different subcategories, their mechanisms of action are diverse. For details, see the specific drug entries.

arsenic trioxide

are-sih-nic try-**ox**-ide
(Trisenox)
Do not confuse Trisenox with Trimox.

CATEGORY AND SCHEDULE

Pregnancy Risk Category: D

MECHANISM OF ACTION

An antineoplastic that produces morphologic changes and DNA fragmentation in promyelocytic leukemia cells. **Therapeutic Effect:** Produces cell death.

AVAILABILITY

Injection: 1 mg/ml.

INDICATIONS AND DOSAGES

▸ **Acute promyelocytic leukemia**

IV

Adults, Elderly. Induction: 0.15 mg/kg/day until myelosuppression occurs. Do not exceed 60 induction doses. Beginning 3–6 wk after completion of induction therapy, 0.15 mg/kg/day for 25 doses over a period of up to 5 wk.

CONTRAINDICATIONS

None known.

INTERACTIONS

Drug

Amphotericin B, diuretics: May produce electrolyte imbalances.
Antiarrhythmics, thioridazine: May prolong QT interval.

Herbal

None known.

Food

None known.

DIAGNOSTIC TEST EFFECTS

May decrease Hgb levels, serum calcium and magnesium levels, and platelet and WBC counts. May increase AST (SGOT) and ALT (SGPT) levels.

IV INCOMPATIBILITIES

Don't mix arsenic trioxide with any other medications.

SIDE EFFECTS

Expected (75%–50%)
Nausea, cough, fatigue, fever, headache, vomiting, abdominal pain, tachycardia, diarrhea, dyspnea
Frequent (43%–30%)
Dermatitis, insomnia, edema, rigors, prolonged QT interval, sore throat, pruritus, arthralgia, paresthesia, anxiety
Occasional (28%–20%)
Constipation, myalgia, hypotension, epistaxis, anorexia, dizziness, sinusitis
Occasional (15%–8%)
Ecchymosis, nonspecific pain, weight gain, herpes simplex, wheezing, flushing, diaphoresis, tremor, hypertension, palpitations, dyspepsia, eye irritation, blurred vision, asthenia, diminished breath sounds, crackles
Rare
Confusion, petechiae, dry mouth, oral candidiasis, incontinence, rhonchi

SERIOUS REACTIONS

! Seizures, GI hemorrhage, renal impairment or failure, pleural or pericardial effusion, hemoptysis, and sepsis occur rarely.
! Prolonged QT interval, complete AV block, unexplained fever, dyspnea, weight gain, and effusion are evidence of arsenic toxicity. If arsenic toxicity is apparent, stop arsenic trioxide treatment and begin steroid treatment as ordered.

NURSING CONSIDERATIONS

Baseline Assessment

• Obtain the patient's blood Hct and Hgb levels, platelet count, and WBC count before and frequently during treatment.

Lifespan Considerations

• Arsenic trioxide is distributed in breast milk and may cause fetal harm. It should not be used by pregnant or breast-feeding women.

Precautions

• Use arsenic cautiously in patients with cardiac abnormalities or renal impairment.

Administration and Handling

IV

◀ALERT▶ A central venous line is not required for administration of arsenic; the drug may be infused through a peripheral line.

• Store the drug at room temperature.

• After withdrawing the drug from ampule, dilute it with 100 to 250 ml D_5W or 0.9% NaCl.

• The diluted solution is stable for 24 hours at room temperature and 48 hours if refrigerated.

• Infuse the solution over 1 to 2 hours. The duration of the infusion may be extended up to 4 hours.

Intervention and Evaluation

• Monitor the patient's CBC, hepatic function test results, and blood chemistry values. Check serum potassium levels (hypokalemia is more common than hyperkalemia) and blood glucose levels (hyperglycemia is more common than hypoglycemia).

• Monitor the patient for signs and symptoms of arsenic toxicity, including confusion, dyspnea, fever, muscle weakness, seizures, and weight gain.

Patient Teaching

• Advise the patient to avoid tasks that require alertness or motor skills until the effects of the drug are known.

• Instruct the patient to contact the physician if fever, vomiting, difficulty breathing, or rapid pulse rate occur.

asparaginase

ah-spa-**raj**-in-ace
(Elspar, Kidrolase[CAN], Leunase[AUS])

Do not confuse asparaginase with pegaspargase.

CATEGORY AND SCHEDULE

Pregnancy Risk Category: C

MECHANISM OF ACTION

An enzyme that inhibits DNA, RNA, and protein synthesis by breaking down asparagine, thus depriving tumor cells of this essential amino acid. Cell cycle–specific for G_1 phase of cell division. **Therapeutic Effect:** Kills leukemic cells.

PHARMACOKINETICS

Metabolized by the reticuloendothelial system through slow sequestration. ***Half-life:*** 39–49 hr IM; 8–30 hr IV.

AVAILABILITY

Powder for Injection: 10,000 international units.

INDICATIONS AND DOSAGES

▸ **Acute lymphocytic leukemia**

IV

Adults, Elderly, Children. 1,000 units/kg/day for 10 days as combination therapy or 200 units/kg/day for 28 days as monotherapy.

IM

Adults, Elderly, Children. 6 to 6,000

units/m^2/dose 3 times a week for 3 wk as combination therapy.

OFF-LABEL USES
Treatment of acute myelocytic leukemia, acute myelomonocytic leukemia, chronic lymphocytic leukemia, Hodgkin's disease, lymphosarcoma, melanosarcoma, and reticulum cell sarcoma

CONTRAINDICATIONS
History of hypersensitivity to asparaginase, pancreatitis

INTERACTIONS
Drug
Antigout medications: May decrease the effects of these drugs.
Live-virus vaccines: May potentiate virus replication, increase vaccine side effects, and decrease the patient's antibody response to the vaccine.
Methotrexate: May block the effects of this drug.
Steroids, vincristine: May increase the risk of neuropathy and disturbances of erythropoiesis; may enhance hyperglycemic effect of asparaginase.
Herbal
None known.
Food
None known.

DIAGNOSTIC TEST EFFECTS
May increase BUN, blood ammonia, and blood glucose levels; serum alkaline phosphatase, bilirubin, uric acid, AST (SGOT), and ALT (SGPT) levels; platelet count, PT; activated partial thromboplastin time; and thrombin time. May decrease blood-clotting factors (including antithrombin, plasma fibrinogen, and plasminogen) as well as serum albumin, calcium, and cholesterol levels.

IV INCOMPATIBILITIES
None known.

SIDE EFFECTS
Frequent
Allergic reaction (rash, urticaria, arthralgia, facial edema, hypotension, respiratory distress) pancreatitis (severe abdominal pain, nausea and vomiting)
Occasional
CNS effects (confusion, drowsiness, depression, anxiety, and fatigue), stomatitis, hypoalbuminemia or uric acid nephropathy (manifested as pedal or lower extremity edema), hyperglycemia
Rare
Hyperthermia (including fever or chills), thrombosis, seizures

SERIOUS REACTIONS
! Hepatotoxicity usually occurs within 2 weeks of initial treatment.
! The risk of an allergic reaction, including anaphylaxis, increases after repeated therapy.
! Myelosuppression may be severe.

NURSING CONSIDERATIONS
Baseline Assessment
◀ALERT▶ Keep antihistamines, epinephrine, IV corticosteroids, and oxygen equipment readily available before administering asparaginase.
• Assess baseline CNS function and expect to obtain comprehensive blood chemistry studies and CBC results before therapy begins and whenever more than 1 week has elapsed between doses.
Lifespan Considerations
• Asparaginase use should be avoided during pregnancy, especially during the first trimester, and in patients who are breast-feeding.
• No age-related precautions have been noted in children or the elderly.

Precautions

• Use asparaginase cautiously in patients with diabetes mellitus, current or recent chickenpox, gout, herpes zoster, infection, or hepatic or renal impairment, and in those who have recently had cytotoxic or radiation therapy.

Administration and Handling

◀ALERT▶ Asparaginase dosage is individualized based on the patient's clinical response and tolerance of the drug's adverse effects. When administering this drug in combination therapy, consult specific protocols for optimum dosage and sequence of drug administration.

◀ALERT▶ Asparaginase may be carcinogenic, mutagenic, or teratogenic. Handle with extreme care during preparation and administration. Treat urine as infectious waste. Asparaginase powder or solution may irritate the skin on contact. Wash the affected area for 15 minutes if contact occurs.

◀ALERT▶ Administer an intradermal test dose (2 international units) before beginning asparginase therapy and when more than 1 week has elapsed between doses. To prepare the test solution, reconstitute 10,000-units vial with 5 ml sterile water for injection or 0.9% NaCl and shake to dissolve. Withdraw 0.1 ml and inject it into another vial containing 9.9 ml of the same diluent to produce a concentration of 20 international units/ml. After injecting the test dose, observe the site for 1 hour for the appearance of erythema or a wheal.

IV

• Refrigerate the powder for the injected form.
• Reconstituted solutions are stable for 8 hours if refrigerated.
• If gelatinous, fiber-like particles develop in the solution, remove them by using a 5-micron filter during administration.
• Reconstitute the 10,000-units vial with 5 ml sterile water for injection or 0.9% NaCl to provide a concentration of 2,000 international units/ml.
• Shake gently to ensure complete dissolution. Vigorous shaking will produce foam and cause some loss of potency.
• For IV injection, administer asparaginase solution into the tubing of free-flowing IV solution of D_5W or 0.9% NaCl over at least 30 minutes.
• For IV infusion, further dilute with up to 1,000 ml D_5W or 0.9% NaCl.

IM

• Add 2 ml 0.9% NaCl to 10,000-units vial to provide a concentration of 5,000 international units/ml.
• Administer no more than 2 ml at any one site.

Intervention and Evaluation

• As appropriate, monitor serum amylase levels frequently during therapy.

◀ALERT▶ Expect to discontinue asparaginase at the first sign or symptom of renal failure (oliguria, anuria) or pancreatitis (abdominal pain, nausea and vomiting, elevated serum amylase and lipase levels).

• Monitor the patient for signs and symptoms of hematologic toxicity, such as excessive fatigue and weakness, ecchymosis, fever, signs of local infection, sore throat, and unusual bleeding from any site.

Patient Teaching

• Advise the patient to drink plenty of fluids to help prevent kidney problems.
• Caution the patient to avoid receiving any immunizations without the physician's approval and coming in contact with those who have recently received a live-virus vaccine.

azacitidine

ay-zah-**sigh**-tih-deen
(Vidaza)

CATEGORY AND SCHEDULE

Pregnancy Risk Category: D

MECHANISM OF ACTION

An antineoplastic agent that exerts a cytotoxic effect on rapidly dividing cells by causing demethylation of DNA in abnormal hematopoietic cells in the bone marrow. **Therapeutic Effect:** Restores normal function to tumor-suppressor genes regulating cellular differentiation and proliferation.

PHARMACOKINETICS

Rapidly absorbed after subcutaneous administration. Metabolized by the liver. Eliminated in urine. ***Half-life:*** 4 hr.

AVAILABILITY

Powder for Injection: 100 mg.

INDICATIONS AND DOSAGES

▸ **Refractory anemia, chronic myelomonocytic leukemia**

Subcutaneous

Adults, Elderly. 75 mg/m^2/day for 7 days every 4 wk. Dosage may be increased to 100 mg/m^2 if initial dose is insufficient and toxicity is manageable.

CONTRAINDICATIONS

Advanced malignant hepatic tumors, hypersensitivity to mannitol

INTERACTIONS

Drug

Bone marrow suppressants: May increase myelosuppression.

Herbal

None known.

Food

None known.

DIAGNOSTIC TEST EFFECTS

May decrease hemoglobin level, hematocrit, and WBC, RBC, and platelet counts. May increase serum creatinine and potassium levels.

SIDE EFFECTS

Frequent (71%–29%)

Nausea, vomiting, fever, diarrhea, fatigue, injection site erythema, constipation, ecchymosis, cough, dyspnea, weakness

Occasional (26%–16%)

Rigors, petechiae, injection site pain, pharyngitis, arthralgia, headache, limb pain, dizziness, peripheral edema, back pain, erythema, epistaxis, weight loss, myalgia

Rare (13%–8%)

Anxiety, abdominal pain, rash, depression, tachycardia, insomnia, night sweats, stomatitis

SERIOUS REACTIONS

! Hematologic toxicity, manifested most commonly as anemia, leukopenia, neutropenia, and thrombocytopenia, is a common adverse effect.

NURSING CONSIDERATIONS

Baseline Assessment

- Obtain blood counts before each dosing cycle to monitor the patient's response and assess for drug toxicity.

Lifespan Considerations

- Azacitidine may be embryotoxic, causing developmental abnormalities in the fetus. Women of childbearing age should avoid becoming pregnant while taking azacitidine.
- Patients should avoid breastfeeding while taking azacitidine.
- The safety and efficacy of azaciti-

dine have not been established in children.
• Age-related renal impairment may increase the risk of renal toxicity in the elderly.

Precautions

• Use azacitidine cautiously in patients with hepatic or renal impairment.

Administration and Handling

Subcutaneous

• Use strict aseptic technique when preparing the drug.
• Store vials at room temperature.
• The reconstituted solution may be stored for up to 1 hour at room temperature or up to 8 hours if refrigerated. After removing from refrigeration, allow the drug solution to return to room temperature and use it within 30 minutes.
• Reconstitute azacitidine with 4 ml sterile water for injection. The reconstituted solution will appear cloudy.
• Use the solution within 1 hour after reconstitution.
• Divide doses greater than 4 ml equally into two syringes.
• To resuspend the contents, invert the syringe 2 or 3 times and roll it between your palms for 30 seconds immediately before administration.
• Rotate injection sites among the abdomen, upper arm, and thigh for each injection.
• Administer each new injection at least 1 inch from a previous injection site.

Intervention and Evaluation

• Protect the patient from infection.
• Monitor the patient for signs and symptoms of hematologic toxicity, including easy bruising, unusual bleeding, fever, signs of local infections, sore throat, and excessive fatigue and weakness.
• Observe the patient's response to the medication. Notify the physician if the patient develops diarrhea, nausea, or vomiting.
• Avoid measures that may induce bleeding, such as taking a rectal temperature.
• Provide the patient and family with emotional support.

Patient Teaching

• Caution the patient to avoid crowds and persons with known infections.
• Urge the patient to immediately report any signs of infection, including fever and flu-like symptoms.
• Advise the patient not to receive immunizations without the physician's approval because azacitidine lowers the body's resistance to infection.
• Instruct the patient to contact the physician if nausea or vomiting continues at home.
• Advise the patient to use barrier contraception while receiving azacitidine.

BCG, intravesical

(Immucyst[AUS], OncoTice[AUS], TheraCys, Tice BCG)

CATEGORY AND SCHEDULE

Pregnancy Risk Category: D

MECHANISM OF ACTION

An antineoplastic that produces a local inflammatory reaction with histiocytic and leukocytic infiltration in the urinary bladder. **Therapeutic Effect:** Decreases superficial cancerous lesions in the urinary bladder.

AVAILABILITY

Parenteral Vials: 50 mg, 81 mg

INDICATIONS AND DOSAGES

▸ Treatment and prevention of bladder carcinoma in situ

Intravesical (TheraCys)

Adults, Elderly. One dose in 50 ml 0.9% NaCl once weekly for 6 wk, then repeated 3, 6, 12, 18, and 24 months after initial treatment. Begin 7-14 days after biopsy or transurethral resection.

Intravesical (Tice BCG)

Adults, Elderly. One dose in 50 ml 0.9% NaCl once weekly for 6 wk; may repeat once. Thereafter, continue monthly for 6–12 mo.

CONTRAINDICATIONS

Compromised immune system, concurrent corticosteroid or immunosuppressive therapy, fever due to infection or undetermined cause, HIV infection, positive Mantoux test, UTI

INTERACTIONS

Drug

Bone marrow depressants, immunosuppressants: May decrease the immune response and increase the risk of osteomyelitis and disseminated BCG infection.

Live-virus vaccines: May potentiate virus replication, increase vaccine side effects, and decrease the patient's antibody response to the vaccine.

Herbal

None known.

Food

None known.

DIAGNOSTIC TEST EFFECTS

None known.

SIDE EFFECTS

Frequent

Dysuria, urinary frequency, hematuria, hypersensitivity reaction (manifested as malaise, fever, chills)

Occasional

Cystitis, urinary urgency, nausea, vomiting, anorexia, diarrhea, myalgia, arthralgia

SERIOUS REACTIONS

! Disseminated BCG infection is usually characterized by a fever higher than 103°F (or persistently higher than 101°F for more than 2 days), chills and severe malaise.

NURSING CONSIDERATIONS

Baseline Assessment

- Establish the patient's baseline renal status.
- Plan to obtain a urine specimen for culture and sensitivity tests to rule out a UTI.
- Determine which medications that the patient is taking concurrently, especially corticosteroids and immunosuppressants.
- Determine if the patient has a compromised immune system, has a fever, or is HIV positive.

Administration and Handling

◂ALERT▸ Be aware that BCG contains live, attenuated mycobacteria. Treat the drug as infectious material, and use protective gear when reconstituting it. Avoid contact with the drug if you are immunocompromised.

Intravesical

- Reconstitute the powder immediately before administration. Discard any unused portion within 2 hours of reconstitution.
- After adding diluent to the powder, gently swirl the solution, or repeatedly inject and withdraw the solution from the vial until the solution is mixed. Avoid vigorous shaking, which could cause foaming.
- Don't give BCG intravenously or subcutaneously; plan to deliver the drug by urethral catheter.

Intervention and Evaluation
• Ensure that the patient doesn't drink fluids within 4 hours of administration. Also have the patient void immediately before the drug is given.
• During the first hour of drug administration, have the patient lie in different positions (supine, prone, and both sides) for 15 minutes each to allow the drug to come in contact with all parts of the bladder. Ask the patient to try to retain the solution for 2 hours.
• Instruct the patient to sit while voiding after instillation to avoid spraying or splashing the infected urine.
• Disinfect all urine expelled within 6 hours of drug instillation with an equal volume of 5% hypochlorite solution (undiluted household bleach), before flushing.
• Diligently monitor the patient's renal status.
• Assess the patient for dysuria, hematuria, and urinary frequency, and obtain urinalysis to check for UTI.
• Monitor the patient for disseminated BCG infection.

Patient Teaching
• Warn the patient to notify the physician if symptoms persist or increase or if he or she experiences blood in urine, chills, fever, frequent or painful urination, joint pain, and nausea or vomiting.
• Urge the patient to avoid receiving immunizations and coming in contact with those who have recently received a live-virus vaccine during BCG treatment.

dacarbazine

day-**car**-bah-zeen
(DTIC[CAN], DTIC-Dome)
Do not confuse dacarbazine with Dicarbosil or procarbazine.

CATEGORY AND SCHEDULE
Pregnancy Risk Category: C

MECHANISM OF ACTION
An alkylating antineoplastic agent that forms methyldiazonium ions, which attack nucleophilic groups in DNA. Cross-links DNA strands. **Therapeutic Effect:** Inhibits DNA, RNA, and protein synthesis.

PHARMACOKINETICS
Minimally crosses the blood-brain barrier. Protein binding: 5%. Metabolized in the liver. Excreted in urine. ***Half-life:*** 5 hr (increased in impaired renal function).

AVAILABILITY
Powder for Injection: 100-mg, 200-mg, 500-mg vials.

INDICATIONS AND DOSAGES
▸ **Malignant melanoma**
IV
Adults, Elderly. 2–4.5 mg/kg/ day for 10 days, repeated q4wk; or 250 mg/m^2 a day for 5 days, repeated q3wk.
▸ **Hodgkin's disease**
IV
Adults, Elderly. 150 mg/m^2/day for 5 days, repeated q4wk; or 375 mg/m^2 once, repeated every 15 days (as combination therapy).
Children. 375 mg/m^2 on days 1 and 15; repeated every 28 days (as combination therapy).

▸ **Solid tumors**
IV
Children. 200–470 mg/m^2/day over 5 days every 21–28 days.
▸ **Neuroblastoma**
IV
Children. 800–900 mg/m^2 as single dose on day 1 of therapy, repeated q3–4wk (as combination therapy).

OFF-LABEL USES
Treatment of islet cell carcinoma, neuroblastoma, soft-tissue sarcoma

CONTRAINDICATIONS
Demonstrated hypersensitivity to dacarbazine

INTERACTIONS
Drug
Bone marrow depressants: May enhance myelosuppression.
Live-virus vaccines: May potentiate virus replication, increase vaccine side effects, and decrease the patient's antibody response to the vaccine.
Herbal
None known.
Food
None known.

DIAGNOSTIC TEST EFFECTS
May increase BUN, serum alkaline phosphatase, AST (SGOT), and ALT (SGPT) levels.

IV INCOMPATIBILITIES
Allopurinol (Aloprim), cefepime (Maxipime), heparin, piperacillin and tazobactam (Zosyn)

IV COMPATIBILITIES
Etoposide (VePesid), granisetron (Kytril), ondansetron (Zofran), paclitaxel (Taxol)

SIDE EFFECTS
Frequent (90%)
Nausea, vomiting, anorexia (occurs within 1 hr of initial dose, may last up to 12 hr)
Occasional
Facial flushing, paresthesia, alopecia, flulike symptoms (fever, myalgia, malaise), dermatologic reactions, confusion, blurred vision, headache, lethargy
Rare
Diarrhea, stomatitis, photosensitivity

SERIOUS REACTIONS
! Myelosuppression may result in blood dyscrasias, such as leukopenia and thrombocytopenia, generally 2–4 weeks after the last dacarbazine dose.
! Hepatotoxicity occurs rarely.

NURSING CONSIDERATIONS
Baseline Assessment
• Hydrate the patient before treatment to avoid dehydration from vomiting.
Lifespan Considerations
• Because of the risk of fetal harm, pregnant women should not take dacarbazine, especially during the first trimester. Breast-feeding women also should not take this drug.
• The safety and efficacy of dacarbazine have not been established in children.
• In the elderly, age-related renal impairment may require a dosage adjustment.
Precautions
• Use dacarbazine cautiously in patients with hepatic impairment.
Administration and Handling
◂ALERT▸ Dacarbazine dosage is individualized based on the patient's clinical response and tolerance of the drug's adverse effects. When administering this drug in combination

therapy, consult specific protocols for optimum dosage and sequence of drug administration.

◀ALERT▶ Give dacarbazine by IV push or IV infusion, as prescribed. Because dacarbazine may be carcinogenic, mutagenic, or teratogenic, handle the drug with extreme care during preparation and administration.

IV

- Refrigerate unopened vials and protect them from light.
- Reconstitute the 100-mg vial with 9.9 ml (or the 200-mg vial with 19.7 ml) sterile water for injection to provide a concentration of 10 mg/ml.
- The reconstituted solution containing 10 mg/ml is stable for up to 8 hours at room temperature or up to 72 hours if refrigerated.
- Give by IV push over 2 to 3 minutes.
- For IV infusion, further dilute with up to 250 ml D_5W or 0.9% NaCl. Solutions further diluted with D_5W or 0.9% NaCl are stable for up to 8 hours at room temperature or up to 24 hours if refrigerated. Infuse the drug over 15 to 30 minutes. Discard it if the color changes from ivory to pink because this indicates decomposition.
- Apply hot packs if the patient develops a burning sensation, irritation, or local pain at the injection site.
- Monitor the injection site for signs and symptoms of extravasation, including coolness, stinging, swelling, and slight or no blood return.

Intervention and Evaluation

- Monitor the patient's erythrocyte, leukocyte, and platelet counts for evidence of myelosuppression.
- Monitor the patient for signs and symptoms of hematologic toxicity, including ecchymosis, fever, signs of local infection, sore throat, and unusual bleeding from any site.

Patient Teaching

- Inform the patient that nausea and vomiting usually diminish after 1 or 2 days of treatment. Advise the patient to notify the physician if these symptoms persist at home.
- Instruct the patient to notify the physician if he or she experiences easy bruising, fever, signs of local infection, sore throat, or unusual bleeding from any site.
- Urge the patient to avoid receiving vaccinations and coming in contact with anyone who has recently received a live-virus vaccine.

erlotinib

er-**low**-tih-nib
(Tarceva)

CATEGORY AND SCHEDULE

Pregnancy Risk Category: D

MECHANISM OF ACTION

A human epidermal growth factor that inhibits tyrosine kinases (TK) associated with transmembrane cell surface receptors found on both normal and cancer cells. One such receptor is epidermal growth factor receptor (EGFR). **Therapeutic Effect:** TK activity appears to be vitally important to cell proliferation and survival.

AVAILABILITY

Tablets: 25 mg, 100 mg, 150 mg.

INDICATIONS AND DOSAGES

▸ **Overactive bladder**

PO

Adults, Elderly. Initially, 7.5 mg once a day. If response is not adequate after a minimum of 2 weeks, dosage may be increased to 15 mg once daily. Do not exceed 7.5 mg once a day in patients with moderate hepatic impairment.

CONTRAINDICATIONS

Pregnancy

INTERACTIONS

Drug

Aminoglutethimide, carbamazepine, nafcillin, nevirapine, phenobarbital, phenytoin: May decrease the levels and effects of erlotinib.
Azole antifungals, ciprofloxacin, clarithromycin, diclofenac, doxycycline, erythromycin, imatinib, isoniazid, nefazodone, nicardipine, propofol, protease inhibitors, quinidine, verapamil: May increase the levels and effects of erlotinib.
Ketoconazole: May increase serum erlotinib concentration.
Rifampin: May decrease serum erlotinib concentration.

Herbal

St. John's wort: May increase metabolism and decrease serum erlotinib concentration.

Food

Give erlotinib at least 1 hr before or 2 hrs after ingestion of food.

DIAGNOSTIC TEST EFFECTS

May increase hepatic enzyme levels.

SIDE EFFECTS

Frequent (35%–21%)
Dry mouth, constipation
Occasional (8%–4%)
Dyspepsia, headache, nausea, abdominal pain
Rare (3%–2%)
Asthenia, diarrhea, dizziness, ocular dryness

SERIOUS REACTIONS

! Urinary tract infection occurs occasionally.

NURSING CONSIDERATIONS

Precautions

• Use erlotinib cautiously in patients with hepatic or severe renal impairment.

Administration and Handling

PO
• Give erlotinib at least 1 hour before or 2 hours after ingestion of food. Swallow extended-release tablets whole; do not crush.

etoposide, VP-16

eh-**toe**-poe-side
(Etopophos, Toposar, VePesid)
Do not confuse VePesid with Pepcid or Versed.

CATEGORY AND SCHEDULE

Pregnancy Risk Category: D

MECHANISM OF ACTION

An epipodophyllotoxin that induces single- and double-stranded breaks in DNA. Cell cycle-dependent and phase-specific; most effective in the S and G_2 phases of cell division. **Therapeutic Effect:** Inhibits or alters DNA synthesis.

PHARMACOKINETICS

Variably absorbed from the GI tract. Rapidly distributed, low concentrations in CSF. Protein binding: 97%. Metabolized in the liver. Primarily excreted in urine. Not removed by hemodialysis. ***Half-life:*** 3–12 hr.

AVAILABILITY

Capsules (VePesid): 50 mg.

Injection (Toposar, VePesid): 20 mg/ml.
Injection (Water-soluble [Etopophos]): 100 mg/ml.

INDICATIONS AND DOSAGES

▸ Refractory testicular tumors
IV
Adults. 50–100 mg/m²/day on days 1 to 5, or 100 mg/m²/day on days 1, 3, 5 (as combination therapy).

▸ Acute myelocytic leukemia
IV
Children. 150 mg/m²/day for 2–3 days and 2–3 cycles.

▸ Brain tumor
IV
Children. 150 mg/m²/day on days 2 and 3 of treatment course.

▸ Neuroblastoma
IV
Children. 100 mg/m²/day on days 1–5 of treatment course; repeated q4wk.

▸ Small-cell lung carcinoma
PO
Adults. Twice the IV dose rounded to nearest 50 mg. Give once a day for doses 400 mg or less, in divided doses for dosages greater than 400 mg.
IV
Adults. 35 mg/m²/day for 4 consecutive days up to 50 mg/m²/day for 5 consecutive days (as combination therapy).

▸ Leukemia, rhabdomyosarcoma
Children. 60–150 mg/m²/day for 2–5 days q3–6wk.

▸ Dosage in renal impairment
Creatinine clearance 10–50 ml/min. 75% of normal dose.
Creatinine clearance less than 10 ml/min. 50% of normal dose.

OFF-LABEL USES

Treatment of acute myelocytic leukemia, AIDS-associated Kaposi's sarcoma, bladder carcinoma, Ewing's sarcoma, Hodgkin's disease, non-Hodgkin's lymphoma

CONTRAINDICATIONS

Pregnancy

INTERACTIONS

Drug

Bone marrow depressants: May increase myelosuppression.
Live-virus vaccines: May potentiate virus replication, increase vaccine side effects, and decrease the patient's antibody response to the vaccine.

Herbal

None known.

Food

None known.

DIAGNOSTIC TEST EFFECTS

None known.

IV INCOMPATIBILITIES

VePesid: cefepime (Maxipime), filgrastim (Neupogen), idarubicin (Idamycin).
Etopophos: amphotericin B (Fungizone), cefepime (Maxipime), chlorpromazine (Thorazine), methylprednisolone (Solu-Medrol), prochlorperazine (Compazine)

IV COMPATIBILITIES

VePesid: carboplatin (Paraplatin), cisplatin (Platinol), cytarabine (Cytosar), daunorubicin (Cerubidine), doxorubicin (Adriamycin), granisetron (Kytril), mitoxantrone (Novantrone), ondansetron (Zofran)
Etopophos: carboplatin (Paraplatin), cisplatin (Platinol), cytarabine (Cytosar), dacarbazine (DTIC-Dome), daunorubicin (Cerubidine), dexamethasone (Decadron), diphenhydramine (Benadryl), doxorubicin (Adriamycin), granisetron (Kytril), magnesium sulfate, mannitol, mito-

xantrone (Novantrone), ondansetron (Zofran), potassium chloride

SIDE EFFECTS

Frequent (66%–43%)
Mild to moderate nausea and vomiting, alopecia
Occasional (13%–6%)
Diarrhea, anorexia, stomatitis
Rare (2% or less)
Hypotension, peripheral neuropathy

SERIOUS REACTIONS

! Myelosuppression may result in hematologic toxicity, manifested as anemia, leukopenia (occurring 7–14 days after drug administration), thrombocytopenia (occurring 9–16 days after administration) and, to lesser extent, pancytopenia. Bone marrow recovery occurs by day 20.
! Hepatotoxicity occurs occasionally.

NURSING CONSIDERATIONS

Baseline Assessment

- Monitor the patient's hematology test results before and frequently during etoposide therapy.
- Administer antiemetics, if ordered, to control nausea and vomiting.

Lifespan Considerations

- Because of the risk of fetal harm, pregnant women should not take etoposide, especially during the first trimester. Breast-feeding women also should not take this drug.
- The safety and efficacy of etoposide have not been established in children.
- In the elderly, age-related renal impairment may require dosage adjustment.

Precautions

- Use etoposide cautiously in patients with myelosuppression or hepatic or renal impairment.

Administration and Handling

◀ **ALERT** ▶ Etoposide dosage is individualized based on the patient's clinical response and tolerance of the drug's adverse effects. Treatment is repeated at 3- to 4-week intervals.
◀ **ALERT** ▶ Administer parenteral etoposide by slow IV infusion. Wear gloves when preparing the solution. If the powder or solution comes in contact with your skin, wash immediately and thoroughly with soap and water. Because etoposide may be carcinogenic, mutagenic, or teratogenic, handle the drug with extreme care during preparation and administration.

PO
- Refrigerate gelatin capsules.

IV (VePesid)
- Store VePesid injection at room temperature before dilution.
- VePesid concentrate for injection normally is clear and yellow.
- Dilute each 100 mg (5 ml) of VePesid with at least 250 ml D_5W or 0.9% NaCl to provide a concentration of 0.4 mg/ml (or 500 ml for a concentration of 0.2 mg/ml).
- Reconstituted VePesid solution is stable at room temperature for up to 96 hours at 0.2 mg/ml and 48 hours at 0.4 mg/ml. Discard VePesid solution if crystallization occurs.
- Infuse VePesid slowly, over 30 to 60 minutes. Rapid IV infusion may produce marked hypotension.
- Monitor the patient receiving VePesid for an anaphylactic reaction manifested as back, chest, or throat pain; chills; diaphoresis; dyspnea; fever; lacrimation; and sneezing.

IV (Etopophos)
- Refrigerate Etopophos vials.
- Reconstitute each 100 mg of Etopophos with 5 to 10 ml sterile water for injection, D_5W, or 0.9% NaCl to provide a concentration of 20 mg/ml or 10 mg/ml, respectively.

• Etopophos may be given without further dilution or may be further diluted with 0.9% NaCl or D_5W to a concentration as low as 0.1 mg/ml.
• After reconstitution, Etopophos is stable for up to 24 hours at room temperature or refrigerated.
• Administer Etopophos over 5 to 210 minutes, as appropriate.

Intervention and Evaluation

• Monitor the patient's blood Hgb and Hct levels and platelet and WBC counts.
• Assess the patient's pattern of daily bowel activity and stool consistency.
• Monitor the patient for signs and symptoms of hematologic toxicity, including excessive fatigue and weakness, ecchymosis, fever, signs of local infection, sore throat, and unusual bleeding from any site.
• Assess the patient for signs and symptoms of paresthesia and peripheral neuropathy.
• Monitor the patient for signs and symptoms of stomatitis.

Patient Teaching

• Warn the patient to notify the physician if he or she experiences easy bruising, fever, signs of local infection, sore throat, or unusual bleeding from any site.
• Urge the patient to avoid receiving vaccinations and coming in contact with anyone who has recently received a live-virus vaccine.
• Inform the patient that alopecia is reversible but that new hair growth may have a different color or texture.

interleukin-2 (aldesleukin)

in-tur-**lew**-kin
(IL-2, Proleukin)
Do not confuse interleukin-2 with interferon 2.

CATEGORY AND SCHEDULE

Pregnancy Risk Category: C

MECHANISM OF ACTION

A biological response modifier that acts like human recombinant interleukin-2, promoting proliferation, differentiation, and recruitment of T and B cells, lymphokine-activated and natural cells, and thymocytes. **Therapeutic Effect:** Enhances cytolytic activity in lymphocytes.

PHARMACOKINETICS

Primarily distributed into plasma, lymphocytes, lungs, liver, kidney, and spleen. Metabolized to amino acids in the cells lining the kidneys. ***Half-life:*** 85 min.

AVAILABILITY

Powder for Injection: 22 million units (1.3 mg).

INDICATIONS AND DOSAGES

▸ Metastatic melanoma, metastatic renal cell carcinoma

IV

Adults 18 yr and older. 600,000 units/kg q8h for 14 doses; followed by 9 days of rest, then another 14 doses for a total of 28 doses per course. Course may be repeated after rest period of at least 7 wk from date of hospital discharge.

OFF-LABEL USES

Treatment of colorectal cancer,

Kaposi's sarcoma, non-Hodgkin's lymphoma

CONTRAINDICATIONS

Abnormal pulmonary function or thallium stress test results, bowel ischemia or perforation, coma or toxic psychosis lasting longer than 48 hr, GI bleeding requiring surgery, intubation lasting more than 72 hr, organ allografts, pericardial tamponade, renal dysfunction requiring dialysis for longer than 72 hr, repetitive or difficult-to-control seizures; retreatment in those who experience any of the following toxicities: angina, MI, recurrent chest pain with EKG changes, sustained ventricular tachycardia, uncontrolled or unresponsive cardiac rhythm disturbances

INTERACTIONS

Drug

Antihypertensives: May increase hypotensive effect.
Cardiotoxic, hepatotoxic, myelotoxic, or nephrotoxic medications: May increase the risk of toxicity.
Glucocorticoids: May decrease the effects of interleukin-2.

Herbal

None known.

Food

None known.

DIAGNOSTIC TEST EFFECTS

May increase BUN and serum alkaline phosphatase, bilirubin, creatinine, AST (SGOT), and ALT (SGPT) levels. May decrease serum calcium, magnesium, phosphorus, potassium, and sodium levels.

IV INCOMPATIBILITIES

Ganciclovir (Cytovene), pentamidine (Pentam), prochlorperazine (Compazine), promethazine (Phenergan)

IV COMPATIBILITIES

Calcium gluconate, dopamine (Intropin), heparin, lorazepam (Ativan), magnesium, potassium

SIDE EFFECTS

Side effects are generally self-limiting and reversible within 2–3 days after discontinuing therapy.

Frequent (89%–48%)
Fever, chills, nausea, vomiting, hypotension, diarrhea, oliguria or anuria, mental status changes, irritability, confusion, depression, sinus tachycardia, pain (abdominal, chest, back), fatigue, dyspnea, pruritus

Occasional (47%–17%)
Edema, erythema, rash, stomatitis, anorexia, weight gain, infection (UTI, injection site, catheter tip), dizziness

Rare (15%–4%)
Dry skin, sensory disorders (vision, speech, taste), dermatitis, headache, arthralgia, myalgia, weight loss, hematuria, conjunctivitis, proteinuria

SERIOUS REACTIONS

! Anemia, thrombocytopenia, and leukopenia occur commonly.
! GI bleeding and pulmonary edema occur occasionally.
! Capillary leak syndrome results in hypotension (systolic pressure less than 90 mm Hg or a 20-mm Hg drop from baseline systolic pressure), extravasation of plasma proteins and fluid into extravascular space, and loss of vascular tone. It may result in cardiac arrhythmias, angina, MI, and respiratory insufficiency.
! Other rare reactions include fatal malignant hyperthermia, cardiac arrest, CVA, pulmonary emboli, bowel perforation, gangrene, and severe depression leading to suicide.

NURSING CONSIDERATIONS

Baseline Assessment

- Treat patients with bacterial infection and those with indwelling central lines with antibiotic therapy before beginning interleukin-2 therapy.
- Confirm that the patient is neurologically stable with a negative CT scan before beginning interleukin-2 therapy.
- Obtain results of blood chemistry studies (including electrolytes), chest x-ray, CBC, and liver and renal function tests results before beginning interleukin-2 therapy and every day thereafter.

Lifespan Considerations

- Interleukin-2 use should be avoided in patients of either sex who don't practice effective contraception.
- The safety and efficacy of interleukin have not been established in children.
- Elderly patients may require cautious use of the drug because of age-related renal impairment. They are also less able to tolerate drug-related toxicities.

Precautions

- Use interleukin-2 extremely cautiously in patients with a history of cardiac or pulmonary disease even if they have normal thallium stress and pulmonary function test results.
- Use the drug cautiously in patients with fixed requirements for large volumes of fluid (such as those with hypercalcemia) or a history of seizures.

Administration and Handling

◀ALERT▶ Withhold the drug in patients who exhibit moderate to severe lethargy or somnolence because continued administration may result in coma.

◀ALERT▶ Restrict interleukin-2 therapy to patients with normal cardiac and pulmonary function as determined by thallium stress testing and pulmonary function testing. Dosage is individualized based on the patient's clinical response and tolerance of the drug's adverse effects.

IV

- Refrigerate—don't freeze—unopened vials.
- Reconstitute the 22-million-unit vial with 1.2 ml sterile water for injection to provide a concentration of 18 million units/ml. Do not use bacteriostatic water for injection or 0.9% NaCl.
- During reconstitution, direct the diluent at the side of vial. Swirl the contents gently—do not shake—to avoid foaming.
- Further dilute the dose in 50 ml D_5W and infuse over 15 minutes. Do not use an in-line filter.
- The reconstituted solution is stable for 48 hours at room temperature or refrigerated (refrigeration is preferred).
- Warm the solution to room temperature before infusion.
- Closely monitor the patient for a drop in mean arterial BP, a sign of capillary leak syndrome. Continued treatment may result in edema, pleural effusion, mental status changes, and significant hypotension (systolic pressure less than 90 mm Hg or a 20-mm Hg drop from baseline systolic pressure).

Intervention and Evaluation

- Monitor the patient's CBC, electrolyte levels, liver and renal function test results, platelet count, pulse oximetry values, and weight.
- Determine the patient's serum amylase concentration frequently during therapy.
- Discontinue interleukin-2 at the first sign of hypotension or moderate

to severe lethargy; the physician will decide whether therapy should continue.
• Assess the patient for mental status changes, such as irritability, confusion, and depression.
• Maintain strict intake and output protocols.
• Assess the patient for extravascular fluid accumulation, as evidenced by dependent edema and crackles.

Patient Teaching

• Inform the patient that nausea and vomiting typically decrease with continued therapy.
• Instruct the patient to drink plenty of fluids to protect against renal impairment.
• Advise the patient to contact the physician if he or she experiences fever, chills, lower back pain, difficulty with urination, unusual bleeding or bruising, black tarry stools, blood in urine, or pinpoint red spots on the skin.
• Warn the patient to avoid exposure to anyone who has an infection.
• Caution the patient to immediately report if he or she experiences symptoms of depression or suicidal ideation.

irinotecan

eye-rin-**oh**-teh-can
(Camptosar)

CATEGORY AND SCHEDULE

Pregnancy Risk Category: C (first trimester), D (second and third trimester)

MECHANISM OF ACTION

A DNA topoisomerase inhibitor that inhibits the action of topoisomerase I, an enzyme that allows DNA replication by producing reversible single-strand breaks in DNA that relieve torsional strain. Irinotecan prevents religation of the DNA strand, resulting in damage to double-strand DNA and cell death. **Therapeutic Effect:** Kills cancer cells.

PHARMACOKINETICS

Metabolized to active metabolite in the liver after IV administration. Protein binding: 95% (metabolite). Excreted in urine and eliminated by biliary route. ***Half-life:*** 6 hr; metabolite, 10 hr.

AVAILABILITY

Injection: 20 mg/ml.

INDICATIONS AND DOSAGES

▸ **Carcinoma of the colon or rectum that has progressed or recurred after treatment with 5-fluorouracil**

IV

Adults, Elderly. Initially, 125 mg/m^2 once weekly for 4 wk, followed by a rest period of 2 wk. Additional courses may be repeated q6wk. Dosage may be adjusted in 25–50 mg/m^2 increments to as high as 150 mg/m^2 or as low as 50 mg/m^2.

CONTRAINDICATIONS

None known.

INTERACTIONS

Drug

Diuretics: May increase the risk of dehydration from vomiting and diarrhea.
Laxatives: May increase the severity of diarrhea.
Live-virus vaccines: May potentiate virus replication, increase vaccine side effects, and decrease the patient's antibody response to the vaccine.

Other bone marrow depressants: May increase the risk of myelosuppression.
Prochlorperazine: May increase akathisia.

Herbal
None known.

Food
None known.

DIAGNOSTIC TEST EFFECTS

May increase serum alkaline phosphatase and AST (SGOT) levels.

IV INCOMPATIBILITIES

Gemcitabine (Gemzar)

SIDE EFFECTS

Expected
Nausea (64%), alopecia (49%), vomiting (45%), diarrhea (32%)
Frequent
Constipation, fatigue (29%); fever (28%); asthenia (25%); skeletal pain (23%); abdominal pain, dyspnea (22%)
Occasional
Anorexia (19%); headache, stomatitis (18%); rash (16%)

SERIOUS REACTIONS

! Myelosuppression characterized as neutropenia occurs in 97% of patients; severe neutropenia—a neutrophil count less than 50/mm^3—occurs in 78% of patients.
! Thrombocytopenia, anemia, and sepsis are common reactions.

NURSING CONSIDERATIONS

Baseline Assessment
- Assess the patient's CBC, serum electrolyte levels, and hydration status before giving each each dose of irinotecan.
- Premedicate the patient with antiemetics on the day of irinotecan treatment, as prescribed, at least 30 minutes before irinotecan administration.

Lifespan Considerations
- Because of the risk of fetal harm, pregnant women should not take irinotecan, especially in the first trimester. It is unknown if irinotecan is distributed in breast milk; however, breast-feeding is not recommended for patients taking this drug.
- The safety and efficacy of irinotecan have not been established in children.
- Elderly patients are at increased risk for diarrhea.

Precautions
- Use irinotecan cautiously in patients who have previously received abdominal or pelvic irradiation because they're at increased risk for myelosuppression.
- Use cautiously in elderly patients older than 65 years of age.

Administration and Handling
◀ALERT▶ As prescribed, begin a new irinotecan course when the patient's granulocyte count recovers to at least 1,500/mm^3, platelet count recovers to at least 100,000/mm^3, and treatment-related diarrhea fully resolves.

IV
- Store vials at room temperature, and protect them from light.
- Dilute the drug in D_5W (the preferred diluent) or 0.9% NaCl to a concentration of 0.12 to 1.1 mg/ml.
- If the solution is reconstituted in D_5W, it remains stable for up to 24 hours at room temperature or 48 hours if refrigerated. However, because the drug contains no preservative, it should be used within 6 hours if kept at room temperature or within 24 hours if refrigerated.
- Do not refrigerate the solution if it's diluted with 0.9% NaCl.
- Administer all doses by IV infusion over 90 minutes.

• Assess the patient for signs and symptoms of extravasation. If extravasation occurs, flush the site with sterile water and apply ice.

Intervention and Evaluation

• Assess the patient for early signs and symptoms of diarrhea, usually preceded by abdominal cramping and complaints of diaphoresis.
• Monitor the patient's blood Hgb levels, CBC, and serum electrolyte levels. Also assess the patient's hydration status, including intake and output.
• Monitor the infusion site for signs and symptoms of inflammation.
• Examine the patient's skin for evidence of rash.
• Offer the patient and family emotional support.

Patient Teaching

• Teach the patient how to recognize signs and symptoms of electrolyte depletion and dehydration.
• Advise the patient to use an antiemetic or antidiarrheal regimen if prescribed.
• Urge the patient to avoid receiving vaccinations and coming in contact with crowds, people with known infections, and anyone who has recently received a live-virus vaccine.
• Inform the patient that hair loss is reversible but that new hair may have a different color or texture.

mitotane

my-tow-tain
(Lysodren)

CATEGORY AND SCHEDULE

Pregnancy Risk Category: C

MECHANISM OF ACTION

A hormonal agent that inhibits activity of the adrenal cortex.
Therapeutic Effect: Suppresses functional and nonfunctional adrenocortical neoplasms by direct cytoxic effect.

AVAILABILITY

Tablets: 500 mg.

INDICATIONS AND DOSAGES

▸ **Adrenocortical carcinomas**

PO

Adults, Elderly. Initially, 2–6 g/day in 3–4 divided doses. Increase by 2–4 g/day every 3–7 days up to 9–10 g/day. Range: 2–16 g/day.

OFF-LABEL USES

Treatment of Cushing's syndrome

CONTRAINDICATIONS

Known hypersensitivity to mitotane

INTERACTIONS

Drug

CNS depressants: May increase CNS depression.

Herbal

None known.

Food

None known.

DIAGNOSTIC TEST EFFECTS

May decrease levels of plasma cortisol, urinary 17-hydroxycorticosteroids, protein-bound iodine, and serum uric acid.

SIDE EFFECTS

Frequent (greater than 15%)

Anorexia, nausea, vomiting, diarrhea, lethargy, somnolence, adrenocortical insufficiency, dizziness, vertigo, maculopapular rash, hypouricemia

Occasional (less than 15%)

Blurred or double vision, retinopathy, hearing loss, excessive salivation, urine abnormalities (hematuria, cystitis, albuminuria), hypertension, orthostatic hypotension, flushing, wheezing, dyspnea, generalized aching, fever

SERIOUS REACTIONS

! Brain damage and functional impairment may occur with long-term, high-dosage therapy.

NURSING CONSIDERATIONS

Baseline Assessment

- Expect to initiate steroid replacement therapy during mitotane therapy.

Precautions

- Use mitotane cautiously in patients with impaired hepatic function.

Administration and Handling

◀ALERT▶

- Mitotane may be carcinogenic, mutagenic, or teratogenic, handle it with extreme care during administration.

Intervention and Evaluation

- Discontinue mitotane therapy immediately after shock or trauma, as prescribed, because the drug produces adrenal suppression.
- Monitor the patient's liver function test results, serum uric acid levels, and urine tests, including urine chemistry and urinalysis.
- Be aware that neurologic and behavioral assessments are performed periodically on patients receiving prolonged therapy (over 2 years).
- Assess the patient's pattern of daily bowel activity and stool consistency.
- Examine the patient's skin for maculopapular rash.

Patient Teaching

- Warn the patient to notify the physician immediately if he or she experiences infection, injury, or other illnesses.
- Caution the patient to notify the physician if he or she experiences darkening of the skin, diarrhea, depression, loss of appetite, or rash.
- Advise the patient to notify the physician if nausea and vomiting continue at home.
- Urge the patient to avoid receiving vaccinations and coming in contact with crowds or people with known infections because mitotane lowers the body's resistance.
- Urge the patient to drink plenty of fluids to help prevent urinary side effects.
- Instruct the patient to avoid tasks that require mental alertness or motor skills because mitotane use may cause dizziness and drowsiness.
- Urge the patient to use effective contraceptive measures during therapy.

mitoxantrone ⚑

my-toe-**zan**-trone
(Novantrone, Onkotrone[AUS])

CATEGORY AND SCHEDULE

Pregnancy Risk Category: D

MECHANISM OF ACTION

An anthracenedione that inhibits B-cell, T-cell, and macrophage proliferation and DNA and RNA synthesis. Active throughout the entire cell cycle. **Therapeutic Effect:** Causes cell death.

PHARMACOKINETICS

Protein binding: 78%. Widely distributed. Metabolized in the liver. Primarily eliminated in feces by the biliary system. Not removed by hemodialysis. ***Half-life:*** 2.3–13 days.

AVAILABILITY

Injection: 2 mg/ml.

INDICATIONS AND DOSAGES

▸ Leukemias

IV

Adults, Elderly, Children 2 yr and older. 12 mg/m²once a day for 2–3 days.

Children younger than 2 yr. 0.4 mg/kg once a day for 3–5 days.

▸ Acute leukemia in relapse

IV

Adults, Elderly, Children older than 2 yr. 8–12 mg/m²once a day for 4–5 days.

▸ Acute nonlymphocytic leukemia

IV

Adults, Elderly, Children older than 2 yr. 10 mg/m²once a day for 3–5 days.

▸ Solid tumors

IV

Adults, Elderly. 12–14 mg/m² once q3–4wk.

Children. 18–20 mg/m² once q3–4wk.

▸ Prostate cancer

IV

Adults, Elderly. 12–14 mg/m² every 21 days.

▸ Multiple sclerosis

IV

Adults, Elderly. 12 mg/m²/dose q3mo.

OFF-LABEL USES

Treatment of breast or hepatic carcinoma, non-Hodgkin's lymphoma

CONTRAINDICATIONS

Baseline left ventricular ejection fraction less than 50%, cumulative lifetime mitoxantrone dose of 140 mg/m² or more, multiple sclerosis with hepatic impairment

INTERACTIONS

Drug

Antigout medications: May decrease the effects of these drugs.

Bone marrow depressants: May increase myelosuppression.

Live-virus vaccines: May potentiate virus replication, increase vaccine side effects, and decrease the patient's antibody response to the vaccine.

Herbal

None known.

Food

None known.

DIAGNOSTIC TEST EFFECTS

May increase serum bilirubin and uric acid, AST (SGOT), and ALT (SGPT) levels.

IV INCOMPATIBILITIES

Heparin, paclitaxel (Taxol), piperacillin and tazobactam (Zosyn)

IV COMPATIBILITIES

Allopurinol (Aloprim), etoposide (VePesid), gemcitabine (Gemzar), granisetron (Kytril), ondansetron (Zofran), potassium chloride

SIDE EFFECTS

Frequent (greater than 10%)

Nausea, vomiting, diarrhea, cough, headache, stomatitis, abdominal discomfort, fever, alopecia

Occasional (9%–4%)

Ecchymosis, fungal infection, conjunctivitis, UTI

Rare (3%)

Arrhythmias

SERIOUS REACTIONS

! Myelosuppression may be severe, resulting in GI bleeding, hematologic toxicity, sepsis, and pneumonia.

! Renal failure, seizures, jaundice, and CHF may occur.

NURSING CONSIDERATIONS

Baseline Assessment

- Assess the patient's baseline body

temperature, CBC, respiratory status (including breath sounds), and pulse quality and rate.

Lifespan Considerations

- Mitoxantrone use should be avoided during pregnancy, especially during the first trimester, because it can cause fetal harm. Breast-feeding also is not recommended for patients taking this drug.
- The safety and efficacy of mitoxantrone have not been established in children.
- No age-related precautions have been noted in the elderly.

Precautions

- Use mitoxantrone cautiously in patients with impaired hepatobiliary function or pre-existing myelosuppression and in those who have previously been treated with cardiotoxic medications.

Administration and Handling

◀ALERT▶ Because mitoxantrone may be carcinogenic, mutagenic, or teratogenic, handle the drug with extreme care during preparation and administration. Dilute the drug before administration, and administer it by IV injection or infusion.

IV

- Store vials at room temperature.
- Dilute with at least 50 ml D_5W or 0.9% NaCl.
- Do not administer by subcutaneous, IM, intrathecal, or intra-arterial injection. Do not give IV push over less than 3 minutes. Give IV bolus over at least 3 minutes or intermittent IV infusion over 15 to 60 minutes. Administer continuous IV infusion of 0.02 to 0.5 mg/ml in D_5W or 0.9% NaCl.

Intervention and Evaluation

- Monitor the patient's hematologic status and liver, renal, and pulmonary function test results.
- Monitor the patient for signs and symptoms of hematologic toxicity (including ecchymosis, fever, signs of local infection, and unusual bleeding from any site) and stomatitis (including burning or erythema of oral mucosa, difficulty swallowing, oral ulcerations, and sore throat).
- Evaluate the patient for signs and symptoms of extravasation, including bluish skin, burning, pain, and swelling.
- Offer the patient and family emotional support.

Patient Teaching

- Inform the patient that urine will appear blue or green and sclera may have a blue tint for 24 hours after mitoxantrone administration.
- Encourage the patient to drink plenty of fluids to protect against renal impairment.
- Urge the patient to avoid receiving vaccinations and coming in contact with crowds and people with known infections.
- Instruct the patient to use contraceptive measures during mitoxantrone therapy.

palifermin

pal-ih-**fur**-min
(Kepivance)

CATEGORY AND SCHEDULE

Pregnancy Risk Category: C

MECHANISM OF ACTION

An antineoplastic adjunct that binds to the keratinocyte growth factor receptor, present on epithelial cells of the buccal mucosa and tongue, resulting in the proliferation, differentiation, and migration of epithelial cells. **Therapeutic Effect:** Reduces incidence and duration of severe oral mucositis.

AVAILABILITY

Injection: 6.25-mg vials.

INDICATIONS AND DOSAGES

▸ Mucositis (premyelotoxic therapy)

IV bolus

Adults, Elderly. 60 mcg/kg/day for 3 consecutive days, with the 3rd dose 24–48 hr before chemotherapy.

▸ Mucositis (post-myelotoxic therapy)

IV

Adults, Elderly. The last 3 doses should be administered after myelotoxic therapy; the first of these doses should be administered after, but on the same day of, hematopoietic stem cell infusion and at least 4 days after the most recent administration of palifermin.

CONTRAINDICATIONS

Patients allergic to *Escherichia coli*–derived proteins

INTERACTIONS

Drug

Heparin: Palifermin binds to heparin.

Myelotoxic chemotherapy: Administration of palifermin during or within 24 hours before or after myelotoxic chemotherapy results in increased severity and duration of oral mucositis.

Herbal

None known.

Food

None known.

DIAGNOSTIC TEST EFFECTS

May elevate serum lipase and amylase levels.

SIDE EFFECTS

Frequent (62%–28%)

Rash, fever, pruritus, erythema, edema

Occasional (17%–10%)

Mouth and tongue thickness or discoloration, altered taste, dysesthesia (hyperesthesia, hypoesthesia, paresthesia), arthralgia

SERIOUS REACTIONS

! Transient hypertension occurs occasionally.

NURSING CONSIDERATIONS

Precautions

• Use palifermin cautiously in women who are pregnant or breast-feeding.

Administration and Handling

IV

• Reconstitute palifermin using aseptic technique. Slowly inject 1.2 ml sterile water for injection to yield a final concentration of 5 mg/ml. Swirl gently to dissolve. Don't shake or agitate the solution. Dissolution takes less than 3 minutes.

• If not used immediately, the reconstituted solution may be stored in the refrigerator for 24 hours. Protect it from light.

• The reconstituted solution may be warmed to room temperature for up to 1 hour before administration. Discard the solution if it's left at room temperature for more than 1 hour or if it becomes discolored or contains particles.

• Administer by IV bolus injection. If heparin is being used to maintain an IV line, use 0.9% NaCl to rinse the IV line before and after palifermin administration.

pegaspargase

peg-ah-spa-**raj**-ace
(Oncaspar)

CATEGORY AND SCHEDULE

Pregnancy Risk Category: C

MECHANISM OF ACTION

An enzyme that breaks down extracellular supplies of the amino acid asparagine, which is necessary for the survival of leukemic cells. Binding to polyethylene glycol decreases the antigenicity of pegaspargase, making it less likely to cause a hypersensitivity reaction. Cell cycle–phase specific for G1 phase of cell division. **Therapeutic Effect:** Interferes with DNA, RNA, and protein synthesis in leukemic cells.

AVAILABILITY

Injection: 7,500 international units/ml.

INDICATIONS AND DOSAGES

▸ Acute lymphocytic leukemia

IV, IM

Adults, Elderly, Children with a body surface area of 0.6 m^2 or more. 2,500 international units/m^2 every 14 days.

Children with a body surface area of less than 0.6 m^2. 82.5 international units/kg every 14 days.

CONTRAINDICATIONS

Previous anaphylactic reaction or significant hemorrhagic event associated with pegaspargase therapy, pancreatitis (current or previous)

INTERACTIONS

Drug

Antigout medications: May decrease the effects of these drugs.

Live-virus vaccine: May potentiate virus replication, increase vaccine side effects, and decrease the patient's antibody response to the vaccine.

Methotrexate: May block the effects of this drug.

Steroids, vincristine: May increase hyperglycemia, risk of neuropathy, and disturbances of erythropoiesis.

Herbal

None known.

Food

None known.

DIAGNOSTIC TEST EFFECTS

May increase BUN, blood ammonia, and blood glucose levels; serum alkaline phosphatase, bilirubin, uric acid, AST (SGOT), and ALT (SGPT) levels; PT; and aPTT. May decrease blood clotting factors (including plasma fibrinogen, antithrombin, and plasminogen) as well as serum albumin, calcium, and cholesterol levels.

SIDE EFFECTS

Frequent

Allergic reaction (including rash, urticaria, arthralgia, facial edema, hypotension, and respiratory distress)

Occasional

CNS effects (including confusion, drowsiness, depression, nervousness, and fatigue), stomatitis, hypoalbuminemia, uric acid nephropathy (manifested as edema of the feet or lower legs), hyperglycemia

Rare

Hyperthermia (fever or chills)

SERIOUS REACTIONS

! The patient may have a hypersensitivity reaction, including anaphylaxis, during therapy.

! Pancreatitis, as evidenced by severe abdominal pain with nausea and vomiting, is a common reaction.

! Hepatotoxicity, as evidenced by

jaundice and abnormal hepatic enzyme test results, may occur, especially in patients with preexisting hepatic impairment.

! An increased risk of hematologic toxicity and coagulation disorders occurs occasionally.

! Seizures occur rarely.

NURSING CONSIDERATIONS

Baseline Assessment

• Keep antihistamines, epinephrine, and corticosteroids readily available before and during pegaspargase administration to ensure an adequate airway and treat any allergic reaction.

• Assess the patient's CBC; bone marrow tests; fibrinogen level; liver, pancreatic, and renal function test results; PT; and aPTT before beginning therapy and whenever a week or more has elapsed between drug doses.

Precautions

• Use pegaspargase cautiously in patients concurrently taking aspirin, NSAIDs, or anticoagulants.

Administration and Handling

◀ **ALERT** ▶ Handle pegaspargase with care because the drug is a contact irritant. Wear gloves, avoid inhaling vapors, and avoid contact with skin or mucous membranes. In case of contact, wash with copious amount of water for at least 15 minutes. Avoid excessive agitation of the vial (do not shake).

◀ **ALERT** ▶ The IM administration route is preferred because it poses less risk of coagulopathy, hepatotoxicity, and GI or renal disorders than the IV route.

• Refrigerate—do not freeze—vials.

• Discard the solution if it's cloudy or contains a precipitate. Also discard it if it has been stored at room temperature for longer than 48 hours or if the vial has been previously frozen because freezing destroys the drug's potency.

• Use one dose per vial; do not re-enter the vial. Discard any unused portion.

IM

• Administer no more than 2 ml at any one IM site. Use multiple injection sites if more than 2 ml is being administered.

IV

• Add 100 ml 0.9% NaCl or D_5W, and administer the drug through an infusion that is already running.

• Infuse over 1 to 2 hours.

Intervention and Evaluation

• Closely monitor the patient after drug administration. Be alert for signs of toxicity.

• Obtain the patient's serum amylase and lipase concentrations frequently during and after therapy for evidence of pancreatitis.

• Monitor the patient's BUN and serum creatinine levels for signs of renal failure.

• Discontinue the drug at the first sign of pancreatitis or renal failure.

• Monitor the patient for signs and symptoms of hematologic toxicity and coagulation disorders, such as excessive fatigue and weakness, ecchymosis, fever, signs of local infection, sore throat, and unusual bleeding from any site.

Patient Teaching

• Inform the patient that nausea may decrease during therapy. Advise the patient to notify the physician if nausea and vomiting continue at home.

• Urge the patient to avoid receiving vaccinations and coming in contact with anyone who has recently received a live-virus vaccine.

• Urge the patient to drink plenty of fluids to protect against renal impairment.

procarbazine hydrochloride

pro-**car**-bah-zeen
(Matulane, Natulan[CAN])
Do not confuse procarbazine with dacarbazine.

CATEGORY AND SCHEDULE

Pregnancy Risk Category: D

MECHANISM OF ACTION

A methylhydrazine derivative that inhibits DNA, RNA, and protein synthesis. May also directly damage DNA. Cell cycle–phase specific for S phase of cell division. **Therapeutic Effect:** Causes cell death.

AVAILABILITY

Capsules: 50 mg.

INDICATIONS AND DOSAGES

▸ Advanced Hodgkin's disease

PO

Adults, Elderly. Initially, 2–4 mg/kg/day as a single dose or in divided doses for 1 wk, then 4–6 mg/kg/day. Maintenance: 1–2 mg/kg/day.
Children. 50–100 mg/m^2/day for 10–14 days of a 28-day cycle. Continue until maximum response occurs, leukocyte count falls below 4,000/mm^3, or platelet count falls below 100,000/mm^3. Maintenance: 50 mg/m^2/day.

OFF-LABEL USES

Treatment of lung carcinoma, malignant melanoma, multiple myeloma, non-Hodgkin's lymphoma, polycythemia vera, primary brain tumors

CONTRAINDICATIONS

Myelosuppression

INTERACTIONS

Drug

Alcohol: May cause a disulfiram-like reaction.
Anticholinergics, antihistamines: May increase the anticholinergic effects of these drugs.
Bone marrow depressants: May increase myelosuppression.
Buspirone, caffeine-containing medications: May increase BP.
Carbamazepine, cyclobenzaprine, MAOIs, maprotiline: May cause hyperpyretic crisis, seizures, or death.
CNS depressants: May increase CNS depression.
Insulin, oral antidiabetics: May increase the effects of these drugs.
Meperidine: May produce coma, seizures, immediate excitation, rigidity, severe hypertension or hypotension, severe respiratory distress, diaphoresis, and vascular collapse.
Sympathomimetics: May increase cardiac stimulant and vasopressor effects.
Tricyclic antidepressants: May increase anticholinergic effects; may cause seizures and hyperpyretic crisis.

Herbal

None known.

Food

Caffeine-containing beverages: May increase BP.

DIAGNOSTIC TEST EFFECTS

None known.

SIDE EFFECTS

Frequent

Severe nausea, vomiting, respiratory disorders (cough, effusion), myalgia, arthralgia, drowsiness, nervousness, insomnia, nightmares, diaphoresis, hallucinations, seizures

Occasional
Hoarseness, tachycardia, nystagmus, retinal hemorrhage, photophobia, photosensitivity, urinary frequency, nocturia, hypotension, diarrhea, stomatitis, paraesthesia, unsteadiness, confusion, decreased reflexes, foot drop
Rare
Hypersensitivity reaction (dermatitis, pruritus, rash, urticaria), hyperpigmentation, alopecia

SERIOUS REACTIONS

! Procarbazine's major toxic effects are myelosuppression manifested as hematologic toxicity (mainly leukopenia, thrombocytopenia, and anemia) and hepatotoxicity manifested as jaundice and ascites.
! UTIs may occur secondary to leukopenia.

NURSING CONSIDERATIONS

Baseline Assessment

• Monitor the patient's WBC count with differential, platelet count, and reticulocyte count. Also, check the patient's bone marrow test results; urinalysis results; BUN level; blood Hct and Hgb levels; and serum alkaline phosphatase, AST (SGOT), and ALT (SGPT) levels before and periodically during procarbazine therapy.

Precautions

• Use procarbazine cautiously in patients with hepatic or renal impairment.

Administration and Handling

• Administer procarbazine with food or fluids if the patient has severe GI side effects or difficulty swallowing.

Intervention and Evaluation

• Monitor the results of the patient's hematologic tests and liver and renal function studies.
• Monitor for the patient for signs and symptoms of anemia, including excessive fatigue and weakness, and hematologic toxicity, including easy ecchymosis, fever, signs of local infection, sore throat, and unusual bleeding from any site.
• Assess the patient for signs and symptoms of stomatitis.
• Expect to discontinue therapy if stomatitis, diarrhea, paraesthesia, neuropathy, confusion, or a hypersensitivity reaction occurs; if the WBC count falls below 4,000/mm^3; or if the platelet count falls below 100,000/mm^3.

Patient Teaching

• Warn the patient to notify the physician if he or she experiences bleeding, easy bruising, fever, or sore throat.
• Caution the patient to avoid consuming alcohol during therapy because it may cause nausea and vomiting, sedation, severe headache, and visual disturbances.

temozolomide ⚑

teh-moe-**zoll**-oh-mide
(Temodal[AUS], Temodar)

CATEGORY AND SCHEDULE

Pregnancy Risk Category: D

MECHANISM OF ACTION

An imidazotetrazine derivative that acts as a prodrug and is converted to a highly active cytotoxic metabolite. Its cytotoxic effect is associated with methylation of DNA. **Therapeutic Effect:** Inhibits DNA replication, causing cell death.

PHARMACOKINETICS

Rapidly and completely absorbed after PO administration. Protein binding: 15%. Peak plasma concentration occurs in 1 hr. Penetrates the blood-brain barrier. Eliminated primarily in urine and, to a much lesser extent, in feces. ***Half-life:*** 1.6–1.8 hr.

AVAILABILITY

Capsules: 5 mg, 20 mg, 100 mg, 250 mg.

INDICATIONS AND DOSAGES

▸ Anaplastic astrocytoma

PO

Adults, Elderly. Initially, 150 mg/m^2/day for 5 consecutive days of a 28-day treatment cycle. Subsequent doses based on platelet count and ANC during previous cycle (ANC greater than 1,500 per microliter and platelet count: more than 100,000 per microliter). Maintenance: 200 mg/m^2/day for 5 days q4wk. Continue until disease progression. Minimum: 100 mg/m^2/day for 5 days q4wk.

CONTRAINDICATIONS

Hypersensitivity to dacarbazine, pregnancy

INTERACTIONS

Drug

Live-virus vaccines: May potentiate virus replication, increase vaccine side effects, and decrease the patient's antibody response to the vaccine.

Valproic acid: Decreases the clearance of temozolomide.

Herbal

None known.

Food

All foods: Decrease the rate of drug absorption.

DIAGNOSTIC TEST EFFECTS

May decrease blood Hgb levels and neutrophil, platelet, and WBC counts.

SIDE EFFECTS

Frequent (53%–33%)

Nausea, vomiting, headache, fatigue, constipation

Occasional (16%–10%)

Diarrhea, asthenia, fever, dizziness, peripheral edema, incoordination, insomnia

Rare (9%–5%)

Paraesthesia, drowsiness, anorexia, urinary incontinence, anxiety, pharyngitis, cough

SERIOUS REACTIONS

! Elderly patients and women are at increased risk for developing severe myelosuppression, characterized by neutropenia and thrombocytopenia and usually occurring within the first few cycles. Neutrophil and platelet counts reach their nadirs approximately 26–28 days after administration and recover within 14 days of the nadir.

NURSING CONSIDERATIONS

Baseline Assessment

- Know that before administration, the patient's absolute neutrophil count (ANC) must be greater than 1,500/mm^3 and the platelet count must be greater than 100,000/mm^3.
- Administer antiemetics, as ordered, to control nausea and vomiting.

Lifespan Considerations

- Temozolomide use should be avoided during pregnancy because the drug may cause fetal harm. Although it's unknown if temozolomide is excreted in breast milk, women taking this drug should avoid breast-feeding.
- The safety and efficacy of temozolomide have not been established in children.
- Patients older than 70 years have a higher risk of developing grade 4

neutropenia and grade 4 thrombocytopenia.

Precautions

• Use temozolomide cautiously in patients with severe hepatic or renal impairment.

Administration and Handling

◀ **ALERT** ▶ Because temozolomide is cytotoxic, avoid touching the contents of an open capsule during preparation and administration.

• Administer temozolomide on an empty stomach because food reduces the rate and extent of drug absorption and increases the risk of nausea and vomiting.

• For best results, give temozolomide at bedtime.

• Have the patient swallow the capsule whole with a glass of water. If the patient can't swallow, open the capsule and mix the contents with applesauce or apple juice.

Intervention and Evaluation

• If ordered, obtain a CBC on day 22 (21 days after the first dose) or within 48 hours of that day and then weekly until the ANC is greater than 1,500/mm^3 and the platelet count is greater than 100,000/mm^3.

• Monitor the patient for signs and symptoms of hematologic toxicity, including excessive fatigue and weakness, ecchymosis, fever, signs of local infection, sore throat, and unusual bleeding from any site.

Patient Teaching

• Advise the patient to take temozolomide on an empty stomach to reduce nausea and vomiting.

• Warn the patient not to touch the ingredients of open capsules because the drug is cytotoxic.

• Warn the patient to notify the physician if he or she experiences easy bruising, fever, signs of local infection, sore throat, or unusual bleeding from any site.

• Caution women of childbearing age to avoid pregnancy while taking temozolomide. Teach the patient about effective contraception methods.

• Urge the patient to avoid receiving vaccinations and coming in contact with crowds and those with known infections.

teniposide

ten-**ih**-poe-side
(Vumon)

CATEGORY AND SCHEDULE

Pregnancy Risk Category: D

MECHANISM OF ACTION

An epipodophyllotoxin that induces single- and double-strand breaks in DNA, inhibiting or altering DNA synthesis. Acts in the late S and early G_2 phases of cell cycle. **Therapeutic Effect:** Prevents cells from entering mitosis.

AVAILABILITY

Injection: 50 mg.

INDICATIONS AND DOSAGES

▸ **Induction therapy in patients with refractory childhood acute lymphoblastic leukemia (in combination with other antineoplastic agents)**

Children. Dosage is individualized based on the patient's clinical response and tolerance of the drug's adverse effects. When used in combination therapy, consult specific protocols for optimum dosage or sequence of drug administration.

CONTRAINDICATIONS

Absolute neutrophil count less than 500/mm^3; hypersensitivity to Cremophor EL (polyoxyethylated castor oil), etoposide, or teniposide; platelet count less than 50,000/mm^3

INTERACTIONS

Drug

Bone marrow depressants: May increase myelosuppression.
Live-virus vaccines: May potentiate virus replication, increase vaccine side effects, and decrease the patient's antibody response to the vaccine.
Methotrexate: May increase intracellular accumulation of this drug.
Vincristine: May increase the severity of peripheral neuropathy.

Herbal

None known.

Food

None known.

DIAGNOSTIC TEST EFFECTS

None significant.

SIDE EFFECTS

Frequent (greater than 30%)
Mucositis, nausea, vomiting, diarrhea, anemia
Occasional (5%–3%)
Alopecia, rash
Rare (less than 3%)
Hepatic dysfunction, fever, renal dysfunction, peripheral neurotoxicity

SERIOUS REACTIONS

! Myelosuppression manifested as hematologic toxicity (principally leukopenia, neutropenia, and thrombocytopenia) may be severe and may increase the risk of infection or bleeding.
! Hypersensitivity reaction may include anaphylaxis (marked by chills, fever, tachycardia, bronchospasm, dyspnea, and facial flushing).

NURSING CONSIDERATIONS

Baseline Assessment

• Assess the patient's hematologic, liver function, and renal function test results before and frequently during teniposide therapy.

Precautions

• Use teniposide cautiously in patients with brain tumors, hepatic dysfunction, Down syndrome, or neuroblastoma (increases the risk of anaphylaxis).

Administration and Handling

◀ **ALERT** ▶ Wear gloves when preparing the solution. If the solution comes in contact with your skin, wash immediately and thoroughly with soap and water.

IV

• Refrigerate unopened ampules, and protect them from light.
• Dilute with 0.9% NaCl or D_5W to provide a concentration of 0.1 to 1 mg/ml.
• Prepare and administer the drug in glass containers or polyolefin plastic bags. Do not use polyvinyl chloride containers.
• Reconstituted solutions are stable for 24 hours at room temperature. They should not be refrigerated.
• Use the 1-mg/ml solution within 4 hours of preparation to reduce the risk of precipitation. Discard the solution if it contains precipitates.
• Infuse teniposide over at least 30 to 60 minutes. Avoid rapid IV injection.

Intervention and Evaluation

• Have appropriate medication and equipment readily available before giving the first dose in case life-threatening anaphylaxis occurs.
• Monitor the patient for signs and symptoms of myelosuppression, including excessive fatigue and weakness, ecchymosis, fever, signs

of local infection, and unusual bleeding or bruising.

Patient Teaching

- Warn the patient to notify the physician if he or she experiences easy bruising, difficulty breathing, fever, signs of infection, or unusual bleeding from any site.
- Caution women of childbearing age to avoid pregnancy during teniposide therapy. Teach contraceptive methods as needed.
- Urge the patient not to receive vaccinations without physician approval and to avoid contact with crowds or people with known infections.
- Inform the patient that hair loss is reversible but that new hair may have a different color or texture.

topotecan

toe-**poh**-teh-can

(Hycamtin)

CATEGORY AND SCHEDULE

Pregnancy Risk Category: D

MECHANISM OF ACTION

A DNA topoisomerase inhibitor that interacts with topoisomerase I, an enzyme that allows DNA replication by producing reversible single-strand breaks in DNA that relieve torsional strain. Topotecan prevents religation of the DNA strand, resulting in damage to double-strand DNA and cell death. **Therapeutic Effect:** Kills cancer cells.

PHARMACOKINETICS

Hydrolyzed to active form after IV administration. Protein binding: 35%. Excreted in urine. ***Half-life:*** 2–3 hr (increased in impaired renal function).

AVAILABILITY

Powder for Injection: 4 mg (single-dose vial).

INDICATIONS AND DOSAGES

▸ **Ovarian carcinoma, small-cell lung cancer**

IV

Adults, Elderly. 1.5 mg/m^2/day over 30 min for 5 consecutive days, beginning on day 1 of a 21-day course. Minimum of four courses recommended. If severe neutropenia (neutrophil count less than 1,500 /mm^2) occurs during treatment, reduce dose for subsequent courses by 0.25 mg/m^2, or administer filgrastim (G-CSF) no sooner than 24 hr after the last dose of topotecan.

▸ **Dosage in renal impairment**

No dosage adjustment is necessary in patients with mild renal impairment (creatinine clearance of 40–60 ml/min). For moderate renal impairment (creatinine clearance of 20–39 ml/min), give 0.75 mg/m^2.

OFF-LABEL USES

Treatment of solid tumors including osteosarcoma, neuroblastoma, pediatric leukemia, rhabdomyosarcoma

CONTRAINDICATIONS

Baseline neutrophil count less than 1,500 cells/mm^3, breast-feeding, pregnancy, severe myelosuppression

INTERACTIONS

Drug

Cisplatin: May increase the severity of myelosuppression.

Live-virus vaccines: May potentiate virus replication, increase vaccine side effects, and decrease the patient's antibody response to the vaccine.

Other bone marrow depressants: May increase the risk of myelosuppression.

Herbal
None known.
Food
None known.

DIAGNOSTIC TEST EFFECTS
May increase serum bilirubin, AST (SGOT), and ALT (SGPT) levels. May decrease RBC, leukocyte, neutrophil, and platelet counts.

IV INCOMPATIBILITIES
Dexamethasone (Decadron), 5-fluorouracil, mitomycin (Mutamycin)

IV COMPATIBILITIES
Carboplatin (Paraplatin), cisplatin (Platinol AQ), cyclophosphamide (Cytoxan), doxorubicin (Adriamycin), etoposide (VePesid), gemcitabine (Gemzar), granisetron (Kytril), ondansetron (Zofran), paclitaxel (Taxol), vincristine (Oncovin)

SIDE EFFECTS
Frequent
Nausea (77%); vomiting (58%); diarrhea, total alopecia (42%); headache (21%); dyspnea (21%)
Occasional
Paraesthesia (9%); constipation, abdominal pain (3%)
Rare
Anorexia, malaise, arthralgia, asthenia, myalgia

SERIOUS REACTIONS
! Severe neutropenia (neutrophil count less than 500 cells/mm^3) occurs in 60% of patients, usually during the first course of therapy. The neutrophil nadir usually occurs at a median of 11 days after starting therapy.
! Thrombocytopenia (platelet count less than 25,000/mm^3) occurs in 26% of patients, and severe anemia (RBC count less than 8 g/dl) occurs in 40% of patients. The platelet and RBC nadirs usually occur at a median of 15 days after starting the first course of therapy.

NURSING CONSIDERATIONS
Baseline Assessment
• Assess the patient's CBC, especially blood Hgb levels, and platelet count before each topotecan dose.
• Know that myelosuppression may precipitate life-threatening anemia, hemorrhage, and infection.
• If the patient's platelet count drops, minimize trauma to the patient (for example, by avoiding IM or rectal drug administration and by gently repositioning the patient).
• Premedicate the patient with antiemetics, if ordered, on the day of treatment, starting at least 30 minutes before topotecan administration.
Lifespan Considerations
• Because of the risk of fetal harm, pregnant women should not take topotecan, especially in the first trimester. It is unknown if topotecan is distributed in breast milk; however, breast-feeding is not recommended for patients taking this drug.
• The safety and efficacy of topotecan have not been established in children.
• In the elderly, age-related renal impairment may require dosage adjustment.
Precautions
• Use topotecan cautiously in patients with hepatic or renal impairment or mild myelosuppression.
Administration and Handling
◀ALERT▶ As prescribed, do not give topotecan if the patient's baseline neutrophil count is less than 1,500 cells/mm^3 and platelet count is less than 100,000/mm^3.

IV

- Store vials at room temperature in original cartons.
- Reconstitute each 4-mg vial with 4 ml sterile water for injection.
- Further dilute with 50 to 100 ml 0.9% NaCl or D_5W.
- Reconstituted vials diluted for infusion are stable at room temperature in ambient lighting for up to 24 hours.
- Administer the drug by IV infusion over 30 minutes.
- Be aware that extravasation is associated with only mild local reactions, such as ecchymosis and erythema.

Intervention and Evaluation

- Monitor the patient's CBC (particularly blood Hgb level and WBC count with differential) and platelet count frequently during topotecan treatment for evidence of myelosuppression.
- Assess the patient for dyspnea, headache, anemia, bleeding, and signs of infection.
- Monitor the patient's serum electrolyte levels, hydration status, and intake and output because diarrhea and vomiting are common side effects of topotecan.
- Assess the patient's therapeutic response to the drug.
- Help the patient manage the drug's side effects, for example, by providing small, frequent meals and antiemetics to help prevent or treat nausea and vomiting.
- Offer emotional support to the patient and family.

Patient Teaching

- Explain that diarrhea may develop late in therapy. Teach the patient to watch for signs and symptoms of dehydration and electrolyte depletion.
- If ordered, provide instructions for using an antiemetic and antidiarrheal.
- Advise the patient to notify the physician if diarrhea and vomiting continue at home.
- Urge the patient to avoid receiving vaccinations and coming in contact with anyone who has recently received a live-virus vaccine.
- Inform the patient that hair loss is reversible but that new hair may have a different color or texture.

21 Angiotensin-Converting Enzyme (ACE) Inhibitors

benazepril
captopril
enalapril maleate
fosinopril
lisinopril
moexipril hydrochloride
perindopril erbumine
quinapril
ramipril
trandolapril

Uses: Angiotensin-converting enzyme (ACE) inhibitors are used to treat hypertension and, as adjuncts, to treat CHF.

Action: ACE inhibitors act primarily by suppressing the renin-angiotensin-aldosterone system. (See the illustration *Site of Action: ACE Inhibitors,* page 434.) They reduce peripheral arterial resistance and increase cardiac output, but produce little or no change in the heart rate.

COMBINATION PRODUCTS

ACCURETIC: quinapril/hydrochlorothiazide (a diuretic) 10 mg/12.5 mg; 20 mg/12.5 mg; 20 mg/25 mg.
CAPOZIDE: captopril/hydrochlorothiazide (a diuretic) 25 mg/15 mg; 25 mg/25 mg; 50 mg/15 mg; 50 mg/25 mg.
LEXXEL: enalapril/felodipine (a calcium channel blocker) 5 mg/2.5 mg; 5 mg/5 mg.
LOTENSIN HCT: benazepril/hydrochlorothiazide (a diuretic) 5 mg/6.25 mg; 10 mg/12.5 mg; 20 mg/12.5 mg; 20 mg/25 mg.
LOTREL: benazepril/amlodipine (a calcium channel blocker) 2.5 mg/10 mg; 5 mg/10 mg; 5 mg/20 mg; 10 mg/20 mg.
PRINZIDE: lisinopril/hydrochlorothiazide (a diuretic) 10 mg/12.5 mg; 20 mg/12.5 mg; 20 mg/25 mg.
TARKA: trandolapril/verapamil (a calcium channel blocker) 1 mg/240 mg; 2 mg/180 mg; 2 mg/240 mg; 4 mg/240 mg.
TECZEM: enalapril/diltiazem (a calcium channel blocker) 5 mg/180 mg.
UNIRETIC: moexipril/hydrochlorothiazide (a diuretic) 7.5 mg/12.5 mg; 15 mg/12.5 mg; 15 mg/25 mg.
VASERETIC: enalapril/hydrochlorothiazide (a diuretic) 5 mg/12.5 mg; 10 mg/25 mg.
ZESTORETIC: lisinopril/hydrochlorothiazide (a diuretic) 10 mg/12.5 mg; 20 mg/12.5 mg; 20 mg/25 mg.

benazepril

be-**naze**-a-pril
(Lotensin)
Do not confuse benazepril with Benadryl, or Lotensin with Loniten or lovastatin.

CATEGORY AND SCHEDULE

Pregnancy Risk Category: C (D if used in second or third trimester)

MECHANISM OF ACTION

An ACE inhibitor that decreases the rate of conversion of angiotensin I to angiotensin II, a potent vasoconstrictor. Reduces peripheral arterial resistance. **Therapeutic Effect:** Lowers BP.

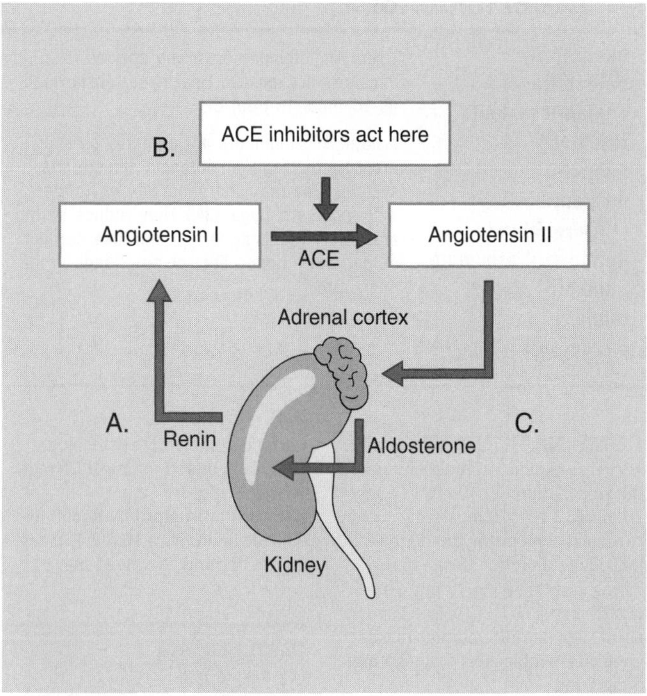

Site of Action: ACE Inhibitors

The renin-angiotensin-aldosterone system plays a major role in regulating BP. Any condition that decreases renal blood flow, reduces BP, or stimulates $beta_1$-adrenergic receptors prompts the kidneys to release renin (A). Renin acts on angiotensinogen, which is converted to angiotensin I, a weak vasoconstrictor. Angiotensin-converting enzyme (ACE) converts angiotensin I to angiotensin II, which causes systemic and renal blood vessels to constrict (B). Systemic vasoconstriction increases peripheral vascular resistance, raising the BP. Renal vasoconstriction decreases glomerular filtration, resulting in sodium and water retention and increasing blood volume and BP. In addition, angiotensin II acts on the adrenal cortex, causing it to release aldosterone (C). This makes the kidneys retain additional sodium and water, which further increases the BP.

ACE inhibitors, such as captopril, enalapril, and lisinopril, block the action of ACE. As a result, angiotensin II can't form, which prevents systemic and renal vasoconstriction and the release of aldosterone.

PHARMACOKINETICS

Route	Onset	Peak	Duration
PO	1 hr	2–4 hr	24 hr

Partially absorbed from the GI tract. Protein binding: 97%. Metabolized in the liver to active metabolite. Primarily excreted in urine. Minimal removal by hemodialysis. ***Half-life:*** 35 min; metabolite 10–11 hr.

AVAILABILITY

Tablets: 5 mg, 10 mg, 20 mg, 40 mg.

INDICATIONS AND DOSAGES

▸ **Hypertension (monotherapy)**

PO

Adults. Initially, 10 mg/day. Maintenance: 20–40 mg/day as single or in 2 divided doses. Maximum: 80 mg/day.

Elderly. Initially, 5–10 mg/day. Range: 20–40 mg/day.

▸ **Hypertension (combination therapy)**

PO

Adults. Discontinue diuretic 2–3 days prior to initiating benazepril, then dose as noted above. If unable to discontinue diuretic, begin benazepril at 5 mg/day.

▸ **Dosage in renal impairment**

For adult patients with creatinine clearance less than 30 ml/min, initially, 5 mg/day titrated up to maximum of 40 mg/day.

OFF-LABEL USES

Treatment of CHF

CONTRAINDICATIONS

History of angioedema from previous treatment with ACE inhibitors

INTERACTIONS

Drug

Alcohol, antihypertensives, diuretics: May increase the effects of benazepril.

Lithium: May increase the lithium blood concentration and risk of lithium toxicity.

NSAIDs: May decrease the effects of benazepril.

Potassium-sparing diuretics, potassium supplements: May cause hyperkalemia.

Herbal

None known.

Food

None known.

DIAGNOSTIC TEST EFFECTS

May increase BUN, serum alkaline phosphatase, serum bilirubin, serum potassium, AST (SGOT), and ALT (SGPT) levels. May decrease serum sodium levels. May cause positive antinuclear antibody titer.

SIDE EFFECTS

Frequent (6%–3%)

Cough, headache, dizziness

Occasional (2%)

Fatigue, somnolence or drowsiness, nausea

Rare (less than 1%)

Rash, fever, myalgia, diarrhea, loss of taste

SERIOUS REACTIONS

! Excessive hypotension ("first-dose syncope") may occur in patients with CHF and in those who are severely salt or volume depleted.

! Angioedema (swelling of the face and lips) and hyperkalemia occur rarely.

! Agranulocytosis and neutropenia may be noted in those with collagen vascular disease, including scleroderma and systemic lupus erythematosus, and impaired renal function.

! Nephrotic syndrome may be noted in patients with history of renal disease.

NURSING CONSIDERATIONS

Baseline Assessment

• Assess the patient's BP immediately before giving each benazepril dose, in addition to regular monitoring. Be alert to fluctuations in BP. If an excessive reduction in BP occurs, place the patient in the supine position with legs elevated.

• As ordered, obtain a CBC and blood chemistry before beginning benazepril therapy, then every 2 weeks for the next 3 months, and periodically thereafter in patients with autoimmune disease, or renal impairment, and in those who are taking drugs that affect immune response or leukocyte count.

Lifespan Considerations

• Benazepril crosses the placenta and it is unknown if it is distributed in breast milk. Benazepril may cause fetal or neonatal morbidity or mortality.

• Safety and efficacy of benazepril have not been established in children.

• The elderly may be more sensitive to the hypotensive effects of benazepril.

Precautions

• Use benazepril cautiously in patients with cerebrovascular or coronary insufficiency, diabetes mellitus, hypovolemia, renal impairment, and sodium depletion.

• Use cautiously in patients on dialysis and in those receiving diuretics.

Administration and Handling

◀ALERT▶ Expect the physician to discontinue diuretics 2 to 3 days before beginning benazepril therapy.

PO

• May give without regard to food.

Intervention and Evaluation

• Assist the patient with ambulation if he or she experiences dizziness.

• Monitor the patient's BP, CBC, and BUN, serum creatinine, and urine protein levels.

Patient Teaching

• Advise the patient to rise slowly from lying to sitting position and to permit legs to dangle from the bed momentarily before standing to reduce the hypotensive effect of benazepril.

• Explain to the patient that the full therapeutic effect of benazepril may take 2 to 4 weeks to appear.

• Caution the patient against noncompliance with drug therapy or skipping drug doses as this may produce severe, rebound hypertension.

captopril

cap-toe-pril

(Acenorm[AUS], Capoten, Captohexal[AUS], Novo-Captoril[CAN], Topace[AUS])

Do not confuse captopril with Capitrol.

CATEGORY AND SCHEDULE

Pregnancy Risk Category: C (D if used in second or third trimester)

MECHANISM OF ACTION

An ACE inhibitor that suppresses the renin-angiotensin-aldosterone system and prevents conversion of angiotensin I to angiotensin II, a potent vasoconstrictor; may also inhibit angiotensin II at local vascular and renal sites. Decreases plasma angiotensin II, increases plasma renin activity, and decreases aldosterone secretion. **Therapeutic Effect:** Reduces peripheral arterial resistance, pulmonary capillary wedge pressure; improves cardiac output and exercise tolerance.

PHARMACOKINETICS

Route	Onset	Peak	Duration
PO	0.25 hr	0.5–1.5 hr	Dose-related

Rapidly, well absorbed from the GI tract (absorption is decreased in the presence of food). Protein binding: 25%–30%. Metabolized in the liver. Primarily excreted in urine. Removed by hemodialysis. ***Half-life:*** less than 3 hr (increased in those with impaired renal function).

AVAILABILITY

Tablets: 12.5 mg, 25 mg, 50 mg, 100 mg.

INDICATIONS AND DOSAGES

▸ **Hypertension**

PO

Adults, Elderly. Initially, 12.5–25 mg 2–3 times a day. After 1–2 wk, may increase to 50 mg 2–3 times a day. Diuretic may be added if no response in additional 1–2 wk. If taken in combination with diuretic, may increase to 100–150 mg 2–3 times a day after 1–2 wk. Maintenance: 25–150 mg 2–3 times a day. Maximum: 450 mg/day.

▸ **CHF**

PO

Adults, Elderly. Initially, 6.25–25 mg 3 times a day. Increase to 50 mg 3 times a day. After at least 2 wk, may increase to 50–100 mg 3 times a day. Maximum: 450 mg/day.

▸ **Post-myocardial infarction, impaired liver function**

PO

Adults, Elderly. 6.25 mg a day, then 12.5 mg 3 times a day. Increase to 25 mg 3 times a day over several days up to 50 mg 3 times a day over several weeks.

▸ **Diabetic nephropathy prevention of kidney failure**

PO

Adults, Elderly. 25 mg 3 times a day.

Children. Initially 0.3–0.5 mg/kg/dose titrated up to a maximum of 6 mg/kg/day in 2–4 divided doses.

Neonates. Initially, 0.05–0.1 mg/kg/dose q8–24h titrated up to 0.5 mg/kg/dose given q6–24h.

▸ **Dosage in renal impairment**

Creatinine clearance 10–50 ml/min. 75% of normal dosage.

Creatinine clearance less than 10 ml/min. 50% of normal dosage.

OFF-LABEL USES

Diagnosis of anatomic renal artery stenosis, hypertensive crisis, rheumatoid arthritis

CONTRAINDICATIONS

History of angioedema from previous treatment with ACE inhibitors

INTERACTIONS

Drug

Alcohol, antihypertensives, diuretics: May increase the effects of captopril.

Lithium: May increase lithium blood concentration and risk of lithium toxicity.

NSAIDs: May decrease the effects of captopril.

Potassium-sparing diuretics, potassium supplements: May cause hyperkalemia.

Herbal

None known.

Food

All food: Food significantly reduces drug absorption by 30% to 40%.

DIAGNOSTIC TEST EFFECTS

May increase BUN, serum alkaline phosphatase, serum bilirubin, serum creatinine, serum potassium, AST (SGOT), and ALT (SGPT) levels. May decrease serum sodium levels. May cause positive antinuclear antibody titer.

SIDE EFFECTS

Frequent (7%–4%)
Rash
Occasional (4%–2%)
Pruritus, dysgeusia (altered taste)
Rare (less than 2%–0.5%)
Headache, cough, insomnia, dizziness, fatigue, paraesthesia, malaise, nausea, diarrhea or constipation, dry mouth, tachycardia

SERIOUS REACTIONS

! Excessive hypotension ("first-dose syncope") may occur in patients with CHF and in those who are severely salt and volume depleted.
! Angioedema (swelling of face and lips) and hyperkalemia occur rarely.
! Agranulocytosis and neutropenia may be noted in those with collagen vascular disease, including scleroderma and systemic lupus erythematosus, and impaired renal function.
! Nephrotic syndrome may be noted in those with history of renal disease.

NURSING CONSIDERATIONS

Baseline Assessment

- Expect to obtain the patient's BP immediately before each captopril dose, in addition to regular monitoring. Be alert to fluctuations in BP. If an excessive reduction in BP occurs, place the patient in the supine position with legs elevated and notify the physician.
- Test the patient's first urine of the day for protein by dipstick method before beginning captopril therapy and periodically thereafter in patients with prior renal disease and in those receiving captopril dosages greater than 150 mg/day.
- As ordered, obtain a CBC and blood chemistry before beginning captopril therapy, then every 2 weeks for the next 3 months, and periodically thereafter in patients with autoimmune disease or renal impairment and in those who are taking drugs that affect immune response or leukocyte count.

Lifespan Considerations

- Captopril crosses the placenta, is distributed in breast milk, and may cause fetal or neonatal morbidity or mortality.
- The safety and efficacy of captopril have not been established in children.
- The elderly may be more sensitive to the hypotensive effects of captopril.

Precautions

- Use captopril cautiously in patients with cerebrovascular or coronary insufficiency, hypovolemia, renal impairment, and sodium depletion.
- Use cautiously in patients on dialysis and in those receiving diuretics.
- Use cautiously in elderly patients.

Administration and Handling

PO

◀ALERT▶ Give captopril 1 hour before meals for maximum absorption because food significantly decreases drug absorption.

- Crush tablets if necessary.

Intervention and Evaluation

- Examine the patient's skin for pruritus and rash.

• Assist the patient with ambulation if he or she experiences dizziness.
• Check the patient's urinalysis test results for proteinuria.
• Assess the patient for anorexia due to altered taste perception.
• Monitor CBC and the BUN, serum creatinine, and serum potassium levels in patients who are also receiving a diuretic.

Patient Teaching

• Explain that the full therapeutic effect of captopril may not occur for several weeks.
• Warn the patient that noncompliance with drug therapy or skipping captopril doses may cause severe, rebound hypertension.
• Urge the patient not to consume alcohol while taking captopril.

enalapril maleate

en-**al**-a-pril
(Alphapril[AUS], Amprace[AUS], Apo-Enalapril[CAN], Auspril[AUS], Renitec[AUS], Vasotec)
Do not confuse enalapril with Anafranil, Eldepryl, or ramipril.

CATEGORY AND SCHEDULE

Pregnancy Risk Category: D (C if used in first trimester)

MECHANISM OF ACTION

This angiotensin-converting enzyme (ACE) inhibitor suppresses the renin-angiotensin-aldosterone system, and prevents conversion of angiotensin I to angiotensin II, a potent vasoconstrictor; may inhibit angiotensin II at local vascular, renal sites. Decreases plasma angiotensin II, increases plasma renin activity, decreases aldosterone secretion. **Therapeutic Effect:** In hypertension, reduces peripheral arterial resistance. In congestive heart failure (CHF), increases cardiac output; decreases peripheral vascular resistance, blood pressure (BP), pulmonary capillary wedge pressure, heart size.

PHARMACOKINETICS

Route	Onset	Peak	Duration
PO	1 hr	4–6 hr	24 hr
IV	15 min	1–4 hr	6 hr

Readily absorbed from the GI tract (not affected by food). Protein binding: 50%–60%. Converted to active metabolite. Primarily excreted in urine. Removed by hemodialysis. ***Half-life:*** 11 hr (half-life is increased in those with impaired renal function).

AVAILABILITY

Tablets: 2.5 mg, 5 mg, 10 mg, 20 mg.
Injection: 1.25 mg/ml.

INDICATIONS AND DOSAGES

▸ **Hypertension alone or in combination with other antihypertensives**

PO

Adults, Elderly. Initially, 2.5–5 mg/day. Range: 10–40 mg/day in 1–2 divided doses.
Children. 0.1 mg/kg/day in 1–2 divided doses. Maximum: 0.5 mg/kg/day.
Neonates. 0.1 mg/kg/day q24h.

IV

Adults, Elderly. 0.625–1.25 mg q6h up to 5 mg q6h.
Children, Neonates. 5–10 mcg/kg/dose q8–24h.

▸ **Adjunctive therapy for CHF**

PO

Adults, Elderly. Initially, 2.5–5

mg/day. Range: 5–20 mg/day in 2 divided doses.

▸ **Dosage in renal impairment**

Dosage is modified based on creatinine clearance.

Creatinine Clearance	% Usual Dose
10–50 ml/min	75–100
less than 10 ml/min	50

OFF-LABEL USES

Treatment of diabetic nephropathy or renal crisis in scleroderma

CONTRAINDICATIONS

History of angioedema from previous treatment with ACE inhibitors

INTERACTIONS

Drug

Alcohol, antihypertensives, diuretics: May increase the effects of enalapril.

Herbal

None known.

Food

None known.

DIAGNOSTIC TEST EFFECTS

May increase BUN and serum alkaline phosphatase, serum bilirubin, serum creatinine, serum potassium, AST (SGOT), and ALT (SGPT) levels. May decrease serum sodium levels. May cause positive ANA titer.

IV INCOMPATIBILITIES

Amphotericin B (Fungizone), amphotericin B complex (Abelcet, AmBisome, Amphotec), cefepime (Maxipime), phenytoin (Dilantin)

IV COMPATIBILITIES

Calcium gluconate, dobutamine (Dobutrex), dopamine (Inotropin), fentanyl (Sublimaze), heparin, lidocaine, magnesium sulfate, morphine, nitroglycerin, potassium chloride, potassium phosphate, propofol (Diprivan)

SIDE EFFECTS

Frequent (7%–5%)

Headache, dizziness

Occasional (3%–2%)

Orthostatic hypotension, fatigue, diarrhea, cough, syncope

Rare (less than 2%)

Angina, abdominal pain, vomiting, nausea, rash, asthenia (loss of strength, energy), syncope

SERIOUS REACTIONS

! Excessive hypotension ("first-dose syncope") may occur in patients with CHF and in those who are severely salt or volume depleted.

! Angioedema (swelling of face, lips) and hyperkalemia occur rarely.

! Agranulocytosis and neutropenia may be noted in patients with collagen vascular diseases, including scleroderma and systemic lupus erythematosus, and impaired renal function.

! Nephrotic syndrome may be noted in those with history of renal disease.

NURSING CONSIDERATIONS

Baseline Assessment

• Assess the patient's BP immediately before each enalapril dose. Be alert to fluctuations in BP.

• As ordered, obtain a CBC and blood chemistry before beginning enalapril therapy, then every 2 weeks for 3 months, and periodically thereafter in patients with autoimmune disease, renal impairment, or those who are taking drugs that affect immune or leukocyte responses.

Lifespan Considerations

• Be aware that enalapril crosses the placenta and is distributed in breast

milk. Enalapril may cause fetal or neonatal morbidity or mortality.
• Be aware that the safety and efficacy of enalapril have not been established in children.
• The elderly may be more susceptible to the hypotensive effects of enalapril.

Precautions
• Use cautiously in patients with cerebrovascular or coronary insufficiency, hypovolemia, renal impairment, and sodium depletion.
• Use cautiously in patients who are receiving dialysis and diuretic therapy.

Intervention and Evaluation
• Assist the patient with ambulation if he or she experiences dizziness.
• Monitor the patient's BP and BUN, serum creatinine, and serum potassium levels.
• Assess the patient's pattern of daily bowel activity and stool consistency.

Patient Teaching
• Advise the patient to rise slowly from a lying to a sitting position and to permit legs to dangle from the bed momentarily before standing to reduce the hypotensive effect of enalapril.
• Explain to the patient that the full therapeutic effect of BP reduction may take several weeks to appear.
• Caution the patient against noncompliance with drug therapy or skipping drug doses because this may produce severe, rebound hypertension.
• Urge the patient to limit consumption of alcohol while taking enalapril.
• Warn the patient to notify the physician if diarrhea, difficulty breathing, excessive perspiration, vomiting, or swelling of the face, lips, or tongue occurs.

fosinopril

fo-**sin**-o-pril
(Monopril)
Do not confuse Monopril with Monurol.

CATEGORY AND SCHEDULE

Pregnancy Risk Category: C (D if used in second or third trimester)

MECHANISM OF ACTION

An ACE inhibitor that suppresses the renin-angiotensin-aldosterone system and prevents conversion of angiotensin I to angiotensin II, a potent vasoconstrictor; may also inhibit angiotensin II at local vascular and renal sites. Decreases plasma angiotensin II, increases plasma renin activity, and decreases aldosterone secretion. **Therapeutic Effect:** Reduces peripheral arterial resistance, pulmonary capillary wedge pressure; improves cardiac output, and exercise tolerance.

PHARMACOKINETICS

Route	Onset	Peak	Duration
PO	1 hr	2–6 hr	24 hr

Slowly absorbed from the GI tract. Protein binding: 97%–98%. Metabolized in the liver and GI mucosa to active metabolite. Primarily excreted in urine. Minimal removal by hemodialysis. ***Half-life:*** 11.5 hr.

AVAILABILITY

Tablets: 10 mg, 20 mg, 40 mg.

INDICATIONS AND DOSAGES

▸ **Hypertension (monotherapy)**
PO
Adults, Elderly. Initially, 10 mg/day.

Maintenance: 20–40 mg/day.
Maximum: 80 mg/day.

▸ **Hypertension (with diuretic)**

PO

Adults, Elderly. Initially, 10 mg/day titrated to patient's needs.

▸ **Heart failure**

PO

Adults, Elderly. Initially, 5–10 mg. Maintenance: 20–40 mg/day.

OFF-LABEL USES

Treatment of diabetic and nondiabetic nephropathy, post-myocardial infarction left ventricular dysfunction, renal crisis in scleroderma

CONTRAINDICATIONS

History of angioedema from previous treatment with ACE inhibitors

INTERACTIONS

Drug

Alcohol, antihypertensives, diuretics: May increase the effects of fosinopril.
Lithium: May increase lithium blood concentration and risk of lithium toxicity.
NSAIDs: May decrease the effects of fosinopril.
Potassium-sparing diuretics, potassium supplements: May cause hyperkalemia.

Herbal

None known.

Food

None known.

DIAGNOSTIC TEST EFFECTS

May increase BUN, serum alkaline phosphatase, serum bilirubin, serum creatinine, serum potassium, AST (SGOT), and ALT (SGPT) levels. May decrease serum sodium levels. May cause positive antinuclear antibody titer.

SIDE EFFECTS

Frequent (12%–9%)
Dizziness, cough
Occasional (4%–2%)
Hypotension, nausea, vomiting, upper respiratory tract infection

SERIOUS REACTIONS

! Excessive hypotension ("first-dose syncope") may occur in patients with CHF and in those who are severely salt and volume depleted.
! Angioedema (swelling of face and lips) and hyperkalemia occur rarely.
! Agranulocytosis and neutropenia may be noted in those with collagen vascular disease, including scleroderma and systemic lupus erythematosus, and impaired renal function.
! Nephrotic syndrome may be noted in those with history of renal disease.

NURSING CONSIDERATIONS

Baseline Assessment

- Obtain the patient's BP immediately before each fosinopril dose in addition to regular monitoring. Be alert to fluctuations in BP. If an excessive reduction in BP occurs, place the patient in the supine position with legs elevated and notify the physician.
- Expect the patient to undergo renal function tests before beginning fosinopril therapy.
- As ordered, obtain a CBC and blood chemistry before beginning fosinopril therapy, then every 2 weeks for 3 months, and periodically thereafter in patients with autoimmune disease, or renal impairment, and in those who are taking drugs that affect immune response or leukocyte count.

Lifespan Considerations

- Fosinopril crosses the placenta, is distributed in breast milk, and may

cause fetal or neonatal morbidity or mortality.
• The safety and efficacy of fosinopril have not been established in children.
• Neonates and infants may be at increased risk for neurologic abnormalities and oliguria.
• The elderly may be more sensitive to the hypotensive effects of fosinopril.

Precautions
• Use fosinopril cautiously in patients with coronary or cerebrovascular insufficiency, hypovolemia, renal impairment, and sodium depletion.
• Use cautiously in patients on dialysis and in those receiving diuretics.

Administration and Handling
◀ALERT▶ Expect to discontinue diuretics 2 to 3 days before beginning fosinopril therapy.
PO
• Give fosinopril without regard to food.
• Crush tablets if necessary.

Intervention and Evaluation
• Assist the patient with ambulation if he or she experiences dizziness.
• Assess the patient's intake and output, as appropriate.
• In patients with CHF, assess for crackles and wheezes.
• Monitor the patient's urinalysis results for proteinuria.
• Monitor BUN, serum creatinine, and serum potassium levels in patients on concurrent diuretic therapy.

Patient Teaching
• Warn the patient to report any signs or symptoms of infection, such as fever or sore throat.
• Explain that the full therapeutic effect of fosinopril may take several weeks to appear.
• Warn the patient that noncompliance with drug therapy or skipping fosinopril doses may cause severe, rebound hypertension.
• Advise the patient to rise slowly from a lying to a sitting position and to permit legs to dangle from the bed momentarily before standing to reduce the hypotensive effect of fosinopril.
• Caution the patient to notify the physician if he or she experiences excessive perspiration, persistent cough, or vomiting.

lisinopril
ly-**sin**-oh-pril
(Apo-Lisinopril[CAN], Fibsol[AUS], Lisodur[AUS], Prinivil, Zestril)
Do not confuse lisinopril with fosinopril; or Prinivil or Zestril with Desyrel, Lioresal, Plendil, Prilosec, Proventil, Restoril, or Zostrix.

CATEGORY AND SCHEDULE
Pregnancy Risk Category: C (D if used in second or third trimester)

MECHANISM OF ACTION
This angiotensin-converting enzyme (ACE) inhibitor suppresses the renin-angiotensin-aldosterone system and prevents conversion of angiotensin I to angiotensin II, a potent vasoconstrictor; may also inhibit angiotensin II at local vascular and renal sites. Decreases plasma angiotensin II, increases plasma renin activity, and decreases aldosterone secretion. **Therapeutic Effect:** Reduces peripheral arterial resistance, BP, afterload, pulmonary capillary wedge pressure (preload), and pulmonary vascular resistance. In those with heart failure, also decreases heart size, increases cardiac output, and exercise tolerance time.

PHARMACOKINETICS

Route	Onset	Peak	Duration
PO	1 hr	6 hr	24 hr

Incompletely absorbed from the GI tract. Protein binding: 25%. Primarily excreted unchanged in urine. Removed by hemodialysis. ***Half-life:*** 12 hr (half-life is prolonged in those with impaired renal function).

AVAILABILITY

Tablets (Prinivil, Zestril): 2.5 mg, 5 mg, 10 mg, 20 mg, 30 mg, 40 mg.

INDICATIONS AND DOSAGES

▸ **Hypertension (used alone)**

PO

Adults. Initially, 10 mg/day. May increase by 5–10 mcg/day at 1- to 2-wk intervals. Maximum: 40 mg/day.

Elderly. Initially, 2.5–5 mg/day. May increase by 2.5–5 mg/day at 1- to 2-wk intervals. Maximum: 40 mg/day.

▸ **Hypertension (used in combination with other antihypertensives)**

PO

Adults. Initially, 2.5–5 mg/day titrated to patient's needs.

▸ **Adjunctive therapy for management of heart failure**

PO

Adults, Elderly. Initially, 2.5–5 mg/day. May increase by no more than 10 mg/day at intervals of at least 2 wk. Maintenance: 5–40 mg/day.

▸ **Improve survival in patients after a myocardial infarction (MI)**

PO

Adults, Elderly. Initially, 5 mg, then 5 mg after 24 hr, 10 mg after 48 hr, then 10 mg/day for 6 wk. For patients with low systolic BP, give 2.5 mg/day for 3 days, then 2.5–5 mg/day.

▸ **Dosage in renal impairment**

Titrate to patient's needs after giving the following initial dose:

Creatinine Clearance	% Normal Dose
10–50 ml/min	50–75
less than 10 ml/min	25–50

OFF-LABEL USES

Treatment of hypertension or renal crises with scleroderma

CONTRAINDICATIONS

History of angioedema from previous treatment with ACE inhibitors

INTERACTIONS

Drug

Alcohol, diuretics, hypotensive agents: May increase the effects of lisinopril.

Lithium: May increase lithium blood concentration and risk of lithium toxicity.

NSAIDs: May decrease the effects of lisinopril.

Potassium-sparing diuretics, potassium supplements: May cause hyperkalemia.

Herbal

None known.

Food

None known.

DIAGNOSTIC TEST EFFECTS

May increase BUN, serum alkaline phosphatase, serum bilirubin, serum creatinine, serum potassium, AST (SGOT), and ALT (SGPT) levels. May decrease serum sodium levels. May cause positive ANA titer.

SIDE EFFECTS

Frequent (12%–5%)
Headache, dizziness, postural hypotension
Occasional (4%–2%)
Chest discomfort, fatigue, rash, abdominal pain, nausea, diarrhea, upper respiratory infection
Rare (1% or less)
Palpitations, tachycardia, peripheral edema, insomnia, paresthesia, confusion, constipation, dry mouth, muscle cramps

SERIOUS REACTIONS

! Excessive hypotension (''first-dose syncope'') may occur in patients with CHF and severe salt and volume depletion.
! Angioedema (swelling of face and lips) and hyperkalemia occur rarely.
! Agranulocytosis and neutropenia may be noted in patients with collagen vascular disease, including scleroderma and systemic lupus erythematosus, and impaired renal function.
! Nephrotic syndrome may be noted in patients with history of renal disease.

NURSING CONSIDERATIONS

Baseline Assessment

- Assess the patient's apical pulse and BP immediately before each lisinopril dose, and regularly throughout therapy. Be alert to fluctuations in apical pulse and BP. If an excessive reduction in BP occurs, place the patient in the supine position with legs elevated and notify the physician.
- Check the results of a CBC and blood chemistry before beginning lisinopril therapy, then every 2 weeks for the next 3 months, and periodically thereafter in patients with autoimmune disease, renal impairment, or who are taking drugs that affect immune response or leukocyte count.

Lifespan Considerations

- Be aware that lisinopril crosses the placenta and that it is unknown if lisinopril is distributed in breast milk. Lisinopril has caused fetal or neonatal morbidity or mortality.
- The safety and efficacy of lisinopril have not been established in children.
- The elderly may be more sensitive to the hypotensive effects of lisinopril.

Precautions

- Use cautiously in patients with cerebrovascular or coronary insufficiency, hypovolemia, renal impairment, severe CHF, and sodium depletion.
- Use cautiously in patients on dialysis or diuretic therapy.

Administration and Handling

◀ALERT▶ Expect to discontinue diuretics, as prescribed, 2 to 3 days before beginning lisinopril therapy.
PO
- Give lisinopril without regard to food.
- Crush tablets if necessary.

Intervention and Evaluation

- Examine the patient for edema.
- Auscultate the patient's lungs for rales.
- Monitor the patient's intake and output and daily weights.
- Assess the patient's pattern of daily bowel activity and stool consistency.
- Assist the patient with ambulation if he or she experiences dizziness.
- Monitor the patient's BP, BUN, serum creatinine, and potassium levels, renal function tests, and WBC count.

Patient Teaching

- Advise the patient to rise slowly from lying to sitting position and to permit legs to dangle from the bed momentarily before standing to reduce the hypotensive effect of lisinopril.

- Urge the patient to limit consumption of alcohol while taking lisinopril.
- Warn the patient to notify the physician if he or she experiences diarrhea, difficulty breathing, excessive perspiration, swelling of the face, lips, or tongue, or vomiting.

moexipril hydrochloride

moe-**ex**-a-prile
(Univasc)

CATEGORY AND SCHEDULE

Pregnancy Risk Category: C (D if used in second or third trimesters)

MECHANISM OF ACTION

An ACE inhibitor that suppresses the renin-angiotensin-aldosterone system and prevents conversion of angiotensin I to angiotensin II, a potent vasoconstrictor; may also inhibit angiotensin II at local vascular and renal sites. **Therapeutic Effect:** Reduces peripheral arterial resistance and lowers BP.

PHARMACOKINETICS

Route	Onset	Peak	Duration
PO	1 hr	3–6 hr	24 hr

Incompletely absorbed from the GI tract. Food decreases drug absorption. Rapidly converted to active metabolite. Protein binding: 50%. Primarily recovered in feces, partially excreted in urine. Unknown if removed by dialysis. ***Half-life:*** 1 hr, metabolite 2–9 hr.

AVAILABILITY

Tablets: 7.5 mg, 15 mg.

INDICATIONS AND DOSAGES

▸ **Hypertension**

PO

Adults, Elderly. For patients not receiving diuretics, initial dose is 7.5 mg once a day 1 hr before meals. Adjust according to BP effect. Maintenance: 7.5–30 mg a day in 1–2 divided doses 1 hr before meals.

▸ **Hypertension in patients with impaired renal function**

PO

Adults, Elderly. 3.75 mg once a day in patients with creatinine clearance of 40 ml/min. Maximum: May titrate up to 15 mg/day.

CONTRAINDICATIONS

History of angioedema from previous treatment with ACE inhibitors

INTERACTIONS

Drug

Alcohol, antihypertensives, diuretics: May increase the effects of moexipril.
Lithium: May increase lithium blood concentration and risk of lithium toxicity.
NSAIDs: May decrease the effects of moexipril.
Potassium-sparing diuretics, potassium supplements: May cause hyperkalemia.

Herbal

None known.

Food

None known.

DIAGNOSTIC TEST EFFECTS

May increase BUN, serum alkaline phosphatase, serum bilirubin, serum creatinine, serum potassium, AST (SGOT), and ALT (SGPT) levels. May decrease serum sodium levels.

May cause positive serum antinuclear antibody titer.

SIDE EFFECTS

Occasional

Cough, headache (6%); dizziness (4%); fatigue (3%)

Rare

Flushing, rash, myalgia, nausea, vomiting

SERIOUS REACTIONS

! Excessive hypotension ("first-dose syncope") may occur in patients with CHF and in those who are severely salt or volume depleted.

! Angioedema (swelling of face and lips) and hyperkalemia occur rarely.

! Agranulocytosis and neutropenia may be noted in those with collagen vascular disease, including scleroderma and systemic lupus erythematosus, and impaired renal function.

! Nephrotic syndrome may be noted in those with history of renal disease.

NURSING CONSIDERATIONS

Baseline Assessment

• Assess the patient's apical pulse and BP immediately before each moexipril dose, and regularly monitoring throughout therapy. Be alert for fluctuations in apical pulse and BP. If an excessive reduction in BP occurs, place the patient in the supine position with legs elevated and notify the physician.

• Expect the patient to have renal function tests done before beginning moexipril therapy.

• As ordered, obtain a CBC and blood chemistry, before beginning moexipril therapy, then every 2 weeks for the next 3 months, and periodically thereafter in patients with autoimmune disease or renal impairment, and in those who are taking drugs that affect immune response or leukocyte count.

Lifespan Considerations

• Moexipril crosses the placenta and it is unknown if it is distributed in breast milk. Moexipril has caused fetal or neonatal morbidity or mortality.

• The safety and efficacy of moexipril have not been established in children.

• In the elderly, age-related renal impairment may require cautious use of moexipril.

Precautions

• Use moexipril cautiously in patients with angina, aortic stenosis, cerebrovascular disease, cerebrovascular or coronary insufficiency, hypovolemia, ischemic heart disease, renal impairment, severe CHF, and sodium depletion.

• Use cautiously in patients on dialysis and in those receiving diuretics.

Administration and Handling

◀ **ALERT** ▶ To reduce the risk of hypotension in patients receiving concurrent diuretic therapy, expect to discontinue the diuretic 2 to 3 days before beginning moexipril therapy. However, if the BP is not controlled, resume diuretic therapy. If diuretics can't be discontinued, administer an initial moexipril dose of 3.75 mg.

PO

• Give moexipril 1 hour before meals.

• Crush tablets if necessary.

Intervention and Evaluation

• Monitor the patient's BP, BUN, serum creatinine, serum potassium levels, and WBC count.

• Assess the patient for hypotension for 1 to 3 hours after the first moexipril dose or after an increase in dose.

• Assess the patient for an irregular heart rate.

• Assist the patient with ambulation if he or she experiences dizziness.

Patient Teaching

• Caution the patient against abruptly discontinuing the drug.
• Warn the patient to notify the physician if he or she experiences chest pain, cough, difficulty breathing, fever, sore throat, or swelling of the eyes, face, feet, hands, lips, or tongue.
• Advise the patient that he or she should stand up slowly from a sitting or lying position to avoid the hypotensive effect of moexipril.
• Tell the patient that he or she may experience arrhythmias during moexipril therapy.

perindopril erbumine

per-**in**-doh-pril
(Aceon)

CATEGORY AND SCHEDULE

Pregnancy Risk Category: C (D if used in second or third trimester)

MECHANISM OF ACTION

An ACE inhibitor that suppresses the renin-angiotensin-aldosterone system and prevents conversion of angiotensin I to angiotensin II, a potent vasoconstrictor; may also inhibit angiotensin II at local vascular and renal sites. **Therapeutic Effect:** Reduces peripheral arterial resistance and BP.

AVAILABILITY

Tablets: 2 mg, 4 mg, 8 mg.

INDICATIONS AND DOSAGES

▸ Hypertension

PO

Adults, Elderly. 2–8 mg/day as single dose or in 2 divided doses. Maximum: 16 mg/day.

OFF-LABEL USES

Management of heart failure

CONTRAINDICATIONS

History of angioedema from previous treatment with ACE inhibitors

INTERACTIONS

Drug

Alcohol, antihypertensives, diuretics: May increase the effects of perindopril.
Lithium: May increase lithium blood concentration and risk of lithium toxicity.
NSAIDs: May decrease the effects of perindopril.
Potassium-sparing diuretics, potassium supplements: May cause hyperkalemia.

Herbal

None known.

Food

None known.

DIAGNOSTIC TEST EFFECTS

May increase BUN, serum alkaline phosphatase, serum bilirubin, serum creatinine, serum potassium, AST (SGOT), and ALT (SGPT) levels. May decrease serum sodium levels. May cause positive antinuclear antibody titer.

SIDE EFFECTS

Occasional (5%–1%)

Cough, back pain, sinusitis, upper extremity pain, dyspepsia, fever, palpitations, hypotension, dizziness, fatigue, syncope

SERIOUS REACTIONS

! Excessive hypotension ("first-dose syncope") may occur in patients with CHF and in those who are severely salt or volume depleted.

! Angioedema (swelling of face and lips) and hyperkalemia occur rarely.
! Agranulocytosis and neutropenia may be noted in those with collagen vascular disease, including scleroderma and systemic lupus erythematosus, and impaired renal function.
! Nephrotic syndrome may be noted in those with history of renal disease.

NURSING CONSIDERATIONS

Baseline Assessment

- Assess the patient's apical pulse and BP immediately before each perindopril dose, and regularly monitoring throughout therapy. Be alert for fluctuations in apical pulse and BP. If an excessive reduction in BP occurs, place the patient in the supine position with legs elevated and notify the physician.
- As ordered, obtain a CBC and blood chemistry before beginning perindopril therapy, then every 2 weeks for the next 3 months, and periodically thereafter in patients with autoimmune disease or renal impairment and in those who are taking drugs that affect immune response or leukocyte count.
- Expect to obtain baseline liver and renal function studies.

Lifespan Considerations

- Perindopril crosses the placenta and it is unknown if it is distributed in breast milk. Perindopril has caused fetal or neonatal morbidity or mortality.
- The safety and efficacy of perindopril have not been established in children.
- In the elderly, age-related renal impairment may require cautious use of perindopril.

Precautions

- Use perindopril cautiously in patients with cerebrovascular insufficiency, coronary insufficiency, hypovolemia, renal impairment, and sodium depletion.
- Use cautiously in patients on dialysis and in those receiving diuretics.

Intervention and Evaluation

- Assist the patient with ambulation if he or she experiences dizziness.
- Monitor the patient's BUN, serum creatinine, serum potassium, AST (SGOT) and ALT (SGPT) levels.
- Assess the patient's pattern of daily bowel activity and stool consistency.

Patient Teaching

- Instruct the patient to rise slowly from a lying to a sitting position and permit legs to dangle from bed momentarily before standing to avoid the hypotensive effect of perindopril.
- Caution the patient that skipping doses or voluntarily discontinuing the drug may produce severe, rebound hypertension.

quinapril

kwin-na-pril
(Accupril, Asig[AUS])
Do not confuse Accupril with Accolate or Accutane.

CATEGORY AND SCHEDULE

Pregnancy Risk Category: C (D if used in second or third trimester)

MECHANISM OF ACTION

An ACE inhibitor that suppresses the renin-angiotensin-aldosterone system and prevents the conversion of angiotensin I to angiotensin II, a potent vasoconstrictor; may also inhibit angiotensin II at local vascular and renal sites. **Therapeutic Effect:** Reduces peripheral arterial resistance, BP, and pulmonary capillary wedge pressure; improves cardiac output.

PHARMACOKINETICS

Route	Onset	Peak	Duration
PO	1 hr	N/A	24 hr

Readily absorbed from the GI tract. Protein binding: 97%. Metabolized in the liver, GI tract, and extravascular tissue to active metabolite. Primarily excreted in urine. Minimal removal by hemodialysis. ***Half-life:*** 1–2 hr; metabolite, 3 hr (increased in those with impaired renal function).

AVAILABILITY

Tablets: 5 mg, 10 mg, 20 mg, 40 mg.

INDICATIONS AND DOSAGES

▸ Hypertension (monotherapy)

PO

Adults. Initially, 10–20 mg/day. May adjust dosage at intervals of at least 2 wk or longer. Maintenance: 20–80 mg/day as single dose or 2 divided doses. Maximum: 80 mg/day.

Elderly. Initially, 2.5–5 mg/day. May increase by 2.5–5 mg q1–2wk.

▸ Hypertension (combination therapy)

PO

Adults. Initially, 5 mg/day titrated to patient's needs.

Elderly. Initially, 2.5–5 mg/day. May increase by 2.5–5 mg q1–2wk.

▸ Adjunct to manage heart failure

PO

Adults, Elderly. Initially, 5 mg twice a day. Range: 20–40 mg/day.

▸ Dosage in renal impairment

Dosage is titrated to the patient's needs after the following initial doses:

Creatinine Clearance	Initial Dose
more than 60 ml/min	10 mg
30–60 ml/min	5 mg
10–29 ml/min	2.5 mg

OFF-LABEL USES

Treatment of hypertension and renal crisis in scleroderma

CONTRAINDICATIONS

Bilateral renal artery stenosis

INTERACTIONS

Drug

Alcohol, antihypertensives, diuretics: May increase the effects of quinapril.

Lithium: May increase lithium blood concentration and risk of lithium toxicity.

NSAIDs: May decrease the effects of quinapril.

Potassium-sparing diuretics, potassium supplements: May cause hyperkalemia.

Herbal

Garlic: May increase antihypertensive effect.

Ginseng, yohimbe: May worsen hypertension.

Food

None known.

DIAGNOSTIC TEST EFFECTS

May increase BUN, serum alkaline phosphatase, serum bilirubin, serum creatinine, serum potassium, AST (SGOT), and ALT (SGPT) levels. May decrease serum sodium levels. May cause positive antinuclear antibody titer.

SIDE EFFECTS

Frequent (7%–5%)

Headache, dizziness

Occasional (4%–2%)

Fatigue, vomiting, nausea, hypotension, chest pain, cough, syncope

Rare (less than 2%)
Diarrhea, cough, dyspnea, rash, palpitations, impotence, insomnia, drowsiness, malaise

SERIOUS REACTIONS

! Excessive hypotension ("first-dose syncope") may occur in patients with CHF and in those who are severely salt or volume depleted.
! Angioedema and hyperkalemia occur rarely.
! Agranulocytosis and neutropenia may be noted in those with collagen vascular disease, including scleroderma and systemic lupus erythematosus, and impaired renal function.
! Nephrotic syndrome may be noted in those with history of renal disease.

NURSING CONSIDERATIONS

Baseline Assessment

- Assess the patient's BP immediately before each quinapril dose and regularly during therapy. Be alert to fluctuations in BP. If an excessive reduction in BP occurs, place the patient in the supine position with legs slightly elevated and notify the physician.
- Monitor the results of the patient's renal function tests before beginning quinapril therapy.
- For patient's with a history of renal disease, test the first urine of the day for protein by dipstick method before beginning quinapril therapy and periodically thereafter.
- As ordered, obtain a CBC and blood chemistry before beginning quinapril therapy, then every 2 weeks for 3 months, and periodically thereafter in patients with autoimmune disease or renal impairment and in those who are taking drugs that affect immune response or leukocyte count.

Lifespan Considerations

- Quinapril crosses the placenta and it is unknown if it is distributed in breast milk. Quinapril may cause fetal or neonatal morbidity or mortality.
- The safety and efficacy of quinapril have not been established in children.
- The elderly may be more sensitive to the hypotensive effect of quinapril.

Precautions

- Use quinapril cautiously in patients with CHF, collagen vascular disease, hyperkalemia, hypovolemia, renal impairment, and renal stenosis.

Administration and Handling

◀ALERT▶ Expect to discontinue diuretics 2 to 3 days before beginning quinapril therapy.

PO
- Give quinapril without regard to food.
- Crush tablets as desired.

Intervention and Evaluation

- Monitor the patient's BUN, serum creatinine and serum potassium levels, and WBC count.
- Assist the patient with ambulation if he or she experiences dizziness.
- Evaluate the patient for headache.
- Give the patient dry toast, noncola carbonated beverages, or unsalted crackers to help relieve nausea.

Patient Teaching

- To reduce the risk of orthostatic hypotension, advise the patient to rise slowly from a lying to a sitting position and to permit legs to dangle from the bed momentarily before standing.
- Explain to the patient that the full therapeutic effect of quinapril may take 1 to 2 weeks to appear.
- Warn the patient to notify the physician if he or she experiences signs or symptoms of infection, including fever and sore throat.

• Caution the patient that discontinuing the drug or skipping doses of quinapril may produce severe, rebound hypertension.
• Urge the patient to avoid tasks that require mental alertness or motor skills until his or her response to the drug has been established.

ramipril

ram-i-pril
(Altace, Ramace[AUS], Tritace[AUS])
Do not confuse Altace with Alteplase or Artane.

CATEGORY AND SCHEDULE

Pregnancy Risk Category: C (D if used in second or third trimester)

MECHANISM OF ACTION

An ACE inhibitor that suppresses the renin-angiotensin-aldosterone system. Decreases plasma angiotensin II, increases plasma renin activity, and decreases aldosterone secretion. **Therapeutic Effect:** Reduces peripheral arterial resistance and BP.

PHARMACOKINETICS

Route	Onset	Peak	Duration
PO	1–2 hr	3–6 hr	24 hr

Well absorbed from the GI tract. Protein binding: 73%. Metabolized in the liver to active metabolite. Primarily excreted in urine. Not removed by hemodialysis. ***Half-life:*** 5.1 hr.

AVAILABILITY

Capsules: 1.25 mg, 2.5 mg, 5 mg, 10 mg.

INDICATIONS AND DOSAGES

▸ **Hypertension (monotherapy)**
PO
Adults, Elderly. Initially, 2.5 mg/day. Maintenance: 2.5–20 mg/day as single dose or in 2 divided doses.
▸ **Hypertension (in combination with other antihypertensives)**
PO
Adults, Elderly. Initially, 1.25 mg/day titrated to patient's needs.
▸ **CHF**
PO
Adults, Elderly. Initially, 1.25–2.5 mg twice a day. Maximum: 5 mg twice a day.
▸ **Risk reduction for myocardial infarction stroke**
PO
Adults, Elderly. Initially, 2.5 mg/day for 7 days, then 5 mg/day for 21 days, then 10 mg/day as a single dose or in divided doses.
▸ **Dosage in renal impairment**
Creatinine clearance equal to or less than 40 ml/min. 25% of normal dose.
Hypertension. Initially, 1.25 mg/day titrated upward.
CHF. Initially, 1.25 mg/day, titrated up to 2.5 mg twice a day.

OFF-LABEL USES

Treatment of hypertension and renal crisis in scleroderma

CONTRAINDICATIONS

Bilateral renal artery stenosis

INTERACTIONS

Drug

Alcohol, antihypertensives, diuretics: May increase the effects of ramipril.
Lithium: May increase lithium blood concentration and risk of lithium toxicity.
NSAIDs: May decrease the effects of ramipril.

Potassium-sparing diuretics, potassium supplements: May cause hyperkalemia.

Herbal

Garlic: May increase antihypertensive effect.

Ginseng, yohimbe: May worsen hypertension.

Food

None known.

DIAGNOSTIC TEST EFFECTS

May increase BUN, serum alkaline phosphatase, serum bilirubin, serum creatinine, serum potassium, AST (SGOT), and ALT (SGPT) levels. May decrease serum sodium levels. May cause positive antinuclear antibody titer.

SIDE EFFECTS

Frequent (12%–5%)

Cough, headache

Occasional (4%–2%)

Dizziness, fatigue, nausea, asthenia (loss of strength)

Rare (less than 2%)

Palpitations, insomnia, nervousness, malaise, abdominal pain, myalgia

SERIOUS REACTIONS

! Excessive hypotension ("first-dose syncope") may occur in patients with CHF and in those who are severely salt or volume depleted.

! Angioedema and hyperkalemia occur rarely.

! Agranulocytosis and neutropenia may be noted in those with collagen vascular disease, including scleroderma and systemic lupus erythematosus, and impaired renal function.

! Nephrotic syndrome may be noted in those with history of renal disease.

NURSING CONSIDERATIONS

Baseline Assessment

- Assess the patient's BP immediately before each ramipril dose and regularly throughout therapy. Be alert to fluctuations in BP. If an excessive reduction in BP occurs, place the patient in the supine position with legs elevated and notify the physician.
- Check the patient's renal function test results and BUN and serum creatinine levels, if ordered, before beginning ramipril therapy.
- For patients with a history of renal disease, test the patient's urine for protein by dipstick method before beginning ramipril therapy and periodically thereafter.
- As ordered, obtain a CBC and blood chemistry before beginning ramipril therapy, then every 2 weeks for 3 months, and periodically thereafter in patients with autoimmune disease or renal impairment and in those who are taking drugs that affect immune response or leukocyte count.

Lifespan Considerations

- Ramipril crosses the placenta, is distributed in breast milk, and may cause fetal or neonatal morbidity or mortality.
- The safety and efficacy of ramipril have not been established in children.
- The elderly may be more sensitive to the hypotensive effect of ramipril.

Precautions

- Use cautiously in patients with CHF, collagen vascular disease, hyperkalemia, hypovolemia, renal impairment, and renal stenosis.

Administration and Handling

◀ALERT▶ Expect to discontinue diuretics 2 to 3 days before beginning ramipril therapy.

PO

- Give ramipril without regard to food.
- Have the patient swallow the

capsules whole and not chew or break them.
- Mix with apple juice, applesauce, or water as needed.

Intervention and Evaluation
- Monitor the patient's BUN, serum creatinine, and serum potassium levels, and WBC count.
- Assess the patient for cough, which frequently occurs.
- Assist the patient with ambulation if he or she experiences dizziness.
- Assess the patient with CHF for crackles and wheezing.
- Monitor the patient's urinalysis for proteinuria.
- Monitor serum potassium levels in patients who are also receiving diuretics.

Patient Teaching
- Caution the patient against discontinuing the drug without physician approval.
- Warn the patient to notify the physician if he or she experiences chest pain, cough, or palpitations.
- Advise the patient that dizziness or light-headedness may occur in the first few days after initiation of ramipril therapy.
- Urge the patient to avoid tasks that require mental alertness or motor skills until his or her response to the drug has been established.

trandolapril

tran-**doe**-la-pril
(Gopten[AUS], Mavik, Odrik[AUS])
Do not confuse trandolapril with tramadol.

CATEGORY AND SCHEDULE
Pregnancy Risk Category: C (D if used in second or third trimester)

MECHANISM OF ACTION
An ACE inhibitor that suppresses the renin-angiotensin-aldosterone system and prevents the conversion of angiotensin I to angiotensin II, a potent vasoconstrictor; may also inhibit angiotensin II at local vascular and renal sites. Decreases plasma angiotensin II, increases plasma renin activity, and decreases aldosterone secretion. **Therapeutic Effect:** Reduces peripheral arterial resistance and pulmonary capillary wedge pressure; improves cardiac output and exercise tolerance.

PHARMACOKINETICS
Slowly absorbed from the GI tract. Protein binding: 80%. Metabolized in the liver and GI mucosa to active metabolite. Primarily excreted in urine. Removed by hemodialysis. ***Half-life:*** 24 hr.

AVAILABILITY
Tablets: 1 mg, 2 mg, 4 mg.

INDICATIONS AND DOSAGES
▸ **Hypertension (without diuretic)**
PO
Adults, Elderly. Initially, 1 mg once a day in nonblack patients, 2 mg once a day in black patients. Adjust dosage at least at 7-day intervals. Maintenance: 2–4 mg/day. Maximum: 8 mg/day.
▸ **CHF**
PO
Adults, Elderly. Initially, 0.5–1 mg, titrated to target dose of 4 mg/day.

CONTRAINDICATIONS
History of angioedema from previous treatment with ACE inhibitors

INTERACTIONS

Drug

Alcohol, antihypertensives, diuretics: May increase the effects of trandolapril.
Lithium: May increase lithium blood concentration and risk of lithium toxicity.
NSAIDs: May decrease the effects of trandolapril.
Potassium-sparing diuretics, potassium supplements: May cause hyperkalemia.

Herbal

None known.

Food

None known.

DIAGNOSTIC TEST EFFECTS

May increase BUN, serum alkaline phosphatase, serum bilirubin, serum creatinine, serum potassium, AST (SGOT), and ALT (SGPT) levels. May decrease serum sodium levels. May cause positive antinuclear antibody titer.

SIDE EFFECTS

Frequent (35%–23%)
Dizziness, cough
Occasional (11%–3%)
Hypotension, dyspepsia (heartburn, epigastric pain, indigestion), syncope, asthenia (loss of strength), tinnitus
Rare (less than 1%)
Palpitations, insomnia, drowsiness, nausea, vomiting, constipation, flushed skin

SERIOUS REACTIONS

! Excessive hypotension ("first-dose syncope") may occur in patients with CHF and in those who are severely salt or volume depleted.
! Angioedema and hyperkalemia occur rarely.
! Agranulocytosis and neutropenia may be noted in those with collagen vascular disease, including scleroderma and systemic lupus erythematosus, and impaired renal function.
! Nephrotic syndrome may be noted in those with history of renal disease.

NURSING CONSIDERATIONS

Baseline Assessment

- Assess the patient's BP immediately before each trandolapril dose, and regularly monitor throughout therapy. Be alert to fluctuations in BP. If an excessive reduction in BP occurs, place the patient in the supine position with legs elevated and notify the physician.
- Check the patient's renal function test results and BUN and serum creatinine levels, if ordered, before beginning trandolapril therapy.
- As ordered, obtain a CBC and blood chemistry before beginning trandolapril therapy, then every 2 weeks for the next 3 months, and periodically thereafter in patients with autoimmune disease or renal impairment and in those who are taking drugs that affect immune response or leukocyte count.

Lifespan Considerations

- Trandolapril crosses the placenta, is distributed in breast milk, and may cause fetal or neonatal morbidity or mortality.
- The safety and efficacy of trandolapril have not been established in children.
- No age-related precautions have been noted in the elderly.

Precautions

- Use cautiously in patients with CHF, hyperkalemia, renal impairment, and valvular stenosis.

Administration and Handling

PO
- Give trandolapril without regard to meals.
- Crush tablets as necessary.

Intervention and Evaluation

- Assist the patient with ambulation if he or she experiences dizziness.
- Evaluate the patient's intake and output and urinary frequency.
- Assess the patient with CHF for crackles and wheezing.
- Monitor the patient's urinalysis for proteinuria.
- Monitor serum potassium levels in patients who are also receiving diuretics.
- Assess the patient's pattern of daily bowel activity and stool consistency.

Patient Teaching

- Caution the patient against abruptly discontinuing the drug.
- Warn the patient to notify the physician if he or she experiences chest pain, cough, diarrhea, difficulty swallowing, fever, palpitations, sore throat, swelling of the face, or vomiting.
- Advise the patient to rise slowly from a lying to a sitting position and to permit legs to dangle from the bed momentarily before standing to reduce the hypotensive effect of trandolapril.
- Stress to the patient that he or she should avoid potassium supplements and salt substitutes during trandolapril therapy.
- Warn the patient to avoid performing tasks that require mental alertness or motor skills until his or her response to the drug has been established.

22 Angiotensin II Receptor Antagonists

candesartan cilexetil
eprosartan
irbesartan
losartan
olmesartan medoxomil
telmisartan
valsartan

Uses: Angiotensin II receptor antagonists (AIIRAs) are used to treat hypertension alone or in combination with other antihypertensives.

Action: AIIRAs block the vasoconstricting and aldosterone-secreting effects of angiotensin II, a potent vasoconstrictor. By selectively blocking the binding of angiotensin II to AT_1 receptors in vascular smooth muscle and the adrenal gland, AIIRAs cause vasodilation, decrease aldosterone effects, and reduce blood pressure.

COMBINATION PRODUCTS

ATACAND HCT: candesartan/hydrochlorothiazide (a diuretic) 16 mg/12.5 mg; 32 mg/12.5 mg.
AVALIDE: irbesartan/hydrochlorothiazide (a diuretic) 150 mg/12.5 mg; 300 mg/12.5 mg.
BENICAR HCT: olmesartan/hydrochlorothiazide (a diuretic) 20 mg/12.5 mg; 40 mg/12.5 mg; 40 mg/25 mg.
DIOVAN HCT: valsartan/hydrochlorothiazide (a diuretic) 80 mg/12.5 mg; 160 mg/12.5 mg; 160 mg/25 mg.
HYZAAR: losartan/hydrochlorothiazide (a diuretic) 50 mg/12.5 mg; 100 mg/25 mg.
MICARDIS HCT: telmisartan/hydrochlorothiazide (a diuretic) 40 mg/12.5 mg; 80 mg/12.5 mg.
TEVETEN HCT: eprosartan/hydrochlorothiazide (a diuretic) 600 mg/12.5 mg; 600 mg/25 mg.

candesartan cilexetil

kan-de-**sar**-tan
(Atacand)

CATEGORY AND SCHEDULE

Pregnancy Risk Category: C (D if used in second or third trimester)

MECHANISM OF ACTION

An angiotensin II receptor, type AT_1, antagonist that blocks the vasoconstrictor and aldosterone-secreting effects of angiotensin II, inhibiting the binding of angiotensin II to the AT_1 receptors. **Therapeutic Effect:** Causes vasodilation, decreases peripheral resistance, and decreases BP.

PHARMACOKINETICS

Route	Onset	Peak	Duration
PO	2–3 hr	6–8 hr	Greater than 24 hr

Rapidly, completely absorbed. Protein binding: greater than 99%. Undergoes minor hepatic metabolism to inactive metabolite. Excreted unchanged in urine and in the feces through the biliary system. Not removed by hemodialysis. ***Half-life:*** 9 hr.

AVAILABILITY

Tablets: 4 mg, 8 mg, 16 mg, 32 mg.

INDICATIONS AND DOSAGES

▸ **Hypertension alone or in combination with other antihypertensives**

PO

Adults, Elderly, Patient with mildly impaired liver or renal function. Initially, 16 mg once a day in those who are not volume depleted. Can be given once or twice a day with total daily doses of 8–32 mg. Give lower dosage in those treated with diuretics or with severely impaired renal function.

OFF-LABEL USES

Treatment of heart failure

CONTRAINDICATIONS

Hypersensitivity to candesartan

INTERACTIONS

Drug

None known.

Herbal

None known.

Food

None known.

DIAGNOSTIC TEST EFFECTS

May increase BUN, serum alkaline phosphatase, serum bilirubin, serum creatinine, AST (SGOT), and ALT (SGPT) levels. May decrease blood Hgb and Hct levels.

SIDE EFFECTS

Occasional (6%–3%)

Upper respiratory tract infection, dizziness, back and leg pain

Rare (2%–1%)

Pharyngitis, rhinitis, headache, fatigue, diarrhea, nausea, dry cough, peripheral edema

SERIOUS REACTIONS

! Overdosage may manifest as hypotension and tachycardia. Bradycardia occurs less often. Institute supportive measures.

NURSING CONSIDERATIONS

Baseline Assessment

- Assess the patient's apical pulse and BP immediately before each candesartan dose, and regularly throughout therapy. Be alert to fluctuations in apical pulse and BP. If an excessive reduction in BP occurs, place the patient in the supine position with feet slightly elevated and notify the physician.
- Determine if the patient is pregnant.
- Determine if the patient has a history of liver or renal impairment or renal artery stenosis.
- Assess the patient's medication history, especially for diuretics.
- Expect to obtain the patient's blood Hgb and Hct and BUN, serum alkaline phosphatase, serum bilirubin, serum creatinine, AST (SGOT), and ALT (SGPT) levels.

Lifespan Considerations

- It is unknown if candesartan is distributed in breast milk. Candesartan may cause fetal or neonatal morbidity or mortality.
- The safety and efficacy of candesartan have not been established in children.
- No age-related precautions have been noted in the elderly.

Precautions

- Use candesartan cautiously in dehydrated patients because they are at risk for developing hypotension.
- Use cautiously in patients with hepatic or renal impairment, renal artery stenosis, or severe CHF.

Administration and Handling

PO

• Give candesartan without regard to food.

Intervention and Evaluation

• Offer the patient fluids frequently to maintain hydration.
• Assess the patient for evidence of an upper respiratory tract infection.
• Assist the patient with ambulation if he or she experiences dizziness.
• Monitor all of the patient's blood levels.
• Assess the patient for hypertension or hypotension.

Patient Teaching

• Advise female patients of the consequences of second- and third-trimester exposure to candesartan. Urge female patients to immediately notify the physician if they become pregnant.
• Warn the patient to avoid tasks that require mental alertness or motor skills until his or her response to the drug has been established.
• Warn the patient to notify the physician if he or she experiences signs and symptoms of infection, including fever and sore throat.
• Explain to the patient that candesartan must be taken for the rest of his or her life to control hypertension.
• Encourage the patient not to exercise outside during hot weather to avoid the risks of dehydration and hypotension.

eprosartan

eh-pro-**sar**-tan
(Teveten)

CATEGORY AND SCHEDULE

Pregnancy Risk Category: C (D if used in second or third trimester)

MECHANISM OF ACTION

An angiotensin II receptor antagonist that blocks the vasoconstrictor and aldosterone-secreting effects of angiotensin II, inhibiting the binding of angiotensin II to the AT_1 receptors. **Therapeutic Effect:** Causes vasodilation, decreases peripheral resistance, and decreases BP.

PHARMACOKINETICS

Rapidly absorbed after PO administration. Protein binding: 98%. Undergoes first-pass metabolism in the liver to active metabolites. Excreted in urine and biliary system. Minimally removed by hemodialysis. ***Half-life:*** 5–9 hr.

AVAILABILITY

Tablets: 400 mg, 600 mg.

INDICATIONS AND DOSAGES

▸ Hypertension

PO

Adults, Elderly. Initially, 600 mg/day. Range: 400–800 mg/day.

CONTRAINDICATIONS

Bilateral renal artery stenosis, hyperaldosteronism

INTERACTIONS

Drug

None known.

Herbal

None known.

Food

None known.

DIAGNOSTIC TEST EFFECTS

May increase BUN, serum alkaline phosphatase, serum bilirubin, serum creatinine, AST (SGOT), and ALT (SGPT) levels. May decrease blood Hgb and Hgb levels.

SIDE EFFECTS

Occasional (5%–2%)
Headache, cough, dizziness
Rare (less than 2%)
Muscle pain, fatigue, diarrhea, upper respiratory tract infection, dyspepsia

SERIOUS REACTIONS

! Overdosage may manifest as hypotension and tachycardia. Bradycardia occurs less often.

NURSING CONSIDERATIONS

Baseline Assessment

- Assess the patient's apical pulse and BP immediately before each eprosartan dose, and regularly throughout therapy. Be alert to fluctuations in apical pulse and BP. If an excessive reduction in BP occurs, place the patient in the supine position with feet slighly elevated and notify the physician.
- Determine if the patient is pregnant or has a history of hepatic or renal impairment or renal artery stenosis.
- Assess the patient's medication history, especially for diuretics.

Lifespan Considerations

- Eprosartan has caused fetal or neonatal morbidity or mortality. Also, because of the potential for adverse effects on the infant, patients taking eprosartan should not breast-feed.
- The safety and efficacy of eprosartan have not been established in children.
- No age-related precautions have been noted in the elderly.

Precautions

- Use cautiously in patients with pre-existing renal insufficiency, significant aortic or mitral stenosis, or unilateral renal artery stenosis.

Administration and Handling

PO

- Give eprosartan without regard to food.
- Do not crush or break tablets.

Intervention and Evaluation

- Monitor the patient's BUN, serum electrolytes, and serum creatinine levels. Also, assess the patient's BP, heart rate for tachycardia, and urinalysis results.

Patient Teaching

- Advise female patients of the consequences of second- and third-trimester exposure to eprosartan.
- Warn the patient to avoid tasks that require mental alertness or motor skills until his or her response to the drug has been established.
- Urge the patient to restrict his or her alcohol and sodium consumption while taking eprosartan, to adhere to the provided diet, and to control weight.
- Explain to the patient that eprosartan must be taken for the rest of his or her life to control hypertension.
- Encourage the patient not to exercise outside during hot weather to avoid the risks of dehydration and hypotension.
- Instruct the patient to check his or her BP regularly.

irbesartan

erb-ba-sar-tan

(Avapro, Karvea[AUS])

CATEGORY AND SCHEDULE

Pregnancy Risk Category: C (D if used in second or third trimester)

MECHANISM OF ACTION

An angiotensin II receptor, type AT_1, antagonist that blocks the vasoconstrictor and aldosterone-secreting effects of angiotensin II, inhibiting the binding of angiotensin II to the AT_1 receptors. **Therapeutic Effect:** Causes vasodilation, decreases peripheral resistance, and decreases BP.

PHARMACOKINETICS

Rapidly and completely absorbed after PO administration. Protein binding: 90%. Undergoes hepatic metabolism to inactive metabolite. Recovered primarily in feces and, to a lesser extent, in urine. Not removed by hemodialysis. ***Half-life:*** 11–15 hr.

AVAILABILITY

Tablets: 75 mg, 150 mg, 300 mg.

INDICATIONS AND DOSAGES

▸ **Hypertension alone or in combination with other antihypertensives**

PO

Adults, Elderly, Children 13 yr and older. Initially, 75–150 mg/day. May increase to 300 mg/day.

Children 6–12 yr. Initially, 75 mg/day. May increase to 150 mg/day.

▸ **Nephropathy**

PO

Adults, Elderly. Target dose of 300 mg/day.

OFF-LABEL USES

Treatment of heart failure

CONTRAINDICATIONS

Bilateral renal artery stenosis, biliary cirrhosis or obstruction, primary hyperaldosteronism, severe hepatic insufficiency

INTERACTIONS

Drug

Hydrochlorothiazide: Further reduces BP.

Herbal

None known.

Food

None known.

DIAGNOSTIC TEST EFFECTS

May slightly increase BUN and serum creatinine levels. May decrease blood Hgb level.

SIDE EFFECTS

Occasional (9%–3%)

Upper respiratory tract infection, fatigue, diarrhea, cough

Rare (2%–1%)

Heartburn, dizziness, headache, nausea, rash

SERIOUS REACTIONS

! Overdosage may manifest as hypotension and tachycardia. Bradycardia occurs less often.

NURSING CONSIDERATIONS

Baseline Assessment

• Assess the patient's apical pulse and BP immediately before each irbesartan dose and regularly throughout therapy. Be alert to fluctuations in apical pulse and BP. If an excessive reduction in BP occurs, place the patient in the supine position with feet slightly elevated and notify the physician.

• Determine if the patient is pregnant before beginning therapy.
• Assess the patient's medication history, especially for diuretics.

Lifespan Considerations

• It is unknown if irbesartan is distributed in breast milk. Irbesartan may cause fetal or neonatal morbidity or mortality.
• The safety and efficacy of irbesartan have not been established in children.
• No age-related precautions have been noted in the elderly.

Precautions

• Use irbesartan cautiously in patients with CHF, coronary artery disease, mild to moderate hepatic dysfunction, sodium or water depletion, or unilateral renal artery stenosis.

Administration and Handling

◀ALERT▶ Irbesartan may be given concurrently with other antihypertensives; if BP is not controlled by irbesartan alone, a diuretic may also be prescribed.

PO

• Give irbesartan without regard to meals.

Intervention and Evaluation

• Offer the patient fluids frequently to maintain hydration.
• Assess the patient for signs and symptoms of an upper respiratory tract infection.
• Assist the patient with ambulation if he or she experiences dizziness.
• Monitor the patient's BP and pulse rate. Also check the results of serum electrolyte tests, liver and renal function tests, and urinalysis.
• Assess the patient for signs and symptoms of hypotension.

Patient Teaching

• Advise female patients of the consequences of second- and third-trimester exposure to irbesartan.
• Warn the patient to avoid tasks that require mental alertness or motor skills until his or her response to the drug has been established.
• Caution the patient to report signs and symptoms of infection, including fever and sore throat.
• Encourage the patient to avoid outdoor exercise during hot weather to avoid the risks of dehydration and hypotension.

losartan

lo-**sar**-tan

(Cozaar)

Do not confuse Cozaar with Zocor.

CATEGORY AND SCHEDULE

Pregnancy Risk Category: C (D if used in second or third trimesters)

MECHANISM OF ACTION

An angiotensin II receptor, type AT_1, antagonist that blocks vasoconstrictor and aldosterone-secreting effects of angiotensin II, inhibiting the binding of angiotensin II to the AT_1 receptors. **Therapeutic Effect:** Causes vasodilation, decreases peripheral resistance, and decreases BP.

PHARMACOKINETICS

Route	Onset	Peak	Duration
PO	N/A	6 hr	24 hr

Well absorbed after PO administration. Protein binding: 98%. Undergoes first-pass metabolism in the liver to active metabolites. Excreted in urine and via the biliary system. Not removed by hemodialysis. ***Half-life:*** 2 hr, metabolite: 6–9 hr.

AVAILABILITY
Tablets: 25 mg, 50 mg, 100 mg.

INDICATIONS AND DOSAGES
▸ Hypertension
PO
Adults, Elderly. Initially, 50 mg once a day. Maximum: May be given once or twice a day, with total daily doses ranging from 25–100 mg.
▸ Nephropathy
PO
Adults, Elderly. Initially, 50 mg/day. May increase to 100 mg/day based on BP response.
▸ Stroke reduction
PO
Adults, Elderly. 50 mg/day. Maximum: 100 mg/day.
▸ Hypertension in patients with impaired hepatic function
PO
Adults, Elderly. Initially, 25 mg/day.

CONTRAINDICATIONS
None known.

INTERACTIONS
Drug
Cimetidine: May increase the effects of losartan.
Ketoconazole, troleandomycin: May inhibit the effects of these drugs.
Lithium: May increase lithium blood concentration and risk of lithium toxicity.
Phenobarbital, rifampin: May decrease the effects of losartan.
Herbal
None known.
Food
Grapefruit juice: May alter the absorption of losartan.

DIAGNOSTIC TEST EFFECTS
May increase BUN, serum alkaline phosphatase, serum bilirubin, serum creatinine, AST (SGOT), and ALT (SGPT) levels. May decrease blood Hgb and Hct levels.

SIDE EFFECTS
Frequent (8%)
Upper respiratory tract infection
Occasional (4%–2%)
Dizziness, diarrhea, cough
Rare (1% or less)
Insomnia, dyspepsia, heartburn, back and leg pain, muscle cramps, myalgia, nasal congestion, sinusitis

SERIOUS REACTIONS
! Overdosage may manifest as hypotension and tachycardia. Bradycardia occurs less often.

NURSING CONSIDERATIONS
Baseline Assessment
• Assess the patient's apical pulse and BP immediately before each dose and regularly throughout therapy. Be alert to fluctuations in apical pulse and BP. If an excessive reduction in BP occurs, place the patient in the supine position with feet slightly elevated and notify the physician.
• Determine if the patient is pregnant.
• Assess the patient's medication history, especially for diuretics.
Lifespan Considerations
• Losartan has caused fetal or neonatal morbidity or mortality and may adversely affect the breast-fed infant. Patients should not breast-feed while taking losartan.
• The safety and efficacy of losartan have not been established in children.
• No age-related precautions have been noted in the elderly.
Precautions
• Use cautiously in patients with hepatic or renal impairment or renal arterial stenosis.

Administration and Handling

PO

- Give losartan without regard to food.
- Do not crush or break tablets.

Intervention and Evaluation

- Offer the patient fluids frequently to maintain hydration.
- Assess the patient for evidence of cough and upper respiratory tract infection.
- Assist the patient with ambulation if he or she experiences dizziness.
- Assess the patient's pattern of daily bowel activity and stool consistency.
- Monitor the patient's BP and pulse rate.

Patient Teaching

- Advise female patients of the consequences of second- and third-trimester exposure to losartan.
- Stress to the female patient that she should immediately notify the physician if she becomes pregnant.
- Warn the patient to avoid tasks that require mental alertness or motor skills until his or her response to the drug has been established.
- Caution the patient to notify the physician if he or she experiences chest pain or signs and symptoms of infection, including fever and sore throat.
- Advise the patient to avoid cold preparations or nasal decongestants while on losartan therapy.
- Caution the patient against abruptly discontinuing the drug.

olmesartan medoxomil

ol-**mess**-er-tan
(Benicar)

CATEGORY AND SCHEDULE

Pregnancy Risk Category: C (D if used in second or third trimester)

MECHANISM OF ACTION

An angiotensin II receptor, type AT_1, antagonist that blocks the vasoconstrictor and aldosterone-secreting effects of angiotensin II, inhibiting the binding of angiotensin II to the AT_1 receptors. **Therapeutic Effect:** Causes vasodilation, decreases peripheral resistance, and decreases BP.

PHARMACOKINETICS

Rapidly and completely absorbed after PO administration. Metabolized in the liver. Recovered primarily in feces and, to a lesser extent, in urine. Not removed by hemodialysis. ***Half-life:*** 13 hr.

AVAILABILITY

Tablets: 5 mg, 20 mg, 40 mg.

INDICATIONS AND DOSAGES

▸ **Hypertension**

PO

Adults, Elderly, Patients with mildly impaired hepatic or renal function. 20 mg once a day in patients who are not volume depleted. After 2 weeks of therapy, if further reduction in BP is needed, may increase dosage to 40 mg/day.

CONTRAINDICATIONS

Bilateral renal artery stenosis

INTERACTIONS

Drug

Diuretics: Further reduces BP.

Herbal

None known.

Food

None known.

DIAGNOSTIC TEST EFFECTS

May increase blood Hgb and Hct levels.

SIDE EFFECTS

Occasional (3%)

Dizziness

Rare (less than 2%)

Headache, diarrhea, upper respiratory tract infection

SERIOUS REACTIONS

! Overdosage may manifest as hypotension and tachycardia. Bradycardia occurs less often.

NURSING CONSIDERATIONS

Baseline Assessment

- Assess the patient's apical pulse and BP immediately before each olmesartan dose and regularly throughout therapy. Be alert to fluctuations in apical pulse and BP. If an excessive reduction in BP occurs, place the patient in the supine position with feet slightly elevated and notify the physician.
- Determine if the patient is pregnant.
- Assess the patient's medication history, especially for diuretics.

Lifespan Considerations

- It is unknown if olmesartan is distributed in breast milk. It may cause fetal or neonatal morbidity or mortality.
- The safety and efficacy of olmesartan have not been established in children.
- No age-related precautions have been noted in the elderly.

Precautions

- Use olmesartan cautiously in patients with hepatic or renal impairment or renal arterial stenosis.

Administration and Handling

PO

- Give olmesartan without regard to meals.

Intervention and Evaluation

- Offer the patient fluids frequently to maintain hydration.
- Assess the patient for signs and symptoms of an upper respiratory tract infection.
- Assist the patient with ambulation if he or she experiences dizziness.
- Monitor the results of the patient's diagnostic tests, such as Hgb and HCT levels and liver function test results.
- Assess the patient for hypertension or hypotension.

Patient Teaching

- Advise female patients of the consequences of second- and third-trimester exposure to olmesartan.
- Urge the patient to avoid tasks that require mental alertness or motor skills until his or her response to the drug has been established.
- Warn the patient to notify the physician if he or she experiences signs or symptoms of infection, including fever and sore throat.
- Explain to the patient that olmesartan must be taken for the rest of his or her life to control hypertension.
- Inform the patient of the importance of diet and exercise.
- Caution the patient against exercising outside during hot weather because of the risks of dehydration and hypotension.

telmisartan

tel-meh-**sar**-tan
(Micardis, Pritor[AUS])

CATEGORY AND SCHEDULE

Pregnancy Risk Category: C (D if used in second or third trimester)

MECHANISM OF ACTION

An angiotensin II receptor, type AT_1, antagonist that blocks vasoconstrictor and aldosterone-secreting effects of angiotensin II, inhibiting the binding of angiotensin II to the AT_1 receptors. **Therapeutic Effect:** Causes vasodilation, decreases peripheral resistance, and decreases BP.

PHARMACOKINETICS

Rapidly and completely absorbed after PO administration. Protein binding: greater than 99%. Undergoes metabolism in the liver to inactive metabolite. Excreted in feces. Unknown if removed by hemodialysis. ***Half-life:*** 24 hr.

AVAILABILITY

Tablets: 20 mg, 40 mg, 80 mg.

INDICATIONS AND DOSAGES

▸ Hypertension

PO

Adults, Elderly. 40 mg once a day. Range: 20–80 mg/day.

OFF-LABEL USES

Treatment of CHF

CONTRAINDICATIONS

None known.

INTERACTIONS

Drug

Digoxin: Increases digoxin plasma concentration.

Warfarin: Slightly decreases warfarin plasma concentration.

Herbal

None known.

Food

None known.

DIAGNOSTIC TEST EFFECTS

May increase serum creatinine level. May decrease blood Hgb and Hct levels.

SIDE EFFECTS

Occasional (7%–3%)

Upper respiratory tract infection, sinusitis, back or leg pain, diarrhea

Rare (1%)

Dizziness, headache, fatigue, nausea, heartburn, myalgia, cough, peripheral edema

SERIOUS REACTIONS

! Overdosage may manifest as hypotension and tachycardia. Bradycardia occurs less often.

NURSING CONSIDERATIONS

Baseline Assessment

• Assess the patient's apical pulse and BP immediately before each telmisartan dose and regularly throughout therapy. Be alert to fluctuations in apical pulse and BP. If an excessive reduction in BP occurs, place the patient in the supine position with feet slightly elevated and notify the physician.
• Assess the patient's medication history, especially for diuretics.
• Determine if the patient has a history of hepatic or renal impairment or renal artery stenosis.
• Monitor the patient's blood Hgb, BUN, and serum creatinine levels. Also monitor BP, pulse rate, and other vital signs.

Lifespan Considerations

• It is unknown if telmisartan is

excreted in breast milk; it may cause fetal harm.
- The safety and efficacy of telmisartan have not been established in children.
- No age-related precautions have been noted in the elderly.

Precautions
- Use telmisartan cautiously in patients with hepatic and renal impairment, renal artery stenosis (bilateral or unilateral), and volume depletion.

Administration and Handling

◀ **ALERT** ▶ May be given concurrently with other antihypertensives. If BP is not controlled by telmisartan alone, a diuretic may be added.

PO
- Give telmisartan without regard to meals.

Intervention and Evaluation
- Monitor the patient's BP, pulse rate, and BUN, serum creatinine, and serum electrolyte levels.
- Monitor the patient for signs and symptoms of hypotension during the initial telmisartan doses.

Patient Teaching
- Encourage the patient to drink fluids frequently to maintain proper hydration.
- Advise female patients of the consequences of second- and third-trimester exposure to telmisartan. Emphasize that they should immediately notify the physician if they become pregnant.
- Urge the patient to avoid tasks that require mental alertness or motor skills until his or her response to the drug has been established.
- Caution the patient to notify the physician if he or she experiences signs or symptoms of infection, including fever and sore throat.
- Explain to the patient that telmisartan must be taken for the rest of his or her life to control hypertension.
- Caution the patient against excessive exertion during hot weather because of the risks of dehydration and hypotension.

valsartan

val-**sar**-tan

(Diovan)

Do not confuse valsartan with Valstan.

CATEGORY AND SCHEDULE

Pregnancy Risk Category: C (D if used in second or third trimester)

MECHANISM OF ACTION

An angiotensin II receptor, type AT_1, antagonist that blocks vasoconstrictor and aldosterone-secreting effects of angiotensin II, inhibiting the binding of angiotensin II to the AT_1 receptors. **Therapeutic Effect:** Causes vasodilation, decreases peripheral resistance, and decreases BP.

PHARMACOKINETICS

Poorly absorbed after PO administration. Food decreases peak plasma concentration. Protein binding: 95%. Metabolized in the liver. Recovered primarily in feces and, to a lesser extent, in urine. Unknown if removed by hemodialysis. ***Half-life:*** 6 hr.

AVAILABILITY

Tablets: 40 mg, 80 mg, 160 mg, 320 mg.

INDICATIONS AND DOSAGES

▸ **Hypertension**

PO

Adults, Elderly. Initially, 80–160 mg/day in patients who are not volume depleted. May increase up to a maximum of 320 mg/day.

▸ **CHF**

PO

Adults, Elderly. Initially, 40 mg twice a day. May increase up to 160 mg twice a day. Maximum: 320 mg/day.

CONTRAINDICATIONS

Bilateral renal artery stenosis, biliary cirrhosis or obstruction, hypoaldosteronism, severe hepatic impairment

INTERACTIONS

Drug

Diuretics: Produces additive hypotensive effects.

Herbal

None known.

Food

All food: Decreases peak plasma concentration of valsartan.

DIAGNOSTIC TEST EFFECTS

May increase AST (SGOT), ALT (SGPT), and serum bilirubin, creatinine, and potassium levels. May decrease blood Hgb and Hct levels.

SIDE EFFECTS

Rare (2%–1%)

Insomnia, fatigue, heartburn, abdominal pain, dizziness, headache, diarrhea, nausea, vomiting, arthralgia, edema

SERIOUS REACTIONS

! Overdosage may manifest as hypotension and tachycardia. Bradycardia occurs less often.

! Viral infection and upper respiratory tract infection (cough, pharyngitis, sinusitis, rhinitis) occur rarely.

NURSING CONSIDERATIONS

Baseline Assessment

- Assess the patient's apical pulse and BP immediately before each valsartan dose and regularly throughout therapy. Be alert to fluctuations in apical pulse and BP. If an excessive reduction in BP occurs, place the patient in the supine position with feet slightly elevated and notify the physician.
- Determine if the patient is pregnant.
- Assess the patient's medication history, especially for diuretics.
- Determine if the patient has a history of hepatic or renal impairment, renal artery stenosis, or severe CHF.
- Monitor the results of the patient's blood Hgb and Hct, BUN, serum alkaline phosphatase, serum bilirubin, serum creatinine, AST, and ALT levels.

Lifespan Considerations

- It is unknown if valsartan is distributed in breast milk; it may cause fetal harm.
- The safety and efficacy of valsartan have not been established in children.
- No age-related precautions have been noted in the elderly.

Precautions

- Use valsartan cautiously in patients also receiving potassium-sparing diuretics or potassium supplements.
- Use cautiously in patients with coronary artery disease, mild to moderate hepatic impairment, or unilateral renal artery stenosis. For patients with severe CHF, monitor for signs and symptoms of impaired renal function, which may develop during valsartan therapy.

Administration and Handling

◂**ALERT**▸ Valsartan may be given concurrently with other antihypertensives. If BP is not controlled by valsartan alone, expect to administer a diuretic, as prescribed.

PO
• Give valsartan without regard to meals.

Intervention and Evaluation

• Offer the patient fluids frequently to maintain hydration.
• Assess the patient for signs and symptoms of an upper respiratory tract infection.
• Monitor the patient's BP, serum electrolyte levels, liver and renal function tests, and urinalysis; regularly assess pulse rate. Observe the patient for signs and symptoms of hypotension.

Patient Teaching

• Advise female patients of the consequences of second- and third-trimester exposure to valsartan.
• Stress to the female patient that she should immediately notify the physician if she becomes pregnant.
• Caution the patient to notify the physician if he or she experiences signs or symptoms of infection, including fever and sore throat.
• Explain to the patient that valsartan must be taken for the rest of his or her life to control hypertension.
• Caution the patient against exercising outside during hot weather because of the risks of dehydration and hypotension.

23 Antiarrhythmic Agents

adenosine
amiodarone hydrochloride
atropine sulfate
disopyramide phosphate
dofetilide
flecainide
ibutilide fumarate
lidocaine hydrochloride
mexiletine hydrochloride
moricizine hydrochloride
procainamide hydrochloride
propafenone hydrochloride
quinidine
tocainide hydrochloride

Uses: Antiarrhythmics are used to prevent and treat cardiac arrhythmias, such as premature ventricular contractions, ventricular tachycardia, premature atrial contractions, paroxysmal atrial tachycardia, atrial fibrillation, and atrial flutter.

Action: Antiarrhythmics affect certain ion channels and receptors on the myocardial cell membrane. They're divided into four classes: Class I drugs are further divided into three subclasses (IA, IB, IC) based on the drugs' electrophysiologic effects. *Class I:* Blocks cardiac sodium channels and slows conduction velocity, prolonging refractoriness and decreasing automaticity of sodium-dependent tissue. *Class IA:* Blocks sodium and potassium channels. *Class IB:* Shortens the repolarization phase. *Class IC:* Doesn't affect the repolarization phase, but slows conduction velocity. *Class II:* Slows sinoatrial (SA) and AV nodal conduction. *Class III:* Blocks cardiac potassium channels, prolonging the repolarization phase of electrical cells. *Class IV:* Inhibits the influx of calcium through its channels, causing slower conduction through the SA and AV nodes.

COMBINATION PRODUCTS

DONNATAL: atropine/hyoscyamine (an anticholinergic)/phenobarbital (a sedative)/scopolamine (an anticholinergic) 0.0194 mg/0.1037 mg/16.2 mg/0.0065 mg.
EMLA: lidocaine/prilocaine (an anesthetic) 2.5%/2.5%.
LIDOCAINE WITH EPINEPHRINE: lidocaine/epinephrine (a vasopressor) 2%/1:50,000; 1%/1:100,000; 1%/1:200,000; 0.5%/1:200,000.
LIDOSITE: lidocaine/epinephrine (a vasopressor) 10%/0.1%.
LOMOTIL: atropine/diphenoxylate (an antidiarrheal) 0.025 mg/2.5 mg.

adenosine

ah-**den**-oh-seen
(Adenocard, Adenocor[AUS], Adenoscan)

CATEGORY AND SCHEDULE

Pregnancy Risk Category: C

MECHANISM OF ACTION

A cardiac agent that slows impulse formation in the SA node and conduction time through the AV node.

Adenosine also acts as a diagnostic aid in myocardial perfusion imaging or stress echocardiography.
Therapeutic Effect: Depresses left ventricular function and restores normal sinus rhythm.

AVAILABILITY

Injection (Adenocard): 3 mg/ml in 2 ml, 4 ml syringes.
Injection (Adenoscan): 3 mg/ml in 20 ml, 30 ml vials.

INDICATIONS AND DOSAGES

▸ Paroxysmal supraventricular tachycardia (PSVT)
Rapid IV Bolus
Adults, Elderly. Initially, 6 mg given over 1–2 sec. If first dose does not convert within 1–2 min, give 12 mg; may repeat 12-mg dose in 1–2 min if no response has occurred.
Children. Initially 0.1 mg/kg (maximum: 6 mg). If ineffective, may give 0.2 mg/kg (maximum: 12 mg).

▸ Diagnostic testing
IV Infusion
Adults. 140 mcg/kg/min for 6 min.

CONTRAINDICATIONS

Atrial fibrillation or flutter, second- or third-degree AV block or sick sinus syndrome (with functioning pacemaker), ventricular tachycardia

INTERACTIONS

Drug

Carbamazepine: May increase degree of heart block caused by adenosine.
Dipyridamole: May increase effect of adenosine.
Methylxanthines (e.g., caffeine, theophylline): May decrease effect of adenosine.

Herbal

None known.

Food

None known.

DIAGNOSTIC TEST EFFECTS

None known.

IV INCOMPATIBILITIES

Any drug or solution other than 0.9% NaCl or D_5W.

SIDE EFFECTS

Frequent (18%–12%)
Facial flushing, dyspnea
Occasional (7%–2%)
Headache, nausea, light-headedness, chest pressure
Rare (1% or less)
Numbness or tingling in arms; dizziness; diaphoresis; hypotension; palpitations; chest, jaw, or neck pain

SERIOUS REACTIONS

! May produce short-lasting heart block.

NURSING CONSIDERATIONS

Baseline Assessment

• Identify the arrhythmia on a 12-lead EKG. Also assess the patient's heart rate and rhythm on a continuous cardiac monitor and evaluate the apical pulse rate, rhythm, and quality.

Precautions

• Use adenosine cautiously in patients with arrhythmias at time of conversion, asthma, heart block, or hepatic or renal failure.

Administration and Handling

IV
• Solution may be stored at room temperature and normally appears clear.
• Crystallization occurs if solution is refrigerated. If crystallization occurs, dissolve crystals by warming to room temperature. Discard unused portion.

• Administer undiluted very rapidly, over 1 to 2 seconds, directly into vein, or if using an IV line, use the port closest to the insertion site. If the IV line is infusing fluid other than 0.9% NaCl, flush the line first before administering adenosine.
• Follow the rapid bolus injection with a rapid 0.9% NaCl flush.

Intervention and Evaluation

• Continue to assess the patient's heart rate and rhythm with continuous cardiac monitoring.
• Monitor the patient's apical pulse rate, rhythm, and strength, BP, and the quality of the respirations.
• Monitor the patient's intake and output; assess the patient for fluid retention.
• Check serum electrolyte levels.

Patient Teaching

• Advise the patient to report unusual signs or symptoms, including chest pain, chest pounding or palpitations, or difficulty breathing or shortness of breath.
• Explain that facial flushing, headache, and nausea may occur and that these symptoms will resolve.

amiodarone hydrochloride

a-**mee**-oh-da-rone
(Aratac[AUS], Cordarone, Cordarone X[AUS], Pacerone)
Do not confuse amiodarone with amiloride, or Cordarone with Cardura.

CATEGORY AND SCHEDULE

Pregnancy Risk Category: D

MECHANISM OF ACTION

A cardiac agent that prolongs duration of myocardial cell action potential and refractory period by acting directly on all cardiac tissue. Decreases AV and sinus node function. **Therapeutic Effect:** Suppresses arrhythmias.

PHARMACOKINETICS

Route	Onset	Peak	Duration
PO	3 days–3 wk	1 wk–5 mo	7–50 days after discontinuation

Slowly, variably absorbed from GI tract. Protein binding: 96%. Extensively metabolized in the liver to active metabolite. Excreted via bile; not removed by hemodialysis. ***Half-life:*** 26–107 days; metabolite, 61 days.

AVAILABILITY

Tablets (Cordarone): 200 mg.
Tablets (Pacerone): 100 mg, 200 mg, 400 mg.
Injection (Cordarone): 50 mg/ml.

INDICATIONS AND DOSAGES

▸ **Life-threatening recurrent ventricular fibrillation or hemodynamically unstable ventricular tachycardia**

PO

Adults, Elderly. Initially, 800–1,600 mg/day in 2–4 divided doses for 1–3 wk. After arrhythmia is controlled or side effects occur, reduce to 600–800 mg/day for about 4 wk. Maintenance: 200–600 mg/day.
Children. Initially, 10–15 mg/kg/day for 4–14 days, then 5 mg/kg/day for several wk. Maintenance: 2.5 mg/kg or lowest effective maintenance dose for 5 of 7 days/wk.

IV Infusion

Adults. Initially, 1,050 mg over 24 hr; 150 mg over 10 min, then 360 mg over 6 hr; then 540 mg over 18 hr. May continue at 0.5 mg/min for up to 2–3 wk regardless of age or renal or left ventricular function.

OFF-LABEL USES

Treatment and prevention of supraventricular arrhythmias and symptomatic atrial flutter refractory to conventional treatment

CONTRAINDICATIONS

Bradycardia-induced syncope (except in the presence of a pacemaker), second- and third-degree AV block, severe hepatic disease, severe sinus-node dysfunction

INTERACTIONS

Drug

Antiarrhythmics: May increase cardiac effects.
Beta blockers, oral anticoagulants: May increase effect of beta blockers and oral anticoagulants.
Digoxin, phenytoin: May increase drug concentration and risk of toxicity of digoxin and phenytoin.

Herbal

None known.

Food

None known.

DIAGNOSTIC TEST EFFECTS

May increase antinuclear antibody titers and AST (SGOT), ALT (SGPT), and serum alkaline phosphatase levels. May cause changes in EKG and thyroid function test results. Therapeutic serum level is 0.5–2.5 mcg/ml; toxic serum level has not been established.

IV INCOMPATIBILITIES

Aminophylline (theophylline), cefazolin (Ancef), heparin, sodium bicarbonate

IV COMPATIBILITIES

Dobutamine (Dobutrex), dopamine (Intropin), furosemide (Lasix), insulin (regular), labetalol (Normodyne), lidocaine, midazolam (Versed), morphine, nitroglycerin, norepinephrine (Levophed), phenylephrine (Neo-Synephrine), potassium chloride, vancomycin

SIDE EFFECTS

Expected

Corneal microdeposits are noted in almost all patients treated for more than 6 months (can lead to blurry vision).

Frequent (greater than 3%)

Parenteral: Hypotension, nausea, fever, bradycardia.
Oral: Constipation, headache, decreased appetite, nausea, vomiting, paresthesias, photosensitivity, muscular incoordination.

Occasional (less than 3%)

Oral: Bitter or metallic taste; decreased libido; dizziness; facial flushing; blue-gray coloring of skin (face, arms, and neck); blurred vision; bradycardia; asymptomatic corneal deposits.

Rare (less than 1%)

Oral: Rash, vision loss, blindness.

SERIOUS REACTIONS

! Serious, potentially fatal pulmonary toxicity (alveolitis, pulmonary fibrosis, pneumonitis, acute respiratory distress syndrome) may begin with progressive dyspnea and cough with crackles, decreased breath sounds, pleurisy, CHF or hepatotoxicity.
! Amiodarone may worsen existing arrhythmias or produce new arrhythmias (called proarrhythmias).

NURSING CONSIDERATIONS

Baseline Assessment

• Expect patient to undergo baseline chest x-ray, EKG, and pulmonary function tests. Also, if ordered, check

the results of baseline liver enzyme tests, and AST, ALT, and serum alkaline phosphatase levels.
• Assess the apical pulse and BP immediately before giving amiodarone. Withhold the medication and notify the physician if the pulse rate is 60 beats/minute or lower or the systolic BP is less than 90 mm Hg.

Lifespan Considerations

• Amiodarone crosses the placenta and is distributed in breast milk; it adversely affects fetal development.
• The safety and efficacy of amiodarone have not been established in children.
• The elderly may be more sensitive to amiodarone's effects on thyroid function and may experience increased incidence of ataxia or other neurotoxic effects.

Precautions

• Use amiodarone cautiously in patients with thyroid disease.

Administration and Handling

PO
• Give with meals to reduce GI distress.
• Tablets may be crushed if necessary.

IV

◀**ALERT**▶ Solution concentrations greater than 3 mg/ml can cause peripheral vein phlebitis.
• Store at room temperature.
• Use glass or polyolefin containers for dilution. Dilute the loading dose of 150 mg in 100 ml D_5W to yield a solution of 1.5 mg/ml. Dilute the maintenance dose of 900 mg in 500 ml D_5W to yield a solution of 1.8 mg/ml.
• Use solutions held in PVC containers within 2 hours of dilution. Use solutions held in glass or polyolefin containers within 24 hours of dilution.
• Give amiodarone through a central venous catheter (CVC) if possible, using an in-line filter. The solution does not need protection from light during administration.
• Give a bolus of 150 mg over 10 minutes (15 mg/minute) not to exceed 30 mg/minute; then 360 mg over 6 hours (1 mg/minute); then 540 mg at a rate of 0.5 mg/minute over 18 hours. For infusions lasting longer than 1 hour, drug concentration should not exceed 2 mg/ml, unless a CVC is used.

Intervention and Evaluation

◀**ALERT**▶ Assess the patient for signs and symptoms of pulmonary toxicity, including progressively worsening cough and dyspnea. Expect to discontinue or reduce the dosage of amiodarone if toxicity occurs.
• Monitor the patient's serum alkaline phosphatase, AST, and ALT levels as well as hepatic and thyroid function tests for evidence of toxicity. Expect to reduce the dosage or discontinue the drug if toxicity is evident or hepatic enzyme levels are elevated.
• Monitor the patient's amiodarone blood level. The drug's therapeutic serum level is 0.5 to 2.5 mcg/ml; the drug's toxic serum level has not been established.
• Assess the patient's pulse rate for bradycardia, an irregular rhythm, and quality. Monitor the patient's EKG for changes such as widening of the QRS complex and prolonged PR and QT intervals. Notify the physician of significant interval changes.
• Assess the patient for signs and symptoms of hyperthyroidism, such as difficulty breathing, bulging eyes (exophthalmos), eyelid edema, frequent urination, hot and dry skin, and weight loss. Also assess the patient for signs and symptoms of hypothyroidism, such as cool and pale skin, lethargy, night cramps, periorbital edema, and pudgy hands and feet.

- Assess the patient for nausea and vomiting.
- Check for bluish discoloration of the skin and cornea in patients receiving amiodarone for longer than 2 months.

Patient Teaching

- Urge the patient not to abruptly discontinue the medication. Explain that compliance with the prescribed therapy is essential to control arrhythmias.
- Teach outpatients to monitor their pulse before taking the drug.
- Instruct the patient to report shortness of breath or cough.
- Warn the patient to limit his or her exposure to sunlight to protect against photosensitivity.
- Inform the patient that the bluish skin and cornea discoloration gradually disappear after the drug is discontinued.
- Recommend the patient seek ophthalmic exams every 6 months. Advise the patient to report any vision changes to the physician.

atropine sulfate

a-troe-peen

(Atropine Sulfate, Atropt[AUS])

Do not confuse atropine with Akarpine or Aplisol.

CATEGORY AND SCHEDULE

Pregnancy Risk Category: C

MECHANISM OF ACTION

An acetylcholine antagonist that inhibits the action of acetylcholine by competing with acetylcholine for common binding sites on muscarinic receptors, which are located on exocrine glands, cardiac and smooth-muscle ganglia, and intramural neurons. This action blocks all muscarinic effects. **Therapeutic Effect:** Decreases GI motility and secretory activity, and GU muscle tone (ureter, bladder); produces ophthalmic cycloplegia, and mydriasis.

AVAILABILITY

Injection: 0.05 mg/ml, 0.1 mg/ml, 0.4 mg/0.5 ml, 0.4 mg/ml, 0.5 mg/ml, 1 mg/ml.

INDICATIONS AND DOSAGES

▸ Asystole, slow pulseless electrical activity

IV

Adults, Elderly. 1 mg; may repeat q3–5min up to total dose of 0.04 mg/kg.

▸ Pre-anesthetic

IV/IM/Subcutaneous

Adults, Elderly. 0.4–0.6 mg 30–60 min pre-op.

Children weighing 5 kg and more. 0.01–0.02 mg/kg/dose to maximum of 0.4 mg/dose.

Children weighing less than 5 kg. 0.02 mg/kg/dose 30–60 min pre-op.

▸ Bradycardia

IV

Adults, Elderly. 0.5–1 mg q5min not to exceed 2 mg or 0.04 mg/kg.

Children. 0.02 mg/kg with a minimum of 0.1 mg to a maximum of 0.5 mg in children and 1 mg in adolescents. May repeat in 5 min. Maximum total dose: 1 mg in children, 2 mg in adolescents.

CONTRAINDICATIONS

Bladder neck obstruction due to prostatic hypertrophy, cardiospasm, intestinal atony, myasthenia gravis in those not treated with neostigmine, narrow-angle glaucoma, obstructive disease of the GI tract, paralytic ileus, severe ulcerative colitis, tachycardia secondary to cardiac insufficiency or thyrotoxicosis, toxic megacolon, unstable cardiovascular status in acute hemorrhage

INTERACTIONS

Drug

Antacids, antidiarrheals: May decrease absorption of atropine.
Anticholinergics: May increase the effects of atropine.
Ketoconazole: May decrease absorption of ketoconazole.
Potassium chloride: May increase severity of GI lesions (wax matrix).

Herbal

None known.

Food

None known.

DIAGNOSTIC TEST EFFECTS

None known.

IV INCOMPATIBILITIES

Pentothal (Thiopental)

IV COMPATIBILITIES

Diphenhydramine (Benadryl), droperidol (Inapsine), fentanyl (Sublimaze), glycopyrrolate (Robinul), heparin, hydromorphone (Dilaudid), midazolam (Versed), morphine, potassium chloride, propofol (Diprivan)

SIDE EFFECTS

Frequent

Dry mouth, nose, and throat that may be severe; decreased sweating, constipation, irritation at subcutaneous or IM injection site

Occasional

Swallowing difficulty, blurred vision, bloated feeling, impotence, urinary hesitancy

Rare

Allergic reaction, including rash and urticaria; mental confusion or excitement, particularly in children; fatigue

SERIOUS REACTIONS

! Overdosage may produce tachycardia, palpitations, hot, dry or flushed skin, absence of bowel sounds, increased respiratory rate, nausea, vomiting, confusion, somnolence, slurred speech, dizziness, and CNS stimulation.
! Overdosage may also produce psychosis as evidenced by agitation, restlessness, rambling speech, visual hallucinations, paranoid behavior, and delusions, followed by depression.

NURSING CONSIDERATIONS

Baseline Assessment

- Instruct the patient to urinate before giving this drug to reduce the risk of urine retention.

Precautions

◀ALERT▶ Use atropine extremely cautiously in patients with autonomic neuropathy, diarrhea, known or suspected GI infections, and mild to moderate ulcerative colitis.
- Use cautiously in patients with CHF, COPD, coronary artery disease, esophageal reflux or hiatal hernia associated with reflux esophagitis, gastric ulcer, hepatic or renal disease, hypertension, hyperthyroidism, and tachyarrhythmias.
- Use atropine cautiously in the elderly and in infants.

Administration and Handling

◀ALERT▶ Notify physician and expect to discontinue atropine immediately if the patient experiences blurred vision, dizziness, or increased pulse rate.

IV
- Give the drug rapidly, to prevent paradoxical slowing of the heart rate.

IM, Subcutaneous
- May be given by IM or subcutaneous injection.

Intervention and Evaluation

- Monitor the patient for changes in the BP, pulse rate, and temperature.
- Monitor the patient with heart disease for signs of tachycardia.
- Assess the patient's skin turgor and mucous membranes to evaluate his or her hydration status. Encourage the patient to drink fluids unless the patient is to have nothing by mouth before surgery.
- Assess the patient's bowel sounds for the presence of peristalsis; be alert for diminished bowel sounds.
- Monitor the patient for fever because patients receiving atropine are at an increased risk for hyperthermia.
- Monitor the patient's intake and output and palpate his or her bladder to assess for urine retention.
- Assess the patient's pattern of daily bowel activity and stool consistency.

Patient Teaching

- Explain to the patient that a warm, dry, flushing feeling may occur upon administration.
- Remind the patient to remain in bed and not to eat or drink anything before surgery.

disopyramide phosphate

dye-soe-**peer**-a-mide
(Norpace, Norpace CR, Rythmodan[CAN])
Do not confuse disopyramide with desipramine, dipyridamole, or Rythmol.

CATEGORY AND SCHEDULE

Pregnancy Risk Category: C

MECHANISM OF ACTION

An antiarrhythmic that prolongs the refractory period of the cardiac cell by direct effect, decreasing myocardial excitability and conduction velocity. **Therapeutic Effect:** Depresses myocardial contractility. Has anticholinergic and negative inotropic effects.

AVAILABILITY

Capsules (Norpace): 100 mg, 150 mg.
Capsules (Extended-Release [Norpace CR]): 100 mg, 150 mg.

INDICATIONS AND DOSAGES

▸ **Suppression and prevention of ventricular ectopy, unifocal or multifocal premature ventricular contractions, paired ventricular contractions (couplets), and episodes of ventricular tachycardia**

PO

Adults, Elderly weighing 50 kg and more. 150 mg q6h (300 mg q12h with extended-release).
Adults, Elderly weighing less than 50 kg. 100 mg q6h (200 mg q12h with extended-release).

▸ **Rapid control of arrhythmias**

PO

◂**ALERT**▸ Do not use extended-release capsules for rapid control.
Adults, Elderly weighing 50 kg and more. Initially, 300 mg, then 150 mg q6h or 300 mg (controlled release) q12h.
Adults, Elderly weighing less than 50 kg. Initially, 200 mg, then 100 mg q6h or 200 mg (controlled release) q12h.

▸ **Severe refractory arrhythmias**

PO

Adults, Elderly. Up to 400 mg q6h.
Children 12–18 yr. 6–15 mg/kg/day in divided doses q6h.
Children 5–11 yr. 10–15 mg/kg/day in divided doses q6h.
Children 1–4 yr. 10–20 mg/kg/day in divided doses q6h.
Children younger than 1 yr. 10–30 mg/kg/day in divided doses q6h.

▸ **Dosage in renal impairment**
With or without loading dose of 150 mg:

Creatinine Clearance	Dosage
40 ml/min and higher	100 mg q6h (extended-release 200 mg q12h)
30–39 ml/min	100 mg q8h
15–29 ml/min	100 mg q12h
less than 15 ml/min	100 mg q24h

▸ **Dosage in liver impairment**
Adults, Elderly weighing 50 kg and more. 100 mg q6h (200 mg q12h with extended-release).
▸ **Dosage in cardiomyopathy, cardiac decompensation**
Adults, Elderly weighing 50 kg and more. No loading dose; 100 mg q6–8h with gradual dosage adjustments.

OFF-LABEL USES
Prophylaxis and treatment of supraventricular tachycardia

CONTRAINDICATIONS
Cardiogenic shock, narrow-angle glaucoma (unless patient is undergoing cholinergic therapy), pre-existing second- or third-degree AV block, pre-existing urinary retention

INTERACTIONS
Drug
Other antiarrhythmics, including diltiazem, propranolol, verapamil: May prolong cardiac conduction, decrease cardiac output.
Pimozide: May increase cardiac arrhythmias.
Herbal
None known.
Food
None known.

DIAGNOSTIC TEST EFFECTS
May decrease blood glucose levels. May cause EKG changes. May increase serum cholesterol and triglyceride levels. Therapeutic serum level is 2 to 8 mcg/ml and the toxic serum level is greater than 8 mcg/ml.

SIDE EFFECTS
Frequent (greater than 9%)
Dry mouth (32%), urinary hesitancy, constipation
Occasional (9%–3%)
Blurred vision, dry eyes, nose, or throat, urinary retention, headache, dizziness, fatigue, nausea
Rare (less than 1%)
Impotence, hypotension, edema, weight gain, shortness of breath, syncope, chest pain, nervousness, diarrhea, vomiting, decreased appetite, rash, itching

SERIOUS REACTIONS
! May produce or aggravate CHF.
! May produce severe hypotension, shortness of breath, chest pain, syncope (especially in patients with primary cardiomyopathy or CHF).
! Hepatotoxicity occurs rarely.

NURSING CONSIDERATIONS
Baseline Assessment
• Have the patient empty his or her bladder before administering disopyramide to reduce the risk of urine retention.
Precautions
• Use cautiously in patients with bundle-branch block, CHF, impaired liver or renal function, myasthenia gravis, prostatic hypertrophy, sick sinus syndrome (sinus bradycardia alternating with tachycardia), and Wolff-Parkinson-White syndrome.
Intervention and Evaluation
• Monitor the patient's EKG for

cardiac changes, particularly widening of the QRS complex and prolongation of the PR and QT intervals.
- Monitor the patient's blood glucose, liver enzyme, and serum alkaline phosphatase, bilirubin, and potassium, AST (SGOT), and ALT (SGPT) levels. Also monitor the patient's BP. Be aware that disopyramide's therapeutic serum level is 2–8 mcg/ml and toxic serum level is greater than 8 mcg/ml.
- Monitor the patient's intake and output for signs of urine retention.
- Assess the patient for signs and symptoms of CHF including cough, dyspnea (particularly on exertion), fatigue, and rales at the base of the lungs.
- Assist the patient with ambulation if he or she experiences dizziness.

Patient Teaching
- Warn the patient to notify the physician if he or she has a productive cough or shortness of breath.
- Explain to the patient that he or she should not take nasal decongestants or OTC cold preparations, especially those containing stimulants, without consulting the physician for approval.
- Encourage the patient to restrict his or her alcohol and salt consumption while taking disopyramide.

dofetilide
doe-**fet**-ill-ide
(Tikosyn)

CATEGORY AND SCHEDULE
Pregnancy Risk Category: C

MECHANISM OF ACTION
A selective potassium channel blocker that prolongs repolarization without affecting conduction velocity by blocking one or more time-dependent potassium currents. Dofetilide has no effect on sodium channels or adrenergic alpha or beta receptors. **Therapeutic Effect:** Terminates reentrant tachyarrhythmias, preventing reinduction.

AVAILABILITY
Capsules: 125 mcg, 250 mcg, 500 mcg.

INDICATIONS AND DOSAGES
▸ **Maintain normal sinus rhythm after conversion from atrial fibrillation or flutter**

PO

Adults, Elderly. Individualized using a seven-step dosing algorithm dependent upon calculated creatinine clearance and QT interval measurements.

CONTRAINDICATIONS
Concurrent use of drugs that prolong the QT interval; concurrent use of amiodarone, megestrol, prochlorperazine, or verapamil; congenital or acquired prolonged QT syndrome; paroxysmal atrial fibrillation; severe renal impairment

INTERACTIONS
Drug

Amiloride, megestrol, metformin, prochlorperazine, triamterene: May increase plasma levels of dofetilide.

Bepridil, phenothiazines, tricyclic antidepressants: May prolong the QT interval.

Cimetidine, verapamil: Increases levels of dofetilide.

Ketoconazole, trimethoprim: Increases plasma concentration of dofetilide.

Herbal

None known.

Food

Grapefruit juice: Can increase dofetilide plasma levels.

DIAGNOSTIC TEST EFFECTS

None known.

SIDE EFFECTS

Occasional (less than 5%)
Headache, chest pain, dizziness, dyspnea, nausea, insomnia, back and abdominal pain, diarrhea, rash

SERIOUS REACTIONS

! Angioedema, bradycardia, cerebral ischemia, facial paralysis, and serious ventricular arrhythmias or various forms of heart block may be noted.

NURSING CONSIDERATIONS

Baseline Assessment
- Be prepared to institute continuous cardiac and BP monitoring.

Administration and Handling
- Administer dofetilde at the same time each day without regard to food.

Intervention and Evaluation
- Monitor the patient's EKG for ventricular arrhythmias and for prolongation of the QT interval.
- Monitor the patient's serum creatinine level for changes.

Patient Teaching
- Explain to the patient that he or she may take dofetilide without regard to food.
- Advise the patient that dofetilide therapy compliance is essential and that the dosing instructions must be followed diligently.
- Warn the patient to notify the physician if he or she experiences dizziness, severe diarrhea, or other adverse effects.

flecainide

fle-kah-nide
(Flecatab[AUS], Tambocor)

CATEGORY AND SCHEDULE

Pregnancy Risk Category: C

MECHANISM OF ACTION

An antiarrhythmic that slows atrial, AV, His-Purkinje, and intraventricular conduction. Decreases excitability, conduction velocity, and automaticity. **Therapeutic Effect:** Controls atrial, supraventricular, and ventricular arrhythmias.

AVAILABILITY

Tablets: 50 mg, 100 mg.

INDICATIONS AND DOSAGES

▸ Life-threatening ventricular arrhythmias, sustained ventricular tachycardia

PO

Adults, Elderly. Initially, 100 mg q12h, increased by 100 mg (50 mg twice a day) every 4 days until effective dose or maximum of 400 mg/day is attained.

▸ Paroxysmal supraventricular tachycardias (PSVT), paroxysmal atrial fibrillation (PAF)

PO

Adults, Elderly. Initially, 50 mg q12h, increased by 100 mg (50 mg twice a day) every 4 days until effective dose or maximum of 300 mg/day is attained.

CONTRAINDICATIONS

Cardiogenic shock, pre-existing second- or third-degree AV block, right bundle-branch block (without presence of a pacemaker)

INTERACTIONS

Drug

Beta blockers: May increase negative inotropic effects.
Digoxin: May increase blood concentration of digoxin.
Other antiarrhythmics: May have additive effects.
Urinary acidifiers: May increase the excretion of flecainide.
Urinary alkalinizers: May decrease the excretion of flecainide.

Herbal

None known.

Food

None known.

DIAGNOSTIC TEST EFFECTS

None significant.

SIDE EFFECTS

Frequent (19%–10%)
Dizziness, dyspnea, headache
Occasional (9%–4%)
Nausea, fatigue, palpitations, chest pain, asthenia (loss of strength, energy), tremor, constipation

SERIOUS REACTIONS

! Flecainide may worsen existing arrhythmias or produce new ones.
! CHF may occur or existing CHF may worsen.
! Overdose may increase QRS duration, prolong QT interval, cause conduction disturbances, reduce myocardial contractility, and cause hypotension.

NURSING CONSIDERATIONS

Baseline Assessment

- Establish the patient's cardiovascular and medication history, especially the use of other antiarrhythmics.
- Make sure that the patient receives continuous cardiac monitoring when initiating flecainide therapy.
- Perform baseline EKG measurements, including QRS duration and QT interval.

Precautions

- Use flecainide cautiously in patients with CHF, impaired myocardial function, second- or third-degree AV block (with pacemaker), or sick sinus syndrome.

Administration and Handling

PO
- Crush scored tablets as needed.

Intervention and Evaluation

- Assess the patient's pulse for irregular rate and quality.
- Monitor the patient's EKG for changes, particularly widening of the QRS complex or prolongation of the QT interval.
- Assess the patient for evidence of CHF, including weight gain, pulmonary crackles, and dyspnea.
- Monitor the patient's intake and output. A decrease in urine output may indicate CHF.
- Monitor the patient for therapeutic serum level, 0.2 to 1 mcg/ml.

Patient Teaching

- Tell the patient that side effects of flecainide therapy generally disappear with continued use or decreased dosage.
- Caution the patient against abruptly discontinuing the medication.
- Warn the patient not to use nasal decongestants or OTC cold preparations without physician approval.
- Instruct the patient to use caution when performing tasks that require mental alertness or motor skills.
- Warn the patient to notify the physician if he or she experiences chest pain, faintness, or palpitations.

ibutilide fumarate

eye-**byoo**-ti-lide
(Corvert)

CATEGORY AND SCHEDULE

Pregnancy Risk Category: C

MECHANISM OF ACTION

An antiarrhythmic that prolongs both atrial and ventricular action potential duration and increases the atrial and ventricular refractory period. Activates slow, inward current (mostly of sodium), produces mild slowing of sinus node rate and AV conduction, and causes dose-related prolongation of QT interval. **Therapeutic Effect:** Converts arrhythmias to sinus rhythm.

PHARMACOKINETICS

After IV administration, highly distributed, rapidly cleared. Protein binding: 40%. Primarily excreted in urine as metabolite. ***Half-life:*** 2–12 hr (average: 6 hr).

AVAILABILITY

Injection: 0.1 mg/ml solution.

INDICATIONS AND DOSAGES

▸ **Rapid conversion of atrial fibrillation or flutter of recent onset to normal sinus rhythm**

IV Infusion

Adults, Elderly weighing 60 kg and more. One vial (1 mg) given over 10 min. If arrhythmia does not stop within 10 min after end of initial infusion, a second 1 mg/10-min infusion may be given.

Adults, Elderly weighing less than 60 kg. 0.01 mg/kg given over 10 min. If arrhythmia does not stop within 10 min after end of initial infusion, a second 0.01 mg/kg, 10-min infusion may be given.

CONTRAINDICATIONS

None known.

INTERACTIONS

Drug

Class IA antiarrhythmics (disopyramide, moricizine, procainamide, quinidine), Class III antiarrhythmics (amiodarone, bretylium, sotalol): Do not give ibutilde with these drugs or give these drugs within 4 hours after infusing ibutilide.

H_1 receptor antagonists, phenothiazines, tricyclic and tetracyclic antidepressants: May prolong QT interval.

Herbal

None known.

Food

None known.

DIAGNOSTIC TEST EFFECTS

None known.

IV INCOMPATIBILITIES

No information is available for Y-site administration.

SIDE EFFECTS

Ibutilde is generally well tolerated.

Occasional

Ventricular extrasystoles (5.1%), ventricular tachycardia (4.9%), headache (3.6%), hypotension, orthostatic hypotension (2%)

Rare

Bundle-branch block, AV block, bradycardia, hypertension

SERIOUS REACTIONS

! Sustained polymorphic ventricular tachycardia, occasionally with QT prolongation (torsades de pointes) occurs rarely.

! Overdose results in CNS toxicity, including CNS depression, rapid gasping breathing, and seizures.

! Expect prolongation of repolarization may be exaggerated.
! Existing arrhythmias may worsen or new arrhythmias may develop.

NURSING CONSIDERATIONS

Baseline Assessment

- For patients with atrial fibrillation lasting more than 3 days, expect to administer an anticoagulant for at least 2 weeks before ibutilide therapy is started.
- Proarrhythmias may develop.

Lifespan Considerations

- Because ibutilide is embryocidal and teratogenic in animals, breast-feeding is not recommended during ibutilde therapy.
- The safety and efficacy of ibutilide have not been established in children.
- No age-related precautions have been noted in the elderly.

Precautions

- Use ibutilde cautiously in patients with abnormal hepatic function or heart block.

Administration and Handling

IV

- Have advanced cardiac life-support equipment, medications, and trained personnel on hand during and after ibutilde administration.
- Ibutilde is compatible with D_5W and 0.9% NaCl. It is also compatible with polyvinyl chloride plastic and polyolefin bag admixtures.
- Admixtures with diluent are stable at room temperature for up to 24 hours or up to 48 hours if refrigerated.
- Give undiluted or may dilute in 50 ml diluent.
- Give over 10 minutes.

Intervention and Evaluation

- Institute continuous EKG monitoring, as ordered, for at least 4 hours following the ibutilide infusion or until the QT interval has returned to baseline. Continue EKG monitoring if the patient develops arrhythmias.
- Monitor the patient's serum electrolyte levels, especially magnesium and potassium, and watch for arrhythmias requiring overdrive cardiac pacing, electrical cardioversion, or defibrillation.

Patient Teaching

- Explain to the patient that his or her BP and EKG will be continuously monitored during therapy.
- Warn the patient to immediately report palpitations or other adverse reactions.

lidocaine hydrochloride

lye-doe-kane
(Lidoderm, Lignocaine Gel[AUS], Xylocaine, Xylocaine Aerosol [AUS], Xylocaine Ointment[AUS], Xylocaine Viscous Topical Solution[AUS], Xylocard[CAN], Zilactin-L[CAN])

CATEGORY AND SCHEDULE

Pregnancy Risk Category: B

MECHANISM OF ACTION

An amide anesthetic that inhibits conduction of nerve impulses. **Therapeutic Effect:** Causes temporary loss of feeling and sensation. Also an antiarrhythmic that decreases depolarization, automaticity, excitability of the ventricle during diastole by direct action. **Therapeutic Effect:** Inhibits ventricular arrhythmias.

PHARMACOKINETICS

Route	Onset	Peak	Duration
IV	30–90 sec	N/A	10–20 min
Local anesthetic	2.5 min	N/A	30–60 min

Completely absorbed after IM administration. Protein binding: 60% to 80%. Widely distributed. Metabolized in the liver. Primarily excreted in urine. Minimally removed by hemodialysis. ***Half-life:*** 1–2 hr.

AVAILABILITY

IM Injection: 300 mg/3 ml.
Direct IV Injection: 10 mg/ml, 20 mg/ml.
IV Admixture Injection: 40 mg/ml, 100 mg/ml, 200 mg/ml.
IV Infusion: 2 mg/ml, 4 mg/ml, 8 mg/ml.
Injection (anesthesia): 0.5%, 1%, 1.5%, 2%, 4%.
Liquid: 2.5%, 5%.
Ointment: 2.5%, 5%.
Cream: 0.5%.
Gel: 0.5%, 2.5%.
Topical Spray: 0.5%.
Topical Solution: 2%, 4%.
Topical Jelly: 2%.
Dermal Patch: 5%.

INDICATIONS AND DOSAGES

▸ **Rapid control of acute ventricular arrhythmias after an MI, cardiac catheterization, cardiac surgery, or digitalis-induced ventricular arrhythmias**

IM

Adults, Elderly. 300 mg (or 4.3 mg/kg). May repeat in 60–90 min.

IV

Adults, Elderly. Initially, 50–100 mg (1 mg/kg) IV bolus at rate of 25–50 mg/min. May repeat in 5 min. Give no more than 200–300 mg in 1 hr. Maintenance: 20–50 mcg/kg/min (1–4 mg/min) as IV infusion.

Children, Infants. Initially, 0.5–1 mg/kg IV bolus; may repeat but total dose not to exceed 3–5 mg/kg. Maintenance: 10–50 mcg/kg/min as IV infusion.

▸ **Dental or surgical procedures, childbirth**

Infiltration, Nerve Block

Adults. Local anesthetic dosage varies with procedure, degree of anesthesia, vascularity, duration. Maximum dose: 4.5 mg/kg. Do not repeat within 2 hr.

▸ **Local skin disorders (minor burns, insect bites, prickly heat, skin manifestations of chickenpox, abrasions), and mucous membrane disorders (local anesthesia of oral, nasal, and laryngeal mucous membranes; local anesthesia of respiratory, urinary tract; relief of discomfort of pruritus ani, hemorrhoids, pruritus vulvae)**

Topical

Adults, Elderly. Apply to affected areas as needed.

▸ **Treatment of shingles-related skin pain**

Topical (Dermal patch)

Adults, Elderly. Apply to intact skin over most painful area (up to 3 applications once for up to 12 hr in a 24-hr period).

CONTRAINDICATIONS

Adams-Stokes syndrome, hypersensitivity to amide-type local anesthetics, septicemia (spinal anesthesia), supraventricular arrhythmias, Wolff-Parkinson-White syndrome

INTERACTIONS

Drug

Anticonvulsants: May increase cardiac depressant effects.

Beta-adrenergic blockers: May increase risk of toxicity.
Other antiarrhythmics: May increase cardiac effects.

Herbal

None known.

Food

None known.

DIAGNOSTIC TEST EFFECTS

IM lidocaine may increase creatine kinase level (used to diagnose acute MI). Therapeutic serum level is 1.5 to 6 mcg/ml; toxic serum level is greater than 6 mcg/ml.

IV INCOMPATIBILITIES

Amphotericin B complex (Abelcet, AmBisome, Amphotec), thiopental

IV COMPATIBILITIES

Aminophylline, amiodarone (Cordarone), calcium gluconate, digoxin (Lanoxin), diltiazem (Cardizem), dobutamine (Dobutrex), dopamine (Intropin), enalapril (Vasotec), furosemide (Lasix), heparin, insulin, nitroglycerin, potassium chloride

SIDE EFFECTS

CNS effects are generally dose-related and of short duration.

Occasional

IM: Pain at injection site
Topical: Burning, stinging, tenderness at application site

Rare

Generally with high dose: Drowsiness; dizziness; disorientation; light-headedness; tremors; apprehension; euphoria; sensation of heat, cold, or numbness; blurred or double vision; ringing or roaring in ears (tinnitus); nausea

SERIOUS REACTIONS

! Although serious adverse reactions to lidocaine are uncommon, high dosage by any route may produce cardiovascular depression, bradycardia, hypotension, arrhythmias, heart block, cardiovascular collapse, and cardiac arrest.
! There is a potential for malignant hyperthermia.
! CNS toxicity may occur, especially with regional anesthesia use, progressing rapidly from mild side effects to tremors, somnolence, seizures, vomiting, and respiratory depression.
! Methemoglobinemia (evidenced by cyanosis) has occurred following topical application of lidocaine for teething discomfort and laryngeal anesthetic spray.

NURSING CONSIDERATIONS

Baseline Assessment

- Determine if the patient has a hypersensitivity to amide anesthetics and lidocaine before beginning drug therapy.
- Obtain the patient's baseline BP, pulse, respirations, EKG, and serum electrolytes.

Lifespan Considerations

- Be aware that lidocaine crosses the placenta and is distributed in breast milk.
- There are no age-related precautions noted in children.
- The elderly are more sensitive to the adverse effects of lidocaine. Lidocaine dose and rate of infusion should be reduced in the elderly.
- In the elderly, age-related renal impairment may require dosage adjustment.

Precautions

- Use cautiously in patients with atrial fibrillation, bradycardia, heart block, hypovolemia, liver disease, marked hypoxia, and severe respiratory depression.

Administration and Handling

◀ALERT▶ Keep resuscitative equipment and drugs, including oxygen, readily available when administering lidocaine by any route.

◀ALERT▶ Know that lidocaine's therapeutic serum level is 1.5–6 mcg/ml and the toxic serum level is greater than 6 mcg/ml.

IV

◀ALERT▶ Use only lidocaine without preservative, clearly marked for IV use.

- Store at room temperature.
- For IV infusion, prepare solution by adding 1 g to 1 L D_5W to provide concentration of 1 mg/ml (0.1%).
- Know that commercially available preparations of 0.2%, 0.4%, and 0.8% may be used for IV infusion. Be aware that the maximum concentration is 4 g/250 ml.
- For IV push, use 1% (10 mg/ml) or 2% (20 mg/ml).
- Administer IV push at rate of 25 to 50 mg/min.
- Administer for IV infusion at rate of 1 to 4 mg/min (1 to 4 ml) and use a volume control IV set.

IM

- Use 10% (100 mg/ml) and clearly identify that the lidocaine preparation is for IM use.
- Give injection in deltoid muscle because the blood level will be significantly higher than if the injection is given in gluteus muscle or lateral thigh.

Topical

- Be aware that the topical form is not for ophthalmic use.
- For skin disorders, apply directly to affected area or put on a gauze or bandage, which is then applied to the skin.
- For mucous membrane use, apply to desired area as per manufacturer's insert.
- Administer the lowest dosage possible that still provides anesthesia.

Intervention and Evaluation

- Monitor the patient's EKG and vital signs closely for cardiac performance during and following lidocaine administration.
- Inform the physician immediately if the patient's EKG shows arrhythmias or prolongation of the PR interval or QRS complex.
- Assess the patient's pulse for its quality and for bradycardia and irregularity.
- Assess the patient's BP for signs of hypotension.
- Monitor the patient for therapeutic serum levels, which is 1.5 to 6 mcg/ml.
- For lidocaine given by all routes, monitor the patient's level of consciousness and vital signs. Be aware that drowsiness may signal high lidocaine blood levels.

Patient Teaching

- Ensure that the patient receiving lidocaine as a local anesthetic understands that he or she will experience a loss of feeling or sensation and will need protection until anesthetic wears off.
- Warn the patient not to chew gum, drink, or eat for 1 hour after oral mucous membrane lidocaine application. The swallowing reflex may be impaired, increasing risk of aspiration; and numbness of tongue or buccal mucosa may lead to trauma.

mexiletine hydrochloride

mex-**il**-e-teen

(Mexitil)

CATEGORY AND SCHEDULE

Pregnancy Risk Category: C

MECHANISM OF ACTION

An antiarrhythmic that shortens duration of action potential, decreases effective refractory period in His-Purkinje system of myocardium by blocking sodium transport across myocardial cell membranes. **Therapeutic Effect:** Suppresses ventricular arrhythmias.

AVAILABILITY

Capsules: 150 mg, 200 mg, 250 mg.

INDICATIONS AND DOSAGES

▸ **Arrhythmias:**

PO

Adults, Elderly. Initially, 200 mg q8h. Adjust dose by 50–100 mg at 2- to 3-day intervals. Maximum: 1,200 mg/day.

OFF-LABEL USES

Treatment of diabetic neuropathy

CONTRAINDICATIONS

Cardiogenic shock, pre-existing second- or third-degree AV block, right bundle branch block without presence of pacemaker

INTERACTIONS

Drug

Antacids: May reduce the absorption of mexiletine.

Cimetidine: May increase the blood concentration of mexiletine.

Metoclopramide: May increase the absorption of mexiletine.

Phenobarbital, phenytoin, rifampin: May increase the blood concentration of mexiletine.

Herbal

None known.

Food

None known.

DIAGNOSTIC TEST EFFECTS

May increase hepatic enzymes. May decrease WBCs and thrombocytes.

SIDE EFFECTS

Frequent (greater than 10%)

Gastrointestinal (GI) distress, including nausea, vomiting, and heartburn, dizziness, light-headedness, tremor

Occasional (10%–1%)

Nervousness, change in sleep habits, headache, visual disturbances, paresthesia, diarrhea or constipation, palpitations, chest pain, rash, respiratory difficulty, edema

SERIOUS REACTIONS

! Mexiletine has the ability to worsen existing arrhythmias or produce new ones.

! May produce or worsen CHF.

NURSING CONSIDERATIONS

Baseline Assessment

- Establish the patient's cardiovascular history and medication history, especially the use of other antiarrhythmics.
- Expect to obtain a baseline EKG.

Precautions

- Use cautiously in patients with CHF, impaired myocardial function, second- or third-degree AV block, with pacemaker, and sick sinus syndrome.

Administration and Handling

◀ **ALERT** ▶ If 300 mg every 8 hours or less controls arrhythmias, may give dose every 12 hours.

PO

- Do not crush, open, or break capsules.

Intervention and Evaluation

- Monitor the patient's EKG and vital signs closely for cardiac side effects.
- Assess the patient's pulse for irregular rate and quality.
- Evaluate the patient for GI disturbances.
- Assess the patient's daily pattern of bowel activity and stool consistency.

- Assess the patient for dizziness and syncope.
- Evaluate the patient's hand movement for evidence of tremor.
- Evaluate the patient for signs and symptoms of CHF.
- Check the patient for therapeutic serum level (0.5 to 2 mcg/ml).

Patient Teaching

- Warn the patient to notify the physician if he or she experiences dark urine, cough, generalized fatigue, nausea, pale stools, severe or persistent abdominal pain, shortness of breath, unexplained sore throat or fever, vomiting, or yellowing of the eyes or skin.
- Caution the patient against using nasal decongestants and OTC cold preparations without physician approval.
- Urge the patient to restrict his or her alcohol and salt intake.

moricizine hydrochloride

mor-**iss**-i-zeen
(Ethmozine)

CATEGORY AND SCHEDULE

Pregnancy Risk Category: B

MECHANISM OF ACTION

An antiarrhythmic that prevents sodium current across myocardial cell membranes. Has potent local anesthetic activity and membrane stabilizing effects. Slows AV and His-Purkinje conduction and decreases action potential duration and effective refractory period.
Therapeutic Effect: Suppresses ventricular arrhythmias.

AVAILABILITY

Tablets: 200 mg, 250 mg, 300 mg.

INDICATIONS AND DOSAGES

▸ **Arrhythmias**

PO

Adults, Elderly. 200–300 mg q8h. May increase by 150 mg/day at no less than 3-day intervals.

OFF-LABEL USES

Atrial arrhythmias, complete and non-sustained ventricular arrhythmias, premature ventricular contractions (PVCs)

CONTRAINDICATIONS

Cardiogenic shock, pre-existing second- or third-degree AV block or right bundle-branch block without pacemaker

INTERACTIONS

Drug

Cimetidine: May increase blood concentration of moricizine.
Theophylline: May decrease blood concentration of theophylline.

Herbal

None known.

Food

None known.

DIAGNOSTIC TEST EFFECTS

May cause EKG changes, such as prolonged PR and QT intervals.

SIDE EFFECTS

Frequent (15%–5%)

Dizziness, nausea, headache, fatigue, dyspnea

Occasional (5%–2%)

Nervousness, paraesthesia, sleep disturbances, dyspepsia, vomiting, diarrhea

SERIOUS REACTIONS

! Moricizine may worsen existing arrhythmias or produce new ones.
! Jaundice with hepatitis occurs rarely.
! Overdosage produces vomiting,

lethargy, syncope, hypotension, conduction disturbances, exacerbation of CHF, MI, and sinus arrest.

NURSING CONSIDERATIONS

Baseline Assessment

- Correct electrolyte imbalances, as prescribed, before administering moricizine.
- Expect to obtain a baseline EKG.
- Measure the PR and QT intervals.

Precautions

- Use moricizine cautiously in patients with CHF, electrolyte imbalance, impaired hepatic or renal function, or sick sinus syndrome.

Administration and Handling

PO

- Moricizine may be given without regard to food but give with food if GI upset occurs.
- Taking drug 30 minutes after a meal decreases absorption and serum level.

Intervention and Evaluation

- Monitor the patient's EKG for cardiac changes, especially increase in PR and QRS intervals.
- Assess the patient's pulse rate for quality and irregularity.
- Evaluate the patient for dizziness, GI upset, headache, and nausea.
- Monitor the patient's electrolyte levels, intake and output, and liver and renal function test results.

Patient Teaching

- Caution the patient against abruptly discontinuing the drug.
- Warn the patient to notify the physician if he or she experiences chest pain or irregular heartbeats.

procainamide hydrochloride

proe-**kane**-a-mide
(Apo-Procainamide[CAN], Procanbid, Procan-SR, Pronestyl)
Do not confuse Procanbid with probenecid, or Pronestyl with Ponstel.

CATEGORY AND SCHEDULE

Pregnancy Risk Category: C

MECHANISM OF ACTION

An antiarrhythmic that increases the electrical stimulation threshold of the ventricles and His-Purkinje system. Decreases myocardial excitability and conduction velocity and depresses myocardial contractility. Exerts direct cardiac effects. **Therapeutic Effect:** Suppresses arrhythmias.

PHARMACOKINETICS

Rapidly, completely absorbed from the GI tract. Protein binding: 15%–20%. Widely distributed. Metabolized in the liver to active metabolite. Primarily excreted in urine. Removed by hemodialysis. ***Half-life:*** 2.5–4.5 hr; metabolite, 6 hr.

AVAILABILITY

Capsules (Pronestyl): 250 mg, 500 mg.
Tablets (Pronestyl): 250 mg, 375 mg, 500 mg.
Tablets (Extended-Release [Pronestyl-SR]): 500 mg.
Tablets (Extended-Release [Procanbid]): 500 mg, 750 mg, 1,000 mg.
Injection (Pronestyl): 100 mg/ml, 500 mg/ml.

INDICATIONS AND DOSAGES AND DOSAGES

▸ Maintenance of normal sinus rhythm after conversion of atrial fibrillation or flutter; treatment of premature ventricular contractions, paroxysmal atrial tachycardia, atrial fibrillation, and ventricular tachycardia

PO

Adults, Elderly. 250–500 mg of immediate-release tablets q3–6h. 0.5–1 g of extended-release tablets (Pronestyl-SR) q6h. 1–2 g of extended-release tablets (Procanbid) q12h.

Children. 15–50 mg/kg/day of immediate-release tablets in divided doses q3–6h. Maximum: 4 g/day.

IV

Adults, Elderly. Loading dose: 50–100 mg. May repeat q5–10min or 15–18 mg/kg (maximum: 1–1.5 g). Then maintenance infusion of 3–4 mg/min. Range: 1–6 mg/min.

Children. Loading dose: 3–6 mg/kg over 5 min (maximum: 100 mg). May repeat q5–10min to maximum total dose of 15 mg/kg. Then maintenance dose of 20–80 mcg/kg/min. Maximum: 2 g/day.

▸ Dosage in renal impairment

Dosage interval is modified based on creatinine clearance.

Creatinine Clearance	Dosage Interval
10–50 ml/min	q6–12h
less than 10 ml/min	q8–24h

OFF-LABEL USES

Conversion and management of atrial fibrillation

CONTRAINDICATIONS

Complete heart block, myasthenia gravis, pre-existing QT prolongation, second-degree heart block, systemic lupus erythematosus, torsades de pointes

INTERACTIONS

Drug

Antihypertensives (IV procainamide), neuromuscular blockers: May increase the effects of these drugs. May decrease antimyasthenic effect on skeletal muscle.

Other antiarrhythmics, pimozide: May increase cardiac effects.

Herbal

None known.

Food

None known.

DIAGNOSTIC TEST EFFECTS

May cause EKG changes and positive ANA titers and Coombs' test. May increase AST (SGOT), ALT (SGPT), serum alkaline phosphatase, serum bilirubin, and serum LDH levels. Therapeutic serum level is 4 to 8 mcg/ml; toxic serum level is greater than 10 mcg/ml.

IV INCOMPATIBILITIES

Milrinone (Primacor)

IV COMPATIBILITIES

Amiodarone (Cordarone), dobutamine (Dobutrex), heparin, lidocaine, potassium chloride

SIDE EFFECTS

Frequent

PO: Abdominal pain or cramping, nausea, diarrhea, vomiting

Occasional

Dizziness, giddiness, weakness, hypersensitivity reaction (rash, urticaria, pruritus, flushing)

IV: Transient, but at times, marked hypotension

Rare

Confusion, mental depression, psychosis

SERIOUS REACTIONS

! Paradoxical, extremely rapid ventricular rate may occur during treatment of atrial fibrillation or flutter.

! Systemic lupus erythematosus–like syndrome (fever, myalgia, pleuritic chest pain) may occur with prolonged therapy.

! Cardiotoxic effects occur most commonly with IV administration and appear as conduction changes (50% widening of QRS complex, frequent ventricular premature contractions, ventricular tachycardia, and complete AV block).

! Prolonged PR and QT intervals and flattened T waves occur less frequently.

NURSING CONSIDERATIONS

Baseline Assessment

• Check the patient's BP and pulse rate for 1 full minute before giving procainamide unless the patient is on a continuous EKG monitor.

Lifespan Considerations

• Procainamide crosses the placenta; it is unknown if it is distributed in breast milk.

• No age-related precautions have been noted in children.

• The elderly are more susceptible to the drug's hypotensive effect.

• Elderly patients with renal impairment may require dosage adjustment.

Precautions

• Use procainamide cautiously in patients with bundle-branch block, CHF, hepatic or renal impairment, marked AV-conduction disturbances, severe digoxin toxicity, or supraventricular tachyarrhythmias.

Administration and Handling

◀ALERT▶ Procainamide dosage and the interval of administration are individualized based on the patient's age, clinical response, renal function, and underlying myocardial disease. Keep in mind that extended-release tablets are used for maintenance therapy.

PO

• Do not crush or break extended-release tablets.

IV, IM

◀ALERT▶ May give procainamide by IV push, IV infusion, or IM injection.

• Solution normally appears clear and colorless to light yellow.

• Discard if solution darkens or appears discolored or if precipitate forms.

• When diluted with D_5W, solution is stable for 24 hours at room temperature or for 7 days if refrigerated.

• For IV push, dilute with 5 to 10 ml D_5W.

• For initial loading IV infusion, add 1 g to 50 ml D_5W to provide a concentration of 20 mg/ml. Infuse 1 ml/min for up to 25 to 30 minutes.

• For IV infusion, add 1 g to 250–500 ml D_5W to provide concentration of 2 to 4 mg/ml.The maximum concentration is 4 g/250 ml. Infuse at 1 to 3 ml/min.

• For IV push, with the patient in the supine position, administer at a rate not exceeding 25 to 50 mg/min.

Intervention and Evaluation

• Check BP every 5 to 10 minutes during IV infusion. If a fall in BP exceeds 15 mm Hg, discontinue infusion and contact the physician.

• Monitor the patient's EKG for cardiac changes, particularly widening of QRS complex and prolongation of PR and QT intervals. Notify the physician of significant interval changes.

• Continuously monitor BP and EKG during IV administration Continuously adjust the rate of infusion to eliminate arrhythmias.

• Assess the patient's pulse rate for quality and irregularity.
• Monitor the patient's intake and output and serum electrolyte levels, including chloride, potassium, and sodium.
• Evaluate the patient for GI upset, headache, dizziness, or myalgia.
• Assess the patient's pattern of daily bowel activity and stool consistency.
• Monitor the patient's BP for signs of hypotension.
• Assess the patient's skin for hypersensitivity reaction, especially in patients receiving high-dose therapy.
• Monitor the patient for a therapeutic serum level of 4 to 8 mcg/ml and a toxic serum level of greater than 10 mcg/ml.

Patient Teaching

• Advise the patient to evenly space oral doses around the clock.
• Warn the patient to notify the physician if he or she experiences fever, joint pain or stiffness, or signs of upper respiratory tract infection.
• Caution the patient against abruptly discontinuing the drug. Explain to the patient that compliance with therapy is essential to control arrhythmias.
• Explain to the patient that he or she should not take nasal decongestants or OTC cold preparations, especially those containing stimulants, without physician approval.
• Warn the patient to avoid performing tasks that require mental alertness or motor skills until his or her response to the drug is established.

propafenone hydrochloride

proe-pa-**fen**-one
(Rythmol, Rythmol SR)

CATEGORY AND SCHEDULE

Pregnancy Risk Category: C

MECHANISM OF ACTION

An antiarrhythmic that decreases the fast sodium current in Purkinje or myocardial cells. Decreases excitability and automaticity; prolongs conduction velocity and the refractory period. **Therapeutic Effect:** Suppresses arrhythmias.

AVAILABILITY

Tablets (Rythmol): 150 mg, 225 mg, 300 mg).
Capsules (Extended-Release [Rythmol SR]): 225 mg, 325 mg, 425 mg.

INDICATIONS AND DOSAGES

▸ **Documented, life-threatening ventricular arrhythmias, such as sustained ventricular tachycardia**

PO (Prompt-Release)
Adults, Elderly. Initially, 150 mg q8h; may increase at 3- to 4-day intervals to 225 mg q8h, then to 300 mg q8h. Maximum: 900 mg/day.
PO (Extended-Release)
Adults, Elderly. Initially, 225 mg q12h. May increase at 5-day intervals. Maximum: 425 mg q12h.

OFF-LABEL USES

Treatment of supraventricular arrhythmias

CONTRAINDICATIONS

Bradycardia; bronchospastic disorders; cardiogenic shock; electrolyte imbalance; sinoatrial, AV, and intraventricular impulse generation or conduction disorders, such as sick sinus syndrome or AV block, without the presence of a pacemaker; uncontrolled CHF

INTERACTIONS

Drug

Digoxin, propranolol: May increase concentrations of these drugs.
Warfarin: May increase warfarin effects.

Herbal

None known.

Food

None known.

DIAGNOSTIC TEST EFFECTS

May cause EKG changes, such as QRS widening and PR interval prolongation, and positive ANA titers.

SIDE EFFECTS

Frequent (13%–7%)

Dizziness, nausea, vomiting, altered taste, constipation

Occasional (6%–3%)

Headache, dyspnea, blurred vision, dyspepsia (heartburn, indigestion, epigastric pain)

Rare (less than 2%)

Rash, weakness, dry mouth, diarrhea, edema, hot flashes

SERIOUS REACTIONS

! Propafenone may produce or worsen existing arrhythmias.
! Overdose may produce hypotension, somnolence, bradycardia, and atrioventricular conduction disturbances.

NURSING CONSIDERATIONS

Baseline Assessment

- Expect to correct patient electrolyte imbalances before beginning propafenone therapy.

Precautions

- Use propafenone cautiously in patients with CHF, conduction disturbances, impaired hepatic or renal function, and recent MI.

Administration and Handling

PO

- Give without regard to meals.

Intervention and Evaluation

- Assess the patient's pulse rate for quality and irregularity.
- Monitor the patient's EKG for cardiac changes and performance, particularly widening of the QRS complex and prolongation of the PR interval.
- Assess the patient for GI upset, headache, or visual disturbances.
- Monitor the patient's serum electrolyte levels.
- Assess the patient's pattern of daily bowel activity and stool consistency.
- Assess the patient for dizziness and unsteadiness.
- Monitor the patient's hepatic enzymes test results.
- Monitor the patient for therapeutic serum level, which is 0.06 to 1 mcg/ml.

Patient Teaching

- Stress to the patient that compliance with the therapy regimen is essential to control arrhythmias.
- Advise the patient that he or she may experience an altered taste sensation while taking this drug.
- Instruct the patient to notify the physician if he or she experiences blurred vision or headache.
- Warn the patient to avoid tasks that require mental alertness or motor skills until his or her response to the drug has been established.

quinidine

kwin-ih-deen

(Apo-Quin-G[CAN], Apo-Quinidine[CAN], BioQuin Durules[CAN], Kinidin Durules[AUS], Quinaglute Dura-Tabs, Quinate[CAN], Quinidex Extentabs)

Do not confuse quinidine with clonidine or quinine.

CATEGORY AND SCHEDULE

Pregnancy Risk Category: C

MECHANISM OF ACTION

An antiarrhythmic that decreases sodium influx during depolarization, potassium efflux during repolarization, and reduces calcium transport across the myocardial cell membrane. Decreases myocardial excitability, conduction velocity, and contractility. **Therapeutic Effect:** Suppresses arrhythmias.

AVAILABILITY

Injection: 80 mg/ml.
Tablets: 200 mg, 300 mg.
Tablets (Extended-Release [Quinidex Extentabs]): 300 mg.
Tablets (Extended-Release [Quinaglute Dura-Tabs]): 324 mg.

INDICATIONS AND DOSAGES

▸ **Maintenance of normal sinus rhythm after conversion of atrial fibrillation or flutter; prevention of premature atrial, AV, and ventricular contractions; paroxysmal atrial tachycardia; paroxysmal AV junctional rhythm; atrial fibrillation; atrial flutter; paroxysmal ventricular tachycardia not associated with complete heart block**

PO
Adults, Elderly. 100–600 mg q4–6h. (Long-acting): 324–972 mg q8–12h.
Children: 30 mg/kg/day in divided doses q4–6h.
IV
Adults, Elderly. 200–400 mg.
Children. 2–10 mg/kg.

OFF-LABEL USES

Treatment of malaria (IV only)

CONTRAINDICATIONS

Complete AV block, intraventricular conduction defects (widening of QRS complex)

INTERACTIONS

Drug

Antimyasthenics: May decrease effects of these drugs on skeletal muscle.
Digoxin: May increase digoxin serum concentration.
Other antiarrhythmics, pimozide: May increase cardiac effects.
Neuromuscular blockers, oral anticoagulants: May increase effects of these drugs.
Urinary alkalizers such as antacids: May decrease quinidine renal excretion.

Herbal

None known.

Food

None known.

DIAGNOSTIC TEST EFFECTS

None known. Therapeutic serum level is 2 to 5 mcg/ml; toxic serum level is greater than 5 mcg/ml.

IV INCOMPATIBILITIES

Furosemide (Lasix), heparin

IV COMPATIBILITIES

Milrinone (Primacor)

SIDE EFFECTS

Frequent

Abdominal pain and cramps, nausea,

diarrhea, vomiting (can be immediate, intense)

Occasional
Mild cinchonism (ringing in ears, blurred vision, hearing loss) or severe cinchonism (headache, vertigo, diaphoresis, light-headedness, photophobia, confusion, delirium)

Rare
Hypotension (particularly with IV administration), hypersensitivity reaction (fever, anaphylaxis, photosensitivity reaction)

SERIOUS REACTIONS

! Cardiotoxic effects occur most commonly with IV administration, particularly at high concentrations, and are observed as conduction changes (50% widening of QRS complex, prolonged QT interval, flattened T waves, and disappearance of P wave), ventricular tachycardia or flutter, frequent premature ventricular contractions (PVCs), or complete AV block.
! Quinidine-induced syncope may occur with the usual dosage.
! Severe hypotension may result from high dosages.
! Patients with atrial flutter and fibrillation may experience a paradoxical, exremely rapid ventricular rate that may be prevented by prior digitalization.
! Hepatotoxicity with jaundice due to drug hypersensitivity may occur.

NURSING CONSIDERATIONS

Baseline Assessment
- Check the patient's BP and pulse rate for 1 full minute before giving quinidine unless the patient is on a continuous cardiac monitor.
- Monitor CBC and BUN, serum alkaline phosphatase, bilirubin, creatinine, AST (SGOT), ALT (SGPT) levels in patients receiving long-term therapy.

Precautions
- Use quinidine cautiously in patients with digoxin toxicity, incomplete AV block, hepatic or renal impairment, myasthenia gravis, myocardial depression, and sick sinus syndrome.

Administration and Handling
◀ALERT▶ Quinidine's therapeutic serum level is 2 to 5 mcg/ml and the toxic level is greater than 5 mcg/ml.
PO
- Ensure that the patient doesn't crush or chew extended-release tablets.
- Give quinidine with food to reduce GI upset.

IV
◀ALERT▶ Continuously monitor the patient's BP and EKG during IV administration; adjust the rate of the infusion as appropriate and as ordered to minimize arrhythmias and hypotension.
- Use only clear, colorless solution.
- Solution is stable for 24 hours at room temperature when diluted with D_5W.
- For IV infusion, dilute 800 mg with 40 ml D_5W to provide concentration of 16 mg/ml. Give at rate of 1 ml (16 mg)/min because a rapid rate may markedly decrease arterial pressure.
- Administer with patient in supine position.

Intervention and Evaluation
- Monitor the patient's EKG for cardiac changes, particularly prolongation of PR or QT interval and widening of the QRS complex. Notify the physician of significant EKG changes.
- Monitor the patient's CBC, intake and output, liver and renal function test results, and serum potassium level.

- Assess the patient's pattern of daily bowel activity and stool consistency.
- Monitor BP for hypotension, especially in patients receiving high-dose therapy.
- Expect to discontinue the drug if the patient develops quinidine-induced syncope.
- Notify the physician immediately if the patient experiences cardiotoxic effects.

Patient Teaching

- Warn the patient to notify the physician if he or she experiences fever, ringing in the ears, or visual disturbances.
- Advise the patient that quinidine may cause a photosensitivity reaction. Urge the patient to avoid direct sunlight or artificial light.

tocainide hydrochloride

toe-**kay**-nide

(Tonocard)

CATEGORY AND SCHEDULE

Pregnancy Risk Category: C

MECHANISM OF ACTION

An amide-type local anesthetic that shortens the action potential duration and decreases the effective refractory period and automaticity in the His-Purkinje system of the myocardium by blocking sodium transport across myocardial cell membranes.

Therapeutic Effect: Suppresses ventricular arrhythmias.

AVAILABILITY

Tablets: 400 mg, 600 mg.

INDICATIONS AND DOSAGES

▸ **Suppression and prevention of ventricular arrhythmias**

PO

Adults, Elderly. Initially, 400 mg q8h. Maintenance: 1.2–1.8 g/day in divided doses q8h. Maximum: 2,400 mg/day.

CONTRAINDICATIONS

Hypersensitivity to local anesthetics, second- or third-degree AV block

INTERACTIONS

Drug

Beta-adrenergic blockers: May increase pulmonary wedge pressure and decrease cardiac index.

Other antiarrhythmics: May increase risk of adverse cardiac effects.

Herbal

None known.

Food

None known.

DIAGNOSTIC TEST EFFECTS

None known.

SIDE EFFECTS

Tocainide is generally well tolerated.

Frequent (10%–3%)

Minor, transient light-headedness, dizziness, nausea, paraesthesia, rash, tremor

Occasional (3%–1%)

Clammy skin, night sweats, myalgia

Rare (less than 1%)

Restlessness, nervousness, disorientation, mood changes, ataxia (muscular incoordination), visual disturbances

SERIOUS REACTIONS

! High dosage may produce bradycardia or tachycardia, hypotension, palpitations, increased ventricular arrhythmias, premature ventricular contractions (PVCs), chest pain, and exacerbation of CHF.

NURSING CONSIDERATIONS

Baseline Assessment

- Assess the patient's baseline EKG and pulse rate for quality and irregularity.

Precautions

- Use tocainide cautiously in patients with bone marrow failure, CHF, hepatic or renal impairment, or pre-existing arrhythmias.

Administration and Handling

IV

◀ALERT▶ When giving tocainide to patients receiving IV lidocaine, give single 600-mg dose 6 hours before cessation of lidocaine and repeat in 6 hours, as prescribed. Then give standard tocainide maintenance doses.

Intervention and Evaluation

◀ALERT▶ Tocainide's therapeutic serum level is 4 to 10 mcg/ml; its toxic serum level has not been established.

- Monitor the patient's EKG for changes, particularly shortening of the QT interval. Notify the physician of significant interval changes.
- Monitor the patient's fluid status and serum electrolyte levels.
- Assess the patient's hand movements for tremor, which is usually the first sign that the maximum dose is being reached.
- Evaluate the sleeping patient for night sweats.
- Monitor the patient for numbness or tingling in the feet or hands.
- Assess the patient's skin for clamminess and rash.
- Observe the patient for CNS disturbances, including disorientation, incoordination, mood changes, and restlessness.
- Assess the patient for signs and symptoms of CHF, including distended neck veins, dyspnea (particularly on exertion or lying down), night cough, and peripheral edema.
- Monitor the patient's intake and output; an increase in weight or decrease in urine output may indicate CHF.
- Monitor blood tests for a therapeutic serum level between 4 and 10 mcg/ml.

Patient Teaching

- Advise the patient to avoid tasks that require mental alertness or motor skills until his or her response to the drug has been established.
- Warn the patient to notify the physician if he or she experiences breathing difficulties, palpitations, or tremor. Explain that side effects usually disappear with continued therapy.
- Tell the patient that tocainide may be taken with food.

24 Antihyperlipidemics

atorvastatin
cholestyramine resin
colesevelam
ezetimibe
fenofibrate
fluvastatin
gemfibrozil
lovastatin
niacin, nicotinic acid
pravastatin
rosuvastatin calcium
simvastatin

Uses: Antihyperlipidemics are used to lower abnormally high blood levels of cholesterol and triglycerides, which are linked with the development and progression of atherosclerosis. Effective management of cholesterol and triglycerides includes dietary modification along with pharmacologic treatment.

Action: Five subclasses of antihyperlipidemics act in different ways. *Bile acid sequestrants,* such as cholestyramine and colesevelam, bind with bile acids in the intestine, preventing their active transport and reabsorption and enhancing their excretion. By depleting hepatic bile acid, these agents increase the conversion of cholesterol to bile acids. *HMG-CoA reductase inhibitors (statins),* such as atorvastatin and lovastatin, inhibit HMG-CoA reductase, an enzyme required for the last regulated step in cholesterol synthesis. This action reduces cholesterol synthesis in the liver. *Niacin (nicotinic acid)* reduces hepatic synthesis of triglycerides and the secretion of VLDLs by inhibiting the mobilization of free fatty acids from peripheral tissues. *Fibric acids,* such as fenofibrate, increase fatty acid oxidation in the liver, resulting in reduced secretion of triglyceride-rich lipoprotein. They also increase lipoprotein lipase activity and fatty acid uptake.

Cholesterol absorption inhibitors, such as ezetimibe, act in the gut wall to prevent cholesterol absorption through the intestinal villi.

COMBINATION PRODUCTS

CADUET: atorvastatin/amlodipine (a calcium channel blocker) 10 mg/5 mg; 10 mg/10 mg; 20 mg/5 mg; 20 mg/10 mg; 40 mg/5 mg; 40 mg/10 mg; 80 mg/5 mg; 80 mg/10 mg.
PRAVIGARD: pravastatin/aspirin (an antiplatelet) 20 mg/81 mg; 20 mg/325 mg; 40 mg/81 mg; 40 mg/325 mg; 80 mg/81 mg; 80 mg/325 mg.
VYTORIN: ezetimibe/simvastatin 10 mg/10 mg; 10 mg/20 mg; 10 mg/40 mg; 10 mg/80 mg.

atorvastatin

ah-tore-**vah**-stah-tin
(Lipitor)
Do not confuse Lipitor with Levatol.

CATEGORY AND SCHEDULE

Pregnancy Risk Category: X

MECHANISM OF ACTION

An antihyperlipidemic that inhibits HMG-CoA reductase, the enzyme that catalyzes the early step in cholesterol synthesis. **Therapeutic Effect:** Decreases LDL and VLDL cholesterol, and plasma triglyceride levels; increases HDL cholesterol concentration.

PHARMACOKINETICS

Poorly absorbed from the GI tract. Protein binding: greater than 98%. Metabolized in the liver. Minimally eliminated in urine. Plasma levels are markedly increased in chronic alcoholic hepatic disease, but are unaffected by renal disease. ***Half-life:*** 14 hr.

AVAILABILITY

Tablets: 10 mg, 20 mg, 40 mg, 80 mg.

INDICATIONS AND DOSAGES

▸ **Hyperlipidemia, Reduction of risk of myocardial infarction (MI), angina revascularization procedures**
PO
Adults, Elderly. Initially, 10–40 mg a day given as a single dose. Dose range: Increase at 2- to 4-wk intervals to maximum of 80 mg/day.
Children 10–17 yr. Initially, 10 mg/day, may increase to 20 mg/day.
▸ **Familial hypercholesterolemia**
PO
Children 10–17 yr. Initially, 10 mg/day. May increase to 20 mg/day.

CONTRAINDICATIONS

Active hepatic disease, lactation, pregnancy, unexplained elevated hepatic function test results

INTERACTIONS

Drug

Antacids, colestipol, propranolol: Decreases atorvastatin activity.
Cyclosporine, erythromycin, gemfibrozil, nicotinic acid: Increases the risk of acute renal failure and rhabdomyolysis with these drugs.
Digoxin, itraconazole, oral contraceptives, warfarin: May increase atorvastatin blood concentration, producing severe muscle inflammation, pain, and weakness.

Herbal

None known.

Food

None known.

DIAGNOSTIC TEST EFFECTS

May increase serum CK and transaminase concentrations.

SIDE EFFECTS

Atorvastatin is generally well tolerated. Side effects are usually mild and transient.

Frequent (16%)
Headache
Occasional (5%–2%)
Myalgia, rash or pruritus, allergy
Rare (2%–1%)
Flatulence, dyspepsia

SERIOUS REACTIONS

! Cataracts may develop, and photosensitivity may occur.

NURSING CONSIDERATIONS

Baseline Assessment

- Determine if the patient is pregnant before beginning atorvastatin therapy. Atorvastatin is pregnancy risk category X.
- Assess the patient's baseline laboratory results and document serum cholesterol and triglyceride levels and hepatic function test results.

Lifespan Considerations

- Atorvastatin is distributed in breast milk. It is contraindicated during

pregnancy because it may produce skeletal malformation.
- Safety and efficacy of atorvastatin have not been established in children.
- No age-related precautions have been noted in the elderly.

Precautions
- Use atorvastatin cautiously in patients with a history of hepatic disease, hypotension, major surgery, severe acute infection, substantial alcohol consumption, or trauma; in those receiving anticoagulant therapy; and in those with severe acute infection, trauma, uncontrolled seizures, or severe endocrine, electrolyte, or metabolic disorders.

Administration and Handling
PO
- May be given without regard to food.
- Do not break film-coated tablets.

Intervention and Evaluation
- Monitor the patient for headache.
- Assess the patient for malaise, pruritus, and rash.
- Monitor the patient's cholesterol and triglyceride values for therapeutic response.

Patient Teaching
- Instruct the patient to follow his or her prescribed diet. Explain that diet is an important part of treatment.
- Advise the patient that periodic laboratory tests are an essential part of therapy.
- Warn the patient not to take other medications without physician approval.

cholestyramine resin

koe-less-**tir**-a-meen
(Novo-Cholamine[CAN], Prevalite, Questran[CAN], Questran Lite[AUS])
Do not confuse Questran with Quarzan.

CATEGORY AND SCHEDULE
Pregnancy Risk Category: B

MECHANISM OF ACTION
An antihyperlipoproteinemic that binds with bile acids in the intestine, forming an insoluble complex. Binding results in partial removal of bile acid from enterohepatic circulation. **Therapeutic Effect:** Removes LDL cholesterol from plasma.

PHARMACOKINETICS
Not absorbed from the GI tract. Decreases in serum LDL apparent in 5 to 7 days and in serum cholesterol in 1 mo. Serum cholesterol returns to baseline levels about 1 mo after drug is discontinued.

AVAILABILITY
Powder for Oral Suspension: 4 g.

INDICATIONS AND DOSAGES
▸ **Primary hypercholesterolemia**
PO
Adults, Elderly. 3–4 g 3–4 times a day. Maximum: 16–32 g/day in 2–4 divided doses.
Children older than 10 yr. 2 g/day. Maximum: 8 g/day in 2 or more divided doses.
Children 10 yr and younger. Initially, 2 g/day. Range: 1–4 g/day.
▸ **Pruritus**
PO
Adults, Elderly. 4 g 1–2 times a day. Maintenance: Up to 24 g/day in divided doses.

OFF-LABEL USES
Treatment of diarrhea (due to bile acids), hyperoxaluria

CONTRAINDICATIONS
Complete biliary obstruction, hypersensitivity to cholestyramine or tartrazine (frequently seen in aspirin hypersensitivity)

INTERACTIONS
Drug
Anticoagulants: May increase effects of these drugs by decreasing level of vitamin K.
Digoxin, folic acid, penicillins, propranolol, tetracyclines, thiazides, thyroid hormones, other medications: May bind and decrease absorption of these drugs.
Oral vancomycin: Binds and decreases the effects of oral vancomycin.
Warfarin: May decrease warfarin absorption.
Herbal
None known.
Food
None known.

DIAGNOSTIC TEST EFFECTS
May increase serum alkaline phosphatase, serum magnesium, AST (SGOT), and ALT (SGPT) levels. May decrease serum calcium, potassium, and sodium levels. May prolong prothrombin time.

SIDE EFFECTS
Frequent
Constipation (may lead to fecal impaction), nausea, vomiting, abdominal pain, indigestion
Occasional
Diarrhea, belching, bloating, headache, dizziness
Rare
Gallstones, peptic ulcer disease, malabsorption syndrome

SERIOUS REACTIONS
! GI tract obstruction, hyperchloremic acidosis, and osteoporosis secondary to calcium excretion may occur.
! High dosage may interfere with fat absorption, resulting in steatorrhea.

NURSING CONSIDERATIONS
Baseline Assessment
- Determine the patient's history of hypersensitivity to aspirin, cholestyramine, and tartrazine before beginning cholsetyramine therapy.
- Check the patient's baseline electrolyte and serum cholesterol and triglyceride levels.

Lifespan Considerations
- Cholestyramine is not systemically absorbed and may interfere with maternal absorption of fat-soluble vitamins.
- No age-related precautions have been noted in children. Cholestyramine use is limited in children younger than 10 years of age.
- The elderly are at increased risk for experiencing adverse nutritional effects and GI side effects.

Precautions
- Use cholestyramine cautiously in patients with bleeding disorders, GI dysfunction (especially constipation), hemorrhoids, or osteoporosis.

Administration and Handling
PO
- Give other drugs at least 1 hour before or 4 to 6 hours after cholestyramine because this drug is capable of binding drugs in the GI tract.
- Don't give cholestyramine in its dry form because it is highly irritating. Mix with 3 to 6 ounces fruit juice, milk, soup, or water.
- Allow the powder to sit on the surface of the liquid for 1 to 2 minutes to prevent lumping; then mix thoroughly.

- When mixing the powder with carbonated beverages, use an extra large glass and stir the liquid slowly to avoid excessive foaming.
- Administer before meals.

Intervention and Evaluation

- Assess the patient's pattern of daily bowel activity and stool consistency.
- Evaluate the patient's abdominal discomfort, flatulence, and food tolerance.
- Monitor the patient's blood chemistry test results.
- Encourage the patient to drink several glasses of water between meals.

Patient Teaching

- Advise the patient to complete a full course of therapy. Caution the patient against omitting or changing drug doses.
- Instruct the patient to take other drugs at least 1 hour before or 4 to 6 hours after cholestyramine.
- Warn the patient never to take cholestyramine in its dry form.
- Teach the patient to mix the powder with 3 to 6 ounces fruit juice, milk, soup, or water. Explain to the patient that he or she should allow the powder to sit on the surface of the liquid for 1 to 2 minutes to prevent lumping and then mix the powder into liquid. Advise the patient who plans to mix the powder with carbonated beverage to use an extra large glass and to stir the liquid slowly to avoid excessive foaming.
- Instruct the patient to take cholestyramine before meals and to drink several glasses of water between meals.
- Encourage the patient to eat high-fiber foods, such as fruits, whole grain cereals, and vegetables to reduce the risk of constipation.

colesevelam

koh-le-**sev**-e-lam

(Welchol)

CATEGORY AND SCHEDULE

Pregnancy Risk Category: B

MECHANISM OF ACTION

A bile acid sequestrant and nonsystemic polymer that binds with bile acids in the intestines, preventing their reabsorption and removing them from the body. **Therapeutic Effect:** Decreases LDL cholesterol.

AVAILABILITY

Tablets: 625 mg.

INDICATIONS AND DOSAGES

▸ To decrease LDL cholesterol level in primary hypercholesterolemia (Fredrickson type IIa)

PO

Adults, Elderly. 3 tablets with meals twice a day or 6 tablets once a day with a meal. May increase daily dose to 7 tablets a day.

CONTRAINDICATIONS

Complete biliary obstruction, hypersensitivity to colesevelam

INTERACTIONS

Drug

Aspirin, clindamycin, digoxin, furosemide, glipizide, hydrocortisone, imipramine, NSAIDs, phenytoin, propranolol, tetracyclines, thiazide diuretics, vitamins A, D, E, K: May decrease the absorption of these drugs.

Herbal

None known.

Food

None known.

DIAGNOSTIC TEST EFFECTS
None known.

SIDE EFFECTS
Frequent (12%–8%)
Flatulence, constipation, infection, dyspepsia (heartburn, epigastric distress)

SERIOUS REACTIONS
! GI tract obstruction may occur.

NURSING CONSIDERATIONS

Baseline Assessment
- Assess the patient's baseline laboratory results for cholesterol and triglyceride levels and liver function.

Lifespan Considerations
- Colesevelam is not absorbed systemically. It may decrease proper maternal vitamin absorption and may affect breast-feeding infants.
- The safety and efficacy of colesevelam have not been established in children.
- No age-related precautions have been noted in the elderly.

Precautions
- Use colesevelam cautiously in patients with dysphagia or severe GI motility disorders.
- Use cautiously in patients who've had major GI tract surgery and in those susceptible to fat-soluble vitamin deficiency.

Administration and Handling
PO
- Administer with meals.
- Give with a liquid.

Intervention and Evaluation
- Monitor the patient's cholesterol and triglyceride levels for therapeutic response.
- Assess the patient's pattern of daily bowel activity and stool consistency.

Patient Teaching
- Advise the patient to follow the prescribed diet and explain that the diet is an important part of treatment.
- Stress to the patient that periodic laboratory tests are an essential part of therapy.
- Explain to the patient that he or she should not take any medications, including OTC drugs, without physician approval.

ezetimibe
eh-**zet**-eh-mibe
(Zetia)
Do not confuse Zetia with Zestril.

CATEGORY AND SCHEDULE
Pregnancy Risk Category: C

MECHANISM OF ACTION
An antihyperlipidemic that inhibits cholesterol absorption in the small intestine, leading to a decrease in the delivery of intestinal cholesterol to the liver. **Therapeutic Effect:** Reduces total serum cholesterol, LDL cholesterol, and triglyceride levels; and increases HDL cholesterol concentration.

PHARMACOKINETICS
Well absorbed following oral administration. Protein binding: greater than 90%. Metabolized in the small intestine and liver. Excreted by the kidneys and bile. ***Half-life:*** 22 hr.

AVAILABILITY
Tablets: 10 mg.

INDICATIONS AND DOSAGES
▸ **Hypercholesterolemia**
PO
Adults, Elderly. Initially, 10 mg once a day, given with or without food. If the patient is also receiving a bile acid sequestrant, give ezetimibe

at least 2 hr before or at least 4 hr after the bile acid sequestrant.

CONTRAINDICATIONS

Concurrent use of an HMG-CoA reductase inhibitor (atorvastatin, fluvastatin, lovastatin, pravastatin, or simvastatin) in patients with active hepatic disease or unexplained persistent elevations in serum transaminase levels, moderate or severe hepatic insufficiency

INTERACTIONS

Drug

Aluminum and magnesium-containing antacids, cyclosporine, fenofibrate, gemfibrozil: Increase ezetimibe plasma concentration.
Cholestyramine: Decreases drug effectiveness.

Herbal

None known.

Food

None known.

DIAGNOSTIC TEST EFFECTS

May increase serum alkaline phosphatase, serum bilirubin, AST (SGOT), and ALT(SGPT) levels.

SIDE EFFECTS

Occasional (4%–3%)
Back pain, diarrhea, arthralgia, sinusitis, abdominal pain

Rare (2%)
Cough, pharyngitis, fatigue

SERIOUS REACTIONS

! None known.

NURSING CONSIDERATIONS

Baseline Assessment

- Assess the patient's blood counts, lipid cholesterol and triglyceride levels, and liver function test results during initial therapy and periodically during treatment. Discontinue treatment if the patient's liver enzyme levels are consistently greater than three times the normal limit.

Lifespan Considerations

- It is unknown if ezetimibe crosses the placenta or is distributed in breast milk.
- Safety and efficacy of ezetimibe have not been established in children 10 years of age and younger.
- In the elderly, age-related mild hepatic impairment requires dosage adjustment. This drug is not recommended for use in elderly patients with moderate or severe hepatic impairment.

Precautions

- Use ezetimibe cautiously in patients with chronic renal failure, diabetes, hypothyroidism, liver function impairment, or obstructive liver disease.

Administration and Handling

PO

- Give ezetimibe without regard to food.

Intervention and Evaluation

- Assess the patient's pattern of daily bowel activity and stool consistency.
- Evaluate the patient for signs and symptoms of abdominal disturbances and back pain.
- Monitor the patient's serum cholesterol and triglyceride concentrations for a therapeutic response.

Patient Teaching:

- Stress to the patient that periodic laboratory tests are an essential part of therapy.
- Caution the patient against discontinuing ezetimibe without physician approval.

fenofibrate

fee-no-**fye**-brate

(Apo-Fenofibrate[CAN], Lafibra, Tricor)

Do not confuse Tricor with Tracleer.

CATEGORY AND SCHEDULE

Pregnancy Risk Category: C

MECHANISM OF ACTION

An antihyperlipidemic that enhances synthesis of lipoprotein lipase and reduces triglyceride-rich lipoproteins and VLDLs. **Therapeutic Effect:** Increases VLDL catabolism and reduces total plasma triglyceride levels.

PHARMACOKINETICS

Well absorbed from the GI tract. Absorption increased when given with food. Protein binding: 99%. Rapidly metabolized in the liver to active metabolite. Excreted primarily in urine; lesser amount in feces. Not removed by hemodialysis. ***Half-life:*** 20 hr.

AVAILABILITY

Capsules (Lafibra): 67 mg, 134 mg, 200 mg.

Tablets (Tricor): 48 mg, 154 mg.

INDICATIONS AND DOSAGES

▸ Reduction of very high serum triglyceride levels in patients at risk for pancreatitis

PO

Adults, Elderly. Initially, 67 mg/day (capsule); may increase to 200 mg/day. Or initially, 48 mg/day (tablet); may increase to 145 mg/day.

▸ Hypercholesterolemia

PO

Adults, Elderly. 200 mg/day (capsule) with meals. Or 145 mg/day (tablet) with meals.

CONTRAINDICATIONS

Gallbladder disease, hypersensitivity to fenofibrate, severe renal or hepatic dysfunction (including primary biliary cirrhosis, unexplained persistent liver function abnormality)

INTERACTIONS

Drug

Anticoagulants: Potentiates effects of these drugs.

Bile acid sequestrants: May impede fenofibrate absorption.

Cyclosporine: Increases risk of nephrotoxicity.

HMG-CoA reductase inhibitors: Increases risk of severe myopathy, rhabdomyolysis, and acute renal failure.

Herbal

None known.

Food

All food: Increases absorption of fenofibrate.

DIAGNOSTIC TEST EFFECTS

May increase BUN and serum CK, AST (SGOT), and ALT (SGPT), levels. May decrease blood Hgb and Hct levels, serum uric acid level, and WBC count.

SIDE EFFECTS

Frequent (8%–4%)

Pain, rash, headache, asthenia or fatigue, flu symptoms, dyspepsia, nausea or vomiting, rhinitis

Occasional (3%–2%)

Diarrhea, abdominal pain, constipation, flatulence, arthralgia, decreased libido, dizziness, pruritus

Rare (less than 2%)

Increased appetite, insomnia, polyuria, cough, blurred vision, eye floaters, earache

SERIOUS REACTIONS

! Fenofibrate may increase excretion of cholesterol into bile, leading to cholelithiasis.
! Pancreatitis, hepatitis, thrombocytopenia, and agranulocytosis occur rarely.

NURSING CONSIDERATIONS

Baseline Assessment

- Check the patient's blood counts, serum lipid cholesterol and triglyceride levels, and liver function test results, including serum ALT (SGPT) level, if ordered, during initial therapy and periodically during treatment. Expect to discontinue fenofibrate if the patient's liver enzyme levels are consistently greater than three times the normal limit.

Lifespan Considerations

- The safety of fenofibrate use during pregnancy has not been established; breast-feeding women should not use this drug.
- The safety and efficacy of fenofibrate have not been established in children.
- No age-related precautions have been noted in the elderly.

Precautions

- Use fenofibrate cautiously in patients who are receiving anticoagulant therapy, have a history of hepatic disease, or consume substantial amounts of alcohol.

Administration and Handling

PO

- Give fenofibrate with meals. Tricor may be given without regard to food.
- Administer fenofibrate 1 hour before or 4 to 6 hours after giving a bile acid sequestrant.

Intervention and Evaluation

- Monitor patients also receiving HMG-CoA reductase inhibitors for signs and symptoms of myopathy, including muscle pain and weakness.
- Monitor the patient's serum CK, cholesterol, and triglyceride levels for a therapeutic response.

Patient Teaching

- Instruct the patient to take fenofibrate with food.
- Advise the patient to notify the physician if constipation, diarrhea, or nausea becomes severe.
- Warn the patient to notify the physician if he or she experiences dizziness, insomnia, muscle pain, rash or skin irritation.

fluvastatin

floo-va-sta-tin
(Lescol, Lescol XL, Vastin[AUS])
Do not confuse fluvastatin with fluoxetine.

CATEGORY AND SCHEDULE

Pregnancy Risk Category: X

MECHANISM OF ACTION

An antihyperlipidemic that inhibits HMG-CoA reductase, the enzyme that catalyzes the early step in cholesterol synthesis. **Therapeutic Effect:** Decreases LDL cholesterol, VLDL, and plasma triglyceride levels. Slightly increases HDL cholesterol concentration.

PHARMACOKINETICS

Well absorbed from the GI tract and is unaffected by food. Does not cross the blood-brain barrier. Protein binding: greater than 98%. Primarily eliminated in feces. ***Half-life:*** 1.2 hr.

AVAILABILITY

Capsules (Lescol): 20 mg, 40 mg.
Tablets (Extended-Release [Lescol XL]): 80 mg.

INDICATIONS AND DOSAGES

▸ Hyperlipoproteinemia

PO

Adults, Elderly. Initially, 20 mg/day (capsule) in the evening. May increase up to 40 mg/day.
Maintenance: 20–40 mg/day in a single dose or divided doses.
Patients requiring more than a 25% decrease in LDL cholesterol. 40 mg (capsule) 1–2 times a day. Or 80 mg tablet once a day.

CONTRAINDICATIONS

Active hepatic disease, unexplained increased serum transaminase levels

INTERACTIONS

Drug

Cyclosporine, erythromycin, gemfibrozil, immunosuppressants, niacin: Increases the risk of acute renal failure and rhabdomyolysis with these drugs.

Herbal

None known.

Food

None known.

DIAGNOSTIC TEST EFFECTS

May increase serum CK and transaminase concentrations

SIDE EFFECTS

Frequent (8%–5%)

Headache, dyspepsia, back pain, myalgia, arthralgia, diarrhea, abdominal cramping, rhinitis

Occasional (4%–2%)

Nausea, vomiting, insomnia, constipation, flatulence, rash, pruritus, fatigue, cough, dizziness

SERIOUS REACTIONS

! Myositis (inflammation of voluntary muscle) with or without increased CK, and muscle weakness, occur rarely. These conditions may progress to frank rhabdomyolysis and renal impairment.

NURSING CONSIDERATIONS

Baseline Assessment

- Determine if the patient is pregnant before beginning fluvastatin therapy.
- Assess the patient's baseline serum cholesterol and triglyceride levels and liver function test results.

Lifespan Considerations

- Fluvastatin use is contraindicated in pregnancy, because the suppression of cholesterol biosynthesis may cause fetal toxicity.
- It is unknown whether fluvastatin is distributed in breast milk; therefore, it is contraindicated during lactation.
- Safety and efficacy of fluvastatin have not been established in children.
- No age-related precautions have been noted in the elderly.

Precautions

- Use fluvastatin cautiously in patients who are receiving anticoagulant therapy, have a history of liver disease, or consume substantial amounts of alcohol.
- Use cautiously in patients experiencing hypotension, major surgery, severe acute infection, renal failure secondary to rhabdomyolysis, uncontrolled seizures, or severe electrolyte, endocrine, or metabolic disorders. Expect to discontinue or withhold fluvastatin if these conditions appear.

Administration and Handling

PO

- Give fluvastatin without regard to food.

Intervention and Evaluation

- Assess the patient's pattern of daily bowel activity and stool consistency.
- Evaluate the patient for dizziness, headache, pruritus, and rash.
- Monitor the patient's serum choles-

terol and triglyceride levels for therapeutic response.

- Assess the patient for malaise and muscle cramping or weakness.

Patient Teaching

- Advise the patient to follow the prescribed diet and explain that the diet is an important part of treatment.
- Stress to the patient that periodic laboratory tests are an essential part of therapy.
- Warn the patient to notify the physician if he or she experiences muscle pain or weakness, especially if accompanied by fever or malaise.

gemfibrozil

gem-**fi**-broe-zil
(Apo-Gemfibrozil[CAN], Ausgem[AUS], Gemfibromax[AUS], Jezil[AUS], Lipazil[AUS], Lopid, Novo-Gemfibrozil[CAN])
Do not confuse Lopid with Lorabid or Levbid.

CATEGORY AND SCHEDULE

Pregnancy Risk Category: C

MECHANISM OF ACTION

A fibric acid derivative that inhibits lipolysis of fat in adipose tissue; decreases liver uptake of free fatty acids and reduces hepatic triglyceride production. Inhibits synthesis of VLDL carrier apolipoprotein B. **Therapeutic Effect:** Lowers serum cholesterol and triglycerides (decreases VLDL, LDL; increases HDL).

PHARMACOKINETICS

Well absorbed from the GI tract. Protein binding: 99%. Metabolized in liver. Primarily excreted in urine. Not removed by hemodialysis. ***Half-life:*** 1.5 hr.

AVAILABILITY

Tablets: 600 mg.
Capsules: 300 mg.

INDICATIONS AND DOSAGES

▸ **Hyperlipidemia**

PO

Adults, Elderly. 1,200 mg/day in 2 divided doses 30 min before breakfast and dinner.

CONTRAINDICATIONS

Liver dysfunction (including primary biliary cirrhosis), pre-existing gallbladder disease, severe renal dysfunction

INTERACTIONS

Drug

Lovastatin: May cause rhabdomyolysis, leading to acute renal failure.
Pioglitazone, repaglinide, warfarin: May increase the effect of these drugs.

Herbal

None known.

Food

None known.

DIAGNOSTIC TEST EFFECTS

May increase serum alkaline phosphatase, serum bilirubin, serum creatinine kinase, serum LDH concentrations, and AST (SGOT) and ALT (SGPT) levels. May decrease blood Hgb and Hct levels, leukocyte counts, and serum potassium levels.

SIDE EFFECTS

Frequent (20%)
Dyspepsia
Occasional (10%–2%)
Abdominal pain, diarrhea, nausea, vomiting, fatigue
Rare (less than 2%)
Constipation, acute appendicitis, vertigo, headache, rash, pruritus, altered taste

SERIOUS REACTIONS

! Cholelithiasis, cholecystitis, acute appendicitis, pancreatitis, and malignancy occur rarely.

NURSING CONSIDERATIONS

Baseline Assessment

- Assess the patient's baseline lab results for blood glucose levels, CBC, serum alkaline phosphatase, bilirubin, cholesterol and triglyceride levels, and AST (SGOT) and ALT (SGPT) levels.

Lifespan Considerations

- Be aware that it is unknown if gemfibrozil crosses the placenta or is distributed in breast milk. Also know that the decision to discontinue breast-feeding or gemfibrozil should be based on the potential for serious adverse effects to the infant.
- Be aware that gemfibrozil use is not recommended in children younger than 2 years of age because cholesterol is necessary for normal development in this age group.
- In the elderly, age-related renal impairment may require dosage adjustment.

Precautions

- Use cautiously in patients with diabetes mellitus, receiving estrogen or anticoagulant therapy, and with hypothyroidism.

Administration and Handling

PO

- Give gemfibrozil 30 minutes before morning and evening meals.

Intervention and Evaluation

- Assess the patient's pattern of daily bowel activity and stool consistency.
- Monitor the patient's serum LDL, VLDL, triglyceride, and cholesterol levels for a therapeutic response.
- Monitor the patient's hematology and liver function test results.
- Assess the patient for pruritus and rash.
- Evaluate the patient for dizziness and headache.
- Assess the patient for pain, especially in the right upper quadrant of the abdomen, because epigastric pain may indicate cholecystitis or cholelithiasis.
- Monitor the blood glucose of patients receiving insulin or oral antihyperglycemics.

Patient Teaching

- Advise the patient to follow the prescribed diet and explain that the diet is an important part of treatment.
- Instruct the patient to take gemfibrozil before meals.
- Stress to the patient that periodic laboratory tests are an essential part of therapy.
- Warn the patient to notify the physician if he or she experiences abdominal pain, diarrhea, dizziness, nausea, or vomiting.

lovastatin

lo-va-sta-tin

(Altoprev, Lotrel, Mevacor)

Do not confuse lovastatin with Leustatin or Livostin, or Mevacor with Mivacron.

CATEGORY AND SCHEDULE

Pregnancy Risk Category: X

MECHANISM OF ACTION

An antihyperlipidemic that inhibits HMG-CoA reductase, the enzyme that catalyzes the early step in cholesterol synthesis. **Therapeutic Effect:** Decreases LDL cholesterol, VLDL cholesterol, plasma triglycerides; increases HDL cholesterol.

PHARMACOKINETICS

Route	Onset	Peak	Duration
PO	3 days	4–6 wk	N/A

Incompletely absorbed from the GI tract (increased on empty stomach). Protein binding: 95%. Hydrolyzed in the liver to active metabolite. Primarily eliminated in feces. Not removed by hemodialysis. ***Half-life:*** 1.1–1.7 hr.

AVAILABILITY

Tablets (Mevacor): 10 mg, 20 mg, 40 mg.
Tablets (Extended-Release [Altoprev]): 20 mg, 40 mg, 60 mg.

INDICATIONS AND DOSAGES

▸ Hyperlipoproteinemia, primary prevention of coronary artery disease

PO

Adults, Elderly. Initially, 20–40 mg/day with evening meal. Increase at 4-wk intervals up to maximum of 80 mg/day. Maintenance: 20–80 mg/day in single or divided doses.

PO (Extended-Release)

Adults, Elderly. Initially, 20 mg/day. May increase at 4-wk intervals up to 60 mg/day.

Children 10–17 yr. 10–40 mg/day with evening meal.

▸ Heterozygous familial hypercholesterolemia

PO

Children 10–17 yr. Initially, 10 mg/day. May increase to 20 mg/day after 8 wk and 40 mg/day after 16 wk if needed.

CONTRAINDICATIONS

Active liver disease, pregnancy, unexplained elevated liver function tests

INTERACTIONS

Drug

Cyclosporine, erythromycin, gemfibrozil, immunosuppressants, niacin: Increases the risk of acute renal failure and rhabdomyolysis.
Erythromycin, itraconazole, ketoconazole: May increase lovastatin blood concentration causing severe muscle inflammation, myalgia, and weakness.

Herbal

None known.

Food

Grapefruit juice: Large amounts of grapefruit juice may increase risk of side effects, such as myalgia and weakness.

DIAGNOSTIC TEST EFFECTS

May increase serum creatine kinase and serum transaminase concentrations.

SIDE EFFECTS

Generally well tolerated. Side effects usually mild and transient.

Frequent (9%–5%)
Headache, flatulence, diarrhea, abdominal pain or cramps, rash and pruritus

Occasional (4%–3%)
Nausea, vomiting, constipation, dyspepsia

Rare (2%–1%)
Dizziness, heartburn, myalgia, blurred vision, eye irritation

SERIOUS REACTIONS

! There is a potential for cataract development.

NURSING CONSIDERATIONS

Baseline Assessment

- Determine if the female patient is pregnant before beginning lovastatin therapy.
- Assess the patient's baseline labo-

ratory test results including serum cholesterol and triglycerides and liver function tests.

Lifespan Considerations

• Lovastatin use is contraindicated in pregnancy, because the suppression of cholesterol biosynthesis may cause fetal toxicity, and lactation.
• It is unknown if lovastatin is distributed in breast milk.
• The safety and efficacy of lovastatin have not been established in children.
• There are no age-related precautions noted in the elderly.

Precautions

• Use cautiously in patients who also use cyclosporine, fibrates, and niacin.
• Use cautiously in patients with a history of heavy or chronic alcohol use and renal impairment.

Administration and Handling

PO
• Give lovastatin with meals.

Intervention and Evaluation

• Assess the patient's daily pattern of bowel activity.
• Evaluate the patient for blurred vision, dizziness, and headache.
• Assess the patient for pruritus and rash.
• Monitor the patient's serum cholesterol and triglyceride levels for a therapeutic response.
• Be alert for the onset of malaise, muscle cramping, or weakness.

Patient Teaching

• Instruct the patient to take lovastatin with meals.
• Encourage the patient to follow the prescribed diet.
• Stress to the patient that the prescribed diet and periodic laboratory tests are essential parts of therapy.
• Urge the patient to avoid consuming grapefruit juice during lovastatin therapy.
• Warn the patient to notify the physician if he or she experiences changes in the color of his or her stool or urine, muscle weakness, myalgia, severe gastric upset, unusual bruising, vision changes, and yellowing of eyes or skin.

niacin, nicotinic acid

nye-a-sin
(Niacor, Niaspan, Nicotinex, Slo-Niacin)
Do not confuse niacin, Niacor, or Niaspan with minocin or Nitro-Bid.

CATEGORY AND SCHEDULE

Pregnancy Risk Category: A
(C if used at dosages above the recommended daily allowance)
OTC

MECHANISM OF ACTION

An antihyperlipidemic, water-soluble vitamin that is a component of two coenzymes needed for tissue respiration, lipid metabolism, and glycogenolysis. Inhibits synthesis of VLDLs. **Therapeutic Effect:** Reduces total, LDL, and VLDL cholesterol levels and triglyceride levels; increases HDL cholesterol concentration.

PHARMACOKINETICS

Readily absorbed from the GI tract. Widely distributed. Metabolized in the liver. Primarily excreted in urine. ***Half-life:*** 45 min.

AVAILABILITY

Capsules (Timed-Release): 125 mg, 250 mg, 400 mg, 500 mg.
Tablets (Niacor): 50 mg, 100 mg, 250 mg, 500 mg.
Tablets (Timed-Release [Slo-Niacin]): 250 mg, 500 mg, 750 mg.

Tablets (Timed-Release [Niaspan]): 500 mg, 750 mg, 1,000 mg.
Elixir (Nicotinex): 50 mg/5 ml.

INDICATIONS AND DOSAGES

Hyperlipidemia

PO (Immediate-Release)
Adults, Elderly. Initially, 50–100 mg twice a day for 7 days. Increase gradually by doubling dose qwk up to 1–1.5 g/day in 2–3 doses. Maximum: 3 g/day.
Children. Initially, 100–250 mg/day (maximum: 10 mg/kg/day) in 3 divided doses. May increase by 100 mg/wk or 250 mg q2–3wks. Maximum: 2,250 mg/day.
PO (Timed-Release)
Adults, Elderly. Initially, 500 mg/day in 2 divided doses for 1 wk; then increase to 500 mg twice a day. Maintenance: 2 g/day.

Nutritional supplement

PO
Adults, Elderly. 10–20 mg/day. Maximum: 100 mg/day.

Pellegra

PO
Adults, Elderly. 50–100 mg 3–4 times a day. Maximum: 500 mg/day.
Children. 50–100 mg 3 times a day.

CONTRAINDICATIONS

Active peptic ulcer disease, arterial hemorrhaging, hepatic dysfunction, hypersensitivity to niacin or tartrazine (frequently seen in patients sensitive to aspirin), severe hypotension

INTERACTIONS

Drug

Alcohol: May increase risk of niacin side effects, such as flushing.
Lovastatin, pravastatin, simvastatin: May increase the risk of acute renal failure and rhabdomyolysis.

Herbal

None known.

Food

None known.

DIAGNOSTIC TEST EFFECTS

May increase serum uric acid level.

SIDE EFFECTS

Frequent

Flushing (especially of the face and neck) occurring within 20 minutes of drug administration and lasting for 30–60 minutes, GI upset, pruritus

Occasional

Dizziness, hypotension, headache, blurred vision, burning or tingling of skin, flatulence, nausea, vomiting, diarrhea

Rare

Hyperglycemia, glycosuria, rash, hyperpigmentation, dry skin

SERIOUS REACTIONS

! Arrhythmias occur rarely.

NURSING CONSIDERATIONS

Baseline Assessment

- Determine if the patient has a history of hypersensitivity to aspirin, niacin, or tartrazine before beginning drug therapy.
- Assess the patient's baseline blood glucose level, serum cholesterol and triglyceride levels, and hepatic function test results.

Lifespan Considerations

- Niacin is not recommended for use during pregnancy and lactation.
- Niacin is distributed in breast milk and is not recommended during lactation.
- No age-related precautions have been noted in children or the elderly.
- Niacin use is not recommended for use in children younger than 2 years of age.

Precautions

• Use niacin cautiously in patients with diabetes mellitus, gallbladder disease, gout, or a history of hepatic disease or jaundice.

Administration and Handling

PO

• Give niacin without regard to meals.
• Administer the drug at bedtime.

Intervention and Evaluation

• Assess the patient's degree of GI discomfort and flushing.
• Evaluate the patient for blurred vision, dizziness, and headache.
• Assess the patient's pattern of daily bowel activity and stool consistency.
• Monitor the patient's blood glucose level; serum alkaline phosphatase, bilirubin, cholesterol, and triglyceride levels; uric acid level; and AST (SGOT) and ALT (SGPT) levels.
• Assess the patient's skin for dryness.

Patient Teaching

• Advise the patient to take the drug at bedtime and to avoid alcohol consumption.
• Advise the patient that itching, flushing of the skin, a sensation of warmth, and tingling may occur.
• Warn the patient to notify the physician if he or she experiences dark urine, dizziness, loss of appetite, nausea, vomiting, weakness, or yellowing of the skin.
• Suggest to the patient to avoid sudden changes in posture to help prevent bouts of dizziness.

pravastatin

prav-i-**sta**-tin
(Pravachol)
Do not confuse pravastatin with Prevacid, or Pravachol with propranolol.

CATEGORY AND SCHEDULE

Pregnancy Risk Category: X

MECHANISM OF ACTION

An HMG-CoA reductase inhibitor that interferes with cholesterol biosynthesis by preventing the conversion of HMG-CoA reductase to mevalonate, a precursor to cholesterol. **Therapeutic Effect:** Lowers serum LDL and VLDL cholesterol and plasma triglyceride levels; increases serum HDL concentration.

PHARMACOKINETICS

Poorly absorbed from the GI tract. Protein binding: 50%. Metabolized in the liver (minimal active metabolites). Primarily excreted in feces via the biliary system. Not removed by hemodialysis. ***Half-life:*** 2.7 hr.

AVAILABILITY

Tablets: 10 mg, 20 mg, 40 mg, 80 mg.

INDICATIONS AND DOSAGES

▸ **Hyperlipidemia, primary and secondary preventionof cardiovascular events in patient with elevated cholesterol levels**

PO

Adults, Elderly. Initially, 40 mg/day. Titrate to desired response. Range: 10–80 mg/day.
Children 14–18 yr. 40 mg/day.
Children 8–13 yr. 20 mg/day.

Dosage in hepatic and renal impairment

For adults, give 10 mg/day initially. Titrate to desired response.

CONTRAINDICATIONS

Active hepatic disease or unexplained, persistent elevations of liver function test results

INTERACTIONS

Drug

Cyclosporine, erythromycin, gemfibrozil, immunosuppressants, niacin: Increases the risk of acute renal failure and rhabdomyolysis.

Herbal

None known.

Food

None known.

DIAGNOSTIC TEST EFFECTS

May increase serum CK and transaminase concentrations.

SIDE EFFECTS

Pravastatin is generally well tolerated. Side effects are usually mild and transient.

Occasional (7%–4%)

Nausea, vomiting, diarrhea, constipation, abdominal pain, headache, rhinitis, rash, pruritus

Rare (3%–2%)

Heartburn, myalgia, dizziness, cough, fatigue, flu-like symptoms

SERIOUS REACTIONS

! Malignancy and cataracts may occur.

! Hypersensitivity occurs rarely.

NURSING CONSIDERATIONS

Baseline Assessment

- Determine if the patient is pregnant before beginning pravastatin therapy.
- Assess the patient's baseline laboratory results including serum cholesterol and triglyceride levels and hepatic function tests.

Lifespan Considerations

- Pravastatin use is contraindicated in pregnancy because suppression of cholesterol biosynthesis may cause fetal toxicity.
- It is unknown if pravastatin is distributed in breast milk; because there is risk of serious adverse reactions in breast-feeding infants, pravastatin is contraindicated during lactation.
- The safety and efficacy of pravastatin have not been established in children.
- No age-related precautions have been noted in the elderly.

Precautions

- Use pravastatin cautiously in patients with a history of hepatic disease, or severe electrolyte, endocrine, or metabolic disorders and in those who consume a substantial amount of alcohol.
- Withholding or discontinuing pravastatin may be necessary when the patient is at risk for renal failure secondary to rhabdomyolysis.

Administration and Handling

◀ALERT▶ Before the patient begins pravastatin therapy, he or she should be on a standard cholesterol-lowering diet for a minimum of 3 to 6 months. The patient should continue the diet throughout pravastatin therapy.

PO

- Give pravastatin without regard to meals and administer in the evening.

Intervention and Evaluation

- Monitor the patient's serum cholesterol and triglyceride levels for a therapeutic response.
- Monitor the patient's serum alkaline phosphatase, bilirubin, AST (SGOT) and ALT (SGPT) levels to assess hepatic function.

• Assess the patient's pattern of daily bowel activity and stool consistency.
• Evaluate the patient for dizziness and headache. Help the patient with ambulation if he or she experiences dizziness.
• Assess the patient for pruritus and rash.
• Assess the patient for malaise and muscle cramping or weakness. If these conditions occur and are accompanied by fever, expect that pravastatin may be discontinued.

Patient Teaching

• Advise the patient to follow the prescribed diet and explain that the diet is an important part of treatment.
• Stress to the patient that periodic laboratory tests are an essential part of therapy.
• Warn the patient to notify the physician if he or she experiences muscle pain or weakness, especially if accompanied by fever or malaise.
• Advise the patient to avoid tasks that require mental alertness or motor skills until his or her response to the drug is established.
• Urge the patient of childbearing years to use nonhormonal contraceptives while taking pravastatin. Explain to the patient that pravastatin is pregnancy risk category X.

rosuvastatin calcium

ross-uh-vah-**stah**-tin
(Crestor)

CATEGORY AND SCHEDULE

Pregnancy Risk Category: X

MECHANISM OF ACTION

An antihyperlipidemic that interferes with cholesterol biosynthesis by inhibiting the conversion of the enzyme HMG-CoA to mevalonate, a precursor to cholesterol. **Therapeutic Effect:** Decreases LDL cholesterol, VLDL, and plasma triglyceride levels, increases HDL concentration.

PHARMACOKINETICS

Protein binding: 88%. Minimal hepatic metabolism. Primarily eliminated in the feces. ***Half-life:*** 19 hr (increased in patients with severe renal dysfunction).

AVAILABILITY

Tablets: 5 mg, 10 mg, 20 mg, 40 mg.

INDICATIONS AND DOSAGES

▸ Hyperlipidemia, dyslipidemia
PO
Adults, Elderly. 5 to 40 mg/day. Usual starting dosage is 10 mg/day, with adjustments based on lipid levels; monitor q2–4wk until desired level is achieved.

▸ Renal impairment (creatinine clearance less than 30 ml/min)
PO
Adults, Elderly. 5 mg/day; do not exceed 10 mg/day.

▸ Concurrent cyclosporine use
PO
Adults, Elderly. 5 mg/day.

▸ Concurrent lipid-lowering therapy
PO
Adults, Elderly. 10 mg/day.

CONTRAINDICATIONS

Active hepatic disease, breast-feeding, pregnancy, unexplained, persistent elevations of serum transaminase levels

INTERACTIONS

Drug

Cyclosporine, gemfibrozil, niacin: Increases the risk of myopathy with cyclosporine, gemfibrozil, and niacin.

Erythromycin: Reduces the plasma concentration of erythromycin.
Ethinylestradiol, norgestrel: Increases the plasma concentrations of ethinylestradiol and norgestrel.
Warfarin: Enhances anticoagulant effect.

Herbal

None known.

Food

None known.

DIAGNOSTIC TEST EFFECTS

May increase serum CK and transaminase concentrations. May produce hematuria and proteinuria.

SIDE EFFECTS

Rosuvastatin is generally well tolerated. Side effects are usually mild and transient.

Occasional (9%–3%)

Pharyngitis, headache, diarrhea, dyspepsia, including heartburn and epigastric distress, nausea

Rare (less than 3%)

Myalgia, asthenia or unusual fatigue and weakness, back pain

SERIOUS REACTIONS

! Lens opacities may occur.
! Hypersensitivity reaction and hepatitis occur rarely.

NURSING CONSIDERATIONS

Baseline Assessment

- Determine if the patient is pregnant before beginning rosuvastatin therapy.
- Assess the patient's baseline serum cholesterol and triglyceride levels and liver function test results.
- Before the patient begins rosuvastatin therapy, he or she should be on a standard cholesterol-lowering diet for a minimum of 3 to 6 months. The patient should continue the diet throughout rosuvastatin therapy.

Lifespan Considerations

- Rosuvastatin use is contraindicated in pregnancy because the suppression of cholesterol biosynthesis may cause fetal toxicity.
- Rosuvastatin is contraindicated during lactation because it carries the risk of serious adverse reactions in breast-feeding infants.
- The safety and efficacy of rosuvastatin have not been established in children.
- No age-related precautions have been noted in the elderly.

Precautions

- Use rosuvastatin cautiously in patients with a history of hepatic disease; hypotension; severe acute infection; severe electrolyte, endocrine, or metabolic imbalances or disorders; trauma; or uncontrolled seizures.
- Use cautiously in patients on anticoagulant therapy, in those who consume a substantial amount of alcohol, and in patients who have had recent major surgery.

Administration and Handling

PO

- Give rosuvastatin without regard to meals and administer in the evening.

Intervention and Evaluation

- Monitor the patient's cholesterol and triglyceride levels for therapeutic response.
- Monitor the patient's hepatic function test results, including serum alkaline phosphatase, bilirubin, AST (SGOT) and ALT (SGPT) levels.
- Assess the patient's daily pattern of bowel activity and stool consistency.
- Evaluate the patient for headache and sore throat.
- Be alert for signs and symptoms of patient muscle aches and weakness.

Patient Teaching

- Instruct the patient to continue following a cholesterol-lowering diet. Explain that the diet is an important part of treatment.

• Tell the patient of childbearing years to use appropriate contraceptive measures during rosuvastatin therapy. Explain to the patient that rosuvastatin is pregnancy risk category X.

• Stress to the patient that periodic laboratory tests are an essential part of therapy.

simvastatin

sim-va-sta-tin
(Apo-Simvastatin[CAN], Lipex[AUS], Zocor)
Do not confuse Zocor with Cozaar.

CATEGORY AND SCHEDULE

Pregnancy Risk Category: X

MECHANISM OF ACTION

A HMG-CoA reductase inhibitor that interferes with cholesterol biosynthesis by inhibiting the conversion of the enzyme HMG-CoA to mevalonate. **Therapeutic Effect:** Decreases serum LDL, cholesterol, VLDL, and plasma triglyceride levels; slightly increases serum HDL concentration.

PHARMACOKINETICS

Route	Onset	Peak	Duration
PO to reduce cholesterol	3 days	14 days	N/A

Well absorbed from the GI tract. Protein binding: 95%. Undergoes extensive first-pass metabolism. Hydrolyzed to active metabolite. Primarily eliminated in feces. Unknown if removed by hemodialysis.

AVAILABILITY

Tablets: 5 mg, 10 mg, 20 mg, 40 mg, 80 mg.

INDICATIONS AND DOSAGES

▸ **To decrease elevated total and LDL cholesterol in hypercholesterolemia (types IIa and IIb), lower triglyceride levels, and increase HDL levels; to reduce risk of death and prevent MI in patients with heart disease and elevated cholesterol level; to reduce risk of revascularization procedures; to decrease risk of stroke or transient ischemic attack; to prevent cardiovascular events.**

PO

Adults. Initially, 10–40 mg/day in evening. Dosage adjusted at 4-wk intervals.

Elderly. Initially, 10 mg/day. May increase by 5–10 mg/day q4wk. Range: 5–80 mg/day. Maximum: 80 mg/day.

CONTRAINDICATIONS

Active hepatic disease or unexplained, persistent elevations of liver function test results, age younger than 18 years, pregnancy

INTERACTIONS

Drug

Cyclosporine, erythromycin, gemfibrozil, immunosuppressants, niacin: Increases the risk of acute renal failure and rhabdomyolysis.

Erythromycin, itraconazole, ketoconazole: May increase simvastatin blood concentration and cause muscle inflammation, myalgia, or weakness.

Herbal

None known.

Food
None known.

DIAGNOSTIC TEST EFFECTS

May increase serum CK and serum transaminase concentrations.

SIDE EFFECTS

Simvastatin is generally well tolerated. Side effects are usually mild and transient.

Occasional (3%–2%)
Headache, abdominal pain or cramps, constipation, upper respiratory tract infection

Rare (less than 2%)
Diarrhea, flatulence, asthenia (loss of strength and energy), nausea or vomiting

SERIOUS REACTIONS

! Lens opacities may occur.
! Hypersensitivity reaction and hepatitis occur rarely.

NURSING CONSIDERATIONS

Baseline Assessment

- Determine if the patient is pregnant or has a history of hypersensitivity to simvastatin before beginning drug therapy.
- Assess the patient's baseline laboratory results, including serum cholesterol, hepatic enzyme, and triglyceride levels.

Lifespan Considerations

- Simvastatin use is contraindicated in pregnancy because suppression of cholesterol biosynthesis may cause fetal toxicity.
- Simvastatin is contraindicated in lactation because there is a risk of serious adverse reactions in breast-feeding infants.
- Safety and efficacy of simvastatin have not been established in children.
- No age-related precautions have been noted in the elderly.

Precautions

- Use simvastatin cautiously in patients with a history of hepatic disease, or severe electrolyte, endocrine, or metabolic disorders and in those who consume substantial amounts of alcohol.
- Withholding or discontinuing simvastatin may be necessary when the patient is at risk for renal failure secondary to rhabdomyolysis.

Administration and Handling

◀ **ALERT** ▶ Before the patient begins simvastatin therapy, he or she should be placed on a standard cholesterol-lowering diet for a minimum of 3 to 6 months. The patient should continue the diet throughout simvastatin therapy.

PO
- Give simvastatin without regard to meals and administer in the evening.

Intervention and Evaluation

- Monitor the patient's serum cholesterol and triglyceride levels and liver function test results, including serum alkaline phosphatase, bilirubin, AST (SGOT) and ALT (SGPT) levels, for a therapeutic response.
- Assess the patient's pattern of daily bowel activity and stool consistency.
- Evaluate the patient for headache.

Patient Teaching

- Advise the patient to use appropriate contraceptive measures while taking simvastatin. Explain that the drug is pregnancy risk category X.
- Stress to the patient that periodic laboratory tests are an essential part of therapy.

25 Beta-Adrenergic Blocking Agents

acebutolol
atenolol
betaxolol
bisoprolol fumarate
carvedilol
esmolol hydrochloride
labetalol hydrochloride
metoprolol tartrate
nadolol
propranolol hydrochloride
sotalol hydrochloride
timolol maleate

Uses: Beta-adrenergic blockers are used to manage hypertension, angina pectoris, arrhythmias, hypertrophic subaortic stenosis, migraine headaches, and glaucoma. They're also used to prevent myocardial infarction.

Action: Beta-adrenergic blockers competitively block $beta_1$-adrenergic receptors, located primarily in the myocardium, and $beta_2$-adrenergic receptors, located primarily in bronchial and vascular smooth muscle. By occupying beta-receptor sites, these agents prevent endogenous or administered epinephrine and norepinephrine from exerting their effects. The results are basically opposite to those of sympathetic stimulation.

Effects of $beta_1$-blockade include slowing the heart rate and decreasing cardiac output and contractility. Effects of $beta_2$-blockade include bronchoconstriction and increased airway resistance in patients with asthma or chronic obstructive pulmonary disease. Beta-adrenergic blockers can affect cardiac rhythm and automaticity, decreasing the sinus rate and sinoatrial and AV conduction and increasing the refractory period in the AV node. These agents decrease systolic and diastolic blood pressure. Although this effect's exact mechanism of action is unknown, it may result from peripheral receptor blockade, decreased sympathetic outflow from the central nervous system, or decreased renin release from the kidneys. All beta-adrenergic blockers mask the tachycardia that occurs with hypoglycemia. When applied to the eyes, they reduce intraocular pressure and aqueous production.

COMBINATION PRODUCTS

CORZIDE: nadolol/bendroflumethiazide (a diuretic) 40 mg/5 mg; 80 mg/5 mg.
COSOPT: timolol/dorzolamide (a carbonic anhydrase inhibitor) 0.5%/2%.
INDERIDE: propranolol/hydrochlorothiazide (a diuretic) 40 mg/25 mg; 80 mg/25 mg.
INDERIDE LA: propranolol/hydrochlorothiazide (a diuretic) 80 mg/50 mg; 120 mg/50 mg; 160 mg/50 mg.
LOPRESSOR HCT: metoprolol/hydrochlorothiazide (a diuretic) 50 mg/25 mg; 100 mg/25 mg; 100 mg/50 mg.

High Alert Drug

NORMOZIDE: labetalol/hydrochlorothiazide (a diuretic) 100 mg/25 mg; 200 mg/25 mg; 300 mg/25 mg.
TENORETIC: atenolol/chlorthalidone (a diuretic) 50 mg/25 mg; 100 mg/25 mg.
TIMOLIDE: timolol/hydrochlorothiazide (a diuretic) 10 mg/25 mg.
ZIAC: bisoprolol/hydrochlorothiazide (a diuretic) 2.5 mg/6.25 mg; 5 mg/6.25 mg; 10 mg/6.25 mg.

acebutolol

a-se-**byoo**-toe-lole
(Monitan[CAN], Novo-Acebutolol[CAN], Rhotral[CAN], Sectral)
Do not confuse Sectral with Factrel or Septra.

CATEGORY AND SCHEDULE

Pregnancy Risk Category: B (D if used in second or third trimester)

MECHANISM OF ACTION

A $beta_1$-adrenergic blocker that competitively blocks $beta_1$-adrenergic receptors in cardiac tissue Reduces the rate of spontaneous firing of the sinus pacemaker and delays AV conduction. **Therapeutic Effect:** Slows heart rate, decreases cardiac output, decreases BP, and exhibits antiarrhythmic activity.

PHARMACOKINETICS

Route	Onset	Peak	Duration
PO (hypotensive)	1–1.5 hr	2–8 hr	24 hr
PO (antiarrhythmic)	1 hr	4–6 hr	10 hr

Well absorbed from the GI tract. Protein binding: 26%. Undergoes extensive first-pass liver metabolism to active metabolite. Eliminated via bile, secreted into GI tract via intestine, and excreted in urine. Removed by hemodialysis. ***Half-life:*** 3–4 hr; metabolite, 8–13 hr.

AVAILABILITY

Capsules: 200 mg, 400 mg.

INDICATIONS AND DOSAGES

▸ Mild to moderate hypertension
PO
Adults. Initially, 400 mg/day in 12 divided doses. Range: Up to 1,200 mg/day in 2 divided doses. Maintenance: 400–800 mg/day.

▸ Ventricular arrhythmias
PO
Adults. Initially, 200 mg q12h. Increase gradually to 600–1,200 mg/day in 2 divided doses.
Elderly. Initially, 200–400 mg/day. Maximum: 800 mg/day.

▸ Dosage in renal impairment
Dosage is modified based on creatinine clearance.

Creatinine Clearance	% of Usual Dosage
less than 50 ml/min	50
less than 25 ml/min	25

OFF-LABEL USES

Treatment of anxiety, chronic angina pectoris, hypertrophic cardiomyopathy, MI, pheochromocytoma, syndrome of mitral valve prolapse, thyrotoxicosis, tremors

CONTRAINDICATIONS

Cardiogenic shock, heart block greater than first degree, overt heart failure, severe bradycardia

INTERACTIONS

Drug

Diuretics, other antihypertensives: May increase hypotensive effect of acebutolol.

Sympathomimetics, xanthines: May mutually inhibit effects of acebutolol; may mask symptoms of hypoglycemia and prolong hypoglycemic effect of insulin and oral hypoglycemics.

Herbal

None known.

Food

None known.

DIAGNOSTIC TEST EFFECTS

May increase antinuclear antibody titer and serum alkaline phosphatase, serum bilirubin, BUN, serum creatinine, LDH, lipoproteins, serum potassium, AST (SGOT), ALT (SGPT), triglyceride, and uric acid levels.

SIDE EFFECTS

Frequent

Hypotension manifested as dizziness, nausea, diaphoresis, headache, cold extremities, fatigue, constipation, or diarrhea

Occasional

Insomnia, urinary frequency, impotence or decreased libido

Rare

Rash, arthralgia, myalgia, confusion (especially in the elderly), altered taste

SERIOUS REACTIONS

! Overdose may produce profound bradycardia and hypotension.

! Abrupt withdrawal may result in diaphoresis, palpitations, headache, and tremors.

! Acebutolol administration may precipitate CHF or MI in patients with heart disease; thyroid storm in those with thyrotoxicosis; or peripheral ischemia in those with existing peripheral vascular disease.

! Hypoglycemia may occur in patients with previously controlled diabetes.

! Signs of thrombocytopenia, such as unusual bleeding or bruising, occur rarely.

NURSING CONSIDERATIONS

Baseline Assessment

• Assess the patient's apical pulse and BP immediately before giving acebutolol. If the pulse rate is 60 beats/minute or lower or systolic BP is less than 90 mm Hg, withhold the medication and notify the physician.

Lifespan Considerations

• Acebutolol readily crosses the placenta and is distributed in breast milk.

• Acebutolol use should be avoided in pregnant women after the first trimester because it may result in low-birth-weight infants. The drug may also produce apnea, bradycardia, hypoglycemia, or hypothermia during childbirth.

• No age-related precautions have been noted in children and dosages have not been established.

• Use cautiously in the elderly, who may have age-related peripheral vascular disease.

Precautions

• Use acebutolol cautiously in patients with bronchospastic disease, diabetes, hyperthyroidism, impaired renal or hepatic function, inadequate cardiac function, or peripheral vascular disease.

Administration and Handling

PO

• Acebutolol may be given without regard to meals.

Intervention and Evaluation

• Monitor the patient's BP for hypotension and assess respiratory status for shortness of breath.

• Assess pulse for quality, rate, and rhythm.

• Monitor the patient's EKG for arrhythmias, shortening of QT interval or prolongation of PR interval.

• Assess the frequency and consistency of the patient's stools.

• Assess for signs and symptoms CHF, such as decreased urine output, distended neck veins, dyspnea (particularly on exertion or lying down), night cough, peripheral edema, and weight gain.

• Assess for diaphoresis, fatigue, headache, and nausea.

Patient Teaching

• Caution the patient against abruptly discontinuing acebutolol. Advise the patient that compliance with the therapy regimen is essential to control hypertension and arrhythmias.

• Instruct the patient to report excessive fatigue, headache, prolonged dizziness, shortness of breath, or weight gain.

• Explain to the patient not to use nasal decongestants or OTC cold preparations (stimulants) without physician approval.

• Suggest to the patient that he or she restrict salt and alcohol intake.

atenolol

a-**ten**-oh-lol

(Apo-Atenol[CAN], AteHexal[AUS], Noten[AUS], Tenolin[CAN], Tenormin, Tensig[AUS])

Do not confuse atenolol with albuterol or timolol.

CATEGORY AND SCHEDULE

Pregnancy Risk Category: D

MECHANISM OF ACTION

A $beta_1$-adrenergic blocker that acts as an antianginal, antiarrhythmic, and antihypertensive agent by blocking $beta_1$-adrenergic receptors in cardiac tissue. **Therapeutic Effect:** Slows sinus node heart rate, decreasing cardiac output and blood pressure (BP). Decreases myocardial oxygen demand.

PHARMACOKINETICS

Route	Onset	Peak	Duration
PO	1 hr	2–4 hr	24 hr

Incompletely absorbed from the GI tract. Protein binding: 6%–16%. Minimal liver metabolism. Primarily excreted unchanged in urine. Removed by hemodialysis. ***Half-life:*** 6–7 hr (increased in impaired renal function).

AVAILABILITY

Tablets: 25 mg, 50 mg, 100 mg.
Injection: 5 mg/10 ml.

INDICATIONS AND DOSAGES

▸ Hypertension

PO

Adults. Initially, 25–50 mg once a day. May increase dose up to 100 mg once a day.

Elderly. Usual initial dose, 25 mg a day.

Children. Initially, 0.8–1 mg/kg/dose given once a day. Range: 0.8–1.5 mg/kg/day. **Maximum:** 2 mg/kg/day or 100 mg/day.

▸ Angina pectoris

PO

Adults. Initially, 50 mg once a day. May increase dose up to 200 mg once a day.

Elderly. Usual initial dose, 25 mg a day.

Acute MI

IV

Adults. Give 5 mg over 5 min; may repeat in 10 min. In those who tolerate full 10-mg IV dose, begin 50-mg tablets 10 min after last IV dose followed by another 50-mg oral dose 12 hr later. Thereafter, give 100 mg once a day or 50 mg twice a day for 6–9 days. Or, for those who do not tolerate full IV dose, give 50 mg orally twice a day or 100 mg once a day for at least 7 days.

Dosage in renal impairment

Dosage interval is modified based on creatinine clearance.

Creatinine Clearance	Dosage Interval
15–35 ml/min	50 mg a day
less than 15 ml/min	50 mg every other day

OFF-LABEL USES

Improved survival in diabetics with heart disease; treatment of hypertrophic cardiomyopathy, pheochromocytoma, and syndrome of mitral valve prolapse; prevention of migraine, thyrotoxicosis, tremors

CONTRAINDICATIONS

Cardiogenic shock, overt heart failure, second- or third-degree heart block, severe bradycardia

INTERACTIONS

Drug

Cimetidine: May increase atenolol blood concentration.
Diuretics, other antihypertensives: May increase hypotensive effect of atenolol.
Insulin, oral hypoglycemics: May mask symptoms of hypoglycemia and prolong hypoglycemic effect of insulin and oral hypoglycemics.
NSAIDs: May decrease antihypertensive effect of atenolol.
Sympathomimetics, xanthines: May mutually inhibit effects.

Herbal

None known.

Food

None known.

DIAGNOSTIC TEST EFFECTS

May increase serum antinuclear antibody titer and BUN, serum creatinine, potassium, lipoprotein, triglyceride, and uric acid levels.

IV INCOMPATIBILITIES

Amphotericin complex (Abelcet, AmBisome, Amphotec)

SIDE EFFECTS

Atenolol is generally well tolerated, with mild and transient side effects.

Frequent

Hypotension manifested as cold extremities, constipation or diarrhea, diaphoresis, dizziness, fatigue, headache, and nausea

Occasional

Insomnia, flatulence, urinary frequency, impotence or decreased libido, depression

Rare

Rash, arthralgia, myalgia, confusion (especially in the elderly), altered taste

SERIOUS REACTIONS

! Overdose may produce profound bradycardia and hypotension.
! Abrupt atenolol withdrawal may result in diaphoresis, palpitations, headache, and tremors.
! Atenolol administration may precipitate CHF or MI in patients with cardiac disease; thyroid storm in those with thyrotoxicosis; and peripheral ischemia in those with existing peripheral vascular disease.
! Hypoglycemia may occur in

patients with previously controlled diabetes.

! Thrombocytopenia, manifested as unusual bruising or bleeding, occurs rarely.

NURSING CONSIDERATIONS

Baseline Assessment

• Assess the patient's apical pulse and BP immediately before giving atenolol. If the pulse rate is 60 beats/minute or lower or systolic BP is less than 90 mm Hg, withhold the medication and notify the physician.

• If atenolol is being given as an antianginal, record the onset, quality (such as dull, sharp, or squeezing), radiation, location, intensity, and duration of anginal pain. Also, document the precipitating factors, such as emotional stress or exertion.

• Obtain the patient's baseline renal and hepatic function test results.

Lifespan Considerations

• Atenolol readily crosses the placenta and is distributed in breast milk.

• Atenolol use should be avoided in pregnant women after the first trimester because it may result in low-birth-weight infants. The drug may also produce apnea, bradycardia, hypoglycemia, or hypothermia during childbirth.

• No age-related precautions have been noted in children.

• Use cautiously in the elderly, who may have age-related peripheral vascular disease and impaired renal function.

Precautions

• Use atenolol cautiously in patients with bronchospastic disease, diabetes, hyperthyroidism, impaired renal or hepatic function, inadequate cardiac function, or peripheral vascular disease.

Administration and Handling

PO

• May give atenolol without regard to meals.

• Crush tablets if necessary.

IV

• Store at room temperature.

• After reconstitution, store parenteral form for up to 48 hours at room temperature.

• Give undiluted or dilute in 10 to 50 ml 0.9% NaCl or D_5W.

• Give IV push over 5 minutes and IV infusion over 15 minutes.

Intervention and Evaluation

• Monitor the patient's BP for hypotension, pulse for bradycardia, and respirations for difficulty breathing.

• Assess the patient's pattern of daily bowel activity and stool consistency.

• Examine the patient for signs and symptoms of CHF, including distended neck veins, dyspnea (particularly on exertion or lying down), night cough, and peripheral edema.

• Monitor the patient's intake and output and weight. An increase in weight or decrease in urine output may indicate CHF.

• Assess the patient's extremities for coldness.

• Assist the patient with ambulation if dizziness occurs.

Patient Teaching

• Warn the patient not to abruptly discontinue atenolol. Advise the patient that compliance with therapy is essential to control angina and hypertension.

• To reduce the drug's orthostatic effects, instruct the patient to rise slowly from a lying to sitting position and to dangle the legs from the bed momentarily before standing.

• Warn the patient to avoid tasks that require alertness or motor skills until his or her response to the drug hs been established.

• Advise the patient to report confusion, depression, dizziness, rash, or unusual bruising or bleeding to the physician.

- Teach outpatients the correct technique for monitoring their BP and pulse before taking atenolol.
- Urge the patient to restrict his or her alcohol and salt intake.
- Advise the patient that the therapeutic antihypertensive effect of atenolol should be noted within 1 to 2 weeks.

betaxolol

bay-**tax**-oh-lol

(Betoptic[AUS], Betoptic-S, Betoquin[AUS], Kerlone)

Do not confuse betaxolol with bethanechol.

CATEGORY AND SCHEDULE

Pregnancy Risk Category: C (D if used in second or third trimester)

MECHANISM OF ACTION

An antihypertensive and antiglaucoma agent that blocks $beta_1$-adrenergic receptors in cardiac tissue. Reduces aqueous humor production. **Therapeutic Effect:** Slows sinus heart rate, decreases BP and reduces intraocular pressure (IOP).

AVAILABILITY

Tablets (Kerlone): 10 mg, 20 mg.
Ophthalmic Solution (Betoptic-S): 0.5%.
Ophthalmic Suspension (Betoptic-S): 0.25%.

INDICATIONS AND DOSAGES

▸ **Hypertension**

PO

Adults. Initially, 5–10 mg/day. May increase to 20 mg/day after 7–14 days.
Elderly. Initially, 5 mg/day.

▸ **Chronic open-angle glaucoma and ocular hypertension**

Ophthalmic (Eye Drops)

Adults, Elderly. 1 drop twice a day.

▸ **Dosage in renal impairment**

For adult and elderly patients who are on dialysis, initially give 5 mg/day; increase by 5 mg/day q2wk. Maximum: 20 mg/day.

OFF-LABEL USES

Treatment of angle-closure glaucoma during or after iridectomy, malignant glaucoma, secondary glaucoma; with miotics, to decrease IOP in acute and chronic angle-closure glaucoma

CONTRAINDICATIONS

Cardiogenic shock, overt cardiac failure, second- or third-degree heart block, sinus bradycardia

INTERACTIONS

Drug

Cimetidine: May increase betaxolol blood concentration.
Diuretics, other antihypertensives: May increase hypotensive effect of betaxolol.
Insulin, oral hypoglycemics: May prolong hypoglycemic effect of these drugs.
NSAIDs: May decrease antihypertensive effect.
Sympathomimetics, xanthines: May mutually inhibit hypotensive effects and may mask symptoms of hypoglycemia.

Herbal

None known.

Food

None known.

DIAGNOSTIC TEST EFFECTS

May increase serum antinuclear antibody titer and BUN, serum lipoprotein, creatinine, potassium, uric acid, and triglyceride levels.

SIDE EFFECTS

Betaxolol is generally well tolerated, with mild and transient side effects.

Frequent

Systemic: Hypotension manifested as dizziness, nausea, diaphoresis, headache, fatigue, constipation or diarrhea, dyspnea
Ophthalmic: Eye irritation, visual disturbances

Occasional

Systemic: Insomnia, flatulence, urinary frequency, impotence or decreased libido
Ophthalmic: Increased light sensitivity, watering of eye

Rare

Systemic: Rash, arrhythmias, arthralgia, myalgia, confusion, altered taste, increased urination
Ophthalmic: Dry eye, conjunctivitis, eye pain

SERIOUS REACTIONS

! Overdose may produce profound bradycardia, hypotension, and bronchospasm.
! Abrupt withdrawal may result in diaphoresis, palpitations, headache, and tremors.
! Betaxolol administration may precipitate CHF or MI in patients with cardiac disease; thyroid storm in those with thyrotoxicosis; and peripheral ischemia in those with existing peripheral vascular disease.
! Hypoglycemia may occur in patients with previously controlled diabetes.
! Ophthalmic overdose may produce bradycardia, hypotension, bronchospasm, and acute cardiac failure.

NURSING CONSIDERATIONS

Baseline Assessment

- Assess the patient's baseline renal and liver function test results.
- Assess the patient's apical pulse and BP immediately before giving betaxolol. If the patient's pulse rate is 60 beats/minute or lower or systolic BP is less than 90 mm Hg, withhold the medication and notify the physician.

Precautions

- Use betaxolol cautiously in patients with diabetes, hyperthyroidism, impaired hepatic or renal function, inadequate cardiac function, or peripheral vascular disease.

Administration and Handling

- To assess the patient's tolerance for betaxolol, obtain a standing systolic BP 1 hour after giving the drug.

Intervention and Evaluation

- Monitor the patient's BP for hypotension.
- Assess the patient's pulse for rate and quality, and for bradycardia.
- Assess the patient's pattern of daily bowel activity and stool consistency.
- Assist the patient with ambulation if he or she experiences dizziness.
- Evaluate the patient for signs and symptoms of CHF including decrease in urine output, distended neck veins, dyspnea (particularly on exertion or lying down), increase in weight, night cough, and peripheral edema.
- Assess the patient for diaphoresis, fatigue, headache, and nausea.

Patient Teaching

- Caution the patient against abruptly discontinuing betaxolol.
- Advise the patient that compliance with the therapy regimen is essential to control glaucoma and hypertension.
- To avoid betaxolol's orthostatic

effects, teach the patient to rise slowly from a lying to sitting position and wait momentarily before standing.
• Advise the patient to avoid tasks that require mental alertness or motor skills until his or her response to the drug has been established.
• Warn the patient to notify the physician if he or she experiences excessive fatigue, headache, prolonged dizziness, or shortness of breath.
• Explain to the patient that he or she should not use nasal decongestants or OTC cold preparations, especially stimulants, without physician approval.
• Urge the patient to limit his or her alcohol and salt intake.

bisoprolol fumarate

bis-**ope**-pro-lal
(Bicor[AUS], Zebeta)
Do not confuse Zebeta with DiaBeta.

CATEGORY AND SCHEDULE
Pregnancy Risk Category: C (D if used in second or third trimester)

MECHANISM OF ACTION
An antihypertensive that blocks $beta_1$-adrenergic receptors in cardiac tissue. **Therapeutic Effect:** Slows sinus heart rate and decreases BP.

PHARMACOKINETICS
Well absorbed from the GI tract. Protein binding: 26%–33%. Metabolized in the liver. Primarily excreted in urine. Not removed by hemodialysis. ***Half-life:*** 9–12 hr (increased in impaired renal function).

AVAILABILITY
Tablets: 5 mg, 10 mg.

INDICATIONS AND DOSAGES
▸ Hypertension
PO
Adults. Initially, 5 mg/day. May increase up to 20 mg/day.
Elderly. Initially, 2.5–5 mg/day. May increase by 2.5–5 mg/day. Maximum: 20 mg/day.
▸ Dosage in hepatic impairment
For adults and elderly patients with cirrhosis or hepatitis whose creatinine clearance is less than 40 ml/minute, initially give 2.5 mg.

OFF-LABEL USES
Angina pectoris, premature ventricular contractions, supraventricular arrhythmias

CONTRAINDICATIONS
Cardiogenic shock, overt cardiac failure, second- or third-degree heart block

INTERACTIONS
Drug
Cimetidine: May increase bisoprolol blood concentration.
Diuretics, other antihypertensives: May increase the hypotensive effect of bisoprolol.
Insulin, oral hypoglycemics: May mask symptoms of hypoglycemia and prolong the hypoglycemic effect of these drugs.
NSAIDs: May decrease antihypertensive effect.
Sympathomimetics, xanthines: May mutually inhibit effects.
Herbal
None known.
Food
None known.

DIAGNOSTIC TEST EFFECTS
May increase antinuclear antibody

titer and BUN, serum lipoprotein, creatinine, potassium, uric acid, and triglyceride levels.

SIDE EFFECTS

Frequent
Hypotension manifested as dizziness, nausea, diaphoresis, headache, cold extremities, fatigue, constipation or diarrhea

Occasional
Insomnia, flatulence, urinary frequency, impotence or decreased libido

Rare
Rash, arthralgia, myalgia, confusion (especially in the elderly), altered taste

SERIOUS REACTIONS

! Overdose may produce profound bradycardia and hypotension.
! Abrupt withdrawal may result in diaphoresis, palpitations, headache, and tremulousness.
! Bisoprolol administration may precipitate CHF and MI in patients with heart disease; thyroid storm in those with thyrotoxicosis; and peripheral ischemia in those with existing peripheral vascular disease.
! Hypoglycemia may occur in patients with previously controlled diabetes.
! Thrombocytopenia, including unusual bruising and bleeding, occurs rarely.

NURSING CONSIDERATIONS

Baseline Assessment

- Assess the patient's baseline renal and liver function test results.
- Assess the patient's apical pulse and BP immediately before giving bisoprolol. If the patient's pulse rate is 60 beats/min or lower or systolic BP is less than 90 mm Hg, withhold the medication and contact the physician.

Lifespan Considerations

- Bisoprolol readily crosses the placenta and is distributed in breast milk.
- Bisoprolol use should be avoided in pregnant women after the first trimester because it may result in low-birth-weight infants. The drug may also produce apnea, bradycardia, hypoglycemia, or hypothermia during childbirth.
- The safety and efficacy of bisoprolol have not been established in children.
- In the elderly, age-related peripheral vascular disease may increase the risk of decreased peripheral circulation.

Precautions

- Use bisoprolol cautiously in patients with bronchospastic disease, diabetes, hyperthyroidism, impaired hepatic or renal function, inadequate cardiac function, or peripheral vascular disease.

Administration and Handling

PO
- Bisoprolol may given without regard to food.
- If necessary, crush scored tablet.

Intervention and Evaluation

- Assess the patient's pulse for rate and quality, and for bradycardia.
- Assist the patient with ambulation if dizziness occurs.
- Assess the patient for peripheral edema. For ambulatory patients, check behind the medial malleolus; for bedridden patients, check the sacral area.
- Assess the patient's pattern of daily bowel activity and stool consistency.

Patient Teaching

- Caution the patient against abruptly discontinuing bisoprolol. Advise the patient that compliance with the therapy regimen is essential to control hypertension.

- Instruct the patient that if he or she experiences dizziness, to sit or lie down immediately.
- Warn the patient to avoid tasks that require mental alertness or motor skills until his or her response to the drug has been established.
- Teach the patient how to properly take his or her pulse before each dose and to report to the physician if he or she experiences dizziness, excessively slow pulse rates (less than 60 beats/minute), or peripheral numbness.
- Advise the patient not to use nasal decongestants and OTC cold preparations, especially those containing stimulants, without physician approval.
- Urge the patient to limit his or her alcohol and salt intake.

carvedilol

kar-**vea**-die-lole
(Coreg, Dilatrend[AUS], Kredex[AUS])
Do not confuse carvedilol with carteolol.

CATEGORY AND SCHEDULE

Pregnancy Risk Category: C (D if used in the second or third trimester)

MECHANISM OF ACTION

An antihypertensive that possesses nonselective beta-blocking and alpha-adrenergic blocking activity. Causes vasodilation. **Therapeutic Effect:** Reduces cardiac output, exercise-induced tachycardia, and reflex orthostatic tachycardia; reduces peripheral vascular resistance.

PHARMACOKINETICS

Route	Onset	Peak	Duration
PO	30 min	1–2 hr	24 hr

Rapidly and extensively absorbed from the GI tract. Protein binding: 98%. Metabolized in the liver. Excreted primarily via bile into feces. Minimally removed by hemodialysis. ***Half-life:*** 7–10 hr. Food delays rate of absorption.

AVAILABILITY

Tablets: 3.125 mg, 6.25 mg, 12.5 mg, 25 mg.

INDICATIONS AND DOSAGES

▸ **Hypertension**

PO

Adults, Elderly. Initially, 6.25 mg twice a day. May double at 7- to 14-day intervals to highest tolerated dosage. Maximum: 50 mg/day.

▸ **CHF**

PO

Adults, Elderly. Initially, 3.125 mg twice a day. May double at 2-wk intervals to highest tolerated dosage. Maximum: For patients weighing more than 85 kg, give 50 mg twice a day, for those weighing 85 kg or less, give 25 mg twice a day.

▸ **Left ventricular dysfunction**

PO

Adults, Elderly. Initially, 3.125–6.25 mg twice a day. May increase at intervals of 3–10 days up to 25 mg twice a day.

OFF-LABEL USES

Treatment of angina pectoris, idiopathic cardiomyopathy

CONTRAINDICATIONS

Bronchial asthma or related bronchospastic conditions, cardiogenic shock, pulmonary edema, second- or third-degree AV block, severe bradycardia

INTERACTIONS

Drug

Calcium blockers: Increase risk of conduction disturbances.
Catapres: May potentiate BP effects.
Cimetidine: May increase carvedilol blood concentration.
Digoxin: Increases concentrations of this drug.
Diuretics, other antihypertensives: May increase hypotensive effect.
Insulin, oral hypoglycemics: May mask symptoms of hypoglycemia and prolong hypoglycemic effect of these drugs.
Rifampin: Decreases carvedilol blood concentration.

Herbal

None known.

Food

None known.

DIAGNOSTIC TEST EFFECTS

None known.

SIDE EFFECTS

Carvedilol is generally well tolerated, with mild and transient side effects.

Frequent (6%–4%)
Fatigue, dizziness
Occasional (2%)
Diarrhea, bradycardia, rhinitis, back pain
Rare (less than 2%)
Orthostatic hypotension, somnolence, UTI, viral infection

SERIOUS REACTIONS

! Overdose may produce profound bradycardia, hypotension, bronchospasm, cardiac insufficiency, cardiogenic shock, and cardiac arrest.
! Abrupt withdrawal may result in diaphoresis, palpitations, headache, and tremors.
! Carvedilol administration may precipitate CHF and MI in patients with heart disease; thyroid storm in those with thyrotoxicosis; and peripheral ischemia in those with existing peripheral vascular disease.
! Hypoglycemia may occur in patients with previously controlled diabetes.

NURSING CONSIDERATIONS

Baseline Assessment

- Assess the patient's apical pulse and BP immediately before giving carvedilol. If the patient's pulse rate is 60 beats/minute or lower or systolic BP is less than 90 mm Hg, withhold the medication and contact the physician.

Lifespan Considerations

- It is unknown if carvedilol crosses the placenta or is distributed in breast milk.
- Carvedilol use should be avoided in pregnant women after the first trimester because it may result in low-birth-weight infants. The drug may also produce apnea, bradycardia, hypoglycemia, or hypothermia during childbirth.
- The safety and efficacy of carvedilol have not been established in children.
- In the elderly, the incidence of dizziness may be increased.

Precautions

- Use carvedilol cautiously in patients undergoing anesthesia and in those with CHF controlled with ACE inhibitor, digoxin or diuretics; diabetes mellitus; hypoglycemia; impaired hepatic function; peripheral vascular disease; and thyrotoxicosis.

Administration and Handling

PO
- Give carvedilol with food to slow

the rate of absorption and reduce the risk of orthostatic hypotension.
• To assess the patient's tolerance for carvedilol, assess a standing systolic BP 1 hour after giving the drug.

Intervention and Evaluation

• Monitor the patient's BP for hypotension and respiratory status for dyspnea.
• Assess the patient's pulse for rate and quality, and for bradycardia.
• Monitor the patient's EKG for arrhythmias.
• Assist the patient with ambulation if he or she experiences dizziness.
• Evaluate the patient for signs and symptoms of CHF, including distended neck veins, dyspnea (particularly on exertion or lying down), night cough, and peripheral edema
• Monitor the patient's intake and output and weight. An increase in weight or a decrease in urine output may indicate CHF.

Patient Teaching

• Caution the patient against abruptly discontinuing carvedilol.
• Advise the patient that compliance with the therapy regimen is essential to control hypertension.
• Explain to the patient that the full antihypertensive effect of carvedilol will be noted in 1 to 2 weeks.
• Advise patients who wear contact lenses that they may experience decreased tearing.
• Teach the patient to take carvedilol with food.
• Advise the patient to avoid tasks that require mental alertness or motor skills until his or her response to the drug has been established.
• Warn the patient to notify the physician if he or she experiences excessive fatigue or prolonged dizziness.
• Advise the patient not to take nasal decongestants and OTC cold preparations, especially those containing stimulants, without physician approval.
• Instruct the patient to check his or her pulse rate and BP before taking the medication.
• Urge the patient to limit his or her alcohol and salt intake.

esmolol hydrochloride

ess-moe-lol
(Brevibloc)

CATEGORY AND SCHEDULE

Pregnancy Risk Category: C

MECHANISM OF ACTION

An antiarrhythmic that selectively blocks $beta_1$-adrenergic receptors. **Therapeutic Effect:** Slows sinus heart rate, decreases cardiac output, reducing BP.

AVAILABILITY

Injection: 10 mg/ml, 250 mg/ml.

INDICATIONS AND DOSAGES

▸ Arrythmias

IV

Adults, Elderly. Initially, loading dose of 500 mcg/kg/min for 1 min, followed by 50 mcg/kg/min for 4 min. If optimum response is not attained in 5 min, give second loading dose of 500 mcg/kg/min for 1 min, followed by infusion of 100 mcg/kg/min for 4 min. Additional loading doses can be given and infusion increased by 50 mcg/kg/min, up to 200 mcg/kg/min, for 4 min. Once desired response is attained, cease loading dose and increase infusion by no more than 25 mcg/kg/min. Interval between doses may be increased to 10 min. Infusion usually administered over 24–48 hr in most patients. Range: 50–200 mcg/kg/min, with average dose of 100 mcg/kg/min.

▸ **Intra-operative tachycardia or hypertension (immediate control)**

IV

Adults, Elderly. Initially, 80 mg over 30 seconds, then 150 mcg/kg/min infusion up to 300 mcg/kg/min.

CONTRAINDICATIONS

Cardiogenic shock, overt cardiac failure, second- and third-degree heart block, sinus bradycardia

INTERACTIONS

Drug

Insulin, oral hypoglycemics: May mask symptoms of hypoglycemia and prolong hypoglycemic effect of these drugs.

MAOIs: May cause significant hypertension.

Sympathomimetics, xanthines: May mutually inhibit effects.

Herbal

None known.

Food

None known.

DIAGNOSTIC TEST EFFECTS

None known.

IV INCOMPATIBILITIES

Amphotericin B complex (Abelcet, AmBisome, Amphotec), furosemide (Lasix)

IV COMPATIBILITIES

Amiodarone (Cordarone), diltiazem (Cardizem), dopamine (Intropin), heparin, magnesium, midazolam (Versed), potassium chloride, propofol (Diprivan)

SIDE EFFECTS

Esmolol is generally well tolerated, with transient and mild side effects.

Frequent

Hypotension (systolic BP less than 90 mm Hg) manifested as dizziness, nausea, diaphoresis, headache, cold extremities, fatigue

Occasional

Anxiety, drowsiness, flushed skin, vomiting, confusion, inflammation at injection site, fever

SERIOUS REACTIONS

! Overdose may produce profound hypotension, bradycardia, dizziness, syncope, drowsiness, breathing difficulty, bluish fingernails or palms of hands, and seizures.

! Esmolol administration may potentiate insulin-induced hypoglycemia in diabetic patients.

NURSING CONSIDERATIONS

Baseline Assessment

- Assess the patient's apical pulse and BP immediately before giving esmolol. If the patient's pulse is 60 beats/minute or lower or systolic BP is less than 90 mm Hg, withhold the medication and contact the physician.

Precautions

- Use esmolol cautiously in patients with bronchial asthma, bronchitis, CHF, diabetes, emphysema, history of allergy, and impaired renal function.

Administration and Handling

◂**ALERT**▸ Give esmolol by IV infusion. Avoid using butterfly needles and very small veins.

IV

- Use only clear and colorless to light yellow solution.
- After dilution, solution is stable for 24 hours.
- Discard solution if it is discolored or if precipitate forms.
- To prevent vein irritation, dilute the 250-mg/ml ampule to a final

concentration not to exceed 10 mg/ml. Don't administer the drug by direct IV injection.
• For IV infusion, remove 20 ml from 500-ml container of D_5W, D_5W in Ringer's solution, D_5W in lactated Ringer's solution, D_5W in 0.9% NaCl, D_5W in 0.45% NaCl, 0.9% NaCl, lactated Ringer's solution, or 0.45% NaCl and dilute the prescribed amount of esmolol 250 mg/ml concentration in the remaining 480 ml of solution to provide a concentration of 10 mg/ml. Maximum concentration: 10 g/250 ml (40 mg/ml).
• Administer by controlled infusion device and titrate according to the patient's tolerance and response.
• Infuse IV loading dose over 1 to 2 minutes.
• Monitor the patient for hypotension (a systolic BP of less than 90 mm Hg), especially during the first 30 minutes of infusion.

Intervention and Evaluation
• Monitor the patient's BP (for hypotension), EKG, and heart and respiratory rates.
• Monitor the patient for diaphoresis and dizziness, the first signs of impending hypotension.
• Assess the patient's pulse for its rate and quality, and for bradycardia.
• Assess the patient's extremities for coldness.
• Assist the patient with ambulation if he or she experiences dizziness.
• Evaluate the patient for diaphoresis, fatigue, headache, and nausea.

Patient Teaching
• Explain to the patient that his or her BP and heart rate will be continuously monitored during esmolol therapy.
• Urge the patient to immediately report cold extremities, dizziness, faintness, or nausea.

labetalol hydrochloride

la-**bet**-a-lole
(Normodyne, Presolol[AUS], Trandate)
Do not confuse Trandate with tramadol or Trental.

CATEGORY AND SCHEDULE
Pregnancy Risk Category: C (D if used in second or third trimester)

MECHANISM OF ACTION
An antihypertensive that blocks alpha$_1$-, beta$_1$-, and beta$_2$- (large doses) adrenergic receptor sites. Large doses increase airway resistance. **Therapeutic Effect:** Slows sinus heart rate; decreases peripheral vascular resistance, cardiac output, and BP.

PHARMACOKINETICS

Route	Onset	Peak	Duration
PO	0.5–2 hr	2–4 hr	8–12 hr
IV	2–5 min	5–15 min	2–4 hr

Completely absorbed from the GI tract. Protein binding: 50%. Undergoes first-pass metabolism. Metabolized in the liver. Primarily excreted in urine. Not removed by hemodialysis. ***Half-life:*** PO, 6–8 hr; IV, 5.5 hr.

AVAILABILITY
Tablets (Normodyne, Trandate): 100 mg, 200 mg, 300 mg.
Injection (Trandate): 5 mg/ml.

INDICATIONS AND DOSAGES
▸ **Hypertension**
PO
Adults. Initially, 100 mg twice a day adjusted in increments of 100 mg twice a day q2–3days. Maintenance:

200–400 mg twice a day. Maximum: 2.4 g/day.
Elderly. Initially, 100 mg 1–2 times a day. May increase as needed.

▸ **Severe hypertension, hypertensive emergency**
IV
Adults. Initially, 20 mg. Additional doses of 20–80 mg may be given at 10-min intervals, up to total dose of 300 mg.
IV Infusion
Adults. Initially, 2 mg/min up to total dose of 300 mg.
PO (after IV therapy)
Adults. Initially, 200 mg; then, 200–400 mg in 6–12 hr. Increase dose at 1-day intervals to desired level.

OFF-LABEL USES

Control of hypotension during surgery, treatment of chronic angina pectoris

CONTRAINDICATIONS

Bronchial asthma, cardiogenic shock, second- or third-degree heart block, severe bradycardia, uncontrolled CHF

INTERACTIONS

Drug

Diuretics, other antihypertensives: May increase hypotensive effect.
Insulin, oral hypoglycemics: May mask symptoms of hypoglycemia and prolong hypoglycemic effect of these drugs.
MAOIs: May produce hypertension.
Sympathomimetics, xanthines: May mutually inhibit effects.

Herbal

None known.

Food

None known.

DIAGNOSTIC TEST EFFECTS

May increase serum antinuclear antibody titer and BUN, serum LDH, lipoprotein, alkaline phosphatase, bilirubin, creatinine, potassium, triglyceride, uric acid, AST (SGOT), and ALT (SGPT) levels.

IV INCOMPATIBILITIES

Amphotericin B complex (Abelcet, AmBisome, Amphotec), ceftriaxone (Rocephin), furosemide (Lasix), heparin, nafcillin (Nafcil), thiopental

IV COMPATIBILITIES

Aminophylline, amiodarone (Cordarone), calcium gluconate, diltiazem (Cardizem), dobutamine (Dobutrex), dopamine (Intropin), enalapril (Vasotec), fentanyl (Sublimaze), hydromorphone (Dilaudid), lidocaine, lorazepam (Ativan), magnesium sulfate, midazolam (Versed), milrinone (Primacor), morphine, nitroglycerin, norepinephrine (Levophed), potassium chloride, potassium phosphate, propofol (Diprivan)

SIDE EFFECTS

Frequent

Drowsiness, difficulty sleeping, unusual fatigue or weakness, diminished sexual ability, transient scalp tingling

Occasional

Dizziness, dyspnea, peripheral edema, depression, anxiety, constipation, diarrhea, nasal congestion, nausea, vomiting, abdominal discomfort

Rare

Altered taste, dry eyes, increased urination, paresthesia

SERIOUS REACTIONS

! Labetolol administration may precipitate or aggravate CHF

because of decreased myocardial stimulation.
! Abrupt withdrawal may precipitate ischemic heart disease, producing sweating, palpitations, headache, and tremor.
! May mask signs and symptoms of acute hypoglycemia (tachycardia, BP changes) in patients with diabetes.

NURSING CONSIDERATIONS

Baseline Assessment

- Assess the patient's baseline liver and renal function test results.
- Assess the patient's apical pulse and BP immediately before giving labetalol. If the patient's pulse is 60 beats/minute or lower or systolic BP is lower than 90 mm Hg, withhold the medication and contact the physician.

Lifespan Considerations

- Labetalol crosses the placenta and is distributed in small amounts in breast milk.
- The safety and efficacy of labetalol have not been established in children.
- In the elderly, age-related peripheral vascular disease may increase susceptibility to decreased peripheral circulation.

Precautions

- Use labetalol cautiously in patients with diabetes mellitus, medication-controlled CHF, impaired cardiac or hepatic function; nonallergic bronchospastic disease, including chronic bronchitis and emphysema; and pheochromocytoma.

Administration and Handling

PO

- Give labetalol without regard to food.
- Crush tablets if necessary.

IV

◀ **ALERT** ▶ Place the patient in a supine position for IV administration and for 3 hours after receiving the medication. Expect a substantial drop in BP if the patient stands within 3 hours following drug administration.

- Store at room temperature.
- After dilution, IV solution is stable for 24 hours.
- Solution normally appears clear and colorless to light yellow; discard solution if precipitate forms or discoloration occurs.
- For IV infusion, dilute 200 mg in 160 ml dextrose 5% in water, 0.9% NaCl, lactated Ringer's solution, or any combination of these solutions to provide a concentration of 1 mg/ml.
- For IV push, give over 2 minutes at 10-minute intervals.
- For IV infusion, administer at a rate of 2 mg/minute (2 ml/minute) initially. Adjust the rate according to the patient's BP.
- Monitor the patient's BP immediately before and every 5 to 10 minutes during IV administration. Maximum effect occurs within 5 minutes.

Intervention and Evaluation

- Monitor the patient's BP for hypotension and EKG for arrhythmias.
- Assess the patient's pulse for bradycardia or an irregular rate.
- Assess the patient's pattern of daily bowel activity and stool consistency.
- Assist the patient with ambulation if he or she experiences dizziness.
- Evaluate the patient for signs and symptoms of CHF, including distended neck veins, dyspnea (particularly on exertion or lying down), night cough, and peripheral edema.
- Monitor the patient's intake and output and weight. An increase in weight or a decrease in urine output may indicate CHF.

Patient Teaching

- Caution the patient against discontinuing the drug except upon the advice of the physician. Explain that

stopping the drug abruptly may precipitate heart failure.
• Stress to the patient that compliance with the therapy regimen is essential to control arrhythmias and hypertension.
• Advise the patient to avoid tasks that require mental alertness or motor skills until his or her response to the drug has been established.
• Warn the patient to notify the physician if he or she experiences excessive fatigue, headache, prolonged dizziness, shortness of breath, or weight gain.
• Advise the patient not to take nasal decongestants and OTC cold preparations, especially those containing stimulants, without physician approval.

metoprolol tartrate

me-**toe**-pro-lole
(Apo-Metoprolol[CAN], Betaloc[CAN], Lopresor[AUS], Lopressor, Metohexal[AUS], Metolol[AUS], Minax[AUS], Nu-Metop[CAN], PMS-Metoprolol [CAN], Toprol XL)
Do not confuse metoprolol with metaproterenol or metolazone.

CATEGORY AND SCHEDULE

Pregnancy Risk Category: C (D if used in second or third trimester)

MECHANISM OF ACTION

An antianginal, antihypertensive, and MI adjunct that selectively blocks $beta_1$-adrenergic receptors; high dosages may block $beta_2$-adrenergic receptors. Decreases oxygen requirements. Large doses increase airway resistance. **Therapeutic Effect:** Slows sinus node heart rate, decreases cardiac output, and reduces BP. Also decreases myocardial ischemia severity.

PHARMACOKINETICS

Route	Onset	Peak	Duration
PO	10–15 min	N/A	6 hr
PO (extended release)	N/A	6–12 hr	24 hr
IV	Immediate	20 min	5–8 hr

Well absorbed from the GI tract. Protein binding: 12%. Widely distributed. Metabolized in the liver (undergoes significant first-pass metabolism). Primarily excreted in urine. Removed by hemodialysis. ***Half-life:*** 3–7 hr.

AVAILABILITY

Tablets (Lopressor): 25 mg, 50 mg, 100 mg.
Tablets (Extended-Release [Toprol XL]): 25 mg, 50 mg, 100 mg, 200 mg.
Injection (Lopressor): 1 mg/ml.

INDICATIONS AND DOSAGES

▸ **Mild to moderate hypertension**
PO
Adults. Initially, 100 mg/day as single or divided dose. Increase at weekly (or longer) intervals. Maintenance: 100–450 mg/day.
Elderly. Initially, 25 mg/day. Range: 25–300 mg/day.
PO (Extended-Release)
Adults. 50–100 mg/day as single dose. May increase at least at weekly intervals until optimum BP attained. Maximum: 200 mg/day.
▸ **Chronic, stable angina pectoris**
PO
Adults. Initially, 100 mg/day as single or divided dose. Increase at weekly (or longer) intervals. Maintenance: 100–450 mg/day.

PO (Extended-Release)
Adults. Initially, 100 mg/day as single dose. May increase at least at weekly intervals until optimum clinical response achieved. Maximum: 200 mg/day.

▸ **Congestive heart failure**
PO (Extended-Release)
Adults. Initially, 25 mg/day. May double dose q2wk. Maximum: 200 mg/day.

▸ **Early treatment of MI**
IV
Adults. 5 mg q2min for 3 doses, followed by 50 mg orally q6h for 48 hr. Begin oral dose 15 min after last IV dose. Or, in patients who do not tolerate full IV dose, give 25–50 mg orally q6h, 15 min after last IV dose.

▸ **Late treatment and maintenance after an MI**
PO
Adults. 100 mg twice a day for at least 3 mo.

OFF-LABEL USES

To increase survival rate in diabetic patients with coronary artery disease (CAD); treatment or prevention of anxiety; cardiac arrhythmias; hypertrophic cardiomyopathy; mitral valve prolapse syndrome; pheochromocytoma; tremors; thyrotoxicosis; vascular headache

CONTRAINDICATIONS

Cardiogenic shock, MI with a heart rate less than 45 beats/minute or systolic BP less than 100 mm Hg, overt heart failure, second- or third-degree heart block, sinus bradycardia

INTERACTIONS

Drug

Cimetidine: May increase metoprolol blood concentration.
Diuretics, other antihypertensives: May increase hypotensive effect.
Insulin, oral hypoglycemics: May mask symptoms of hypoglycemia and prolong hypoglycemic effect of these drugs.
NSAIDs: May decrease antihypertensive effect.
Sympathomimetics, xanthines: May mutually inhibit effects.

Herbal

None known.

Food

None known.

DIAGNOSTIC TEST EFFECTS

May increase serum antinuclear antibody titer and BUN, serum lipoprotein, serum LDH, serum alkaline phosphatase, serum bilirubin, serum creatinine, serum potassium, serum uric acid, AST (SGOT), ALT (SGPT), and serum triglyceride levels.

IV INCOMPATIBILITIES

Amphotericin B complex (Abelcet, AmBisome, Amphotec)

IV COMPATIBILITIES

Alteplase (Activase)

SIDE EFFECTS

Metoprolol is generally well tolerated, with transient and mild side effects.

Frequent
Diminished sexual function, drowsiness, insomnia, unusual fatigue or weakness

Occasional
Anxiety, nervousness, diarrhea, constipation, nausea, vomiting, nasal congestion, abdominal discomfort, dizziness, difficulty breathing, cold hands or feet

Rare
Altered taste, dry eyes, nightmares, paraesthesia, allergic reaction (rash, pruritus)

SERIOUS REACTIONS

! Overdose may produce profound bradycardia, hypotension, and bronchospasm.
! Abrupt withdrawal of metoprolol may result in diaphoresis, palpitations, headache, tremulousness, exacerbation of angina, MI, and ventricular arrhythmias.
! Metoprolol administration may precipitate CHF and MI in patients with heart disease; thyroid storm in those with thyrotoxicosis; and peripheral ischemia in those with existing peripheral vascular disease.
! Hypoglycemia may occur in patients with previously controlled diabetes.

NURSING CONSIDERATIONS

Baseline Assessment

• Assess the patient's baseline liver and renal function test results.
• Assess the patient's apical pulse and BP immediately before giving metoprolol. If the patient's pulse rate is 60 beats/minute or lower, or systolic BP is less than 90 mm Hg, withhold the medication and contact the physician.
• In patients receiving metoprolol for treatment of angina, record the onset, type (sharp, dull, squeezing), radiation, location, intensity, and duration of anginal pain and its precipitating factors, including exertion and emotional stress.

Lifespan Considerations

• Metoprolol crosses the placenta and is distributed in breast milk.
• Metoprolol use should be avoided in pregnant women after the first trimester because it may result in low-birth-weight infants. The drug may also produce apnea, bradycardia, hypoglycemia, or hypothermia during childbirth.
• The safety and efficacy of metoprolol have not been established in children.
• In the elderly, age-related peripheral vascular disease may increase susceptibility to decreased peripheral circulation.

Precautions

• Use metoprolol cautiously in patients with bronchospastic disease, diabetes, hyperthyroidism, impaired renal function, inadequate cardiac function, and peripheral vascular disease.

Administration and Handling

PO
• Crush tablets if necessary; do not crush or break extended-release tablets.
• Give at same time each day.
• Give with or immediately after meals to enhance absorption.

IV
• Store at room temperature.
• Give undiluted as necessary.
• Administer IV injection over 1 minute.
• Monitor the patient's EKG and BP during administration.

Intervention and Evaluation

• Measure the patient's BP near the end of the dosing interval to determine whether the BP is controlled throughout day.
• Monitor the patient's BP for hypotension and respirations for dyspnea.
• Assess the patient's pulse for rate and quality, and for bradycardia.
• Evaluate the patient for signs and symptoms of CHF, including distended neck veins, dyspnea (particularly on exertion or lying down), night cough, and peripheral edema.
• Monitor the patient's intake and output and weight. An increase in weight or a decrease in urine output may indicate CHF.
• Expect the therapeutic response to hypertension to be noted in 1 to 2 weeks.

Patient Teaching

• Caution the patient against discontinuing the drug. Stress to the patient that compliance with the therapy regimen is essential to control arrhythmias and hypertension.
• Instruct the patient that if a dose is missed, he or she should take the next scheduled dose and should not double the dose.
• Teach the patient to rise slowly from a lying to a sitting position and to wait momentarily before standing to avoid the drug's hypotensive effect.
• Warn the patient to notify the physician if he or she experiences dizziness or excessive fatigue.
• Advise the patient not to take nasal decongestants and OTC cold preparations, especially those containing stimulants, without physician approval.
• Warn the patient not to perform tasks that require mental alertness or motor skills until his or her response to the drug has been established.
• Instruct outpatients to monitor their BP and pulse before taking the medication.
• Urge the patient to limit alcohol and salt intake.

nadolol

nay-**doe**-lole
(Apo-Nadol[CAN], Corgard, Novo-Nadolol[CAN])

CATEGORY AND SCHEDULE

Pregnancy Risk Category: C (D if used in second or third trimester)

MECHANISM OF ACTION

A nonselective beta-blocker that blocks $beta_1$- and $beta_2$-adrenergic receptors. Large doses increase airway resistance. **Therapeutic Effect:** Slows sinus heart rate, decreases cardiac output and BP. Decreases myocardial ischemia severity by decreasing oxygen requirements.

AVAILABILITY

Tablets: 20 mg, 40 mg, 80 mg, 120 mg, 160 mg.

INDICATIONS AND DOSAGES

▸ **Mild to moderate hypertension, angina**

PO

Adults. Initially, 40 mg/day. May increase by 40–80 mg at 3- to 7-day intervals. Maximum: 240–360 mg/day.

Elderly. Initially, 20 mg/day. May increase gradually. Range: 20–240 mg/day.

▸ **Dosage in renal impairment**

Dosage is modified based on creatinine clearance.

Creatinine Clearance	% Usual Dosage
10–50 ml/min	50
less than 10 ml/min	25

OFF-LABEL USES

Treatment of arrhythmias, hypertrophic cardiomyopathy, MI, mitral valve prolapse syndrome, neuroleptic-induced akathisia, pheochromocytoma, tremors, thyrotoxicosis, vascular headaches

CONTRAINDICATIONS

Bronchial asthma, cardiogenic shock, CHF secondary to tachyarrhythmias, COPD, patients receiving MAOI therapy, second- or third-degree heart block, sinus bradycardia, uncontrolled cardiac failure

INTERACTIONS

Drug

Cimetidine: May increase nadolol blood concentration.
Diuretics, other antihypertensives: May increase hypotensive effect.
Insulin, oral hypoglycemics: May mask symptoms of hypoglycemia and prolong the hypoglycemic effect of insulin and oral hypoglycemics.
NSAIDs: May decrease antihypertensive effect.
Sympathomimetics, xanthines: May mutually inhibit effects.

Herbal

None known.

Food

None known.

DIAGNOSTIC TEST EFFECTS

May increase serum antinuclear antibody titer and BUN, serum LDH, serum lipoprotein, serum alkaline phosphatase, serum bilirubin, serum creatinine, serum potassium, serum uric acid, AST (SGOT), ALT (SGPT), and serum triglyceride levels.

SIDE EFFECTS

Nadolol is generally well tolerated, with transient and mild side effects.

Frequent

Diminished sexual ability, drowsiness, unusual fatigue or weakness

Occasional

Bradycardia, difficulty breathing, depression, cold hands or feet, diarrhea, constipation, anxiety, nasal congestion, nausea, vomiting

Rare

Altered taste, dry eyes, itching

SERIOUS REACTIONS

! Overdose may produce profound bradycardia and hypotension.
! Abrupt withdrawal of nadolol may result in diaphoresis, palpitations, headache, tremors, exacerbation of angina, MI, and ventricular arrhythmias.
! Nadolol administration may precipitate CHF and MI in patients with cardiac disease; thyroid storm in those with thyrotoxicosis; and peripheral ischemia in those with existing peripheral vascular disease.
! Hypoglycemia may occur in patients with previously controlled diabetes.

NURSING CONSIDERATIONS

Baseline Assessment

- Assess the patient's baseline hepatic and renal function test results.
- Assess the patient's apical pulse and BP immediately before giving nadolol. If the patient's pulse rate is 60 beats/minute or lower, or systolic BP is less than 90 mm Hg, withhold the medication and contact the physician.
- Record the onset, type (sharp, dull, or squeezing), radiation, location, intensity, and duration of anginal pain and its precipitating factors, such as exertion and emotional stress.

Precautions

- Use nadolol cautiously in patients with diabetes mellitus, hyperthyroidism, impaired hepatic or renal function, or inadequate cardiac function.

Administration and Handling

PO

- Give nadolol without regard to meals.
- Tablets may be crushed.

Intervention and Evaluation

- Monitor the patient's BP for hypotension and respiration for dyspnea.
- Assess the patient's pulse for rate and quality, and for bradycardia.
- Assess the patient's hands and feet for coldness, numbness, and tingling.
- Evaluate the patient for signs and symptoms of CHF, including dis-

tended neck veins, dyspnea (particularly on exertion or lying down), night cough, and peripheral edema.
• Monitor the patient's intake and output and weight. An increase in weight or a decrease in urine output may indicate CHF.

Patient Teaching

• Caution the patient against abruptly discontinuing the drug because this action may precipitate angina.
• Warn the patient to notify the physician if he or she experiences confusion, depression, difficulty breathing, dizziness, fever, night cough, rash, slow pulse, sore throat, swelling of arms and legs, or unusual bleeding or bruising.
• Advise the patient to avoid tasks that require mental alertness or motor skills until his or her response to the drug has been established.

propranolol hydrochloride ⚑

proe-**pran**-oh-lole
(Apo-Propranolol[CAN], Deralin[AUS], Inderal, Inderal LA, InnoPran XL, Nu-Propranolol [CAN], Propranolol Intensol)
Do not confuse Inderal with Adderall or Isordil, or propranolol with Pravachol.

CATEGORY AND SCHEDULE

Pregnancy Risk Category: C (D if used in second or third trimester)

MECHANISM OF ACTION

An antihypertensive, antianginal, antiarrhythmic, and antimigraine agent that blocks $beta_1$- and $beta_2$-adrenergic receptors. Decreases oxygen requirements. Slows AV conduction and increases refractory period in AV node. Large doses increase airway resistance.
Therapeutic Effect: Slows sinus heart rate; decreases cardiac output, BP, and myocardial ischemia severity. Exhibits antiarrhythmic activity.

PHARMACOKINETICS

Route	Onset	Peak	Duration
PO	1–2 hr	N/A	6 hr

Well absorbed from the GI tract. Protein binding: 93%. Widely distributed. Metabolized in the liver. Primarily excreted in urine. Not removed by hemodialysis. ***Half-life:*** 3–5 hr.

AVAILABILITY

Tablets (Inderal): 10 mg, 20 mg, 40 mg, 60 mg, 80 mg.
Capsules (Extended-Release [Inderal LA]): 60 mg, 80 mg, 120 mg, 160 mg.
Capsules (Extended-Release [InnoPran XL]): 80 mg, 120 mg.
Oral Solution (Inderal): 4 mg/ml.
Oral Concentrate (Propranolol Intensol): 80 mg/ml.
Injection (Inderal): 1 mg/ml.

INDICATIONS AND DOSAGES

▸ **Hypertension**

PO

Adults, Elderly. Initially, 40 mg twice a day. May increase dose q3–7 days. Range: Up to 320 mg/day in divided doses. Maximum: 640 mg/day.
Children. Initially, 0.5–1 mg/kg/day in divided doses q6–12h. May increase at 3- to 5-day intervals. Usual dose: 1–5 mg/kg/day. Maximum: 16 mg/kg/day.

▸ **Angina**

PO

Adults, Elderly. 80–320 mg/day in

divided doses. (long acting): Initially, 80 mg/day. Maximum: 320 mg/day.

▸ **Arrhythmias**

IV

Adults, Elderly. 1 mg/dose. May repeat q5min. Maximum: 5 mg total dose.

Children. 0.01–0.1 mg/kg. Maximum: infants, 1 mg; children, 3 mg.

PO

Adults, Elderly. Initially, 10–20 mg q6–8h. May gradually increase dose. Range: 40–320 mg/day.

Children. Initially, 0.5–1 mg/kg/day in divided doses q6–8h. May increase q3–5 days. Usual dosage: 2–4 mg/kg/day. Maximum: 16 mg/kg/day or 60 mg/day.

▸ **Life-threatening arrhythmias**

IV

Adults, Elderly. 0.5–3 mg. Repeat once in 2 min. Give additional doses at intervals of at least 4 hr.

Children. 0.01–0.1 mg/kg.

▸ **Hypertrophic subaortic stenosis**

PO

Adults, Elderly. 20–40 mg in 3–4 divided doses. Or 80–160 mg/day as extended-release capsule.

▸ **Adjunct to alpha-blocking agents to treat pheochromocytoma**

PO

Adults, Elderly. 60 mg/day in divided doses with alpha-blocker for 3 days before surgery. Maintenance (inoperable tumor): 30 mg/day with alpha-blocker.

▸ **Migraine headache**

PO

Adults, Elderly. 80 mg/day in divided doses. Or 80 mg once daily as extended-release capsule. Increase up to 160–240 mg/day in divided doses.

Children. 0.6–1.5 mg/kg/day in divided doses q8h. Maximum: 4 mg/kg/day.

▸ **Reduction of cardiovascular mortality and reinfarction in patients with previous MI**

PO

Adults, Elderly. 180–240 mg/day in divided doses.

▸ **Essential tremor**

PO

Adults, Elderly. Initially, 40 mg twice a day increased up to 120–320 mg/day in 3 divided doses.

OFF-LABEL USES

Treatment adjunct for anxiety, mitral valve prolapse syndrome, thyrotoxicosis

CONTRAINDICATIONS

Asthma, bradycardia, cardiogenic shock, COPD, heart block, Raynaud's syndrome, uncompensated CHF

INTERACTIONS

Drug

Diuretics, other antihypertensives: May increase hypotensive effect.

Insulin, oral hypoglycemics: May mask symptoms of hypoglycemia and prolong the hypoglycemic effect of insulin and oral hypoglycemics.

IV phenytoin: May increase cardiac depressant effect.

NSAIDs: May decrease antihypertensive effect.

Sympathomimetics, xanthines: May mutually inhibit effects.

Herbal

None known.

Food

None known.

DIAGNOSTIC TEST EFFECTS

May increase serum antinuclear antibody titer and BUN, serum LDH, serum lipoprotein, serum alkaline phosphatase, serum bilirubin, serum creatinine, serum potassium, serum uric acid, AST (SGOT), ALT (SGPT), and serum triglyceride levels.

IV INCOMPATIBILITIES

Amphotericin B complex (Abelcet, AmBisome, Amphotec)

IV COMPATIBILITIES

Alteplase (Activase), heparin, milrinone (Primacor), potassium chloride, propofol (Diprivan)

SIDE EFFECTS

Frequent

Diminished sexual ability, drowsiness, difficulty sleeping, unusual fatigue or weakness

Occasional

Bradycardia, depression, sensation of coldness in extremities, diarrhea, constipation, anxiety, nasal congestion, nausea, vomiting

Rare

Altered taste, dry eyes, pruritus, paraesthesia

SERIOUS REACTIONS

! Overdose may produce profound bradycardia and hypotension.

! Abrupt withdrawal may result in sweating, palpitations, headache, and tremors.

! Propranolol administration may precipitate CHF and MI in patients with cardiac disease; thyroid storm in those with thyrotoxicosis; and peripheral ischemia in those with existing peripheral vascular disease.

! Hypoglycemia may occur in patients with previously controlled diabetes.

NURSING CONSIDERATIONS

Baseline Assessment

• Assess the patient's baseline hepatic and renal function test results.
• Assess the patient's apical pulse and BP immediately before giving propranolol. If the patient's pulse rate is 60 beats/minute or lower or systolic BP is less than 90 mm Hg, withhold the medication and contact the physician.
• Document the onset, type (sharp, dull, or squeezing), radiation, location, intensity, and duration of the patient's anginal pain and its precipitating factors, such as exertion and emotional stress.

Lifespan Considerations

• Propranolol crosses the placenta and is distributed in breast milk.
• Propranolol use should be avoided in pregnant women after the first trimester because it may result in low-birth-weight infants. The drug may also produce apnea, bradycardia, hypoglycemia, and hypothermia during childbirth.
• No age-related precautions have been noted in children.
• In the elderly, age-related peripheral vascular disease may increase susceptibility to decreased peripheral circulation.

Precautions

• Use propranolol cautiously in patients who are also receiving calcium channel blockers, especially when giving propranolol IV.
• Use cautiously in patients with diabetes or hepatic or renal impairment.

Administration and Handling

PO

• Crush scored tablets if necessary.
• Give at same time each day.

IV

• Store at room temperature.
• Give undiluted for IV push.
• For IV infusion, may dilute each 1 mg in 10 ml D_5W.
• Do not exceed 1 mg/minute injection rate.
• For IV infusion, give 1 mg over 10 to 15 minutes.

Intervention and Evaluation

- Assess the patient's pulse for bradycardia and an irregular rate and EKG for arrhythmias.
- Examine the patient's fingers for lack of color and numbness, which may indicate Raynaud's syndrome.
- Evaluate the patient for signs and symptoms of CHF, including distended neck veins, dyspnea (particularly on exertion or lying down), night cough, and peripheral edema.
- Monitor the patient's intake and output and weight. An increase in weight or a decrease in urine output may indicate CHF.
- Assess the patient for behavioral changes, fatigue, and rash.
- The therapeutic response ranges from a few days to several weeks.
- Measure the patient's BP near the end of the dosing interval to determine if BP is controlled throughout the day.

Patient Teaching

- Caution the patient against discontinuing the drug. Stress to the patient that compliance with the therapy regimen is essential to control anginal pain, arrhythmias, and hypertension.
- Instruct the patient that if a dose is missed he or she should take the next scheduled dose and should not double the dose.
- Teach the patient to rise slowly from a lying to sitting position, and wait momentarily before standing, to avoid the drug's hypotensive effect.
- Advise the patient not to take nasal decongestants and OTC cold preparations, especially those containing stimulants, without physician approval.
- Urge the patient to limit alcohol and salt intake.
- Advise the patient to avoid tasks that require mental alertness or motor skills until his or her response to the drug is established.
- Warn the patient to report dizziness, excessively slow pulse rate (less than 60 beats/minute), or peripheral numbness.

sotalol hydrochloride

soe-ta-lole

(Apo-Sotalol[CAN], Betapace, Betapace AF, Cardol[AUS], Novo-Sotalol[CAN], PMS-Sotalol[CAN], Solavert[AUS], Sorine, Sotab[AUS], Sotacor[AUS], Sotahexal[AUS])

Do not confuse sotalol with Stadol.

CATEGORY AND SCHEDULE

Pregnancy Risk Category: B (D if used in second or third trimester)

MECHANISM OF ACTION

A beta-adrenergic blocking agent that prolongs action potential, effective refractory period, and QT interval. Decreases heart rate and AV node conduction; increases AV node refractoriness. **Therapeutic Effect:** Produces antiarrhythmic activity.

PHARMACOKINETICS

Well absorbed from the GI tract. Protein binding: None. Widely distributed. Primarily excreted unchanged in urine. Removed by hemodialysis. ***Half-life:*** 12 hr (increased in the elderly and patients with impaired renal function).

AVAILABILITY

Tablets (Betapace): 80 mg, 120 mg, 160 mg, 240 mg.
Tablets (Betapace AF): 80 mg, 120 mg, 160 mg.

Tablets (Sorine): 80 mg, 120 mg, 160 mg, 240 mg.

INDICATIONS AND DOSAGES

▸ Documented, life-threatening arrhythmias

PO

Adults, Elderly. Initially, 80 mg twice a day. May increase gradually at 2- to 3-day intervals. Range: 240–320 mg/day.

▸ Dosage in renal impairment

Dosage interval is modified based on creatinine clearance.

Creatinine Clearance	Dosage Interval
31–60 ml/min	24 hr
10–30 ml/min	36–48 hr
less than 10 ml/min	Individualized

OFF-LABEL USES

Maintenance of normal heart rhythm in chronic or recurring atrial fibrillation or flutter; treatment of anxiety, chronic angina pectoris, hypertension, hypertrophic cardiomyopathy, MI, mitral valve prolapse syndrome, pheochromocytoma, thyrotoxicosis, tremors

CONTRAINDICATIONS

Bronchial asthma, cardiogenic shock, prolonged QT syndrome (unless functioning pacemaker is present), second- and third-degree heart block, sinus bradycardia, uncontrolled cardiac failure

INTERACTIONS

Drug

Antiarrhythmics, phenothiazine, tricyclic antidepressants: May prolong QT interval.

Calcium channel blockers: May increase effect on AV conduction and BP.

Clonidine: May potentiate rebound hypertension after clonidine is discontinued.

Digoxin: May increase risk of proarrhythmias.

Insulin, oral hypoglycemics: May mask signs of hypoglycemia and prolong the effects of insulin and oral hypoglycemics.

Sympathomimetics: May inhibit the effects of sympathomimetics.

Herbal

None known.

Food

None known.

DIAGNOSTIC TEST EFFECTS

May increase blood glucose, serum alkaline phosphatase, serum LDH, serum lipoprotein, AST (SGOT), ALT (SGPT), and serum triglyceride levels.

SIDE EFFECTS

Frequent

Diminished sexual function, drowsiness, insomnia, unusual fatigue or weakness

Occasional

Depression, cold hands or feet, diarrhea, constipation, anxiety, nasal congestion, nausea, vomiting

Rare

Altered taste, dry eyes, itching, numbness of fingers, toes, or scalp

SERIOUS REACTIONS

! Bradycardia, CHF, hypotension, bronchospasm, hypoglycemia, prolonged QT interval, torsades de pointes, ventricular tachycardia, and premature ventricular complexes may occur.

NURSING CONSIDERATIONS

Baseline Assessment

• As ordered, institute continuous cardiac monitoring when beginning sotalol therapy. If the patient's pulse rate is 60 beats/minute or less, consult the physician before beginning sotalol therapy.

Lifespan Considerations

• Sotalol crosses the placenta and is excreted in breast milk.
• The safety and efficacy of sotalol have not been established in children.
• In the elderly, age-related peripheral vascular disease may increase susceptibility to decreased peripheral circulation.

Precautions

• Use sotalol cautiously in patients with cardiomegaly, CHF, diabetes mellitus, excessive QT-interval prolongation, history of ventricular tachycardia, hypokalemia, hypomagnesemia, severe and prolonged diarrhea, sick sinus syndrome, or ventricular fibrillation.
• Use cautiously in patients at risk for developing thyrotoxicosis.

Administration and Handling

◀ **ALERT** ▶ Some patients may require 480–640 mg/day. Sotalol has a long half-life and administering the drug more than 2 times a day is usually not necessary. Avoid abrupt withdrawal.

PO
• Give sotalol without regard to food.

Intervention and Evaluation

• Diligently monitor the patient for arrhythmias.
• Assess the patient's BP for hypotension and pulse for bradycardia.
• Evaluate the patient for signs and symptoms of CHF, including decreased urine output, distended neck veins, dyspnea, jugular vein distention, peripheral edema, rales in lungs, and weight gain.

Patient Teaching

• Caution the patient against abruptly discontinuing the drug without physician approval.
• Warn the patient to avoid tasks that require mental alertness or motor skills until his or her response to the drug has been established.
• Explain to the patient that periodic laboratory tests and EKGs are a necessary part of therapy.

timolol maleate

tim-oh-lole
(Apo-Timol[CAN], Apo-Timop[CAN], Betimol, Blocadren, Gen-Timolol[CAN], Istadol, Optimol[AUS], PMS-Timolol [CAN], Tenopt[AUS], Timoptic, Timoptic OccuDose, Timoptic XE, Timoptol[AUS], Timoptol XE [AUS])

Do not confuse timolol with atenolol, or Timoptic with Viroptic.

CATEGORY AND SCHEDULE

Pregnancy Risk Category: C (D if used in second or third trimester)

MECHANISM OF ACTION

An antihypertensive, antimigraine, and antiglaucoma agent that blocks $beta_1$- and $beta_2$-adrenergic receptors. **Therapeutic Effect:** Reduces intraocular pressure (IOP) by reducing aqueous humor production, lowers BP, slows the heart rate, and decreases myocardial contractility.

PHARMACOKINETICS

Route	Onset	Peak	Duration
PO	15–45 min	0.5–2.5 hr	4 hr
Ophthalmic	30 min	1–2 hr	12–24 hr

Well absorbed from the GI tract. Protein binding: 60%. Minimal absorption after ophthalmic administration. Metabolized in the liver. Primarily excreted in urine. Not removed by hemodialysis. ***Half-life:*** 4 hr. Systemic absorption may occur with ophthalmic administration.

AVAILABILITY

Tablets (Blocadren): 5 mg, 10 mg, 20 mg.
Ophthalmic Gel (Timoptic-XE): 0.25%, 0.5%.
Ophthalmic Solution (Betimol, Timoptic, Timoptic OccuDose): 0.25%, 0.5%.

INDICATIONS AND DOSAGES

▸ Mild to moderate hypertension
PO
Adults, Elderly. Initially, 10 mg twice a day, alone or in combination with other therapy. Gradually increase at intervals of not less than 1 wk. Maintenance: 20–60 mg/day in 2 divided doses.

▸ Reduction of cardiovascular mortality in definite or suspected acute MI
PO
Adults, Elderly. 10 mg twice a day, beginning 1–4 wk after infarction.

▸ Migraine prevention
PO
Adults, Elderly. Initially, 10 mg twice a day. Range: 10–30 mg/day.

▸ Reduction of IOP in open-angle glaucoma, aphakic glaucoma, ocular hypertension, and secondary glaucoma
Ophthalmic
Adults, Elderly, Children. 1 drop of 0.25% solution in affected eye(s) twice a day. May be increased to 1 drop of 0.5% solution in affected eye(s) twice a day. When IOP is controlled, dosage may be reduced to 1 drop once a day. If patient is switched to timolol from another antiglaucoma agent, administer concurrently for 1 day. Discontinue other agent on following day.
Ophthalmic (Timoptic XE)
Adults, Elderly. 1 drop/day.
Ophthalmic (Istalol)
Adults, Elderly. Apply once daily.

OFF-LABEL USES

Systemic: Treatment of anxiety, cardiac arrhythmias, chronic angina pectoris, hypertrophic cardiomyopathy, migraine, pheochromocytoma, thyrotoxicosis, tremors
Ophthalmic: To decrease IOP in acute or chronic angle-closure glaucoma, treatment of angle-closure glaucoma during and after iridectomy, malignant glaucoma, secondary glaucoma

CONTRAINDICATIONS

Bronchial asthma, cardiogenic shock, CHF unless secondary to tachyarrhythmias, COPD, patients receiving MAOI therapy, second- or third-degree heart block, sinus bradycardia, uncontrolled cardiac failure

INTERACTIONS

Drug
Diuretics, other antihypertensives: May increase hypotensive effect.
Insulin, oral hypoglycemics: May mask symptoms of hypoglycemia and prolong hypoglycemic effects of these drugs.
NSAIDs: May decrease antihypertensive effect.
Sympathomimetics, xanthines: May mutually inhibit effects.
Herbal
None known.
Food
None known.

DIAGNOSTIC TEST EFFECTS

May increase antinuclear antibody titer and BUN, serum LDH, serum lipoprotein, serum alkaline phosphatase, serum bilirubin, serum creatinine, serum potassium, serum uric acid, AST (SGOT), ALT (SGPT), and serum triglyceride levels.

SIDE EFFECTS

Frequent

Diminished sexual function, drowsiness, difficulty sleeping, unusual tiredness or weakness

Ophthalmic: Eye irritation, visual disturbances

Occasional

Depression, cold hands or feet, diarrhea, constipation, anxiety, nasal congestion, nausea, vomiting

Rare

Altered taste, dry eyes, itching, numbness of fingers, toes, or scalp

SERIOUS REACTIONS

! Overdose may produce profound bradycardia, hypotension, and bronchospasm.

! Abrupt withdrawal may result in diaphoresis, palpitations, headache, and tremors.

! Timolol administration may precipitate CHF and MI in patients with cardiac disease; thyroid storm in those with thyrotoxicosis; and peripheral ischemia in those with existing peripheral vascular disease.

! Hypoglycemia may occur in patients with previously controlled diabetes.

! Ophthalmic overdose may produce bradycardia, hypotension, bronchospasm, and acute cardiac failure.

NURSING CONSIDERATIONS

Baseline Assessment

• Assess the patient's apical pulse and BP immediately before giving timolol. If the patient's pulse rate is 60 beats/minute or lower or systolic BP is less than 90 mm Hg, withhold the medication and contact the physician.

Lifespan Considerations

• Timolol is distributed in breast milk and is not for use in breast-feeding women because of the potential for serious adverse effects in the breast-fed infant.

• Timolol use should be avoided in pregnant women after the first trimester because it may result in low-birth-weight infants. The drug may also produce apnea, bradycardia, hypoglycemia, or hypothermia during childbirth.

• The safety and efficacy of timolol have not been established in children.

• In the elderly, age-related peripheral vascular disease increases susceptibility to decreased peripheral circulation.

Precautions

• Use timolol cautiously in patients with hyperthyroidism, impaired hepatic or renal function, or inadequate cardiac function. Precautions apply to both oral and ophthalmic administration because of the possible systemic absorption of ophthalmic timolol.

Administration and Handling

PO

• Give timolol without regard to meals.

• Tablets may be crushed.

Ophthalmic

◀ALERT▶ When administering gel, invert container and shake once before each use.

• For ophthalmic administration, place a gloved finger on the patient's lower eyelid and pull it out until pocket is formed between the eye and lower lid. Hold the dropper above the pocket and place the prescribed number of drops or amount of prescribed gel into pocket. Instruct the patient to close eyes gently so that medication will not be squeezed out of the sac. Apply gentle digital pressure to the patient's lacrimal sac at the inner canthus for 1 minute after installation to lessen the risk of systemic absorption.

Intervention and Evaluation

- Assess the patient's pulse for rate and quality, and for bradycardia.
- Monitor the patient's EKG for arrhythmias, particularly premature ventricular contractions.
- Assess the patient's pattern of daily bowel activity and stool consistency.
- Monitor the patient's BP, heart rate, IOP (with ophthalmic preparation), and liver and renal function test results.

Patient Teaching

- Caution the patient against abruptly discontinuing timolol. Stress that compliance with the therapy regimen is essential to control angina, arrhythmias, glaucoma, and hypertension.
- Advise the patient to avoid tasks that require mental alertness or motor skills until his or her response to the drug has been established.
- Warn the patient to notify the physician if he or she experiences excessive fatigue, prolonged dizziness or headache, or shortness of breath.
- Advise the patient not to use nasal decongestants and OTC cold preparations, especially those containing stimulants, without physician approval.
- Urge the patient to limit alcohol and salt intake.
- Teach the patient using the ophthalmic form the correct way to instill drops and obtain his or her pulse. Advise the patient that transient discomfort or stinging may occur upon instillation.

26 Calcium Channel Blockers

amlodipine
diltiazem hydrochloride
felodipine
isradipine
nicardipine hydrochloride
nifedipine
nimodipine
verapamil hydrochloride

Uses: Calcium channel blockers are used to treat essential hypertension, to prevent and treat angina pectoris (including vasospastic, chronic stable, and unstable forms), to prevent and control supraventricular tachyarrhythmias, and to prevent neurologic damage caused by subarachnoid hemorrhage.

Action: Calcium channel blockers inhibit the flow of extracellular calcium ions across cell membranes in cardiac and vascular tissue. They relax arterial smooth muscle, depress the rate of firing in the sinus node (the heart's normal pacemaker), slow AV conduction, and decrease the heart rate. Although they also produce negative inotropic effects, these effects are rarely seen clinically because of the reflex response. Calcium channel blockers decrease coronary vascular resistance, increase coronary blood flow, and reduce myocardial oxygen demand. The degree of action varies with the specific drug.

COMBINATION PRODUCTS

CADUET: amlodipine/atorvastatin (an HMG-CoA reductase inhibitor) 5 mg/10mg; 10 mg/10 mg; 5 mg/20 mg; 10 mg/20 mg; 5 mg/40 mg; 10 mg/40 mg; 5 mg/80 mg; 10 mg/80 mg.
LEXXEL: felodipine/enalapril (an ACE inhibitor) 2.5 mg/5 mg; 5 mg/5 mg.
LOTREL: amlodipine/benazepril (an ACE inhibitor) 2.5 mg/10 mg; 5 mg/10 mg; 5 mg/20 mg; 10 mg/20 mg.
TARKA: verapamil/trandolapril (an ACE inhibitor) 240 mg/1 mg; 180 mg/2 mg; 240 mg/2 mg; 240 mg/4 mg.
TECZEM: diltiazem/enalapril (an ACE inhibitor) 180 mg/5 mg.

amlodipine

am-**low**-di-peen
(Norvasc)
Do not confuse amlodipine with amiloride, or Norvasc with Navane or Vascor.

CATEGORY AND SCHEDULE

Pregnancy Risk Category: C

MECHANISM OF ACTION

A calcium channel blocker that inhibits calcium movement across cardiac and vascular smooth-muscle cell membranes. **Therapeutic Effect:** Relieves angina by dilating coronary arteries, peripheral arteries, and arterioles. Decreases total peripheral vascular resistance and BP by vasodilation.

PHARMACOKINETICS

Route	Onset	Peak	Duration
PO	0.5–1 hr	6–12 hr	24 hr

Slowly absorbed from the GI tract. Protein binding: 93%. Undergoes first-pass metabolism in the liver. Excreted primarily in urine. Not removed by hemodialysis. ***Half-life:*** 30–50 hr (increased in the elderly and those with liver cirrhosis).

AVAILABILITY

Tablets: 2.5 mg, 5 mg, 10 mg.

INDICATIONS AND DOSAGES

▸ **Hypertension**

PO

Adults. Initially, 5 mg/day as a single dose. Maximum: 10 mg/day.
Small-Frame, Fragile, Elderly. Initially, 2.5 mg/day as a single dose.

▸ **Angina (chronic stable or vasospastic)**

PO

Adults. 5–10 mg/day as a single dose.
Elderly, Patients with hepatic insufficiency: 5 mg/day as a single dose.

▸ **Dosage in renal impairment**

For adults and elderly patients, give 2.5 mg/day.

CONTRAINDICATIONS

Severe hypotension

INTERACTIONS

Drug

None known.

Herbal

None known.

Food

Grapefruit, grapefruit juice: May increase amlodipine blood concentration and hypotensive effects.

DIAGNOSTIC TEST EFFECTS

None known.

SIDE EFFECTS

Frequent (greater than 5%)

Peripheral edema, headache, flushing

Occasional (less than 5%)

Dizziness, palpitations, nausea, unusual fatigue or weakness (asthenia)

Rare (less than 1%)

Chest pain, bradycardia, orthostatic hypotension

SERIOUS REACTIONS

! Overdose may produce excessive peripheral vasodilation and marked hypotension with reflex tachycardia.

NURSING CONSIDERATIONS

Baseline Assessment

• Assess the patient's apical pulse, BP, and renal and hepatic function test results.

Lifespan Considerations

• It is unknown if amlodipine crosses the placenta or is distributed in breast milk.
• The safety and efficacy of amlodipine have not been established in children.
• The elderly are more sensitive to amlodipine's hypotensive effects and its half-life may be increased in the elderly.

Precautions

• Use amlodipine cautiously in patients with aortic stenosis, CHF, and impaired hepatic function.

Administration and Handling

PO

◂ **ALERT** ▸ Expect to increase amlodipine dosage slowly over 7 to 14 days based on the patient's response.
• Amlodipine may given without regard to food.
• Avoid giving drug with grapefruit

juice, which may increase amlodipine blood concentration.

Intervention and Evaluation

- Assess the patient's BP. If the patient's systolic BP is less than 90 mm Hg, withhold the medication and notify the physician .
- Assess the patient's skin for flushing and peripheral edema, especially behind the medial malleolus and the sacral area.
- Determine if the patient is experiencing asthenia or headache.

Patient Teaching

- Caution the patient against abruptly discontinuing amlodipine. Explain that compliance with therapy is essential to control hypertension.
- Warn the patient to avoid tasks that require alertness and motor skills until his or her response to the drug has been established.
- Urge the patient to avoid drinking grapefruit juice while taking this drug.

diltiazem hydrochloride

dil-**tye**-a-zem

(Apo-Diltiaz[CAN], Auscard[AUS], Cardcal[AUS], Cardizem, Cardizem CD, Cardizem LA, Cardizem SR, Cartia, Coras [AUS], Dilacor XR, Diltahexal[AUS], Diltia XT, Diltiamax[AUS], Dilzem[AUS], Novo-Diltiazem[CAN], Taztia XT, Tiazac, Vasocardal CD[AUS])

Do not confuse Cardizem with Cardene or Cardene SR, or Tiazac with Ziac.

CATEGORY AND SCHEDULE

Pregnancy Risk Category: C

MECHANISM OF ACTION

An antianginal, antihypertensive, and antiarrhythmic agent that inhibits calcium movement across cardiac and vascular smooth-muscle cell membranes. This action causes the dilation of coronary arteries, peripheral arteries, and arterioles. **Therapeutic Effect:** Decreases heart rate and myocardial contractility, slows SA and AV conduction and decreases total peripheral vascular resistance by vasodilation.

PHARMACOKINETICS

Route	Onset	Peak	Duration
PO	0.5–1 hr	N/A	N/A
PO (extended-release)	2–3 hr	N/A	N/A
IV	3 min	N/A	N/A

Well absorbed from the GI tract. Protein binding: 70%–80%. Undergoes first-pass metabolism in the liver to active metabolite. Primarily excreted in urine. Not removed by hemodialysis. ***Half-life:*** 3–8 hr.

AVAILABILITY

Capsules (Sustained-Release [Cardizem SR]): 60 mg, 90 mg, 120 mg.
Capsules (Extended-Release [Cardizem CD]): 120 mg, 180 mg, 240 mg, 300 mg, 360 mg.
Capsules (Extended-Release [Cartia XT]): 120 mg, 180 mg, 240 mg, 300 mg.
Capsules (Extended-Release [Dilacor XR]) 120 mg, 180 mg, 240 mg.
Capsules (Extended-Release [Diltia XT]): 120 mg, 180 mg, 240 mg.
Capsules (Extended-Release [Taztia XT]): 120 mg, 180 mg, 240 mg, 300 mg, 360 mg.
Caspules (Extended-Release [Tiazac]): 120 mg, 180 mg, 240 mg, 300 mg, 360 mg, 420 mg.
Tablets (Cardizem): 30 mg, 60 mg, 90 mg, 120 mg.

Tablets (Extended-Release [Cardizem LA]): 120 mg, 180 mg, 240 mg, 300 mg, 360 mg, 420 mg.
Injection (Ready-to-Hang Infusion): 1 mg/ml.

INDICATIONS AND DOSAGES

▸ Angina related to coronary artery spasm (Prinzmetal's variant), chronic stable angina (effort-associated)

PO
Adults, Elderly. Initially, 30 mg 4 times a day. Increase up to 180–360 mg/day in 3–4 divided doses at 1- to 2-day intervals.
PO (Cardizem LA)
Adults, Elderly. Initially, 180 mg/day. May increase at intervals of 7–14 days up to 360 mg/day.
PO (Cardizem CD)
Adults, Elderly. Initially, 120–180 mg/day; titrate over 7–14 days. Range: Up to 480 mg/day.

▸ Essential hypertension

PO (Cardizem CD, Cartia XT)
Adults, Elderly. Initially, 180–240 mg once a day. May increase at 2 week intervals. Maintenance 240–360 mg/day. Maximum: 480 mg once a day.
PO (Cardizem SR)
Adults, Elderly. Initially, 60–120 mg twice a day. May increase at 2 week intervals. Maintenance: 240–360 mg/day.
PO (Cardizem LA)
Adults, Elderly. Initially, 180–240 mg once a day. May increase at 2 week intervals. Maintenance: 120–540 mg/day.
PO (Dilacor XR)
Adults, Elderly. 180–240 mg once a day.
PO (Dilacor XT)
Adults, Elderly. Initially, 180–240 mg a day. May increase at 2 week intervals. Maximum: 540 mg once a day.
PO (Taztia XT)
Adults, Elderly. Initially, 120–240 mg once a day. May increase at 2 week intervals. Maximum: 540 mg once a day.

▸ Temporary control of rapid ventricular rate in atrial fibrillation or flutter, rapid conversion of paroxysmal supraventricular tachycardia to normal sinus rhythm.

IV Push
Adults, Elderly. Initially, 0.25 mg/kg actual body weight over 2 min. May repeat in 15 min at dose of 0.35 mg/kg actual body weight. Subsequent doses individualized.
IV Infusion
Adults, Elderly. After initial bolus injection, may begin infusion at 5–10 mg/hr; may increase by 5 mg/hr up to a maximum of 15 mg/hr. Infusion duration should not exceed 24 hr.

CONTRAINDICATIONS

Acute MI, pulmonary congestion, severe hypotension (less than 90 mm Hg, systolic), sick sinus syndrome, second- or third-degree AV block (except in the presence of a pacemaker)

INTERACTIONS

Drug

Beta blockers: May have additive effect.
Carbamazepine, quinidine, theophylline: May increase diltiazem blood concentration and risk of toxicity.
Digoxin: May increase serum digoxin concentration.
Procainamide, quinidine: May increase risk of QT-interval prolongation.

Herbal

None known.

Food

None known.

DIAGNOSTIC TEST EFFECTS
PR interval may be increased.

IV INCOMPATIBILITIES
Acetazolamide (Diamox), acyclovir (Zovirax), aminophylline, ampicillin, ampicillin/sulbactam (Unasyn), cefoperazone (Cefobid), diazepam (Valium), furosemide (Lasix), heparin, insulin, nafcillin, phenytoin (Dilantin), rifampin (Rifadin), sodium bicarbonate

IV COMPATIBILITIES
Albumin, aztreonam (Azactam), bumetanide (Bumex), cefazolin (Ancef), cefotaxime (Claforan), ceftazidime (Fortaz), ceftriaxone (Rocephin), cefuroxime (Zinacef), cimetidine (Tagamet), ciprofloxacin (Cipro), clindamycin (Cleocin), digoxin (Lanoxin), dobutamine (Dobutrex), dopamine (Intropin), gentamicin (Garamycin), hydromorphone (Dilaudid), lidocaine, lorazepam (Ativan), metoclopramide (Reglan), metronidazole (Flagyl), midazolam (Versed), morphine, multivitamins, nitroglycerin, norepinephrine (Levophed), potassium chloride, potassium phosphate, tobramycin (Nebcin), vancomycin (Vancocin)

SIDE EFFECTS
Frequent (10%–5%)

Peripheral edema, dizziness, lightheadedness, headache, bradycardia, asthenia (loss of strength, weakness)

Occasional (5%–2%)

Nausea, constipation, flushing, EKG changes

Rare (less than 2%)

Rash, micturition disorder (polyuria, nocturia, dysuria, frequency of urination), abdominal discomfort, somnolence

SERIOUS REACTIONS
! Abrupt withdrawal may increase frequency or duration of angina.
! CHF and second- and third-degree AV block occur rarely.
! Overdose produces nausea, somnolence, confusion, slurred speech, and profound bradycardia.

NURSING CONSIDERATIONS
Baseline Assessment
- Concurrent sublingual nitroglycerin therapy may be used for relief of anginal pain.
- Document the onset, type (sharp, dull, or squeezing), radiation, location, intensity, and duration of anginal pain and its precipitating factors, such as exertion and emotional stress.
- Assess the patient's liver and renal function test results.
- Assess the patient's apical pulse and BP immediately before diltiazem administration.

Lifespan Considerations
- It is unclear if diltiazem crosses the placenta. It should be used during pregnancy only if the benefit to the mother outweighs the risk to the fetus. Diltiazem is distributed in breast milk.
- No age-related precautions have been noted in children.
- In the elderly, age-related renal impairment may require cautious use.

Precautions
- Use diltiazem cautiously in patients with CHF or impaired hepatic or renal function.

Administration and Handling
PO
- Give diltiazem before meals and at bedtime.
- Crush tablets as needed.
- Do not crush or open sustained-release capsules.

IV

◀ALERT▶ Refer to manufacturer's information for dose concentration and infusion rates.

- Refrigerate vials.
- After dilution, solution is stable for 24 hours.
- Add 125 mg to 100 ml D_5W or 0.9% NaCl to provide a concentration of 1 mg/ml. Add 250 mg to 250 or 500 ml diluent to provide a concentration of 0.83 mg/ml or 0.45 mg/ml, respectively. The maximum concentration is 1.25 g/250 ml or 5 mg/ml.
- Infuse per dilution or rate chart provided by manufacturer.

Intervention and Evaluation

- Assist the patient with ambulation if he or she experiences dizziness.
- Assess the patient for peripheral edema behind the medial malleolus in ambulatory patients or in the sacral area in bedridden patients.
- Monitor the patient's pulse for bradycardia.
- For patients receiving IV diltiazem, assess BP, EKG, and liver and renal function test results.
- Assess the patient for signs and symptoms of asthenia or headache.

Patient Teaching

- Caution the patient against abruptly discontinuing diltiazem. Stress to the patient that compliance with the treatment regimen is essential to control anginal pain.
- Instruct the patient to rise slowly from a lying to a sitting position and wait momentarily before standing to avoid diltiazem's hypotensive effect.
- Warn the patient to avoid tasks that require mental alertness or motor skills until his or her response to the drug has been established.
- Warn the patient to notify the physician if he or she experiences constipation, irregular heartbeat, nausea, pronounced dizziness, or shortness of breath.

felodipine

fell-**o**-da-peen

(AGON SR[AUS], Felodur ER[AUS], Plendil, Plendil ER[AUS], Renedil[CAN])

Do not confuse Plendil with Pletal, or Renedil with Prinivil.

CATEGORY AND SCHEDULE

Pregnancy Risk Category: C

MECHANISM OF ACTION

An antihypertensive and antianginal agent that inhibits calcium movement across cardiac and vascular smooth-muscle cell membranes. Potent peripheral vasodilator (does not depress SA or AV nodes). **Therapeutic Effect:** Increases myocardial contractility, heart rate, and cardiac output; decreases peripheral vascular resistance and BP.

PHARMACOKINETICS

Route	Onset	Peak	Duration
PO	2–5 hr	N/A	N/A

Rapidly, completely absorbed from the GI tract. Protein binding: greater than 99%. Undergoes first-pass metabolism in the liver. Primarily excreted in urine. Not removed by hemodialysis. ***Half-life:*** 11–16 hr.

AVAILABILITY

Tablets (Extended-Release): 2.5 mg, 5 mg, 10 mg.

INDICATIONS AND DOSAGES

▸ Hypertension

PO

Adults. Initially, 5 mg/day as single dose.

Elderly, Patients with impaired hepatic function. Initially, 2.5 mg/day. Adjust dosage at no less than 2-wk intervals. Maintenance: 2.5–10 mg/day.

OFF-LABEL USES

Treatment of CHF, chronic angina pectoris, Raynaud's phenomenon

CONTRAINDICATIONS

None known.

INTERACTIONS

Drug

Beta blockers: May have additive effect.

Digoxin: May increase digoxin blood concentration.

Erythromycin: May increase felodipine blood concentration and risk of toxicity.

Hypokalemia-producing agents (such as fursosemide and certain other diuretics): May increase risk of arrhythmias.

Procainamide, quinidine: May increase risk of QT-interval prolongation.

Herbal

DHEA: May increase felodipine blood concentration.

Food

Grapefruit, grapefruit juice: May increase the absorption and blood concentration of felodipine.

DIAGNOSTIC TEST EFFECTS

None known.

SIDE EFFECTS

Frequent (22%–18%)

Headache, peripheral edema

Occasional (6%–4%)

Flushing, respiratory infection, dizziness, light-headedness, asthenia (loss of strength, weakness)

Rare (less than 3%)

Paresthesia, abdominal discomfort, nervousness, muscle cramping, cough, diarrhea, constipation

SERIOUS REACTIONS

! Overdose produces nausea, somnolence, confusion, slurred speech, hypotension, and bradycardia.

NURSING CONSIDERATIONS

Baseline Assessment

- Assess the patient's apical pulse and BP immediately before beginning felodipine administration. If the patient's pulse rate is 60 beats/minute or lower or systolic BP is less than 90 mm Hg, withhold the medication and contact the physician.

Lifespan Considerations

- It is unknown if felodipine crosses the placenta or is distributed in breast milk.
- The safety and efficacy of felodipine drug have not been established in children.
- The elderly may experience a greater hypotensive response and constipation may be more problematic in the elderly.

Precautions

- Use felodipine cautiously in patients with CHF, edema, hepatic or renal impairment, hypertrophic cardiomyopathy, or severe left ventricular dysfunction and in those currently receiving beta-blockers or digoxin.

Administration and Handling

PO

- Give felodipine without regard to food.
- Do not crush or break tablets.

Intervention and Evaluation

- Assist the patient with ambulation if he or she experiences dizziness or light-headedness.
- Assess for peripheral edema behind the media malleolus in ambulatory patients or the sacral area in bedridden patients.
- Monitor the patient's liver function test results, and pulse for bradycardia.
- Examine the patient's skin for flushing.
- Evaluate the patient for asthenia and headache.

Patient Teaching

- Caution the patient against abruptly discontinuing felodipine. Stress that compliance with the therapy regimen is essential to control hypertension.
- Instruct the patient to rise slowly from a lying to a sitting position and wait momentarily before standing to avoid felodipine's hypotensive effect.
- Advise the patient to avoid tasks that require mental alertness or motor skills until his or her response to the drug has been established.
- Warn the patient to notify the physician if he or she experiences an irregular heartbeat, nausea, prolonged dizziness, or shortness of breath.
- Teach the patient to swallow felodipine tablets whole. Explain to the patient the he or she should not crush or chew felodipine tablets.
- Urge the patient to avoid grapefruit and grapefruit juice because these foods increase the blood concentration and effects of felodipine.

isradipine

is-**rad**-i-peen
(DynaCirc, DynaCirc CR)
Do not confuse DynaCirc with Dynabac or Dynacin.

CATEGORY AND SCHEDULE

Pregnancy Risk Category: C

MECHANISM OF ACTION

An antihypertensive that inhibits calcium movement across cardiac and vascular smooth-muscle cell membranes. Potent peripheral vasodilator that does not depress SA or AV nodes. **Therapeutic Effect:** Produces relaxation of coronary vascular smooth muscle and coronary vasodilation. Increases myocardial oxygen delivery to those with vasospastic angina.

PHARMACOKINETICS

Route	Onset	Peak	Duration
PO	2–3 hr	2–4 wk (with multiple doses) 8-16 hr (with single dose)	N/A
PO (Controlled-release)	2 hr	8-10 hr	N/A

Well absorbed from the GI tract. Protein binding: 95%. Metabolized in the liver (undergoes first-pass effect). Primarily excreted in urine. Not removed by hemodialysis. ***Half-life:*** 8 hr.

AVAILABILITY

Capsules (DynaCirc): 2.5 mg, 5 mg.

Capsules (Controlled-Release [DynaCirc-CR]): 5 mg, 10 mg.

INDICATIONS AND DOSAGES

▸ Hypertension

PO

Adults, Elderly. Initially 2.5 mg twice a day. May increase by 2.5 mg at 2- to 4-wk intervals. Range: 5–20 mg/day

OFF-LABEL USES

Treatment of chronic angina pectoris, Raynaud's phenomenon

CONTRAINDICATIONS

Cardiogenic shock, CHF, heart block, hypotension, sinus bradycardia, ventricular tachycardia

INTERACTIONS

Drug

Beta blockers: May have additive effect.

Herbal

None known.

Food

Grapefruit, grapefruit juice: May increase the absorption of isradipine.

DIAGNOSTIC TEST EFFECTS

None known.

SIDE EFFECTS

Frequent (7%–4%)

Peripheral edema, palpitations (higher frequency in females)

Occasional (3%)

Facial flushing, cough

Rare (2%–1%)

Angina, tachycardia, rash, pruritus

SERIOUS REACTIONS

! Overdose produces nausea, drowsiness, confusion, and slurred speech.

! CHF occurs rarely.

NURSING CONSIDERATIONS

Baseline Assessment

- Assess the patient's liver and renal function test results.
- Assess the patient's apical pulse and BP immediately before giving isradipine. If the patient's pulse rate is 60 beats/minute or lower or systolic BP is less than 90 mm Hg, withhold the medication and contact the physician.

Lifespan Considerations

- It is unknown if isradipine crosses the placenta or is distributed in breast milk.
- The safety and efficacy of isradipine have not been established in children.
- In the elderly, age-related renal impairment may require cautious use.

Precautions

- Use isradipine cautiously in patients with edema, hepatic disease, severe left ventricular dysfunction, or sick sinus syndrome and in those concurrently receiving beta blockers.

Administration and Handling

PO

- Do not crush, open, or break capsules.

Intervention and Evaluation

- Assess for peripheral edema behind the medial malleolus in ambulatory patients or in the sacral area in bedridden patients.
- Monitor the patient's BP for hypotension and pulse for bradycardia.
- Observe the patient for signs and symptoms of CHF and examine the patient's skin for flushing.

Patient Teaching

- Caution the patient against abruptly discontinuing isradipine. Stress that compliance with the treatment regimen is essential to control hypertension.
- Instruct the patient to rise slowly

from a lying to a sitting position and wait momentarily before standing to avoid isradipine's hypotensive effect.

- Warn the patient to notify the physician if he or she experiences an irregular heartbeat, nausea, pronounced dizziness, or shortness of breath.
- Urge the patient to avoid grapefruit and grapefruit juice because these foods may increase the absorption of isradipine.

nicardipine hydrochloride

nye-**card**-i-peen
(Cardene, Cardene IV, Cardene SR)
Do not confuse nicardipine with nifedipine, Cardene with codeine, or Cardene SR with Cardizem SR or codeine.

CATEGORY AND SCHEDULE

Pregnancy Risk Category: C

MECHANISM OF ACTION

An antianginal and antihypertensive agent that inhibits calcium ion movement across cell membranes, depressing contraction of cardiac and vascular smooth muscle. **Therapeutic Effect:** Increases heart rate and cardiac output. Decreases systemic vascular resistance and BP.

PHARMACOKINETICS

Route	Onset	Peak	Duration
PO	N/A	1–2 hr	8 hr

Rapidly, completely absorbed from the GI tract. Protein binding: 95%. Undergoes first-pass metabolism in the liver. Primarily excreted in urine. Not removed by hemodialysis. ***Half-life:*** 2–4 hr.

AVAILABILITY

Capsules (Cardene): 20 mg, 30 mg.
Capsules (Sustained-Release [Cardene SR]): 30 mg, 45 mg, 60 mg.
Injection (Cardene IV): 2.5 mg/ml.

INDICATIONS AND DOSAGES

▸ **Chronic stable (effort-associated) angina**

PO

Adults, Elderly. Initially, 20 mg 3 times a day. Range: 20–40 mg 3 times a day.

▸ **Essential hypertension**

PO

Adults, Elderly. Initially, 20 mg 3 times a day. Range: 20–40 mg 3 times a day.

PO (Sustained-Release)

Adults, Elderly. Initially, 30 mg twice a day. Range: 30–60 mg twice a day.

▸ **Short-term treatment of hypertension when oral therapy isn't feasible or desirable (substitute for oral nicardipine)**

IV

Adults, Elderly. 0.5 mg/hr (for patient receiving 20 mg PO q8h); 1.2 mg/hr (for patient receiving 30 mg PO q8h); 2.2 mg/hr (for patient receiving 40 mg PO q8h).

▸ **Patients not already receiving nicardipine**

IV

Adults, Elderly (gradual BP decrease). Initially, 5 mg/hr. May increase by 2.5 mg/hr q15min. After BP goal is achieved, decrease rate to 3 mg/hr.

Adults, Elderly (rapid BP decrease). Initially, 5 mg/hr. May increase by 2.5 mg/hr q5min. Maximum: 15 mg/hr until desired BP attained.

After BP goal achieved, decrease rate to 3 mg/hr.

▸ **Changing from IV to oral antihypertensive therapy**

Adults, Elderly. Begin antihypertensives other than nicardipine when IV has been discontinued; for nicardipine, give first dose 1 hr before discontinuing IV.

▸ **Dosage in hepatic impairment**

For adults and elderly patients, initially give 20 mg twice a day; then titrate.

▸ **Dosage in renal impairment**

For adults and elderly patients, initially give 20 mg q8h (30 mg twice a day [sustained-release capsules]); then titrate.

OFF-LABEL USES

Treatment of associated neurologic deficits, Raynaud's phenomenon, subarachnoid hemorrhage, vasospastic angina

CONTRAINDICATIONS

Atrial fibrillation or flutter associated with accessory conduction pathways, cardiogenic shock, CHF, second- or third-degree heart block, severe hypotension, sinus bradycardia, ventricular tachycardia, within several hours of IV beta-blocker therapy

INTERACTIONS

Drug

Beta blockers: May have additive effect.

Digoxin: May increase nicardipine blood concentration.

Hypokalemia-producing agents (such as furosemide and certain other diuretics): May increase risk of arrhythmias.

Procainamide, quinidine: May increase risk of QT-interval prolongation.

Herbal

None known.

Food

Grapefruit, grapefruit juice: May alter absorption of nicardipine.

DIAGNOSTIC TEST EFFECTS

None known.

IV INCOMPATIBILITIES

Furosemide (Lasix), heparin, thiopental (Pentothal)

IV COMPATIBILITIES

Diltiazem (Cardizem), dobutamine (Dobutrex), dopamine (Intropin), epinephrine, hydromorphone (Dilaudid), labetalol (Trandate), lorazepam (Ativan), midazolam (Versed), milrinone (Primacor), morphine, nitroglycerin, norepinephrine (Levophed)

SIDE EFFECTS

Frequent (10%–7%)

Headache, facial flushing, peripheral edema, light-headedness, dizziness

Occasional (6%–3%)

Asthenia (loss of strength, energy), palpitations, angina, tachycardia

Rare (less than 2%)

Nausea, abdominal cramps, dyspepsia, dry mouth, rash

SERIOUS REACTIONS

! Overdose produces confusion, slurred speech, somnolence, marked hypotension, and bradycardia.

NURSING CONSIDERATIONS

Baseline Assessment

- Concurrent administration of sublingual nitroglycerin therapy may be used for relief of anginal pain.
- Record the onset, type (sharp, dull, or squeezing), radiation, location, intensity, and duration of anginal pain and its precipitating factors,

such as exertion and emotional stress.

Lifespan Considerations

• It is unclear if nicardipine crosses the placenta. It should only be administered when the benefit to the mother exceeds the risk to the fetus. It is unknown if nicardipine is distributed in breast milk.

• The safety and efficacy of nicardipine have not been established in children.

• In the elderly, age-related renal impairment may require cautious use.

Precautions

• Use nicardipine cautiously in patients with cardiomyopathy, edema, hepatic or renal impairment, severe left ventricular dysfunction, or sick sinus syndrome and in those concurrently receiving beta blockers or digoxin.

Administration and Handling

PO

• Do not crush, open, or break sustained-release capsules.

• Give nicardipine without regard to food.

IV

• Store at room temperature.

• Store diluted IV solution for up to 24 hours at room temperature.

• Dilute each 25-mg ampule with 250 ml D_5W, 0.9% NaCl, 0.45% NaCl, or any combination thereof to provide a concentration of 1 mg/10 ml. Maximum concentration is 4 mg/10 ml.

• Give by slow IV infusion.

• Change IV site every 12 hours if drug is administered by a peripheral rather than a central venous catheter line.

Intervention and Evaluation

• Monitor the patient's BP during and following the IV infusion.

• Assess for peripheral edema behind the medial malleolus.

• Examine the patient's skin for dermatitis, facial flushing, and rash.

• Evaluate the patient for asthenia and headache.

• Monitor the patient's liver function test results.

• Assess the patient's EKG and pulse for tachycardia.

Patient Teaching

• Instruct the patient to take nicardipine's sustained-release form with food and not to crush or open the capsules.

• Urge the patient to avoid alcohol and limit caffeine while taking nicardipine.

• Warn the patient to notify the physician if he or she experiences anginal pain not relieved by the medication, constipation, dizziness, irregular heartbeat, nausea, shortness of breath, or swelling, or symptoms of hypotension such as lightheadedness.

nifedipine

nye-**fed**-i-peen

(Adalat 5[AUS], Adalat 10[AUS], Adalat 20[AUS], Adalat CC, Adalat Oros[AUS], Apo-Nifed[CAN], Nifecard[AUS], Nifedicol XL, Nifehexal[AUS], Novo-Nifedin[CAN], Nyefax[AUS], Procardia, Procardia XL)

Do not confuse nifedipine with nicardipine or nimodipine.

CATEGORY AND SCHEDULE

Pregnancy Risk Category: C

MECHANISM OF ACTION

An antianginal and antihypertensive agent that inhibits calcium ion movement across cell membranes, depressing contraction of cardiac and vascular smooth muscle.

Therapeutic Effect: Increases heart rate and cardiac output. Decreases systemic vascular resistance and BP.

PHARMACOKINETICS

Route	Onset	Peak	Duration
Sublingual	1–5 min	N/A	N/A
PO	20–30 min	N/A	4–8 hr
PO (extended release)	2 hr	N/A	24 hr

Rapidly, completely absorbed from the GI tract. Protein binding: 92%–98%. Undergoes first-pass metabolism in the liver. Primarily excreted in urine. Not removed by hemodialysis. ***Half-life:*** 2–5 hr.

AVAILABILITY

Capsules (Procardia): 10 mg.
Tablets (Extended-Release [Adalat CC, Procardia XL]): 30 mg, 60 mg, 90 mg.
Tablets (Extended-Release [Nifedical XL]): 30 mg, 60 mg.

INDICATIONS AND DOSAGES

▸ **Prinzmetal's variant angina, chronic stable (effort-associated) angina**

PO

Adults, Elderly. Initially, 10 mg 3 times a day. Increase at 7- to 14-day intervals. Maintenance: 10 mg 3 times a day up to 30 mg 4 times a day.

PO (Extended-Release)

Adults, Elderly. Initially, 30–60 mg/day. Maintenance: Up to 120 mg/day.

▸ **Essential hypertension**

PO (Extended-Release)

Adults, Elderly. Initially, 30–60 mg/day. Maintenance: Up to 120 mg/day.

OFF-LABEL USES

Treatment of Raynaud's phenomenon

CONTRAINDICATIONS

Advanced aortic stenosis, severe hypotension

INTERACTIONS

Drug

Beta blockers: May have additive effect.
Digoxin: May increase digoxin blood concentration.
Hypokalemia-producing agents (such as furosemide and certain other diuretics): May increase risk of arrhythmias.

Herbal

None known.

Food

Grapefruit, grapefruit juice: May increase nifedipine plasma concentration.

DIAGNOSTIC TEST EFFECTS

May cause positive ANA and direct Coombs' test.

SIDE EFFECTS

Frequent (30%–11%)
Peripheral edema, headache, flushed skin, dizziness
Occasional (12%–6%)
Nausea, shakiness, muscle cramps and pain, somnolence, palpitations, nasal congestion, cough, dyspnea, wheezing
Rare (5%–3%)
Hypotension, rash, pruritus, urticaria, constipation, abdominal discomfort, flatulence, sexual difficulties

SERIOUS REACTIONS

! Nifedipine may precipitate CHF and MI in patients with cardiac disease and peripheral ischemia.
! Overdose produces nausea,

somnolence, confusion, and slurred speech.

NURSING CONSIDERATIONS

Baseline Assessment

- Concurrent sublingual nitroglycerin therapy may be used for relief of anginal pain.
- Record the onset, type (sharp, dull, or squeezing), radiation, location, intensity, and duration of anginal pain and its precipitating factors, such as exertion and emotional stress.
- Assess the patient's BP for hypotension immediately before nifedipine administration.

Lifespan Considerations

- It is unclear if nifedipine crosses the placenta. It should be administered only when the benefit to the mother outweighs the risk to the fetus. An insignificant amount of nifedipine is distributed in breast milk.
- The safety and efficacy of nifedipine have not been established in children.
- In the elderly, age-related renal impairment may require cautious use.

Precautions

- Use nifedipine cautiously in patients with impaired hepatic or renal function.

Administration and Handling

PO

- Do not crush or break extended-release tablets.
- Give nifedipine without regard to meals.
- Grapefruit juice may alter absorption.

Sublingual

◀**ALERT**▶ May give 10–20 mg of nifedipine sublingually as needed for acute attack of angina.

- Capsule must be punctured with a sterile pin or needle and squeezed to express liquid under the tongue.

Intervention and Evaluation

- Assist the patient with ambulation if he or she experiences dizziness or light-headedness.
- Assess for peripheral edema behind the medial malleolus in ambulatory patients or in the sacral area in bedridden patients.
- Examine the patient's skin for flushing.
- Monitor the patient's liver function test results.

Patient Teaching

- Instruct the patient to rise slowly from a lying to a sitting position and to permit legs to dangle from bed momentarily before standing to reduce nifedipine's hypotensive effect.
- Warn the patient to notify the physician if he or she experiences irregular heartbeat, prolonged dizziness, nausea, or shortness of breath.
- Urge the patient to avoid alcohol, grapefruit, and grapefruit juice.

nimodipine

nye-**mode**-i-peen

(Nimotop)

Do not confuse nimodipine with nifedipine.

CATEGORY AND SCHEDULE

Pregnancy Risk Category: C

MECHANISM OF ACTION

A cerebral vasospasm agent that inhibits movement of calcium ions across vascular smooth-muscle cell membranes. **Therapeutic Effect:** Produces favorable effect on severity of neurologic deficits due to cerebral vasospasm. Exerts greatest effect on cerebral arteries; may prevent cerebral spasm.

PHARMACOKINETICS

Rapidly absorbed from the GI tract. Protein binding: 95%. Metabolized in the liver. Excreted in urine; eliminated in feces. Not removed by hemodialysis. ***Half-life:*** terminal, 3 hr.

AVAILABILITY

Capsules: 30 mg.

INDICATIONS AND DOSAGES

▸ Improvement neurologic deficits after subarachnoid hemorrhage from ruptured congenital aneurysms

PO

Adults, Elderly. 60 mg q4h for 21 days. Begin within 96 hr of subarachnoid hemorrhage.

OFF-LABEL USES

Treatment of chronic and classic migraine, chronic cluster headaches

CONTRAINDICATIONS

Atrial fibrillation or flutter, cardiogenic shock, CHF, heart block, sinus bradycardia, ventricular tachycardia, within several hours of IV beta-blocker therapy

INTERACTIONS

Drug

Beta blockers: May prolong SA and AV conduction, which may lead to severe hypotension, bradycardia, and cardiac failure.
Erythromycin, itraconazole, ketoconazole, protease inhibitors: May inhibit the metabolism of nimodipine.
Rifabutin, rifampin: May increase the metabolism of nimodipine.

Herbal

Garlic: May increase antihypertensive effect.
Ginseng, yohimbe: May worsen hypertension.

Food

Grapefruit juice: May increase nimodipine blood concentration and risk of toxicity.

DIAGNOSTIC TEST EFFECTS

None known.

SIDE EFFECTS

Occasional (6%–2%)

Hypotension, peripheral edema, diarrhea, headache

Rare (less than 2%)

Allergic reaction (rash, hives), tachycardia, flushing of skin

SERIOUS REACTIONS

! Overdose produces nausea, weakness, dizziness, somnolence, confusion, and slurred speech.

NURSING CONSIDERATIONS

Baseline Assessment

- Monitor the patient's liver function test results.
- Assess the patient's LOC and neurologic response, initially and throughout nimodipine therapy.
- Assess the patient's apical pulse and BP immediately before giving nimodipine. If the patient's pulse rate is 60 beats/minute or lower or systolic BP is less than 90 mm Hg, withhold the medication and contact physician.

Lifespan Considerations

- It is unknown if nimodipine crosses the placenta or is distributed in breast milk.
- The safety and efficacy of nimodipine have not been established in children.
- In the elderly, age-related renal impairment may require cautious use. The elderly may also experience

greater hypotensive response and constipation.

Precautions

• Use nimodipine cautiously in patients with impaired hepatic or renal function.

Administration and Handling

PO

• If the patient is unable to swallow, place a hole in both ends of a capsule with an 18-gauge needle to extract contents into a syringe.
• Empty contents of syringe into an NG tube; flush tube with 30 ml normal saline.

Intervention and Evaluation

• Monitor the patient's BP, CNS response, and heart rate for signs and symptoms of CHF and hypotension.

Patient Teaching

• Instruct the patient not to crush or chew capsules.
• Warn the patient to notify the physician if he or she experiences constipation, dizziness, irregular heartbeat, nausea, shortness of breath, or swelling.

verapamil hydrochloride

ver-**ap**-a-mill

(Anpec[AUS], Apo-Verap[CAN], Calan, Calan SR, Chronovera[CAN], Cordilox SR[AUS], Covera-HS, Isoptin[AUS], Isoptin SR, Novo-Veramil[CAN], Novo-Veramil SR[CAN], Veracaps SR[AUS], Verahexal[AUS], Verelan, Verelan PM)

Do not confuse Isoptin with Intropin; or Verelan with Virilon, Vivarin, or Voltaren.

CATEGORY AND SCHEDULE

Pregnancy Risk Category: C

MECHANISM OF ACTION

A calcium channel blocker and antianginal, antiarrhythmic, and antihypertensive agent that inhibits calcium ion entry across cardiac and vascular smooth-muscle cell membranes. This action causes the dilation of coronary arteries, peripheral arteries, and arterioles. **Therapeutic Effect:** Decreases heart rate and myocardial contractility and slows SA and AV conduction. Decreases total peripheral vascular resistance by vasodilation.

PHARMACOKINETICS

Route	Onset	Peak	Duration
PO	30 min	1–2 hr	6–8 hr
PO (Extended-Release)	30 min	N/A	N/A
IV	1–2 min	3–5 min	10–60 min

Well absorbed from the GI tract. Protein binding: 90% (60% in neonates.) Undergoes first-pass metabolism in the liver to active metabolite. Primarily excreted in urine. Not removed by hemodialysis. ***Half-life:*** 2–8 hr.

AVAILABILITY

Caplet (Calan SR): 120 mg, 180 mg, 240 mg.
Capsules (Extended-Release [Verelan PM]): 100 mg, 200 mg, 300 mg.
Capsules (Sustained-Release [Verelan]): 120 mg, 180 mg, 240 mg, 360 mg.
Tablets (Calan): 40 mg, 80 mg, 120 mg.
Tablets (Extended-Release [Covera HS]): 180 mg, 240 mg.
Tablets (Sustained-Release [Isoptin SR]): 120 mg, 180 mg, 240 mg.
Injection: 2.5 mg/ml.

INDICATIONS AND DOSAGES

▸ **Supraventricular tachyarrhythmias, temporary control of rapid ventricular rate with atrial fibrillation or flutter**

IV

Adults, Elderly. Initially, 5–10 mg; repeat in 30 min with 10-mg dose.
Children 1 to 15 yr. 0.1 mg/kg. May repeat in 30 min up to a maximum second dose of 10 mg. Not recommended in children younger than 1 yr.

▸ **Arrhythmias, including prevention of recurrent paroxysmal supraventricular tachycardia and control of ventricular resting rate in chronic atrial fibrillation or flutter (with digoxin)**

PO

Adults, Elderly. 240–480 mg/day in 3–4 divided doses.

▸ **Vasospastic angina (Prinzmetal's variant), unstable (crescendo or preinfarction) angina, chronic stable (effort-associated) angina**

PO

Adults. Initially, 80–120 mg 3 times a day. For elderly patients and those with hepatic dysfunction, 40 mg 3 times a day. Titrate to optimal dose. Maintenance: 240–480 mg/day in 3–4 divided doses.

PO (Covera-HS)

Adults, Elderly. 180–480 mg/day at bedtime.

▸ **Hypertension**

PO

Adults, Elderly. Initially, 40–80 mg 3 times a day. Maintenance: 480 mg or less a day.

PO (Covera-HS)

Adults, Elderly. 180–480 mg/day at bedtime.

PO (Extended-Release)

Adults, Elderly. 120–240 mg/day. May give 480 mg or less a day in 2 divided doses.

PO (Verelan PM)

Adults, Elderly. 100–300 mg/day.

OFF-LABEL USES

Treatment of hypertrophic cardiomyopathy, vascular headaches

CONTRAINDICATIONS

Atrial fibrillation or flutter and an accessory bypass tract, cardiogenic shock, heart block, sinus bradycardia, ventricular tachycardia

INTERACTIONS

Drug

Beta blockers: May have additive effect.
Carbamazepine, quinidine, theophylline: May increase verapamil blood concentration and risk of toxicity.
Digoxin: May increase digoxin blood concentration.
Disopyramide: May increase negative inotropic effect.
Procainamide, quinidine: May increase risk of QT-interval prolongation.

Herbal

None known.

Food

Grapefruit, grapefruit juice: May increase verapamil blood concentration.

DIAGNOSTIC TEST EFFECTS

EKG waveform may show increased PR interval. Therapeutic serum level is 0.08–0.3 mcg/ml.

IV INCOMPATIBILITIES

Amphotericin B complex (Abelcet, AmBisome, Amphotec), nafcillin (Nafcil), propofol (Diprivan), sodium bicarbonate

IV COMPATIBILITIES

Amiodarone (Cordarone), calcium chloride, calcium gluconate, dexamethasone (Decadron), digoxin (Lanoxin), dobutamine (Dobutrex), dopamine (Intropin), furosemide (Lasix), heparin, hydromorphone (Dilaudid), lidocaine, magnesium sulfate, metoclopramide (Reglan), milrinone (Primacor), morphine, multivitamins, nitroglycerin, norepinephrine (Levophed), potassium chloride, potassium phosphate, procainamide (Pronestyl), propranolol (Inderal)

SIDE EFFECTS

Frequent (7%)
Constipation
Occasional (4%–2%)
Dizziness, light-headedness, headache, asthenia (loss of strength, energy), nausea, peripheral edema, hypotension
Rare (less than 1%)
Bradycardia, dermatitis or rash

SERIOUS REACTIONS

! Rapid ventricular rate in atrial flutter or fibrillation, marked hypotension, extreme bradycardia, CHF, asystole, and second- and third-degree AV block occur rarely.

NURSING CONSIDERATIONS

Baseline Assessment

- Record the onset, type (such as sharp, dull, or squeezing), radiation, location, intensity, and duration of the patient's anginal pain and its precipitating factors, such as exertion and emotional stress.
- Before verapamil administration, assess the patient's BP for hypotension and pulse rate for bradycardia.

Lifespan Considerations

- Verapamil crosses the placenta and is distributed in breast milk. Breastfeeding is not recommended for patients taking this drug.
- No age-related precautions have been noted in children.
- In the elderly, age-related renal impairment may require cautious use.

Precautions

- Use verapamil cautiously in patients with CHF, hepatic or renal impairment, or sick sinus syndrome and in those concurrently receiving beta blockers or digoxin.

Administration and Handling

PO

- Do not give verapamil with grapefruit juice.
- Give tablets that are not sustained-release with or without food. Sustained-release form should be given on an empty stomach.
- Have patient swallow extended-release or sustained-released preparations whole and without chewing or crushing.
- If needed, open sustained-release capsules and sprinkle contents on applesauce. Have the patient swallow the applesauce immediately, without chewing.

IV

- Store vials at room temperature.
- Give undiluted, if desired.
- Administer IV push over more than 2 minutes for adults and children and over more than 3 minutes for the elderly.
- Continuous EKG monitoring during IV injection is required for children and recommended for adults.
- Monitor the patient's EKG for asystole, extreme bradycardia, heart block, PR-interval prolongation, and rapid ventricular rates. Notify the physician of significant EKG changes.
- Monitor the patient's BP every 5–10 minutes, or as ordered.
- Keep the patient in a recumbent

position for at least 1 hour after IV administration.

Intervention and Evaluation

• Assess the patient's pulse for rate, rhythm, and quality.

◀ **ALERT** ▶ Monitor the patient's EKG for changes, particularly PR-interval prolongation. Notify the physician of significant PR-interval or other EKG changes.

• Assist the patient with ambulation if he or she experiences dizziness.

• Assess for peripheral edema behind the medial malleolus in ambulatory patients or in the sacral area in bedridden patients.

• For patients taking the oral form of verapamil, assess stool consistency and frequency.

• Keep in mind that the therapeutic serum level for verapamil is 0.08 to 0.3 mcg/ml.

Patient Teaching

• Caution the patient against abruptly discontinuing verapamil. Stress that compliance with the treatment regimen is essential to control anginal pain.

• To avoid the orthostatic effects of verapamil, instruct the patient to rise slowly from a lying to a sitting position and to wait momentarily before standing.

• Advise the patient to avoid tasks that require mental alertness or motor skills until his or her response to the drug has been established.

• Urge the patient to avoid consuming grapefruit or grapefruit juice and to limit caffeine intake while taking verapamil.

• Warn the patient to notify the physician if he or she experiences anginal pain not reduced by the drug, constipation, dizziness, irregular heartbeat, nausea, shortness of breath, or swelling of the hands and feet.

27 Cardiac Glycosides

digoxin
milrinone lactate

Uses: Cardiac glycosides are used to treat CHF, atrial fibrillation, paroxysmal atrial tachycardia, and cardiogenic shock with pulmonary edema.

Action: Cardiac glycosides act directly on the myocardium to increase the force of contraction, which leads to increased stroke volume and cardiac output. These agents also depress the firing of the SA node, decrease conduction time through the AV node, and decrease electrical impulses caused by a slow heart rate from vagal stimulation. Their ability to increase myocardial contractility may result from the improved transport of calcium, sodium, and potassium ions across cell membranes.

digoxin

di-**jox**-in
(Digitek, Lanoxicaps, Lanoxin, Sigmaxin[AUS])
Do not confuse digoxin with Desoxyn or doxepin, or Lanoxin with Levsinex or Lonox.

CATEGORY AND SCHEDULE

Pregnancy Risk Category: C

MECHANISM OF ACTION

A cardiac glycoside that increases the influx of calcium from extracellular to intracellular cytoplasm. **Therapeutic Effect:** Potentiates the activity of the contractile cardiac muscle fibers and increases the force of myocardial contraction. Slows the heart rate by decreasing conduction through the SA and AV nodes.

PHARMACOKINETICS

Route	Onset	Peak	Duration
PO	0.5–2 hr	28 hr	3–4 days
IV	5–30 min	1–4 hr	3–4 days

Readily absorbed from the GI tract. Widely distributed. Protein binding: 30%. Partially metabolized in the liver. Primarily excreted in urine. Minimally removed by hemodialysis. ***Half-life:*** 36–48 hr (increased with impaired renal function and in the elderly).

AVAILABILITY

Capsules (Lanoxicaps): 50 mcg, 100 mcg, 200 mcg.
Elixir (Lanoxin): 50 mcg/ml.
Tablets (Digitek, Lanoxin): 125 mcg, 250 mcg.
Injection (Lanoxin): 250 mcg/ml, 100 mcg/ml.

INDICATIONS AND DOSAGES

▸ Rapid loading dose for the management and treatment of CHF; control of ventricular rate in patients with atrial fibrillation; treatment and prevention of recurrent paroxysmal atrial tachycardia

PO

Adults, Elderly. Initially, 0.5–0.75 mg, additional doses of 0.125–0.375 mg at 6- to 8-hr intervals. Range: 0.75–1.25 mg.
Children 10 yr and older. 10–15 mcg/kg.
Children 5–9 yr. 20–35 mcg/kg.
Children 2–4 yr. 30–40 mcg/kg.
Children 1–23 mo. 35–60 mcg/kg.
Neonate, full-term. 25–35 mcg/kg.
Neonate, premature. 20–30 mcg/kg.

IV

Adults, Elderly. 0.6–1 mg.
Children 10 yr and older. 8–12 mcg/kg.
Children 5–9 yr. 15–30 mcg/kg.
Children 2–4 yr. 25–35 mcg/kg.
Children 1–23 mo. 30–50 mcg/kg.
Neonates, full-term. 20–30 mcg/kg.
Neonates, premature. 15–25 mcg/kg.

▸ Maintenance dosage for CHF; control of ventricular rate in patients with atrial fibrillation; treatment and prevention of recurrent paroxysmal atrial tachycardia

PO, IV

Adults, Elderly. 0.125–0.375 mg/day.
Children. 25%–35% loading dose (20%–30% for premature neonates).

▸ Dosage in renal impairment

Dosage adjustment is based on creatinine clearance. Total digitalizing dose: decrease by 50% in end-stage renal disease.

Creatinine Clearance	Dosage
10–50 ml/min	25%–75% usual
less than 10 ml/min	10%–25% usual

CONTRAINDICATIONS

Ventricular fibrillation, ventricular tachycardia unrelated to CHF

INTERACTIONS

Drug

Amiodarone: May increase digoxin blood concentration and risk of toxicity; may have an additive effect on the SA and AV nodes.
Amphotericin, glucocorticoids, potassium-depleting diuretics: May increase risk of toxicity due to hypokalemia.
Antiarrhythmics, parenteral calcium, sympathomimetics: May increase risk of arrhythmias.
Antidiarrheals, cholestyramine, colestipol, sucralfate: May decrease absorption of digoxin.
Diltiazem, fluoxetine, quinidine, verapamil: May increase digoxin blood concentration.
Parenteral magnesium: May cause cardiac conduction changes and heart block.

Herbal

Siberian ginseng: May increase serum digoxin levels.

Food

None known.

DIAGNOSTIC TEST EFFECTS

None known.

IV INCOMPATIBILITIES

Amphotericin B complex (Abelcet, Amphotec, AmBisome), fluconazole (Diflucan), foscarnet (Foscavir), propofol (Diprivan)

IV COMPATIBILITIES

Cimetidine (Tagamet), diltiazem (Cardizem), furosemide (Lasix), heparin, insulin (regular), lidocaine, midazolam (Versed), milrinone (Primacor), morphine, potassium chloride, propofol (Diprivan)

SIDE EFFECTS

None known. However, there is a very narrow margin of safety between a therapeutic and toxic result. Long-term therapy may produce mammary gland enlargement in women but is reversible when drug is withdrawn.

SERIOUS REACTIONS

! The most common early manifestations of digoxin toxicity are GI disturbances (anorexia, nausea, vomiting) and neurologic abnormalities (fatigue, headache, depression, weakness, drowsiness, confusion, nightmares).

! Facial pain, personality change, and ocular disturbances (photophobia, light flashes, halos around bright objects, yellow or green color perception) may be noted.

NURSING CONSIDERATIONS

Baseline Assessment

- Assess the patient's apical pulse for 60 seconds, or 30 seconds if the patient is receiving maintenance therapy. If the pulse rate is 60 beats/minute or lower in adults or 70 beats/minute or less in children, withhold the drug and contact the physician.
- Expect to obtain blood samples for digoxin level 6 to 8 hours after digoxin administration or just before administration of next digoxin dose.

Lifespan Considerations

- Digoxin crosses the placenta and is distributed in breast milk. Premature infants are more susceptible to toxicity.
- Keep in mind that infants and children experience signs of overdose differently than adults. The first sign of overdose in children is usually an arrhythmia, such as bradycardia, followed by nausea, vomiting, diarrhea, anorexia, and CNS disturbances.
- In the elderly, age-related hepatic or renal function impairment may require dosage adjustment. Also, there is an increased risk of loss of appetite in this age group.

Precautions

- Use digoxin cautiously in patients with acute MI, advanced cardiac disease, cor pulmonale, hypokalemia, hypothyroidism, impaired hepatic or renal function, incomplete AV block, or pulmonary disease.

Administration and Handling

◀ALERT▶ Avoid giving digoxin by the IM route because the drug may cause severe local irritation and is erratically absorbed. If no other route is possible, give deep into the muscle followed by massage. Give no more than 2 ml at any one site.

◀ALERT▶ Expect to adjust the digoxin dosage in elderly patients and those with renal dysfunction. Know that larger digoxin doses are often required for adequate control of ventricular rate in patients with atrial fibrillation or flutter. Administer digoxin loading dosage in several doses at 4- to 8-hour intervals, as prescribed.

PO

- May give without regard to meals.
- Crush tablets if necessary.

IV

- Give undiluted or dilute with at least a four-fold volume of sterile water for injection, or D_5W because using less than this amount may cause a precipitate to form. Use immediately.
- Give IV slowly over at least 5 minutes.

Intervention and Evaluation

- Monitor the patient's pulse for bradycardia and EKG for arrhythmias for 1 to 2 hours after digoxin

administration. Excessive slowing of the patient's pulse may be the first sign of toxicity.
• Assess the patient for signs and symptoms of digoxin toxicity, including GI disturbances and neurologic abnormalities, every 2 to 4 hours during loading dose and daily during maintenance therapy.
• Monitor the patient's serum potassium and magnesium levels. The therapeutic serum level is 0.8 to 2 ng/ml and toxic serum level is greater than 2 ng/ml.

Patient Teaching
• Stress to the patient the importance of follow-up visits and blood tests.
• Teach the patient to take the apical pulse correctly and to notify the physician of a pulse rate of 60 beats/minute or less or a rate less than that indicated by the physician.
• Instruct the patient to recognize the signs and symptoms of toxicity and to notify the physician if these occur.
• Advise the patient to carry or wear identification that he or she is receiving digoxin and to inform dentists and other physicians about digoxin therapy.
• Caution the patient not to increase or skip digoxin doses.
• Explain to the patient that he or she should not take OTC medications without physician approval.
• Warn the patient to notify the physician if decreased appetite, diarrhea, nausea, visual changes, or vomiting occurs.

milrinone lactate
mill-re-none
(Primacor)

CATEGORY AND SCHEDULE
Pregnancy Risk Category: C

MECHANISM OF ACTION
A cardiac inotropic agent that inhibits phosphodiesterase, which increases cyclic adenosine monophosphate and potentiates the delivery of calcium to myocardial contractile systems. **Therapeutic Effect:** Relaxes vascular muscle, causing vasodilation. Increases cardiac output; decreases pulmonary capillary wedge pressure and vascular resistance.

PHARMACOKINETICS

Route	Onset	Peak	Duration
IV	5–15 min	N/A	N/A

Protein binding: 70%. Primarily excreted unchanged in urine. ***Half-life:*** 2.4 hr.

AVAILABILITY
Injection: 1 mg/ml, 10-ml single-dose vial, 20-mg single-dose vial, 50-ml single-dose vial, 5-ml sterile cartridge unit.
Injection (Premix): 200 mcg/ml.

INDICATIONS AND DOSAGES
▸ **Short-term management of CHF**
IV
Adults. Initially, 50 mcg/kg over 10 min. Continue with maintenance infusion rate of 0.375–0.75 mcg/kg/min based on hemodynamic and clinical response. Total daily dosage: 0.59–1.13 mg/kg.

Dosage in renal impairment
For patients with severe renal impairment, reduce dosage to 0.2–0.43 mcg/kg/min.

CONTRAINDICATIONS
None known.

INTERACTIONS
Drug
Other cardiac glycosides: Produces additive inotropic effects.
Herbal
None known.
Food
None known.

DIAGNOSTIC TEST EFFECTS
None known.

IV INCOMPATIBILITIES
Furosemide (Lasix)

IV COMPATIBILITIES
Calcium gluconate, digoxin (Lanoxin), diltiazem (Cardizem), dobutamine (Dobutrex), dopamine (Intropin), heparin, lidocaine, magnesium, midazolam (Versed), nitroglycerin, potassium, propofol (Diprivan)

SIDE EFFECTS
Occasional (3%–1%)
Headache, hypotension
Rare (less than 1%)
Angina, chest pain

SERIOUS REACTIONS
! Supraventricular and ventricular arrhythmias (12%), nonsustained ventricular tachycardia (2%), and sustained ventricular tachycardia (1%) may occur.

NURSING CONSIDERATIONS
Baseline Assessment
- Offer the patient emotional support, especially if he or she has become anxious as a result of experiencing difficulty breathing.
- Assess the patient's apical pulse and BP before beginning treatment and during IV therapy.
- Assess the patient's breath sounds for crackles and rhonchi and check the patient's skin for edema.

Lifespan Considerations
- It is unknown if milrinone crosses the placenta or is distributed in breast milk.
- The safety and efficacy of milrinone have not been established in children.
- In the elderly, age-related renal impairment may require dosage adjustment.

Precautions
- Use milrinone cautiously in patients with atrial fibrillation or flutter, history of ventricular arrhythmias, impaired renal function, or severe obstructive aortic or pulmonic valvular disease.

Administration and Handling
IV
- Store at room temperature.
- For IV infusion, dilute 20-mg (20-ml) vial with 80 or 180 ml diluent (0.9% NaCl, D_5W) or 10-mg (10-ml) vial with 40 or 90 ml diluent to provide concentration of 200 or 100 mcg/ml, respectively. Maximum concentration: 100 mg/250 ml.
- For a loading dose IV injection, administer milrinone undiluted slowly over 10 minutes.
- Monitor the patient for arrhythmias and hypotension during IV therapy. If one or both of these conditions occur, reduce or temporarily discontinue infusion until condition stabilizes.

Intervention and Evaluation

• Monitor the patient's BP, cardiac output, EKG, heart rate, renal function, and serum potassium levels.
• Assess the patient for signs and symptoms of CHF.

Patient Teaching

• Warn the patient to immediately report palpitations or chest pain.
• Explain to the patient that milrinone is not a cure for CHF but will help relieve symptoms.

28 Sympatholytics

clonidine
doxazosin mesylate
methyldopa
prazosin hydrochloride
terazosin hydrochloride

Uses: Sympatholytics, also called adrenergic inhibitors, are used to treat mild to severe hypertension. Because these agents effectively control BP, they help prevent the development and progression of serious cardiovascular complications.

Action: Sympatholytics can act centrally or peripherally. (See the illustration *Sites of Action: Sympatholytics,* page 576.) Central-acting agents, such as clonidine and methyldopa, stimulate alpha$_2$-adrenergic receptors in the cardiovascular centers of the CNS, reducing sympathetic outflow and producing antihypertensive effects. *Peripheral-acting agents,* such as doxazosin and prazosin, block alpha$_1$-adrenergic receptors in arterioles and veins, inhibiting vasoconstriction and decreasing peripheral vascular resistance, which reduces BP.

COMBINATION PRODUCTS

ALDORIL: methyldopa/hydrochlorothiazide (a diuretic) 250 mg/15 mg; 250 mg/25 mg; 500 mg/30 mg; 500 mg/50 mg.
COMBIPRES: clonidine/chlorthalidone (a diuretic) 0.1 mg/15 mg; 0.2 mg/15 mg; 0.3 mg/15 mg.
MINIZIDE: prazosin/polythiazide (a diuretic) 1 mg/0.5 mg; 2 mg/0.5 mg; 5 mg/0.5 mg.

clonidine

klon-ih-deen
(Catapres, Catapres TTS, Dixarit[CAN], Duraclon)
Do not confuse clonidine with clomiphene, Klonopin, or quinidine; or Catapres with with Cetapred.

CATEGORY AND SCHEDULE

Pregnancy Risk Category: C

MECHANISM OF ACTION

An antiadrenergic, sympatholytic agent that prevents pain signal transmission to the brain and produces analgesia at pre- and post-alpha-adrenergic receptors in the spinal cord. **Therapeutic Effect:** Reduces peripheral resistance; decreases BP and heart rate.

PHARMACOKINETICS

Route	Onset	Peak	Duration
PO	0.5–1 hr	2–4 hr	Up to 8 hr

Well absorbed from the GI tract. Transdermal best absorbed from the chest and upper arm; least absorbed from the thigh. Protein binding: 20%–40%. Metabolized in the liver. Primarily excreted in urine. Minimally removed by hemodialysis. ***Half-life:*** 12–16 hr (increased with impaired renal function).

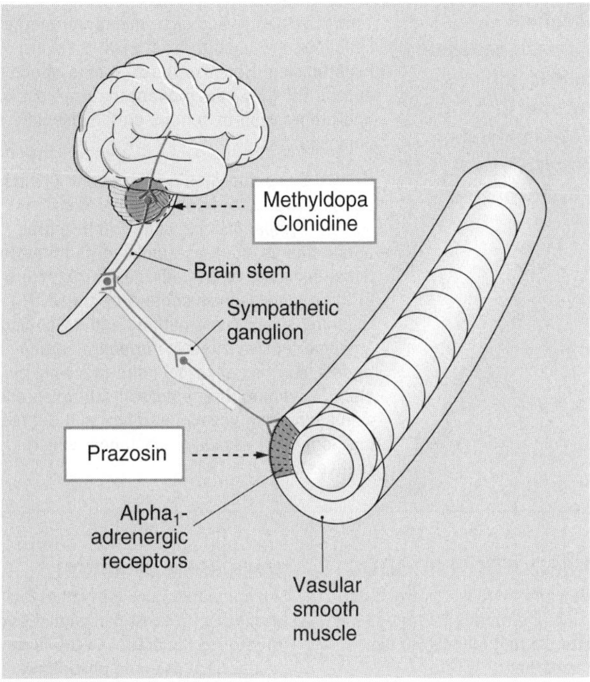

Sites of Action: Sympatholytics

Sympatholytics inhibit sympathetic nervous system (SNS) activity, which plays a major role in regulating BP. Normally when the SNS is stimulated, nerve impulses travel from the cardiovascular center of the CNS to the sympathetic ganglia. From there, the impulses travel along postganglionic fibers to specific effector organs, such as the heart and blood vessels. SNS stimulation also triggers the release of norepinephrine, which acts primarily at alpha-adrenergic receptors.

Sympatholytics fall into two subclasses: central-acting alpha$_2$ agonists and peripheral-acting alpha$_1$-adrenergic antagonists. Central-acting alpha$_2$ agonists, such as methyldopa and clonidine, stimulate alpha$_2$-adrenergic receptors in the cardiovascular center of the CNS and reduce activity in the vasomotor center of the brain, interfering with sympathetic stimulation of the heart and blood vessels. This causes blood vessel dilation and decreased cardiac output, which leads to reduced BP.

Peripheral-acting alpha$_1$-adrenergic antagonists, such as prazosin, inhibit the stimulation of alpha$_1$-adrenergic receptors by norepinephrine in vascular smooth muscle, interfering with SNS-induced vasoconstriction. As a result, the blood vessels dilate, reducing peripheral vascular resistance and venous return to the heart. These effects, in turn, lead to decreased BP.

AVAILABILITY

Tablets (Catapres): 0.1 mg, 0.2 mg, 0.3 mg.
Transdermal Patch (Catapres TTS): 2.5 mg (release at 0.1 mg/24 hr), 5 mg (release at 0.2 mg/24 hr), 7.5 mg (release at 0.3 mg/24 hr).
Injection (Duraclon): 100 mcg/ml, 500 mcg/ml.

INDICATIONS AND DOSAGES

▸ Hypertension

PO
Adults. Initially, 0.1 mg twice a day. Increase by 0.1–0.2 mg q2–4days. Maintenance: 0.2–1.2 mg/day in 2–4 divided doses up to maximum of 2.4 mg/day.
Elderly. Initially, 0.1 mg at bedtime. May increase gradually.
Children. 5–25 mcg/kg/day in divided doses q6h. Increase at 5- to 7-day intervals. Maximum: 0.9 mg/day.
Transdermal
Adults, Elderly. System delivering 0.1 mg/24 hr up to 0.6 mg/24 hr q7days.

▸ Attention deficit hyperactivity disorder (ADHD)

PO
Children. Initially 0.05 mg/day. May increase by 0.05 mg/day q3–7days. Maximum: 0.3–0.4 mg/day.

▸ Severe pain

Epidural
Adults, Elderly. 30–40 mcg/hr.
Children. Initially, 0.5 mcg/kg/hr, not to exceed adult dose.

OFF-LABEL USES

ADHD, diagnosis of pheochromocytoma, opioid withdrawal, prevention of migraine headaches, treatment of dysmenorrhea, menopausal flushing

CONTRAINDICATIONS

Epidural contraindicated in those patients with bleeding diathesis or infection at the injection site, and in those receiving anticoagulation therapy

INTERACTIONS

Drug

Beta blockers: Discontinuing these drugs may increase risk of clonidine-withdrawal hypertensive crisis.
Tricyclic antidepressants: May decrease effect of clonidine.

Herbal

None known.

Food

None known.

DIAGNOSTIC TEST EFFECTS

None known.

IV INCOMPATIBILITIES

None known.

IV COMPATIBILITIES

Bupivacaine (Marcaine, Sensorcaine), fentanyl (Sublimaze), heparin, ketamine (Ketalar), lidocaine, lorazepam (Ativan)

SIDE EFFECTS

Frequent
Dry mouth (40%), somnolence (33%), dizziness (16%), sedation, constipation (10%)
Occasional (5%–1%)
Tablets, injection: Depression, swelling of feet, loss of appetite, decreased sexual ability, itching eyes, dizziness, nausea, vomiting, nervousness
Transdermal: Itching, reddening or darkening of skin
Rare (less than 1%)
Nightmares, vivid dreams, cold feeling in fingers and toes

SERIOUS REACTIONS

! Overdose produces profound hypotension, irritability, bradycardia, respiratory depression, hypothermia, miosis (pupillary constriction), arrhythmias, and apnea.

! Abrupt withdrawal may result in rebound hypertension associated with nervousness, agitation, anxiety, insomnia, hand tingling, tremor, flushing, and diaphoresis.

NURSING CONSIDERATIONS

Baseline Assessment

- Obtain the patient's BP immediately before giving each dose, in addition to regular monitoring. Be alert for BP fluctuations.

Lifespan Considerations

- Clonidine crosses the placenta and is distributed in breast milk.
- Children are more sensitive to clonidine's effects. Use clonidine with caution in children.
- The elderly may be more sensitive to the hypotensive effect of clonidine.
- Age-related renal impairment may require dosage adjustment in the elderly.

Precautions

- Use clonidine cautiously in patients with cerebrovascular disease, chronic renal failure, Raynaud's disease, recent MI, severe coronary insufficiency, or thromboangiitis obliterans.

Administration and Handling

PO

- Give clonidine without regard to food.
- Tablets may be crushed.
- Give last oral dose just before bedtime.

Transdermal

- Apply transdermal system to dry, hairless area of intact skin on upper arm or chest.
- Rotate sites to prevent skin irritation.
- Do not trim patch to adjust dose.

Intervention and Evaluation

- Assess the patient's pattern of daily bowel activity and stool consistency.
- Expect to discontinue concurrent beta-blocker therapy several days before discontinuing clonidine therapy to prevent clonidine-withdrawal hypertensive crisis. Also, expect to slowly reduce clonidine dosage over 2 to 4 days.

Patient Teaching

- Recommend sips of tepid water and sugarless gum to the patient to help relieve dry mouth.
- Instruct the patient to rise slowly from a lying to a sitting position and permit legs to dangle momentarily before standing to avoid clonidine's hypotensive effect.
- Warn the patient that skipping doses or voluntarily discontinuing clonidine may produce severe, rebound hypertension.
- Advise the patient that clonidine's side effects tend to diminish during therapy.

doxazosin mesylate

dox-**ay**-zoe-sin

(Cardura)

Do not confuse doxazosin with doxapram, doxepin, or doxorubicin; or Cardura with Cardene, Cordarone, Coumadin, K-Dur, or Ridaura.

CATEGORY AND SCHEDULE

Pregnancy Risk Category: C

MECHANISM OF ACTION

An antihypertensive that selectively blocks $alpha_1$-adrenergic receptors, decreasing peripheral vascular resistance. **Therapeutic Effect:** Causes peripheral vasodilation and lowers

BP. Also relaxes smooth muscle of bladder and prostate.

PHARMACOKINETICS

Route	Onset	Peak	Duration
PO	N/A	2–6 hr	24 hr

Well absorbed from the GI tract. Protein binding: 98%–99%. Metabolized in the liver. Primarily eliminated in feces. Not removed by hemodialysis. ***Half-life:*** 19–22 hr.

AVAILABILITY

Tablets: 1 mg, 2 mg, 4 mg, 8 mg.

INDICATIONS AND DOSAGES

▸ **Mild to moderate hypertension**

PO

Adults. Initially, 1 mg once a day. May increase to a maximum of 16 mg/day.

Elderly. Initially, 0.5 mg once a day.

▸ **Benign prostatic hyperplasia, alone or in combination with finasteride (Proscar)**

PO

Adults, Elderly. Initially, 1 mg/day. May increase q1–2wk. Maximum: 8 mg/day.

CONTRAINDICATIONS

None known.

INTERACTIONS

Drug

Estrogen, NSAIDs: May decrease the effect of doxazosin.

Hypotension-producing medications, such as antihypertensives and diuretics: May increase the effect of doxazosin.

Herbal

None known.

Food

None known.

DIAGNOSTIC TEST EFFECTS

None known.

SIDE EFFECTS

Frequent (20%–10%)

Dizziness, asthenia, headache, edema

Occasional (9%–3%)

Nausea, pharyngitis, rhinitis, pain in extremities, somnolence

Rare (3%–1%)

Palpitations, diarrhea, constipation, dyspnea, myalgia, altered vision, dizziness, nervousness

SERIOUS REACTIONS

! First-dose syncope (hypotension with sudden loss of consciousness) may occur 30 to 90 minutes following initial dose of 2 mg or greater, a too-rapid increase in dosage, or addition of another antihypertensive agent to therapy. First-dose syncope may be preceded by tachycardia (pulse rate of 120–160 beats/minute).

NURSING CONSIDERATIONS

Baseline Assessment

- Give first dose of doxazosin at bedtime. If the initial dose is given during the day, keep the patient recumbent for 3 to 4 hours.
- Assess the patient's BP and pulse immediately before each dose, and every 15 to 30 minutes thereafter until BP is stabilized. Be alert for fluctuations in BP.

Lifespan Considerations

- It is unknown if doxazosin crosses the placenta or is distributed in breast milk.
- The safety and efficacy of doxazosin have not been established in children.
- The elderly may be more sensitive to the hypotensive effects of doxazosin.

Precautions
- Use doxazosin cautiously in patients with chronic renal failure or impaired hepatic function.

Administration and Handling
PO
- Give doxazosin without regard to food.

Intervention and Evaluation
- Monitor the patient's pulse frequently because first-dose syncope may be preceded by a rapid pulse rate.
- Assess the patient for edema and headache.
- Assist the patient with ambulation if he or she experiences dizziness or light-headedness.

Patient Teaching
- Advise the patient that the full therapeutic effect of doxazosin may not appear for 3 to 4 weeks.
- Explain to the patient that doxazosin use may cause fainting or syncope.
- Warn the patient to avoid performing tasks that require mental alertness or motor skills until his or her response to doxazosin has been established.

methyldopa
meth-ill-**doe**-pa
(Aldomet, Apo-Methyldopa[CAN], Hydopa[AUS], Novomedopa[CAN], Nudopa[AUS])
Do not confuse Aldomet with Anzemet.

CATEGORY AND SCHEDULE
Pregnancy Risk Category: B

MECHANISM OF ACTION
An antihypertensive agent that stimulates central inhibitory alpha-adrenergic receptors, lowers arterial pressure, and reduces plasma renin activity. **Therapeutic Effect:** Reduces BP.

AVAILABILITY
Tablets: 250 mg, 500 mg.
Injection: 50 mg/ml.

INDICATIONS AND DOSAGES
▸ Moderate to severe hypertension
PO
Adults. Initially, 250 mg 2–3 times a day for 2 days. Adjust dosage at intervals of 2 days (minimum).
Elderly. Initially, 125 mg 1–2 times a day. May increase by 125 mg q2–3days. Maintenance: 500 mg to 2 g/day in 2–4 divided doses.
Children. Initially, 10 mg/kg/day in 2–4 divided doses. Adjust dosage at intervals of 2 days (minimum). Maximum: 65 mg/kg/day or 3 g/day, whichever is less.
IV
Adults. 250–1,000 mg q6–8h. Maximum: 4 g/day.
Children. Initially, 2–4 mg/kg/dose. May increase to 5–10 mg/kg/dose in 4–6h if no response. Maximum: 65 mg/kg/day or 3 g/day, whichever is less.

CONTRAINDICATIONS
Hepatic disease, pheochromocytoma

INTERACTIONS
Drug
Hypotensive-producing medications, such as antihypertensives and diuretics: May increase the effects of methyldopa.
Lithium: May increase the risk of lithium toxicity.
MAOIs: May cause hyperexcitability.
NSAIDs, tricyclic antidepressants: May decrease the effects of methyldopa.

Other sympathomimetics: May decrease the effects of sympathomimetics.

Herbal

None known.

Food

None known.

DIAGNOSTIC TEST EFFECTS

May increase BUN and serum prolactin, alkaline phosphatase, bilirubin, creatinine, potassium, sodium, uric acid, AST (SGOT), and ALT (SGPT) levels. May produce false-positive Coombs' test and prolong prothrombin time.

SIDE EFFECTS

Frequent

Peripheral edema, somnolence, headache, dry mouth

Occasional

Mental changes (such as anxiety, depression), decreased sexual function or libido, diarrhea, swelling of breasts, nausea, vomiting, lightheadedness, paraesthesia, rhinitis

SERIOUS REACTIONS

! Hepatotoxicity (abnormal liver function test results, jaundice, hepatitis), hemolytic anemia, unexplained fever and flu-like symptoms may occur. If these conditions appear, discontinue the medication and contact the physician.

NURSING CONSIDERATIONS

Baseline Assessment

• Obtain the patient's BP, pulse, and weight.

Precautions

• Use methyldopa cautiously in patients with renal impairment.

Administration and Handling

IV

• Inspect the drug vial for particulate matter and discoloration, and discard if present.

• For IV infusion, add the prescribed dose to 100 ml D_5W and infuse over 30–60 minutes. Alternatively, add the prescribed dose to D_5W to make a final concentration of 100 mg per 10 ml and infuse over 30–60 minutes.

Intervention and Evaluation

• Assess the patient's BP and pulse closely every 30 minutes until stabilized.

• Monitor the patient's weight daily at the start of therapy.

• Monitor the patient's liver function test results, including serum alkaline phosphatase, bilirubin, AST (SGOT), and ALT (SGPT) levels.

• Assess the patient for peripheral edema.

Patient Teaching

• Warn the patient to avoid tasks requiring mental alertness and motor skills until his or her response to the drug has been established.

prazosin hydrochloride

pra-zoe-sin

(Minipress, Prasig[AUS], Pratisol[AUS], Pressin[AUS])

CATEGORY AND SCHEDULE

Pregnancy Risk Category: C

MECHANISM OF ACTION

An antidote, antihypertensive, and vasodilator that selectively blocks $alpha_1$-adrenergic receptors, decreasing peripheral vascular resistance.

Therapeutic Effect: Produces vasodilation of veins and arterioles, decreases total peripheral resistance, and relaxes smooth muscle in bladder neck and prostate.

AVAILABILITY

Capsules: 1 mg, 2 mg, 5 mg.

INDICATIONS AND DOSAGES

▸ Mild to moderate hypertension

PO

Adults, Elderly. Initially, 1 mg 2–3 times a day. Maintenance: 3–15 mg/day in divided doses. Maximum: 20 mg/day.

Children. 5 mcg/kg/dose q6h. Gradually increase up to 25 mcg/kg/dose.

OFF-LABEL USES

Treatment of benign prostate hyperplasia, CHF, ergot alkaloid toxicity, pheochromocytoma, Raynaud's phenomenon

CONTRAINDICATIONS

None known.

INTERACTIONS

Drug

Estrogen, NSAIDs, other sympathomimetics: May decrease the effects of prazosin.

Hypotension-producing medications, such as antihypertensives and diuretics: May increase the effects of prazosin.

Herbal

Licorice: Causes sodium and water retention and potassium loss.

Food

None known.

DIAGNOSTIC TEST EFFECTS

None known.

SIDE EFFECTS

Frequent (10%–7%)

Dizziness, somnolence, headache, asthenia (loss of strength, energy)

Occasional (5%–4%)

Palpitations, nausea, dry mouth, nervousness

Rare (less than 1%)

Angina, urinary urgency

SERIOUS REACTIONS

! First-dose syncope (hypotension with sudden loss of consciousness) may occur 30 to 90 minutes following initial dose of more than 2 mg, a too-rapid increase in dosage, or addition of another antihypertensive agent to therapy. First-dose syncope may be preceded by tachycardia (pulse rate of 120–160 beats/minute).

NURSING CONSIDERATIONS

Baseline Assessment

- Give the first prazosin dose at bedtime. If the initial dose is given during the day, keep the patient recumbent for 3 to 4 hours.
- Assess the patient's BP and pulse immediately before each dose and every 15 to 30 minutes thereafter until BP is stabilized. Be alert for BP fluctuations.

Precautions

- Use prazosin cautiously in patients with chronic renal failure or impaired hepatic function.

Administration and Handling

PO

- Give prazosin without regard to food.
- Administer the first dose at bedtime to minimize the risk of fainting from first-dose syncope.

Intervention and Evaluation

- Monitor the patient's BP and pulse frequently because first-dose syncope may be preceded by tachycardia.
- Assess the patient's pattern of daily bowel activity and stool consistency.
- Assist the patient with ambulation if he or she experiences dizziness.

Patient Teaching

- Warn the patient to avoid tasks that require mental alertness or motor skills until his or her response the drug is established.
- Warn the patient to use caution

when driving or operating machinery and when rising from a sitting or lying position.
• Advise the patient to notify the physician if dizziness or palpitations become bothersome.

terazosin hydrochloride

ter-**a**-zoe-sin
(Apo-Terazosin[CAN], Hytrin, Novo-Terazosin [CAN])

CATEGORY AND SCHEDULE
Pregnancy Risk Category: C

MECHANISM OF ACTION
An antihypertensive and benign prostatic hyperplasia agent that blocks alpha-adrenergic receptors. Produces vasodilation, decreases peripheral resistance, and targets receptors around bladder neck and prostate. **Therapeutic Effect:** In hypertension, decreases BP. In benign prostatic hyperplasia, relaxes smooth muscle and improves urine flow.

PHARMACOKINETICS

Route	Onset	Peak	Duration
PO	15 min	1–2 hr	12–24 hr

Rapidly, completely absorbed from the GI tract. Protein binding: 90%–94%. Metabolized in the liver to active metabolite. Primarily eliminated in feces via biliary system; excreted in urine. Not removed by hemodialysis. ***Half-life:*** 12 hr.

AVAILABILITY
Capsules: 1 mg, 2 mg, 5 mg, 10 mg.
Tablets: 1 mg, 2 mg, 5 mg, 10 mg.

INDICATIONS AND DOSAGES
▸ **Mild to moderate hypertension**
PO
Adults, Elderly. Initially, 1 mg at bedtime. Slowly increase dosage to desired levels. Range: 1–5 mg/day as single or 2 divided doses. Maximum: 20 mg.
▸ **Benign prostatic hyperplasia**
PO
Adults, Elderly. Initially, 1 mg at bedtime. May increase up to 10 mg/day. Maximum: 20 mg/day.

CONTRAINDICATIONS
None known.

INTERACTIONS
Drug
Estrogen, NSAIDs, other sympathomimetics: May decrease the effects of terazosin.
Hypotension-producing medications, such as antihypertensives and diuretics: May increase the effects of terazosin.
Herbal
Dong quai, ginseng, garlic, yohimbe: May decrease the effects of terazosin.
Food
None known.

DIAGNOSTIC TEST EFFECTS
May decrease blood Hgb and Hct levels, serum albumin level, total serum protein level, and WBC count.

SIDE EFFECTS
Frequent (9%–5%)
Dizziness, headache, unusual tiredness
Rare (less than 2%)
Peripheral edema, orthostatic hypotension, myalgia, arthralgia, blurred vision, nausea, vomiting, nasal congestion, somnolence

SERIOUS REACTIONS

! First-dose syncope (hypotension with sudden loss of consciousness) may occur 30 to 90 minutes after initial dose of 2 mg or more, a too-rapid increase in dosage, or addition of another antihypertensive agent to therapy. First-dose syncope may be preceded by tachycardia (pulse rate of 120–160 beats/minute).

NURSING CONSIDERATIONS

Baseline Assessment

- Give first terazosin dose at bedtime. If the initial dose is given during the day, keep the patient recumbent for 3 to 4 hours.
- Assess the patient's BP and pulse immediately before each terazosin dose and every 15 to 30 minutes thereafter until BP is stabilized. Be alert for BP fluctuations.

Lifespan Considerations

- It is unknown if terazosin crosses the placenta or is distributed in breast milk.
- The safety and efficacy of terazosin have not been established in children.
- No age-related precautions have been noted in the elderly, but this age-group may be more sensitive to the drug's hypotensive effects.

Precautions

- Use terazosin cautiously in patients with confirmed or suspected coronary artery disease.

Administration and Handling

◀ **ALERT** ▶ If terazosin is discontinued for several days, expect to restart therapy with a 1-mg dose at bedtime.

PO

- Give terazosin without regard to food.
- Tablets may be crushed.
- Administer first dose at bedtime to minimize the risk of fainting due to first-dose syncope.

Intervention and Evaluation

- Monitor the patient's pulse frequently because first-dose syncope may be preceded by tachycardia.
- Assist the patient with ambulation if he or she experiences dizziness.
- Assess for peripheral edema.
- Monitor the patient's BP and assess for GU symptoms.

Patient Teaching

- Suggest to the patient that consuming dry toast, noncola carbonated beverages, and unsalted crackers may relieve nausea.
- Inform the patient that nasal congestion may occur.
- Advise the patient that the full therapeutic effect of terazosin may not occur for 3 to 4 weeks.
- Advise the patient to use caution when driving, performing tasks requiring mental alertness, and rising from a sitting or lying position.
- Warn the patient to notify the physician if he or she experiences dizziness or palpitations.

29 Vasodilators

bosentan
epoprostenol sodium, prostacyclin
fenoldopam
hydralazine hydrochloride
isosorbide dinitrate, isosorbide mononitrate
minoxidil
nesiritide
nitroglycerin
nitroprusside sodium

Uses: Vasodilators are used primarily to treat essential hypertension, angina pectoris, heart failure, and MI. Some of these agents are also used to manage peripheral vascular disease and to produce controlled hypotension during surgery. In addition, minoxidil is used as a hair growth stimulant.

Action: For vasodilators, the exact mechanism of action isn't known. These agents directly relax smooth muscle, which reduces vascular resistance. Some of them act primarily on arterioles, others affect veins, and still others work on both types of vessels.

COMBINATION PRODUCTS

APRESAZIDE: hydralazine/hydrochlorothiazide (a diuretic) 25 mg/25 mg; 50 mg/50 mg; 100 mg/50 mg.

bosentan

bo-sen-tan
(Tracleer)
Do not confuse Tracleer with Tricor.

CATEGORY AND SCHEDULE

Pregnancy Risk Category: X

MECHANISM OF ACTION

An endothelin receptor antagonist that blocks endothelin-1, the neurohormone that constricts pulmonary arteries. **Therapeutic Effect:** Improves exercise ability and slows clinical worsening of pulmonary arterial hypertension (PAH).

PHARMACOKINETICS

Highly bound to plasma proteins, mainly albumin. Metabolized in the liver. Eliminated by biliary excretion. ***Half-life:*** Approximately 5 hr.

AVAILABILITY

Tablets: 62.5 mg, 125 mg.

INDICATIONS AND DOSAGES

▸ **PAH in those with World Health Organization Class III or IV symptoms**

PO

Adults, Elderly. 62.5 mg twice a day for 4 wk; then increase to maintenance dosage of 125 mg twice a day.
Children weighing less than 40 kg. 62.5 mg twice a day.

CONTRAINDICATIONS

Administration with cyclosporine or glyburide, pregnancy

INTERACTIONS

Drug

Atorvastatin, glyburide, hormonal contraceptives (including oral, injectable, and implantable), lovastatin, simvastatin, warfarin: May decrease the plasma concentrations of these drugs.

Cyclosporine, ketoconazole: May increase plasma concentration of bosentan.

Herbal

None known.

Food

None known.

DIAGNOSTIC TEST EFFECTS

May increase serum bilirubin, AST (SGOT), and ALT (SGPT) levels. May decrease blood Hgb and Hct levels.

SIDE EFFECTS

Occasional

Headache, nasopharyngitis, flushing

Rare

Dyspepsia (heartburn, epigastric distress), fatigue, pruritus, hypotension

SERIOUS REACTIONS

! Abnormal hepatic function, lower extremity edema, and palpitations occur rarely.

NURSING CONSIDERATIONS

Baseline Assessment

• Because pregnancy must be avoided during bosentan therapy, determine if the patient is pregnant before the start of therapy. A negative result from a urine or serum pregnancy test performed during the first 5 days of a normal menstrual period and at least 11 days after the last act of sexual intercourse must be obtained before drug therapy begins. Expect the patient to undergo monthly pregnancy tests during bosentan therapy.

Lifespan Considerations

• Bosentan administration may induce atrophy of seminiferous tubules of the testes, cause male infertility, or reduce sperm count.

• Bosentan causes fetal harm and has teratogenic effects on the fetus, including malformations of the face, head, large vessels, and mouth. Also, breast-feeding is not recommended for patients taking bosentan.

• The safety and efficacy of bosentan have not been established in children.

• Use cautiously in the elderly because the higher frequency of decreased cardiac, hepatic, and renal function is more common in this age-group.

Precautions

• Use bosentan extremely cautiously in patients with moderate to severe hepatic function impairment, and use cautiously in patients with mild hepatic impairment.

Administration and Handling

• Give bosentan in the morning and evening, with or without food.

• Do not break or crush film-coated tablets. Have the patient swallow the film-coated tablets whole and avoid chewing them.

Intervention and Evaluation

• Assess the patient's hepatic enzyme levels [serum aminotransferase, serum alkaline phosphatase, bilirubin, AST (SGOT), and ALT (SGPT)] before bosentan therapy begins and monthly thereafter. Expect to initiate changes in monitoring and treatment if an elevation in hepatic enzyme levels occurs. Expect to stop treatment if clinical symptoms of hepatic injury, including abdominal pain, fatigue, jaundice, nausea, and vomiting, occur or if the patient's bilirubin level increases.

• Monitor the patient's blood Hgb level at 1 and 3 months after treatment begins and every 3 months thereafter. A decrease in blood Hct and Hgb levels signifies anemia.

Patient Teaching

• Discuss with the patient the importance of pregnancy testing and the avoidance of pregnancy while taking bosentan. Teach the patient about the various methods of effective contraception.

epoprostenol sodium, prostacyclin

e-poe-**pros**-ten-ol
(Flolan)

CATEGORY AND SCHEDULE

Pregnancy Risk Category: B

MECHANISM OF ACTION

An antihypertensive that directly dilates pulmonary and systemic arterial vascular beds and inhibits platelet aggregation. **Therapeutic Effect:** Reduces right and left ventricular afterload; increases cardiac output and stroke volume.

AVAILABILITY

Injection, Powder for Reconstitution: 0.5 mg, 1.5 mg.

INDICATIONS AND DOSAGES

▸ **Long-term treatment of New York Heart Association Class III and IV primary pulmonary hypertension**

IV Infusion

Adults, Elderly. Procedure to determine dose range: Initially, 2 ng/kg/min, increased in increments of 2 ng/kg/min q15min until dose-limiting adverse effects occur. Chronic infusion: Start at 4 ng/kg/min less than the maximum dose rate tolerated during acute dose ranging (or one half of the maximum rate if rate was less than 5 ng/kg/min).

OFF-LABEL USES

Cardiopulmonary bypass surgery; hemodialysis; pulmonary hypertension associated with acute respiratory distress syndrome, systemic lupus erythematosus, or congenital heart disease; neonatal pulmonary hypertension, refractory CHF; severe community-acquired pneumonia

CONTRAINDICATIONS

Long-term use in patients with CHF (severe ventricular systolic dysfunction)

INTERACTIONS

Drug

Acetate in dialysis fluids, other vasodilators: May increase hypotensive effect.
Anticoagulants, antiplatelets: May increase the risk of bleeding.
Vasoconstrictors: May decrease effects of epoprostenol.

Herbal

None known.

Food

None known.

DIAGNOSTIC TEST EFFECTS

None known.

IV INCOMPATIBILITIES

Don't mix epoprostenol with other medications.

SIDE EFFECTS

Frequent

Acute phase: Flushing (58%), headache (49%), nausea (32%), vomiting (32%), hypotension (16%), anxiety (11%), chest pain (11%), dizziness (8%)
Chronic phase (greater than 20%): Dyspnea, asthenia, dizziness, headache, chest pain, nausea, vomiting, palpitations, edema, jaw pain, tachycardia, flushing, myalgia, nonspecific muscle pain, paresthesia, diarrhea, anxiety, chills, fever, or flu-like symptoms

Occasional
Acute phase (5%–2%): Bradycardia, abdominal pain, muscle pain, dyspnea, back pain
Chronic phase (20%–10%): Rash, depression, hypotension, pallor, syncope, bradycardia, ascites
Rare
Acute phase: Paresthesia
Chronic phase (less than 2%): Diaphoresis, dyspepsia, tachycardia

SERIOUS REACTIONS

! Overdose may cause hyperglycemia or ketoacidosis manifested as increased urination, thirst, and fruit-like breath odor.
! Angina, MI, and thrombocytopenia occur rarely.
! Abrupt withdrawal, including a large reduction in dosage or interruption in drug delivery, may produce rebound pulmonary hypertension as evidenced by dyspnea, dizziness, and asthenia.

NURSING CONSIDERATIONS

Baseline Assessment

- Before beginning therapy, obtain a backup infusion pump and IV infusion sets to avoid interruptions in therapy.
- Make sure the patient has a central venous catheter in place.
- Take baseline vital signs for later comparison.

Lifespan Considerations

- Use epoprostenol cautiously in elderly patients.

Precautions

- Avoid interruptions in the IV infusion because even a short break in the infusion can result in rebounding pulmonary hypertension.
- Closely monitor the patient during initiation of therapy.

Administration and Handling

◀ALERT▶ Infuse epoprostenol continuously through an indwelling central venous catheter. If necessary and on a temporary basis, infuse through a peripheral vein.

IV

- Store unopened vial at room temperature. Do not freeze.
- Reconstituted solutions are stable for up to 48 hours if refrigerated.

◀ALERT▶ Use only the diluent provided by the manufacturer.

- Follow instructions of manufacturer for dilution to specific concentrations.
- Give as pump infusion only.

Intervention and Evaluation

- Monitor the patient's standing and supine BP for several hours after a dosage adjustment.
- Assess the patient for a therapeutic response as evidenced by decreased chest pain, dyspnea on exertion, fatigue, pulmonary arterial pressure, pulmonary vascular resistance, and syncope, and improved pulmonary function.

Patient Teaching

- Teach the patient how to reconstitute and administer epoprostenol and how to care for the permanent central venous catheter.
- Advise the patient that brief interruptions in drug delivery may result in rapidly, worsening symptoms.
- Explain to the patient that epoprostenol therapy will be necessary for a prolonged period, possibly years.

fenoldopam

fhe-**knowl**-doh-pam
(Corlopam)

CATEGORY AND SCHEDULE

Pregnancy Risk Category: B

MECHANISM OF ACTION

A rapid-acting vasodilator. An agonist for D_1-like dopamine receptors; also produces vasodilation in coronary, renal, mesenteric, and peripheral arteries. **Therapeutic Effect:** Reduces systolic and diastolic BP and increases heart rate.

PHARMACOKINETICS

After IV administration, metabolized in the liver. Primarily excreted in urine. Unknown if removed by hemodialysis. ***Half-life:*** Approximately 5 min.

AVAILABILITY

Injection: 10 mg/ml.

INDICATIONS AND DOSAGES

▸ **Short-term management of severe hypertension when rapid, but quickly reversible emergency reduction of BP is clinically indicated, including malignant hypertension with deteriorating end-organ function**

IV Infusion (continuous)

Adults. Initially, 0.1 mcg/kg/min. May increase in increments of 0.05–0.2 mcg/kg/min until target blood pressure is achieved. Usual length of treatment is 1–6 hours with tapering of dose q15–30min. Average rate: 0.25–0.5 mcg/kg/min.

CONTRAINDICATIONS

None known.

INTERACTIONS

Drug

Beta blockers: May produce excessive hypotension.

Herbal

None known.

Food

None known.

DIAGNOSTIC TEST EFFECTS

May elevate BUN, blood glucose, serum LDH, and serum transaminase levels. May decrease serum potassium levels.

IV INCOMPATIBILITIES

Do not mix fenoldopam with other medications. Specific IV incompatibilities are not available.

SIDE EFFECTS

Expected

Beta blockers may cause unforeseen hypotension.

Occasional

Headache (7%), flushing (3%), nausea (4%), hypotension (2%)

Rare (2% or less)

Nervousness or anxiety, vomiting, constipation, nasal congestion, diaphoresis, back pain

SERIOUS REACTIONS

! Excessive hypotension occurs occasionally.

! Substantial tachycardia may lead to ischemic cardiac events or worsened heart failure.

! Allergic-type reactions, including anaphylaxis and life-threatening asthmatic exacerbation, may occur in patients with sulfite sensitivity.

NURSING CONSIDERATIONS

Baseline Assessment

- Obtain the patient's apical pulse and BP before therapy begins.
- Assess the patient's medication history, especially beta blocker use.
- Obtain the patient's serum electrolyte levels, particularly potassium, as ordered, and periodically monitor the patient's electrolyte levels during the fenoldopam infusion.
- Determine if asthmatic patients have a history of sulfite sensitivity.
- Be sure to check with the physician

for the desired BP range parameter for each patient.

Lifespan Considerations

- It is unknown if fenoldopam is distributed in breast milk.
- The safety and efficacy of fenoldopam have not been established in children.
- No age-related precautions have been noted in the elderly.

Precautions

- Use fenoldopam cautiously in patients with glaucoma, hypokalemia, hypotension, intraocular hypertension, sulfite sensitivity, or tachycardia.

Administration and Handling

IV

◀ALERT▶ Give fenoldopam only by continuous IV infusion and not as a bolus injection.

- Store ampules at room temperature.
- Each 10 mg (1 ml) must be diluted with 250 ml 0.9% NaCl or D_5W to provide a concentration of 40 mcg/ml.
- Diluted solution is stable for 24 hours. Discard any solution not used within 24 hours.
- Use an infusion pump and administer as an IV infusion at an initial rate of 0.1 mcg/kg/minute.

Intervention and Evaluation

- Monitor the infusion rate frequently.
- Diligently monitor the patient's BP during the infusion to assess for signs of hypotension and to avoid a too-rapid decrease in BP.
- Monitor the patient's EKG for tachycardia (which may lead to angina, ischemic heart disease, MI, extrasystoles, or worsening heart failure).
- Observe the patient closely for symptomatic hypotension.

Patient Teaching

- Warn patient to change positions slowly to avoid orthostasis.
- Tell the patient that he or she will most likely require an oral antihypertensive when fenoldopam therapy has been completed.

hydralazine hydrochloride

hye-**dral**-a-zeen

(Alphapress[AUS], Apresoline, Novohylazin[CAN])

Do not confuse hydralazine with hydroxyzine.

CATEGORY AND SCHEDULE

Pregnancy Risk Category: C

MECHANISM OF ACTION

An antihypertensive with direct vasodilating effects on arterioles. **Therapeutic Effect:** Decreases BP and systemic resistance.

PHARMACOKINETICS

Route	Onset	Peak	Duration
PO	20–30 min	N/A	2–4 hr
IV	5–20 min	N/A	2–6 hr

Well absorbed from the GI tract. Widely distributed. Protein binding: 85%–90%. Metabolized in the liver to active metabolite. Primarily excreted in urine. Not removed by hemodialysis. ***Half-life:*** 3–7 hr (increased with impaired renal function).

AVAILABILITY

Tablets: 10 mg, 25 mg, 50 mg, 100 mg.

Injection: 20 mg/ml.

INDICATIONS AND DOSAGES

▸ Moderate to severe hypertension

PO

Adults. Initially, 10 mg 4 times a day. May increase by 10–25 mg/dose q2–5days. Maximum: 300 mg/day.
Children. Initially, 0.75–1 mg/kg/day in 2–4 divided doses, not to exceed 25 mg/dose. May increase over 3–4 wk. Maximum: 7.5 mg/kg/day (5 mg/kg/day in infants).

IV, IM

Adults, Elderly. Initially, 10–20 mg/dose q4–6h. May increase to 40 mg/ dose.
Children. Initially, 0.1–0.2 mg/kg/dose (maximum: 20 mg) q4–6h, as needed, up to 1.7–3.5 mg/kg/day in divided doses q4–6h.

▸ Dosage in renal impairment

Dosage interval is based on creatinine clearance.

Creatinine Clearance	Dosage Interval
10–50 ml/min	q8h
less than 10 ml/min	q8–24h

OFF-LABEL USES

Treatment of CHF, hypertension secondary to eclampsia and preeclampsia, primary pulmonary hypertension

CONTRAINDICATIONS

Coronary artery disease, lupus erythematosus, rheumatic heart disease

INTERACTIONS

Drug

Diuretics, other antihypertensives: May increase hypotensive effect.

Herbal

None known.

Food

None known.

DIAGNOSTIC TEST EFFECTS

May produce positive direct Coombs' test.

IV INCOMPATIBILITIES

Aminophylline, ampicillin (Polycillin), furosemide (Lasix)

IV COMPATIBILITIES

Dobutamine (Dobutrex), heparin, hydrocortisone (Solu-Cortef), nitroglycerin, potassium

SIDE EFFECTS

Frequent

Headache, palpitations, tachycardia (generally disappears in 7–10 days)

Occasional

GI disturbance (nausea, vomiting, diarrhea), paraesthesia, fluid retention, peripheral edema, dizziness, flushed face, nasal congestion

SERIOUS REACTIONS

! High dosage may produce lupus erythematosus-like reaction, including fever, facial rash, muscle and joint aches, and splenomegaly.
! Severe orthostatic hypotension, skin flushing, severe headache, myocardial ischemia, and cardiac arrhythmias may develop.
! Profound shock may occur with severe overdosage.

NURSING CONSIDERATIONS

Baseline Assessment

- Obtain the patient's BP and pulse immediately before each hydralazine dose, in addition to regular BP monitoring. Be alert for BP fluctuations.

Lifespan Considerations

- Hydralazine crosses the placenta; it is unknown if it is distributed in breast milk.
- Hematomas, leukopenia, petechial bleeding, and thrombocytopenia

have occurred in newborns; these conditions resolve within 1 to 3 weeks.
- No age-related precautions have been noted in children.
- The elderly are more sensitive to the drug's hypotensive effects.
- In the elderly, age-related renal impairment may require dosage adjustment.

Precautions
- Use hydralazine cautiously in patients with cerebrovascular disease and impaired renal function.

Administration and Handling
PO
- Hydralazine is best given with food or regularly spaced meals.
- Crush tablets if necessary.

IV
- Store drug at room temperature.
- Give undiluted if necessary.
- Give single dose over 1 minute.

Intervention and Evaluation
- Monitor the patient for headache, palpitations, and tachycardia.
- Assess for peripheral edema of the hands and feet.
- Assess the patient's pattern of daily bowel activity and stool consistency.

Patient Teaching
- Instruct the patient to rise slowly from a lying to a sitting position and to permit legs to dangle from the bed momentarily before standing to reduce the hypotensive effect of hydralazine.
- Suggest to the patient that consuming dry toast or unsalted crackers may relieve nausea.
- Warn patients who are receiving high doses of hydralazine to notify the physician if they experience fever (lupus-like reaction) or joint and muscle aches.

isosorbide dinitrate
eye-sew-**sore**-bide
(Apo-ISDN[CAN], Cedocard[CAN], Dilatrate, Isogen[AUS], Isordil, Sorbidin[AUS])

isosorbide mononitrate
(Duride[AUS], Imdur, Imdur Durules[AUS], Imtrate[AUS], ISMO, Monodur Durules[AUS], Monoket)
Do not confuse Isordil with Isuprel or Plendil, or Imdur with Inderal or K-Dur.

CATEGORY AND SCHEDULE
Pregnancy Risk Category: C

MECHANISM OF ACTION
A nitrate that stimulates intracellular cyclic guanosine monophosphate. **Therapeutic Effect:** Relaxes vascular smooth muscle of both arterial and venous vasculature. Decreases preload and afterload.

PHARMACOKINETICS

Route	Onset	Peak	Duration
Dinitrate			
Sublingual	2–5 min	N/A	1–2 hr
Oral (Chewable)	2–5 min	N/A	1–2 hr
Oral	15–40 min	N/A	4–6 hr
Oral (Sustained-Release)	30 min	N/A	12 hr
Mononitrate			
Oral (Extended-Release)	60 min	N/A	N/A

Dinitrate is poorly absorbed and metabolized in the liver to its active metabolite isosorbide mononitrate. Mononitrate is well absorbed after

PO administration. Excreted in urine and feces. ***Half-life:*** Dinitrate, 1–4 hr; mononitrate, 4 hr.

AVAILABILITY

Capsules (Sustained-Release [Dilatrate]): 40 mg.
Tablets (Isordil): 5 mg, 10 mg, 20 mg, 30 mg, 40 mg.
Tablets (Ismo, Monoket): 10 mg, 20 mg.
Tablets (Chewable): 5 mg, 10 mg.
Tablets (Extended-Release [Imdur]): 30 mg, 60 mg, 120 mg.
Tablets (Sublingual [Isordil]): 10 mg.

INDICATIONS AND DOSAGES

▸ **Angina**

PO (isosorbide dinitrate)
Adults, Elderly. 5–40 mg 4 times a day. Sustained-release: 40 mg q8–12h.
PO (isosorbide mononitrate)
Adults, Elderly. 5–10 mg twice a day given 7 hours apart. Sustained-release: Initially, 30–60 mg/day in morning as a single dose. May increase dose at 3-day intervals. Maximum: 240 mg/day.

OFF-LABEL USES

CHF, dysphagia, pain relief, relief of esophageal spasm with gastroesophageal reflux

CONTRAINDICATIONS

Closed-angle glaucoma, GI hypermotility or malabsorption (extended-release tablets), head trauma, hypersensitivity to nitrates, increased intracranial pressure, orthostatic hypotension, severe anemia (extended-release tablets)

INTERACTIONS

Drug

Alcohol, antihypertensives, vasodilators: May increase risk of orthostatic hypotension.

Herbal

None known.

Food

None known.

DIAGNOSTIC TEST EFFECTS

May increase urine catecholamine and urine vanillylmandelic acid levels.

SIDE EFFECTS

Frequent

Burning and tingling at oral point of dissolution (sublingual), headache (possibly severe) occurs mostly in early therapy, diminishes rapidly in intensity, and usually disappears during continued treatment, transient flushing of face and neck, dizziness (especially if patient is standing immobile or is in a warm environment), weakness, orthostatic hypotension, nausea, vomiting, restlessness

Occasional

GI upset, blurred vision, dry mouth

SERIOUS REACTIONS

! Blurred vision or dry mouth may occur (drug should be discontinued).
! Isosorbide administration may cause severe orthostatic hypotension manifested by fainting, pulselessness, cold or clammy skin, and diaphoresis.
! Tolerance may occur with repeated, prolonged therapy, but may not occur with the extended-release form. Minor tolerance may be seen with intermittent use of sublingual tablets.
! High dosage tends to produce severe headache.

NURSING CONSIDERATIONS

Baseline Assessment

• Record the onset, type (sharp, dull, or squeezing), radiation, location, intensity, and duration of anginal pain and its precipitating factors, such as exertion and emotional stress.

Lifespan Considerations

• It is unknown if isosorbide crosses the placenta or is distributed in breast milk.
• The safety and efficacy of isosorbide have not been established in children.
• The elderly may be more sensitive to the drug's hypotensive effects.
• In the elderly, age-related decreased renal function may require cautious use.

Precautions

• Use isosorbide cautiously in patients with acute MI, blood volume depletion from therapy, glaucoma (contraindicated in closed-angle glaucoma), hepatic or renal disease, or systolic BP less than 90 mm Hg.

Administration and Handling

PO

• Best if taken on an empty stomach; however, administer isosorbide with meals if the patient experiences a headache.
• Oral tablets, except the extended-release form, may be crushed.
• Do not crush or break extended-release form.
• Do not crush chewable form before administering.

Sublingual

• Do not crush or have patient chew sublingual tablets.
• Have patient dissolve tablets under tongue without swallowing.

Intervention and Evaluation

• Monitor and document the number of anginal episodes and the patient's orthostatic BP.
• Assist the patient with ambulation if he or she experiences dizziness or light-headedness.
• Assess the patient for facial or neck flushing.

Patient Teaching

• Teach the patient to take sublingual tablets while sitting down. Explain to the patient that he or she should not chew or crush sublingual, extended-release, or sustained-release forms. Instruct the patient to dissolve sublingual tablets under the tongue and not to swallow them.
• Instruct the patient to take isosorbide at the first sign or symptom of angina. Explain to the patient that if angina is not relieved within 5 minutes, he or she can dissolve a second tablet under the tongue and then repeat the dosage 5 minutes later if he or she still feels no relief. Caution patient to take no more than 3 tablets within 15 to 30 minutes.
• Warn the patient to seek immediate emergency assistance if anginal pain persists.
• Advise the patient that after anginal pain is completely relieved, he or she should expel any remaining sublingual tablet from under the tongue.
• Instruct the patient to rise slowly from a lying to a sitting position and dangle legs momentarily before standing.
• Teach the patient to take the oral form on an empty stomach unless headache occurs during management therapy. Advise the patient to take the oral form with meals if headache occurs.
• Caution the patient against changing from one brand of drug to another.
• Urge the patient to avoid alcohol during isosorbide therapy because alcohol intensifies the drug's hypotensive effect. Explain to the patient

that if alcohol is ingested soon after taking nitrates, he or she may experience an acute hypotensive episode marked by pallor, vertigo, and a drop in BP.

minoxidil

min-**nox**-i-dill

(Apo-Gain[CAN], Loniten, Milnox [CAN], Regaine[AUS], Rogaine, Rogaine Extra Strength)

Do not confuse Loniten with Lotensin.

CATEGORY AND SCHEDULE

Pregnancy Risk Category: C

OTC (topical solution)

MECHANISM OF ACTION

An antihypertensive and hair growth stimulant that has direct action on vascular smooth muscle, producing vasodilation of arterioles. **Therapeutic Effect:** Decreases peripheral vascular resistance and BP; increases cutaneous blood flow; stimulates hair follicle epithelium and hair follicle growth.

PHARMACOKINETICS

Route	Onset	Peak	Duration
PO	0.5 hr	2–8 hr	2–5 days

Well absorbed from the GI tract; minimal absorption after topical application. Protein binding: None. Widely distributed. Metabolized in the liver to active metabolite. Primarily excreted in urine. Removed by hemodialysis. ***Half-life:*** 4.2 hr.

AVAILABILITY

Tablets (Loniten): 2.5 mg, 10 mg.

Topical Solution (Rogaine): 2% (20 mg/ml).

Topical Solution (Rogaine Extra Strength): 5% (50 mg/ml).

INDICATIONS AND DOSAGES

▸ **Severe symptomatic hypertension, hypertension associated with organ damage, hypertension that has failed to respond to maximal therapeutic dosages of a diuretic or two other antihypertensives**

PO

Adults. Initially, 5 mg/day. Increase with at least 3-day intervals to 10 mg, then 20 mg, then up to 40 mg/day in 1–2 doses.

Elderly. Initially, 2.5 mg/day. May increase gradually. Maintenance: 10–40 mg/day. Maximum: 100 mg/day.

Children. Initially, 0.1–0.2 mg/kg (5 mg maximum) daily. Gradually increase at a minimum of 3-day intervals. Maintenance: 0.25–1 mg/kg/day in 1–2 doses. Maximum: 50 mg/day.

▸ **Hair regrowth**

Topical

Adults. 1 ml to affected areas of scalp 2 times a day. Total daily dose not to exceed 2 ml.

CONTRAINDICATIONS

Pheochromocytoma

INTERACTIONS

Drug

Parenteral antihypertensives: May increase hypotensive effect.

NSAIDs: May decrease the hypotensive effects of minoxidil.

Herbal

None known.

Food

None known.

DIAGNOSTIC TEST EFFECTS

May increase plasma renin activity

and BUN, serum alkaline phosphatase, serum creatinine, and serum sodium levels. May decrease blood Hgb and Hct levels and erythrocyte count.

SIDE EFFECTS

Frequent

PO: Edema with concurrent weight gain, hypertrichosis (elongation, thickening, increased pigmentation of fine body hair; develops in 80% of patients within 3–6 weeks after beginning therapy)

Occasional

PO: T-wave changes (usually revert to pretreatment state with continued therapy or drug withdrawal)
Topical: Pruritus, rash, dry or flaking skin, erythema

Rare

PO: Breast tenderness, headache, photosensitivity reaction
Topical: Allergic reaction, alopecia, burning sensation at scalp, soreness at hair root, headache, visual disturbances

SERIOUS REACTIONS

! Tachycardia and angina pectoris may occur because of increased oxygen demands associated with increased heart rate and cardiac output.

! Fluid and electrolyte imbalance and CHF may occur, especially if a diuretic is not given concurrently with minoxidil.

! Too rapid reduction in BP may result in syncope, CVA, MI, and ocular or vestibular ischemia.

! Pericardial effusion and tamponade may be seen in patients with impaired renal function who are not on dialysis.

NURSING CONSIDERATIONS

Baseline Assessment

• Assess the patient's BP on both arms and take the patient's pulse for 1 full minute immediately before giving the medication. If the patient's pulse rate increases 20 beats/minute or more over baseline, or systolic or diastolic BP decreases more than 20 mm Hg, withhold minoxidil and contact the physician.

Lifespan Considerations

• Minoxidil crosses the placenta and is distributed in breast milk.
• No age-related precautions have been noted in children.
• The elderly are more sensitive to the drug's hypotensive effects.
• In the elderly, age-related renal impairment may require dosage adjustment.

Precautions

• Use minoxidil cautiously in patients with chronic CHF, coronary artery disease, recent MI (within 1 month), or severe renal impairment.

Administration and Handling

PO
• Give drug without regard to food. Can give with food if GI upset occurs.
• Crush tablets if necessary.

Topical
• Shampoo and dry patient's hair before applying medication. Wash hands immediately after application.
• Do not use a hair dryer to dry the patient's hair after application (reduces effectiveness).

Intervention and Evaluation

• Monitor the patient's BP, weight, and serum electrolyte levels.
• Assess the patient for peripheral edema.
• Assess the patient for signs and symptoms of CHF, including cool extremities, cough, dyspnea on

exertion, and crackles at the base of the lungs.

• Auscultate the patient's heart sounds. Distant or muffled heart sounds may indicate pericardial effusion or tamponade.

Patient Teaching

• Advise the patient that maximum BP response occurs 3 to 7 days after initiation of minoxidil therapy and reversible growth of fine body hair may begin 3 to 6 weeks after the start of treatment.

• Explain to the patient that when minoxidil is used topically for stimulation of hair growth, treatment must continue on a permanent basis and that any cessation of treatment will reverse new hair growth.

• Warn the patient to avoid exposure to sunlight and artificial light sources.

nesiritide

neh-**sir**-i-tide

(Natrecor)

CATEGORY AND SCHEDULE

Pregnancy Risk Category: C

MECHANISM OF ACTION

A brain natriuretic peptide that facilitates cardiovascular homeostasis and fluid status through counter-regulation of the renin-angiotensin-aldosterone system, stimulating cyclic guanosine monophosphate, thereby leading to smooth-muscle cell relaxation. **Therapeutic Effect:** Promotes vasodilation, natriuresis, and diuresis, correcting CHF.

PHARMACOKINETICS

Route	Onset	Peak	Duration
IV	15–30 min	1–2 hr	4 hr

Excreted primarily in the heart by the left ventricle. Metabolized by the natriuretic neutral endopeptidase enzymes on the vascular luminal surface. ***Half-life:*** 18–23 min.

AVAILABILITY

Injection Powder for Reconstitution: 1.5 mg/5-ml vial.

INDICATIONS AND DOSAGES

▸ **Treatment of acutely decompensated CHF in patients with dyspnea at rest or with minimal activity**

IV Bolus

Adults, Elderly. 2 mcg/kg followed by a continuous IV infusion of 0.01 mcg/kg/min. May be incrementally increased q3h to a maximum of 0.03 mcg/kg/min.

CONTRAINDICATIONS

Cardiogenic shock, systolic BP less than 90 mm Hg

INTERACTIONS

Drug

ACE inhibitors, IV nitroglycerin, milrinone, nitroprusside: May increase risk of hypotension.

Herbal

None known.

Food

None known.

DIAGNOSTIC TEST EFFECTS

None known.

IV INCOMPATIBILITIES

Sodium metabisulfite, bumetanide (Bumex), enalapril (Vasotec), ethacrynic acid (Edecrin), furosemide

(Lasix), heparin, hydralazine (Apresoline), insulin

SIDE EFFECTS

Frequent (11%)
Hypotension
Occasional (8%–2%)
Headache, nausea, bradycardia
Rare (1% or less)
Confusion, paresthesia, somnolence, tremor

SERIOUS REACTIONS

! Ventricular arrhythmias, including ventricular tachycardia, atrial fibrillation, AV node conduction abnormalities, and angina pectoris occur rarely.

NURSING CONSIDERATIONS

Baseline Assessment

- Obtain the patient's BP immediately before each nesiritide dose, in addition to regular monitoring. Be alert to BP fluctuations. Place the patient in the supine position with legs elevated if he or she experiences an excessive reduction in BP.

Lifespan Considerations

- It is unknown if nesiritide crosses the placenta or is distributed in breast milk.
- The safety and efficacy of nesiritide have not been established in children.
- No age-related precautions have been noted in the elderly.

Precautions

- Use nesiritide cautiously in patients with atrial conduction defects, constrictive pericarditis, hypotension, hepatic impairment, pericardial tamponade, renal impairment, restrictive or obstructive cardiomyopathy, significant valvular stenosis, suspected low cardiac filling pressures, or ventricular conduction defects.

Administration and Handling

◀ ALERT ▶ Do not mix with other injections or infusions. Do not give IM.

IV

- Store vial at room temperature. Once reconstituted, store at room temperature or refrigerate; use within 24 hours.
- Reconstitute one 1.5-mg vial with 5 ml D_5W, 0.9% NaCl, 0.2% NaCl, or any combination thereof. Swirl or rock gently, and add to 250-ml bag D_5W, 0.9% NaCl, 0.2% NaCl, or any combination thereof yielding a solution of 6 mcg/ml.
- Give initially as an IV bolus over approximately 60 seconds, followed by continuous IV infusion.

Intervention and Evaluation

- Frequently monitor the patient's BP for hypotension and pulse rate for abnormalities.
- Establish parameters with the physician for adjusting the rate or stopping the infusion.
- Maintain accurate patient intake and output records; assess the patient's urine output frequently.
- Immediately notify the physician of cardiac arrhythmias, decreased urine output, or a significant decrease in BP or heart rate.

Patient Teaching

- Explain to the patient that nesiritide is not a cure for CHF but that it will help relieve symptoms.
- Caution the patient to immediately report chest pain or palpitations.

nitroglycerin

nye-troe-**gli**-ser-in
(Anginine[AUS], Minitran, Nitradisc[AUS], Nitrek, Nitro-Bid, Nitro-Dur, Nitrogard, Nitroject [CAN], Nitrolingual, Nitrolingual Spray[AUS], Nitrong-SR, NitroQuick, Nitrostat, Nitro-Tab, Rectogesic[AUS], Transiderm Nitro[AUS], Trinipatch[CAN])
Do not confuse nitroglycerin with nitroprusside; Nitro-Bid with Nicobid; Nitro-Dur with Nicoderm; Nitrostat with Hyperstat, Nilstat, or Nystatin; or Nitrong-SR with Nizoral.

CATEGORY AND SCHEDULE

Pregnancy Risk Category: B

MECHANISM OF ACTION

A nitrate that decreases myocardial oxygen demand. Reduces left ventricular preload and afterload. **Therapeutic Effect:** Dilates coronary arteries and improves collateral blood flow to ischemic areas within myocardium. IV form produces peripheral vasodilation.

PHARMACOKINETICS

Route	Onset	Peak	Duration
Sublingual	1–3 min	4–8 min	30–60 min
Translingual spray	2 min	4–10 min	30–60 min
Buccal Tablet	2–5 min	4–10 min	2 hr
PO (Extended-Release)	20–45 min	45–120 min	4–8 hr
Topical	15–60 min	30–120 min	2–12 hr
Transdermal Patch	40–60 min	60–180 min	18–24 hr
IV	1–2 min	Immediate	3–5 min

Well absorbed after PO, sublingual, and topical administration. Undergoes extensive first-pass metabolism. Metabolized in the liver and by enzymes in the bloodstream. Primarily excreted in urine. Not removed by hemodialysis. ***Half-life:*** 1–4 min.

AVAILABILITY

Capsules (Extended-Release [NitroBid]): 2.5 mg, 6.5 mg, 9 mg.
Tablets (Buccal [Nitrogard]): 2 mg, 3 mg.
Tablets (Sublingual [NitroQuick, Nitrostat, Nitro-Tab]): 0.4 mg, 0.6 mg.
Spray (Translingual [Nitrolingual]): 0.4 mg/spray.
Infusion Solution: 0.1 mg/ml, 0.2 mg/ml, 0.4 mg/ml.
Topical Ointment (Nitro-Bid, Nitrol): 2%.
Transdermal Patch (Minitran): 0.1 mg/h, 0.2 mg/h, 0.3 mg/h, 0.4 mg/h.
*Transdermal Patch (NitroDur):*0.1 mg/h, 0.2 mg/h, 0.3 mg/h, 0.4 mg/h, 0.6 mg/h, 0.8 mg/h.
Transdermal Patch (Nitrek): 0.2 mg/h, 0.4 mg/h, 0.6 mg/h.

INDICATIONS AND DOSAGES

▸ **Acute relief of angina pectoris, acute prophylaxis**
Lingual Spray
Adults, Elderly. 1 spray onto or under tongue q3–5min until relief is noted (no more than 3 sprays in 15-min period).
Sublingual
Adults, Elderly. 0.4 mg q5min until relief is noted (no more than 3 doses in 15-min period). Use prophylactically 5–10 min before activities that may cause an acute attack.
▸ **Long-term prophylaxis of angina**
PO (Extended-Release)
Adults, Elderly. 2.5–9 mg q8–12h.
Topical
Adults, Elderly. Initially, ½ inch

q8h. Increase by ½ inch with each application. Range: 1–2 inches q8h up to 4–5 inches q4h.
Transdermal Patch
Adults, Elderly. Initially, 0.2–0.4 mg/hr. Maintenance: 0.4–0.8 mg/hr. Consider patch on for 12–14 hr, patch off for 10–12 hr (prevents tolerance).

▸ **CHF associated with acute MI**
IV
Adults, Elderly. Initially, 5 mcg/min via infusion pump. Increase in 5-mcg/min increments at 3- to 5-min intervals until BP response is noted or until dosage reaches 20 mcg/min; then increase as needed by 10 mcg/min. Dosage may be further titrated according to clinical, therapeutic response up to 200 mcg/min.
Children. Initially, 0.25–0.5 mcg/kg/min; titrate by 0.5–1 mcg/kg/min up to 20 mcg/kg/min.

CONTRAINDICATIONS

Allergy to adhesives (transdermal), closed-angle glaucoma, constrictive pericarditis (IV), early MI (sublingual), GI hypermotility or malabsorption (extended-release), head trauma, hypotension (IV), inadequate cerebral circulation (IV), increased intracranial pressure, nitrates, orthostatic hypotension, pericardial tamponade (IV), severe anemia, uncorrected hypovolemia (IV)

INTERACTIONS

Drug

Alcohol, other antihypertensives, vasodilators: May increase risk of orthostatic hypotension.
Sildenafil, tadalafil, vardenafil: Concurrent use of these drugs produces significant hypotension.

Herbal

None known.

Food

None known.

DIAGNOSTIC TEST EFFECTS

May increase blood methemoglobin , urine catecholamine, and urine vanillylmandelic acid concentrations.

IV INCOMPATIBILITIES

Alteplase (Activase)

IV COMPATIBILITIES

Amiodarone (Cordarone), diltiazem (Cardizem), dobutamine (Dobutrex), dopamine (Intropin), epinephrine, famotidine (Pepcid), fentanyl (Sublimaze), furosemide (Lasix), heparin, hydromorphone (Dilaudid), insulin, labetalol (Trandate), lidocaine, lorazepam (Ativan), midazolam (Versed), milrinone (Primacor), morphine, nicardipine (Cardene), nitroprusside (Nipride), norepinephrine (Levophed), propofol (Diprivan)

SIDE EFFECTS

Frequent

Headache (possibly severe; occurs mostly in early therapy, diminishes rapidly in intensity, and usually disappears during continued treatment), transient flushing of face and neck, dizziness (especially if patient is standing immobile or is in a warm environment), weakness, orthostatic hypotension
Sublingual: Burning, tingling sensation at oral point of dissolution
Ointment: Erythema, pruritus

Occasional

GI upset
Transdermal: Contact dermatitis

SERIOUS REACTIONS

! Nitroglycerin should be discontinued if blurred vision or dry mouth occurs.
! Severe orthostatic hypotension may occur, manifested by fainting, pulselessness, cold or clammy skin, and diaphoresis.
! Tolerance may occur with re-

peated, prolonged therapy; minor tolerance may occur with intermittent use of sublingual tablets.

! High doses of nitroglycerin tend to produce severe headache.

NURSING CONSIDERATIONS

Baseline Assessment

- Document the onset, type (sharp, dull, or squeezing), radiation, location, intensity, and duration of anginal pain and its precipitating factors, such as exertion and emotional stress.
- Assess the patient's apical pulse and BP before administration and periodically after the dose has been given.

Lifespan Considerations

- It is unknown if nitroglycerin crosses the placenta or is distributed in breast milk.
- The safety and efficacy of nitroglycerin have not been established in children.
- The elderly are more susceptible to the hypotensive effects of nitroglycerin.
- In the elderly, age-related renal impairment may require cautious use.

Precautions

- Use nitroglycerin cautiously in patients with acute MI, blood volume depletion from diuretic therapy, glaucoma (contraindicated in closed-angle glaucoma), hepatic or renal disease, or systolic BP less than 90 mm Hg.

Administration and Handling

◀ALERT▶ The cardioverter or defibrillator must not be discharged through a paddle electrode overlying a nitroglycerin system as this may cause burns to the patient or damage the paddle via arching.

◀ALERT▶ Do not give nitrates if the patient has recently taken Cialis, Levitra, or Viagra.

PO

- Instruct the patient to swallow extended-release capsules whole. Capsules should not be chewed or crushed.
- Do not shake aerosol canister before lingual spraying.

Sublingual

- Have the patient dissolve the sublingual form under the tongue and avoid swallowing.
- Administer while the patient is seated.
- To lessen the burning sensation under the tongue, place the tablet in the buccal pouch.
- Keep sublingual tablets in their original container.

Topical

- Spread a thin layer on clean, dry, hairless skin of the upper arm or body, and not below the knee or elbow, using the applicator or dose-measuring papers. Do not use fingers; do not rub or massage into skin.

Transdermal

- Apply patch on clean, dry, hairless skin of the upper arm or body and not below the knee or elbow.

IV

- Store at room temperature.
- The IV form is available in ready-to-use injectable containers.
- Dilute vials in 250 or 500 ml D_5W or 0.9% NaCl to a maximum concentration of 250 mg/250 ml.
- Use microdrop or infusion pump.

Intervention and Evaluation

◀ALERT▶ Remove the transdermal patch before cardioversion or defibrillation because the electrical current may cause arcing which can burn the patient and damage the paddles.

- Monitor the patient's BP and heart rate.

• Continuously monitor the patient's EKG during IV administration.
• Examine the patient for facial or neck flushing.

Patient Teaching

• Teach the patient to take oral nitroglycerin on an empty stomach. Advise the patient to take the medication with meals if he or she experiences headache during therapy.
• Teach the patient to use the translingual spray only when lying down.
• Teach the patient to dissolve sublingual nitroglycerin tablets under the tongue. Stress to the patient that he or she should not swallow sublingual tablets.
• Instruct the patient to take sublingual tablets at the first sign of angina. Explain that if anginal pain is not relieved within 5 minutes of the first dose, that he or she may dissolve a second tablet under the tongue. Then, advise the patient that if the second dose does not relive his or her anginal pain within 5 minutes, he or she may dissolve a third tablet under the tongue. Warn the patient that if anginal pain continues, with no relief from the third tablet, that he or she should immediately notify the physician or seek emergency medical help.
• Teach the patient using nitroglycerin lingual aerosol to spray it on or under the tongue. Explain that the patient should avoid inhaling or swallowing the lingual aerosol.
• Teach the patient to place transmucosal tablets under the upper lip or buccal pouch, which is between the cheek and gum. Advise the patient to avoid chewing or swallowing transmucosal tablets.
• Instruct the patient to expel any remaining intrabuccal, buccal, lingual, or sublingual tablets after the anginal pain is completely relieved.
• Teach the patient to keep the drug container away from heat and moisture.
• Caution the patient against changing brands of nitroglycerin.
• Instruct the patient to rise slowly from a lying to a sitting position and dangle legs momentarily before standing to avoid the drug's hypotensive effect.
• Urge the patient to avoid alcohol during nitroglycerin therapy. Explain that alcohol intensifies the drug's hypotensive effect. Warn the patient that alcohol ingested soon after taking nitroglycerin can cause an acute hypotensive episode noted by vertigo, pallor, and a marked drop in BP.

nitroprusside sodium

nye-troe-**pruss**-ide
(Nipride[CAN], Nitropress)
Do not confuse nitroprusside with nitroglycerin or Nitrostat.

CATEGORY AND SCHEDULE

Pregnancy Risk Category: C

MECHANISM OF ACTION

A potent vasodilator used to treat emergent hypertensive conditions; acts directly on arterial and venous smooth muscle. Decreases peripheral vascular resistance, preload and afterload; improves cardiac output. **Therapeutic Effect:** Dilates coronary arteries, decreases oxygen consumption, and relieves persistent chest pain.

PHARMACOKINETICS

Route	Onset	Peak	Duration
IV	1–10 min	Dependent on infusion rate	Dissipates rapidly after stopping IV

Reacts with Hgb in erythrocytes, producing cyanmethemoglobin, and cyanide ions. Primarily excreted in urine. ***Half-life:*** less than 10 min.

AVAILABILITY

Injection: 25 mg/ml.
Powder for Injection: 50 mg.

INDICATIONS AND DOSAGES

▸ Immediate reduction of BP in hypertensive crisis; to produce controlled hypotension in surgical procedures to reduce bleeding; treatment of acute CHF

IV

Adults, Elderly, Children. Initially, 0.3 mcg/kg/min. Range: 0.5–10 mcg/kg/min. Do not exceed 10 mcg/kg/min (risk of precipitous drop in BP).

OFF-LABEL USES

Control of paroxysmal hypertension before and during surgery for pheochromocytoma, peripheral vasospasm caused by ergot alkaloid overdose, treatment adjunct for MI, valvular regurgitation

CONTRAINDICATIONS

Compensatory hypertension (atrioventricular [AV] shunt or coarctation of aorta), inadequate cerebral circulation, moribund patients

INTERACTIONS

Drug

Dobutamine: May increase cardiac output and decrease pulmonary wedge pressure.
Hypotension-producing medications: May increase hypotensive effect.

Herbal

None known.

Food

None known.

DIAGNOSTIC TEST EFFECTS

None known.

IV INCOMPATIBILITIES

Cisatracurium (Nimbex)

IV COMPATIBILITIES

Diltiazem (Cardizem), dobutamine (Dobutrex), dopamine (Intropin), enalapril (Vasotec), heparin, insulin, labetalol (Normodyne, Trandate), lidocaine, midazolam (Versed), milrinone (Primacor), nitroglycerin, propofol (Diprivan)

SIDE EFFECTS

Occasional

Flushing of skin, increased intracranial pressure, rash, pain or redness at injection site

SERIOUS REACTIONS

! A too-rapid IV infusion rate reduces BP too quickly.
! Nausea, vomiting, diaphoresis, apprehension, headache, restlessness, muscle twitching, dizziness, palpitations, retrosternal pain, and abdominal pain may occur. Symptoms disappear rapidly if rate of administration is slowed or drug is temporarily discontinued.
! Overdose produces metabolic acidosis and tolerance to therapeutic effect.

NURSING CONSIDERATIONS

Baseline Assessment

- Obtain the patient's baseline BP and EKG.
- Determine, with the physician, the desired BP level. BP is normally maintained at about 30% to 40% below pretreatment levels.

Lifespan Considerations

- It is unknown if nitroprusside crosses the placenta or is distributed in breast milk.
- The safety and efficacy of nitroprusside have not been established in children.
- The elderly are more sensitive to the drug's hypotensive effect.
- In the elderly, age-related renal impairment may require cautious use.

Precautions

- Use nitroprusside cautiously in patients with hyponatremia, hypothyroidism, or severe hepatic or renal impairment.
- Use cautiously in elderly patients.

Administration and Handling

IV

- Protect solution from light.
- Inspect solution, which normally appears as very faint brown. A color change from brown to blue, green, or dark red indicates drug deterioration.
- Use only freshly prepared solution. Once the solution has been prepared, it must be used within 24 hours; do not keep it for longer than 24 hours. Discard unused portion.
- Reconstitute 50-mg vial with 2–3 ml D_5W or sterile water for injection without preservative.
- Further dilute with 250 to 1,000 ml D_5W to provide a concentration of 200 mcg/ml to 50 mcg/ml, respectively, up to a maximum concentration of 200 mg/250 ml.
- Wrap infusion bottle in aluminum foil immediately after mixing.
- Give by IV infusion only using infusion rate chart provided by manufacturer or facility protocol.
- Administer using IV infusion pump and lock in rate.

Intervention and Evaluation

- Monitor the rate of infusion frequently.
- Continuously monitor the patient's BP and EKG.

◀ALERT▶ Be alert for extravasation, which produces severe pain and sloughing.

- Monitor the patient's blood acid-base balance, electrolyte levels, intake and output, and laboratory results.
- Assess the patient for signs and symptoms of metabolic acidosis, including disorientation, headache, hyperventilation, nausea, vomiting, and weakness.
- Assess the patient for therapeutic response. Expect to discontinue nitroprusside if the therapeutic response is not achieved within 10 minutes after IV infusion at 10 mcg/kg/min is initiated.
- Monitor the patient's BP for potential rebound hypertension after the infusion has been discontinued.

Patient Teaching

- Advise the patient to immediately report dizziness, headache, nausea, palpitations, or other unusual signs or symptoms.
- Warn the patient to immediately report pain, redness, or swelling at the IV insertion site.

30 Vasopressors

dobutamine hydrochloride
dopamine hydrochloride
epinephrine
midodrine
norepinephrine bitartrate
phenylephrine hydrochloride

Uses: Different groups of vasopressors are used for different effects. *Alpha$_1$-receptor stimulators,* such as midodrine and phenylephrine, are used to induce vasoconstriction primarily in the skin and mucous membranes, to provide nasal decongestion, and to delay local anesthetic absorption. They're also used to increase BP in certain hypotensive states and to produce mydriasis, facilitating eye examinations and ocular surgery. Many vasopressors, however, produce their effects by working on a combination of adrenergic receptors. In most cases, the site of action depends on the drug dose. For example, at low doses, dopamine stimulates dopaminergic receptors, dilating renal arteries. But at much higher doses, the drug stimulates alpha$_1$ receptors, causing vasoconstriction. The chart below shows how vasopressors stimulate particular receptors and produce the corresponding therapeutic effects.

Name	Receptor Specificity	Uses	Dosage Range
Dobutamine	Beta$_1$, beta$_2$, alpha$_1$	Inotropic support in cardiac decompensation	2.5–10 mcg/kg/min IV
Dopamine	Beta$_1$, alpha$_1$, dopaminergic	Vasopressor, cardiac stimulant	Dopaminergic: 0.5–3 mcg/kg/min IV Beta$_1$: 2–10 mcg/kg/min IV Alpha$_1$: greater than 10 mcg/kg/min IV
Epinephrine	Beta$_1$, beta$_2$, alpha$_1$	Cardiac arrest, anaphylactic shock	Vasopressor: 1–10 mcg/min IV Cardiac arrest: 1 mg q3–5min IV during resuscitation
Midodrine	Alpha$_1$	Vasopressor, orthostatic hypotension	10 mg PO, 3 times daily
Norepinephrine	Beta$_1$, alpha$_1$	Vasopressor	0.5–1 mcg/min up to 2–12 mcg/min IV
Phenylephrine	Alpha$_1$	Vasopressor	Initially, 10–180 mcg/min, then 40–60 mcg/min IV

Action: The sympathetic nervous system (SNS) maintains homeostasis, including the regulation of heart rate, cardiac contractility, BP, bronchial airway tone, and carbohydrate and fatty acid metabolism. The SNS is mediated by neurotransmitters (primarily norepinephrine, epinephrine, and dopamine) that act on adrenergic receptors, which include $alpha_1$, $alpha_2$, $beta_1$, $beta_2$, and dopaminergic receptors. Vasopressors differ widely in their actions based on their specificity for these receptors:

- $Alpha_1$-receptor stimulation causes constriction of arterioles and veins.
- $Beta_1$-receptor stimulation increases the rate, force of contraction, and conduction velocity of the heart and releases renin from the kidneys.
- $Beta_2$-receptor stimulation dilates arterioles.
- Dopamine-receptor stimulation dilates renal vessels.

COMBINATION PRODUCTS

AC GEL: epinephrine/cocaine (an anesthetic).

LIDOCAINE WITH EPINEPHRINE: lidocaine (an anesthetic)/epinephrine 2%/1:50,000; 1%/1:100,000; 1%/1:200,000; 0.5%/1:2,000,000.

LIDOSITE: epinephrine/lidocaine (an anesthetic) 0.1%/10%.

PHENERGAN VC: phenylephrine/promethazine (an antihistamine) 5 mg/5 mg.

PHENERGAN VC WITH CODEINE: phenylephrine/promethazine (an antihistamine)/codeine (an analgesic) 6.25 mg/5 mg/10 mg.

TAC: epinephrine/tetracaine (an anesthetic)/cocaine (an anesthetic).

dobutamine hydrochloride

doe-**byoo**-ta-meen

(Dobutrex)

Do not confuse dobutamine with Dopamine.

CATEGORY AND SCHEDULE

Pregnancy Risk Category: B

MECHANISM OF ACTION

A direct-acting inotropic agent acting primarily on $beta_1$-adrenergic receptors. **Therapeutic Effect:** Decreases preload and afterload, and enhances myocardial contractility, stroke volume, and cardiac output. Improves renal blood flow and urine output.

PHARMACOKINETICS

Route	Onset	Peak	Duration
IV	1–2 min	10 min	Length of infusion

Metabolized in the liver. Primarily excreted in urine. Not removed by hemodialysis. ***Half-life:*** 2 min.

AVAILABILITY

Infusion (ready-to-use): 1 mg/ml, 2 mg/ml, 4 mg/ml.
Injection: 12.5-mg/ml vial.

INDICATIONS AND DOSAGES

▸ Short-term management of cardiac decompensation
IV Infusion
Adults, Elderly, Children. 2.5–15 mcg/kg/min. Rarely, drug can be infused at a rate of up to 40 mcg/kg/min to increase cardiac output.
Neonates. 2–15 mcg/kg/min.

CONTRAINDICATIONS

Hypovolemia patients, idiopathic hypertrophic subaortic stenosis, sulfite sensitivity

INTERACTIONS

Drug
Beta blockers: May antagonize the effects of dobutamine.
Digoxin: May increase the risk of arrhythmias and enhance the inotropic effect of both drugs.
MAOIs, oxytocics, tricyclic antidepressants: May increase the adverse effects of dobutamine, such as arrhythmias and hypertension.
Herbal
None known.
Food
None known.

DIAGNOSTIC TEST EFFECTS

Decreases serum potassium level

IV INCOMPATIBILITIES

Acyclovir (Zovirax), alteplase (Activase), amphotericin B complex (Abelcet, AmBisome, Amphotec), bumetanide (Bumex), cefepime (Maxipime), foscarnet (Foscavir), furosemide (Lasix), heparin, piperacillin/tazobactam (Zosyn)

IV COMPATIBILITIES

Amiodarone (Cordarone), calcium chloride, calcium gluconate, diltiazem (Cardizem), dopamine (Intropin), enalapril (Vasotec), famotidine (Pepcid), hydromorphone (Dilaudid), insulin (regular), lidocaine, lorazepam (Ativan), magnesium sulfate, midazolam (Versed), milrinone (Primacor), morphine, nitroglycerin, norepinephrine (Levophed), potassium chloride, propofol (Diprivan)

SIDE EFFECTS

Frequent (greater than 5%)
Increased heart rate, increased BP
Occasional (5%–3%)
Pain at injection site
Rare (3%–1%)
Nausea, headache, anginal pain, shortness of breath, fever

SERIOUS REACTIONS

! Overdose may produce a marked increase in heart rate (by 30 beats/minute or higher) marked increase in BP (by 50 mm Hg or higher), anginal pain, and premature ventricular contractions (PVCs).

NURSING CONSIDERATIONS

Baseline Assessment
• Perform continuous cardiac monitoring of the patient to check for arrhythmias.
• Determine the patient's body weight in kilograms for dosage calculation.

• Obtain the patient's initial BP, heart rate, and respiration rate.
• Correct hypovolemia before beginning dobutamine therapy.

Lifespan Considerations

• It is unknown if dobutamine crosses the placenta or is distributed in breast milk; therefore, it is not administered to pregnant women.
• No age-related precautions have been noted in children or the elderly.

Precautions

• Use dobutamine cautiously in patients with atrial fibrillation or hypertension.

Administration and Handling

◀ **ALERT** ▶ Dobutamine dosage is determined by the patient's response to the drug.

◀ **ALERT** ▶ Plan to correct hypovolemia with volume expanders before dobutamine infusion. Expect to administer digoxin to patients with atrial fibrillation before infusion. Administer by IV infusion only.

IV

• Store at room temperature because freezing produces crystallization.
• Pink discoloration of the solution, caused by oxidation, does not indicate loss of potency if the solution is used within the recommended time period.
• Further diluted solution for infusion must be used within 24 hours.
• Dilute 250-mg ampule with 10 ml sterile water for injection or D_5W for injection; the resulting solution is 25 mg/ml. Add additional 10 ml of diluent if contents of ampule are not completely dissolved; the resulting solution is 12.5 mg/ml.
• Further dilute 250-mg vial with D_5W or 0.9% NaCl. Maximum concentration is 3.125 g/250 ml, or 12.5 mg/ml.
• Use infusion pump to control flow rate.
• Titrate dosage to individual response, as prescribed.

Intervention and Evaluation

• Continuously monitor the patient for arrhythmias or changes in the heart rate.
• Establish parameters with the physician for adjusting the drug rate or stopping infusion.
• Watch for signs and symptoms of infiltration of the IV solution, which can cause local inflammatory changes and possible dermal necrosis.
• Maintain accurate intake and output records. Measure the patient's urine output frequently.
• Assess the patient's serum potassium and dobutamine plasma levels. Keep in mind that dobutamine's therapeutic range is 40 to 190 ng/ml.
• Continuously monitor the patient's BP. Keep in mind that high BP is a greater risk in patients with preexisting hypertension.
• Check the patient's cardiac output and pulmonary wedge pressure or central venous pressure frequently.
• Immediately notify the physician if the patient experiences cardiac arrhythmias, decreased urine output, or a significant increase or decrease in BP or heart rate.

Patient Teaching

• Tell the patient to report chest pain or palpitations during the infusion or pain or burning at the IV site.

dopamine hydrochloride

doe-pa-meen
(Dopamine Injection[AUS], Intropin)
Do not confuse dopamine with dobutamine or Dopram, or Intropin with Isoptin.

CATEGORY AND SCHEDULE
Pregnancy Risk Category: C

MECHANISM OF ACTION
A sympathomimetic (adrenergic agonist) that stimulates adrenergic receptors. Effects are dose dependent. Low dosages (less than 5 mcg/kg/min) stimulate dopaminergic receptors, causing renal vasodilation. Low to moderate dosages (10 mcg/kg/min or less) have a positive inotropic effect by direct action and release of norepinephrine. High dosages (greater than 10 mcg/kg/min) stimulate alpha-receptors. **Therapeutic Effect:** With low dosages, increases renal blood flow, urine flow, and sodium excretion. With low to moderate dosages, increases myocardial contractility, stroke volume, and cardiac output. With high dosages, increases peripheral resistance, renal vasoconstriction, and systolic and diastolic BP.

PHARMACOKINETICS

Route	Onset	Peak	Duration
IV	1–2 min	N/A	less than 10 min

Widely distributed. Does not cross blood-brain barrier. Metabolized in the liver, kidney, and plasma. Primarily excreted in urine. Not removed by hemodialysis. ***Half-life:*** 2 min.

AVAILABILITY
Injection: 40 mg/ml, 80 mg/ml, 160 mg/ml.
Injection (Premix with dextrose): 80 mg/100 ml, 160 mg/100 ml, 320 mg/100 ml.

INDICATIONS AND DOSAGES
▸ **Treatment and prevention of acute hypotension; shock (associated with cardiac decompensation, MI, open heart surgery, renal failure, or trauma), treatment of low cardiac output, treatment of CHF**
IV
Adults, Elderly. 1 mcg/kg/min up to 50 mcg/kg/min titrated to desired response.
Children. 1–20 mcg/kg/min. Maximum: 50 mcg/kg/min.
Neonates. 1–20 mcg/kg/min.

CONTRAINDICATIONS
Pheochromocytoma, sulfite sensitivity, uncorrected tachyarrhythmias, ventricular fibrillation

INTERACTIONS
Drug
Beta blockers: May decrease the effects of dopamine.
Digoxin: May increase the risk of arrhythmias.
Ergot alkaloids: May increase vasoconstriction.
MAOIs: May increase cardiac stimulation and vasopressor effects.
Tricyclic antidepressants: May increase cardiovascular effects.
Herbal
None known.
Food
None known.

DIAGNOSTIC TEST EFFECTS
None known.

IV INCOMPATIBILITIES
Acyclovir (Zovirax), amphotericin B

complex (Abelcet, AmBisome, Amphotec), cefepime (Maxipime), furosemide (Lasix), insulin, sodium bicarbonate

IV COMPATIBILITIES

Amiodarone (Cordarone), calcium chloride, diltiazem (Cardizem), dobutamine (Dobutrex), enalapril (Vasotec), heparin, hydromorphone (Dilaudid), labetalol (Trandate), levofloxacin (Levaquin), lidocaine, lorazepam (Ativan), methylprednisolone (Solu-Medrol), midazolam (Versed), milrinone (Primacor), morphine, nicardipine (Cardene), nitroglycerin, norepinephrine (Levophed), piperacillin/tazobactam (Zosyn), potassium chloride, propofol (Diprivan)

SIDE EFFECTS

Frequent

Headache, ectopic beats, tachycardia, anginal pain, palpitations, vasoconstriction, hypotension, nausea, vomiting, dyspnea

Occasional

Piloerection or goose bumps, bradycardia, widening of QRS complex.

SERIOUS REACTIONS

! High doses may produce ventricular arrhythmias.

! Patients with occlusive vascular disease are at high-risk for further compromise of circulation to the extremities, which may result in gangrene.

! Tissue necrosis with sloughing may occur with extravasation of IV solution.

NURSING CONSIDERATIONS

Baseline Assessment

• Determine if the patient has been on MAOI therapy within the last 2 to 3 weeks. If he or she has received MAOIs within this time frame, dopamine dosage will have to be reduced.

• Expect to place the patient on a continuous cardiac monitor to assess for arrhythmias.

• Determine the patient's weight for dosage calculation.

• Obtain the patient's initial BP, heart rate, and respiration rates.

Lifespan Considerations

• It is unknown if dopamine crosses the placenta or is distributed in breast milk.

• Closely monitor children because gangrene due to extravasation has been reported.

• No age-related precautions have been noted in the elderly.

Precautions

• Use dopamine cautiously in patients with ischemic heart disease or occlusive vascular disease.

Administration and Handling

◀ALERT▶ Expect to correct blood volume depletion before administering dopamine. Blood volume replacement may occur simultaneously with dopamine infusion.

IV

• Do not use solutions darker than slightly yellow or solutions that have discolored to brown or pink to purple because these discolorations indicate decomposition of drug.

• Dopamine is stable for 24 hours after dilution.

• Dilute 200–400 mg ampule in 250–500 ml 0.9% NaCl, D_5W/0.45 NaCl, D_5W/0.45 NaCl, D_5W/lactated Ringer's or lactated Ringer's. Keep in mind the concentration is dependent on the dosage and the patient's fluid requirements. Remember that a 200 mg/250 ml solution yields 800 mcg/ml, and a 200 mg/500 ml solution yields 400 mcg/ml. The maximum concentration is 3.2 g/250 ml

or 12.8 mg/ml. The drug is available prediluted in 250 or 500 ml of D_5W.
• Administer into large vein, such as the antecubital or subclavian vein, to prevent drug extravasation.
• Use an infusion pump to control rate of flow.
• Titrate dosage to the desired hemodynamic values or optimum urine flow, as prescribed.

Intervention and Evaluation

• Continuously monitor the patient for cardiac arrhythmias.
• Measure the patient's urine output frequently.
• If extravasation occurs, immediately infiltrate the affected tissue with 10 to 15 ml 0.9% NaCl solution containing 5 to 10 mg phentolamine mesylate, as ordered.
• Monitor the patient's BP, heart rate, and respiration rates at least every 15 minutes during dopamine administration.
• Assess the patient's cardiac output and pulmonary wedge pressure or central venous pressure frequently.
• Examine the patient's peripheral circulation by palpating pulses and noting the color and temperature of extremities.
• Immediately notify the physician if the patient experiences arrhythmias, decreased peripheral circulation (marked by cold, pale, or mottled extremities), decreased urine output, or significant changes in BP or heart rate. Also notify the physician if the patient fails to respond to increase or decrease in infusion rate.
• Taper the dopamine dosage before discontinuing the drug because abrupt cessation of dopamine therapy may result in marked hypotension.
• Be alert to excessive vasoconstriction as evidenced by decreased urine output, disproportionate increase in diastolic BP, and increased arrhythmias or heart rate. Slow or temporarily stop the dopamine infusion and notify the physician if excessive vasoconstriction occurs.

Patient Teaching

• Tell the patient to report chest pain or palpitations during the infusion or pain or burning at the IV site.

epinephrine

ep-i-**nef**-rin
(Adrenalin, Adrenaline Injection[AUS], EpiPen, EpiPen Jr. 0.15 Adrenaline Autoinjector[AUS], Primatene)
Do not confuse epinephrine with ephedrine.

CATEGORY AND SCHEDULE

Pregnancy Risk Category: C

MECHANISM OF ACTION

A sympathomimetic, adrenergic agonist that stimulates alpha-adrenergic receptors causing vasoconstriction and pressor effects, $beta_1$-adrenergic receptors, resulting in cardiac stimulation, and $beta_2$-adrenergic receptors, resulting in bronchial dilation and vasodilation. With ophthalmic form, increases outflow of aqueous humor from anterior eye chamber. **Therapeutic Effect:** Relaxes smooth muscle of the bronchial tree, produces cardiac stimulation, and dilates skeletal muscle vasculature. The ophthalmic form dilates pupils and constricts conjunctival blood vessels.

PHARMACOKINETICS

Route	Onset	Peak	Duration
IM	5–10 min	20 min	1–4 hr
Subcutaneous	5–10 min	20 min	1–4 hr
Inhalation	3–5 min	20 min	1–3 hr
Ophthalmic	1 hr	4–8 hr	12–24 hr

Well absorbed after parenteral administration; minimally absorbed after inhalation. Metabolized in the liver, other tissues, and sympathetic nerve endings. Excreted in urine. The ophthalmic form may be systemically absorbed as a result of drainage into nasal pharyngeal passages. Mydriasis occurs within several min and persists several hr; vasoconstriction occurs within 5 min, and lasts less than 1 hr.

AVAILABILITY

Injection: 0.1 mg/ml, 1 mg/ml.
Injection (Epi-Pen): 0.3 mg/0.3 ml, 0.15 mg/0.3 ml.
Inhalation Aerosol (Primatene Mist): 0.2 mg/inhalation.
Inhalation Solution: 1%, 2.25%.
Ophthalmic Solution (Epifrin): 0.5%, 1%, 2%.

INDICATIONS AND DOSAGES

▸ **Asystole**
IV
Adults, Elderly. 1 mg q3–5min up to 0.1 mg/kg q3–5min.
Children. 0.01 mg/kg (0.1 ml/kg of 1:10,000 solution). May repeat q3–5min. Subsequent doses of 0.1 mg/kg (0.1 ml/kg) of a 1:1000 solution q3–5min.

▸ **Bradycardia**
IV Infusion
Adults, Elderly. 1–10 mcg/min titrated to desired effect.
IV
Children. 0.01 mg/kg (0.1 mg/kg of 1:10,000 solution) q3–5min. Maximum: 1 mg/10 ml.

▸ **Bronchodilation**
IM, Subcutaneous
Adults, Elderly. 0.1–0.5 mg (1:1000) q10–15min to 4 hrs.
Subcutaneous
Children. 10 mcg/kg (0.01 ml/kg of 1:1,000) Maximum: 0.5 mg or suspension (1:200) 0.005 ml/kg/dose (0.025 mg/kg/dose) to a maximum of 0.15 ml (0.75 mg for single dose) q8–12h.

▸ **Hypersensitivity reaction**
IM, Subcutaneous
Adults, Elderly. 0.3–0.5 mg q15–20min.
Subcutaneous
Children. 0.01 mg/kg q15min for 2 doses, then q4h. Maximum single dose: 0.5 mg.
Inhalation
Adults, Elderly, Children 4 yr and older. 1 inhalation, may repeat in at least 1 min. Give subsequent doses no sooner than 3 hr.
Nebulizer
Adults, Elderly, Children 4 yr and older. 1–3 deep inhalations. Give subsequent doses no sooner than 3 hr.

▸ **Glaucoma**
Ophthalmic
Adults, Elderly. 1–2 drops 1–2 times a day.

OFF-LABEL USES

Systemic: Treatment of gingival or pulpal hemorrhage, priapism
Ophthalmic: Treatment of conjunctival congestion during surgery, secondary glaucoma

CONTRAINDICATIONS

Cardiac arrhythmias, cerebrovascular insufficiency, hypertension, hyperthyroidism, ischemic heart disease, narrow-angle glaucoma, shock

INTERACTIONS

Drug

Beta blockers: May decrease the effects of beta blockers.
Digoxin, sympathomimetics: May increase risk of arrhythmias.
Ergonovine, methergine, oxytocin: May increase vasoconstriction.
MAOIs, tricyclic antidepressants: May increase cardiovascular effects.

Herbal

None known.

Food

None known.

DIAGNOSTIC TEST EFFECTS

May decrease serum potassium level.

IV INCOMPATIBILITIES

Ampicillin (Omnipen, Polycillin)

IV COMPATIBILITIES

Calcium chloride, calcium gluconate, diltiazem (Cardizem), dobutamine (Dobutrex), dopamine (Intropin), fentanyl (Sublimaze), heparin, hydromorphone (Dilaudid), lorazepam (Ativan), midazolam (Versed), milrinone (Primacor), morphine, nitroglycerin, norepinephrine (Levophed), potassium chloride, propofol (Diprivan)

SIDE EFFECTS

Frequent

Systemic: Tachycardia, palpitations, nervousness
Ophthalmic: Headache, eye irritation, watering of eyes

Occasional

Systemic: Dizziness, lightheadedness, facial flushing, headache, diaphoresis, increased BP, nausea, trembling, insomnia, vomiting, fatigue
Ophthalmic: Blurred or decreased vision, eye pain

Rare

Systemic: Chest discomfort or pain, arrhythmias, bronchospasm, dry mouth or throat

SERIOUS REACTIONS

! Excessive doses may cause acute hypertension or arrhythmias.
! Prolonged or excessive use may result in metabolic acidosis due to increased serum lactic acid concentrations. Metabolic acidosis may cause disorientation, fatigue, hyperventilation, headache, nausea, vomiting, and diarrhea.

NURSING CONSIDERATIONS

Baseline Assessment

- Obtain vital signs, especially heart rate and BP.
- Obtain a EKG to monitor the patient for arrhythmias.

Lifespan Considerations

- Epinephrine crosses the placenta and is distributed in breast milk.
- No age-related precautions have been noted in children or the elderly; however, use caution when administering to elderly patients suspected of having an underlying cardiac, vascular, neurologic, or other disorder.

Precautions

- Use epinephrine cautiously in patients with angina pectoris, diabetes mellitus, hypoxia, MI, psychoneurotic disorders, tachycardia, or severe hepatic or renal impairment.

Administration and Handling

IV

- Store parenteral forms at room temperature.
- Do not use if solution appears pink or brown or contains a precipitate.
- For injection, dilute each 1 mg of 1:1,000 solution with 10 ml 0.9% NaCl to provide 1:10,000 solution, and inject each 1 mg or fraction thereof over more than 1 minute.
- For infusion, further dilute with 250 to 500 D_5W. Maximum concen-

tration is 64 mg/250 ml. Give at 1 to 10 mcg/min, and titrate to desired response.
Subcutaneous
- Shake ampule thoroughly.
- Use tuberculin syringe for injection into lateral deltoid region.
- Massage injection site to minimize vasoconstriction effect.

Intervention and Evaluation
- Monitor the patient for changes in vital signs.
- Assess the patient's breath sounds for crackles, rhonchi, and wheezing.
- Monitor the patient's ABGs.
- Monitor the EKG and the patient's condition, especially in the patient with cardiac arrest.

Patient Teaching
- Urge the patient to avoid consuming excessive amounts of caffeine derivatives such as chocolate, cocoa, coffee, cola, and tea.
- Explain to the patient receiving the ophthalmic solution that he or she will feel a slight burning or stinging when the drug is initially administered. Warn the patient to immediately report any new symptoms such as dizziness, shortness of breath, and tachycardia because they may be a sign of systemic absorption.

midodrine

mid-o-dreen
(Amatine, ProAmatine)
Do not confuse Amatine or ProAmantine with amantadine or protamine.

CATEGORY AND SCHEDULE
Pregnancy Risk Category: C

MECHANISM OF ACTION
A vasopressor that forms the active metabolite desglymidodrine, an $alpha_1$-agonist, activating alpha receptors of the arteriolar and venous vasculature. **Therapeutic Effect:** Increases vascular tone and BP.

AVAILABILITY
Tablets: 2.5 mg, 5 mg, 10 mg.

INDICATIONS AND DOSAGES
▸ **Orthostatic hypotension**
PO
Adults, Elderly. 10 mg 3 times a day. Give during the day when patient is upright, such as upon arising, midday, and late afternoon. Do not give later than 6 p.m.
▸ **Dosage in renal impairment**
For adults and elderly patients, give 2.5 mg 3 times a day; increase gradually, as tolerated.

CONTRAINDICATIONS
Acute renal function impairment, persistent hypertension, pheochromocytoma, severe cardiac disease, thyrotoxicosis, urine retention

INTERACTIONS
Drug
Digoxin: May have additive bradycardia effects.
Sodium-retaining steroids (such as fludrocortisone): May increase sodium retention.
Vasoconstrictors: May have an additive vasocontricting effect.
Herbal
None known.
Food
None known.

DIAGNOSTIC TEST EFFECTS
None known.

SIDE EFFECTS
Frequent (20%–7%)
Paresthesia, piloerection, pruritus, dysuria, supine hypertension

Occasional (less than 7%–1%)
Pain, rash, chills, headache, facial flushing, confusion, dry mouth, anxiety

SERIOUS REACTIONS

! None known.

NURSING CONSIDERATIONS

Baseline Assessment

• Assess the patient's hypersensitivity to midodrine, and determine if he or she is taking other medications, especially digoxin, sodium-retaining steroids, and vasoconstrictors.
• Assess the patient's medical problems, including acute renal function impairment, severe hypertension, and cardiac disease.

Precautions

• Use midodrine cautiously in patients with a history of vision problems and renal or hepatic impairment.

Intervention and Evaluation

• Monitor the patient's BP and liver or renal function test results.

Patient Teaching

• Tell the patient not to take the last dose of the day after the evening meal or less than 4 hours before bedtime and caution him or her not to take the medication while lying down.
• Advise the patient to use OTC medications, such as cough, cold, and diet preparations, cautiously because they may affect BP.

norepinephrine bitartrate

nor-ep-i-**nef**-rin
(Levophed)
Do not confuse Levophed with Levid, or norepinephrine with epinephrine.

CATEGORY AND SCHEDULE

Pregnancy Risk Category: C

MECHANISM OF ACTION

A sympathomimetic that stimulates $beta_1$-adrenergic receptors and alpha-adrenergic receptors, increasing peripheral resistance. Enhances contractile myocardial force, increases cardiac output. Constricts resistance and capacitance vessels. **Therapeutic Effect:** Increases systemic BP and coronary blood flow.

PHARMACOKINETICS

Route	Onset	Peak	Duration
IV	Rapid	1–2 min	N/A

Localized in sympathetic tissue. Metabolized in the liver. Primarily excreted in urine.

AVAILABILITY

Injection: 1-mg/ml ampules.

INDICATIONS AND DOSAGES

▸ Acute hypotension unresponsive to fluid volume replacement
IV
Adults, Elderly. Initially, administer at 0.5–1 mcg/min. Adjust rate of flow to establish and maintain desired BP (40 mm Hg below preexisting systolic pressure). Average maintenance dose: 8–12 mcg/min.
Children. Initially, 0.05–0.1 mcg/

kg/min; titrate to desired effect. Maximum: 1–2 mcg/kg/min. Range: 0.5–3 mcg/min.

CONTRAINDICATIONS

Hypovolemic states (unless as an emergency measure), mesenteric or peripheral vascular thrombosis, profound hypoxia

INTERACTIONS

Drug

Beta blockers: May have mutually inhibitory effects.
Digoxin: May increase risk of arrhythmias.
Ergonovine, oxytocin: May increase vasoconstriction.
Maprotiline, tricyclic antidepressants: May increase cardiovascular effects.
Methyldopa: May decrease the effects of methyldopa.

Herbal

None known.

Food

None known.

DIAGNOSTIC TEST EFFECTS

None known.

IV INCOMPATIBILITIES

Regular insulin

IV COMPATIBILITIES

Amiodarone (Cordarone), calcium gluconate, diltiazem (Cardizem), dobutamine (Dobutrex), dopamine (Intropin), epinephrine, esmolol (Brevibloc), fentanyl (Sublimaze), furosemide (Lasix), haloperidol (Haldol), heparin, hydromorphone (Dilaudid), labetalol (Trandate), lorazepam (Ativan), magnesium, midazolam (Versed), milrinone (Primacor), morphine, nicardipine (Cardene), nitroglycerin, potassium chloride, propofol (Diprivan)

SIDE EFFECTS

Norepinephrine produces less pronounced and less frequent side effects than epinephrine.

Occasional (5%–3%)

Anxiety, bradycardia, palpitations

Rare (2%–1%)

Nausea, anginal pain, shortness of breath, fever

SERIOUS REACTIONS

! Extravasation may produce tissue necrosis and sloughing.

! Overdose is manifested as severe hypertension with violent headache (which may be the first clinical sign of overdose), arrhythmias, photophobia, retrosternal or pharyngeal pain, pallor, excessive sweating, and vomiting.

! Prolonged therapy may result in plasma volume depletion. Hypotension may recur if plasma volume is not restored.

NURSING CONSIDERATIONS

Baseline Assessment

- Assess the patient's BP and EKG continuously. Be alert to precipitous drops in BP.

Lifespan Considerations

- Norepinephrine readily crosses the placenta and may produce fetal anoxia due to constriction of uterine blood vessels and uterine contraction.
- No age-related precautions have been noted in children or the elderly.

Precautions

- Use norepinephrine cautiously in patients with hypertension, hypothyroidism, or severe cardiac disease.
- Use cautiously in patients on concurrent MAOI therapy.

Administration and Handling

◀ALERT▶ Expect to restore blood and fluid volume before administering norepinephrine.

IV

- Do not use if solution is brown or contains precipitate.
- Store ampules at room temperature.
- Add 4 ml (4 mg) to 1 liter of D_5W for a 4-mcg/ml solution. Maximum concentration: 128 mcg/ml.
- Administer infusion through a central venous catheter, if available, to avoid extravasation.
- Closely monitor the infusion flow rate with a microdrip or infusion pump.
- Monitor the patient's BP every 2 minutes during the infusion until desired therapeutic response is achieved, then every 5 minutes during the remainder of the infusion.
- Never leave the patient unattended during the infusion.
- Be alert to any patient complaint of headache.
- Plan to maintain BP at 80 to 100 mm Hg in previously normotensive patients, and 30 to 40 mm Hg below pre-existing BP in previously hypertensive patients.
- Reduce the infusion gradually, as prescribed. Avoid abrupt withdrawal.
- Check the peripherally inserted catheter IV site frequently for signs of extravasation, including blanching, coldness, hardness, and pallor to the extremity.

Intervention and Evaluation

- Monitor the patient's IV flow rate diligently.
- Assess the patient for extravasation. If extravasation occurs, expect to infiltrate the affected area with 10 to 15 ml sterile saline containing 5 to 10 mg phentolamine. Know that phentolamine does not alter the pressor effects of norepinephrine.
- Assess the patient's capillary refill, and the strength of his or her peripheral pulses, to monitor circulation.
- Monitor the patient's intake and output hourly, or as ordered. In patients with a urine output of less than 30 ml/hour, expect to stop the infusion unless the systolic BP falls below 80 mm Hg.

Patient Teaching

- Instruct the patient to immediately report burning, pain, or coolness at the IV site.

phenylephrine hydrochloride

fen-ill-**eh**-frin

(AK-Dilate, AD-Nephrin, Isopto Frin[AUS], Mydfrin, Neo-Synephrine, Neo-Synephrine Ophthalmic Viscous 10%[AUS], Prefrin)

CATEGORY AND SCHEDULE

Pregnancy Risk Category: C

OTC (nasal solution, nasal spray, ophthalmic solution)

MECHANISM OF ACTION

A sympathomimetic, alpha receptor stimulant that acts on the alpha-adrenergic receptors of vascular smooth muscle. Causes vasoconstriction of arterioles of nasal mucosa or conjunctiva, activates dilator muscle of the pupil to cause contraction, produces systemic arterial vasoconstriction. **Therapeutic Effect:** Decreases mucosal blood flow and relieves congestion and increases systolic BP.

PHARMACOKINETICS

Route	Onset	Peak	Duration
IV	Immediate	N/A	15–20 min
IM	10–15 min	N/A	0.5–2 hr
Subcutaneous	10–15 min	N/A	1 hr

Minimal absorption after intranasal and ophthalmic administration. Metabolized in the liver and GI tract. Primarily excreted in urine. ***Half-life:*** 2.5 hr.

AVAILABILITY

Injection: 1% (10 mg/ml).
Nasal Solution Drops (Neosynephrine): 0.5%, 1%.
Nasal Spray (Neosynephrine): 0.25%, 0.5%, 1%.
Ophthalmic Solution (Ak-Nephrin): 0.12%.
Ophthalmic Solution (AK-Dilate): 2.5%, 10%.
Ophthalmic Solution (Mydfrin, Neosynephrine): 2.5%.

INDICATIONS AND DOSAGES

▸ **Nasal decongestant**
Nasal Spray, Nasal Solution
Adults, Elderly, Children 12 yr and older. 2–3 drops or 1–2 sprays of 0.25%–0.5% solution into each nostril.
Children 6–11 yr. 2–3 drops or 1–2 sprays of 0.25% solution into each nostril.
Children younger than 6 yr. 2–3 drops of 0.125% solution (dilute 0.5% solution with 0.9% NaCl to achieve 0.125%) in each nostril. Repeat q4h as needed. Do not use for more than 3 days.

▸ **Conjunctival congestion, itching, and minor irritation; whitening of sclera**
Ophthalmic
Adults, Elderly, Children 12 yr and older. 1–2 drops of 0.12% solution q3–4h.

▸ **Hypotension, shock**
IM, Subcutaneous
Adults, Elderly. 2–5 mg/dose q1–2h.
Children. 0.1 mg/kg/dose q1–2h.
IV Bolus
Adults, Elderly. 0.1–0.5 mg/dose q10–15min as needed.
Children. 5–20 mcg/kg/dose q10–15min.
IV Infusion
Adults, Elderly. 100–180 mcg/min.
Children. 0.1–0.5 mcg/kg/min. Titrate to desired effect.

CONTRAINDICATIONS

Acute pancreatitis, heart disease, hepatitis, narrow-angle glaucoma, pheochromocytoma, severe hypertension, thrombosis, ventricular tachycardia

INTERACTIONS

Drug

Beta blockers: May have mutually inhibitory effects.
Digoxin: May increase risk of arrhythmias.
Ergonovine, oxytocin: May increase vasoconstriction.
MAOIs: May increase vasopressor effects.
Maprotiline, tricyclic antidepressants: May increase cardiovascular effects.
Methyldopa: May decrease effects of methyldopa.

Herbal

None known.

Food

None known.

DIAGNOSTIC TEST EFFECTS

None known.

IV INCOMPATIBILITIES

Thiopentothal (Pentothal)

IV COMPATIBILITIES

Amiodarone (Cordarone), dobutamine (Dobutrex), lidocaine, potassium chloride, propofol (Diprivan)

SIDE EFFECTS

Frequent

Nasal: Rebound nasal congestion due

to overuse, especially when used longer than 3 days

Occasional

Mild CNS stimulation (restlessness, nervousness, tremors, headache, insomnia, particularly in those hypersensitive to sympathomimetics, such as elderly patients)

Nasal: Stinging, burning, drying of nasal mucosa

Ophthalmic: Transient burning or stinging, brow ache, blurred vision

SERIOUS REACTIONS

! Large doses may produce tachycardia and palpitations (particularly in those with cardiac disease), light-headedness, nausea, and vomiting.

! Overdose in those older than 60 years may result in hallucinations, CNS depression, and seizures.

! Prolonged nasal use may produce chronic swelling of nasal mucosa and rhinitis.

NURSING CONSIDERATIONS

Baseline Assessment

- Be sure to obtain vital signs, including apical heart rate and BP.
- Assess the patient for irritation of nasal mucosa before administering nasal preparation.

Lifespan Considerations

- Phenylephrine crosses the placenta and is distributed in breast milk.
- Children may exhibit increased absorption and toxicity with nasal preparation.
- No age-related precautions have been noted with systemic use in children.
- The elderly are more likely to experience adverse effects.

Precautions

- Use phenylephrine cautiously in patients with bradycardia, heart block, hyperthyroidism, or severe arteriosclerosis.
- If phenylephrine 10% ophthalmic is instilled into denuded or damaged corneal epithelium, corneal clouding may result.

Administration and Handling

Nasal

- Have the patient blow his or her nose before giving the medication. Tilt back the patient's head and instill the drops in one nostril, as prescribed. Have the patient remain in the same position; wait 5 minutes before applying drops in other nostril.
- Administer nasal spray into each nostril with the patient's head erect. Have the patient sniff briskly while squeezing container; then instruct him or her to wait 3 to 5 minutes before blowing nose gently.
- Rinse tip of spray bottle.

Ophthalmic

- Have the patient tilt head backward and look up.
- With a gloved finger, gently pull the patient's lower eyelid down to form a pouch; instill medication into the pouch.
- Do not touch tip of applicator to eyelids or any surface.
- When lower eyelid is released, have patient keep eye open without blinking for at least 30 seconds.
- Apply gentle finger pressure to lacrimal sac, which is located at the bridge of the nose at inside corner of the eye, for 1 to 2 minutes.
- Remove excess solution around eye with tissue. Wash hands immediately to remove medication on hands.

IV

- Store vials at room temperature.
- For IV push, dilute 1 ml of 10-mg/ml solution with 9 ml sterile water for injection to provide a concentration of 1 mg/ml. Give over 20 to 30 seconds.

• For IV infusion, dilute 10-mg vial with 500 ml D_5W or 0.9% NaCl to provide a concentration of 2 mcg/ml. Maximum concentration: 500 mg/ 250 ml. Titrate as prescribed

Intervention and Evaluation

• Monitor the patient's BP and heart rate.

Patient Teaching

• Instruct the patient not to use the drug for nasal decongestion longer than 5 days because of the risk of rebound nasal congestion.

• Strongly advise the patient to immediately contact the physician and discontinue the drug if dizziness, feeling of irregular heartbeat, insomnia, tremor, or weakness occurs.

• Explain to the patient the different preparations of the drug and the common side effects associated with each.

• Warn the patient to discontinue ophthalmic medication and notify the physician if redness or swelling of eyelids or itching occurs.

31 Miscellaneous Cardiovascular Agents

alfuzosin hydrochloride
alprostadil (prostaglandin E_1; PGE_1)
digoxin immune FAB
eplerenone
sodium polystyrene sulfonate
tamsulosin hydrochloride

Uses: Several miscellaneous agents are used primarily for their cardiovascular therapeutic effects. Although *alfuzosin* and *tamsulosin* are chemically related to other cardiovascular agents, they're used to improve urine flow and relieve symptoms of benign prostatic hyperplasia. *Alprostadil* is used to maintain patency of the ductus arteriosus until surgery can be performed; it's also used to treat erectile dysfunction. *Digoxin immune FAB* is used as an antidote for digoxin intoxication. *Eplerenone* may be used alone or with other antihypertensives to control hypertension. *Sodium polystyrene sulfonate* is used to correct hyperkalemia, which can cause serious or life-threatening arrhythmias.

Action: Each of the cardiovascular agents in this section acts in a different way. *Alfuzosin* and *tamsulosin* block $alpha_1$-adrenergic receptors in the lower urinary tract, causing relaxation of smooth muscle in the bladder neck and prostate. As a prostaglandin, *alprostadil* directly affects vascular and ductus arteriosus smooth muscle and relaxes trabecular smooth muscle. *Digoxin immune FAB* binds with digoxin molecules, preventing them from binding at their sites of action. *Eplerenone* binds to mineralocorticoid receptors in the kidneys, heart, blood vessels, and brain, blocking the binding of aldosterone. Because *sodium polystyrene sulfonate* is a cation exchange resin, it releases sodium ions in exchange primarily for potassium ions and promotes potassium excretion from the body; this action prevents serious complications, such as life-threatening arrhythmias.

alfuzosin hydrochloride

ale-few-**zoe**-sin
(Uroxatral)

CATEGORY AND SCHEDULE

Pregnancy Risk Category: B

MECHANISM OF ACTION

An $alpha_1$ antagonist that targets receptors around bladder neck and prostate capsule. **Therapeutic Effect:** Relaxes smooth muscle and improves urinary flow and symptoms of prostatic hyperplasia.

PHARMACOKINETICS

Rapidly absorbed and widely distributed. Protein binding: 90%. Extensively metabolized in the liver. Primarily excreted in urine. ***Half-life:*** 3–9 hr.

AVAILABILITY

Tablets (Extended-Release): 10 mg.

INDICATIONS AND DOSAGES

▸ Benign prostatic hyperplasia

PO

Adults. 10 mg once a day, approximately 30 min after same meal each day.

CONTRAINDICATIONS

History of hypersensitivity to alfuzosin

INTERACTIONS

Drug

Cimetidine: May increase alfuzosin blood concentration.

Other alpha blockers, such as doxazosin, prazosin, tamsulosin, and terazosin: May increase the alpha-blockade effects of both drugs.

Herbal

None known.

Food

None known.

DIAGNOSTIC TEST EFFECTS

None known.

SIDE EFFECTS

Frequent (7%–6%)

Dizziness, headache, malaise

Occasional (4%)

Dry mouth

Rare (3%–2%)

Nausea, dyspepsia (such as heartburn, and epigastric discomfort), diarrhea, orthostatic hypotension, tachycardia, drowsiness

SERIOUS REACTIONS

! Ischemia-related chest pain may occur rarely.

NURSING CONSIDERATIONS

Baseline Assessment

• Determine the patient's sensitivity to alfuzosin. Also ask about use of other alpha-blockers, including doxazosin, prazosin, tamsulosin, and terazosin.

Lifespan Considerations

• Alfuzosin is not indicated for use in women and children.

• No age-related precautions have been noted in the elderly.

Precautions

• Use alfuzosin cautiously in patients with coronary artery disease, hepatic impairment, or orthostatic hypotension.

• Use cautiously in patients under general anesthesia.

Administration and Handling

PO

• Give after the same meal each day. The extended-release tablet should not be crushed or chewed.

Intervention and Evaluation

• Assist the patient with ambulation if he experiences dizziness.

Patient Teaching

- Instruct the patient to take alfuzosin after the same meal each day.
- Caution the patient to avoid performing tasks that require mental alertness or motor skills until his response to the drug has been established.
- Warn the patient to notify the physician if he experiences headache.
- Teach the patient not to chew or crush extended-release tablets.

alprostadil (prostaglandin E_1; PGE_1)

al-**pros**-ta-dil
(Caverject, Edex, Muse, Prostin VR[AUS], Prostin VR Pediatric)

CATEGORY AND SCHEDULE

Pregnancy Risk Category: C

MECHANISM OF ACTION

A prostaglandin that directly affects vascular and ductus arteriosus smooth muscle and relaxes trabecular smooth muscle. **Therapeutic Effect:** Causes vasodilation; dilates cavernosal arteries, allowing blood flow to and entrapment in the lacunar spaces of the penis.

AVAILABILITY

Injection (Prostin VR Pediatric): 500 mcg/ml.
Powder for Injection (Caverject, Edex): 10 mcg, 20 mcg, 40 mcg.
Urethral Pellet (Muse): 125 mcg, 250 mcg, 500 mcg, 1,000 mcg.

INDICATIONS AND DOSAGES

▸ **Maintain patency of ductus arteriosus**

IV Infusion
Neonates. Initially, 0.05–0.1 mcg/kg/min. Maintenance: 0.01–0.4 mcg/kg/min. Maximum: 0.4 mcg/kg/min.

▸ **Impotence**

Pellet, Intracavernosal
Adults. Dosage is individualized.

OFF-LABEL USES

Treatment of atherosclerosis, gangrene, pain due to severe peripheral arterial occlusive disease

CONTRAINDICATIONS

Conditions predisposing to anatomic deformation of penis, hyaline membrane disease, penile implants, priapism, respiratory distress syndrome

INTERACTIONS

Drug

Anticoagulants, including heparin, thrombolytics: May increase risk of bleeding.
Sympathomimetics: May decrease effect of alprostadil.
Vasodilators: May increase risk of hypotension.

Herbal

None known.

Food

None known.

DIAGNOSTIC TEST EFFECTS

May increase blood bilirubin levels. May decrease glucose, serum calcium, and serum potassium levels.

IV INCOMPATIBILITIES

No information available.

SIDE EFFECTS

Frequent

Intracavernosal (4%–1%): Penile

pain (37%), prolonged erection, hypertension, localized pain, penile fibrosis, injection site hematoma or ecchymosis, headache, respiratory infection, flulike symptoms
Intraurethral (3%): Penile pain (36%), urethral pain or burning, testicular pain, urethral bleeding, headache, dizziness, respiratory infection, flulike symptoms
Systemic (greater than 1%): Fever, seizures, flushing, bradycardia, hypotension, tachycardia, apnea, diarrhea, sepsis

Occasional

Intracavernosal (less than 1%): Hypotension, pelvic pain, back pain, dizziness, cough, nasal congestion
Intraurethral (less than 3%): Fainting, sinusitis, back and pelvic pain
Systemic (less than 1%): Anxiety, lethargy, myalgia, arrhythmias, respiratory depression, anemia, bleeding, thrombocytopenia, hematuria

SERIOUS REACTIONS

! Overdose is manifested as apnea, flushing of the face and arms, and bradycardia.

! Cardiac arrest and sepsis occur rarely.

NURSING CONSIDERATIONS

Precautions

- Use alprostadil cautiously in patients with coagulation defects, leukemia, multiple myeloma, polycythemia, severe hepatic disease, sickle cell disease, or thrombocythemia.

Administration and Handling

◀ALERT▶ Doses greater than 40 mcg (Edex) or 60 mcg (Caverject) are not recommended.

- Urethral pellet
- Refrigerate pellet unless used within 14 days.

IV

◀ALERT▶ Give by continuous IV infusion or through umbilical artery catheter placed at ductal opening.

- Store the parenteral form in refrigerator.
- Dilute drug before administration. Prepare fresh dose every 24 hours and discard unused portions.
- Prepare continuous IV infusion by diluting 1 ml alprostadil, containing 500 mcg, with D_5W or 0.9% NaCl to yield a solution containing 2 to 20 mcg/ml. Diluting volumes can range from 25 to 250 ml, depending on the patient and the available infusion device.
- Infuse the lowest possible dose over the shortest possible time.
- Decrease the infusion rate immediately if a significant decrease in arterial pressure is noted via auscultation, Doppler transducer, or umbilical artery catheter.
- Discontinue the infusion immediately if signs and symptoms of overdose, such as apnea and bradycardia, occur.

Intervention and Evaluation

- For patients with patent ductus arteriosus, monitor arterial pressure by auscultation, Doppler transducer, or umbilical artery catheter. Decrease the infusion rate immediately if a significant decrease in arterial pressure occurs. Expect to maintain continuous cardiac monitoring. Also, frequently assess the patient's heart sounds, femoral pulse (to monitor lower extremity circulation), and respiratory status.
- For patients with patent ductus arteriosus, monitor the patient for signs and symptoms of hypotension and assess BP, ABG values, and temperature. If apnea or bradycardia occurs, discontinue infusion immediately and notify the physician.

Patient Teaching

- For the patients with patent ductus arteriosus, explain to his or her parents the purpose of this palliative therapy.
- For the patient with impotence, inform him that his erection should occur within 2 to 5 minutes of administration.
- For the patient with impotence, warn him not to use alprostadil if his female sexual partner is pregnant, unless the couple is using a condom barrier.
- For the patient with impotence, advise him to notify the physician if his erection lasts longer than 4 hours or becomes painful.

digoxin immune FAB

di-**jox**-in
(Digibind, DigiFab)
Do not confuse digoxin with Desoxyn or doxepin.

CATEGORY AND SCHEDULE

Pregnancy Risk Category: C

MECHANISM OF ACTION

An antidote that binds molecularly to digoxin in the extracellular space. **Therapeutic Effect:** Makes digoxin unavailable for binding at its site of action on cells in the body.

PHARMACOKINETICS

Route	Onset	Peak	Duration
IV	30 min	N/A	3–4 days

Widely distributed into extracellular space. Excreted in urine. ***Half-life:*** 15–20 hr.

AVAILABILITY

Powder for Injection (Digibind): 38-mg vial.
Powder for Injection (DigiFab): 40-mg vial.

INDICATIONS AND DOSAGES

▸ Potentially life-threatening digoxin overdose

IV

Adults, Elderly, Children. Dosage varies according to amount of digoxin to be neutralized. Refer to manufacturer's dosing guidelines.

CONTRAINDICATIONS

None known.

INTERACTIONS

Drug

None known.

Herbal

None known.

Food

None known.

DIAGNOSTIC TEST EFFECTS

May alter serum potassium level. Serum digoxin concentration may increase precipitously and persist for up to 1 week until FAB/digoxin complex is eliminated from the body.

IV INCOMPATIBILITIES

None known.

SIDE EFFECTS

None known.

SERIOUS REACTIONS

! Hyperkalemia may occur as a result of digitalis toxicity. Signs and symptoms of hyperkalemia include diarrhea, paresthesia of extremities, heaviness of legs, decreased BP, cold skin, grayish pallor, hypotension, mental confusion, irritability, flaccid paralysis, tented T waves, widening QRS interval, and ST depression.

! Hypokalemia may develop rapidly when the effect of digitalis is reversed. Signs and symptoms of hypokalemia include muscle cramping, nausea, vomiting, hypoactive bowel sounds, abdominal distention, difficulty breathing, and orthostatic hypotension.
! Low cardiac output and CHF may occur rarely.

NURSING CONSIDERATIONS

Baseline Assessment

- Obtain the patient's serum digoxin level before administering the drug. If the serum digoxin level was drawn less than 6 hours before the last digoxin dose, the serum digoxin level may be unreliable.
- Patients with impaired renal function may require more than 1 week before serum digoxin assay is reliable.
- Assess the patient's mental status and muscle strength.

Lifespan Considerations

- It is unknown if digoxin immune FAB crosses the placenta or is distributed in breast milk.
- No age-related precautions have been noted in children.
- In the elderly, age-related renal impairment may require cautious use.

Precautions

- Use digoxin immune FAB cautiously in patients with impaired cardiac or renal function.

Administration and Handling

IV

- Refrigerate vials.
- After reconstitution, use the solution immediately. If it's not used immediately, store the solution in the refrigerator for up to 4 hours.
- Reconstitute each 38-mg vial with 4 ml sterile water for injection to provide a concentration of 9.5 mg/ml. Reconstitute each 40-mg vial with 4 ml of sterile water for injection to provide a concentration of 10 mg/ml.
- Further dilute with 50 ml 0.9% NaCl.
- Infuse over 30 minutes. It is recommended that the solution be infused through a 0.22-micron filter.
- If cardiac arrest is imminent, may give drug by IV push.

Intervention and Evaluation

- Closely monitor the patient's BP, EKG, serum potassium level, and temperature during and after drug administration.
- Observe the patient for changes from the initial assessment. Hypokalemia may result in cardiac arrhythmias, changes in mental status, muscle cramps, muscle strength changes, or tremor. Hyperkalemia may result in cold and clammy skin, confusion, and diarrhea.
- Assess for signs and symptoms of an arrhythmia (such as palpitations), or heart failure (such as dyspnea and edema) if the digoxin level falls below the therapeutic level.

Patient Teaching

- Before discharge, review the digoxin dosages carefully with the patient, and make sure he or she knows how to take the drug as prescribed.
- Instruct the patient about any follow-up care, including monitoring serum digoxin level.
- Make sure the patient knows the signs and symptoms of digoxin toxicity, including anorexia, nausea, and vomiting, as well as visual changes.

eplerenone
e-**plear**-a-nown
(Inspra)

CATEGORY AND SCHEDULE
Pregnancy Risk Category: B

MECHANISM OF ACTION
An aldosterone receptor antagonist that binds to the mineralocorticoid receptors in the kidney, heart, blood vessels, and brain, blocking the binding of aldosterone. **Therapeutic Effect:** Reduces BP.

PHARMACOKINETICS
Absorption unaffected by food. Protein binding: 50%. No active metabolites. Excreted in the urine with a lesser amount eliminated in the feces. Not removed by hemodialysis. ***Half-life:*** 4–6 hr.

AVAILABILITY
Tablets: 25 mg, 50 mg.

INDICATIONS AND DOSAGES
▸ **Hypertension**

PO

Adults, Elderly. 50 mg once a day. If 50 mg once a day produces an inadequate BP response, may increase dosage to 50 mg twice a day. If patient is concurrently receiving erythromycin, saquinavir, verapamil, or fluconazole, reduce initial dose to 25 mg once a day.

▸ **CHF following MI**

PO

Adults, Elderly. Initially, 25 mg once a day. If tolerated, titrate up to 50 mg once a day within 4 wk.

CONTRAINDICATIONS
Concurrent use of potassium supplements or potassium-sparing diuretics (such as amiloride, spironolactone, and triamterene), or strong inhibitors of the cytochrome P450 3A4 enzyme system (including ketoconazole and itraconazole), creatinine clearance less than 50 ml/min, serum creatinine level greater than 2 mg/dl in males or 1.8 mg/dl in females, serum potassium level greater than 5.5 mEq/L, type 2 diabetes mellitus with microalbuminuria

INTERACTIONS
Drug

ACE inhibitors, angiotensin II antagonists, erythromycin, fluconazole, saquinavir, verapamil: Increases risk of hyperkalemia.

Herbal

St. John's wort: Decreases eplerenone effectiveness.

Food

Grapefruit, grapefruit juice: Produces small increase in serum potassium level.

DIAGNOSTIC TEST EFFECTS
May increase serum potassium level. May decrease serum sodium level.

SIDE EFFECTS
Rare (3%–1%)

Dizziness, diarrhea, cough, fatigue, flu-like symptoms, abdominal pain

SERIOUS REACTIONS
! Hyperkalemia may occur, particularly in patients with type 2 diabetes mellitus and microalbuminuria.

NURSING CONSIDERATIONS
Baseline Assessment

• Obtain the patient's apical heart rate and BP immediately before each dose, in addition to regular monitoring. Be alert to BP fluctuations. If an excessive reduction in BP occurs, place the patient in the supine position with feet slightly elevated, and notify the physician.

Lifespan Considerations

• It is unknown if eplerenone crosses the placenta or is distributed in breast milk.
• The safety and efficacy of eplerenone have not been established in children.
• No age-related precautions have been noted in the elderly.

Precautions

• Use eplerenone cautiously in patients with hyperkalemia or hepatic impairment.

Administration and Handling

PO

• Film-coated tablets should not be broken, crushed, or chewed.

Intervention and Evaluation

• Assist the patient with ambulation if he or she experiences dizziness.
• Monitor the patient's serum potassium and sodium levels.
• Assess the patient's BP for hypertension or hypotension.
• Assess the patient's pattern of daily bowel activity and stool consistency.
• Evaluate the patient for flu-like symptoms.

Patient Teaching

• Warn the patient to avoid tasks that require mental alertness or motor skills until his or her response to the drug has been established.
• Explain to the patient that eplerenone will have to be taken for the rest of his or her life to control hypertension.
• Tell the patient not to break, crush, or chew film-coated tablets
• Caution the patient against exercising outside during hot weather because of the risks of dehydration and hypotension.

sodium polystyrene sulfonate

pol-ee-**stye**-reen
(Kayexelate, Kionex, PMS-Sodium Polystyrene Sulfonate [CAN], Resonium A[AUS], SPS)

CATEGORY AND SCHEDULE

Pregnancy Risk Category: C

MECHANISM OF ACTION

An ion exchange resin that releases sodium ions in exchange primarily for potassium ions. **Therapeutic Effect:** Moves potassium from the blood into the intestine so it can be expelled from the body.

AVAILABILITY

Suspension (SPS): 15 g/60 ml.
Powder for Suspension (Kayexelate, Kionex): 454 g.

INDICATIONS AND DOSAGES

▸ **Hyperkalemia**

PO

Adults, Elderly. 60 ml (15 g) 1–4 times a day.
Children. 1 g/kg/dose q6h.

Rectal

Adults, Elderly. 30–50 g as needed q6h.
Children. 1 g/kg/dose q2–6h.

CONTRAINDICATIONS

Hypernatremia, intestinal obstruction or perforation

INTERACTIONS

Drug

Cation-donating antacids, laxatives (such as magnesium hydroxide): May decrease effect of sodium polystyrene sulfonate, and cause systemic alkalosis in patients with renal impairment.

Herbal
None known.
Food
None known.

DIAGNOSTIC TEST EFFECTS

May decrease serum calcium and magnesium levels.

SIDE EFFECTS

Frequent
High dosage: Anorexia, nausea, vomiting, constipation
High dosage in elderly: Fecal impaction characterized by severe stomach pain with nausea or vomiting
Occasional
Diarrhea, sodium retention marked by decreased urination, peripheral edema, and increased weight

SERIOUS REACTIONS

! Potassium deficiency may occur. Early signs of hypokalemia include confusion, delayed thought processes, extreme weakness, irritability, and EKG changes (including prolonged QT interval; widening, flattening, or inversion of T wave; and prominent U waves).
! Hypocalcemia, manifested by abdominal or muscle cramps, occurs occasionally.
! Arrhythmias and severe muscle weakness may be noted.

NURSING CONSIDERATIONS

Baseline Assessment
- Because sodium polystyrene sulfonate does not rapidly correct severe hyperkalemia (it may take hours to days), consider other measures, such as dialysis, IV glucose and insulin, IV calcium, and IV sodium bicarbonate to correct severe hyperkalemia in a medical emergency.

Lifespan Considerations
- It is unknown if sodium polystyrene sulfonate crosses the placenta or is distributed in breast milk.
- No age-related precautions have been noted in children.
- The elderly may be at increased risk for fecal impaction.

Precautions
- Use sodium polystyrene sulfonate cautiously in patients with edema, hypertension, or severe CHF.

Administration and Handling
PO
- Give with 20 to 100 ml sorbitol to aid in potassium removal, facilitate passage of resin through intestinal tract, and prevent constipation.
- Do not mix this drug with foods or liquids containing potassium.

Rectal
- After initial cleansing enema, insert large rubber tube well into sigmoid colon and tape in place.
- Introduce suspension with 100 ml sorbitol by gravity.
- Flush with 50 to 100 ml fluid and clamp.
- Have patient retain the solution for several hours, if possible.
- Irrigate colon with a non–sodium-containing solution to remove resin.

Intervention and Evaluation
- Monitor the patient's serum potassium level frequently. Also monitor serum calcium and magnesium levels.
- Assess the patient's clinical condition and EKG, which is valuable in determining when treatment should be discontinued.
- Assess the patient's pattern of daily bowel activity and stool consistency. Fecal impaction may occur in patients receiving high dosages of sodium polystyrene sulfonate, particularly the elderly.
- Plan to consult a dietician to provide dietary counseling.

Patient Teaching
- Instruct the patient to drink the

entire amount of the resin for best results.
- Urge the patient receiving the drug rectally to try to retain the solution for several hours, if possible.
- Instruct the patient about which foods are rich in potassium.

tamsulosin hydrochloride

tam-**sool**-o-sin
(Flomax)
Do not confuse Flomax with Fosamax or Volmax.

CATEGORY AND SCHEDULE

Pregnancy Risk Category: B (Not indicated for use in women.)

MECHANISM OF ACTION

An $alpha_1$ antagonist that targets receptors around bladder neck and prostate capsule. **Therapeutic Effect:** Relaxes smooth muscle and improves urinary flow and symptoms of prostatic hyperplasia.

PHARMACOKINETICS

Well absorbed and widely distributed. Protein binding: 94%–99%. Metabolized in the liver. Primarily excreted in urine. Unknown if removed by hemodialysis. ***Half-life:*** 9–13 hr.

AVAILABILITY

Capsules: 0.4 mg.

INDICATIONS AND DOSAGES

▸ Benign prostatic hyperplasia
PO
Adults. 0.4 mg once a day, approximately 30 min after same meal each day. May increase dosage to 0.8 mg if inadequate response in 2–4 wk.

CONTRAINDICATIONS

History of sensitivity to tamsulosin

INTERACTIONS

Drug
Other alpha-adrenergic blocking agents (such as cimetidine, doxazosin, prazosin, terazosin): May increase the alpha-blockade effects of both drugs.
Warfarin: May alter the effects of warfarin.
Herbal
None known.
Food
None known.

DIAGNOSTIC TEST EFFECTS

None known.

SIDE EFFECTS

Frequent (9%–7%)
Dizziness, somnolence
Occasional (5%–3%)
Headache, anxiety, insomnia, orthostatic hypotension
Rare (less than 2%)
Nasal congestion, pharyngitis, rhinitis, nausea, vertigo, impotence

SERIOUS REACTIONS

! First-dose syncope (hypotension with sudden loss of consciousness) may occur within 30 to 90 minutes after administration of initial dose and may be preceded by tachycardia (pulse rate of 120–160 beats/minute).

NURSING CONSIDERATIONS

Baseline Assessment
- Determine if the patient is hypersensitive to tamsulosin and if he is using other alpha-adrenergic blocking agents or warfarin.

Lifespan Considerations
- Tamsulosin is not indicated for use in women or children.

- No age-related precautions have been noted in the elderly.

Precautions

- Use tamsulosin cautiously in patients with renal impairment.

Administration and Handling

PO

- Give at the same time each day, 30 minutes after the same meal.
- Do not crush or open capsule unless directed by the physician.

Intervention and Evaluation

- Assist the patient with ambulation if he experiences dizziness.
- Monitor the patient's BP and renal function.

Patient Teaching

- Instruct the patient to take tamsulosin at the same time each day, 30 minutes after the same meal. Teach the patient not to chew, crush, or open the capsules.
- Advise the patient to use caution when getting up from a sitting or lying position.
- Warn the patient to avoid tasks that require mental alertness or motor skills until his response to the drug has been established.

32 Antianxiety Agents

alprazolam
buspirone hydrochloride
chlordiazepoxide
clorazepate dipotassium
diazepam
doxepin hydrochloride
hydroxyzine
lorazepam
midazolam hydrochloride
oxazepam

Uses: Antianxiety agents are used to treat anxiety. In addition, some benzodiazepines are used as hypnotics to induce sleep, as anticonvulsants to prevent delirium tremors during alcohol withdrawal, and as adjunctive therapy for relaxation of skeletal muscle spasms. Midazolam, a short-acting benzodiazepine, is used for preoperative sedation and relief of anxiety in short diagnostic endoscopic procedures.

Action: Although their exact mechanism of action is unknown, antianxiety agents may increase the inhibiting effect of gamma-aminobutyric acid (GABA), an inhibitory neurotransmitter. Benzodiazepines, the largest and most frequently prescribed group of antianxiety agents, may inhibit nerve impulse transmission by binding to specific benzodiazepine receptors in various areas of the CNS. (See the illustration *Mechanism of Action: Benzodiazepines,* page 633.)

COMBINATION PRODUCTS

LIBRAX: chlordiazepoxide/clidinium (an anticholinergic) 5 mg/2.5 mg.
LIMBITROL: chlordiazepoxide/amitriptyline (an antidepressant) 5 mg/12.5 mg; 10 mg/25 mg.

alprazolam

al-**pray**-zoe-lam
(Alprax[AUS], Apo-Alpraz[CAN], Kalma[AUS], Novo-Alprazol[CAN], Xanax, Xanax XR)
Do not confuse alprazolam with lorazepam, or Xanax with Tenex or Zantac.

CATEGORY AND SCHEDULE

Pregnancy Risk Category: D
Controlled Substance: Schedule IV

MECHANISM OF ACTION

A benzodiazepine that enhances the action of the inhibitory neurotransmitter gamma-aminobutyric acid in the brain. **Therapeutic Effect:** Produces anxiolytic effect from its CNS depressant action.

PHARMACOKINETICS

Well absorbed from GI tract. Protein binding: 80%. Metabolized in the liver. Primarily excreted in urine. Minimal removal by hemodialysis. ***Half-life:*** 11–16 hr.

AVAILABILITY

Oral Solution (Xanax): 1 mg/ml.
Tablets: 0.25 mg, 0.5 mg, 1 mg, 2 mg.
Tablets (Extended-Release [Xanax XR]): 0.5 mg, 1 mg, 2 mg, 3 mg.

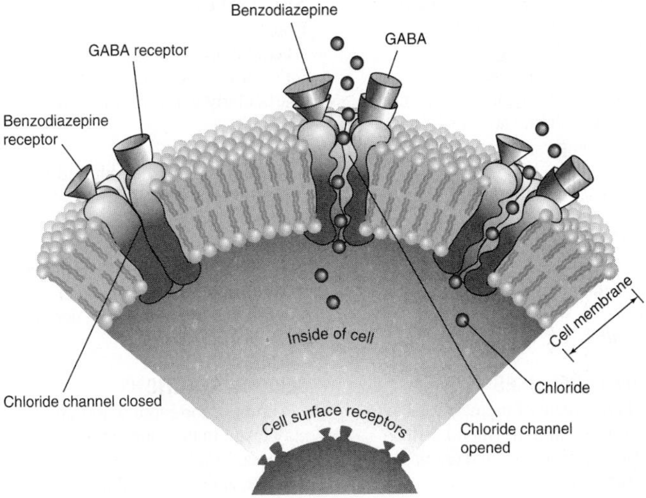

Mechanism of Action: Benzodiazepines

Benzodiazepines reduce anxiety by stimulating the action of the inhibitory neurotransmitter gamma-aminobutyric acid (GABA) in the limbic system. The limbic system plays an important role in the regulation of human behavior. Dysfunction of GABA neurotransmission in the limbic system may be linked to the development of certain anxiety disorders.

The limbic system contains a highly dense area of benzodiazepine receptors that may be linked to the antianxiety effects of benzodiazepines. These benzodiazepine receptors are located on the surface of neuronal cell membranes and are adjacent to GABA receptors. The binding of a benzodiazepine to its receptor enhances the affinity of a GABA receptor for GABA. In the absence of a benzodiazepine, the binding of GABA to its receptor causes the chloride channel in the cell membrane to open, which increases the influx of chloride into the cell. This influx of chloride results in hyperpolarization of the neuronal cell membrane and reduces the neuron's ability to fire, which is why GABA is considered an inhibitory neurotransmitter.

A benzodiazepine acts only in the presence of GABA. When it binds to a benzodiazepine receptor, it prolongs the time that the chloride channel remains open. This results in greater depression of neuronal function and a reduction in anxiety.

INDICATIONS AND DOSAGES

▸ Anxiety disorders

PO (Immediate-Release)

Adults. Initially, 0.25–0.5 mg 3 times a day. May titrate q3–4 days. Maximum: 4 mg/day in divided doses.

Elderly, Debilitated patients, Patients with hepatic disease or low serum albumin. Initially, 0.25 mg 2–3 times a day. Gradually increase to optimum therapeutic response.

▸ Panic disorder

PO (Immediate-Release)

Adults. Initially, 0.5 mg 3 times a

day. May increase at 3- to 4-day intervals. Range: 5–6 mg/day. Maximum: 10 mg/day.
PO (Extended-Release)
Adults. Initially, 0.5–1 mg once a day. May titrate at 3- to 4-day intervals. Range: 3–6 mg/day. Maximum: 10 mg/day.
Elderly. Initially, 0.125–0.25 mg 2 times a day; may increase in 0.125–mg increments until desired effect attained.

▸ **Premenstrual syndrome**
PO
Adults. 0.25 mg 3 times a day.

OFF-LABEL USES

Management of premenstrual syndrome symptoms (mood disturbances, insomnia, and cramps), irritable bowel syndrome

CONTRAINDICATIONS

Acute alcohol intoxication with depressed vital signs, acute angle-closure glaucoma, concurrent use of itraconazole or ketoconazole, myasthenia gravis, severe COPD

INTERACTIONS

Drug

Alcohol, other CNS depressants: Potentiate effects of alprazolam and may increase sedation.
Fluvoxamine, itraconazole, ketoconazole, nefazodone: May inhibit metabolism and increase serum concentrations of alprazolam.

Herbal

Kava kava, valerian: May increase CNS depressant effect of alprazolam.

Food

Grapefruit, grapefruit juice: May inhibit alprazolam's metabolism.

DIAGNOSTIC TEST EFFECTS

None known.

SIDE EFFECTS

Frequent

Ataxia; light-headedness; transient, mild somnolence; slurred speech (particularly in elderly or debilitated patients)

Occasional

Confusion, depression, blurred vision, constipation, diarrhea, dry mouth, headache, nausea

Rare

Behavioral problems such as anger; impaired memory; paradoxical reactions such as insomnia, nervousness, or irritability

SERIOUS REACTIONS

! Abrupt or too-rapid withdrawal may result in pronounced restlessness, irritability, insomnia, hand tremors, abdominal and muscle cramps, diaphoresis, vomiting, and seizures.
! Overdose results in somnolence, confusion, diminished reflexes, and coma.
! Blood dyscrasias have been reported rarely.

NURSING CONSIDERATIONS

Baseline Assessment

- Assess the patient for motor responses, such as agitation, tension, and trembling, and autonomic responses, such as cold, clammy hands and diaphoresis.

Lifespan Considerations

- Alprazolam crosses the placenta and is distributed in breast milk.
- Chronic use of alprazolam during pregnancy may produce withdrawal symptoms in the patient and CNS depression in the neonate.
- The safety and efficacy of alprazolam have not been established in children.
- Expect to give elderly patients small doses initially and to increase

dosage gradually to avoid excessive sedation or ataxia.

Precautions

- Use alprazolam cautiously in patients with impaired renal or hepatic function.

Administration and Handling

PO

- Give alprazolam without regard to food.
- Crush tablets as needed.

PO (Extended-Release)

- Administer once a day.
- Swallow tablets whole. Do not break, chew, or crush tablets.

Intervention and Evaluation

- Expect to perform blood tests periodically to assess hepatic and renal function in patients receiving long-term therapy.
- Assess the patient for paradoxical CNS reactions, particularly early in therapy.
- Evaluate the patient for the desired therapeutic response, including a calm facial expression and decreased insomnia and restlessness.
- Offer emotional support to the anxious patient.

Patient Teaching

- Caution the patient not to stop taking alprazolam abruptly after long-term therapy.
- Inform the patient that drowsiness usually disappears with continued therapy.
- Instruct the patient to change positions slowly—from recumbent, to sitting, before standing—to prevent dizziness.
- Caution the patient to avoid tasks that require mental alertness or motor skills until his or her response to the drug has been established.
- Advise the patient not to take other medications, including OTC drugs, without consulting the physician.
- Urge the patient to avoid alcohol during therapy.
- Encourage the patient to stop smoking because smoking reduces alprazolam's effectiveness.
- Urge the female patient on long-term therapy to use effective contraception during therapy and to notify the physician immediately if she becomes or may be pregnant.
- Inform the patient that sour hard candy, gum, or sips of tepid water may relieve dry mouth.

buspirone hydrochloride

byoo-**spir**-own
(BuSpar, Buspirex[CAN], Bustab[CAN])

Do not confuse buspirone with bupropion.

CATEGORY AND SCHEDULE

Pregnancy Risk Category: B

MECHANISM OF ACTION

Although its exact mechanism of action is unknown, this nonbarbiturate is thought to bind to serotonin and dopamine receptors in the CNS. The drug may also increase norepinephrine metabolism in the locus ceruleus. **Therapeutic Effect:** Produces anxiolytic effect.

PHARMACOKINETICS

Rapidly and completely absorbed from the GI tract. Protein binding: 95%. Undergoes extensive first-pass metabolism. Metabolized in the liver to active metabolite. Primarily excreted in urine. Not removed by hemodialysis. ***Half-life:*** 2–3 hr.

AVAILABILITY

Tablets: 5 mg, 7.5 mg, 10 mg, 15 mg, 30 mg.

INDICATIONS AND DOSAGES

▸ Short-term management (up to 4 weeks) of anxiety disorders

PO

Adults. 5 mg 2–3 times a day or 7.5 mg twice a day. May increase by 5 mg/day every 2–4 days. Maintenance: 15–30 mg/day in 2–3 divided doses. Maximum: 60 mg/day.

Elderly. Initially, 5 mg twice a day. May increase by 5 mg/day every 2–3 days. Maximum: 60 mg/day.

Children. Initially, 5 mg/day. May increase by 5 mg/day at weekly intervals. Maximum: 60 mg/day.

OFF-LABEL USES

Management of panic attack, premenstrual syndrome (aches, pain, fatigue, irritability)

CONTRAINDICATIONS

Concurrent use of MAOIs, severe hepatic or renal impairment

INTERACTIONS

Drug

Alcohol, other CNS depressants: Potentiates effects of buspirone and may increase sedation.

Erythromycin, itraconazole: May increase buspirone blood concentration and risk of toxicity.

MAOIs: May increase BP.

Herbal

Kava kava: May increase sedation.

Food

Grapefruit, grapefruit juice: May increase buspirone blood concentration and risk of toxicity.

DIAGNOSTIC TEST EFFECTS

None known.

SIDE EFFECTS

Frequent (12%–6%)

Dizziness, somnolence, nausea, headache

Occasional (5%–2%)

Nervousness, fatigue, insomnia, dry mouth, lightheadedness, mood swings, blurred vision, poor concentration, diarrhea, paraesthesia

Rare

Muscle pain and stiffness, nightmares, chest pain, involuntary movements

SERIOUS REACTIONS

! Buspirone does not appear to cause drug tolerance, psychological or physical dependence, or withdrawal syndrome.

! Overdose may produce severe nausea, vomiting, dizziness, drowsiness, abdominal distention, and excessive pupil contraction.

NURSING CONSIDERATIONS

Baseline Assessment

- Assess the patient for autonomic responses, such as, cold, clammy hands and diaphoresis, and motor responses, such as agitation, trembling, and tension.

Lifespan Considerations

- It is unknown if buspirone crosses the placenta or is distributed in breast milk.
- The safety and efficacy of buspirone have not been established in children.
- No age-related precautions have been noted in the elderly.

Precautions

- Use buspirone cautiously in patients with hepatic or renal impairment.

Administration and Handling

PO

- Give buspirone without regard to food.
- Crush tablets as needed.

Intervention and Evaluation

- Expect to perform blood tests periodically to assess hepatic and

renal function in patients on long-term therapy.
• Assist the patient with ambulation if he or she experiences drowsiness or light-headedness.
• Evaluate the patient for evidence of a therapeutic response, including a calm facial expression and decreased restlessness and insomnia.
• Offer emotional support to the anxious patient.

Patient Teaching

• Inform the patient that he or she may notice an improvement within 7–10 days of starting therapy, but that the optimum therapeutic effect generally takes 3 to 4 weeks to appear.
• Tell the patient that drowsiness usually disappears with continued therapy.
• Instruct the patient to change positions slowly—from recumbent to sitting before standing—to avoid dizziness.
• Advise the patient to avoid tasks that require mental alertness and motor skills until his or her response to buspirone has been established.
• Caution the patient not to take buspirone with grapefruit juice because doing so may increase the risk of drug toxicity.

chlordiazepoxide

klor-dye-az-e-**pox**-ide
(Apo-Chlordiazepoxide[CAN], Librium, Novopoxide[CAN])
Do not confuse Librium with Librax.

CATEGORY AND SCHEDULE

Pregnancy Risk Category: D

MECHANISM OF ACTION

A benzodiazepine that enhances the action of the inhibitory neurotransmitter gamma-aminobutyric acid in the CNS. **Therapeutic Effect:** Produces anxiolytic effect.

AVAILABILITY

Capsules: 5 mg, 10 mg, 25 mg.
Injection Powder for Reconstitution. 100 mg.

INDICATIONS AND DOSAGES

▸ Alcohol withdrawal symptoms

PO

Adults, Elderly. 50–100 mg. May repeat q2–4h. Maximum: 300 mg/24 hr.

▸ Anxiety

PO

Adults. 15–100 mg/day in 3–4 divided doses.
Elderly. 5 mg 2–4 times a day.

IV, IM

Adults. Initially, 50–100 mg, then 25–50 mg 3–4 times a day as needed.

OFF-LABEL USES

Treatment of panic disorder, tension headache, tremors

CONTRAINDICATIONS

Acute alcohol intoxication, acute angle-closure glaucoma

INTERACTIONS

Drug

Alcohol, other CNS depressants: May increase CNS depression.

Herbal

Kava kava, valerian: May increase CNS depression.

Food

None known.

DIAGNOSTIC TEST EFFECTS

None known. Therapeutic serum drug level is 1–3 mcg/ml; toxic serum drug level is greater than 5 mcg/ml.

SIDE EFFECTS

Frequent

Pain at IM injection site; somnolence, ataxia, dizziness, confusion with oral dose (particularly in elderly or debilitated patients)

Occasional

Rash, peripheral edema, GI disturbances

Rare

Paradoxical CNS reactions, such as hyperactivity or nervousness in children and excitement or restlessness in the elderly (generally noted during first 2 weeks of therapy, particularly in presence of uncontrolled pain)

SERIOUS REACTIONS

! IV administration may produce pain, swelling, thrombophlebitis, and carpal tunnel syndrome.

! Abrupt or too-rapid withdrawal may result in pronounced restlessness, irritability, insomnia, hand tremors, abdominal or muscle cramps, diaphoresis, vomiting, and seizures.

! Overdose results in somnolence, confusion, diminished reflexes, and coma.

NURSING CONSIDERATIONS

Baseline Assessment

• Assess the patient's BP, pulse rate, and respiratory rate, rhythm, and depth immediately before giving chlordiazepoxide.

• Assess the patient for autonomic responses, such as cold, clammy hands or diaphoresis, and motor responses, such as agitation, trembling, and tension.

Precautions

• Use chlordiazepoxide cautiously in patients with impaired hepatic or renal function.

Administration and Handling

◀ **ALERT** ▶ Expect to use the smallest effective chlordiazepoxide dose in elderly or debilitated patients and patients with hepatic disease or a low serum albumin level.

• Keep the patient recumbent for up to 3 hours after parenteral administration to reduce the drug's hypotensive effect.

Intervention and Evaluation

• Assess pediatric and elderly patients for paradoxical CNS reactions, particularly early in therapy.

• Assist the patient with ambulation if he or she experiences ataxia or drowsiness.

• Know that the therapeutic serum level for chlordiazepoxide is 1–3 mcg/ml, and the toxic serum level is greater than 5 mcg/ml.

Patient Teaching

• Caution the patient not to discontinue the drug abruptly after long-term therapy.

• Inform the patient that IM injection may produce discomfort.

• Explain that drowsiness usually disappears with continued therapy.

• Instruct the patient to change positions slowly—from recumbent to sitting before standing—to prevent dizziness.

• Urge the patient to stop smoking during therapy because smoking reduces the drug's effectiveness.

• Warn the patient to avoid alcohol consumption while taking this drug.

clorazepate dipotassium

klor-**az**-e-pate

(Novoclopate[CAN], Tranxene, Tranxene SD, Tranxene SD Half-Strength, T-Tab)

Do not confuse clorazepate with clofibrate.

CATEGORY AND SCHEDULE

Pregnancy Risk Category: D

MECHANISM OF ACTION

A benzodiazepine that depresses all levels of the CNS, including limbic and reticular formation, by binding to benzodiazepine receptor sites on the gamma-aminobutyric acid (GABA) receptor complex. Modulates GABA, a major inhibitory neurotransmitter in the brain. **Therapeutic Effect:** Produces anxiolytic effect, suppresses seizure activity.

AVAILABILITY

Tablets (Tranxene, T-Tab): 3.75 mg, 7.5 mg, 15 mg.
Tablets (Extended-Release [Tranxene SD]): 22.5 mg.
Tablets (Extended-Release [Tranxene SD Half-Strength]): 11.25 mg.

INDICATIONS AND DOSAGES

▸ **Anxiety**

PO (Regular-Release)
Adults, Elderly. 7.5–15 mg 2–4 times a day.
PO (Sustained-Release)
Adults, Elderly. 11.25 mg or 22.5 mg once a day at bedtime.

▸ **Anticonvulsant**

PO
Adults, Elderly, Children older than 12 yr. Initially, 7.5 mg 2–3 times a day. May increase by 7.5 mg at weekly intervals. Maximum: 90 mg/day.
Children 9–12 yr. Initially, 3.75–7.5 mg twice a day. May increase by 2.75 mg at weekly intervals. Maximum: 60 mg/day.

▸ **Alcohol withdrawal**

PO
Adults, Elderly. Initially, 30 mg, then 15 mg 2–4 times a day on first day. Gradually decrease dosage over subsequent days. Maximum: 90 mg/day.

CONTRAINDICATIONS

Acute narrow-angle glaucoma

INTERACTIONS

Drug

Alcohol, other CNS depressants: May increase CNS depressant effects.

Herbal

Kava kava, valerian: May increase CNS depression.

Food

None known.

DIAGNOSTIC TEST EFFECTS

None known. Therapeutic serum drug level is 0.12–1.5 mcg/ml; toxic serum drug level is greater than 5 mcg/ml.

SIDE EFFECTS

Frequent

Somnolence

Occasional

Dizziness, GI disturbances, nervousness, blurred vision, dry mouth, headache, confusion, ataxia, rash, irritability, slurred speech

Rare

Paradoxical CNS reactions, such as hyperactivity or nervousness in children and excitement or restlessness in the elderly or debilitated (generally noted during first 2 weeks of therapy, particularly in presence of uncontrolled pain)

SERIOUS REACTIONS

! Abrupt or too-rapid withdrawal may result in pronounced restlessness, irritability, insomnia, hand tremors, abdominal or muscle cramps, diaphoresis, vomiting, and seizures.

! Overdose results in somnolence, confusion, diminished reflexes, and coma.

NURSING CONSIDERATIONS

Baseline Assessment

- Assess the anxious patient for autonomic responses, such as cold or clammy hands and diaphoresis, and motor responses, such as agitation, trembling, and tension.
- In seizure patients, assess LOC and review the history of the seizure disorder, including the duration, intensity, and frequency of seizures.

Precautions

- Use clorazepate cautiously in patients with acute alcohol intoxication or renal or hepatic impairment.

Administration and Handling

◀ALERT▶ If the patient must change to another anticonvulsant, plan to decrease clorazepate dosage gradually as low-dose therapy begins with the replacement drug.

Intervention and Evaluation

- For the patient with seizures, initiate seizure precautions and observe the patient frequently for recurrence of seizure activity.
- Assess the patient for paradoxical CNS reactions, particularly early in therapy.
- Assist the patient with ambulation if he or she experiences dizziness and drowsiness.
- Evaluate the patient for a therapeutic response, characterized by a calm facial expression and decreased restlessness in anxious patients and a decrease in intensity or frequency of seizures in patients with seizure disorder.
- Monitor the patient's serum drug level. The therapeutic peak serum level is 0.12–1.5 mcg/ml; the toxic serum level is greater than 5 mcg/ml.
- Offer emotional support to the anxious patient.

Patient Teaching

- Caution the patient against abruptly stopping the medication after long-term use because this may precipitate seizures. Explain that strict compliance with the drug regimen is essential for seizure control.
- Inform the patient that drowsiness usually disappears with continued therapy.
- Advise the patient to avoid tasks that require mental alertness or motor skills until his or her response to the drug has been established.
- Instruct the patient to change positions slowly—from recumbent to sitting before standing—to prevent dizziness.
- Urge the female patient on long-term therapy to use effective contraception during therapy and to notify the physician immediately if she becomes or may be pregnant.
- Urge the patient to stop smoking and consuming alcoholic beverages during clorazepate therapy. Explain that smoking reduces the drug's effectiveness and alcohol may increase sedation.

diazepam

dye-**az**-e-pam
(Antenex[AUS], Apo-Diazepam[CAN], Diastat, Diazemuls[CAN], Dizac, Ducene[AUS], Valium, Valpam[AUS], Vivol[CAN])
Do not confuse diazepam with diazoxide or Ditropan, or Valium with Valcyte.

CATEGORY AND SCHEDULE

Pregnancy Risk Category: D
Controlled Substance: Schedule IV

MECHANISM OF ACTION

A benzodiazepine that depresses all levels of the CNS by enhancing the action of gamma-aminobutyric acid, a major inhibitory neurotransmitter in the brain. **Therapeutic Effect:** Produces anxiolytic effect, elevates the seizure threshold, produces skeletal muscle relaxation.

PHARMACOKINETICS

Route	Onset	Peak	Duration
PO	30 min	1–2 hr	2–3 hr
IV	1–5 min	15 min	15–60 min
IM	15 min	30–90 min	30–90 min

Well absorbed from the GI tract. Widely distributed. Protein binding: 98%. Metabolized in the liver to active metabolite. Excreted in urine. Minimally removed by hemodialysis. ***Half-life:*** 20–70 hr (increased in hepatic dysfunction and the elderly).

AVAILABILITY

Oral Concentrate (Diazepam Intensol): 5 mg/ml.
Oral Solution: 5 mg/5 ml.
Tablets (Valium): 2 mg, 5 mg, 10 mg.
Injection: 5 mg/ml.
Rectal Gel (Diastat): 5 mg/ml.

INDICATIONS AND DOSAGES

▸ Anxiety, skeletal muscle relaxation

PO

Adults. 2–10 mg 2–4 times a day.
Elderly. 2.5 mg twice a day.
Children. 0.12–0.8 mg/kg/day in divided doses q6–8h.

IV, IM

Adults. 2–10 mg repeated in 3–4 hr.
Children. 0.04–0.3 mg/kg/dose q2–4h. Maximum: 0.5 mg/kg in an 8-hr period.

▸ Preanesthesia

IV

Adults, Elderly. 5–15 mg 5–10 min before procedure.
Children. 0.2–0.3 mg/kg. Maximum: 10 mg.

▸ Alcohol withdrawal

PO

Adults, Elderly. 10 mg 3–4 times during first 24 hr, then reduced to 5–10 mg 3–4 times a day as needed.

IV, IM

Adults, Elderly. Initially, 10 mg, followed by 5–10 mg q3–4h.

▸ Status epilepticus

IV

Adults, Elderly. 5–10 mg q10–15min up to 30 mg/8 hr.
Children 5 yr and older. 0.05–0.3 mg/kg/dose q15–30min. Maximum: 10 mg/dose.
Children 1 mo to younger than 5 yr. 0.05–0.3 mg/kg/dose q15–30min. Maximum: 5 mg/dose.

▸ **Control of increased seizure activity in patients with refractory epilepsy who are on stable regimens of anticonvulsants**
Rectal Gel
Adults, Children 12 yr and older. 0.2 mg/kg; may be repeated in 4–12 hr.
Children 6–11 yr. 0.3 mg/kg; may be repeated in 4–12 hr.
Children 2–5 yr. 0.5 mg/kg; may be repeated in 4–12 hr.

OFF-LABEL USES
Treatment of panic disorder, tension headache, tremors

CONTRAINDICATIONS
Angle-closure glaucoma, coma, pre-existing CNS depression, respiratory depression, severe, uncontrolled pain

INTERACTIONS
Drug
Alcohol, other CNS depressants: May increase CNS depression.
Herbal
Kava kava, valerian: May increase CNS depression.
Food
None known.

DIAGNOSTIC TEST EFFECTS
May elevate serum LDH, alkaline phosphatase, bilirubin, AST (SGOT), and ALT (SGPT) levels. May produce abnormal renal function test results. Therapeutic serum drug level is 0.5–2 mcg/ml; toxic serum drug level is greater than 3 mcg/ml.

IV INCOMPATIBILITIES
Amphotericin B complex (Abelcet, AmBisome, Amphotec), cefepime (Maxipime), diltiazem (Cardizem), fluconazole (Diflucan), foscarnet (Foscavir), heparin, hydrocortisone (Solu-Cortef), hydromorphone (Dilaudid), meropenem (Merrem IV), potassium chloride, propofol (Diprivan), vitamins

IV COMPATIBILITIES
Dobutamine (Dobutrex), fentanyl, morphine

SIDE EFFECTS
Frequent
Pain with IM injection, somnolence, fatigue, ataxia
Occasional
Slurred speech, orthostatic hypotension, headache, hypoactivity, constipation, nausea, blurred vision
Rare
Paradoxical CNS reactions, such as hyperactivity or nervousness in children and excitement or restlessness in the elderly or debilitated (generally noted during first 2 weeks of therapy, particularly in presence of uncontrolled pain)

SERIOUS REACTIONS
! IV administration may produce pain, swelling, thrombophlebitis, and carpal tunnel syndrome.
! Abrupt or too-rapid withdrawal may result in pronounced restlessness, irritability, insomnia, hand tremor, abdominal or muscle cramps, diaphoresis, vomiting, and seizures.
! Abrupt withdrawal in patients with epilepsy may produce an increase in the frequency or severity of seizures.
! Overdose results in somnolence, confusion, diminished reflexes, and coma.

NURSING CONSIDERATIONS
Baseline Assessment
• Assess the patient's BP, pulse rate, and respiratory rate, rhythm, and depth immediately before giving diazepam.

• Assess the anxious patient for autonomic responses, including cold, clammy hands and diaphoresis, and motor responses, such as agitation, trembling, and tension.
• For patients being treated for musculoskeletal spasm, record the duration, location, onset, and type of pain, and check for immobility, stiffness, and swelling.
• For patients being treated for seizures, assess LOC and review the history of the seizure disorder, including the duration, frequency, and intensity of seizures. Initiate seizure precautions and observe the patient frequently for a recurrence of seizure activity.

Lifespan Considerations

• Diazepam crosses the placenta and is distributed in breast milk. Diazepam may increase the risk of fetal abnormalities if administered during the first trimester of pregnancy.
• Chronic diazepam use during pregnancy may produce withdrawal symptoms in the patient and CNS depression in the neonate.
• For children and the elderly, expect to administer a reduced dose initially and to increase dosage gradually to prevent ataxia and excessive sedation.

Precautions

• Use diazepam cautiously in patients with hypoalbuminemia or hepatic or renal impairment and in those who are taking other CNS depressants.

Administration and Handling

PO

• Give diazepam without regard to food.
• Crush tablets as needed, but don't crush or break capsules.
• Dilute the oral concentrate with juice, water, or a carbonated beverage or mix it with a semisolid food, such as applesauce or pudding.

IV

• Store unopened vials at room temperature.
• Administer IV push into the tubing of a free-flowing IV solution as close to the vein insertion point as possible.
• Administer directly into a large vein to reduce the risk of phlebitis and thrombosis. Don't use small veins, such as those of the wrist or dorsum of hand.
• Administer IV at a rate not exceeding 5 mg/minute. For children, give over a 3-minute period because a too-rapid IV may result in hypotension and respiratory depression.
• Monitor respirations every 5–15 minutes for 2 hours.
• Keep the patient recumbent for up to 3 hours after parenteral administration to reduce the drug's hypotensive effect.

IM

• Inject the IM dose deep into the deltoid muscle. IM injection may be painful.

Rectal

◂ALERT▸ Don't administer the rectal gel more often than once every 5 days or 5 times a month.

Intervention and Evaluation

• Monitor the patient's BP, heart rate, and respiratory rate.
• Assess pediatric and elderly patients for paradoxical CNS reactions, particularly early in therapy.
• Evaluate the patient for evidence of a therapeutic response; in patients with seizure disorder, a decrease in the frequency or intensity of seizures; in patients with anxiety, a calm facial expression and decreased restlessness; in patients with musculoskeletal spasm, decreased intensity of skeletal muscle pain.
• Monitor the patient's serum drug level. The therapeutic serum level for diazepam is 0.5 to 2 mcg/ml, and the

toxic serum level is greater than 3 mcg/ml.

Patient Teaching

- Caution the patient not to discontinue diazepam abruptly after prolonged use.
- Explain to the patient that diazepam may be habit forming.
- Urge the patient to avoid consuming alcohol and to limit caffeine intake during diazepam therapy.
- Warn the patient to avoid tasks that require mental alertness and motor skills until his or her response to the drug has been established.
- Urge the female patient on long-term therapy to use effective contraception during therapy and to notify the physician immediately if she becomes or may be pregnant.
- Instruct the patient not to take the rectal form of the drug more than once every 5 days or more than 5 times a month.

doxepin hydrochloride

dox-eh-pin
(Deptran[AUS], Novo-Doxepin[CAN], Prudoxin, Sinequan, Zonalon)
Do not confuse doxepin with doxapram, doxazosin, or Doxidan; or Sinequan with saquinavir.

CATEGORY AND SCHEDULE

Pregnancy Risk Category: C (B for topical form)

MECHANISM OF ACTION

A tricyclic antidepressant, antianxiety agent, antineuralgic agent, antipruritic, and antiulcer agent that increases synaptic concentrations of norepinephrine and serotonin. **Therapeutic Effect:** Produces antidepressant and anxiolytic effects.

PHARMACOKINETICS

Rapidly and well absorbed from the GI tract. Protein binding: 80%–85%. Metabolized in the liver to active metabolite. Primarily excreted in urine. Not removed by hemodialysis. ***Half-life:*** 6–8 hr. Topical: Absorbed through the skin. Distributed to body tissues. Metabolized to active metabolite. Excreted in urine.

AVAILABILITY

Capsules (Sinequan): 10 mg, 25 mg, 50 mg, 75 mg, 100 mg, 150 mg.
Oral Concentrate (Sinequan): 10 mg/ml.
Cream (Prudoxin, Zonalon): 5%.

INDICATIONS AND DOSAGES

▸ **Depression, anxiety**

PO

Adults. 30–150 mg/day at bedtime or in 2–3 divided doses. May increase to 300 mg/day.
Elderly. Initially, 10–25 mg at bedtime. May increase by 10–25 mg/day every 3–7 days. Maximum: 75 mg/day.
Adolescents. Initially, 25–50 mg/day as a single dose or in divided doses. May increase to 100 mg/day.
Children 12 yr and younger. 1–3 mg/kg/day.

▸ **Pruritus associated with eczema**

Topical

Adults, Elderly. Apply thin film 4 times a day.

OFF-LABEL USES

Treatment of neurogenic pain, panic disorder; prevention of vascular headache, pruritus in idiopathic urticaria

CONTRAINDICATIONS

Angle-closure glaucoma, hypersensitivity to other tricyclic antidepressants, urine retention

INTERACTIONS

Drug

Alcohol, other CNS depressants: May increase CNS and respiratory depression and the hypotensive effects of doxepin.
Antithyroid agents: May increase the risk of agranulocytosis.
Cimetidine: May increase doxepin blood concentration and risk of toxicity.
Clonidine, guanadrel: May decrease the effects of these drugs.
MAOIs: May increase the risk of seizures, hyperpyrexia, and hypertensive crisis..
Phenothiazines: May increase the anticholinergic and sedative effects of doxepin.
Sympathomimetics: May increase cardiac effects.

Herbal

None known.

Food

None known.

DIAGNOSTIC TEST EFFECTS

May alter blood glucose levels and EKG readings. Therapeutic serum drug level is 110–250 ng/ml; toxic serum drug level is greater than 300 ng/ml.

SIDE EFFECTS

Frequent

Oral: Orthostatic hypotension, somnolence, dry mouth, headache, increased appetite, weight gain, nausea, unusual fatigue, unpleasant taste
Topical: Edema, increased itching, eczema, burning, or stinging at application site; altered taste; dizziness; somnolence; dry skin; dry mouth; fatigue; headache; thirst

Occasional

Oral: Blurred vision, confusion, constipation, hallucinations, difficult urination, eye pain, irregular heartbeat, fine muscle tremors, nervousness, impaired sexual function, diarrhea, diaphoresis, heartburn, insomnia
Topical: Anxiety, skin irritation or cracking, nausea

Rare

Oral: Allergic reaction, alopecia, tinnitus, breast enlargement
Topical: Fever, photosensitivity

SERIOUS REACTIONS

! Overdose may produce confusion; seizures; severe somnolence; fast, slow, or irregular heartbeat; fever; hallucinations; agitation; dyspnea; vomiting; and unusual fatigue or weakness.
! Abrupt withdrawal after prolonged therapy may produce headache, malaise, nausea, vomiting, and vivid dreams.

NURSING CONSIDERATIONS

Baseline Assessment

- Assess the patient's BP and pulse rate.
- Monitor the EKG of patients with a history of cardiovascular disease.

Lifespan Considerations

- Doxepin crosses the placenta and is distributed in breast milk.
- The safety and efficacy of this drug have not been established in children.
- Lower doxepin dosages are recommended for the elderly because they're at increased risk for toxicity.

Precautions

- Use doxepin cautiously in patients with cardiac disease, diabetes mellitus, glaucoma, hiatal hernia, history of seizures, history of urinary obstruction or urine retention, hyperthyroidism, increased intraocular pressure, renal or hepatic disease, benign prostatic hyperplasia or schizophrenia.

Administration and Handling

PO

- Give doxepin with food or milk if GI distress occurs.
- Dilute the oral concentrate in 8 oz fruit juice (such as grapefruit, orange, pineapple, or prune), milk, or water. Avoid diluting in carbonated drinks because they are incompatible with the doxepin.

Intervention and Evaluation

- Monitor the patient's BP, pulse rate, and weight.
- Closely supervise suicidal patients during early therapy. As depression lessens, the patient's energy level generally improves, which increases the suicide potential.
- Assess the patient's appearance, behavior, level of interest, mood, and speech pattern.
- Monitor the patient for therapeutic serum drug levels. The therapeutic serum level for doxepin is 110–250 ng/ml; the toxic serum level is greater than 300 ng/ml.

Patient Teaching

- Inform the patient that he or she may notice an improvement within 2 to 5 days of starting therapy but that the maximum therapeutic effect usually takes 2 to 3 weeks to appear.
- Warn the patient to avoid tasks that require mental alertness and motor skills until his or her response to the drug has been established.
- Warn the patient to change positions slowly, especially early in therapy, to avoid dizziness.
- Urge the patient to avoid alcohol and limit caffeine intake while taking doxepin.
- Inform the patient that doxepin may cause dry mouth and increased appetite.
- Caution the patient to avoid exposure to sunlight or artificial light sources.

hydroxyzine

hye-**drox**-i-zeen

(Apo-Hydroxyzine[CAN], Atarax, Novohydroxyzin[CAN], Vistaril)

Do not confuse hydroxyzine with hydralazine or hydroxyurea.

CATEGORY AND SCHEDULE

Pregnancy Risk Category: C

MECHANISM OF ACTION

A piperazine derivative that competes with histamine for receptor sites in the GI tract, blood vessels, and respiratory tract. May exert CNS depressant activity in subcortical areas. Diminishes vestibular stimulation and depresses labyrinthine function. **Therapeutic Effect:** Produces anxiolytic, anticholinergic, antihistaminic, and analgesic effects; relaxes skeletal muscle; controls nausea and vomiting.

PHARMACOKINETICS

Route	Onset	Peak	Duration
PO	15–30 min	N/A	4–6 hr

Well absorbed from the GI tract and after parenteral administration. Metabolized in the liver. Primarily excreted in urine. Not removed by hemodialysis. ***Half-life:*** 20–25 hr (increased in the elderly).

AVAILABILITY

Capsules (Vistaril): 25 mg, 50 mg, 100 mg.

Oral Suspension (Vistaril): 25 mg/5 ml.
Syrup (Atarax): 10 mg/5 ml.
Tablets (Atarax): 10 mg, 25 mg, 50 mg, 100 mg.
Injection (Vistaril): 25 mg/ml, 50 mg/ml.

INDICATIONS AND DOSAGES

▸ Anxiety
PO
Adults, Elderly. 25–100 mg 4 times a day. Maximum: 600 mg/day.

▸ Nausea and vomiting
IM
Adults, Elderly. 25–100 mg/dose q4–6h.

▸ Pruritus
PO
Adults, Elderly. 25 mg 3–4 times a day.

▸ Preoperative sedation
PO
Adults, Elderly. 50–100 mg.
IM
Adults, Elderly. 25–100 mg.

▸ Usual pediatric dosage
PO
Children. 2 mg/kg/day in divided doses q6–8h.
IM
Children. 0.5–1 mg/kg/dose q4–6h.

CONTRAINDICATIONS

None known.

INTERACTIONS

Drug

Alcohol, other CNS depressants: May increase CNS depressant effects.
MAOIs: May increase anticholinergic and CNS depressant effects.

Herbal

None known.

Food

None known.

DIAGNOSTIC TEST EFFECTS

May cause false-positive urine 17-hydroxycorticosteroid determinations.

SIDE EFFECTS

Side effects are generally mild and transient.

Frequent

Somnolence, dry mouth, marked discomfort with IM injection

Occasional

Dizziness, ataxia, asthenia, slurred speech, headache, agitation, increased anxiety

Rare

Paradoxical CNS reactions, such as hyperactivity or nervousness in children and excitement or restlessness in elderly or debilitated patients (generally noted during first 2 weeks of therapy, particularly in presence of uncontrolled pain)

SERIOUS REACTIONS

! A hypersensitivity reaction, including wheezing, dyspnea, and chest tightness, may occur.

NURSING CONSIDERATIONS

Baseline Assessment

• Assess the anxious patient for autonomic responses, including cold or clammy hands and diaphoresis, and motor responses, such as agitation, trembling, and tension.
• Assess the patient with severe vomiting for signs and symptoms of dehydration, including dry mucous membranes, longitudinal furrows in the tongue, and poor skin turgor.

Lifespan Considerations

• It is unknown if hydroxyzine crosses the placenta or is distributed in breast milk.
• Hydroxyzine use is not recommended for neonates or premature

infants because they're at increased risk for anticholinergic effects.
• Children may experience paradoxical excitement.
• Elderly patients are at increased risk for confusion, dizziness, sedation, hypotension, and hyperexcitability.

Precautions
• Use hydroxyzine cautiously in patients with asthma, bladder neck obstruction, COPD, angle-closure glaucoma, or benign prostatic hyperplasia.

Administration and Handling
PO
• Crush scored tablets as needed, but don't crush or break capsules.
• Shake the oral suspension thoroughly.
IM
◀ALERT▶ Don't give hydroxyzine by the subcutaneous, intra-arterial, or IV route because doing so can cause significant tissue damage, thrombosis, and gangrene.
• The IM form may be given undiluted.
• Inject the drug deep into the gluteus maximus or midlateral thigh in adults and the midlateral thigh in children. Use the Z-track technique of injection to prevent subcutaneous infiltration.

Intervention and Evaluation
• Plan to perform CBC and blood chemistry tests periodically for patients on long-term therapy.
• Monitor the patient's breath sounds for signs of a hypersensitivity reaction, such as wheezing.
• Monitor serum electrolyte levels in patients with severe vomiting.
• Assess the patient for paradoxical CNS reactions, particularly early in therapy.
• Assist the patient with ambulation if he or she experiences drowsiness or dizziness.
• Offer emotional support to the anxious patient.

Patient Teaching
• Inform the patient that IM injection may cause marked discomfort.
• Tell the patient that drowsiness usually diminishes with continued therapy.
• Warn the patient to avoid tasks that require mental alertness and motor skills until his or her response to the drug has been established.
• Recommend taking sips of tepid water and chewing sugarless gum to help relieve dry mouth.

lorazepam
lor-**a**-ze-pam
(Apo-Lorazepam[CAN], Ativan, Lorazepam Intensol, Novolorazepam[CAN])
Do not confuse lorazepam with Alprazolam.

CATEGORY AND SCHEDULE
Pregnancy Risk Category: D
Controlled Substance: Schedule IV

MECHANISM OF ACTION
A benzodiazepine that enhances the action of the inhibitory neurotransmitter gamma-aminobutyric acid in the CNS, affecting memory, as well as motor, sensory, and cognitive function. **Therapeutic Effect:** Produces anxiolytic, anticonvulsant, sedative, muscle relaxant, and antiemetic effects.

PHARMACOKINETICS

Route	Onset	Peak	Duration
PO	60 min	N/A	8–12 hr
IV	15–30 min	N/A	8–12 hr
IM	30–60 min	N/A	8–12 hr

Well absorbed after PO and IM administration. Protein binding: 85%. Widely distributed. Metabolized in the liver. Primarily excreted in urine. Not removed by hemodialysis. ***Half-life:*** 10–20 hr.

AVAILABILITY

Tablets (Ativan): 0.5 mg, 1 mg, 2 mg.
Injection (Ativan): 2 mg/ml, 4 mg/ml.
Oral solution (Lorazepam Intensol): 2 mg/ml.

INDICATIONS AND DOSAGES

▸ **Anxiety**
PO
Adults. 1–10 mg/day in 2–3 divided doses. Average: 2–6 mg/day.
Elderly. Initially, 0.5–1 mg/day. May increase gradually. Range: 0.5–4 mg.
IV
Adults, Elderly. 0.02–0.06 mg/kg q2–6h.
IV Infusion
Adults, Elderly. 0.01–0.1 mg/kg/h.
PO, IV
Children. 0.05 mg/kg/dose q4–8h. Range: 0.02–0.1 mg/kg. Maximum: 2 mg/dose.

▸ **Insomnia due to anxiety**
PO
Adults. 2–4 mg at bedtime.
Elderly. 0.5–1 mg at bedtime.

▸ **Preoperative sedation**
IV
Adults, Elderly. 0.044 mg/kg 15–20 min before surgery. Maximum total dose: 2 mg.
IM
Adults, Elderly. 0.05 mg/kg 2 hr before procedure. Maximum total dose: 4 mg.

▸ **Status epilepticus**
IV
Adults, Elderly. 4 mg over 2–5 min. May repeat in 10–15 min. Maximum: 8 mg in 12-hr period.
Children. 0.1 mg/kg over 2–5 min. May give second dose of 0.05 mg/kg in 15–20 min. Maximum: 4 mg.
Neonates. 0.05 mg/kg. May repeat in 10–15 min.

OFF-LABEL USES

Treatment of alcohol withdrawal, panic disorders, skeletal muscle spasms, chemotherapy-induced nausea or vomiting, tension headache, tremors; adjunctive treatment before endoscopic procedures (diminishes patient recall)

CONTRAINDICATIONS

Angle-closure glaucoma; preexisting CNS depression; severe hypotension; severe uncontrolled pain

INTERACTIONS

Drug

Alcohol, other CNS depressants: May increase CNS depression.

Herbal

Kava kava, valerian: May increase CNS depression.

Food

None known.

DIAGNOSTIC TEST EFFECTS

None known. Therapeutic serum drug level is 50–240 ng/ml; toxic serum drug level is unknown.

IV INCOMPATIBILITIES

Aldesleukin (Proleukin), aztreonam (Azactam), idarubicin (Idamycin), ondansetron (Zofran), sufentanil (Sufenta)

IV COMPATIBILITIES

Bumetanide (Bumex), cefepime (Maxipime), diltiazem (Cardizem), dobutamine (Dobutrex), dopamine (Intropin), heparin, labetalol (Normodyne, Trandate), milrinone (Primacor), norepinephrine (Levophed), piperacillin and tazobactam (Zosyn), potassium, propofol (Diprivan)

SIDE EFFECTS

Frequent

Somnolence (initially in the morning), ataxia, confusion

Occasional

Blurred vision, slurred speech, hypotension, headache

Rare

Paradoxical CNS restlessness or excitement in elderly or debilitated

SERIOUS REACTIONS

! Abrupt or too-rapid withdrawal may result in pronounced restlessness, irritability, insomnia, hand tremor, abdominal or muscle cramps, diaphoresis, vomiting, and seizures.

! Overdose results in somnolence, confusion, diminished reflexes, and coma.

NURSING CONSIDERATIONS

Baseline Assessment

• Assess the patient for autonomic responses, such as cold and clammy hands and diaphoresis and motor responses, such as agitation, trembling, and tension.

Lifespan Considerations

• Lorazepam may cross the placenta and be distributed in breast milk.

• Lorazepam may increase the risk of fetal abnormalities if administered during the first trimester of pregnancy.

• Chronic lorazepam use during pregnancy may produce withdrawal symptoms in the patient and CNS depression in the neonate.

• The safety and efficacy of this drug have not been established in children younger than 12 years.

• In the elderly, expect to give small doses initially and to increase dosage gradually to avoid ataxia and excessive sedation.

Precautions

• Use lorazepam cautiously in neonates; in patients with pulmonary, hepatic, or renal impairment; and in those using other CNS depressants concurrently.

Administration and Handling

PO

• Give lorazepam with food.

• Crush tablets as needed.

IV

• Refrigerate—don't freeze—parenteral form.

• Don't use the solution it it appears discolored or contains a precipitate.

• Dilute with an equal volume of sterile water for injection, 0.9% NaCl, or D_5W. To dilute a prefilled syringe, remove air from a half-filled syringe, aspirate an equal volume of diluent, pull the plunger back slightly to allow for mixing, and gently invert the syringe several times—don't shake vigorously.

• Give by IV push into the tubing of a free-flowing IV infusion of 0.9% NaCl or D_5W at a rate not exceeding 2 mg/minute.

• Keep the patient recumbent for up to 8 hours after parenteral administration to reduce the drug's hypotensive effect.

IM

• Inject the drug deep into a large muscle mass, such as gluteus maximus.

Intervention and Evaluation

• Monitor the patient's BP, heart rate, respiratory rate, CBC with differential, and hepatic function. For those on long-term therapy, expect blood chemistry studies and hepatic and renal function tests to be performed periodically.

• Assess the patient for paradoxical

CNS reactions, particularly early in therapy.
- Evaluate the patient for a therapeutic response, such as a calm facial expression, and decreased restlessness and insomnia.
- Monitor the patient's serum drug level. The therapeutic serum level for lorazepam is 50–240 ng/ml; the toxic serum level is unknown.
- Offer emotional support to the anxious patient.

Patient Teaching
- Caution the patient not to stop taking lorazepam abruptly after long-term therapy.
- Inform the patient that drowsiness usually disappears with continued therapy.
- Warn the patient to avoid tasks that require mental alertness or motor skills until his or her response to the drug has been established.
- Urge the patient to avoid smoking, drinking alcoholic beverages, and taking other CNS depressants. Explain that smoking reduces the effectiveness of lorazepam, and alcohol and CNS depressants increase sedation.
- Urge the female patient on long-term therapy to use effective contraception during therapy and to notify the physician immediately if she becomes or may be pregnant.

midazolam hydrochloride

mid-**az**-zoe-lam
(Apo-Midazolam[CAN], Hypnovel[AUS], Versed)
Do not confuse Versed with VePesid.

CATEGORY AND SCHEDULE
Pregnancy Risk Category: D
Controlled Substance: Schedule IV

MECHANISM OF ACTION
A benzodiazepine that enhances the action of gamma-aminobutyric acid, one of the major inhibitory neurotransmitters in the brain.
Therapeutic Effect: Produces anxiolytic, hypnotic, anticonvulsant, muscle relaxant, and amnestic effects.

PHARMACOKINETICS

Route	Onset	Peak	Duration
PO	10–20 min	N/A	N/A
IV	1–5 min	5–7 min	20–30 min
IM	5–15 min	15–60 min	2–6 hr

Well absorbed after IM administration. Protein binding: 97%. Metabolized in the liver to active metabolite. Primarily excreted in urine. Not removed by hemodialysis. ***Half-life:*** 1–5 hr.

AVAILABILITY
Syrup: 2 mg/ml.
Injection: 1 mg/ml, 5 mg/ml.

INDICATIONS AND DOSAGES
▸ **Preoperative sedation**
PO
Children. 0.25–0.5 mg/kg. Maximum: 20 mg.

IV
Children 6–12 yr. 0.025–0.05 mg/kg.
Children 6 mo–5 yr. 0.05–0.1 mg/kg.
IM
Adults, Elderly. 0.07–0.08 mg/kg 30–60 min before surgery.
Children. 0.1–0.15 mg/kg 30–60 min before surgery. Maximum: 10 mg.

▸ Conscious sedation for diagnostic, therapeutic, and endoscopic procedures
IV
Adults, Elderly. 1–2.5 mg over 2 min. Titrate as needed. Maximum total dose: 2.5–5 mg.

▸ Conscious sedation during mechanical ventilation
IV
Adults, Elderly. 0.01–0.05 mg/kg; may repeat q10–15min until adequately sedated. Then continuous infusion at initial rate of 0.02–0.1 mg/kg/hr (1–7 mg/hr).
Children older than 32 wk. Initially, 1 mcg/kg/min as continuous infusion.
Children 32 wk and younger. Initially, 0.5 mcg/kg/min as continuous infusion.

▸ Status epilepticus
IV
Children older than 2 mo. Loading dose of 0.15 mg/kg followed by continuous infusion of 1 mcg/kg/min. Titrate as needed. Range: 1–18 mcg/kg/min.

CONTRAINDICATIONS

Acute alcohol intoxication, acute angle-closure glaucoma, coma, shock

INTERACTIONS

Drug

Alcohol, other CNS depressants: May increase CNS and respiratory depression and hypotensive effects of midazolam.
Hypotension-producing medications: May increase hypotensive effects of midazolam.

Herbal

Kava kava, valerian: May increase CNS depression.

Food

Grapefruit, grapefruit juice: Increases the oral absorption and systemic availability of midazolam.

DIAGNOSTIC TEST EFFECTS

None known.

IV INCOMPATIBILITIES

Albumin, ampicillin and sulbactam (Unasyn), amphotericin B complex (Abelcet, AmBisome, Amphotec), ampicillin (Polycillin), bumetanide (Bumex), co-trimoxazole (Bactrim), dexamethasone (Decadron), fosphenytoin (Cerebyx), furosemide (Lasix), hydrocortisone (Solu-Cortef), methotrexate, nafcillin (Nafcil), sodium bicarbonate, sodium pentothal (Thiopental)

IV COMPATIBILITIES

Amiodarone (Cordarone), atropine, calcium gluconate, diltiazem (Cardizem), diphenhydramine (Benadryl), dobutamine (Dobutrex), dopamine (Intropin), etomidate (Amidate), fentanyl (Sublimaze), glycopyrrolate (Robinul), heparin, hydromorphone (Dilaudid), hydroxyzine (Vistaril), insulin, lorazepam (Ativan), milrinone (Primacor), morphine, nitroglycerin, norepinephrine (Levophed), potassium chloride, propofol (Diprivan)

SIDE EFFECTS

Frequent (10%–4%)

Decreased respiratory rate, tenderness at IM or IV injection site, pain during injection, oxygen desaturation, hiccups

Occasional (3%–2%)
Hypotension, paradoxical CNS reaction
Rare (less than 2%)
Nausea, vomiting, headache, coughing

SERIOUS REACTIONS

! Inadequate or excessive dosage or improper administration may result in cerebral hypoxia, agitation, involuntary movements, hyperactivity, and combativeness.
! A too-rapid IV rate, excessive doses, or a single large dose increases the risk of respiratory depression or arrest.
! Respiratory depression or apnea may produce hypoxia and cardiac arrest.

NURSING CONSIDERATIONS

Baseline Assessment

• Obtain the patient's vital signs before administering midazolam.

Lifespan Considerations

• Midazolam crosses the placenta; it is unknown if midazolam is distributed in breast milk.
• Neonates are more likely to experience respiratory depression.
• In the elderly, age-related renal impairment may require dosage adjustment.

Precautions

• Use midazolam cautiously in patients with acute illness; CHF; pulmonary, renal, or hepatic impairment; severe fluid or electrolyte imbalance; and treated angle-closure glaucoma.

Administration and Handling

◀ALERT▶ Midazolam dosage is individualized based on the patient's age, underlying disease, and medications and on the desired effect.
IV
• Store vials at room temperature.
• Midazolam may be given undiluted or as an infusion.
• Ensure that resuscitative supplies, such as endotracheal tubes, suction equipment, and oxygen, are readily available.
• Administer the drug by slow IV injection in incremental doses. Give each incremental dose over 2 minutes or more and wait at least 2 minutes between doses.
• Reduce the IV rate in patients older than 60 years, debilitated patients, and those with chronic diseases or impaired pulmonary function.
• A too-rapid IV rate, excessive doses, or a single large dose increases the risk of respiratory depression or arrest.
IM
• Inject the drug deep into a large muscle mass, such as the gluteus maximus.

Intervention and Evaluation

• Monitor the patient's respiratory rate and oxygen saturation continuously during parenteral administration to detect apnea and respiratory depression.
• Monitor the patient's level of sedation every 3 to 5 minutes, and assess vital signs during the recovery period.

Patient Teaching

• Inform the patient before the procedure that midazolam produces an amnesic effect.
• Urge the female patient on long-term therapy to use effective contraception during therapy and to notify the physician immediately if she becomes or may be pregnant.

oxazepam

ox-**a**-ze-pam
(Alepam[AUS], Apo-Oxazepam[CAN], Murelax[AUS], Serax, Serepax[AUS])
Do not confuse oxazepam with oxaprozin, or Serax with Eurax or Xerac.

CATEGORY AND SCHEDULE

Pregnancy Risk Category: D
Controlled Substance: Schedule IV

MECHANISM OF ACTION

A benzodiazepine that potentiates the effects of gamma-aminobutyric acid and other inhibitory neurotransmitters by binding to specific receptors in the CNS. **Therapeutic Effect:** Produces anxiolytic effect and skeletal muscle relaxation.

PHARMACOKINETICS

Well absorbed from the GI tract. Protein binding: 97%. Metabolized in the liver. Primarily excreted in urine. Not removed by hemodialysis. ***Half-life:*** 5–20 hr.

AVAILABILITY

Capsules: 10 mg, 15 mg, 30 mg.
Tablet: 15 mg.

INDICATIONS AND DOSAGES

▸ **Mild to moderate anxiety**

PO

Adults. 10–15 mg 3–4 times a day.

▸ **Severe anxiety**

PO

Adults. 15–30 mg 3–4 times a day.

▸ **Alcohol withdrawal**

PO

Adults. 15–30 mg 3–4 times a day.
Elderly. Initially, 10–20 mg 3 times a day. May gradually increase up to 30–45 mg/day.

CONTRAINDICATIONS

Angle-closure glaucoma; preexisting CNS depression; severe, uncontrolled pain

INTERACTIONS

Drug

Alcohol, other CNS depressants: May potentiate CNS depression.

Herbal

Kava kava, valerian: May increase CNS depression.

Food

None known.

DIAGNOSTIC TEST EFFECTS

May elevate serum alkaline phosphatase, bilirubin, LDH, AST (SGOT), and ALT (SGPT) levels. May produce abnormal renal function test results. Therapeutic serum drug level is 0.2–1.4 mcg/ml; toxic serum drug level has not been established.

SIDE EFFECTS

Frequent

Mild, transient somnolence at beginning of therapy

Occasional

Dizziness, headache

Rare

Paradoxical CNS reactions, such as hyperactivity or nervousness in children and excitement or restlessness in the elderly or debilitated (generally noted during the first 2 weeks of therapy)

SERIOUS REACTIONS

! Abrupt or too-rapid withdrawal may result in pronounced restlessness, irritability, insomnia, hand tremor, abdominal or muscle cramps, diaphoresis, vomiting, and seizures.

! Overdose results in somnolence, confusion, diminished reflexes, and coma.

NURSING CONSIDERATIONS

Baseline Assessment

• Assess the patient for autonomic responses, such as cold or clammy hands and diaphoresis, and motor responses, such as agitation, trembling, and tension.

Precautions

• Use oxazepam cautiously in patients with a history of drug dependence.

Administration and Handling

◀ **ALERT** ▶ Plan to use the smallest effective dose in elderly or debilitated patients and in those with hepatic disease or a low serum albumin level.

Intervention and Evaluation

• Monitor the patient's CBC and blood chemistry studies periodically to assess hepatic and renal function, especially during long-term therapy.
• Assess the patient for paradoxical CNS reactions, particularly early in therapy.
• Assist the patient with ambulation if he or she experiences drowsiness or dizziness.
• Evaluate the patient for evidence of a therapeutic response, such as a calm facial expression and decreased restlessness and diminished insomnia.
• Monitor the patient's serum drug levels. The therapeutic serum level for oxazepam is 0.2-1.4 mcg/ml; the toxic serum level is not established.
• Offer emotional support to the anxious patient.

Patient Teaching

• Caution the patient not to stop taking oxazepam abruptly after long-term use.
• Urge the patient to avoid alcohol and other CNS depressants while taking oxazepam.
• Inform the patient that oxazepam may cause drowsiness. Advise the patient to avoid tasks requiring mental alertness or motor skills until his or her response to the drug has been established.
• Urge the female patient on long-term therapy to use effective contraception during therapy and to notify the physician immediately if she becomes or may be pregnant.

33 Anticonvulsants

carbamazepine
clonazepam
clorazepate dipotassium
diazepam
fosphenytoin
gabapentin
lamotrigine
levetiracetam
oxcarbazepine
phenobarbital
phenytoin
primidone
tiagabine
topiramate
valproic acid, valproate sodium, divalproex sodium
zonisamide

Uses: Anticonvulsants are used to treat seizure disorders. Seizures can be divided into two broad categories: partial seizures and generalized seizures. Partial seizures begin focally in the cerebral cortex and spread to limited areas. Simple partial seizures don't involve loss of consciousness (unless they evolve into generalized seizures) and typically last less than 1 minute. Complex partial seizures involve an alteration in consciousness and usually last longer than 1 minute. Generalized seizures may be convulsive or nonconvulsive and usually produce immediate loss of consciousness.

Action: Anticonvulsants can prevent or reduce excessive discharge by neurons with seizure foci or decrease the spread of excitation from neurons with seizure foci to normal neurons. Although their exact mechanism of action is unknown, these agents may act by suppressing sodium influx, suppressing calcium influx, or increasing the action of gamma-aminobutyric acid (GABA), which inhibits neurotransmitters in the brain. (See the illustration *Mechanism of Action: Phenytoin,* page 657.)

COMBINATION PRODUCTS

BELLERGAL-S: phenobarbital/ergotamine (an antimigraine)/belladonna (an anticholinergic) 40 mg/0.6 mg/0.2 mg.
DONNATAL: phenobarbital/atropine (an anticholinergic)/hyoscyamine (an anticholinergic)/scopolamine (an anticholinergic) 16.2 mg/0.0194 mg/0.1037 mg/0.0065 mg.
DILANTIN WITH PB: phenytoin/phenobarbital 100 mg/15 mg; 100 mg/30 mg.
CLORAZEPATE (TRANXENE): See antianxiety agents
DIAZEPAM: See antianxiety agents

carbamazepine

kar-ba-**maz**-e-peen
(Apo-Carbamazepine[CAN], Carbatrol, Epitol, Equetro, Tegretol, Tegretol CR[AUS], Tegretol XR, Teril[AUS])
Do not confuse Tegretol with Cartrol, Toradol, or Trental.

CATEGORY AND SCHEDULE

Pregnancy Risk Category: D

MECHANISM OF ACTION

An iminostilbene derivative that decreases sodium and calcium ion influx into neuronal membranes, reducing post-tetanic potentiation at

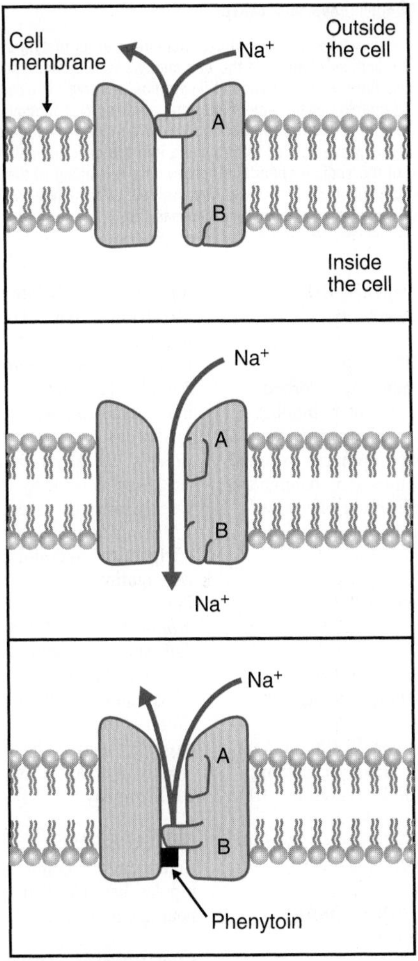

Mechanism of Action: Phenytoin

Phenytoin, which is used to treat tonic-clonic seizures, acts in the motor cortex and brain stem where the tonic phase of tonic-clonic seizures originates. By altering sodium transport across neuronal cel membranes, phenytoin stabilizes the cell membrane, reduces repetitive firing of the neurons, and halts or limits the spread of seizures.

Continued

Mechanism of Action: Phenytoin, cont'd

The first illustration shows a neuronal cell membrane in its resting state. The activation gate (A) of the sodium channel in the cell membrane is closed and blocks sodium (Na^+) from entering the cell. In the second illustration, a nerve impulse has caused depolarization and opening of the activation gate, allowing Na^+ to move into the cell. In the third illustration, depolarization continues and an inactivation gate (B) moves into the channel. This prevents Na^+ from moving into the cell. Phenytoin prolongs the inactivated state of the sodium channel by preventing reopening of the inactivation gate. By further preventing Na^+ from entering the cell, phenytoin slows impulse transmission, and thus slows the rate at which neurons fire.

---

synapses. **Therapeutic Effect:** Reduces seizure activity.

PHARMACOKINETICS

Slowly and completely absorbed from the GI tract. Protein binding: 75%. Metabolized in the liver to active metabolite. Primarily excreted in urine. Not removed by hemodialysis. ***Half-life:*** 25–65 hr (decreased with chronic use).

AVAILABILITY

Capsules (Extended-Release [Carbatrol]): 100 mg, 200 mg, 400 mg.
Capsules (Extended-Release [Equetro]): 100 mg, 200 mg, 300 mg.
Suspension (Tegretol): 100 mg/5 ml.
Tablets (Epitol, Tegretol): 200 mg.
Tablets (Chewable [Tegretol]): 100 mg.
Tablets (Extended-Release [Tegretol XR]): 100 mg, 200 mg, 400 mg.

INDICATIONS AND DOSAGES

▸ **Seizure control**

PO

Adults, Children older than 12 yr. Initially, 200 mg twice a day. May increase dosage by 200 mg/day at weekly intervals. Range: 400–1,200 mg/day in 2–4 divided doses. Maximum: 1.6–2.4 g/day.
Children 6–12 yr. Initially, 100 mg twice a day. May increase by 100 mg/day at weekly intervals. Range: 20–30 mg/kg/day. Maxiumum: 1,000 mg/day.
Children younger than 6 yr. Initially 5 mg/kg/day. May increase at weekly intervals to 10 mg/kg/day up to 20 mg/kg/day.
Elderly. Initially 100 mg 1–2 times a day. May increase by 100 mg/day at weekly intervals. Usual dose 400–1,000 mg/day.

▸ **Trigeminal neuralgia, diabetic neuropathy**

PO

Adults. Initially, 100 mg twice a day. May increase by 100 mg twice a day up to 400–800 mg/day. Maxiumum: 1,200 mg/day.
Elderly. Initially 100 mg 1–2 times a day. May increase by 100 mg/day at weekly intervals. Usual dose 400–1,000 mg/day.

OFF-LABEL USES

Treatment of alcohol withdrawal, bipolar disorder, diabetes insipidus, neurogenic pain, psychotic disorders

CONTRAINDICATIONS

Concomitant use of MAOIs, history of myelosuppression, hypersensitivity to tricyclic antidepressants

INTERACTIONS

Drug

Anticoagulants, clarithromycin, diltiazem, erythromycin, estrogens, propoxyphene, quinidine, steroids: May decrease the effects of these drugs.
Antipsychotics, haloperidol, tricyclic antidepressants: May increase CNS depressant effects.
Cimetidine: May increase carbamazepine blood concentration and risk of toxicity.
Isoniazid: May increase metabolism of isoniazid; may increase carbamazepine blood concentration and risk of toxicity.
MAOIs: May cause seizures and hypertensive crisis.
Other anticonvulsants, barbiturates, benzodiazepines, valproic acid: May increase the metabolism of these drugs.
Verapamil: May increase the toxicity of carbamazepine.

Herbal

None known.

Food

Grapefruit, grapefruit juice: May increase the absorption and blood concentration of carbamazepine.

DIAGNOSTIC TEST EFFECTS

May increase BUN and blood glucose levels and serum alkaline phosphatase, bilirubin, AST (SGOT), ALT (SGPT), protein, cholesterol, HDL, and triglyceride levels. May decrease serum calcium and thyroid hormone (T_3, T_4, T_4 index) levels. Therapeutic serum level is 4–12 mcg/ml; toxic serum level is greater than 12 mcg/ml.

SIDE EFFECTS

Frequent

Drowsiness, dizziness, nausea, vomiting

Occasional

Visual abnormalities (spots before eyes, difficulty focusing, blurred vision), dry mouth or pharynx, tongue irritation, headache, fluid retention, diaphoresis, constipation or diarrhea, behavioral changes in children

SERIOUS REACTIONS

! Toxic reactions may include blood dyscrasias (such as aplastic anemia, agranulocytosis, thrombocytopenia, leukopenia, leukocytosis, and eosinophilia), cardiovascular disturbances (such as CHF, hypotension or hypertension, thrombophlebitis and arrhythmias), and dermatologic effects (such as rash, urticaria, pruritus, and photosensitivity).
! Abrupt withdrawal may precipitate status epilepticus.

NURSING CONSIDERATIONS

Baseline Assessment

• Assess the patient's LOC and review the history of the seizure disorder, including the duration, frequency, and intensity of seizures. Initiate seizure precautions.
• Expect to obtain BUN level, CBC, serum iron determination, and urinalysis before and periodically during carbamazepine therapy.

Lifespan Considerations

• Be aware that carbamazepine crosses the placenta and accumulates in fetal tissue. It is also distributed in breast milk.
• Children are more likely than adults to develop behavioral changes.
• The elderly are more susceptible to agitation, AV block, bradycardia, confusion, and syndrome of inappropriate antidiuretic hormone secretion.

Precautions

• Use carbamazepine cautiously in patients with impaired cardiac, hepatic, or renal function.

Administration and Handling

◀ALERT▶ If the patient must change to another anticonvulsant, plan to decrease the carbamazepine dose gradually as therapy begins with a low dose of the replacement drug. When transferring from tablets to suspension, expect to divide the total daily tablet dose into smaller, more frequent doses of suspension. Also plan to administer extended-release tablets in 2 divided doses.

PO

• Store the tablets, capsules, and oral suspension at room temperature.
• Give carbamazepine with meals to reduce the risk of GI distress.
• Shake the oral suspension well. Don't administer it simultaneously with any other liquid medicine.
• Don't crush extended-release tablets.

Intervention and Evaluation

• Provide the patient with a quiet, dark environment and institute safety precautions.
• Observe the seizure patient frequently for recurrence of seizure activity.
• Monitor the patient for therapeutic serum levels of carbamazepine (4–12 mcg/ml).
• Assess the seizure patient for evidence of clinical improvement, such as a decrease in the frequency and intensity of seizures.
• Assess the patient for early signs of toxicity, such as ecchymosis, fever, joint pain, mouth ulcerations, sore throat, and unusual bleeding from any site.
• Encourage the neuralgia patient to avoid anything that could trigger tic douloureux, such as cold or hot foods or liquids, and jarring bed.

Patient Teaching

• Instruct the patient not to take the oral suspension of carbamazepine simultaneously with other liquid medicines.
• Caution the patient not to take the drug with grapefruit juice because this juice may increase drug's blood concentration.
• Caution the patient against abruptly discontinuing carbamazepine after long-term use because this may precipitate seizures. Explain that strict maintenance of drug therapy is essential for seizure control.
• Inform the patient that drowsiness usually disappears with continued therapy.
• Caution the patient to avoid tasks that require mental alertness or motor skills until his or her response to the drug is established.
• Instruct the patient to notify the physician if he or she experiences visual disturbances.
• Inform the patient that blood tests will be repeated frequently during the first 3 months of therapy and monthly thereafter for 2 to 3 years.
• Advise the patient to always carry an identification card or wear an identification bracelet that displays his or her seizure disorder and anticonvulsant therapy.

clonazepam

kloe-**na**-zi-pam

(Apo-Clonazepam[CAN], Clonapam[CAN], Klonopin, Paxam[AUS], Rivotril[CAN])

Do not confuse clonazepam with clonidine or lorazepam.

CATEGORY AND SCHEDULE

Pregnancy Risk Category: D

MECHANISM OF ACTION

A benzodiazepine that depresses all levels of the CNS; inhibits nerve impulse transmission in the motor cortex and suppresses abnormal discharge in petit mal seizures. **Therapeutic Effect:** Produces anxiolytic and anticonvulsant effects.

PHARMACOKINETICS

Well absorbed from the GI tract. Protein binding: 85%. Metabolized in the liver. Excreted in urine. Not removed by hemodialysis. ***Half-life:*** 18–50 hr.

AVAILABILITY

Tablets: 0.5 mg, 1 mg, 2 mg.
Tablets (Disintegrating): 0.125 mg, 0.25 mg, 0.5 mg, 1 mg, 2 mg.

INDICATIONS AND DOSAGES

▸ **Adjunctive treatment of Lennox-Gastaut syndrome (petit mal variant) and akinetic, myoclonic, and absence (petit mal) seizures**

PO

Adults, Elderly, Children 10 yr and older. 1.5 mg/day; may be increased in 0.5- to 1-mg increments every 3 days until seizures are controlled. Don't exceed maintenance dosage of 20 mg/day.

Infants, Children younger than 10 yr or weighing less than 30 kg. 0.01–0.03 mg/kg/day in 2–3 divided doses; may be increased by up to 0.5 mg every 3 days until seizures are controlled. Don't exceed maintenance dosage of 0.2 mg/kg/day.

▸ **Panic disorder**

PO

Adults, Elderly. Initially, 0.25 mg twice a day; increased in increments of 0.125–0.25 mg twice a day every 3 days. Maximum: 4 mg/day.

OFF-LABEL USES

Adjunctive treatment of seizures; treatment of simple, complex partial, and tonic-clonic seizures

CONTRAINDICATIONS

Narrow-angle glaucoma, significant hepatic disease

INTERACTIONS

Drug

Alcohol, other CNS depressants: May increase CNS depressant effect.

Herbal

Kava kava: May increase sedation.

Food

None known.

DIAGNOSTIC TEST EFFECTS

None known.

SIDE EFFECTS

Frequent

Mild, transient drowsiness; ataxia; behavioral disturbances (aggression, irritability, agitation), especially in children

Occasional

Rash, ankle or facial edema, nocturia, dysuria, change in appetite or weight, dry mouth, sore gums, nausea, blurred vision

Rare

Paradoxical CNS reactions, including hyperactivity or nervousness in children and excitement or restlessness in the elderly (particularly in the presence of uncontrolled pain).

SERIOUS REACTIONS

! Abrupt withdrawal may result in pronounced restlessness, irritability, insomnia, hand tremors, abdominal or muscle cramps, diaphoresis, vomiting, and status epilepticus.

! Overdose results in somnolence, confusion, diminished reflexes, and coma.

NURSING CONSIDERATIONS

Baseline Assessment

- Assess the seizure patient's LOC, and review the history of the seizure disorder, including the duration, frequency, and intensity of seizures. Initiate seizure precautions.
- Assess the panic disorder patient for autonomic responses, such as cold or clammy hands and diaphoresis, and motor responses, such as agitation, trembling, and tension.

Lifespan Considerations

- Clonazepam crosses the placenta and may be distributed in breast milk.
- Chronic clonazepam use during pregnancy may produce withdrawal symptoms and CNS depression in neonates.
- Long-term clonazepam use may adversely affect the mental and physical development of children.
- Elderly patients are usually more sensitive to clonazepam's CNS effects, such as ataxia, dizziness, and oversedation. Expect to give them a lower dosage and increase it gradually.

Precautions

- Use clonazepam cautiously in patients with chronic respiratory disease or impaired renal or hepatic function.

Administration and Handling

◀ALERT▶ If the patient must switch to another anticonvulsant, expect to decrease the clonazepam dose gradually as therapy begins with a low dose of the replacement drug.

PO

- Give clonazepam without regard to meals.
- Crush tablets as needed.

Intervention and Evaluation

- Assess pediatric and elderly patients for paradoxical CNS reactions, particularly early in therapy.
- Observe seizure pateints frequently for a recurrence of seizure activity and implement safety measures.
- Assist the patient with ambulation if he or she experiences ataxia or drowsiness.
- For patients on long-term clonazepam therapy, obtain CBC and blood chemistry tests periodically to assess hepatic and renal function.
- Evaluate the patient for evidence of a therapeutic response to the drug, such as a decrease in the frequency or intensity of seizures in seizure patients and a calm facial expression and decreased restlessness in patients with panic disorder.

Patient Teaching

- Caution the patient against abruptly stopping clonazepam after long-term therapy.
- Explain that strict maintenance of drug therapy is essential for seizure control.
- Inform the patient that drowsiness usually diminishes with continued therapy.
- Warn the patient to avoid tasks that require mental alertness or motor skills until his or her response to the drug is established.
- Urge the patient to stop smoking and to avoid alcohol. Explain that smoking reduces the drug's effectiveness and alcohol increases sedation.
- Advise the patient to always carry an identification card or wear an identification bracelet that displays his or her seizure disorder and anticonvulsant therapy.

---

clorazepate dipotassium (Tranxene)

See Antianxiety Agents

diazepam (Valium)
See Antianxiety Agents

fosphenytoin
fos-**phen**-ih-toyn
(Cerebyx)
Do not confuse Cerebyx with Celebrex or Celexa.

CATEGORY AND SCHEDULE
Pregnancy Risk Category: D

MECHANISM OF ACTION
A hydantoin anticonvulsant that stabilizes neuronal membranes by decreasing sodium and calcium ion influx into the neurons. Also decreases post-tetanic potentiation and repetitive discharge. **Therapeutic Effect:** Decreases seizure activity.

PHARMACOKINETICS
Completely absorbed after IM administration. Protein binding: 95%–99%. Rapidly and completely hydrolyzed to phenytoin after IM or IV administration. Time of complete conversion to phenytoin: 4 hr after IM injection; 2 hr after IV infusion. ***Half-life:*** 8–15 min (for conversion to phenytoin).

AVAILABILITY
Injection: 75 mg/ml (equivalent to 50 mg/ml phenytoin)

INDICATIONS AND DOSAGES
▸ **Status epilepticus**
IV
Adults. Loading dose: 15–20 mg phenytoin equivalent (PE)/kg infused at rate of 100–150 mg PE/min.
▸ **Nonemergent seizures**
IV, IM
Adults. Loading dose: 10–20 mg PE/kg. Maintenance: 4–6 mg PE/kg/day.
▸ **Short term substitution for oral phenytoin**
IV, IM
Adults. May substitute for oral phenytoin at same total daily dose.

CONTRAINDICATIONS
Adams-Stokes syndrome, hypersensitivity to fosphenytoin or phenytoin, second- or third-degree AV block, severe bradycardia, sinoatrial block

INTERACTIONS
Drug
Alcohol, other CNS depressants: May increase CNS depression.
Amiodarone, anticoagulants, cimetidine, disulfiram, fluoxetine, isoniazid, sulfonamides: May increase fosphenytoin blood concentration, effects, and risk of toxicity.
Antacids: May decrease fosphenytoin absorption.
Fluconazole, ketoconazole, miconazole: May increase fosphenytoin blood concentration.
Glucocorticoids: May decrease the effects of glucocorticoids.
Lidocaine, propranolol: May increase cardiac depressant effects.
Valproic acid: May increase the blood concentration and decrease the metabolism of fosphenytoin.
Xanthines: May increase the metabolism of xanthines.
Herbal
None known.
Food
None known.

DIAGNOSTIC TEST EFFECTS
May increase blood glucose, serum GGT, and serum alkaline phosphatase levels.

IV INCOMPATIBILITIES
Midazolam (Versed)

IV COMPATIBILITIES

Lorazepam (Ativan), phenobarbital, potassium chloride

SIDE EFFECTS

Frequent
Dizziness, paresthesia, tinnitus, pruritus, headache, somnolence
Occasional
Morbilliform rash

SERIOUS REACTIONS

! An elevated fosphenytoin blood concentration may produce ataxia, nystagmus, diplopia, lethargy, slurred speech, nausea, vomiting, and hypotension. As the drug level increases, extreme lethargy may progress to coma.

NURSING CONSIDERATIONS

Baseline Assessment

- Assess the patient's LOC and review the history of the seizure disorder, including the duration, frequency, and intensity of seizures. Initiate seizure precautions.
- Obtain the patient's vital signs and medication history, especially the use of phenytoin or other anticonvulsants.

Lifespan Considerations

- Fosphenytoin use during pregnancy may increase the frequency of seizures in the mother and the risk of congenital malformations in the fetus.
- It is unknown if fosphenytoin is excreted in breast milk.
- The safety of this drug has not been established in children.
- A lower fosphenytoin dosage is recommended for the elderly.

Precautions

- Use fosphenytoin cautiously in patients with hypoalbuminemia, hypotension, hepatic or renal disease, porphyria, or severe myocardial insufficiency.

Administration and Handling

◀ALERT▶ Know that 150 mg fosphenytoin yields 100 mg phenytoin and that the dose, concentration solution, and infusion rate of fosphenytoin are expressed in terms of phenytoin equivalents (PE). Keep in mind that elderly patients may require lower, less frequent dosing and that the drug is not approved for use in children.

IV

- Refrigerate unopened vials. Don't store the drug at room temperature for longer than 48 hours. Discard vials that contain particulate matter. After dilution, the solution is stable for 8 hours at room temperature or 24 hours if refrigerated.
- Dilute the drug in D_5W or 0.9% NaCl to a concentration of 1.5 to 25 mg PE/ml.
- Administer at less than 150 mg PE/minute to decrease the risk of hypotension and arrhythmias.

IM

- Refrigerate unopened vials. Don't store at room temperature for longer than 48 hours. Discard vials that contain particulate matter.

Intervention and Evaluation

- Monitor the patient's BP, EKG, and cardiac and respiratory function during and for 10–20 minutes after the infusion.
- Discontinue the infusion, as ordered, if the patient develops a rash.
- Expect to interrupt the infusion or decrease the infusion rate if the patient experiences arrhythmias or hypotension.
- Assess the patient after the infusion for ataxia, dizziness, or drowsiness.
- Assess the patient's blood level of fosphenytoin 2 hours after IV infusion or 4 hours after IM injection.

Patient Teaching

- Teach the patient about the seizure condition, and explain his or her role in seizure management.
- If noncompliance with therapy was a factor in causing acute seizures, try to resolve the patient's reasons for noncompliance.
- Advise the patient to always carry an identification card or wear an identification bracelet that displays his or her seizure disorder and anticonvulsant therapy.
- Caution the patient to avoid performing tasks that require mental alertness or motor skills until his or her response to the drug has been established.

gabapentin

ga-ba-pen-tin
(Gantin[AUS], Neurontin, Pendine [AUS])
Do not confuse Neurontin with Noroxin.

CATEGORY AND SCHEDULE

Pregnancy Risk Category: C

MECHANISM OF ACTION

An anticonvulsant and antineuralgic agent whose exact mechanism unknown. May increase the synthesis or accumulation of gamma-aminobutyric acid by binding to as-yet-undefined receptor sites in brain tissue. **Therapeutic Effect:** Reduces seizure activity and neuropathic pain.

PHARMACOKINETICS

Well absorbed from the GI tract (not affected by food). Protein binding: less than 5%. Widely distributed. Crosses the blood-brain barrier. Primarily excreted unchanged in urine. Removed by hemodialysis. ***Half-life:*** 5–7 hr (increased in impaired renal function and the elderly).

AVAILABILITY

Capsules: 100 mg, 300 mg, 400 mg.
Oral Solution: 250 mg/5 ml.
Tablets: 600 mg, 800 mg.

INDICATIONS AND DOSAGES

▸ **Adjunctive therapy for seizure control**

PO

Adults, Elderly, Children older than 12 yr. Initially, 300 mg 3 times a day. May titrate dosage. Range: 900–1,800 mg/day in 3 divided doses. Maximum: 3,600 mg/day.

Children 3–12 yr. Initially, 10–15 mg/kg/day in 3 divided doses. May titrate up to 25–35 mg/kg/day (for children 5–12 yr) and 40 mg/kg/day (for children 3–4 yr). Maximum: 50 mg/kg/day.

▸ **Adjunctive therapy for neuropathic pain**

PO

Adults, Elderly. Initially, 100 mg 3 times a day; may increase by 300 mg/day at weekly intervals. Maximum: 3,600 mg/day in 3 divided doses.

Children. Initially, 5 mg/kg/dose at bedtime, followed by 5 mg/kg/dose for 2 doses on day 2, then 5 mg/kg/dose for 3 doses on day 3. Range: 8–35 mg/kg/day in 3 divided doses.

▸ **Postherpetic neuralgia**

PO

Adults, Elderly. 300 mg on day 1, 300 mg twice a day on day 2, and 300 mg 3 times a day on day 3. Titrate up to 1,800 mg/day.

Dosage in renal impairment
Dosage and frequency are modified based on creatinine clearance:

Creatinine Clearance	Dosage
60 ml/min or higher	400 mg q8h
30–59 ml/min	300 mg q12h
16–29 ml/min	300 mg daily
less than 16 ml/min	300 mg every other day
Hemodialysis	200–300 mg after each 4-hr hemodialysis session

OFF-LABEL USES
Treatment of essential tremor, hot flashes, hyperhidrosis, migraines, psychiatric disorders

CONTRAINDICATIONS
None known.

INTERACTIONS
Drug
None known.
Herbal
None known.
Food
None known.

DIAGNOSTIC TEST EFFECTS
May decrease serum WBC count.

SIDE EFFECTS
Frequent (19%–10%)
Fatigue, somnolence, dizziness, ataxia
Occasional (8%–3%)
Nystagmus, tremor, diplopia, rhinitis, weight gain
Rare (less than 2%)
Nervousness, dysarthria, memory loss, dyspepsia, pharyngitis, myalgia

SERIOUS REACTIONS
! Abrupt withdrawal may increase seizure frequency.
! Overdosage may result in diplopia, slurred speech, drowsiness, lethargy, and diarrhea.

NURSING CONSIDERATIONS
Baseline Assessment
- Assess the seizure patient's LOC and review the history of the seizure disorder, including the onset, duration, frequency, intensity, and type of seizures. Initiate seizure precautions.
- Routine laboratory monitoring of serum gabapentin levels is not necessary for the drug's safe use.

Lifespan Considerations
- It is unknown whether gabapentin is distributed in breast milk.
- The safety and efficacy of this drug have not been established in children 3 years and younger.
- In the elderly, age-related renal impairment may require dosage adjustment.

Precautions
- Use gabapentin cautiously in patients with renal impairment.

Administration and Handling
◀ALERT▶ Keep in mind that the interval between drug doses should not exceed 12 hours.

PO
- Gabapentin may be given with food to reduce GI upset.
- If gabapentin treatment will be discontinued or another anticonvulsant will be added to the treatment regimen, expect to make the changes gradually over at least 1 week to prevent loss of seizure control.

Intervention and Evaluation
- Institute safety measures as needed.
- Monitor the patient's weight, renal function, and behavior (in children). Also monitor seizure duration and frequency.

Patient Teaching
- Instruct the patient to take gabapentin only as prescribed.

• Caution the patient not to discontine the drug abruptly because this may increase seizure frequency.
• Warn the patient to avoid tasks requiring mental alertness or motor skills until his or her response to the drug is established.
• Urge the patient to avoid alcohol while taking gabapentin.
• Advise the patient to always carry an identification card or wear an identification bracelet that displays his or her seizure disorder and anticonvulsant therapy.

lamotrigine

la-moe-**trih**-jeen
(Lamictal)
Do not confuse lamotrigine with lamivudine.

CATEGORY AND SCHEDULE

Pregnancy Risk Category: C

MECHANISM OF ACTION

An anticonvulsant whose exact mechanism is unknown. May block voltage-sensitive sodium channels, thus stabilizing neuronal membranes and regulating presynaptic transmitter release of excitatory amino acids. **Therapeutic Effect:** Reduces seizure activitiy.

AVAILABILITY

Tablets: 25 mg, 100 mg, 150 mg, 200 mg.
Tablets (Chewable): 2 mg, 5 mg, 25 mg.

INDICATIONS AND DOSAGES

▸ Seizure control in patients receiving enzyme-inducing antiepileptic drug (EIAEDs), but not valproate acid

PO

Adults, Elderly, Children 12 yr and older. Recommended as add–on therapy: 50 mg once a day for 2 wk, followed by 100 mg/day in 2 divided doses for 2 wk. Maintenance: Dosage may be increased by 100 mg/day every week, up to 300–500 mg/day in 2 divided doses.
Children 2–12 yr. 0.6 mg/kg/day in 2 divided doses for 2 wk, then 1.2 mg/kg/day in 2 divided doses for wk 3 and 4. Maintenance: 5–15 mg/kg/day. Maximum: 400 mg/day.

▸ Seizure control in patients receiving combination therapy of EIAEDs and valproic acid

PO

Adults, Elderly, Children 12 yr and older. 25 mg every other day for 2 wk, followed by 25 mg once a day for 2 wk. Maintenance: Dosage may be increased by 25–50 mg/day q1–2wk, up to 150 mg/day in 2 divided doses.
Children 2–12 yr. 0.15 mg/kg/day in 2 divided doses for 2 wk, then 0.3 mg/kg/day in 2 divided doses for wk 3 and 4. Maintenance: 1–5 mg/kg/day in 2 divided doses. Maximum: 200 mg/day.

▸ Conversion to monotherapy

PO

Adults, Children 12 yr and older. Add lamotrigine 50 mg/day for 2 wk; then 100 mg/day during wk 3 and 4. Increase by 100 mg/day q1–2wk until maintenance dosage (300–500 mg/day in 2 divided doses) is achieved. Gradually discontinue other EIAEDs over 4 wk once maintenance dose is achieved.

▸ Bipolar disorder

PO

Adults, Elderly. Initially, 25 mg/day. May double dose after wk 2, 4, and 5. Target dose: 200 mg/day.

Discontinuation therapy

Adults, Children older than 12 yr. A dosage reduction of approximately 50% per week over at least 2 wk is recommended.

CONTRAINDICATIONS

None known.

INTERACTIONS

Drug

Carbamazepine, phenobarbital, phenytoin, primidone, valproic acid: Decrease lamotrigine blood concentration.

Carbamazepine, valproic acid: May increase serum levels of these drugs.

Herbal

None known.

Food

None known.

DIAGNOSTIC TEST EFFECTS

None known.

SIDE EFFECTS

Frequent

Dizziness (38%), diplopia (28%), headache (29%), ataxia (22%), nausea (19%), blurred vision (16%), somnolence, rhinitis (14%)

Occasional (10%–5%)

Rash, pharyngitis, vomiting, cough, flulike symptoms, diarrhea, dysmenorrhea, fever, insomnia, dyspepsia

Rare

Constipation, tremor, anxiety, pruritus, vaginitis, hypersensitivity reaction

SERIOUS REACTIONS

! Abrupt withdrawal may increase seizure frequency.

NURSING CONSIDERATIONS

Baseline Assessment

- Assess the patient's LOC and review the drug history, including use of other anticonvulsants; the history of the seizure disorder, including duration, frequency, intensity, onset, and type of seizure; and other medical conditions, such as renal impairment.
- Provide the patient with a quiet, dark environment and institute safety precautions.

Precautions

- Use lamotrigine cautiously in patients with cardiac, hepatic, or renal impairment.

Administration and Handling

◀ALERT▶ If the patient is currently taking valproic acid, expect to reduce the lamotrigine dosage to less than half the normal dosage.

◀ALERT▶ Be aware that a decreased dosage may be effective in patients with significant renal impairment.

PO

- Give lamotrigine without regard to food.

Intervention and Evaluation

- Notify the physician promptly if the patient experiences a rash, and expect to discontinue the drug.
- Assist the patient with ambulation if he or she experiences ataxia or dizziness.
- Assess the patient for signs of clinical improvement, including a decrease in the frequency and intensity of seizures.
- Assess the patient for headache and visual abnormalities.

Patient Teaching

- Instruct the patient to take lamotrigine only as prescribed and not to discontinue the drug abruptly after long-term therapy. Explain that strict maintenance of drug therapy is essential for seizure control.
- Warn the patient to avoid alcohol and tasks that require mental alertness or motor skills until his or her response to the drug is established.

• Advise the patient to notify the physician at the first sign of fever, rash, or swollen glands.
• Instruct the patient to avoid exposure to sunlight and artificial light because lamotrigine may cause a photosensitivity reaction.
• Advise the patient to always carry an identification card or wear an identification bracelet that displays his or her seizure disorder and anticonvulsant therapy.

levetiracetam

leva-tir-**ass**-eh-tam
(Keppra)
Do not confuse Keppra with Kaletra.

CATEGORY AND SCHEDULE

Pregnancy Risk Category: C

MECHANISM OF ACTION

An anticonvulsant that inhibits burst firing without affecting normal neuronal excitability. **Therapeutic Effect:** Prevents seizure activity.

AVAILABILITY

Liquid: 100 mg/ml.
Tablets: 250 mg, 500 mg, 750 mg.

INDICATIONS AND DOSAGES

▸ Partial-onset seizures

PO

Adults, Elderly. Initially, 500 mg q12h. May increase by 1,000 mg/day q2wk. Maximum: 3,000 mg/day.
Children 4–16 yr. 10–20 mg/kg/day in 2 divided doses. May increase at weekly intervals by 10–20 mg/kg. Maximum: 60 mg/kg.

▸ Dosage in renal impairment

Dosage is modified based on creatinine clearance.

Creatinine Clearance (ml/min)	Dosage
Higher than 80 ml/min	500–1,500 mg q12h
50–80 ml/min	500–1,000 mg q12h
30–50 ml/min	250–750 mg q12h
less than 30 ml/min	250–500 mg q12h
End stage renal disease using dialysis	500–1,000 mg q12h, after dialysis, a 250- to 500-mg supplemental dose is recommended.

CONTRAINDICATIONS

Hypersensitivity reaction

INTERACTIONS

Drug

None known.

Herbal

None known.

Food

None significant.

DIAGNOSTIC TEST EFFECTS

May increase blood Hgb level, Hct, and RBC and WBC counts.

SIDE EFFECTS

Frequent (15%–10%)

Somnolence, asthenia, headache, infection

Occasional (9%–3%)

Dizziness, pharyngitis, pain, depression, nervousness, vertigo, rhinitis, anorexia

Rare (less than 3%)

Amnesia, anxiety, emotional lability, cough, sinusitis, anorexia, diplopia

SERIOUS REACTIONS

! None known.

NURSING CONSIDERATIONS

Baseline Assessment

• Assess the patient's LOC and

review the history of the seizure disorder, including the duration, frequency, and intensity of seizures. Initiate seizure precautions.

- Assess the patient for hypersensitivity to levetiracetam.
- Obtain the patient's BUN and serum creatinine levels to assess renal function.

Precautions

- Use levetiracetam cautiously in patients with renal impairment.

Intervention and Evaluation

- Observe the patient for recurrence of seizures.
- Assess the patient for signs of clinical improvement, such as a decrease in the frequency or intensity of seizures.
- Monitor the patient's renal function test results.
- Assist the patient with ambulation if he or she experiences dizziness.

Patient Teaching

- Caution the patient against discontinuing levetiracetam therapy abruptly because this may precipitate seizures. Explain that strict maintenance of drug therapy is essential for seizure control.
- Inform the patient that dizziness and somnolence usually diminish with continued therapy.
- Warn the patient to avoid tasks that require mental alertness or motor skills until his or her response to the drug is established.
- Advise the patient to always carry an identification card or wear an identification bracelet that displays his or her seizure disorder and anticonvulsant therapy.

oxcarbazepine

oks-kar-**bays**-uh-peen
(Trileptal)

CATEGORY AND SCHEDULE

Pregnancy Risk Category: C

MECHANISM OF ACTION

An anticonvulsant that blocks sodium channels, resulting in stabilization of hyperexcited neural membranes, inhibition of repetitive neuronal firing, and diminishing synaptic impulses. **Therapeutic Effect:** Prevents seizures.

PHARMACOKINETICS

Completely absorbed from GI tract and extensively metabolized in the liver to active metabolite. Protein binding: 40%. Primarily excreted in urine. ***Half-life:*** 2 hr; metabolite, 6–10 hr.

AVAILABILITY

Oral Suspension: 300 mg/5 ml.
Tablets: 150 mg, 300 mg, 600 mg.

INDICATIONS AND DOSAGES

▸ **Adjunctive treatment of seizures**

PO

Adults, Elderly. Initially, 600 mg/day in 2 divided doses. May increase by up to 600 mg/day at weekly intervals. Maximum: 2,400 mg/day.
Children 4–16 yr. 8–10 mg/kg. Maximum: 600 mg/day. Maintenance (based on weight): 1,800 mg/day for children weighing more than 39 kg; 1,200 mg/day for children weighing 29.1–39 kg; and 900 mg/day for children weighing 20–29 kg.

▸ **Conversion to monotherapy**

PO

Adults, Elderly. 600 mg/day in 2 divided doses (while decreasing concomitant anticonvulsant over 3–6 wk). May increase by 600 mg/day at weekly intervals up to 2,400 mg/day. *Children.* Initially, 8–10 mg/kg/day in 2 divided doses with simultaneous initial reduction of dose of concomitant antiepileptic.

▸ **Initiation of monotherapy**

PO

Adults, Elderly. 600 mg/day in 2 divided doses. May increase by 300 mg/day every 3 days up to 1,200 mg/day.
Children. Initially, 8–10 mg/kg/day in 2 divided doses. Increase at 3 day intervals by 5 mg/kg/day to achieve maintenance dose by weight; (70 kg): 1,500–2,100 mg/day; (60–69 kg): 1,200–2,100 mg/day; (50–59 kg): 1,200–1,800 mg/day; (41–49 kg): 1,200–1,500 mg/day; (35–40 kg): 900–1,500 mg/day; (25–34 kg): 900–1,200 mg/day; (20–24 kg): 600–900 mg/day.

▸ **Dosage in renal impairment**

For patients with creatinine clearance less than 30 ml/min, give 50% of normal starting dose, then titrate slowly to desired dose.

OFF-LABEL USES

Atypical panic disorder

CONTRAINDICATIONS

None known.

INTERACTIONS

Drug

Carbamazepine, phenobarbital, phenytoin, valproic acid, verapamil: May decrease the blood concentration and effects of oxcarbazepine.
Felodipine, oral contraceptives: May decrease the effectiveness of these drugs.
Phenobarbital, phenytoin: May increase the blood concentration and risk of toxicity of these drugs.

Herbal

None known.

Food

None known.

DIAGNOSTIC TEST EFFECTS

May increase GGT level and other hepatic function test results. May increase or decrease blood glucose level. May decrease serum calcium, potassium, and sodium levels.

SIDE EFFECTS

Frequent (22%–13%)
Dizziness, nausea, headache
Occasional (7%–5%)
Vomiting, diarrhea, ataxia, nervousness, heartburn, indigestion, epigastric pain, constipation
Rare (4%)
Tremor, rash, back pain, epistaxis, sinusitis, diplopia

SERIOUS REACTIONS

! Clinically significant hyponatremia may occur.

NURSING CONSIDERATIONS

Baseline Assessment

- Assess the patient's LOC and review the history of the seizure disorder, including the duration, frequency, intensity, onset, and type of seizures, and the drug history, especially the use of other anticonvulsants.
- Provide the patient with a quiet, dark environment.

Lifespan Considerations

- Oxcarbazepine crosses the placenta and is distributed in breast milk.
- No age-related precautions have been noted in children older than 4 years.
- In the elderly, age-related renal impairment may require dosage adjustment.

Precautions
• Use oxcarbazepine cautiously in patients with renal impairment or a hypersensitivity to carbamazepine.
Administration and Handling
PO
◀ **ALERT** ▶ Plan to give all doses in a twice-daily regimen.
• Give oxcarbazepine without regard to food.
Intervention and Evaluation
• Assist the patient with ambulation if he or she experiences ataxia or dizziness.
• Assess the patient for headache and visual abnormalities.
• Monitor the patient's serum sodium levels. Assess the patient for signs and symptoms of hyponatremia including confusion, headache, lethargy, malaise, and nausea.
• Assess the patient for signs of clinical improvement, such as a decrease in the frequency or intensity of seizures.
Patient Teaching
• Caution the patient against discontinuing oxcarbazepine abruptly because doing so may increase seizure frequency.
• Warn the patient to notify the physician if he or she experiences dizziness, headache, nausea, and rash.
• Inform the patient that periodic blood tests may be necessary.
• Advise the patient to always carry an identification card or wear an identification bracelet that displays his or her seizure disorder and anticonvulsant therapy.

phenobarbital
fee-noe-**bar**-bi-tal
(Luminal, Phenobarbitone[AUS])
Do not confuse phenobarbital with pentobarbital, or Luminal with Tuinal.

CATEGORY AND SCHEDULE
Pregnancy Risk Category: D
Controlled Substance Schedule IV

MECHANISM OF ACTION
A barbiturate that enhances the activity of gamma-aminobutyric acid (GABA) by binding to the GABA receptor complex. **Therapeutic Effect:** Depresses CNS activity.

PHARMACOKINETICS

Route	Onset	Peak	Duration
PO	20–60 min	N/A	6–10 hr
IV	5 min	30 min	4–10 hr

Well absorbed after PO or parenteral administration. Protein binding: 35%–50%. Rapidly and widely distributed. Metabolized in the liver. Primarily excreted in urine. Removed by hemodialysis. ***Half-life:*** 53–118 hr.

AVAILABILITY
Elixir: 20 mg/5 ml.
Tablets: 30 mg, 100 mg.
Injection: 60 mg/ml, 130 mg/ml.

INDICATIONS AND DOSAGES
▶ **Status epilepticus**
IV
Adults, Elderly, Children, Neonates. Loading dose of 15–20 mg/kg as a single dose or in divided doses.

▸ **Seizure control**
PO, IV
Adults, Elderly, Children older than 12 yr. 1–3 mg/kg/day.
Children 6–12 yr. 4–6 mg/kg/day.
Children 1–5 yr. 6–8 mg/kg/day.
Children younger than 1 yr. 5–6 mg/kg/day.
Neonates. 3–4 mg/kg/day.

▸ **Sedation**
PO, IM
Adults, Elderly. 30–120 mg/day in 2–3 divided doses.
Children. 2 mg/kg 3 times a day.

▸ **Hypnotic**
PO, IV, IM, Subcutaneous
Adults, Elderly. 100–320 mg at bedtime.
Children. 3–5 mg/kg at bedtime.

OFF-LABEL USES
Prevention and treatment of hyperbilirubinemia

CONTRAINDICATIONS
Porphyria, pre-existing CNS depression, severe pain, severe respiratory disease

INTERACTIONS
Drug
Alcohol, other CNS depressants: May increase the effects of phenobarbital.
Carbamazepine: May increase the metabolism of carbamazepine.
Digoxin, glucocorticoids, metronidazole, oral anticoagulants, quinidine, tricyclic antidepressants: May decrease the effects of these drugs.
Valproic acid: Increases the blood concentration and risk of toxicity of phenobarbital.
Herbal
None known.
Food
None known.

DIAGNOSTIC TEST EFFECTS
May decrease serum bilirubin level. Therapeutic serum level is 10–40 mcg/ml; toxic serum level is greater than 40 mcg/ml.

IV INCOMPATIBILITIES
Amphotericin B complex (Abelcet, AmBisome, Amphotec), hydrocortisone (Solu-Cortef), hydromorphone (Dilaudid), insulin

IV COMPATIBILITIES
Calcium gluconate, enalapril (Vasotec), fentanyl (Sublimaze), fosphenytoin (Cerebyx), morphine, propofol (Diprivan)

SIDE EFFECTS
Occasional (3%–1%)
Somnolence
Rare (less than 1%)
Confusion; paradoxical CNS reactions, such as hyperactivity or nervousness in children and excitement or restlessness in the elderly (generally noted during first 2 weeks of therapy, particularly in presence of uncontrolled pain)

SERIOUS REACTIONS
! Abrupt withdrawal after prolonged therapy may produce increased dreaming, nightmares, insomnia, tremor, diaphoresis, and vomiting, hallucinations, delirium, seizures, and status epilepticus.
! Skin eruptions may be a sign of a hypersensitivity reaction.
! Blood dyscrasias, hepatic disease, and hypocalcemia occur rarely.
! Overdose produces cold or clammy skin, hypothermia, severe CNS depression, cyanosis, tachycardia, and Cheyne-Stokes respirations.
! Toxicity may result in severe renal impairment.

NURSING CONSIDERATIONS

Baseline Assessment

• Assess the patient's BP, pulse rate, and respiratory rate immediately before giving phenobarbital.
• For the patient using the drug as a hypnotic, provide conditions conducive to sleep, such as a quiet environment with low lighting. Raise the bed rails as a safety precaution.
• Review the seizure patient's history of the seizure disorder, including the duration, frequency, and intensity of seizures. Initiate seizure precautions, and observe the patient frequently for a recurrence of seizure activity.

Lifespan Considerations

• Phenobarbital readily crosses the placenta and is distributed in breast milk.
• Phenobarbital use lowers serum bilirubin concentrations in neonates, produces respiratory depression in neonates during labor, and may increase the risk of maternal bleeding and neonatal hemorrhage in during delivery.
• Neonates born to women who use barbiturates during the last trimester of pregnancy may experience withdrawal symptoms.
• Phenobarbital use may cause paradoxical excitement in children.
• Elderly patients taking phenobarbital may exhibit confusion, excitement, and mental depression.

Precautions

• Use phenobarbital cautiously in patients with hepatic or renal impairment.

Administration and Handling

PO
• Give phenobarbital without regard to food.
• Crush tablets as needed.
• The elixir may be mixed with fruit juice, milk, or water.

IV
• Store vials at room temperature.
• Phenobarbital may be given undiluted or may be diluted with NaCl, D_5W, or lactated Ringer's solution.
• Expect to adequately hydrate the patient before and immediately after infusion to decrease the risk of adverse renal effects.
◀ ALERT ▶ Expect to administer the maintenance dose 12 hours after the loading dose.
• Don't exceed an injection rate of 30 mg/minute for children and 60 mg/minute for adults. Injecting too rapidly may produce marked respiratory depression and severe hypotension.
• Be aware that inadvertent intra-arterial injection may result in arterial spasm with severe pain and tissue necrosis and that extravasation in subcutaneous tissue may produce redness, tenderness, and tissue necrosis. If either occurs, inject 0.5% procaine solution into the affected area and apply moist heat, as ordered.

IM
• Don't inject more than 5 ml in any one injection site because doing so may cause tissue irritation.
• Inject the drug deep intramuscularly into large muscle mass.

Intervention and Evaluation

• Monitor the patient's BP, heart rate, respiratory rate, CNS status, renal and hepatic function, and seizure activity.
• Monitor the patient for a therapeutic serum drug level of 10–40 mcg/ml. The toxic serum drug level is greater than 40 mcg/ml.

Patient Teaching

• Caution the patient against discontinuing phenobarbital abruptly.
• Urge the patient to avoid alcohol consumption and to limit caffeine intake while taking phenobarbital.

• Inform the patient that phenobarbital may be habit forming.
• Warn the patient to avoid tasks that require mental alertness or motor skills until his or her response to the drug is established.
• Advise the patient to always carry an identification card or wear an identification bracelet that displays his or her seizure disorder and anticonvulsant therapy.

phenytoin

phen-ih-toyn
(Dilantin, Epamin, Phenytek)
Do not confuse phenytoin with mephenytoin, or Dilantin with Dilaudid.

CATEGORY AND SCHEDULE

Pregnancy Risk Category: D

MECHANISM OF ACTION

A hydantoin anticonvulsant that stabilizes neuronal membranes in the motor cortex by decreasing sodium and calcium ion influx into the neurons. Also acts as an antiarrhythmic agent by decreasing abnormal ventricular automaticity and shortening the refractory period, QT interval, and action potential duration. **Therapeutic Effect:** Limits the spread of seizure activity. Restores normal cardiac rhythm.

PHARMACOKINETICS

Slowly and variably absorbed after PO administration; slowly but completely absorbed after IM administration. Protein binding: 90%–95%. Widely distributed. Metabolized in the liver. Primarily excreted in urine. Not removed by hemodialysis. ***Half-life:*** 22 hr.

AVAILABILITY

Capsules (Prompt-Release): 100 mg.
Capsules (Extended-Release [Dilantin]): 30 mg.
Capsules (Extended-Release [Phenytek]): 200 mg, 300 mg.
Oral Suspension (Dilantin): 125 mg/5 ml.
Tablets (Chewable [Dilantin]): 50 mg.
Injection: 50 mg/ml.

INDICATIONS AND DOSAGES

▸ **Status epilepticus**

IV

Adults, Elderly, Children. 15–18 mg/kg. Maintenance dose: 300 mg/day in 2–3 divided doses for adults and elderly; 6–7 mg/kg/day for children 10–16 yr; 7–8 mg/kg/day for children 7–9 yr; 7.5–9 mg/kg/day for children 4–6 yr; 8–10 mg/kg/day for children 6 mo–3 yr.
Neonates. Loading dose: 15–20 mg/kg. Maintenance dose: 5–8 mg/kg/day.

▸ **Seizure control**

PO

Adults, Elderly, Children. Loading dose: 15–20 mg/kg in 3 divided doses 2–4 hr apart. Maintenance dose: Same as for status epilepticus.

▸ **Arrhythmias**

PO

Adults, Elderly. Loading dose: 250 mg 4 times a day for 1 day, then 250 mg twice a day for 2 days. Maintenance Dose: 300–400 mg/day 1–4 times a day.
Children. Maintenance dose: 5–10 mg/kg/day in 2–3 divided doses.

IV

Adults, Elderly, Children. Loading dose: 1.25 mg/kg q5min. May repeat up to total dose of 15 mg/kg.
Children. Maintenance dose: 5–10 mg/kg/day in 2–3 divided doses.

OFF-LABEL USES
Adjunctive treatment of tricyclic antidepressant toxicity; treatment of muscle hyperirritability, digoxin-induced arrhythmias, and trigeminal neuralgia

CONTRAINDICATIONS
Hypersensitivity to hydantoins, seizures due to hypoglycemia
IV: Adam-Stokes syndrome, second- and third-degree AV block, sinoatrial block, sinus bradycardia

INTERACTIONS
Drug
Alcohol, other CNS depressants: May increase CNS depression.
Amiodarone, anticoagulants, cimetidine, disulfiram, fluoxetine, isoniazid, sulfonamides: May increase phenytoin blood concentration, effects, and risk of toxicity.
Antacids: May decrease phenytoin absorption.
Fluconazole, ketoconazole, miconazole: May increase phenytoin blood concentration.
Glucocorticoids: May decrease the effects of glucocorticoids.
Lidocaine, propranolol: May increase cardiac depressant effects.
Valproic acid: May decrease the metabolism and increase the blood concentration of phenytoin.
Xanthine: May increase the metabolism of these drugs.
Herbal
None known.
Food
None known.

DIAGNOSTIC TEST EFFECTS
May increase blood glucose level and serum GGT and alkaline phosphatase levels. Therapeutic serum level is 10–20 mcg/ml; toxic serum level is greater than 20 mcg/ml.

IV INCOMPATIBILITIES
Diltiazem (Cardizem), dobutamine (Dobutrex), enalapril (Vasotec), heparin, hydromorphone (Dilaudid), insulin, lidocaine, morphine, nitroglycerin, norepinephrine (Levophed), potassium chloride, propofol (Diprivan)

SIDE EFFECTS
Frequent
Drowsiness, lethargy, confusion, slurred speech, irritability, gingival hyperplasia, hypersensitivity reaction (including fever, rash, and lymphadenopathy), constipation, dizziness, nausea
Occasional
Headache, hirsutism, coarsening of facial features, insomnia, muscle twitching

SERIOUS REACTIONS
! Abrupt withdrawal may precipitate status epilepticus.
! Blood dyscrasias, lymphadenopathy, and osteomalacia (caused by impaired vitamin D metabolism) may occur.
! Toxic phenytoin blood concentration (25 mcg/ml or more) may produce ataxia, nystagmus, or diplopia. As the level increases, extreme lethargy may lead to coma.

NURSING CONSIDERATIONS
Baseline Assessment
• Assess the seizure patient's LOC, and review the history of the seizure disorder, including the duration, frequency, and intensity of seizures. Initiate seizure precautions.
• Perform a CBC and blood chemistry tests to assess hepatic function before and periodically during phenytoin therapy. Repeat the CBC 2 weeks after beginning phenytoin therapy and 2 weeks after the

phenytoin maintenance dose is established.

Lifespan Considerations

- Phenytoin crosses the placenta and is distributed in small amounts in breast milk. Fetal hydantoin syndrome, marked by craniofacial abnormalities, digital or nail hypoplasia, and prenatal growth deficiency, has been reported.
- Pregnant women may experience more frequent seizures because of altered drug absorption and metabolism.
- Phenytoin use may increase the risk of neonatal hemorrhage and maternal bleeding during delivery.
- Children are more susceptible to coarsening of facial hair, hirsutism, and gingival hyperplasia.
- Lower dosages are recommended for the elderly, although no age-related precautions have been noted for this age-group.

Precautions

- Use IV phenytoin extremely cautiously in patients with CHF, myocardial damage, MI, or respiratory depression.
- Use phenytoin cautiously in patients with hyperglycemia, hypotension, hepatic or renal impairment, or severe myocardial insufficiency.

Administration and Handling

PO

- Give phenytoin with food if GI distress occurs.
- Don't let the patient chew, open, or break capsules. Tablets may be chewed.
- Shake the oral suspension well before using.

IV

◀**ALERT**▶ Give phenytoin by IV push. Remember that the maintenance dose is usually given 12 hours after the loading dose.

- If refrigerated, the solution may form a precipitate that dissolves at room temperature. Don't use the solution if it's not clear. A slight yellow discoloration of the solution won't affect its potency.
- Phenyton may be given undiluted or may be diluted with 0.9% NaCl.
- Don't exceed an injection rate of 50 mg/minute for adults to avoid cardiovascular collapse and severe hypotension. For elderly patients, administer 50 mg over 2 to 3 minutes. For neonates, don't exceed 1–3 mg/kg/minute.
- To minimize pain from chemical irritation of the vein, flush the catheter with sterile saline solution after each bolus dose of phenytoin.

Intervention and Evaluation

- Monitor the patient for a therapeutic serum drug level of 10–20 mcg/ml. The toxic serum drug level is greater than 20 mcg/ml.
- Be alert for signs of IV phenytoin toxicity, such as cardiovascular collapse and CNS depression.
- Monitor the patient's BP (with IV use), CBC, and renal and hepatic function test results.
- Observe the patient frequently for recurrence of seizure activity.
- Assess the patient for signs of clinical improvement, such as a decrease in the frequency or intensity of seizures.
- Assist the patient with ambulation if he or she experiences drowsiness, dizziness, or lethargy.

Patient Teaching

- Caution the patient against abruptly discontinuing phenytoin after long-term use because doing so may precipitate seizures. Explain that strict maintenance of drug therapy is essential for control of seizures and arrhythmias.
- Inform the patient that IV injection may cause pain.
- Encourage the patient to maintain good oral hygiene, including gum

massage and regular dental visits, to prevent gingival hyperplasia, marked by bleeding, swelling, and tenderness of gums.
- Instruct the patient to undergo a CBC every month for 1 year after the maintenance dose is established and every 3 months thereafter.
- Warn the patient to avoid tasks that require mental alertness or motor skills until his or her response to the drug is established. Inform the patient that drowsiness usually diminishes with continued therapy.
- Advise the patient to notify the physician if he or she experiences fever, swollen glands, sore throat, a skin reaction, or signs of hematologic toxicity (such as a bleeding tendency, bruising, fatigue, or fever).
- Urge the patient to avoid alcohol while taking phenytoin.
- Advise the patient to always carry an identification card or wear an identification bracelet that displays his or her seizure disorder and anticonvulsant therapy.

primidone

pri-mi-done
(Apo-Primidone[CAN], Mysoline)
Do not confuse primidone with prednisone.

CATEGORY AND SCHEDULE

Pregnancy Risk Category: D

MECHANISM OF ACTION

A barbiturate that decreases motor activity from electrical and chemical stimulation and stabilizes the seizure threshold against hyperexcitability. **Therapeutic Effect:** Reduces seizure activity.

AVAILABILITY

Tablets: 50 mg, 250 mg.

INDICATIONS AND DOSAGES

▸ Seizure control

PO

Adults, Elderly, Children 8 yr and older. 125–150 mg/day at bedtime. May increase by 125–250 mg/day every 3–7 days. Maximum: 2 g/day.
Children younger than 8 yr. Initially, 50–125 mg/day at bedtime. May increase by 50–125 mg/day every 3–7 days. Usual dose: 10–25 mg/kg/day in divided doses.
Neonates. 12–20 mg/kg/day in divided doses.

OFF-LABEL USES

Treatment of essential tremor

CONTRAINDICATIONS

History of bronchopneumonia, porphyria

INTERACTIONS

Drug

Alcohol, other CNS depressants: May increase the effects of primidone.
Carbamazepine: May increase the metabolism of carbamazepine.
Digoxin, glucocorticoids, metronidazole, oral anticoagulants, quinidine, tricyclic antidepressants: May decrease the effects of these drugs.
Valproic acid: Increases the blood concentration and risk of toxicity of primidone.

Herbal

None known.

Food

None known.

DIAGNOSTIC TEST EFFECTS

May decrease serum bilirubin level. Therapeutic serum level is 4–12 mcg/ml; toxic serum level is greater than 12 mcg/ml.

SIDE EFFECTS

Frequent

Ataxia, dizziness

Occasional

Anorexia, drowsiness, mental changes, nausea, vomiting, paradoxical excitement

Rare

Rash

SERIOUS REACTIONS

! Abrupt withdrawal after prolonged therapy may produce effects ranging from increased dreaming, nightmares, insomnia, tremor, diaphoresis, and vomiting to hallucinations, delirium, seizures, and status epilepticus.

! Skin eruptions may may be a sign of a hypersensitivity reaction.

! Blood dyscrasias, hepatic disease, and hypocalcemia occur rarely.

! Overdose produces cold or clammy skin, hypothermia, and severe CNS depression, followed by high fever and coma.

NURSING CONSIDERATIONS

Baseline Assessment

- Assess the patient's LOC, and review the history of the seizure disorder, including the duration, frequency, and intensity of seizures. Initiate seizure precautions, and observe the patient frequently for a recurrence of seizure activity.

Precautions

- Use primidone cautiously in patients with hepatic or renal impairment.

Administration and Handling

- Administer primidone at the same time each day.

Intervention and Evaluation

- Monitor the patient's CBC, neurologic status (including duration, frequency, and severity of seizures), and serum concentrations of primidone.
- Monitor the patient for a therapeutic serum drug level of 4–12 mcg/ml. The toxic serum drug level is greater than 12 mcg/ml.

Patient Teaching

- Caution the patient against abruptly discontinuing primidone after long-term use because this may precipitate seizures. Explain that strict maintenance of drug therapy is essential for seizure control.
- Warn the patient to avoid tasks that require mental alertness or motor skills until his or her response to the drug is established. Inform the patient that drowsiness usually disappears with continued therapy.
- Instruct the patient to change positions slowly—from recumbent to sitting position before standing—if he or she experiences dizziness.
- Urge the patient to avoid alcohol while taking primidone.
- Advise the patient to always carry an identification card or wear an identification bracelet that displays his or her seizure disorder and anticonvulsant therapy.

tiagabine

ti-ah-**ga**-bean

(Gabitril)

CATEGORY AND SCHEDULE

Pregnancy Risk Category: C

MECHANISM OF ACTION

An anticonvulsant that enhances the activity of gamma-aminobutyric acid, the major inhibitory neurotransmitter in the CNS. **Therapeutic Effect:** Inhibits seizures.

AVAILABILITY

Tablets: 2 mg, 4 mg, 12 mg, 16 mg.

INDICATIONS AND DOSAGES

▸ Adjunctive treatment of partial seizures

PO

Adults, Elderly. Initially, 4 mg once a day. May increase by 4–8 mg/day at weekly intervals. Maximum: 56 mg/day.

Children 12–18 yr. Initially, 4 mg once a day. May increase by 4 mg at week 2 and by 4–8 mg at weekly intervals thereafter. Maximum: 32 mg/day.

CONTRAINDICATIONS

None known.

INTERACTIONS

Drug

Carbamazepine, phenobarbital, phenytoin: May increase tiagabine clearance.

Valproic acid: May alter the effects of valproic acid.

Herbal

None known.

Food

None known.

DIAGNOSTIC TEST EFFECTS

None known.

SIDE EFFECTS

Frequent (34%–20%)

Dizziness, asthenia, somnolence, nervousness, confusion, headache, infection, tremor

Occasional

Nausea, diarrhea, abdominal pain, impaired concentration

SERIOUS REACTIONS

! Overdose is characterized by agitation, confusion, hostility, and weakness. Full recovery occurs within 24 hours.

NURSING CONSIDERATIONS

Baseline Assessment

• Assess the patient's LOC, and review the history of the seizure disorder, including the duration, frequency, and intensity of seizures. Initiate seizure precautions, and observe the patient frequently for a recurrence of seizures.

Precautions

• Use tiagabine cautiously in patients with hepatic impairment and in those who take other CNS depressants concurrently.

Intervention and Evaluation

• For patients on long-term therapy, expect to perform periodic CBCs and blood chemistry tests to assess hepatic and renal function.
• Assist the patient with ambulation if he or she experiences dizziness.
• Assess the patient for signs of clinical improvement, such as a decrease in the frequency or intensity of seizures.

Patient Teaching

• Instruct the patient to change positions slowly—from recumbent to sitting position before standing—if he or she experiences dizziness.
• Warn the patient to avoid tasks that require mental alertness or motor skills until his or her response to the drug is established.
• Urge the patient to avoid alcohol while taking tiagabine.
• Advise the patient to always carry an identification card or wear an identification bracelet that displays his or her seizure disorder and anticonvulsant therapy.

topiramate

toe-**peer**-a-mate
(Topamax)
Do not confuse topiramate or Topamax with Toprol XL.

CATEGORY AND SCHEDULE

Pregnancy Risk Category: C

MECHANISM OF ACTION

An anticonvulsant that blocks repetitive, sustained firing of neurons by enhancing the ability of gamma-aminobutyric acid to induce an influx of chloride ions into the neurons; may also block sodium channels. **Therapeutic Effect:** Decreases seizure activity.

PHARMACOKINETICS

Rapidly absorbed after PO administration. Protein binding: 13%–17%. Not extensively metabolized. Primarily excreted unchanged in urine. Removed by hemodialysis. ***Half-life:*** 21 hr.

AVAILABILITY

Capsules (Sprinkle): 15 mg, 25 mg.
Tablets: 25 mg, 50 mg, 100 mg, 200 mg.

INDICATIONS AND DOSAGES

▸ Adjunctive treatment of partial seizures, Lennox-Gastant Syndrome
PO
Adults, Elderly, Children older than 17 yr. Initially, 25–50 mg for 1 wk. May increase by 25–50 mg/day at weekly intervals. Maximum: 1,600 mg/day.
Children 2–16 yr. Initially, 1–3 mg/kg/day to maximum of 25 mg. May increase by 1–3 mg/kg/day at weekly intervals. Maintenance: 5–9 mg/kg/day in 2 divided doses.

▸ Tonic-clonic seizures
PO
Adults, Elderly, Children. Dosage is individualized and titrated.

▸ Migraine prevention
PO
Adults, Elderly. 100 mg/day in 2 divided doses.

▸ Dosage in renal impairment
Expect to reduce drug dosage by 50% in patients with tonic-clonic seizures who have a creatinine clearance of less than 70 ml/min.

OFF-LABEL USES

Prevention of migraine headaches, treatment of alcohol dependence

CONTRAINDICATIONS

None known.

INTERACTIONS

Drug

Alcohol, other CNS depressants: May increase CNS depression.
Carbamazepine, phenytoin, valproic acid: May decrease topiramate blood concentration.
Carbonic anhydrase inhibitors: May increase the risk of renal calculi.
Oral contraceptives: May decrease the effectiveness of oral contraceptives.

Herbal

None known.

Food

None known.

DIAGNOSTIC TEST EFFECTS

None known.

SIDE EFFECTS

Frequent (30%–10%)
Somnolence, dizziness, ataxia, nervousness, nystagmus, diplopia, paresthesia, nausea, tremor
Occasional (9%–3%)
Confusion, breast pain, dysmenor-

rhea, dyspepsia, depression, asthenia, pharyngitis, weight loss, anorexia, rash, musculoskeletal pain, abdominal pain, difficulty with coordination, sinusitis, agitation, flulike symptoms
Rare (3%–2%)
Mood disturbances, such as irritability and depression; dry mouth; aggressive behavior

SERIOUS REACTIONS

! Psychomotor slowing, impaired concentration, language problems (such as word-finding difficulties), and memory disturbances occur occasionally. These reactions are generally mild to moderate but may be severe enough to require discontinuation of drug therapy.

NURSING CONSIDERATIONS

Baseline Assessment

• Assess the patient's LOC, and review the history of the seizure disorder, including the duration, frequency, and intensity of seizures.
• Provide the patient with a quiet, dark environment and institute seizure precautions.
• Determine if the patient is pregnant, sensitive to topiramate, or using other anticonvulsants, especially carbamazepine, carbonic anhydrase inhibitors, phenytoin, or valproic acid.
• Obtain the patient's BUN and serum creatinine levels to assess renal function.

Lifespan Considerations

• It is unknown if topiramate is distributed in breast milk.
• No age-related precautions have been noted in children older than 2 years.
• In the elderly, age-related renal impairment may require dosage adjustment.

Precautions

• Use topiramate cautiously in patients with impaired hepatic or renal function, predisposition to renal calculi, or hypersensitivity to topiramate.

Administration and Handling

PO
• Don't break tablets because they have a bitter taste.
• Give topiramate without regard to food.
• Capsules may be swallowed whole or contents sprinkled on a teaspoonful of soft food and swallowed immediately. They should not be chewed.

Intervention and Evaluation

• Institute seizure precautions, and observe the patient frequently for a recurrence of seizure activity.
• Assess the patient for signs of clinical improvement, such as a decrease in the frequency and intensity of seizures.
• Monitor the patient's serum renal function test results, including BUN and serum creatinine levels.
• Assist the patient with ambulation if he or she experiences dizziness.

Patient Teaching

• Instruct the patient not to break tablets to avoid their bitter taste.
• Caution the patient against abruptly discontinuing topiramate because this may precipitate seizures. Explain that strict maintenance of drug therapy is essential for seizure control.
• Because topiramate may cause dizziness, drowsiness, or impaired thinking, warn the patient to avoid tasks that require mental alertness or motor skills until his or her response to the drug is established. Tell the patient that drowsiness usually diminishes with continued therapy.
• Urge the patient to avoid alcohol

and other CNS depressants while on topiramate therapy.
- Urge the patient to drink plenty of fluids to decrease the risk of kidney stones.
- Advise the patient to notify the physician if he or she experiences blurred vision or or other visual changes.
- Instruct the patient to use additional or alternative means of contraception if she takes oral contraceptives because topiramate decreases contraceptive effectiveness.
- Advise the patient to always carry an identification card or wear an identification bracelet that displays his or her seizure disorder and anticonvulsant therapy.

valproic acid

val-**pro**-ick
(Depakene)

valproate sodium

(Depakene Syrup, Epilim[AUS], Valpro[AUS])

divalproex sodium

(Depacon, Depakote, Depakote ER, Depakote Sprinkle)

CATEGORY AND SCHEDULE

Pregnancy Risk Category: D

MECHANISM OF ACTION

An anticonvulsant, antimanic, and antimigraine agent that directly increases concentration of the inhibitory neurotransmitter gamma-aminobutyric acid. **Therapeutic Effect:** Reduces seizure activity.

PHARMACOKINETICS

Well absorbed from the GI tract. Protein binding: 80%–90%. Metabolized in the liver. Primarily excreted in urine. Not removed by hemodialysis. ***Half-life:*** 6–16 hr (may be increased in hepatic impairment, the elderly, and children younger than 18 mo).

AVAILABILITY

Capsules (Depakene): 250 mg.
Syrup (Depakene): 250 mg/5 ml.
Tablets (Delayed-Release [Depakote]): 125 mg, 250 mg, 500 mg.
Tablets (Extended-Release [Depakote ER]): 500 mg.
Capsules (Sprinkles [Depakote Sprinkle]): 125 mg.
Injection (Depacon): 100 mg/ml.

INDICATIONS AND DOSAGES

▸ Seizures

PO

Adults, Elderly, Children 10 yr and older. Initially, 10–15 mg/kg/day in 1–3 divided doses. May increase by 5–10 mg/kg/day at weekly intervals up to 30–60 mg/kg/day. Usual adult dosage: 1,000–2,500 mg/day.

IV

Adults, Elderly, Children. Same as oral dose but given q6h.

▸ Manic episodes

PO

Adults, Elderly. Initially, 750 mg/day in divided doses. Maximum: 60 mg/kg/day.

▸ Prevention of migraine headaches

PO (Extended-Release)

Adults, Elderly. Initially, 500 mg/day for 7 days. May increase up to 1,000 mg/day.

PO (Delayed-Release)

Adults, Elderly. Initially, 250 mg twice a day. May increase up to 1,000 mg/day.

OFF-LABEL USES

Treatment of myoclonic, simple partial, and tonic-clonic seizures

CONTRAINDICATIONS

Active hepatic disease

INTERACTIONS

Drug

Alcohol, other CNS depressants: May increase CNS depressant effects.
Amitriptyline, primidone: May increase the blood concentration of these drugs.
Anticoagulants, heparin, platelet aggregation inhibitors, thrombolytics: May increase the risk of bleeding.
Carbamazepine: May decrease valproic acid blood concentration.
Hepatotoxic medications: May increase the risk of hepatotoxicity.
Phenytoin: May increase the risk of phenytoin toxicity and decrease the effects of valproic acid.

Herbal

None known.

Food

None known.

DIAGNOSTIC TEST EFFECTS

May increase serum LDH, bilirubin, AST (SGOT), and ALT (SGPT) levels. Therapeutic serum level is 50–100 mcg/ml; toxic serum level is greater than 100 mcg/ml.

IV INCOMPATIBILITIES

Do not mix valproic acid with any other medications.

SIDE EFFECTS

Frequent

Epilepsy: Abdominal pain, irregular menses, diarrhea, transient alopecia, indigestion, nausea, vomiting, tremors, weight gain or loss
Mania (22%–19%): Nausea, somnolence

Occasional

Epilepsy: Constipation, dizziness, drowsiness, headache, skin rash, unusual excitement, restlessness
Mania (12%–6%): Asthenia, abdominal pain, dyspepsia (heartburn, indigestion, epigastric distress), rash

Rare

Epilepsy: Mood changes, diplopia, nystagmus, spots before eyes, unusual bleeding or ecchymosis

SERIOUS REACTIONS

! Hepatotoxicity may occur, particularly in the first 6 months of valproic acid therapy. It may be preceded by loss of seizure control, malaise, weakness, lethargy, anorexia, and vomiting rather than abnormal serum liver function test results.
! Blood dyscrasias may occur.

NURSING CONSIDERATIONS

Baseline Assessment

- Assess the seizure patient's LOC, and review the history of the seizure disorder, including the duration, frequency, and intensity of seizures.
- Initiate seizure precautions, and provide the patient with a dark, quiet environment.
- For seizure patients, obtain a CBC and platelet count before beginning valproic acid therapy, 2 weeks later, and again 2 weeks after the maintenance dose has been established.
- Assess the manic patient's appearance, behavior, emotional status, response to environment, speech pattern, and thought content.
- Determine the duration, location, onset. and precipitating factors of the patient's migraine headaches.

Lifespan Considerations

- Valproic acid crosses the placenta and is distributed in breast milk.
- Children younger than 2 years are at increased risk for hepatotoxicity.
- Lower dosages are recommended for the elderly, although no age-

related precautions have been noted for this age-group.

Precautions

• Use valproic acid cautiously in patients with bleeding abnormalities or a history of hepatic disease.

Administration and Handling

PO

◀ALERT▶ Regular-release and delayed-release formulations are given in 2–4 divided doses daily; extended-release formulations are given once a day.

• Give valproic acid without regard to food. Don't administer it with carbonated drinks.

• Capsule contents may be sprinkled on applesauce and given immediately; however, don't break, chew, or crush the sprinkle beads.

• Give delayed-release or extended-release tablets whole.

IV

• Store vials at room temperature.

• Diluted solutions are stable for 24 hours.

• Discard unused portion.

• Dilute each single dose with at least 50 ml D_5W, 0.9% NaCl, or lactated Ringer's solution.

• Infuse over 5–10 minutes.

• Don't exceed an infusion rate of 3 mg/kg/minute (5-minute infusion) or 1.5 mg/kg/min (10-minute infusion). Too-rapid infusion increases the likelihood of side effects.

Intervention and Evaluation

• Monitor the patient's CBC and serum alkaline phosphatase, ammonia, bilirubin, AST (SGOT), and ALT (SGPT) levels.

• Assess the seizure patient's skin for ecchymosis and petechiae, and observe the patient frequently for recurrence of seizure activity.

• Monitor the seizure patient for evidence of clinical improvement, such as a decrease in the frequency or intensity of seizures.

• Assess the manic patient for a therapeutic response, such as an improved ability to concentrate, increased interest in surroundings, and a relaxed facial expression.

• Evaluate migraine patients for relief of migraine headache and associated symptoms, such as nausea, vomiting, phonophobia, and photophobia.

• Monitor the patient's valproic acid serum level. The therapeutic serum level is 50–100 mcg/ml, and the toxic serum level is greater than 100 mcg/ml.

Patient Teaching

• Caution the patient against abruptly discontinuing valproic acid after long-term use because this may precipitate seizures. Explain that strict maintenance of drug therapy is essential for seizure control.

• Urge the patient to notify the physician if he or she experiences abdominal pain, altered mental status, bleeding, easy bruising, lethargy, loss of appetite, nausea, vomiting, weakness, or yellowing of skin.

• Warn the patient to avoid tasks that require mental alertness or motor skills until his or her response to the drug is established. Inform the patient that drowsiness usually disappears with continued therapy.

• Urge the patient to avoid alcohol while taking valproic acid.

• Advise the patient to always carry an identification card or wear an identification bracelet that displays his or her seizure disorder and anticonvulsant therapy.

zonisamide

zoh-**nis**-a-mide

(Zonegran)

CATEGORY AND SCHEDULE

Pregnancy Risk Category: C

MECHANISM OF ACTION

A succinimide that may stabilize neuronal membranes and suppress neuronal hypersynchronization by blocking sodium and calcium channels. **Therapeutic Effect:** Reduces seizure activity.

PHARMACOKINETICS

Well absorbed after PO administration. Extensively bound to RBCs. Protein binding: 40%. Primarily excreted in urine. ***Half-life:*** 63 hr (plasma), 105 hr (RBCs).

AVAILABILITY

Capsules: 25 mg, 50 mg, 100 mg.

INDICATIONS AND DOSAGES

▸ Partial seizures

PO

Adults, Elderly, Children older than 16 yr. Initially, 100 mg/day for 2 wk. May increase by 100 mg/day at intervals of 2 wk or longer. Range: 100–600 mg/day.

OFF-LABEL USES

Treatment of obesity, weight loss

CONTRAINDICATIONS

Allergy to sulfonamides

INTERACTIONS

Drug

Alcohol, other CNS depressants: May increase zonisamide's sedative effect.

Carbamazepine, phenobarbital, phenytoin, valproic acid: May increase the metabolism and decrease the effect of zonisamide.

Herbal

None known.

Food

None known.

DIAGNOSTIC TEST EFFECTS

May increase BUN and serum creatinine levels.

SIDE EFFECTS

Frequent (17%–9%)

Somnolence, dizziness, anorexia, headache, agitation, irritability, nausea

Occasional (8%–5%)

Fatigue, ataxia, confusion, depression, impaired memory or concentration, insomnia, abdominal pain, diplopia, diarrhea, speech difficulty

Rare (4%–3%)

Paresthesia, nystagmus, anxiety, rash, dyspepsia, weight loss

SERIOUS REACTIONS

! Overdose is characterized by bradycardia, hypotension, respiratory depression, and coma.

! Leukopenia, anemia, and thrombocytopenia occur rarely.

NURSING CONSIDERATIONS

Baseline Assessment

- Assess the seizure patient's LOC, and review the history of the seizure disorder, including the duration, frequency, and intensity of seizures. Initiate seizure precautions.
- Expect to perform a CBC and blood chemistry tests to assess renal and hepatic function before and periodically during therapy.

Lifespan Considerations

- It is unknown if zonisamide is distributed in breast milk.
- The safety and efficacy of this drug

have not been established in children younger than 16 years.

• Lower dosages are recommended for the elderly, although no age-related precautions have been noted for this age-group.

Precautions

• Use zonisamide cautiously in patients with renal impairment.

Administration and Handling

PO

• Give zonisamide without regard to food.

• Have the patient swallow the capsules whole.

• Don't give this drug to patients allergic to sulfonamides.

Intervention and Evaluation

• Assess the patient for evidence of clinical improvement, such as a decrease in the frequency or intensity of seizures, and be alert for a recurrence of seizure activity.

• Assist the patient with ambulation if he or she experiences dizziness.

Patient Teaching

• Caution the patient against abruptly discontinuing zonisamide after long-term use because this may precipitate seizures. Explain that strict maintenance of drug therapy is essential for seizure control.

• Instruct the patient to notify the physician if he or she experiences abdominal or back pain, blood in urine, easy bruising, fever, rash, sore throat, or ulcers in the mouth.

• Warn the patient to avoid tasks that require mental alertness or motor skills until his or her response to the drug is established.

• Urge the patient to avoid alcohol and CNS depressants while taking zonisamide.

• Advise the patient to always carry an identification card or wear an identification bracelet that displays his or her seizure disorder and anticonvulsant therapy.

34 Antidepressants

amitriptyline hydrochloride
bupropion
citalopram hydrobromide
clomipramine hydrochloride
desipramine hydrochloride
doxepin hydrochloride
duloxetine
escitalopram
fluoxetine hydrochloride
imipramine
mirtazapine
nefazodone hydrochloride
nortriptyline hydrochloride
paroxetine hydrochloride
phenelzine sulfate
sertraline hydrochloride
tranylcypromine sulfate
trazodone hydrochloride
venlafaxine

Uses: Antidepressants are used primarily to treat depression. In addition, amitriptyline is also used for pain relief, bupropion for smoking cessation, and imipramine for childhood enuresis. Clomipramine is used only for obsessive-compulsive disorder. Monoamine oxidase inhibitors (MAOIs) are rarely prescribed as initial therapy, except for patients who don't respond to, or who have contraindications for, other antidepressants.

Action: Antidepressants are classified as tricyclic antidepressants, MAOIs, or second-generation antidepressants, which include selective serotonin reuptake inhibitors (SSRIs) and atypical antidepressants. Depression may result from decreased amounts (or effects at the receptor sites) of monoamine neurotransmitters, such as norepinephrine, serotonin, and dopamine, in the CNS. Antidepressants block the metabolism of monoamine neurotransmitters, increasing their levels and effects at receptor sites. These agents also change the responsiveness and sensitivity of presynaptic and postsynaptic receptor sites. (See the illustration *Mechanisms of Action: Antidepressants,* page 689.)

COMBINATION PRODUCTS

ETRAFON: amitriptyline/perphenazine (an antipsychotic) 10 mg/2 mg; 25 mg/2 mg; 10 mg/4 mg; 25 mg/4 mg; 50 mg/4 mg.
LIMBITROL: amitriptyline/chlordiazepoxide (an antianxiety agent) 12.5 mg/5 mg; 25 mg/ 10 mg.
SYMBYAX: fluoxetine/olanzapine (an antipsychotic) 25 mg/6 mg; 50 mg/6 mg; 25 mg/12 mg; 50 mg/12 mg.
TRIAVIL: amitriptyline/perphenazine (an antipsychotic) 10 mg/2 mg; 25

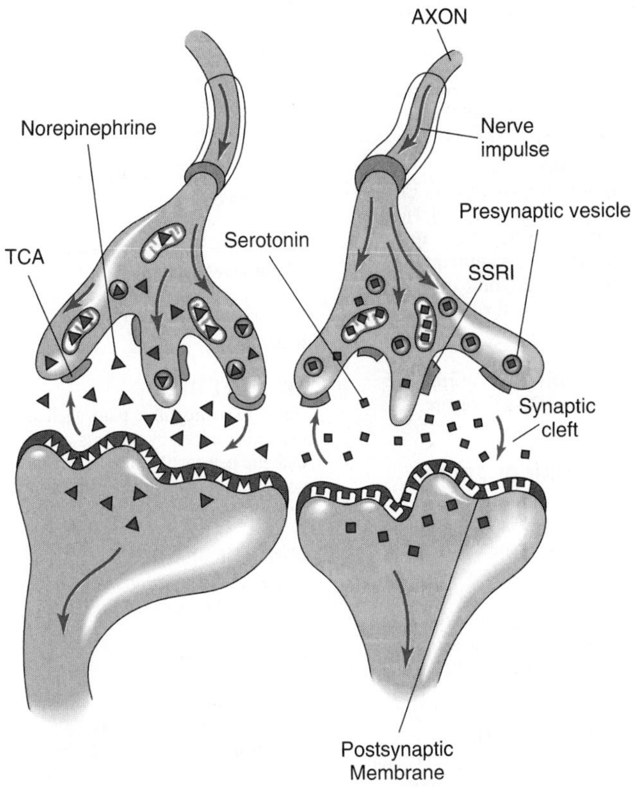

Mechanisms of Action: Antidepressants

Depression is thought to occur when levels of neurotransmitters, such as norepinephrine and serotonin, are reduced at postsynaptic receptor sites. These neurotransmitters affect a wide array of functions, including mood, obsessions, appetite, and anxiety. Antidepressants work by increasing the availability of these neurotransmitters at postsynaptic membranes and by enhancing and prolonging their effects. As a result, these agents improve mood, reduce anxiety, and minimize obsessions.

Antidepressants typically are classified as tricyclic antidepressants (TCAs), monoamine oxidase inhibitors (not shown), selective serotonin reuptake inhibitors (SSRIs), and atypical antidepressants (not shown). TCAs, such as amitriptyline and desipramine, primarily block norepinephrine reuptake at presynaptic membranes, thereby increasing the norepinephrine concentration at synapses and making more available at postsynaptic receptors (A).

SSRIs, such as fluoxetine and paroxetine, selectively inhibit serotonin uptake at presynaptic membranes. This action leads to increased serotonin availability at postsynaptic receptors (B).

mg/2 mg; 10 mg/4 mg; 25 mg/4 mg; 50 mg/4 mg.

amitriptyline hydrochloride

a-mee-**trip**-ti-leen
(Apo-Amitriptyline[CAN], Elavil, Endep[AUS], Levate[CAN], Novo-Triptyn[CAN], Tryptanol[AUS])
Do not confuse amitriptyline with aminophylline or nortriptyline, or Elavil with Equanil or Mellaril.

CATEGORY AND SCHEDULE

Pregnancy Risk Category: C

MECHANISM OF ACTION

A tricyclic antidepressant that blocks the reuptake of neurotransmitters, including norepinephrine and serotonin, at presynaptic membranes, thus increasing their availability at postsynaptic receptor sites. Also has strong anticholinergic activity. **Therapeutic Effect:** Relieves depression.

PHARMACOKINETICS

Rapidly and well absorbed from the GI tract. Protein binding: 90%. Undergoes first-pass metabolism in the liver. Primarily excreted in urine. Minimal removal by hemodialysis. ***Half-life:*** 10–26 hr.

AVAILABILITY

Tablets: 10 mg, 25 mg, 50 mg, 75 mg, 100 mg, 150 mg.
Injection: 10 mg/ml.

INDICATIONS AND DOSAGES

▸ **Depression**

PO

Adults. 30–100 mg/day as a single dose at bedtime or in divided doses. May gradually increase up to 300 mg/day. Titrate to lowest effective dosage.

Elderly. Initially, 10–25 mg at bedtime. May increase by 10–25 mg at weekly intervals. Range: 25–150 mg/day.

Children 6–12 yr. 1–5 mg/kg/day in 2 divided doses.

IM

Adults. 20–30 mg 4 times a day.

▸ **Pain management**

PO

Adults, Elderly. 25–100 mg at bedtime.

OFF-LABEL USES

Relief of neuropathic pain, such as that experienced by patients with diabetic neuropathy or postherpetic neuralgia; treatment of bulimia nervosa

CONTRAINDICATIONS

Acute recovery period after MI, use within 14 days of MAOIs

INTERACTIONS

Drug

Antithyroid agents: May increase the risk of agranulocytosis.
Cimetidine, valproic acid: May increase amitriptyline blood concentration and risk of toxicity.
Clonidine, guanadrel: May decrease the effects of these drugs.
CNS depressants (including alcohol, anticonvulsants, barbiturates, phenothiazines, and sedative-hypnotics): May increase CNS and respiratory depression and the hypotensive effects of amitriptyline.
MAOIs: May increase the risk of neuroleptic malignant syndrome, seizures, hypertensive crisis, and hyperpyresis.

Phenothiazines: May increase the sedative and anticholinergic effects of amitriptyline.
Sympathomimetics: May increase the risk of cardiac effects.

Herbal

None known.

Food

None known.

DIAGNOSTIC TEST EFFECTS

May alter blood glucose levels and EKG readings. Therapeutic serum drug level is 120–250 ng/ml; toxic serum drug level is greater than 500 ng/ml.

SIDE EFFECTS

Frequent

Dizziness, somnolence, dry mouth, orthostatic hypotension, headache, increased appetite, weight gain, nausea, unusual fatigue, unpleasant taste

Occasional

Blurred vision, confusion, constipation, hallucinations, delayed micturition, eye pain, arrhythmias, fine muscle tremors, parkinsonian syndrome, anxiety, diarrhea, diaphoresis, heartburn, insomnia

Rare

Hypersensitivity, alopecia, tinnitus, breast enlargement, photosensitivity

SERIOUS REACTIONS

! Overdose may produce confusion, seizures, severe somnolence, arrhythmias, fever, hallucinations, agitation, dyspnea, vomiting, and unusual fatigue or weakness.

! Abrupt discontinuation after prolonged therapy may produce headache, malaise, nausea, vomiting, and vivid dreams.

! Blood dyscrasias and cholestatic jaundice occur rarely.

NURSING CONSIDERATIONS

Baseline Assessment

- Observe and document the patient's appearance, behavior, interest in the environment, mood, and sleep pattern.
- Expect to obtain a CBC and blood chemistry profile before and periodically during therapy, especially with long-term use.

Lifespan Considerations

- Amitriptyline crosses the placenta and is minimally distributed in breast milk.
- Children are more sensitive to an acute overdose and are at increased risk for amitriptyline toxicity.
- Elderly patients are more sensitive to the drug's anticholinergic effects and are at increased risk for amitriptyline toxicity.

Precautions

- Use amitriptyline cautiously in patients with cardiovascular disease, diabetes mellitus, glaucoma, hiatal hernia, history of seizures, history of urine retention or urinary obstruction, hyperthyroidism, increased IOP, hepatic or renal disease, benign prostatic hyperplasia, or schizophrenia.

Administration and Handling

◀ **ALERT** ▶ Make sure at least 14 days elapse between the use of MAOIs and amitriptyline.

PO

- Give amitriptyline tablets with food or milk if GI distress occurs.

IM

- Give the drug by IM injection only if oral administration is not feasible.
- If crystals form in the ampule, immerse it in hot water for 1 minute.
- Slowly inject drug deep into a large muscle, such as the gluteus maximus, to minimize pain at the injec-

tion site. Avoid the lateral aspect of the thigh.

Intervention and Evaluation

- Closely supervise patients at risk for suicide during early therapy. As depression lessens, the patient's energy level improves, increasing the likelihood of suicide attempts.
- Assess the patient's appearance, behavior, level of interest, mood, and sleep pattern to determine the drug's therapeutic effect.
- Expect to monitor the patient's BP and pulse rate to detect arrhythmias and hypotension.

Patient Teaching

- Caution the patient not to discontinue the drug abruptly.
- Inform the patient that the drug's full therapeutic effect may be noted in 2 to 4 weeks.
- Advise the patient to change positions slowly to prevent dizziness.
- Inform the patient that he or she will develop a tolerance to the drug's hypotensive, sedative, and anticholinergic effects during early therapy.
- Inform the patient that he or she may develop sensitivity to sunlight.
- Urge the patient to report any visual disturbances.
- Warn the patient to avoid tasks that require alertness or motor skills until his or her response to the drug has been established.
- Suggest that the patient sip tepid water or chew sugarless gum to relieve dry mouth.

bupropion

byoo-**proe**-pee-on
(Wellbutrin, Wellbutrin SR, Wellbutrin XL, Zyban, Zyban sustained release[AUS])

Do not confuse bupropion with buspirone, Wellbutrin with Wellcovorin or Wellferon, or Zyban with Zagam.

CATEGORY AND SCHEDULE

Pregnancy Risk Category: B

MECHANISM OF ACTION

An aminoketone that blocks the reuptake of neurotransmitters, including serotonin and norepinephrine at CNS presynaptic membranes, increasing their availability at postsynaptic receptor sites. Also reduces the firing rate of noradrenergic neurons. **Therapeutic Effect:** Relieves depression and nicotine withdrawal symptoms.

PHARMACOKINETICS

Rapidly absorbed from the GI tract. Protein binding: 84%. Crosses the blood-brain barrier. Undergoes extensive first-pass metabolism in the liver to active metabolite. Primarily excreted in urine. ***Half-life:*** 14 hr.

AVAILABILITY

Tablets (Wellbutrin): 75 mg, 100 mg.
Tablets (Extended-Release [Wellbutrin XL]): 150 mg, 300 mg.
Tablets (Sustained-Release [Wellbutrin SR]): 100 mg, 150 mg, 200 mg.
Tablets (Sustained-Release [Zyban]): 150 mg.

INDICATIONS AND DOSAGES

▸ Depression

PO (Immediate-Release)

Adults. Initially, 100 mg twice a day. May increase to 100 mg 3 times a day no sooner than 3 days after beginning therapy. Maximum: 450 mg/day.

Elderly. 37.5 mg twice a day. May increase by 37.5 mg q3–4days. Maintenance: Lowest effective dosage.

PO (Sustained-Release)

Adults. Initially, 150 mg/day as a single dose in the morning. May increase to 150 mg twice a day as early as day 4 after beginning therapy. Maximum: 400 mg/day.

Elderly. 50–100 mg/day. May increase by 50–100 mg/day q3–4days. Maintenance: Lowest effective dosage.

PO (Extended-Release)

Adults. 150 mg once a day. May increase to 300 mg once a day. Maximum: 450 mg a day.

▸ Smoking cessation

PO

Adults. Initially, 150 mg a day for 3 days; then 150 mg twice a day for 7–12 wk.

OFF-LABEL USES

Treatment of attention deficit hyperactivity disorder in adults and children

CONTRAINDICATIONS

Current or prior diagnosis of anorexia nervosa or bulimia, seizure disorder, use within 14 days of MAOIs

INTERACTIONS

Drug

Alcohol, lithium, ritonavir, trazodone, tricyclic antidepressants: May increase the risk of seizures.

MAOIs: May increase the risk of neuroleptic malignant syndrome and acute bupropion toxicity.

Herbal

None known.

Food

None known.

DIAGNOSTIC TEST EFFECTS

May decrease serum WBC count.

SIDE EFFECTS

Frequent (32%–18%)

Constipation, weight gain or loss, nausea, vomiting, anorexia, dry mouth, headache, diaphoresis, tremor, sedation, insomnia, dizziness, agitation

Occasional (10%–5%)

Diarrhea, akinesia, blurred vision, tachycardia, confusion, hostility, fatigue

SERIOUS REACTIONS

! The risk of seizures increases in patients taking more than 150 mg/dose of bupropion, in patients with a history of bulimia or seizure disorders and in patients discontinuing drugs that may lower the seizure threshold.

NURSING CONSIDERATIONS

Baseline Assessment

- Expect to obtain blood chemistry studies before and periodically during long-term therapy to assess hepatic and renal function.
- Observe and record the patient's appearance, behavior, level of interest, mood, and sleep pattern.

Lifespan Considerations

- It is unknown if bupropion crosses the placenta or is distributed in breast milk.
- The safety and efficacy of bupropion have not been established in children younger than 18 years.

• The elderly are more sensitive to the drug's anticholinergic, cardiovascular, and sedative effects. They may also require a dosage adjustment because of age-related renal impairment.

Precautions

• Use bupropion cautiously in patients with impaired hepatic or renal function, those with a history of cranial trauma or seizures, and those who are currently taking other antidepressants or antipsychotics.

Administration and Handling

◀ALERT▶ Make sure at least 14 days elapse between the use of MAOIs and bupropion.

PO

◀ALERT▶ Expect to increase bupropion dosage gradually to minimize agitation, insomnia, and motor restlessness.

• Give bupropion with food to reduce GI irritation.
• Don't crush sustained-release tablets.
• Avoid bedtime administration to decrease the risk of insomnia.
• Expect to space doses 4 hours apart for immediate-onset tablets and 8 hours apart for sustained-release and extended-release tablets to avoid seizures.
• Be aware that sustained-release bupropion causes fewer side effects than other forms of the drug.

Intervention and Evaluation

• Closely supervise suicidal patients during early therapy. As depression lessens, the patient's energy level generally improves, increasing the suicide potential.
• Assess the patient's appearance, behavior, level of interest, mood, and sleep pattern to determine the drug's therapeutic effect.

Patient Teaching

• Inform the patient that bupropion's full therapeutic effect may take 4 weeks to appear.
• Warn the patient to avoid tasks that require mental alertness or motor skills until his or her response to the drug has been established.
• Suggest taking sips of tepid water or chewing sugarless gum to relieve dry mouth.

citalopram hydrobromide

sy-**tal**-oh-pram

(Celexa, Cipramil[AUS], Talam[AUS])

Do not confuse Celexa with Celebrex, Zyprexa, or Cerebyx.

CATEGORY AND SCHEDULE

Pregnancy Risk Category: C

MECHANISM OF ACTION

A selective serotonin reuptake inhibitor that blocks the uptake of the neurotransmitter serotonin at CNS presynaptic neuronal membranes, increasing its availability at postsynaptic receptor sites. **Therapeutic Effect:** Relieves depression.

PHARMACOKINETICS

Well absorbed after PO administration. Protein binding: 80%. Primarily metabolized in the liver. Primarily excreted in feces with a lesser amount eliminated in urine. ***Half-life:*** 35 hr.

AVAILABILITY

Oral Solution: 10 mg/5 ml.
Tablets: 10 mg, 20 mg, 40 mg.

INDICATIONS AND DOSAGES

▸ **Depression**

PO

Adults. Initially, 20 mg once a day in the morning or evening. May increase in 20-mg increments at

intervals of no less than 1 wk. Maximum: 60 mg/day.
Elderly, Patients with hepatic impairment. 20 mg/day. May titrate to 40 mg/day only for nonresponding patients.

OFF-LABEL USES

Treatment of alcohol abuse, dementia, diabetic neuropathy, obsessive-compulsive disorder, smoking cessation

CONTRAINDICATIONS

Sensitivity to citalopram, use within 14 days of MAOIs

INTERACTIONS

Drug

Antifungals, cimetidine, macrolide antibiotics: May increase the citalopram plasma level.
Carbamazepine: May decrease the citalopram plasma level.
MAOIs: May cause serotonin syndrome, marked by autonomic hyperactivity, coma, diaphoresis, excitement, hyperthermia, and rigidity, and neuroleptic malignant syndrome.
Metoprolol: Increases the metoprolol plasma level.

Herbal

None known.

Food

None known.

DIAGNOSTIC TEST EFFECTS

May reduce serum sodium level.

SIDE EFFECTS

Frequent (21%–11%)
Nausea, dry mouth, somnolence, insomnia, diaphoresis
Occasional (8%–4%)
Tremor, diarrhea, abnormal ejaculation, dyspepsia, fatigue, anxiety, vomiting, anorexia
Rare (3%–2%)
Sinusitis, sexual dysfunction, menstrual disorder, abdominal pain, agitation, decreased libido

SERIOUS REACTIONS

! Overdose is manifested as dizziness, drowsiness, tachycardia, somnolence, confusion, and seizures.

NURSING CONSIDERATIONS

Baseline Assessment

- As ordered, obtain a CBC and blood chemistry tests before and periodically during therapy for patients on long-term therapy.
- Observe and record the patient's appearance, behavior, interest in the environment, mood, sleep pattern, and thought content.

Lifespan Considerations

- Citalopram is distributed in breast milk.
- Citalopram use in children may increase anticholinergic effects and hyperexcitability.
- The elderly are more sensitive to the drug's anticholinergic effects, such as dry mouth, and are more likely to experience confusion, dizziness, hyperexcitability, and sedation.

Precautions

- Use citalopram cautiously in patients with hepatic or renal impairment and in those with a history of hypomania, mania, or seizures.

Administration and Handling

◀ **ALERT** ▶ Make sure at least 14 days elapse between the use of MAOIs and citalopram.

PO

- Give citalopram without regard to food.
- Crush scored tablets if necessary.

Intervention and Evaluation

- Closely supervise the suicidal patient during early therapy; as

depression lessens, the patient's energy level improves, increasing the risk of suicide.
- Assess the patient's appearance, behavior, level of interest, mood, and sleep pattern to determine the drug's therapeutic effect.

Patient Teaching

- Caution the patient against discontinuing citalopram abruptly or increasing the dosage.
- Urge the patient to avoid alcohol while taking citalopram.
- Warn the patient to avoid tasks that require mental alertness or motor skills until his or her response to the drug has been established.
- Inform the patient that sipping tepid water and chewing sugarless gum may help relieve dry mouth.

clomipramine hydrochloride

klom-**ip**-ra-meen
(Anafranil, Apo-Clomipramine[CAN], Clopram[AUS], Novo-Clopamine[CAN], Placil[AUS])
Do not confuse clomipramine with chlorpromazine or clomiphene; or Anafranil with alfentanil, enalapril, or nafarelin.

CATEGORY AND SCHEDULE

Pregnancy Risk Category: C

MECHANISM OF ACTION

A tricyclic antidepressant that blocks the reuptake of neurotransmitters, such as norepinephrine and serotonin, at CNS presynaptic membranes, increasing their availability at postsynaptic receptor sites. **Therapeutic Effect:** Reduces obsessive-compulsive behavior.

AVAILABILITY

Capsules: 25 mg, 50 mg, 75 mg.

INDICATIONS AND DOSAGES

▸ Obsessive-compulsive disorder
PO
Adults, Elderly. Initially, 25 mg/day. May gradually increase to 100 mg/day in the first 2 wk. Maximum: 250 mg/day.
Children 10 yr and older. Initially, 25 mg/day. May gradually increase up to maximum of 200 mg/day.

OFF-LABEL USES

Treatment of bulimia nervosa, cataplexy associated with narcolepsy, mental depression, neurogenic pain, panic disorder

CONTRAINDICATIONS

Acute recovery period after MI, use within 14 days of MAOIs

INTERACTIONS

Drug

Alcohol, other CNS depressants: May increase CNS and respiratory depression and the hypotensive effects of clomipramine.
Antithyroid agents: May increase the risk of agranulocytosis.
Cimetidine: May increase clomipramine blood concentration and risk of toxicity.
Clonidine, guanadrel: May decrease the effects of these drugs.
MAOIs: May increase the risk of neuroleptic malignant syndrome, seizures, hyperpyresis, and hypertensive crisis.
Phenothiazines: May increase the anticholinergic and sedative effects of clomipramine.
Sympathomimetics: May increase the risk of cardiac effects.

Herbal

None known.

Food

None known.

DIAGNOSTIC TEST EFFECTS

May alter the blood glucose level and EKG readings.

SIDE EFFECTS

Frequent

Somnolence, fatigue, dry mouth, blurred vision, constipation, sexual dysfunction (42%), ejaculatory failure (20%), impotence, weight gain (18%), delayed micturition, orthostatic hypotension, diaphoresis, impaired concentration, increased appetite, urine retention

Occasional

GI disturbances (such as nausea, GI distress, and metallic taste), asthenia, aggressiveness, muscle weakness

Rare

Paradoxical reactions (agitation, restlessness, nightmares, insomnia), extrapyramidal symptoms, (particularly fine hand tremor), laryngitis, seizures

SERIOUS REACTIONS

! Overdose may produce seizures; cardiovascular effects, such as severe orthostatic hypotension, dizziness, tachycardia, palpitations, and arrhythmias; and altered temperature regulation, including hyperpyrexia or hypothermia.

! Abrupt discontinuation after prolonged therapy may produce headache, malaise, nausea, vomiting, and vivid dreams.

! Anemia and agranulocytosis have been noted.

NURSING CONSIDERATIONS

Baseline Assessment

- Plan to perform blood tests, including CBC, before and periodically during therapy to assess for abnormalities, including anemia and agranulocytosis.

Lifespan Considerations

- Clomipramine is minimally distributed in breast milk.
- Clomipramine use is not recommended for children younger than 10 years.
- Expect to administer a lower dosage to elderly patients because they're at increased risk for drug toxicity.

Precautions

- Use clomipramine cautiously in patients with cardiac disease, diabetes mellitus, glaucoma, hiatal hernia, history of seizures, history of urinary obstruction or urine retention, hyperthyroidism, increased IOP, benign prostatic hyperplasia, renal or hepatic disease, and schizophrenia.

Administration and Handling

◀ALERT▶ Make sure at least 14 days elapse between the use of MAOIs and clomipramine.

PO

- Give clomipramine with food or milk if GI distress occurs.

Intervention and Evaluation

- Closely supervise suicidal patients during early therapy. As depression lessens, the patient's energy level improves, increasing the likelihood of suicide attempts.
- Assess the patient's appearance, behavior, level of interest, mood, and sleep pattern to determine the drug's therapeutic effect.
- Monitor CBC to detect signs of anemia and agranulocytosis.
- Monitor EKG tracings to detect arrhythmias.

Patient Teaching

- Caution the patient against abruptly discontinuing clomipramine.
- Explain that the drug's full therapeutic effect may be noted in 2 to 4 weeks.

• Inform the patient that clomipramine may cause blurred vision, constipation, and dry mouth.
• Instruct the patient to change positions slowly, especially early in therapy, to help prevent dizziness.
• Advise the patient that he or she will develop a tolerance to the drug's hypotensive, anticholinergic, and sedative effects during early therapy.
• Warn the patient to avoid tasks that require mental alertness or motor skills until his or her response to the drug has been established.
• Urge the patient to avoid alcohol while taking clomipramine.

desipramine hydrochloride

dess-**ip**-ra-meen
(Apo-Desipramine[CAN], Norpramin, Novo-Desipramine[CAN], Pertofran[AUS])
Do not confuse desipramine with disopyramide or imipramine.

CATEGORY AND SCHEDULE

Pregnancy Risk Category: C

MECHANISM OF ACTION

A tricyclic antidepressant that blocks the reuptake of neurotransmitters, such as norepinephrine and serotonin, at presynaptic membranes, increasing their availability at postsynaptic receptor sites. Also has strong anticholinergic activity. **Therapeutic Effect:** Relieves depression.

PHARMACOKINETICS

Rapidly, and well absorbed from the GI tract. Protein binding: 90%. Metabolized in the liver. Primarily excreted in urine. Minimally removed by hemodialysis. ***Half-life:*** 12–27 hr.

AVAILABILITY

Tablets: 10 mg, 25 mg, 50 mg, 75 mg, 100 mg, 150 mg.

INDICATIONS AND DOSAGES

▸ Depression

PO

Adults. 75 mg/day. May gradually increase to 150–200 mg/day. Maximum: 300 mg/day.
Elderly. Initially, 10–25 mg/day. May gradually increase to 75–100 mg/day. Maximum: 300 mg/day.
Children older than 12 yr. Initially, 25–50 mg/day. May gradually increase to 100 mg/day. Maximum: 150 mg/day.
Children 6–12 yr. 1–3 mg/kg/day. Maximum: 5 mg/kg/day.

OFF-LABEL USES

Treatment of attention deficit hyperactivity disorder, bulimia nervosa, cataplexy associated with narcolepsy, cocaine withdrawal, neurogenic pain, panic disorder

CONTRAINDICATIONS

Angle-closure glaucoma, use within 14 days of MAOIs

INTERACTIONS

Drug

Alcohol, other CNS depressants: May increase CNS and respiratory depression and the hypotensive effects of desipramine.
Antithyroid agents: May increase the risk of agranulocytosis.
Cimetidine: May increase desipramine blood concentration and risk of toxicity.
Clonidine, guanadrel: May decrease the effects of these drugs.
MAOIs: May increase the risk of neuroleptic malignant syndrome,

hyperpyrexia, hypertensive crisis, and seizures.
Phenothiazines: May increase the anticholinergic and sedative effects of desipramine.
Phenytoin: May decrease the desipramine blood concentration.
Sympathomimetics: May increase the risk of cardiac effects.

Herbal

St. John's wort: May increase desipramine's pharmacologic effects and risk of toxicity.

Food

None known.

DIAGNOSTIC TEST EFFECTS

May alter blood glucose level and EKG readings. Therapeutic serum drug level is 115–300 ng/ml; toxic serum drug level is greater than 400 ng/ml.

SIDE EFFECTS

Frequent

Somnolence, fatigue, dry mouth, blurred vision, constipation, delayed micturition, orthostatic hypotension, diaphoresis, impaired concentration, increased appetite, urine retention

Occasional

GI disturbances (such as nausea, GI distress, metallic taste)

Rare

Paradoxical reactions (agitation, restlessness, nightmares, insomnia), extrapyramidal symptoms (particularly fine hand tremor)

SERIOUS REACTIONS

! Overdose may produce confusion, seizures, somnolence, arrhythmias, fever, hallucinations, dyspnea, vomiting, and unusual fatigue or weakness.
! Abrupt discontinuation after prolonged therapy may produce severe headache, malaise, nausea, vomiting, and vivid dreams.

NURSING CONSIDERATIONS

Baseline Assessment

- Plan to perform a CBC and blood chemistry tests before and periodically during long-term therapy to assess hepatic and renal function.
- Plan to perform a baseline EKG if the patient is at risk for arrhythmias.

Lifespan Considerations

- Desipramine crosses the placenta and is minimally distributed in breast milk.
- Desipramine use is not recommended for children younger than 6 years.
- Expect to administer lower dosages to elderly patients because they're at increased risk for drug toxicity.

Precautions

- Use desipramine cautiously in patients with cardiac conduction disturbances, cardiovascular disease, hyperthyroidism, seizure disorders, or urine retention and in patients taking thyroid replacement therapy.

Administration and Handling

◀ALERT▶ Make sure at least 14 days elapse between the use of MAOIs and desipramine.

PO

- Give desipramine with food or milk if GI distress occurs.

Intervention and Evaluation

- Closely monitor suicidal patients during early therapy. As depression lessens, the patient's energy level improves, increasing the likelihood of suicide attempts.
- Assess the patient's appearance, behavior, level of interest, mood, and sleep pattern to determine the drug's therapeutic effect.
- Monitor the patient for therapeutic desipramine serum levels. The therapeutic serum level for desipramine is 115 to 300 ng/ml, and the toxic serum level is greater than 400 ng/ml.

• Monitor the patient's EKG if he or she has a history of arrhythmias.

Patient Teaching

• Caution the patient against abruptly discontinuing desipramine.
• Inform the patient that the drug's full therapeutic effect may be noted in 2 to 4 weeks.
• Instruct the patient to change positions slowly to help prevent dizziness.
• Explain to the patient that he or she will develop a tolerance to the drug's anticholinergic, sedative, and hypotensive effects during early therapy.

doxepin hydrochloride (Sinequan)

See Antianxiety Agents

duloxetine

dew-**lox**-ah-teen
(Cymbalta)

CATEGORY AND SCHEDULE

Pregnancy Risk Category: C

MECHANISM OF ACTION

An antidepressant that appears to inhibit serotonin and norepinephrine reuptake at central nervous system (CNS) neuronal presynaptic membranes, less potent inhibitor of dopamine reuptake. **Therapeutic Effect:** Produces antidepressant effect.

PHARMACOKINETICS

Well absorbed from the GI tract. Protein binding: greater than 90%. Extensively metabolized to active metabolites. Excreted primarily in urine with a lesser amount eliminated in feces. ***Half-life:*** 8–17 hr.

AVAILABILITY

Capsules: 20 mg, 30 mg, 60 mg.

INDICATIONS AND DOSAGES

▸ **Major depressive disorder**

PO

Adults. 40 mg/day, given as 20 mg twice a day, up to 60 mg/day, given either once a day or as 30 mg twice a day.

CONTRAINDICATIONS

End-stage renal disease (creatinine clearance less than 30 ml/min), recent (within 14 days) MAOI ingestion, severe hepatic impairment, uncontrolled narrow-angle glaucoma

INTERACTIONS

Drug

Alcohol: Increases the risk of hepatic injury.
Fluoxetine, fluvoxamine, paroxetine, quinidine, quinolone antimicrobials: May increase duloxetine concentration.
MAOIs: May cause serotonergic syndrome characterized by autonomic hyperactivity, coma, diaphoresis, excitement, hyperthermia, and rigidity.
Thioridazine: Concurrent use may produce ventricular arrhythmias.
Warfarin: May increase the concentration of warfarin.

Herbal

St John's wort: May increase adverse effects.

Food

None known.

DIAGNOSTIC TEST EFFECTS

May increase hepatic serum bilirubin, AST (SGOT), ALT (SGPT), and transaminase levels.

SIDE EFFECTS

Frequent (20%–11%)

Nausea, dry mouth, constipation, insomnia

Occasional (9%–5%)
Dizziness, fatigue, diarrhea, somnolence, anorexia, diaphoresis, vomiting
Rare (4%–2%)
Blurred vision, erectile dysfunction, delayed or failed ejaculation, anorgasmia, anxiety, decreased libido, hot flashes

SERIOUS REACTIONS

! Duloxetine use may slightly increase the patient's heart rate.
! Colitis, dysphagia, gastritis, and irritable bowel syndrome occur rarely.

NURSING CONSIDERATIONS

Baseline Assessment

• Assess the patient's appearance, behavior, level of interest, mood, sleep pattern, and speech.

Lifespan Considerations

• Be aware that duloxetine use in pregnant women may produce neonatal adverse reactions including constant crying, feeding difficulty, hyperreflexia, and irritability.
• Be aware that it is unknown if duloxetine is distributed in breast milk. Breastfeeding is not recommended in this patient population.
• Be aware that the safety and efficacy of duloxetine have not been established in children.
• Exercise caution when increasing duloxetine doses in elderly patients.

Precautions

• Use cautiously in patients with conditions that may slow gastric emptying, hepatic impairment, history of anemia, history of seizures, renal impairment, and those with suicidal ideation and behavior.

Administration and Handling

PO
• Give without regard to meals.
• Give with food or milk if GI distress occurs.
• Do not crush or chew enteric-coated capsules.
• Do not sprinkle capsule contents on food or mix with liquids.

Intervention and Evaluation

• Obtain periodic blood serum chemistry profiles for those patients on long-term duloxetine therapy to assess hepatic function.
• Closely supervise patients at risk for suicide during early therapy. As the patient's depression lessens, his or her energy level will improve, increasing the potential that he or she will attempt suicide.

Patient Teaching

• Advise the patient that the therapeutic effects of duloxetime will be noted within 1 to 4 weeks.
• Caution the patient against abruptly discontinuing duloxetine.
• Warn the patient to avoid tasks that require mental alertness or motor skills until his or her response to the drug is established.
• Tell the female patient to inform the physician if she becomes or intends to become pregnant.
• Urge the patient to report to the physician any feelings of anxiety, agitation, panic, or worsening depression.
• Suggest that the patient avoid consuming large amounts of alcohol to avoid severe hepatic injury.

escitalopram

es-sy-**tal**-oh-pram
(Lexapro)

CATEGORY AND SCHEDULE

Pregnancy Risk Category: C

MECHANISM OF ACTION

A selective serotonin reuptake inhibitor that blocks the uptake of the neurotransmitter serotonin at neuronal presynaptic membranes, increasing its availability at postsynaptic receptor sites. **Therapeutic Effect:** Relieves depression.

PHARMACOKINETICS

Well absorbed after PO administration. Primarily metabolized in the liver. Primarily excreted in feces with a lesser amount eliminated in urine. ***Half-life:*** 35 hr.

AVAILABILITY

Oral Solution: 5 mg/5 ml.
Tablets: 5 mg, 10 mg, 20 mg.

INDICATIONS AND DOSAGES

▸ Depression, general anxiety disorder (GAD)

PO

Adults. Initially, 10 mg once a day in the morning or evening. May increase to 20 mg after a minimum of 1 wk.

Elderly, Patients with hepatic impairment. 10 mg/day.

CONTRAINDICATIONS

Breast-feeding, use within 14 days of MAOIs

INTERACTIONS

Drug

Alcohol, other CNS suppressants: May increase CNS depression.

Antifungals, cimetidine, macrolide antibiotics: May increase plasma level of escitalopram.

Carbamazepine: May decrease plasma level of escitalopram.

MAOIs: May cause serotonin syndrome, marked by autonomic hyperactivity, coma, diaphoresis, excitement, hyperthermia, and rigidity, and neuroleptic malignant syndrome.

Metoprolol: Increases plasma level of metoprolol.

Herbal

None known.

Food

None known.

DIAGNOSTIC TEST EFFECTS

May reduce serum sodium level.

SIDE EFFECTS

Frequent (21%–11%)

Nausea, dry mouth, somnolence, insomnia, diaphoresis

Occasional (8%–4%)

Tremor, diarrhea, abnormal ejaculation, dyspepsia, fatigue, anxiety, vomiting, anorexia

Rare (3%–2%)

Sinusitis, sexual dysfunction, menstrual disorder, abdominal pain, agitation, decreased libido

SERIOUS REACTIONS

! Overdose is manifested as dizziness, drowsiness, tachycardia, somnolence, confusion, and seizures.

NURSING CONSIDERATIONS

Baseline Assessment

- As ordered, perform a CBC and liver and renal function tests before and periodically during long-term therapy.
- Observe and record the patient's behavior, appearance, interest in the environment, mood, sleep pattern, and thought content.

Lifespan Considerations

- Escitalopram is distributed in breast milk.
- Escitalopram use may increase anticholinergic effects and hyperexcitability in children.
- The elderly are more sensitive to the drug's anticholinergic effects, such as dry mouth and are more likely to experience confusion, dizziness, hyperexcitability, and sedation.

Precautions

• Use escitalopram cautiously in patients with hepatic or renal impairment; those with a history of hypomania, mania, or seizures; and patients concurrently using CNS depressants.

Administration and Handling

◀ **ALERT** ▶ Make sure at least 14 days elapse between the use of MAOIs and escitalopram.

PO

• Give escitalopram without regard to food.

• Don't crush film-coated tablets.

Intervention and Evaluation

• Closely supervise suicidal patients during early therapy. As depression lessens, the patient's energy level generally improves, increasing the suicide potential.

• Assess the patient's appearance, behavior, level of interest, mood, and sleep pattern to determine the drug's therapeutic effect.

Patient Teaching

• Caution the patient against discontinuing escitalopram or increasing the dosage.

• Urge the patient to avoid alcohol while taking escitalopram.

• Warn the patient to avoid tasks that require mental alertness or motor skills until his or her response to the drug has been established.

fluoxetine hydrochloride

floo-**ox**-e-teen

(Auscap[AUS], Fluohexal[AUS], Lovan[AUS], Novo-Fluoxetine[CAN], Prozac, Prozac Weekly, Sarafem, Zactin[AUS])

Do not confuse fluoxetine with fluvastatin; Prozac with Prilosec, Proscar, or ProSom; or Sarafem with Serophene.

CATEGORY AND SCHEDULE

Pregnancy Risk Category: C

MECHANISM OF ACTION

A psychotherapeutic agent that selectively inhibits serotonin uptake in the CNS, enhancing serotonergic function. **Therapeutic Effect:** Relieves depression; reduces obsessive-compulsive and bulimic behavior.

PHARMACOKINETICS

Well absorbed from the GI tract. Crosses the blood-brain barrier. Protein binding: 94%. Metabolized in the liver to active metabolite. Primarily excreted in urine. Not removed by hemodialysis. ***Half-life:*** 2–3 days; metabolite 7–9 days.

AVAILABILITY

Capsules (Prozac): 10 mg, 20 mg, 40 mg.

Capsules (Sarafem): 10 mg, 20 mg.

Capsules (Delayed-Release [Prozac Weekly]): 90 mg.

Oral Solution (Prozac): 20 mg/5 ml.

Tablets (Prozac): 10 mg, 20 mg.

INDICATIONS AND DOSAGES

▸ **Depression, obsessive-compulsive disorder**

PO

Adults. Initially, 20 mg each morning. If therapeutic improvement does

not occur after 2 wk, gradually increase to maximum of 80 mg/day in 2 equally divided doses in morning and at noon. Prozac Weekly: 90 mg/wk, begin 7 days after last dose of 20 mg.
Elderly. Initially, 10 mg/day. May increase by 10-20 mg q2wk.
Children 7–17 yr. Initially, 5–10 mg/day. Titrate upward as needed. Usual dosage is 20 mg/day.

▸ **Panic disorder**
PO
Adults, Elderly. Initially, 10 mg/day. May increase to 20 mg/day after 1 week. Maximum: 60 mg/day.

▸ **Bulimia nervosa**
PO
Adults. 60 mg each morning.

▸ **Premenstrual dysphoric disorder**
PO
Adults. 20 mg/day.

OFF-LABEL USES
Treatment of hot flashes

CONTRAINDICATIONS
Use within 14 days of MAOIs

INTERACTIONS
Drug
Alcohol, other CNS depressants: May increase CNS depression.
Highly protein-bound medications (including oral anticoagulants): May increase adverse effects.
MAOIs: May produce serotonin syndrome and neuroleptic malignant syndrome.
Phenytoin: May increase phenytoin blood concentration and risk of toxicity.
Herbal
St. John's wort: May increase fluoxetine's pharmacologic effects and risk of toxicity.
Food
None known.

DIAGNOSTIC TEST EFFECTS
None known.

SIDE EFFECTS
Frequent (more than 10%)
Headache, asthenia, insomnia, anxiety, nervousness, somnolence, nausea, diarrhea, decreased appetite
Occasional (9%–2%)
Dizziness, tremor, fatigue, vomiting, constipation, dry mouth, abdominal pain, nasal congestion, diaphoresis, rash
Rare (less than 2%)
Flushed skin, light-headedness, impaired concentration

SERIOUS REACTIONS
! Overdose may produce seizures, nausea, vomiting, agitation, and restlessness.

NURSING CONSIDERATIONS
Baseline Assessment
• Expect to perform a CBC and liver and renal function tests before and periodically during long-term therapy.
Lifespan Considerations
• It is unknown if fluoxetine crosses the placenta or is distributed in breast milk.
• Children may be more sensitive to the drug's behavioral side effects, such as insomnia and restlessness.
• No age-related precautions have been noted in the elderly.
Precautions
• Use fluoxetine cautiously in patients with cardiac dysfunction, diabetes, or seizure disorder and in patients at high risk for suicide.
Administration and Handling
◀ **ALERT** ▶ Make sure at least 14 days elapse between the use of MAOIs and fluoxetine.
PO
◀ **ALERT** ▶ Expect to decrease dosage

or frequency in elderly patients, patients with hepatic or renal impairment or a pre-existing disease, and in those who take multiple medications.

• Give fluoxetine with food or milk if GI distress occurs.

• Avoid administration at night.

Intervention and Evaluation

• Closely supervise suicidal patients during early therapy. As depression lessens, the patient's energy level improves, increasing the suicide potential.

• Assess the patient's appearance, behavior, level of interest, mood, and sleep pattern before and during therapy.

• Assess the patient's pattern of daily bowel activity and stool consistency.

• Examine the patient's skin for a rash.

• Monitor the patient's blood glucose level and serum alkaline phosphatase, bilirubin, sodium, AST (SGOT) and ALT (SGPT) levels.

Patient Teaching

• Instruct the patient to take the last dose of the drug before 4 p.m. to avoid insomnia.

• Caution the patient against discontinuing fluoxetine abruptly.

• Inform the patient that the drug's full therapeutic response may require 4 weeks or more of therapy.

• Warn the patient to avoid tasks that require mental alertness or motor skills until his or her response to the drug has been established.

• Urge the patient to avoid alcohol while taking fluoxetine.

imipramine

ih-**mih**-prah-meen

(Apo-Imipramine[CAN], Melipramine[AUS], Tofranil, Tofranil-PM)

Do not confuse imipramine with desipramine.

CATEGORY AND SCHEDULE

Pregnancy Risk Category: D

MECHANISM OF ACTION

A tricyclic antidepressant, antibulimic, anticataplectic, antinarcoleptic, antineuralgic, antineuritic, and antipanic agent that blocks the reuptake of neurotransmitters, such as norepinephrine and serotonin, at presynaptic membranes, increasing their concentration at postsynaptic receptor sites. **Therapeutic Effect:** Relieves depression and controls nocturnal enuresis.

AVAILABILITY

Tablets: 10 mg, 25 mg, 50 mg.
Capsules: 75 mg, 100 mg, 125 mg, 150 mg.

INDICATIONS AND DOSAGES

▸ Depression

PO

Adults. Initially, 75–100 mg/day. May gradually increase to 300 mg/day for hospitalized patients, or 200 mg/day for outpatients; then reduce dosage to effective maintenance level, 50–150 mg/day.

Elderly. Initially, 10–25 mg/day at bedtime. May increase by 10–25 mg every 3–7 days. Range: 50–150 mg/day.

Children. 1.5 mg/kg/day. May increase by 1 mg/kg every 3–4 days. Maximum: 5 mg/kg/day.

▸ **Enuresis**

PO

Children older than 6 yr. Initially, 10–25 mg at bedtime. May increase by 25 mg/day. Maximum: 50 mg for children older than 12 yr.

OFF-LABEL USES

Treatment of attention-deficit hyperactivity disorder, cataplexy associated with narcolepsy, neurogenic pain, panic disorder

CONTRAINDICATIONS

Acute recovery period after MI, use within 14 days of MAOIs

INTERACTIONS

Drug

Alcohol, other CNS depressants: May increase the hypotensive effects and CNS and respiratory depression caused by imipramine.

Antithyroid agents: May increase the risk of agranulocytosis.

Cimetidine: May increase imipramine blood concentration and risk of toxicity.

Clonidine, guanadrel: May decrease the effects of these drugs.

MAOIs: May increase the risk of neuroleptic malignant syndrome, hyperpyrexia, hypertensive crisis, and seizures.

Phenothiazines: May increase the anticholinergic and sedative effects of imipramine.

Phenytoin: May decrease the imipramine blood concentration.

Sympathomimetics: May increase the risk of cardiac effects.

Herbal

Ginkgo biloba: May decrease seizure threshold.

St. John's wort: May increase imipramine's pharmacologic effects and risk of toxicity.

Food

None known.

DIAGNOSTIC TEST EFFECTS

May alter blood glucose levels and EKG readings. Therapeutic serum drug level is 225–300 ng/ml; toxic serum drug level is greater than 500 ng/ml.

SIDE EFFECTS

Frequent

Somnolence, fatigue, dry mouth, blurred vision, constipation, delayed micturition, orthostatic hypotension, diaphoresis, impaired concentration, increased appetite, urine retention, photosensitivity.

Occasional

GI disturbances (nausea, metallic taste).

Rare

Paradoxical reactions, (agitation, restlessness, nightmares, insomnia), extrapyramidal symptoms (particularly fine hand tremor).

SERIOUS REACTIONS

! Overdose may produce seizures; cardiovascular effects, such as severe orthostatic hypotension, dizziness, tachycardia, palpitations, and arrhythmias; and altered temperature regulation, including hyperpyrexia or hypothermia.

! Abrupt discontinuation after prolonged therapy may produce headache, malaise, nausea, vomiting, and vivid dreams.

NURSING CONSIDERATIONS

Baseline Assessment

• Expect to perform a CBC, blood serum chemistry tests (specifically to assess the blood glucose level), and liver and renal function tests before and periodically during long-term therapy.

• Plan to perform a baseline EKG if the patient is at risk for arrhythmias.

Lifespan Considerations

- Imipramine is minimally distributed in breat milk.
- Imipramine use is not recommended for children younger than 6 years.
- Expect to administer a lower dosage to elderly patients because they're at increased risk for drug toxicity.

Precautions

- Use imipramine cautiously in patients with cardiac disease, diabetes mellitus, glaucoma, hiatal hernia, history of seizures, history of urinary obstruction or retention, hyperthyroidism, increased IOP, benign prostatic hyperplasia, renal or hepatic disease, or schizophrenia.

Administration and Handling

◀ **ALERT** ▶ Make sure at least 14 days elapse between the use of MAOIs and imipramine.

PO

- Give imipramine with food or milk if GI distress occurs.
- Don't crush or break film-coated tablets.

Intervention and Evaluation

- Closely monitor suicidal patients during early therapy. As depression lessens, the patient's energy level generally improves, increasing the likelihood of suicide attempts.
- Assess the patient's appearance, behavior, level of interest, mood, and sleep pattern before and during therapy.
- Assess the patient's pattern of daily bowel activity and stool consistency.
- Monitor the patient's BP and pulse rate to detect hypotension and arrhythmias.
- Palpate the patient's bladder for evidence of urine retention.
- Monitor the patient's therapeutic serum drug level. The therapeutic serum level for imipramine is 225 to 300 ng/ml; the toxic serum level is greater than 500 ng/ml.

Patient Teaching

- Caution the patient against abruptly discontinuing imipramine.
- Inform the patient that improvement may occur 2 to 5 days after starting therapy but that the full therapeutic effect will likely occur within 2 to 3 weeks.
- Instruct the patient to change positions slowly to help prevent dizziness.
- Explain to the patient that he or she will develop a tolerance to the drug's anticholinergic, hypotensive, and sedative effects during early therapy.
- Warn the patient to avoid tasks that require mental alertness or motor skills until his or her response to the drug has been established.
- Inform the patient that taking sips of tepid water and chewing sugarless gum may relieve dry mouth.

mirtazapine

mir-**taz**-a-peen

(Avanza[AUS], Mirtazon[AUS], Remeron, Remeron Soltab)

Do not confuse Remeron with Premarin.

CATEGORY AND SCHEDULE

Pregnancy Risk Category: C

MECHANISM OF ACTION

A tetracyclic compound that acts as an antagonist at presynaptic alpha$_2$-adrenergic receptors, increasing both norepinephrine and serotonin neurotransmission. Has low anticholinergic activity. **Therapeutic Effect:** Relieves depression and produces sedative effects.

PHARMACOKINETICS
Rapidly and completely absorbed after PO administration; absorption not affected by food. Protein binding: 85%. Metabolized in the liver. Primarily excreted in urine. Unknown if removed by hemodialysis. ***Half-life:*** 20–40 hr (longer in males [37 hr] than females [26 hr]).

AVAILABILITY
Tablets: 7.5 mg, 15 mg, 30 mg, 45 mg.
Tablets (Disintegrating): 15 mg, 30 mg, 45 mg.

INDICATIONS AND DOSAGES
▸ Depression
PO
Adults. Initially, 15 mg at bedtime. May increase by 15 mg/day q1–2wk. Maximum: 45 mg/day.
Elderly. Initially, 7.5 mg at bedtime. May increase by 7.5–15 mg/day q1–2wk. Maximum: 45 mg/day.

CONTRAINDICATIONS
Use within 14 days of MAOIs

INTERACTIONS
Drug
Alcohol, diazepam: May increase impairment of cognition and motor skills.
MAOIs: May increase the risk of neuroleptic malignant syndrome, hypertensive crisis, and severe seizures.
Herbal
None known.
Food
None known.

DIAGNOSTIC TEST EFFECTS
May increase serum cholesterol, triglyceride, AST (SGOT), and ALT (SGPT) levels.

SIDE EFFECTS
Frequent
Somnolence (54%), dry mouth (25%), increased appetite (17%), constipation (13%), weight gain (12%)
Occasional
Asthenia (8%), dizziness (7%), flu-like symptoms (5%), abnormal dreams (4%)
Rare
Abdominal discomfort, vasodilation, paresthesia, acne, dry skin, thirst, arthralgia

SERIOUS REACTIONS
! Mirtazapine poses a higher risk of seizures than tricyclic antidepressants, especially in those with no previous history of seizures.
! Overdose may produce cardiovascular effects, such as severe orthostatic hypotension, dizziness, tachycardia, palpitations, and arrhythmias.
! Abrupt discontinuation after prolonged therapy may produce headache, malaise, nausea, vomiting, and vivid dreams.
! Agranulocytosis occurs rarely.

NURSING CONSIDERATIONS
Baseline Assessment
• Plan to obtain a CBC and serum alkaline phosphatase, bilirubin, AST (SGOT), and ALT (SGPT) levels before and periodically during therapy to assess hepatic and renal function in patients on long-term therapy.
• Expect to perform a baseline EKG if the patient is at risk for arrhythmias.
• Assess the patient's appearance, behavior, level of interest, mood, and sleep pattern.
Lifespan Considerations
• It is unknown if mirtazapine is distributed in breast milk.

• The safety and efficacy of this drug have not been established in children.
• In the elderly, age-related renal impairment may require cautious use.

Precautions

• Use mirtazapine cautiously in patients with cardiovascular disorders, GI disorders, angle-closure glaucoma, benign prostatic hyperplasia, hepatic or renal impairment, or urine retention.

Administration and Handling

◀ALERT▶ Make sure at least 14 days elapse between the use of MAOIs and mirtazapine.

PO

• Give mirtazapine without regard to food.
• Scored tablets may be crushed or broken if needed.

Intervention and Evaluation

• Closely supervise suicidal patients during early therapy. As depression lessens, the patient's energy level improves, increasing the suicide potential.
• Monitor the patient for signs and symptoms of hypotension and arrhythmias.
• Assess the patient's appearance, behavior, level of interest, mood, and sleep pattern to determine the drug's therapeutic effect.

Patient Teaching

• Instruct the patient to take mirtazapine as a single bedtime dose.
• Urge the patient to avoid alcohol and other sedating medications during therapy.
• Warn the patient to avoid tasks that require mental alertness or motor skills until his or her response to the drug has been established.

nefazodone hydrochloride

neh-**faz**-oh-doan

CATEGORY AND SCHEDULE

Pregnancy Risk Category: C

MECHANISM OF ACTION

Exact mechanism is unknown. Appears to inhibit neuronal uptake of serotonin and norepinephrine and to antagonize alpha$_1$-adrenergic receptors. **Therapeutic Effect:** Relieves depression.

PHARMACOKINETICS

Rapidly and completely absorbed from the GI tract; food delays absorption. Protein binding: 99%. Widely distributed in body tissues, including CNS. Extensively metabolized to active metabolites. Excreted in urine and eliminated in feces. Unknown if removed by hemodialysis. ***Half-life:*** 2–4 hr.

AVAILABILITY

Tablets: 50 mg, 100 mg, 150 mg, 200 mg, 250 mg.

INDICATIONS AND DOSAGES

▸ **Depression, prevention of relapse of acute depressive episode**

PO

Adults. Initially, 200 mg/day in 2 divided doses. Gradually increase by 100–200 mg/day at intervals of at least 1 wk. Range: 300–600 mg/day.
Elderly. Initially, 100 mg/day in 2 divided doses. Subsequent dosage titration based on clinical response. Range: 200–400 mg/day.
Children. 300–400 mg/day.

CONTRAINDICATIONS

Use within 14 days of MAOIs

INTERACTIONS

Drug

Alprazolam, triazolam: May increase the blood concentration and risk of toxicity of these drugs.
MAOIs: May produce severe reactions.

Herbal

St. John's wort: May increase the risk of adverse effects.

Food

None known.

DIAGNOSTIC TEST EFFECTS

None known.

SIDE EFFECTS

Frequent

Headache (36%); dry mouth, somnolence (25%); nausea (22%); dizziness (17%); constipation (14%); insomnia, asthenia, light-headedness (10%).

Occasional

Dyspepsia, blurred vision (9%); diarrhea, infection (8%); confusion, abnormal vision (7%); pharyngitis (6%); increased appetite (5%); orthostatic hypotension, flushing, feeling of warmth (4%); peripheral edema, cough, flu-like symptoms (3%).

SERIOUS REACTIONS

! Serious reactions, such as hyperthermia, rigidity, myoclonus, extreme agitation, delirium, and coma, will occur if the patient takes an MAOI concurrently or fails to let enough time elapse when switching from an MAOI to nefazodone or vice versa.

NURSING CONSIDERATIONS

Baseline Assessment

- Determine if the patient has a history of sensitivity to nefazodone, trazodone, or other medications, especially alprazolam, triazolam, and MAOIs.
- Determine if the patient has a history of cardiovascular or cerebrovascular disease, hypomania, mania, or seizures.

Lifespan Considerations

- It is unknown if nefazodone crosses the placenta or is distributed in breast milk.
- The safety and efficacy of this drug have not been established in children.
- Elderly and debilitated patients are more susceptible to side effects.
- Lower dosages are recommended for the elderly, although no age-related precautions have been noted for this age-group.

Precautions

- Use nefazodone cautiously in patients with cerebrovascular or cardiovascular disease, recent MI, dehydration, hypovolemia, cirrhosis, a history of hypomania or mania, or a history of seizures.

Administration and Handling

◀ **ALERT** ▶ Allow at least 14 days to elapse before switching the patient from an MAOI to nefazodone and at least 7 days to elapse before switching the patient from nefazodone to an MAOI.

PO

- Give nefazodone without regard to food.

Intervention and Evaluation

- Monitor the patient's BP and pulse rate.
- Closely supervise suicidal patients during early therapy. As depression lessens, the patient's energy level generally improves, increasing the suicide potential.
- Assess the patient's appearance, behavior, level of interest, mood, and sleep pattern before and during therapy.
- Assist the patient with ambulation

if dizziness or light-headedness occurs.

• Assess the patient's pattern of daily bowel activity and stool consistency.

Patient Teaching

• Inform the patient that the drug's full therapeutic response may require several weeks of nefazodone therapy.

• Advise the patient to notify the physician if he or she experiences headache, nausea, or visual disturbances.

• Inform the patient that nefazodone may cause dizziness and light-headedness. Warn the patient to avoid tasks that require mental alertness or motor skills until his or her response to the drug has been established.

• Urge the patient to avoid alcohol while taking nefazodone.

• Suggest that the patient take sips of tepid water or chew sugarless gum to help relieve dry mouth.

nortriptyline hydrochloride

nor-**trip**-ti-leen

(Allegron[AUS], Aventyl, Norventyl, Pamelor)

Do not confuse nortriptyline with amitriptyline, or Aventyl with Ambenyl or Bentyl.

CATEGORY AND SCHEDULE

Pregnancy Risk Category: D

MECHANISM OF ACTION

A tricyclic antidepressant that blocks reuptake of the neurotransmitters norepinephrine and serotonin at neuronal presynaptic membranes, increasing their availability at post-synaptic receptor sites. **Therapeutic Effect:** Relieves depression.

AVAILABILITY

Capsules (Aventyl): 10 mg, 25 mg.
Capsules (Pamelor): 10 mg, 25 mg, 75 mg.
Oral Solution (Aventyl, Pamelor): 10 mg/5 ml.

INDICATIONS AND DOSAGES

▸ **Depression**

PO

Adults. 75–100 mg/day in 1–4 divided doses until therapeutic response is achieved. Reduce dosage gradually to effective maintenance level.
Elderly. Initially, 10–25 mg at bed-time. May increase by 25 mg every 3–7 days. Maximum: 150 mg/day.
Children 12 yr and older. 30–50 mg/day in 3–4 divided doses.
Children 6–11 yr. 10–20 mg/day in 3–4 divided doses.

▸ **Enuresis**

PO

Children 12 yr and older. 25–35 mg/day.
Children 8–11 yr. 10–20 mg/day.
Children 6–7 yr. 10 mg/day.

OFF-LABEL USES

Treatment of neurogenic pain, panic disorder; prevention of migraine headache

CONTRAINDICATIONS

Acute recovery period after MI, use within 14 days of MAOIs

INTERACTIONS

Drug

Alcohol, other CNS depressants: May increase CNS and respiratory depression and the hypotensive effects of nortriptyline.
Antithyroid agents: May increase the risk of agranulocytosis.
Cimetidine: May increase the blood concentration and risk of toxicity of nortriptyline.

Clonidine, guanadrel: May decrease the effects of these drugs.
MAOIs: May increase the risk of neuroleptic malignant syndrome, seizures, hyperpyrexia, and hypertensive crisis.
Phenothiazines: May increase the anticholinergic and sedative effects of nortriptyline.
Sympathomimetics: May increase the risk of cardiac effects.

Herbal

None known.

Food

None known.

DIAGNOSTIC TEST EFFECTS

May alter blood glucose level and EKG readings. The therapeutic peak serum level is 6–10 mcg/ml; the therapeutic trough serum level is 0.5–2 mcg/ml. The toxic peak serum level is greater than 12 mcg/ml; the toxic trough serum level is greater than 2 mcg/ml.

SIDE EFFECTS

Frequent

Somnolence, fatigue, dry mouth, blurred vision, constipation, delayed micturition, orthostatic hypotension, diaphoresis, impaired concentration, increased appetite, urine retention

Occasional

GI disturbances (nausea, GI distress, metallic taste), photosensitivity

Rare

Paradoxical reactions (agitation, restlessness, nightmares, insomnia), extrapyramidal symptoms (particularly fine hand tremor)

SERIOUS REACTIONS

! Overdose may produce seizures; cardiovascular effects, such as severe orthostatic hypotension, dizziness, tachycardia, palpitations, and arrhythmias; and altered temperature regulation, such as hyperpyrexia or hypothermia.

! Abrupt discontinuation after prolonged therapy may produce headache, malaise, nausea, vomiting, and vivid dreams.

NURSING CONSIDERATIONS

Baseline Assessment

- Plan to perform a CBC, blood chemistry tests (specifically to assess the blood glucose level), and hepatic and renal function tests before and periodically during long-term therapy.
- Plan to perform a baseline EKG if the patient is at risk for arrhythmias.

Precautions

- Use nortriptyline cautiously in patients with cardiac disease, diabetes mellitus, glaucoma, hiatal hernia, history of seizures, history of urinary obstruction or urine retention, hyperthyroidism, increased IOP, prostatic hypertrophy, hepatic or renal disease, or schizophrenia.

Administration and Handling

◀ **ALERT** ▶ Make sure at least 14 days elapse between the use of MAOIs and nortriptyline.

PO

- Give nortriptyline with food or milk if GI distress occurs.

Intervention and Evaluation

- Closely supervise patients at risk for suicide during early therapy. As depression lessens, the patient's energy level improves, increasing the likelihood of suicide attempts.
- Assess the patient's appearance, behavior, level of interest, mood, and speech pattern before and during therapy.
- Assess the patient's pattern of daily bowel activity and stool consistency. Encourage the patient to eat high-fiber foods and drink plenty of fluids to help prevent constipation.

• Monitor the patient's BP and pulse rate, and EKG to detect hypotension and arrhythmias.
• Palpate the patient's bladder for signs of urine retention, and monitor urine output.
• Monitor the patient's therapeutic serum drug levels. Nortriptyline's therapeutic peak serum level is 6–10 mcg/ml and therapeutic trough serum level is 0.5–2 mcg/ml. Nortriptyline's toxic peak serum level is greater than 12 mcg/ml and toxic trough serum level is greater than 2 mcg/ml.

Patient Teaching

• Caution the patient against abruptly discontinuing nortriptyline.
• Inform the patient that nortriptyline's therapeutic effect may be noted in 2 weeks or longer.
• Instruct the patient to change positions slowly to avoid dizziness.
• Inform the patient that he or she will develop a tolerance to the drug's anticholinergic, hypotensive, and sedative effects during early therapy.
• Warn the patient to avoid tasks that require mental alertness or motor skills until his or her response to the drug has been established.
• Advise the patient to notify the physician if he or she experiences visual disturbances.
• Encourage the patient to use sunscreens and wear protective clothing because the drug may cause photosensitivity to sunlight.
• Suggest that the patient take sips of tepid water or chew sugarless gum to relieve dry mouth.

paroxetine hydrochloride

par-**ox**-e-teen
(Aropax 20[AUS], Paxeva, Paxil, Paxil CR, Paxtine[AUS])
Do not confuse paroxetine with pyridoxine, or Paxil with Doxil or Taxol.

CATEGORY AND SCHEDULE

Pregnancy Risk Category: C

MECHANISM OF ACTION

An antidepressant, anxiolytic, and antiobsessional agent that selectively blocks uptake of the neurotransmitter serotonin at neuronal presynaptic membranes, thereby increasing its availability at postsynaptic receptor sites. **Therapeutic Effect:** Relieves depression, reduces obsessive-compulsive behavior, decreases anxiety.

PHARMACOKINETICS

Well absorbed from the GI tract. Protein binding: 95%. Widely distributed. Metabolized in the liver. Excreted in urine. Not removed by hemodialysis. ***Half-life:*** 24 hr.

AVAILABILITY

Oral Suspension (Paxil): 10 mg/5 ml.
Tablets (Paxil, Pexeva): 10 mg, 20 mg, 30 mg, 40 mg.
Tablets (Controlled-Release [Paxil CR]): 12.5 mg, 25 mg, 37.5 mg.

INDICATIONS AND DOSAGES

▸ **Depression**

PO

Adults. Initially, 20 mg/day. May increase by 10 mg/day at intervals of more than 1 wk. Maximum: 50 mg/day.

PO (Controlled-Release)
Adults. Initially, 25 mg/day. May increase by 12.5 mg/day at intervals of more than 1 wk. Maximum: 62.5 mg/day.

▸ **Generalized anxiety disorder**
PO
Adults. Initially, 20 mg/day. May increase by 10 mg/day at intervals of more than 1 wk. Range: 20–50 mg/day.

▸ **Obsessive compulsive disorder**
PO
Adults. Initially, 20 mg/day. May increase by 10 mg/day at intervals of more than 1 wk. Range: 20–60 mg/day.

▸ **Panic disorder**
PO
Adults. Initially, 10–20 mg/day. May increase by 10 mg/day at intervals of more than 1 wk. Range: 10–60 mg/day.

▸ **Social anxiety disorder**
PO
Adults. Initially 20 mg/day. Range: 20–60 mg/day.

▸ **Posttraumatic stress disorder**
PO
Adults. Initially, 20 mg/day. May increase by 10 mg/day at intervals of more than 1 wk. Range: 20–50 mg/day.

▸ **Premenstrual dysphoric disorder**
PO (Paxil CR)
Adults. Initially, 12.5 mg/day. May increase by 12.5 mg at weekly intervals to a maximum of 25 mg/day.

▸ **Usual elderly dosage**
PO: Initially, 10 mg/day. May increase by 10 mg/day at intervals of more than 1 wk. Maximum: 40 mg/day.
PO (Controlled-Release): Initially, 12.5 mg/day. May increase by 12.5 mg/day at intervals of more than 1 wk. Maximum: 50 mg/day.

CONTRAINDICATIONS

Use within 14 days of MAOIs

INTERACTIONS

Drug

Cimetidine: May increase paroxetine blood concentration.
MAOIs: May cause serotonin syndrome, marked by excitement, diaphoresis, rigidity, hyperthermia, autonomic hyperactivity, and coma, and neuroleptic malignant syndrome.
Phenytoin: May decrease paroxetine blood concentration.
Risperidone: May increase risperidone blood concentration and cause extrapyramidal symptoms.

Herbal

St. John's wort: May increase paroxetine's pharmacologic effects and risk of toxicity.

Food

None known.

DIAGNOSTIC TEST EFFECTS

May increase serum hepatic enzyme levels. May decrease blood Hgb level, Hct, and WBC count.

SIDE EFFECTS

Frequent

Nausea (26%); somnolence (23%); headache, dry mouth (18%); asthenia (15%); constipation (15%); dizziness, insomnia (13%); diarrhea (12%); diaphoresis (11%); tremor (8%)

Occasional

Decreased appetite, respiratory disturbance (such as increased cough) (6%); anxiety, nervousness (5%); flatulence, paresthesia, yawning (4%); decreased libido, sexual dysfunction, abdominal discomfort (3%)

Rare

Palpitations, vomiting, blurred vision, altered taste, confusion

SERIOUS REACTIONS

! None known.

NURSING CONSIDERATIONS

Baseline Assessment

- Assess the patient's appearance, behavior, level of interest, mood, and sleep pattern.
- Monitor the patient's liver function test results, Hgb level, Hct, and WBC count.

Lifespan Considerations

- Paroxetine use may impair reproductive function; it is not distributed in breast milk.
- The safety and efficacy of this drug have not been established in children.
- In the elderly, age-related renal impairment may require dosage adjustment.

Precautions

- Use paroxetine cautiously in patients with a suicidal tendency, cardiac disease, a history of seizures, impaired platelet aggregation, mania, or hepatic or renal impairment; in volume-depleted patients; and in those using diuretics.

Administration and Handling

◀ALERT▶ Make sure at least 14 days elapse between the use of MAOIs and paroxetine.

◀ALERT▶ Expect to reduce paroxetine dosage in the elderly and patients with severe hepatic or renal impairment. Keep in mind that dosage changes should occur at intervals of 1 week or longer.

PO

- Give paroxetine as a single morning dose. Give it with food or milk if GI distress occurs.
- Scored tablets may be crushed or broken.

Intervention and Evaluation

- Perform a CBC and hepatic and renal function tests periodically, as ordered, for patients on long-term therapy.
- Closely supervise suicidal patients during early therapy. As depression lessens, the patient's energy level improves, increasing the suicide potential.
- Assess the patient's appearance, behavior, level of interest, mood, and sleep pattern to determine the drug's therapeutic effect.

Patient Teaching

- Inform the patient that paroxetine's full therapeutic effect may be noted within 1 to 4 weeks.
- Caution the patient against abruptly discontinuing paroxetine.
- Warn the patient to avoid tasks that require mental alertness or motor skills until his or her response to the drug has been established.
- Instruct the patient to notify the physician if she is or intends to become pregnant.
- Suggest that the patient take sips of tepid water or chew sugarless gum to help relieve dry mouth.
- Urge the patient to avoid alcohol and St. John's wort while taking paroxetine.

phenelzine sulfate

fen-el-zeen

(Nardil)

CATEGORY AND SCHEDULE

Pregnancy Risk Category: C

MECHANISM OF ACTION

An MAOI that inhibits the activity of the enzyme monoamine oxidase at CNS storage sites, leading to increased levels of the neurotransmitters epinephrine, norepinephrine, serotonin, and dopamine at neuronal receptor sites. **Therapeutic Effect:** Relieves depression.

AVAILABILITY

Tablets: 15 mg.

INDICATIONS AND DOSAGES

▸ Depression refractory to other antidepressants or electroconvulsive therapy

PO

Adults. 15 mg 3 times a day. May increase to 60–90 mg/day.

Elderly. Initially, 7.5 mg/day. May increase by 7.5–15 mg/day q3–4wk up to 60 mg/day in divided doses.

OFF-LABEL USES

Treatment of panic disorder, vascular or tension headaches

CONTRAINDICATIONS

Cardiovascular or cerebrovascular disease, hepatic or renal impairment, pheochromocytoma

INTERACTIONS

Drug

Alcohol, other CNS depressants: May increase CNS depression.

Buspirone: May increase BP.

Caffeine-containing medications: May increase the risk of cardiac arrhythmias and hypertension.

Carbamazepine, cyclobenzaprine, maprotiline, other MAOIs: May precipitate hypertensive crisis.

Dopamine, tryptophan: May cause sudden, severe hypertension.

Fluoxetine, trazodone, tricyclic antidepressants: May cause serotonin syndrome.

Insulin, oral antidiabetics: May increase the effects of these drugs.

Meperidine, other opioid analgesics: May produce diaphoresis, immediate excitation, rigidity, and severe hypertension or hypotension, sometimes leading to severe respiratory distress, vascular collapse, seizures, coma, and death.

Methylphenidate: May increase the CNS stimulant effects of methylphenidate.

Sympathomimetics: May increase the cardiac stimulant and vasopressor effects of phenelzine.

Herbal

None known.

Food

Caffeine, chocolate, tyramine-containing foods (such as aged cheese): May cause sudden, severe hypertension.

DIAGNOSTIC TEST EFFECTS

None known.

SIDE EFFECTS

Frequent

Orthostatic hypotension, restlessness, GI upset, insomnia, dizziness, headache, lethargy, asthenia, dry mouth, peripheral edema

Occasional

Flushing, diaphoresis, rash, urinary frequency, increased appetite, transient impotence

Rare

Visual disturbances

SERIOUS REACTIONS

! Hypertensive crisis occurs rarely and is marked by severe hypertension, occipital headache radiating frontally, neck stiffness or soreness, nausea, vomiting, diaphoresis, fever or chilliness, clammy skin, dilated pupils, palpitations, tachycardia or bradycardia, and constricting chest pain.

NURSING CONSIDERATIONS

Baseline Assessment

• Plan to perform hepatic function tests periodically in patients taking high doses or undergoing prolonged therapy.

Precautions

• Use phenelzine cautiously within several hours of ingestion of a contraindicated substance, such as tyramine-containing foods.

• Use phenelzine cautiously in patients with cardiac arrhythmias, frequent or severe headaches, hypertension, and suicidal tendencies.

Administration and Handling

PO

• Store phenelzine tablets at room temperature. Don't freeze.

• Administer the drug with food or milk to alleviate GI symptoms.

• If patient has difficulty swallowing the tablets whole, crush them and give with food or fluids.

Intervention and Evaluation

• Assess the patient's appearance, behavior, level of interest, mood, and sleep pattern to determine the drug's therapeutic effect.

• Closely supervise suicidal patients during early therapy. As depression lessens, the patient's energy level improves, increasing the suicide potential.

• Monitor the patient for occipital headache radiating frontally and neck stiffness or soreness, which may be the first symptoms of an impending hypertensive crisis. If hypertensive crisis occurs, administer phentolamine 5–10 mg IV, as prescribed.

• Monitor the patient's BP, heart rate, diet, and weight.

Patient Teaching

• Tell the patient that depression may start to lift during the first week of therapy but that phenelzine's full therapeutic effect may require 2 to 6 weeks of therapy.

• Caution the patient to notify the physician immediately if he or she experiences headache or neck soreness or stiffness.

• Urge the patient to avoid foods that require bacteria or molds for their preparation or preservation (such as yogurt and aged cheese); foods containing tyramine (including avocados, bananas, broad beans, figs, papayas, raisins, sour cream, soy sauce, beer, wine, yeast extracts, meat tenderizers, liver, and smoked or pickled meats and fish); and excessive amounts of caffeine-containing foods or beverages (such as chocolate, coffee, and tea).

• Tell the patient to avoid using OTC preparations for colds, hay fever, and weight reduction.

sertraline hydrochloride

sir-trall-een

(Apo-Sertraline[CAN], Novo-Sertraline[CAN], PMS-Sertraline [CAN], Zoloft)

Do not confuse sertraline with Serentil.

CATEGORY AND SCHEDULE

Pregnancy Risk Category: B

MECHANISM OF ACTION

An antidepressant, anxiolytic, and obsessive-compulsive disorder adjunct that blocks the reuptake of the neurotransmitter serotonin at CNS neuronal presynaptic membranes, increasing its availability at postsynaptic receptor sites. **Therapeutic Effect:** Relieves depression, reduces obsessive-compulsive behavior, decreases anxiety.

PHARMACOKINETICS

Incompletely and slowly absorbed

from the GI tract; food increases absorption. Protein binding: 98%. Widely distributed. Undergoes extensive first-pass metabolism in the liver to active compound. Excreted in urine and feces. Not removed by hemodialysis. ***Half-life:*** 26 hr.

AVAILABILITY

Oral Concentrate: 20 mg/ml.
Tablets: 25 mg, 50 mg, 100 mg.

INDICATIONS AND DOSAGES

▸ Depression, obsessive-compulsive disorder

PO

Adults, Children 13–17 yr. Initially, 50 mg/day with morning or evening meal. May increase by 50 mg/day at 7-day intervals.

Elderly, Children 6–12 yr. Initially, 25 mg/day. May increase by 25–50 mg/day at 7-day intervals.

Maximum: 200 mg/day.

▸ Panic disorder, posttraumatic stress disorder, social anxiety disorder

PO

Adults, Elderly. Initially, 25 mg/day. May increase by 50 mg/day at 7-day intervals. Range: 50–200 mg/day.

Maximum: 200 mg/day.

▸ Premenstrual dysphoric disorder

PO

Adults. Initially, 50 mg/day. May increase up to 150 mg/day in 50-mg increments.

CONTRAINDICATIONS

User within 14 days of MAOIs

INTERACTIONS

Drug

Highly protein-bound medications (such as, digoxin and warfarin): May increase the blood concentration and risk of toxicity of these drugs.

MAOIs: May cause neuroleptic malignant syndrome, hypertensive crisis, hyperpyrexia, seizures, and serotonin syndrome (marked by diaphoresis, diarrhea, fever, mental changes, restlessness, and shivering).

Herbal

St. John's wort: May increase the risk of adverse effects.

Food

None known.

DIAGNOSTIC TEST EFFECTS

May increase serum total cholesterol, triglyceride, AST (SGOT), and ALT (SGPT) levels. May decrease serum uric acid level.

SIDE EFFECTS

Frequent (26%–12%)

Headache, nausea, diarrhea, insomnia, somnolence, dizziness, fatigue, rash, dry mouth

Occasional (6%–4%)

Anxiety, nervousness, agitation, tremor, dyspepsia, diaphoresis, vomiting, constipation, abnormal ejaculation, visual disturbances, altered taste

Rare (less than 3%)

Flatulence, urinary frequency, paraesthesia, hot flashes, chills

SERIOUS REACTIONS

! None known.

NURSING CONSIDERATIONS

Baseline Assessment

- Plan to perform a CBC and liver and renal function tests before and periodically during long-term therapy.

Lifespan Considerations

- It is unknown if sertraline crosses the placenta or is distributed in breast milk.
- No age-related precautions have been noted in children older than 6 years.

• Lower initial sertraline dosages are recommended for the elderly, although no age-related precautions have been noted in this age-group.

Precautions

• Use sertraline cautiously in patients with cardiac disease, heaptic impairment, or seizure disorders; in patients who have had a recent MI; and in suicidal patients.

Administration and Handling

◀ **ALERT** ▶ Make sure at least 14 days elapse between the use of MAOIs and sertraline.

PO

• Give sertraline with food or milk if GI distress occurs.

Intervention and Evaluation

• Closely supervise suicidal patients during early therapy. As depression lessens, the patient's energy level improves, increasing the suicide potential.

• Assess the patient's appearance, behavior, level of interest, mood, and sleep pattern before and during therapy.

• Monitor the patient's pattern of daily bowel activity and stool consistency.

• Assist the patient with ambulation if he or she experiences dizziness.

Patient Teaching

• Advise the patient to take sertraline with food if he or she experiences nausea.

• Caution the femal pateint to notify the physician if she becomes pregnant.

• Instruct the patient to report fatigue, headache, sexual dysfunction, or tremor.

• Caution the patient to avoid tasks that require mental alertness or motor skills until his or her response to the drug has been established.

• Urge the patient to avoid alcohol while taking sertraline.

• Urge the patient not to take OTC medications without consulting the physician.

• Suggest that the patient take sips of tepid water or chew sugarless gum to relieve dry mouth.

tranylcypromine sulfate

tran-ill-**sip**-roe-meen

(Parnate)

CATEGORY AND SCHEDULE

Pregnancy Risk Category: C

MECHANISM OF ACTION

An MAOI that inhibits the activity of the enzyme monoamine oxidase at CNS storage sites, leading to increased levels of the neurotransmitters epinephrine, norepinephrine, serotonin, and dopamine at neuronal receptor sites. **Therapeutic Effect:** Relieves depression.

AVAILABILITY

Tablets: 10 mg.

INDICATIONS AND DOSAGES

▸ **Depression refractory to or intolerant of other therapy**

PO

Adults, Elderly. Initially, 10 mg twice a day. May increase by 10 mg/day at 1- to 3-wk intervals up to 60 mg/day in divided doses.

CONTRAINDICATIONS

CHF, children younger than 16 years, pheochromocytoma, severe hepatic or renal impairment, uncontrolled hypertension

INTERACTIONS

Drug

Alcohol, other CNS depressants: May increase CNS depressant effects.

Buspirone: May increase BP.
Caffeine-containing medications: May increase the risk of cardiac arrhythmias and hypertension.
Carbamazepine, cyclobenzaprine, maprotiline, other MAOIs: May precipitate hypertensive crisis.
Dopamine, tryptophan: May cause sudden, severe hypertension.
Fluoxetine, trazodone, tricyclic antidepressants: May cause serotonin syndrome and neuroleptic malignant syndrome.
Insulin, oral antidiabetics: May increase the effects of these drugs.
Meperidine, other opioid analgesics: May produce diaphoresis, immediate excitation, rigidity, and severe hypertension or hypotension, sometimes leading to severe respiratory distress, vascular collapse, seizures, coma, and death.

Herbal

None known.

Food

Caffeine, chocolate, tyramine-containing foods (such as aged cheese): May cause sudden, severe hypertension.

DIAGNOSTIC TEST EFFECTS

None known.

SIDE EFFECTS

Frequent

Orthostatic hypotension, restlessness, GI upset, insomnia, dizziness, lethargy, weakness, dry mouth, peripheral edema

Occasional

Flushing, diaphoresis, rash, urinary frequency, increased appetite, transient impotence

Rare

Visual disturbances

SERIOUS REACTIONS

! Hypertensive crisis occurs rarely and is marked by severe hypertension, occipital headache radiating frontally, neck stiffness or soreness, nausea, vomiting, diaphoresis, fever or chills, clammy skin, dilated pupils, palpitations, tachycardia or bradycardia, and constricting chest pain.

NURSING CONSIDERATIONS

Baseline Assessment

- Plan to perform baseline and periodic serum hepatic and renal function tests.
- Assess the patient for sensitivity to tranylcypromine.
- Determine the patients medical conditions, especially alcoholism, arrhythmias, cardiovascular disease, congestive heart failure, hypertension, pheochromocytoma, and suicidal tendencies.
- Determine the patient's medication history. Ask the patient if he or she takes CNS depressants, meperidine, and other antidepressants. Tranylcypromine should not be used within 14 days of taking selective serotonin reuptake inhibitors (SSRIs).

Precautions

- Use tranylcypromine cautiously within several hours of ingestion of a contraindicated substance, such as tyramine-containing food.
- Use tranylcypromine cautiously in patients with cardiac arrhythmias, frequent or severe headaches, hypertension, and suicidal tendencies.

Administration and Handling

◀ **ALERT** ▶ Make sure at least 14 days elapse between the use of tranylcypromine and a selective serotonin reuptake inhibitor.

Intervention and Evaluation

- Assess the patient's appearance, behavior, level of interest, mood, and sleep pattern before and during therapy.
- Closely supervise suicidal patients

during early therapy. As depression lessens, the patient's energy level improves, increasing the suicide potential.
• Monitor the patient's BP, temperature, and weight.
• Evaluate the patient for an occipital headache radiating frontally and neck stiffness or soreness, which may be the first symptoms of an impending hypertensive crisis. If hypertensive crisis occurs, administer phentolamine 5 to 10 mg IV, as prescribed.
• Expect to discontinue tranylcypromine immediately if the patient experiences frequent headaches or palpitations.

Patient Teaching

• Instruct the patient to take the second daily dose no later than 4 p.m. to avoid insomnia.
• Tell the patient that depression may start to lift during the first week of therapy and that the drug's full therapeutic benefit will occur within 3 weeks.
• Warn the patient to notify the physician immediately if he or she experiences headache and neck soreness or stiffness.
• Instruct the patient to change positions slowly and to dangle the legs momentarily before standing to avoid dizziness.
• Urge the patient to avoid foods that require bacteria or molds for their preparation or preservation (such as yogurt and aged cheese); foods containing tyramine (such as avocados, bananas, broad beans, meat tenderizers, liver, smoked or pickled meats and fish, papayas, figs, raisins, sour cream, soy sauce, beer, wine, and yeast extracts); and excessive amounts of caffeine-containing foods or beverages (including chocolate, coffee, and tea).
• Urge the patient to avoid OTC preparations for allergies, colds, hay fever, and weight reduction.

trazodone hydrochloride

tra-zoh-doan

(Apo-Trazodone[CAN], Desyrel, Novo-Trazodone[CAN], PMS-Trazodone[CAN])

Do not confuse Desyrel with Delsym or Zestril.

CATEGORY AND SCHEDULE

Pregnancy Risk Category: C

MECHANISM OF ACTION

An antidepressant that blocks the reuptake of serotonin at neuronal presynaptic membranes, increasing its availability at postsynaptic receptor sites. **Therapeutic Effect:** Relieves depression.

PHARMACOKINETICS

Well absorbed from the GI tract. Protein binding: 85%–95%. Metabolized in the liver. Primarily excreted in urine. Unknown if removed by hemodialysis. ***Half-life:*** 5–9 hr.

AVAILABILITY

Tablets: 50 mg, 100 mg, 150 mg, 300 mg.

INDICATIONS AND DOSAGES

▸ **Depression**

PO

Adults. Initially, 150 mg/day in equally divided doses. Increase by 50 mg/day at 3- to 4-day intervals until therapeutic response is achieved. Maximum: 600 mg/day.

Elderly. Initially, 25–50 mg at bedtime. May increase by 25–50 mg every 3–7 days. Range: 75–150 mg/day.

Children 6–18 yr. Initially, 1.5–2 mg/kg/day in divided doses. May increase gradually to 6 mg/kg/day in 3 divided doses.

OFF-LABEL USES

Treatment of neurogenic pain

CONTRAINDICATIONS

None known.

INTERACTIONS

Drug

Alcohol, CNS depression-producing medications: May increase CNS depression.
Antihypertensives: May increase the effects of antihypertensives.
Digoxin, phenytoin: May increase the blood concentration of these drugs.
Indinavir, ketoconazole, ritonavir: May increase the blood concentration and toxicity of trazodone.

Herbal

St. John's wort: May increase the adverse effects of trazodone.

Food

None known.

DIAGNOSTIC TEST EFFECTS

May decrease serum WBC and neutrophil counts.

SIDE EFFECTS

Frequent (9%–3%)
Somnolence, dry mouth, lightheadedness, dizziness, headache, blurred vision, nausea, vomiting
Occasional (3%–1%)
Nervousness, fatigue, constipation, generalized aches and pains, mild hypotension
Rare
Photosensitivity reaction

SERIOUS REACTIONS

! Priapism, diminished or improved libido, retrograde ejaculation, and impotence occur rarely.

! Trazodone appears to be less cardiotoxic than other antidepressants, although arrhythmias may occur in patients with preexisting cardiac disease.

NURSING CONSIDERATIONS

Baseline Assessment

- Plan to perform a CBC and liver and renal function tests before and periodically during long-term therapy.

Lifespan Considerations

- Trazodone crosses the placenta and is minimally distributed in breast milk.
- The safety and efficacy of trazodone have not been established in children younger than 6 years.
- Lower dosages are recommended for the elderly, who are more likely to experience hypotensive or sedative effects.

Precautions

- Use trazodone cautiously in patients with arrhythmias or cardiac disease.

Administration and Handling

PO
- Give trazodone shortly after a meal or snack to reduces the risk of dizziness or light-headedness.
- Crush tablets, as needed.

Intervention and Evaluation

- Closely supervise suicidal patients during early therapy. As depression lessens, the patient's energy level generally improves, increasing the suicide potential.
- Assess the patient's appearance, behavior, level of interest, mood, and sleep pattern before and during therapy.
- Monitor the patient's serum neutrophil and WBC counts. Discontinue the drug, as ordered, if these counts drop.
- Assist the patient with ambulation

if he or she experiences dizziness or light-headedness.
- Monitor the EKG for arrhythmias.

Patient Teaching
- Advise the patient to take trazodone after a meal or snack to help prevent dizziness and light-headedness.
- Instruct the patient to take trazodone at bedtime if he or she experiences drowsiness while taking the drug.
- Explain that most patients develop a tolerance to the drug's anticholinergic and sedative effects early in therapy.
- Caution the patient against abruptly discontinuing the drug.
- Instruct the patient to change positions slowly to avoid the drug's hypotensive effect.
- Warn the patient to avoid tasks that require mental alertness or motor skills until his or her response to the drug has been established.
- Warn the male patient to immediately notify the physician if he experiences a painful, prolonged penile erection.
- Inform the patient that he or she may develop a photosensitivity to sunlight during trazodone therapy.
- Advise the patient to notify the physician if visual disturbances occur.
- Urge the patient to avoid alcohol while taking trazodone.
- Suggest that the patient take sips of tepid water or chew sugarless gum to relieve dry mouth.

venlafaxine

ven-la-**fax**-een
(Effexor, Effexor XR)

CATEGORY AND SCHEDULE
Pregnancy Risk Category: C

MECHANISM OF ACTION
A phenethylamine derivative that potentiates CNS neurotransmitter activity by inhibiting the reuptake of serotonin, norepinephrine, and, to a lesser degree, dopamine.
Therapeutic Effect: Relieves depression.

PHARMACOKINETICS
Well absorbed from the GI tract. Protein binding: 25%–30%. Metabolized in the liver to active metabolite. Primarily excreted in urine. Not removed by hemodialysis. ***Half-life:*** 3–7 hr; metabolite, 9–13 hr (increased in hepatic or renal impairment).

AVAILABILITY
Capsules (Extended-Release [Effexor XL]): 37.5 mg, 75 mg, 150 mg.
Tablets (Effexor): 25 mg, 37.5 mg, 50 mg, 75 mg, 100 mg.

INDICATIONS AND DOSAGES
▸ **Depression**

PO

Adults, Elderly. Initially, 75 mg/day in 2–3 divided doses with food. May increase by 75 mg/day at intervals of 4 days or longer. Maximum: 375 mg/day in 3 divided doses.

PO (Extended-Release)

Adults, Elderly. 75 mg/day as a single dose with food. May increase by 75 mg/day at intervals of 4 days or longer. Maximum: 225 mg/day.

▸ **Anxiety disorder**

PO (Extended-Release)

Adults. 37.5–225 mg/day.

▸ **Dosage in renal and hepatic impairment**

Expect to decrease venlafaxine dosage by 50% in patients with moderate hepatic impairment, 25% in patients with mild to moderate renal impairment, and 50% in patients on dialysis (withhold dose until completion of dialysis).

OFF-LABEL USES

Prevention of relapses of depression; treatment of attention-deficit hyperactivity disorder, autism, chronic fatigue syndrome, obsessive-compulsive disorder

CONTRAINDICATIONS

Use within 14 days of MAOIs

INTERACTIONS

Drug

MAOIs: May cause neuroleptic malignant syndrome, autonomic instability (including rapid fluctuations of vital signs), extreme agitation, hyperthermia, mental status changes, myoclonus, rigidity, and coma.

Herbal

St. John's wort: May increase the sedative-hypnotic effect of venlafaxine.

Food

None known.

DIAGNOSTIC TEST EFFECTS

May increase BUN level and serum alkaline phosphatase, bilirubin, cholesterol, uric acid, AST (SGOT), and ALT (SGPT) levels. May decrease serum phosphate and sodium levels. May alter blood glucose and serum potassium levels.

SIDE EFFECTS

Frequent (greater than 20%)

Nausea, somnolence, headache, dry mouth

Occasional (20%–10%)

Dizziness, insomnia, constipation, diaphoresis, nervousness, asthenia, ejaculatory disturbance, anorexia

Rare (less than 10%)

Anxiety, blurred vision, diarrhea, vomiting, tremor, abnormal dreams, impotence

SERIOUS REACTIONS

! A sustained increase in diastolic BP of 10–15 mm Hg occurs occasionally.

NURSING CONSIDERATIONS

Baseline Assessment

- Obtain the patient's baseline BP and weight.
- Assess the patient's appearance, behavior, level of interest, mood, and sleep pattern.

Lifespan Considerations

- It is unknown if venlafaxine is excreted in breast milk.
- The safety and efficacy of venlafaxine have not been established in children.
- No age-related precautions have been noted in the elderly.

Precautions

- Use venlafaxine cautiously in suicidal patients and patients with abnormal platelet function, CHF, volume depletion, hyperthyroidism, mania, angle-closure glaucoma, hepatic or renal impairment, or seizure disorder.

Administration and Handling

◀ALERT▶ When discontinuing venlafaxine, plan to taper the dosage slowly over 2 weeks.

◀ALERT▶ Allow at least 14 days to elapse before switching the patient from an MAOI to venlafaxine and at least 7 days to elapse before switching the patient from venlafaxine to an MAOI.

PO

- Administer venlafaxine with food or milk if the patient experiences GI distress.
- Crush scored tablets if needed.
- Do not break, open, or crush extended-release capsules.

Intervention and Evaluation

- Closely supervise the suicidal patient during early therapy. As depression lessens, the patient's energy level improves, increasing the suicide potential.

- Assess the patient's appearance, behavior, level of interest, mood, and sleep patterns for evidence of a therapeutic response.
- Monitor the patient's BP and weight.
- If the patient experiences anxiety, dizziness, or somnolence, provide assistance as necessary.

Patient Teaching

- Instruct the patient to take venlafaxine with food to minimize GI distress.
- Caution the patient against abruptly discontinuing the drug or decreasing or increasing the dosage.
- Warn the patient to avoid tasks that require mental alertness or motor skills until his or her response to the drug has been established.
- Instruct the patient to notify the physician if she is breast-feeding, pregnant, or planning to become pregnant.
- Urge the patient to avoid alcohol while taking venlafaxine.

35 Antiemetics

aprepitant
chlorpromazine
dimenhydrinate
dolasetron
dronabinol
granisetron
meclizine
metoclopramide
ondansetron hydrochloride
palonosetron hydrochloride
prochlorperazine
scopolamine
trimethobenzamide hydrochloride

Uses: Antiemetics are used to suppress vomiting (emesis). Resulting from chemotherapy, motion sickness, and other causes, emesis is a complex reflex caused by activation of the vomiting center in the medulla oblongata.

Action: Each subclass of antiemetics has a different mechanism of action. *Serotonin antagonists,* such as ondansetron, block serotonin receptors peripherally on vagal nerve terminals and centrally in the chemoreceptor trigger zone (CTZ). *Dopamine antagonists,* such as chlorpromazine, block dopamine receptors in the CTZ. *Cannabinoids,* such as dronabinol, act by an unknown mechanism. *Anticholinergics,* such as scopolamine, block muscarinic receptors in the pathway from the inner ear to the vomiting center. *Antihistamines,* such as dimenhydrinate, block histamine (H_1) and muscarinic receptors in the pathway from the inner ear to the vomiting center. In addition, *aprepitant* antagonizes neurokinin receptors in the CTZ, and *palonosetron* antagonizes serotonin subtype 3 ($5HT_3$) receptors in the CTZ and peripherally.

COMBINATION PRODUCTS

DONNATAL: scopolamine/atropine (an anticholinergic)/hyoscyamine (an anticholinergic)/phenobarbital (an anticonvulsant) 0.0065 mg/0.0194 mg/0.1037 mg/16.2 mg.

aprepitant

ah-**prep**-ih-tant
(Emend)

CATEGORY AND SCHEDULE

Pregnancy Risk Category: B

MECHANISM OF ACTION

A selective human substance P and neurokinin-1 (NK_1) receptor antagonist that inhibits chemotherapy-induced nausea and vomiting centrally in the chemoreceptor trigger zone. **Therapeutic Effect:** Prevents the acute and delayed phases of chemotherapy-induced emesis, including vomiting caused by high-dose cisplatin.

PHARMACOKINETICS

Crosses the blood-brain barrier. Extensively metabolized in the liver. Eliminated primarily by liver metabolism (not excreted renally). ***Half-life:*** 9–13 hr.

AVAILABILITY

Capsules: 80 mg, 125 mg.

INDICATIONS AND DOSAGES

▸ **Prevention of chemotherapy-induced nausea and vomiting**
PO
Adults, Elderly: 125 mg 1 hr before

chemotherapy on day 1 and 80 mg once a day in the morning on days 2 and 3.

CONTRAINDICATIONS

Breast-feeding, concurrent use of pimozide (Orap)

INTERACTIONS

Drug

Alprazolam, docetaxel, etoposide, ifosfamide, imatinib, irinotecan, midazolam, paclitaxel, triazolam, vinblastine, vincristine, vinorelbine: May increase the plasma concentrations of these drugs.
Antifungals, clarithromycin, diltiazem, nefazodone, nelfinavir, ritonavir: Increase aprepitant plasma concentration.
Carbamazepine, phenytoin, rifampin: Decrease aprepitant plasma concentration.
Contraceptives: May decrease the effectiveness of contraceptives.
Paroxetine: May decrease the effectiveness of either drug.
Steroids: Increases the blood levels and effects of steroids.
Warfarin: May decrease the effectiveness of warfarin.

Herbal

None known.

Food

None known.

DIAGNOSTIC TEST EFFECTS

May increase BUN level and serum creatinine, AST (SGOT), and ALT (SGPT) levels. May produce proteinuria.

SIDE EFFECTS

Frequent (17%–10%)
Fatigue, nausea, hiccups, diarrhea, constipation, anorexia
Occasional (8%–4%)
Headache, vomiting, dizziness, dehydration, heartburn
Rare (3% or less)
Abdominal pain, epigastric discomfort, gastritis, tinnitus, insomnia

SERIOUS REACTIONS

! Neutropenia and mucous membrane disorders occur rarely.

NURSING CONSIDERATIONS

Baseline Assessment

- Assess the patient who experiences severe vomiting for signs and symptoms of dehydration, including dry mucous membranes, longitudinal furrow in the tongue, and poor skin turgor.

Lifespan Considerations

- It is unknown if aprepitant crosses the placenta or is distributed in breast milk.
- The safety and efficacy of aprepitant have not been established in children.
- No age-related precautions have been noted in the elderly.

Administration and Handling

PO

◀ **ALERT** ▶ As prescribed, give aprepitant with 12 mg dexamethasone PO and 32 mg ondansetron IV on day 1, and with 8 mg dexamethasone PO on days 2 to 4.

- Give aprepitant without regard to food.
- If the patient is also receiving a steroid, expect to reduce the IV steroid dose by 25% and the oral dose by 50%.

Intervention and Evaluation

- Assist the patient with ambulation if he or she experiences dizziness.
- Assess the patient's pattern of daily bowel activity and stool consistency. Also auscultate bowel sounds for peristalsis and record time of evacuation.
- Offer the patient emotional support.

Patient Teaching

• Inform the patient nausea and vomiting should be relieved shortly after drug administration.
• Instruct the patient to notify the physician if he or she experiences headache or persistent vomiting.

chlorpromazine

klor-**proe**-ma-zeen
(Chlorpromanyl[CAN], Largactil[CAN], Thorazine)
Do not confuse chlorpromazine with chlorpropamide, clomipramine, or prochlorperazine; or Thorazine with thiamide or thioridazine.

CATEGORY AND SCHEDULE

Pregnancy Risk Category: C

MECHANISM OF ACTION

A phenothiazine that blocks dopamine neurotransmission at postsynaptic dopamine receptor sites. Possesses strong anticholinergic, sedative, and antiemetic effects; moderate extrapyramidal effects; and slight antihistamine action. **Therapeutic Effect:** Relieves nausea and vomiting; improves psychotic conditions; controls intractable hiccups and porphyria.

PHARMACOKINETICS

Rapidly absorbed after oral or IM administration. Protein binding: 92%–97%. Metabolized in the liver. Excreted in urine. ***Half-life:*** 6 hr.

AVAILABILITY

Oral Concentrate: 30 mg/ml, 100 mg/ml.
Syrup: 10 mg/5 ml.
Tablets: 10 mg, 25 mg, 50 mg, 100 mg, 200 mg.
Capsules (Sustained-Release): 30 mg, 75 mg, 150 mg.
Injection (Thorazine): 25 mg/ml.
Suppositories: 25 mg, 100 mg.

INDICATIONS AND DOSAGES

▸ Severe nausea or vomiting
PO
Adults, Elderly. 10–25 mg q4–6h.
Children. 0.5–1 mg/kg q4–6h.
IM, IV
Adults, Elderly. 25–50 mg q4–6h.
Children. 0.5–1 mg/kg q6–8h.
Rectal
Adults, Elderly. 50–100 mg q6–8h.
Children. 1 mg/kg q6–8h.

▸ Psychotic disorders
PO
Adults, Elderly. 30–800 mg/day in 1–4 divided doses.
Children older than 6 mo. 0.5–1 mg/kg q4–6h.
IV, IM
Adults, Elderly. Initially, 25 mg; may repeat in 1–4 hr. May gradually increase to 400 mg q4–6h. Maximum: 300–800 mg/day.
Children older than 6 mo. 0.5–1 mg/kg q6–8h. Maximum: 75 mg/day for children 5–12 yr; 40 mg/day for children younger than 5 yr.

▸ Intractable hiccups
PO, IV, IM
Adults. 25–50 mg 3 times a day.

▸ Porphyria
PO
Adults. 25–50 mg 3–4 times a day.
IM
Adults, Elderly. 25 mg 3–4 times a day.

OFF-LABEL USES

Treatment of choreiform movement of Huntington's disease

CONTRAINDICATIONS

Comatose states, myelosuppression, severe cardiovascular disease, severe

CNS depression, subcortical brain damage

INTERACTIONS

Drug

Alcohol, other CNS depressants: May increase respiratory depression and the hypotensive effects of chlorpromazine.
Antithyroid agents: May increase the risk of agranulocytosis.
Extrapyramidal symptom-producing medications: Increased risk of extrapyramidal symptoms.
Hypotensives: May increase hypotension.
Levodopa: May decrease the effects of levodopa.
Lithium: May decrease the absorption of chlorpromazine and produce adverse neurologic effects.
MAOIs, tricyclic antidepressants: May increase the anticholinergic and sedative effects of chlorpromazine.

Herbal

None known.

Food

None known.

DIAGNOSTIC TEST EFFECTS

May produce false-positive pregnancy and phenylketonuria (PKU) test results. May cause EKG changes, including Q- and T-wave disturbances. Therapeutic serum drug level is 50–300 mcg/ml; toxic serum drug level is greater than 750 mcg/ml.

SIDE EFFECTS

Frequent

Somnolence, blurred vision, hypotension, color vision or night vision disturbances, dizziness, decreased sweating, constipation, dry mouth, nasal congestion

Occasional

Urinary retention, photosensitivity, rash, decreased sexual function, swelling or pain in breasts, weight gain, nausea, vomiting, abdominal pain, tremors

SERIOUS REACTIONS

! Extrapyramidal symptoms appear to be dose related and are divided into three categories: akathisia (including inability to sit still, tapping of feet), parkinsonian symptoms (such as masklike face, tremors, shuffling gait, hypersalivation), and acute dystonias (including torticollis, opisthotonos, and oculogyric crisis). A dystonic reaction may also produce diaphoresis and pallor.
! Tardive dyskinesia, including tongue protrusion, puffing of the cheeks, and puckering of the mouth is a rare reaction that may be irreversible.
! Abrupt discontinuation after long-term therapy may precipitate nausea, vomiting, gastritis, dizziness, and tremors.
! Blood dyscrasias, particularly agranulocytosis and mild leukopenia, may occur.
! Chlorpromazine may lower the seizure threshold.

NURSING CONSIDERATIONS

Baseline Assessment

- Avoid skin contact with solution to prevent contact dermatitis.
- Assess the patient for signs and symptoms of dehydration including dry mucous membranes, longitudinal furrows in the tongue, and poor skin turgor.
- Assess the appearance, behavior, emotional status, response to the environment, speech pattern, and thought content of the patient being treated for psychotic disorders.

Precautions

- Use chlorpromazine cautiously in patients with alcoholism; glaucoma;

history of seizures; hypocalcemia (increases susceptibility to dystonias); impaired cardiac, hepatic, renal, or respiratory function; benign prostatic hyperplasia, or urine retention.

Administration and Handling

• Avoid skin contact with the oral concentrate and syrup to prevent contact dermatitis.
• A slight yellow color in the oral concentrate or syrup won't affect the drug's potency. However, discard the drug if it is markedly discolored or contains precipitate.
• Dilute each dose of oral concentrate immediately before administration with 60 ml or more of water, coffee, tea, milk, carbonated beverage, tomato or fruit juice, simple syrup, orange syrup, soup, or pudding. Use immediately and discard any remaining mixture.

IM

◀ **ALERT** ▶ Do not give chlorpromazine by the subcutaneous route because severe tissue necrosis may occur.

• To prevent irritation at the injection site, dilute the injection solution with sodium chloride for injection or add 2% procaine, as prescribed.

Intervention and Evaluation

• Monitor the patient's BP for hypotension.
• Monitor the patient for signs of tardive dyskinesia, such as tongue protrusion, and for extrapyramidal symptoms.
• Regularly check the patient's CBC, as ordered, for evidence of blood dyscrasias.
• Monitor serum calcium levels to detect hypocalcemia.
• Supervise the suicidal psychotic patient closely during early therapy; as depression lessens, the patient's energy level improves, increasing the risk of suicide.
• Assess the psychotic patient for a therapeutic response, including increased ability to concentrate and interest in surroundings, improvement in self-care, and a relaxed facial expression.
• Monitor the patient's serum drug level. The therapeutic serum level for chlorpromazine is 50 to 300 mcg/ml, and the toxic serum level is greater than 750 mcg/ml.

Patient Teaching

• Inform the patient that the drug's full therapeutic benefit may require up to 6 weeks to appear.
• Caution the patient against abruptly discontinuing the drug after long-term drug therapy.
• Advise the patient that urine may darken.
• Instruct the patient to notify the physician if visual disturbances occur.
• Inform the patient that drowsiness generally subsides with continued therapy.
• Warn the patient to avoid tasks that require mental alertness or motor skills until his or her response to the drug has been established.
• Urge the patient to avoid alcohol and excessive exposure to sunlight while taking chlorpromazine.

dimenhydrinate

dye-men-**hye**-dri-nate
(Dramamine)

CATEGORY AND SCHEDULE

Pregnancy Risk Category: B

MECHANISM OF ACTION

An antihistamine and anticholinergic that competes for H_1 receptor sites on effector cells of the GI tract, blood vessels, and respiratory tract.

The anticholinergic action diminishes vestibular stimulation and depresses labyrinthine function. **Therapeutic Effect:** Prevents symptoms of motion sickness.

AVAILABILITY

Tablets (Chewable): 50 mg.
Tablets: 50 mg.

INDICATIONS AND DOSAGES

▸ Motion sickness

PO

Adults, Elderly, Children older than 12 yr. 50–100 mg q4–6h. Maximum: 400 mg/day.
Children 6–12 yr. 25–50 mg q6–8h. Maximum: 150 mg/day.
Children 2–5 yr. 12.5–25 mg q6–8h. Maximum: 75 mg/day.

CONTRAINDICATIONS

None significant.

INTERACTIONS

Drug

Alcohol, other CNS suppressants: May increase CNS depression.
Aminoglycosides: Masks signs and symptoms of ototoxicity associated with aminoglycosides.
Other anticholinergics: Increases anticholinergic effect.

Herbal

None known.

Food

None known.

DIAGNOSTIC TEST EFFECTS

None known.

SIDE EFFECTS

Frequent

Dry mouth

Occasional

Hypotension, palpitations, tachycardia, headache, somnolence, dizziness, paradoxical stimulation (especially in children), anorexia, constipation, dysuria, blurred vision, tinnitus, wheezing, chest tightness

Rare

Photosensitivity, rash, urticaria

SERIOUS REACTIONS

! None significant.

NURSING CONSIDERATIONS

Baseline Assessment

- Assess the patient's other medical conditions, such as asthma, glaucoma, benign prostatic hyperplasia, and seizures.
- Obtain the patient's medication history, especially concurrent use of other anticholinergics and CNS depressants.

Precautions

- Use dimenhydrinate cautiously in patients with asthma, bladder neck obstruction, history of seizures, angle-closure glaucoma, or benign prostatic hyperplasia.

Administration and Handling

PO

- Tablets may be swallowed whole, chewed, or allowed to dissolve.
- For motion sickness, give dimenhydrinate 1 to 2 hours before the activity that may cause motion sickness.

Intervention and Evaluation

- Monitor the patient's BP, and be alert for paradoxical reactions, especially in children, and signs and symptoms of motion sickness.

Patient Teaching

- Inform the patient that dimenhydrinate may cause drowsiness, dizziness, and dry mouth.
- Warn the patient to avoid tasks requiring mental alertness or motor skills until his or her response to the drug has been established.
- Urge the patient to avoid alcohol during dimenhydrinate therapy.
- Caution the patient to avoid pro-

longed sun exposure because the drug may cause a photosensitivity reaction.

dolasetron

doe-**lass**-eh-tron
(Anzemet)
Do not confuse Anzemet with Aldomet.

CATEGORY AND SCHEDULE

Pregnancy Risk Category: B

MECHANISM OF ACTION

A 5-HT_3 receptor antagonist that acts centrally in the chemoreceptor trigger zone and peripherally at the vagal nerve terminals. **Therapeutic Effect:** Prevents nausea and vomiting.

PHARMACOKINETICS

Readily absorbed from the GI tract after PO administration. Protein binding: 69%–77%. Metabolized in the liver. Primarily excreted in urine. Unknown if removed by hemodialysis. ***Half-life:*** 5–10 hr.

AVAILABILITY

Tablets: 50 mg, 100 mg.
Injection: 20 mg/ml in single use 0.625 ml amps, 0.625 ml fill in 2 ml Carpuject and 5 ml vials.

INDICATIONS AND DOSAGES

▸ Prevention of chemotherapy-induced nausea and vomiting

PO

Adults. 100 mg within 1 hr of chemotherapy.
Children 2–16 yr. 1.8 mg/kg within 1 hr of chemotherapy. Maximum: 100 mg.

IV

Adults, Children 1–16 yr. 1.8 mg/kg as a single dose 30 min before chemotherapy. Maximum: 100 mg.

▸ Treatment or prevention of postoperative nausea or vomiting

PO

Adults. 100 mg within 2 hr of surgery.
Children 2–16 yr. 1.2 mg/kg within 2 hr of surgery. Maximum: 100 mg.

IV

Adults. 12.5 mg 15 min before cessation of anesthesia or as soon as nausea occurs.
Children 2–16 yr. 0.35 mg/kg 15 min before cessation of anesthesia or as soon as nausea occurs. Maximum: 12.5 mg.

OFF-LABEL USES

Radiation therapy–induced nausea and vomiting

CONTRAINDICATIONS

None known.

INTERACTIONS

Drug
None known.
Herbal
None known.
Food
None known.

DIAGNOSTIC TEST EFFECTS

May transiently increase AST (SGOT) and ALT (SGPT) levels.

IV INCOMPATIBILITIES

No information available for Y-site administration.

SIDE EFFECTS

Frequent (10%–5%)
Headache, diarrhea, fatigue
Occasional (5%–1%)
Fever, dizziness, tachycardia, dyspepsia

SERIOUS REACTIONS

! Overdose may produce a combination of CNS stimulant and depressant effects.

NURSING CONSIDERATIONS

Baseline Assessment

- Assess the patient who experiences severe vomiting for signs and symptoms of dehydration, including dry mucous membranes, longitudinal furrows in the tongue, and poor skin turgor.

Lifespan Considerations

- It is unknown if dolasetron is distributed in breast milk.
- The safety and efficacy of this drug have not been established in children younger than 2 years.
- No age-related precautions have been noted in the elderly.

Precautions

- Use dolasetron cautiously in patients with congenital prolonged QT interval syndrome, hypokalemia, hypomagnesemia, or prolonged cardiac conduction intervals.
- Use dolasetron cautiously in patients taking diuretics with the potential to cause electrolyte disturbances, antiarrhythmics that may lead to prolonged QT interval, or high doses of anthracyclines.

Administration and Handling

PO

- Do not cut, break, or chew film-coated tablets.
- For children 2–16 years, injection form may be mixed in apple or apple-grape juice and given orally, if needed, at a dosage of 1.8 mg/kg up to a maximum of 100 mg.

IV

- Store vials at room temperature.
- After dilution, store solution for up to 24 hours at room temperature or up to 48 hours if refrigerated.
- Dilute the injection in 0.9% NaCl, D_5W, dextrose 5% in 0.45% NaCl, lactated Ringer's (LR) solution, D_5LR, or 10% mannitol injection to 50 ml.
- After dilution, the solution may be stored for up to 24 hours at room temperature or up to 48 hours if refrigerated.
- Administer by IV push as rapidly as 100 mg/30 second or by intermittent or piggyback IV infusion over 15 minutes.

Intervention and Evaluation

- Assess the patient for relief of nausea and vomiting.
- Monitor the EKG of high-risk patients.
- Maintain a quiet, supportive atmosphere.
- Offer the patient emotional support.

Patient Teaching

- Instruct the patient not to cut, break, or chew film-coated tablets.
- Advise the postoperative patient to report nausea as soon as it occurs because prompt administration of the drug increases its effectiveness.
- Teach the patient other methods of reducing nausea, such as lying quietly and avoiding strong odors.

dronabinol

droe-**nab**-i-nol

(Marinol)

Do not confuse dronabinol with droperidol.

CATEGORY AND SCHEDULE

Pregnancy Risk Category: C

Controlled Substance: Schedule III

MECHANISM OF ACTION

An antiemetic and appetite stimulant that may act by inhibiting vomiting control mechanisms in the medulla oblongata. **Therapeutic Effect:** Inhibits vomiting and stimulates appetite.

AVAILABILITY

Capsules (Gelatin): 2.5 mg, 5 mg, 10 mg.

INDICATIONS AND DOSAGES

▸ Prevention of chemotherapy-induced nausea and vomiting

PO

Adults, Children. Initially, 5 mg/m^2 1–3 hr before chemotherapy, then q2–4h after chemotherapy for total of 4–6 doses a day. May increase by 2.5 mg/m^2 up to 15 mg/m^2 per dose.

▸ Appetite stimulant

PO

Adults. Initially, 2.5 mg twice a day (before lunch and dinner). Range: 2.5–20 mg/day.

CONTRAINDICATIONS

Treatment of nausea and vomiting not caused by chemotherapy

INTERACTIONS

Drug

Alcohol, other CNS suppressants: May increase CNS depression.

Herbal

None known.

Food

None known.

DIAGNOSTIC TEST EFFECTS

None known.

SIDE EFFECTS

Frequent (24%–3%)

Euphoria, dizziness, paranoid reaction, somnolence

Occasional (3%–1%)

Asthenia, ataxia, confusion, abnormal thinking, depersonalization

Rare (less than 1%)

Diarrhea, depression, nightmares, speech difficulties, headache, anxiety, tinnitus, flushed skin

SERIOUS REACTIONS

! Mild intoxication may produce increased sensory awareness (including taste, smell, and sound), altered time perception, reddened conjunctiva, dry mouth, and tachycardia.

! Moderate intoxication may produce memory impairment and urine retention.

! Severe intoxication may produce lethargy, decreased motor coordination, slurred speech, and orthostatic hypotension.

NURSING CONSIDERATIONS

Baseline Assessment

- Assess the patient who experiences severe vomiting for signs and symptoms of dehydration, including dry mucous membranes, low urine output, and poor skin turgor.

Lifespan Considerations

- Dronabinol use is not recommended for children.

Precautions

- Use dronabinol cautiously in patients with heart disease, hypertension, depression, mania, or schizophrenia.

Intervention and Evaluation

- Observe the patient closely for serious behavioral and mood reactions.
- Monitor the patient's BP and heart rate.

Patient Teaching

- If the patient is taking dronabinol to stimulate appetite, instruct him or her to take it before lunch and dinner.
- Inform the patient that relief from nausea or vomiting generally occurs within 15 minutes of drug administration.

• Urge the patient to avoid alcohol, barbiturates, and other CNS depressants while taking dronabinol.
• Warn the patient to avoid tasks that require mental alertness or motor skills until his or her response to the drug has been established.

granisetron

gra-**ni**-se-tron
(Kytril)

CATEGORY AND SCHEDULE

Pregnancy Risk Category: B

MECHANISM OF ACTION

A 5-HT_3 receptor antagonist that acts centrally in the chemoreceptor trigger zone or peripherally at the vagal nerve terminals. **Therapeutic Effect:** Prevents nausea and vomiting.

PHARMACOKINETICS

Route	Onset	Peak	Duration
IV	1–3 min	N/A	24 hr

Rapidly and widely distributed to tissues. Protein binding: 65%. Metabolized in the liver to active metabolite. Eliminated in urine and feces. ***Half-life:*** 10–12 hr (increased in the elderly).

AVAILABILITY

Oral Solution: 1 mg/5 ml.
Tablets: 1 mg.
Injection: 0.1 mg/ml, 1 mg/ml.

INDICATIONS AND DOSAGES

▸ **Prevention of chemotherapy-induced nausea and vomiting**
PO
Adults, Elderly. 2 mg once a day up to 1 hr before chemotherapy or 1 mg twice a day.
IV
Adults, Elderly, Children 2 yr and older. 10 mcg/kg/dose (or 1 mg/dose) within 30 min of chemotherapy.

▸ **Prevention of radiation-induced nausea and vomiting**
PO
Adults, Elderly. 2 mg once a day given 1 hr before radiation therapy.

▸ **Postoperative nausea or vomiting**
PO
Adults, Elderly, Children 4 yr and older. 20–40 mcg/kg as a single postoperative dose.
IV
Adults, Elderly. 1 mg as a single postoperative dose.
Children older than 4 yr. 20–40 mcg/kg. Maximum: 1 mg.

OFF-LABEL USES

PO: Prophylaxis of nausea or vomiting associated with radiation therapy

CONTRAINDICATIONS

None known.

INTERACTIONS

Drug
Hepatic enzyme inducers: May decrease the effects of granisetron.
Herbal
None known.
Food
None known.

DIAGNOSTIC TEST EFFECTS

May increase AST (SGOT) and ALT (SGPT) levels.

IV INCOMPATIBILITIES

Amphotericin B (Fungizone)

IV COMPATIBILITIES

Allopurinol (Aloprim), bumetanide (Bumex), calcium gluconate, carboplatin (Paraplatin), cisplatin (Platinol), cyclophosphamide (Cytoxan), cytarabine (Ara-C), dacarbazine (DTIC-Dome), dexamethasone (Decadron), diphenhydramine (Benadryl), docetaxel (Taxotere), doxorubicin (Adriamycin), etoposide (VePesid), gemcitabine (Gemzar), magnesium, mitoxantrone (Novantrone), paclitaxel (Taxol), potassium

SIDE EFFECTS

Frequent (21%–14%)
Headache, constipation, asthenia
Occasional (8%–6%)
Diarrhea, abdominal pain
Rare (less than 2%)
Altered taste, hypersensitivity reaction

SERIOUS REACTIONS

! None known.

NURSING CONSIDERATIONS

Baseline Assessment

• Assess the patient for nausea and vomiting, and auscultate bowel sounds before and during drug therapy.

Lifespan Considerations

• It is unknown if granisetron is distributed in breast milk.
• The safety and efficacy of granisetron have not been established in children younger than 2 years.
• No age-related precautions have been noted in the elderly.

Precautions

• Use granisetron cautiously in patients younger than 2 years.

Administration and Handling

◀ ALERT ▶
• Administer only on days of chemotherapy, as prescribed.
• Administer oral granisetron to the patient within 1 hour and the IV form within 30 minutes before starting chemotherapy.

PO
• Keep the bottle of oral solution tightly closed. Protect the bottle from light, and store it in an upright position.

IV
• Store vials at room temperature.
• The solution normally appears clear and colorless. Inspect it for particles and discoloration.
• Administer granisetron undiluted or dilute it with 20 to 50 ml 0.9% NaCl or D_5W. Don't mix it with other medications.
• After dilution, the solution is stable for at least 24 hours at room temperature.
• Administer the undiluted drug by IV push over 30 seconds.
• For IV piggyback, infuse over 5 to 20 minutes, depending on the volume of diluent used.

Intervention and Evaluation

• Monitor the patient for therapeutic effect.
• Assess the patient for headache.
• Assess the patient's pattern of daily bowel activity and stool consistency.

Patient Teaching

• Inform the patient that granisetron is effective shortly after administration in preventing nausea and vomiting.
• Explain to the patient that the drug may affect the sense of taste temporarily.
• Teach the patient other methods of reducing nausea and vomiting, such as lying quietly and avoiding strong odors.

meclizine

mek-li-zeen
(Antivert, Bonamine[CAN], Bonine)
Do not confuse Antivert with Axert.

CATEGORY AND SCHEDULE

Pregnancy Risk Category: B

MECHANISM OF ACTION

An anticholinergic that reduces labyrinthine excitability and diminishes vestibular stimulation of the labyrinth, affecting the chemoreceptor trigger zone. **Therapeutic Effect:** Reduces nausea, vomiting, and vertigo.

PHARMACOKINETICS

Route	Onset	Peak	Duration
PO	30–60 min	N/A	12–24 hr

Well absorbed from the GI tract. Widely distributed. Metabolized in the liver. Primarily excreted in urine. ***Half-life:*** 6 hr.

AVAILABILITY

Tablets (Antivert): 12.5 mg, 25 mg, 50 mg.
Tablets (Chewable [Bonine]): 25 mg.

INDICATIONS AND DOSAGES

▸ **Motion sickness**

PO

Adults, Elderly, Children 12 yr and older. 12.5–25 mg 1 hr before travel. May repeat q12–24h. May require a dose of 50 mg.

▸ **Vertigo**

PO

Adults, Elderly, Children 12 yr and older. 25–100 mg/day in divided doses, as needed.

CONTRAINDICATIONS

None known.

INTERACTIONS

Drug

Alcohol, CNS depression-producing medications: May increase CNS depressant effect.

Herbal

None known.

Food

None known.

DIAGNOSTIC TEST EFFECTS

May produce false-negative results in antigen skin testing unless meclizine is discontinued 4 days before testing.

SIDE EFFECTS

Frequent

Drowsiness

Occasional

Blurred vision; dry mouth, nose, or throat

SERIOUS REACTIONS

! A hypersensitivity reaction, marked by eczema, pruritus, rash, cardiac disturbances, and photosensitivity, may occur.
! Overdose may produce CNS depression (manifested as sedation, apnea, cardiovascular collapse, or death) or severe paradoxical reactions (such as hallucinations, tremor, and seizures).
! Children may experience paradoxical reactions, including restlessness, insomnia, euphoria, nervousness, and tremors.
! Overdose in children may result in hallucinations, seizures, and death.

NURSING CONSIDERATIONS

Lifespan Considerations

• It is unknown if meclizine crosses the placenta or is distributed in breast

milk: Meclizine use may produce irritability in breast-feeding infants.
• Children and the elderly may be more sensitive to the drug's anticholinergic effects, such as dry mouth.

Precautions
• Use meclizine cautiously in patients with angle-closure glaucoma or obstructive diseases of the GI or GU tract.

Administration and Handling

◀ALERT▶
• Elderly patients (older than 60 years) are at increased risk for developing agitation, disorientation, dizziness, sedation, hypotension, confusion, and psychotic-like symptoms.

PO
• Give meclizine without regard to food.
• Crush scored tablets if needed.

Intervention and Evaluation
• Monitor the patient's BP, especially in elderly patients, who are at increased risk for hypotension.
• Monitor children closely for paradoxical reactions.
• Monitor serum electrolyte levels of patients experiencing severe vomiting.
• Assess the patient's mucous membranes and skin turgor to evaluate hydration status.

Patient Teaching
• Inform the patient that meclizine commonly causes dizziness, drowsiness, and dry mouth.
• Tell the patient that coffee or tea may help reduce drowsiness. Explain that he or she will probably develop a tolerance to the drug's sedative effect.
• Warn the patient to avoid tasks that require mental alertness or motor skills until his or her response to the drug has been established.
• Urge the patient to avoid alcohol during meclizine therapy.
• Suggest taking sips of tepid water and chewing sugarless gum to help relieve dry mouth.

metoclopramide

met-oh-kloe-**pra**-mide
(Apo-Metoclop[CAN], Maxolon [AUS], Pramin[AUS], Reglan)
Do not confuse Reglan with Renagel.

CATEGORY AND SCHEDULE
Pregnancy Risk Category: B

MECHANISM OF ACTION
A dopamine receptor antagonist that stimulates motility of the upper GI tract and decreases reflux into the esophagus. Also raises the threshold of activity in the chemoreceptor trigger zone. **Therapeutic Effect:** Accelerates intestinal transit and gastric emptying; relieves nausea and vomiting.

PHARMACOKINETICS

Route	Onset	Peak	Duration
PO	30–60 min	N/A	N/A
IV	1–3 min	N/A	N/A
IM	10–15 min	N/A	N/A

Well absorbed from the GI tract. Metabolized in the liver. Protein binding: 30%. Primarily excreted in urine. Not removed by hemodialysis. ***Half-life:*** 4–6 hr.

AVAILABILITY
Syrup: 5 mg/5 ml.
Tablets: 5 mg, 10 mg.
Injection: 5 mg/ml.

INDICATIONS AND DOSAGES

▸ Prevention of chemotherapy-induced nausea and vomiting

IV

Adults, Elderly, Children. 1–2 mg/kg 30 min before chemotherapy; repeat q2h for 2 doses, then q3h as needed.

▸ Postoperative nausea and vomiting

IV

Adults, Elderly, Children 15 yr and older. 10 mg; repeat q6–8h as needed.

Children 14 yr and younger. 0.1–0.2 mg/kg/dose; repeat q6–8h as needed.

▸ Diabetic gastroparesis

PO, IV

Adults. 10 mg 30 min before meals and at bedtime for 2–8 wk.

PO

Elderly. Initially, 5 mg 30 min before meals and at bedtime. May increase to 10 mg.

IV

Elderly. 5 mg over 1–2 min. May increase to 10 mg.

▸ Symptomatic gastroesophageal reflux

PO

Adults. 10–15 mg up to 4 times a day, or single doses up to 20 mg as needed.

Elderly. Initially, 5 mg 4 times a day. May increase to 10 mg.

Children. 0.4–0.8 mg/kg/day in 4 divided doses.

▸ To facilitate small bowel intubation (single dose)

IV

Adults, Elderly. 10 mg as a single dose.

Children 6–14 yr. 2.5–5 mg as a single dose.

Children younger than 6 yr. 0.1 mg/kg as a single dose.

▸ Dosage in renal impairment

Dosage is modified based on creatinine clearance.

Creatinine Clearance	% of normal dose
40–50 ml/min	75%
10–40 ml/min	50%
less than 10 ml/min	25%–50%

OFF-LABEL USES

Prevention of aspiration pneumonia; treatment of drug-related postoperative nausea and vomiting, persistent hiccups, slow gastric emptying, vascular headaches

CONTRAINDICATIONS

Concurrent use of medications likely to produce extrapyramidal reactions, GI hemorrhage, GI obstruction or perforation, history of seizure disorders, pheochromocytoma

INTERACTIONS

Drug

Alcohol, other CNS suppressants: May increase CNS depressant effect.

Herbal

None known.

Food

None known.

DIAGNOSTIC TEST EFFECTS

May increase serum aldosterone and prolactin concentrations.

IV INCOMPATIBILITIES

Allopurinol (Aloprim), cefepime (Maxipime), doxorubicin liposomal (Doxil), furosemide (Lasix), propofol (Diprivan)

IV COMPATIBILITIES

Dexamethasone, diltiazem (Cardizem), diphenhydramine (Benadryl), fentanyl (Sublimaze), heparin, hydromorphone (Dilaudid), morphine, potassium chloride

SIDE EFFECTS

Frequent (10%)
Somnolence, restlessness, fatigue, lethargy
Occasional (3%)
Dizziness, anxiety, headache, insomnia, breast tenderness, altered menstruation, constipation, rash, dry mouth, galactorrhea, gynecomastia
Rare (less than 3%)
Hypotension or hypertension, tachycardia

SERIOUS REACTIONS

! Extrapyramidal reactions occur most commonly in children and young adults (18–30 years) receiving large doses (2 mg/kg) during chemotherapy and are usually limited to akathisia (involuntary limb movement and facial grimacing).

NURSING CONSIDERATIONS

Baseline Assessment

• Assess the patient taking metoclopramide as an antiemetic for signs of dehydration, such as dry mucous membranes, longitudinal furrows in the tongue, and poor skin turgor.

Lifespan Considerations

• Metoclopramide crosses the placenta and is distributed in breast milk.
• Children are more susceptible to dystonic reactions.
• Elderly patients are more likely to have parkinsonian reactions and dyskinesias after long-term therapy.

Precautions

• Use metoclopramide cautiously in patients with cirrhosis, CHF, or renal impairment.

Administration and Handling

◀ALERT▶ Metoclopramide may be given by PO and IM routes and by IV push or IV infusion.
◀ALERT▶ Doses of 2 mg/kg or more or prolonged therapy may increase the incidence of side effects.

PO
• Give metoclopramide 30 minutes before meals and at bedtime.
• Crush tablets as needed.

IV
• Store vials at room temperature.
• Dilute doses greater than 10 mg in 50 ml D_5W, 0.9% NaCl, or lactated Ringer's solution.
• After dilution, IV piggyback infusion is stable for 48 hours.
• Infuse over 15 minutes.
• Give slow IV push of 10 mg over 1 to 2 minutes.
• Too-rapid IV injection may produce intense anxiety or restlessness, followed by drowsiness.

Intervention and Evaluation

• Monitor the patient for anxiety, extrapyramidal symptoms, and restlessness during IV administration.
• Assess the patient's pattern of daily bowel activity and stool consistency.
• Assess the patient's skin for rash.
• Evaluate the patient with gastroparesis for a therapeutic response, such as relief of bloating, nausea, and vomiting.
• Monitor the patient's BP, heart rate, and BUN and serum creatinine levels to assess renal function.

Patient Teaching

• Warn the patient to avoid tasks that require mental alertness or motor skills until his or her response to the drug has established.
• Instruct the patient to notify the physician if he or she experiences involuntary eye, facial, or limb movement.
• Urge the patient to avoid alcohol during metoclopramide therapy.

ondansetron hydrochloride

on-dan-**seh**-tron
(Zofran, Zofran ODT)
Do not confuse Zofran with Zantac or Zosyn.

CATEGORY AND SCHEDULE

Pregnancy Risk Category: B

MECHANISM OF ACTION

An antiemetic that blocks serotonin, both peripherally on vagal nerve terminals and centrally in the chemoreceptor trigger zone. **Therapeutic Effect:** Prevents nausea and vomiting.

PHARMACOKINETICS

Readily absorbed from the GI tract. Protein binding: 70%–76%. Metabolized in the liver. Primarily excreted in urine. Unknown if removed by hemodialysis. ***Half-life:*** 4 hr.

AVAILABILITY

Oral Solution (Zofran): 4 mg/5 ml.
Tablets (Zofran): 4 mg, 8 mg, 24 mg.
Tablets (Orally-Disintegrating [Zofran ODT]): 4 mg, 8 mg.
Injection (Zofran): 2 mg/ml.
Injection (Premix): 32 mg/50 ml.

INDICATIONS AND DOSAGES

▸ Prevention of chemotherapy-induced nausea and vomiting

PO

Adults, Elderly, Children older than 11 yr. 24 mg as a single dose 30 min before starting chemotherapy. Or 8 mg 30 min before chemotherapy and again 8 hr after first dose, then q12h for 1–2 days.

Children 4–11 yr. 4 mg 30 min before chemotherapy and again 4 and 8 hr after chemotherapy, then q8h for 1–2 days.

IV

Adults, Elderly, Children 4–18 yr. 32 mg as a single dose or 0.15 mg/kg/dose 30 min before chemotherapy, then 4 and 8 hr after chemotherapy.

▸ Prevention of radiation-induced nausea and vomiting

PO

Adults, Elderly. 8 mg 3 times a day.

▸ Prevention of postoperative nausea and vomiting

IV, IM

Adults, Elderly. 4 mg undiluted over 2–5 min.

Children weighing less than 40 kg. 0.1 mg/kg.

Children weighing 10 kg and more. 4 mg.

OFF-LABEL USES

Treatment of postoperative nausea and vomiting

CONTRAINDICATIONS

None known.

INTERACTIONS

Drug

None known.

Herbal

None known.

Food

None known.

DIAGNOSTIC TEST EFFECTS

May transiently increase serum bilirubin, AST (SGOT), and ALT (SGPT) levels.

IV INCOMPATIBILITIES

Acyclovir (Zovirax), allopurinol (Aloprim), aminophylline, amphotericin B (Fungizone), amphotericin B complex (Abelcet, AmBisome, Amphotec), ampicillin (Polycillin), ampicillin and sulbactam (Unasyn), cefepime (Maxipime), cefoperazone (Cefobid), 5-fluorouracil, lorazepam

(Ativan), meropenem (Merrem IV), methylprednisolone (Solu-Medrol)

IV COMPATIBILITIES

Carboplatin (Paraplatin), cisplatin (Platinol), cyclophosphamide (Cytoxan), cytarabine (Cytosar), dacarbazine (DTIC-Dome), daunorubicin (Cerubidine), dexamethasone (Decadron), diphenhydramine (Benadryl), docetaxel (Taxotere), dopamine (Intropin), etoposide (VePesid), gemcitabine (Gemzar), heparin, hydromorphone (Dilaudid), ifosfamide (Ifex), magnesium, mannitol, mesna (Mesnex), methotrexate, metoclopramide(Reglan), mitomycin (Mutamycin), mitoxantrone (Novantrone), morphine, paclitaxel (Taxol), potassium chloride, teniposide (Vumon), topotecan (Hycamtin), vinblastine (Velban), vincristine (Oncovin), vinorelbine (Navelbine)

SIDE EFFECTS

Frequent (13%–5%)
Anxiety, dizziness, somnolence, headache, fatigue, constipation, diarrhea, hypoxia, urine retention
Occasional (4%–2%)
Abdominal pain, xerostomia, fever, feeling of cold, redness and pain at injection site, paresthesia, asthenia
Rare (1%)
Hypersensitivity reaction (including rash and pruritus), blurred vision

SERIOUS REACTIONS

! Overdose may produce a combination of CNS stimulant and depressant effects.

NURSING CONSIDERATIONS

Baseline Assessment

• Assess the patient who experiences severe vomiting for signs and symptoms of dehydration, including dry mucous membranes, longitudinal furrows in the tongue, and poor skin turgor.
• Monitor serum bilirubin, AST (SGOT), and ALT (SGPT) levels.

Lifespan Considerations

• It is unknown if ondansetron crosses the placenta or is distributed in breast milk.
• The safety and efficacy of ondansetron have not been established in children.
• No age-related precautions have been noted in the elderly.

Administration and Handling

PO
◀ **ALERT** ▶ Give all oral doses 30 minutes before chemotherapy and repeat at 8-hour intervals, as prescribed.
• Give ondansetron without regard to food.
IV
• Store vials at room temperature.
• Ondansetron may be given undiluted as an IV push over 2 to 5 minutes.
• For IV infusion, dilute with 50 ml D_5W or 0.9% NaCl before administration, and infuse over 15 minutes.
• The solution is stable for 48 hours after dilution.

Intervention and Evaluation

• Assess and record the patient's pattern of daily bowel activity and stool consistency, and auscultate bowel sounds for peristalsis.
• Offer the patient emotional support.

Patient Teaching

• Inform the patient that nausea and vomiting should be relieved shortly after drug administration. Advise the patient to notify the physician if vomiting persists.
• Inform the patient that ondansetron may cause dizziness or drowsiness.
• Urge the patient to avoid alcohol and barbiturates while taking ondansetron.

• Teach the patient other methods of reducing nausea and vomiting, including lying quietly and avoiding strong odors.
• Warn the patient to avoid performing tasks that require mental alerness or motor skills until his or her response to ondansetron has been established.

palonosetron hydrochloride

pal-oh-**noe**-seh-tron
(Aloxi)

CATEGORY AND SCHEDULE

Pregnancy Risk Category: B

MECHANISM OF ACTION

A 5-HT_3 receptor antagonist that acts centrally in the chemoreceptor trigger zone and peripherally at the vagal nerve terminals. **Therapeutic Effect:** Prevents nausea and vomiting associated with chemotherapy.

PHARMACOKINETICS

Protein binding: 52%. Eliminated in urine. ***Half-life:*** 40 hr.

AVAILABILITY

Injection: 0.25 mg/5 ml.

INDICATIONS AND DOSAGES

▸ Chemotherapy-induced nausea and vomiting

IV

Adults, Elderly. 0.25 mg as a single dose 30 min before starting chemotherapy.

CONTRAINDICATIONS

None known.

INTERACTIONS

Drug

None known.

Herbal

None known.

Food

None known.

DIAGNOSTIC TEST EFFECTS

May transiently increase serum bilirubin, AST (SGOT), and ALT (SGPT) levels.

IV INCOMPATIBILITIES

Don't mix palonosetron with any other drugs.

SIDE EFFECTS

Occasional (9%–5%)

Headache, constipation

Rare (less than 1%)

Diarrhea, dizziness, fatigue, abdominal pain, insomnia

SERIOUS REACTIONS

! Overdose may produce a combination of CNS stimulant and depressant effects.

NURSING CONSIDERATIONS

Baseline Assessment

• Assess the patient who experiences severe vomiting for signs and symptoms of dehydration, including dry mucous membranes, longitudinal furrows in the tongue, and poor skin turgor.

Lifespan Considerations

• It is unknown if palonosetron is excreted in breast milk.
• The safety and efficacy of palonosetron have not been established in children.
• No age-related precautions have been noted in the elderly.

Precautions

• Use palonosetron cautiously in

patients with a history of cardiovascular disease.

Administration and Handling

IV

- Store vials at room temperature.
- The solution normally appears clear and colorless. Discard it if it appears cloudy or contains precipitate.
- Give the drug undiluted as an IV push over 30 seconds. Flush the IV line with 0.9% NaCl before and after administration.

Intervention and Evaluation

- Assess the patient's pattern of daily bowel activity and stool consistency, and record time of evacuation.
- Provide emotional support to the patient.

Patient Teaching

- Inform the patient that nausea and vomiting should be relieved shortly after drug administration. Advise the patient to notify the physician if vomiting persists.
- Urge the patient to avoid alcohol and barbiturates during palonosetron therapy.
- Teach the patient other methods of reducing nausea and vomiting, including lying quietly and avoiding strong odors.

prochlorperazine

proe-klor-**per**-a-zeen

(Compazine, Stemetil[CAN], Stemzine[AUS])

Do not confuse prochlorperazine with chlorpromazine, or Compazine with Copaxone.

CATEGORY AND SCHEDULE

Pregnancy Risk Category: C

MECHANISM OF ACTION

A phenothiazine that acts centrally to inhibit or block dopamine receptors in the chemoreceptor trigger zone and peripherally to block the vagus nerve in the GI tract. **Therapeutic Effect:** Relieves nausea and vomiting and improves psychotic conditions.

PHARMACOKINETICS

Route	Onset*	Peak	Duration
Tablets, oral solution	30–40 min	N/A	3–4 hr
Capsules (Extended-Release)	30–40 min	N/A	10–12 hr
Rectal	60 min	N/A	3–4 hr

*As an antiemetic

Variably absorbed after PO administration. Widely distributed. Metabolized in the liver and GI mucosa. Primarily excreted in urine. Unknown if removed by hemodialysis. ***Half-life:*** 23 hr.

AVAILABILITY

Capsules (Extended-Release): 10 mg, 15 mg.
Oral Solution: 5 mg/5ml.
Tablets: 5 mg, 10 mg.
Suppositories: 2.5 mg, 5 mg, 25 mg.
Injection (Compazine): 5 mg/ml.

INDICATIONS AND DOSAGES

▸ Nausea and vomiting

PO

Adults, Elderly. 5–10 mg 3–4 times a day.

Children. 0.4 mg/kg/day in 3–4 divided doses.

PO (Extended-Release)

Adults, Elderly. 10 mg twice a day or 15 mg once a day.

IV
Adults, Elderly. 2.5–10 mg. May repeat q3–4h.
Children. 0.1–0.15 mg/kg/dose q8–12h. Maximum: 40 mg/day.
IM
Adults, Elderly. 5–10 mg q3–4h.
Children. 0.1–0.15 mg/kg/dose q8–12h. Maximum: 40 mg/day.
Rectal
Adults, Elderly. 25 mg twice a day.
Children. 0.4 mg/kg/day in 3–4 divided doses.

▸ **Psychosis**
PO
Adults, Elderly. 5–10 mg 3–4 times a day. Maximum: 150 mg/day.
Children. 2.5 mg 2–3 times a day. Maximum: 25 mg for children 6–12 yr; 20 mg for children 2–5 yr.
IM
Adults, Elderly. 10–20 mg q4h.
Children. 0.13 mg/kg/dose.

CONTRAINDICATIONS

Angle-closure glaucoma, CNS depression, coma, myelosuppression, severe cardiac or hepatic impairment, severe hypotension or hypertension

INTERACTIONS

Drug

Alcohol, other CNS depressants: May increase CNS and respiratory depression and the hypotensive effects of prochlorperazine.
Antihypertensives: May increase hypotension.
Antithyroid agents: May increase the risk of agranulocytosis.
Extrapyramidal symptom–producing medications: May increase extrapyramidal symptoms.
Levodopa: May decrease the effects of levodopa.
Lithium: May decrease the absorption of prochlorperazine and produce adverse neurologic effects.
MAOIs, tricyclic antidepressants: May increase the anticholinergic and sedative effects of prochlorperazine.

Herbal

None known.

Food

None known.

DIAGNOSTIC TEST EFFECTS

None known.

IV INCOMPATIBILITIES

Atropine, furosemide (Lasix), midazolam (Versed)

IV COMPATIBILITIES

Calcium gluconate, diphenhydramine (Benadryl), fentanyl, glycopyrrolate (Robinul), heparin, hydromorphone (Dilaudid), morphine, metoclopramide (Reglan), nalbuphine (Nubain), potassium chloride, promethazine (Phenergan), propofol (Diprivan)

SIDE EFFECTS

Frequent

Somnolence, hypotension, dizziness, fainting (commonly occurring after first dose, occasionally after subsequent doses, and rarely with oral form)

Occasional

Dry mouth, blurred vision, lethargy, constipation, diarrhea, myalgia, nasal congestion, peripheral edema, urine retention

SERIOUS REACTIONS

! Extrapyramidal symptoms appear to be dose related and are divided into three categories: akathisia (marked by inability to sit still, tapping of feet), parkinsonian symptoms (including mask-like face, tremors, shuffling gait, hypersalivation), and acute dystonias (such as torticollis, opisthotonos, and oculogyric crisis). A dystonic reaction may also produce diaphoresis or pallor.

! Tardive dyskinesia, manifested as tongue protrusion, puffing of the cheeks, and puckering of the mouth, is a rare reaction that may be irreversible.

! Abrupt withdrawal after long-term therapy may precipitate nausea, vomiting, gastritis, dizziness, and tremors.

! Blood dyscrasias, particularly agranulocytosis and mild leukopenia, may occur.

! Prochlorperazine use may lower the seizure threshold.

NURSING CONSIDERATIONS

Baseline Assessment

- Assess the patient who experiences severe vomiting for signs and symptoms of dehydration, including dry mucous membranes, longitudinal furrows in the tongue, and poor skin turgor.
- Assess the psychotic patient's appearance, behavior, emotional status, response to the environment, speech pattern, and thought content.

Lifespan Considerations

- Prochlorperazine crosses the placenta and is distributed in breast milk.
- The safety and efficacy of this drug have not been established in children younger than 2 years or weighing less than 9 kg.
- A decreased prochlorperazine dosage is recommended for elderly patients, who are more susceptible to the drug's sedative, anticholinergic, extrapyramidal, and hypotensive effects.

Precautions

- Use prochlorperazine cautiously in patients with Parkinson's disease or seizures and in children younger than 2 years.

Administration and Handling

PO

- Give prochlorperazine without regard to food.
- Avoid skin contact with prochlorperazine oral solution because it may cause contact dermatitis.

Parenteral

- Keep the patient recumbent—head low and legs raised—for 30 to 60 minutes after drug administration to minimize the drug's hypotensive effect.

Rectal

- Moisten the suppository with cold water before inserting it well into the rectum.

IV

- Store prochlorperazine at room temperature and protect from light.
- Solution should be clear or slightly yellow.
- May give by IV push slowly over 5 to 10 minutes.
- May give by IV infusion over 30 minutes

Intervention and Evaluation

- Monitor the patient's BP for hypotension.
- Assess the patient for extrapyramidal symptoms.
- Monitor the patient's CBC for blood dyscrasias.
- Observe the patient for rapid tongue movement, which may be an early sign of tardive dyskinesia.
- Closely supervise the suicidal psychotic patient during early therapy. As depression lessens, the patient's energy level generally improves, which increases the suicide potential.
- Assess the psychotic patient for a therapeutic response, including improvement in self-care, increased ability to concentrate and interest in surroundings, and a relaxed facial expression.

Patient Teaching

- Urge the patient to avoid alcohol and limit caffeine intake while taking prochlorperazine.
- Warn the patient to avoid tasks that require mental alertness or motor skills until his or her response to the drug has been established.

scopolamine

skoe-**pol**-a-meen
(Trans-Derm Scop, Transderm-V)

CATEGORY AND SCHEDULE

Pregnancy Risk Category: C

MECHANISM OF ACTION

An anticholinergic that reduces excitability of labyrinthine receptors, depressing conduction in the vestibular cerebellar pathway. **Therapeutic Effect:** Prevents motion-induced nausea and vomiting.

AVAILABILITY

Transdermal System: 1.5 mg.

INDICATIONS AND DOSAGES

▸ Prevention of motion sickness
Transdermal
Adults. 1 system q72h.

▸ Post-operative nause or vomiting
Transdermal
Adults, Elderly. 1 system no sooner than 1 h before surgery and removed 24 h after surgery.

CONTRAINDICATIONS

Angle-closure glaucoma, GI or GU obstruction, myasthenia gravis, paralytic ileus, tachycardia, thyrotoxicosis

INTERACTIONS

Drug

Antihistamines, tricyclic antidepressants: May increase the anticholinergic effects of scopolamine.
CNS depressants: May increase CNS depression.

Herbal

None known.

Food

None known.

DIAGNOSTIC TEST EFFECTS

May interfere with gastric secretion test.

SIDE EFFECTS

Frequent (greater than 15%)
Dry mouth, somnolence, blurred vision
Rare (5%–1%)
Dizziness, restlessness, hallucinations, confusion, difficulty urinating, rash

SERIOUS REACTIONS

! None known.

NURSING CONSIDERATIONS

Baseline Assessment

- Determine if the patient uses other CNS depressants or drugs with anticholinergic action or has a history of angle-closure glaucoma.

Precautions

- Use scopolamine cautiously in patients with cardiac disease, renal or hepatic impairment, psychoses, or seizures.

Administration and Handling

Transdermal

- Apply patch to the hairless area behind one ear.
- Replace the patch after 72 hours or if it becomes dislodged.

Intervention and Evaluation

- Monitor the patient's BUN level; blood chemistry test results; and serum alkaline phosphatase, bilirubin, creatinine, AST (SGOT), and

ALT (SGPT) levels to assess hepatic and renal function.

Patient Teaching

- Teach the patient how to properly apply the patch. Instruct him or her to use only one patch at a time and not to cut it.
- Advise the patient to wash his or her hands after applying the patch.
- Warn the patient to avoid tasks requiring mental alertness or motor skills until his or her response to the drug has been established.

trimethobenzamide hydrochloride

trye-meth-oh-**ben**-za-mide

(Tigan)

CATEGORY AND SCHEDULE

Pregnancy Risk Category: C

MECHANISM OF ACTION

An anticholinergic that acts at the chemoreceptor trigger zone in the medulla oblongata. **Therapeutic Effect:** Relieves nausea and vomiting.

PHARMACOKINETICS

Route	Onset	Peak	Duration
PO	10–40 min	N/A	3–4 hr
IM	15–30 min	N/A	2–3 hr

Partially absorbed from the GI tract. Distributed primarily to the liver. Metabolic fate unknown. Excreted in urine. ***Half-life:*** 7–9 hr.

AVAILABILITY

Capsules: 100 mg, 300 mg.
Injection: 100 mg/ml.
Suppositories: 100 mg, 200 mg.

INDICATIONS AND DOSAGES

▸ Nausea and vomiting

PO

Adults, Elderly. 300 mg 3–4 times a day.

Children weighing 30–100 lb. 100–200 mg 3–4 times a day.

IM

Adults, Elderly. 200 mg 3–4 times a day.

Rectal

Adults, Elderly. 200 mg 3–4 times a day.

Children weighing 30–100 lb. 100–200 mg 3–4 times a day.

Children weighing less than 30 lb. 100 mg 3–4 times a day.

CONTRAINDICATIONS

Hypersensitivity to benzocaine or similar local anesthetics; use of parenteral form in children or suppositories in premature infants or neonates

INTERACTIONS

Drug

CNS depressants: May increase CNS depression.

Herbal

None known.

Food

None known.

DIAGNOSTIC TEST EFFECTS

None known.

SIDE EFFECTS

Frequent

Somnolence

Occasional

Blurred vision, diarrhea, dizziness, headache, muscle cramps

Rare

Rash, seizures, depression, opisthotonos, parkinsonian syndrome, Reye's syndrome (marked by vomiting, seizures)

SERIOUS REACTIONS

! A hypersensitivity reaction, manifested as extrapyramidal symptoms such as muscle rigidity and allergic skin reactions, occurs rarely.
! Children may experience paradoxical reactions, marked by restlessness, insomnia, euphoria, nervousness, and tremor.
! Overdose may produce CNS depression (manifested as sedation, apnea, cardiovascular collapse, and death) or severe paradoxical reactions (such as hallucinations, tremor, and seizures).

NURSING CONSIDERATIONS

Baseline Assessment

- Assess the patient who experiences severe vomiting.

Lifespan Considerations

- It is unknown if trimethobenzamide crosses the placenta or is distributed in breast milk.
- No age-related precautions have been noted in children or the elderly.
- Don't administer the parenteral form to children or the suppositories to neonates.

Precautions

- Use trimethobenzamide cautiously in debilitated or elderly patients and in patients with dehydration, electrolyte imbalances, or high fever.

Administration and Handling

◀ALERT▶ Elderly patients (older than 60 years) are at increased risk for developing agitation, disorientation, confusion, and psychotic-like symptoms.

◀ALERT▶ Don't administer trimethobenzamide by the IV route because it produces severe hypotension.

PO

- Give trimethobenzamide without regard to food.
- Don't crush, open, or break the capsules.

IM

- Inject the drug deep into a large muscle mass.

Rectal

- If the suppository is too soft, refrigerate it for 30 minutes or run cold water over the foil wrapper.
- Moisten the suppository with cold water before inserting it well into the rectum.

Intervention and Evaluation

- Monitor the patient's BP, especially in elderly patients, who are at an increased risk for hypotension.
- Assess children closely for signs of a paradoxical reaction.
- Monitor serum electrolyte levels in patients with severe vomiting.
- Measure the patient's intake and output; assess any vomitus.
- Assess the patient's mucous membranes and skin turgor to evaluate hydration status.
- Observe the patient for extrapyramidal symptoms, which may signal a as hypersensitivity reaction.

Patient Teaching

- Tell the patient that relief from nausea or vomiting generally occurs within 30 minutes of drug administration.
- Inform the patient that trimethobenzamide causes drowsiness. Warn the patient to avoid tasks that require mental alertness or motor skills until his or her response to the drug has been established.
- Advise the patient to notify the physician if he or she experiences headache, visual disturbances, restlessness, or involuntary muscle movements.
- Teach the patient other methods of relieving nausea and vomiting, including lying quietly and avoiding strong odors.

36 Antimigraine Agents

almotriptan malate
dihydroergotamine
eletriptan
ergotamine tartrate
frovatriptan
naratriptan
rizatriptan benzoate
sumatriptan
zolmitriptan

Uses: Antimigraine agents are used to treat migraine headaches with aura (also called classic migraine) or without aura (also called common migraine) in patients age 18 or older. The goal of treatment includes relief of the headache and accompanying symptoms and a return to baseline functioning. Antimigraine agents are commonly used with nondrug measures, such as lifestyle modification and avoidance of headache triggers.

Action: Two groups of antimigraine agents work by different mechanisms. *Triptans,* such as sumatriptan and zolmitriptan, selectively stimulate serotonin (5-HT) receptors that inhibit neuropeptide release and vasodilation. As a result, cerebral inflammation is reduced and blood vessels constrict. Both actions are believed to reduce the pain associated with vascular headaches. *Ergot alkaloids,* such as ergotamine and dihydroergotamine, interact with neurotransmitter receptors, including serotonergic, dopaminergic, and alpha-adrenergic receptors. More specifically, they may stimulate specific subtypes of serotonin receptors. However, their exact mechanism of action is unknown.

COMBINATION PRODUCTS

BELLERGAL-S: ergotamine/belladonna (an anticholinergic)/phenobarbital (a sedative-hypnotic) 0.6 mg/0.2 mg/40 mg.
CAFERGOT, WIGRAINE: ergotamine/caffeine (a stimulant) 1 mg/100 mg; 2 mg/100 mg.

almotriptan malate

al-moe-**trip**-tan
(Axert)
Do not confuse Axert with Antivert.

CATEGORY AND SCHEDULE

Pregnancy Risk Category: C

MECHANISM OF ACTION

A serotonin receptor agonist that binds selectively to vascular receptors, producing a vasoconstrictive effect on cranial blood vessels. **Therapeutic Effect:** Produces relief of migraine headache.

PHARMACOKINETICS
Well absorbed after PO administration. Metabolized by the liver, excreted in urine. ***Half-life:*** 3–4 hr.

AVAILABILITY
Tablets: 6.5 mg, 12.5 mg.

INDICATIONS AND DOSAGES
▸ Migraine headache

PO

Adults, Elderly. 6.25–12.5 mg. If headache improves but then returns, dose may be repeated after 2 hr. Maximum: 2 doses/24 hr.

▸ Dosage in renal impairment

For adult and elderly patients, recommended initial dose is 6.25 mg and maximum daily dose is 12.5 mg.

CONTRAINDICATIONS
Arrhythmias associated with conduction disorders, hemiplegic or basilar migraine, ischemic heart disease (including angina pectoris, history of MI, silent ischemia, and Prinzmetal's angina), uncontrolled hypertension, use within 24 hours of ergotamine-containing preparation or another serotonin receptor antagonist, use within 14 days of MAOIs,Wolff-Parkinson-White syndrome

INTERACTIONS
Drug
Ergotamine-containing medications: May produce a vasospastic reaction.

Erythromycin, itraconazole, ketoconazole, MAOIs, ritonavir: May increase the almotriptan plasma level.

Fluoxetine, fluvoxamine, paroxetine, sertraline: May produce weakness, hyperreflexia, and incoordination.

Herbal
None known.

Food
None known.

DIAGNOSTIC TEST EFFECTS
None known.

SIDE EFFECTS
Frequent
Nausea, dry mouth, paresthesia, flushing

Occasional
Changes in temperature sensation, asthenia, dizziness

SERIOUS REACTIONS
! Excessive dosage may produce tremor, red extremities, reduced respirations, cyanosis, seizures, and chest pain.

! Serious arrhythmias occur rarely, particularly in patients with hypertension or diabetes, obese patients, smokers, and those with a strong family history of coronary artery disease.

NURSING CONSIDERATIONS
Baseline Assessment
- Determine if the patient has a history of peripheral vascular disease.
- Determine the onset, location, and duration of the patient's migraines and possible precipitating factors.

Lifespan Considerations
- It is unknown if almotriptan is distributed in breast milk.
- The safety and efficacy of almotriptan have not been established in children younger than 12 years.
- No age-related precautions have been noted in the elderly.

Precautions
- Use almotriptan cautiously in patients with controlled hypertension, a history of CVA, mild to moderate hepatic or renal impairment, or cardiovascular risk factors.

Administration and Handling

◀ALERT▶ Don't administer erythromycin, itraconazole, ketoconazole, or ritonavir during the last 7 days of almotriptan therapy.

PO

- Have the patient swallow tablets whole with a full glass of water.

Intervention and Evaluation

- Evaluate the patient for relief of migraines and associated symptoms, including nausea and vomiting, photophobia, and phonophobia (sound sensitivity).

Patient Teaching

- Instruct the patient to take a single dose of almotriptan as soon migraine symptoms appear.
- Explain that this drug is intended to relieve migraines, not to prevent them or reduce the number of attacks.
- Advise the patient to lie down in a quiet, dark room for additional benefit after taking this drug.
- Warn the patient to avoid tasks that require mental alertness or motor skills until his or her response to the drug has been established.
- Warn the patient to notify the physician immediately if he or she experiences palpitations, pain or tightness in the chest or throat, or pain or weakness in the extremities.

dihydroergotamine

(Migranal)

See ergotamine.

eletriptan

el-eh-**trip**-tan

(Relpax)

CATEGORY AND SCHEDULE

Pregnancy Risk Category: C

MECHANISM OF ACTION

A serotonin receptor agonist that binds selectively to vascular receptors, producing a vasoconstrictive effect on cranial blood vessels. **Therapeutic Effect:** Relieves migraine headache.

PHARMACOKINETICS

Well absorbed after PO administration. Metabolized by the liver to inactive metabolite. Eliminated in urine. ***Half-life:*** 4.4 hr (increased in hepatic impairment and the elderly [older than 65 yr]).

AVAILABILITY

Tablets: 20 mg, 40 mg.

INDICATIONS AND DOSAGES

▶ **Acute migraine headache**

PO

Adults, Elderly. 20–40 mg. If headache improves but then returns, dose may be repeated after 2 hr. Maximum: 80 mg/day.

CONTRAINDICATIONS

Arrhythmias associated with conduction disorders, coronary artery disease, ischemic heart disease, severe hepatic impairment, uncontrolled hypertension

INTERACTIONS

Drug

Clarithromycin, itraconazole, ketoconazole, nefazodone, nelfinavir, ritonavir: May decrease eletriptan metabolism.
Ergotamine-containing medications: May produce a vasospastic reaction.
Sibutramine: May produce serotonin syndrome (marked by altered LOC, CNS irritability, motor weakness, myoclonus, and shivering).

Herbal

None known.

Food

None known.

DIAGNOSTIC TEST EFFECTS

None known.

SIDE EFFECTS

Occasional (6%–5%)
Dizziness, somnolence, asthenia, nausea
Rare (3%–2%)
Paresthesia, headache, dry mouth, warm or hot sensation, dyspepsia, dysphagia

SERIOUS REACTIONS

! Cardiac reactions (including ischemia, coronary artery vasospasm, and MI) and noncardiac vasospasm-related reactions (such as hemorrhage and CVA) occur rarely, particularly in patients with hypertension, diabetes, or a strong family history of coronary artery disease; obese patients; smokers; males older than 40 years; and postmenopausal women.

NURSING CONSIDERATIONS

Baseline Assessment

• Determine the onset, location, and duration of the patient's migraines and possible precipitating factors.
• Obtain the patient's baseline BP for evidence of uncontrolled hypertension, which is a contraindication.

Lifespan Considerations

• Eletriptan is distributed in breast milk and may suppress ovulation.
• The safety and efficacy of eletriptan have not been established in patients younger than 18 years.
• Patients older than 65 years are at increased risk for hypertension.

Precautions

• Use eletriptan cautiously in patients with controlled hypertension, mild to moderate hepatic or renal impairment, or a history of CVA.

Administration and Handling

◀ALERT▶ Don't administer clarithromycin, erythromycin, itraconazole, ketoconazole, nefazodone, nelfinavir, or ritonavir during the last 7 days of eletriptan therapy.
PO
• Administer film-coated tablets whole; don't crush or break them.

Intervention and Evaluation

• Assess the patient for relief of the migraine and associated symptoms, including nausea and vomiting, photophobia, and phonophobia (sound sensitivity).

Patient Teaching

• Instruct the patient to swallow the tablets whole, not to crush or break them.
• Instruct the patient to take a single dose of eletriptan as soon as migraine symptoms appear.
• Explain that this drug is intended to relieve migraines, not to prevent them or reduce the number of attacks.
• Warn the patient to avoid tasks that require mental alertness or motor skills until his or her response to the drug has been established.
• Instruct the patient to notify the physician immediately if he or she experiences palpitations, pain or

tightness in the chest or throat, pain or weakness in the extremities, or sudden or severe abdominal pain.
• Caution female patients who are planning pregnancy that the drug may suppress ovulation.
• Encourage the patient to lie down in dark, quiet room for additional benefit after taking eletriptan.

ergotamine tartrate

er-**got**-a-meen
(Cafergot[CAN], Ergodryl Mono[AUS], Ergomar, Ergostat, Gynergen)

dihydroergotamine

(D.H.E. 45, Dihydergot[AUS], Dihydroergotamine Sandoz[CAN], Migranal)

CATEGORY AND SCHEDULE

Pregnancy Risk Category: X

MECHANISM OF ACTION

An ergotamine derivative and alpha-adrenergic blocker that directly stimulates vascular smooth muscle, resulting in peripheral and cerebral vasoconstriction. May also have antagonist effects on serotonin. **Therapeutic Effect:** Suppresses vascular headaches.

PHARMACOKINETICS

Slowly and incompletely absorbed from the GI tract; rapidly and extensively absorbed after rectal administration. Protein binding: greater than 90%. Undergoes extensive first-pass metabolism in the liver to active metabolite. Eliminated in feces by the biliary system. ***Half-life:*** 21 hr.

AVAILABILITY

Tablets (Sublingual [Ergomar]): 2 mg.
Injection (DHE 45): 1 mg/ml.
Nasal Spray (Migranal): 0.5 mg/spray.
Suppositories (ergotamine and caffeine): 2 mg, with 100 mg caffeine.

INDICATIONS AND DOSAGES

▸ **Vascular headaches**

PO (Cafergot [fixed-combination of ergotamine and caffeine])
Adults, Elderly. 2 mg at onset of headache, then 1–2 mg q30min. Maximum: 6 mg/episode; 10 mg/wk.
PO, Sublingual
Children. 1 mg at onset of headache, then 1 mg q30min. Maximum: 3 mg/episode.
IV
Adults, Elderly. 1 mg at onset of headache; may repeat hourly. Maximum: 2 mg/day; 6 mg/wk.
Sublingual
Adults, Elderly. 1 tablet at onset of headache, then 1 tablet q30min. Maximum: 3 tablets/24 hr; 5 tablets/wk.
IM, Subcutaneous (dihydroergotamine)
Adults, Elderly. 1 mg at onset of headache; may repeat hourly. Maximum: 3 mg/day; 6 mg/wk.
Intranasal
Adults, Elderly. 1 spray (0.5 mg) into each nostril; may repeat in 15 min. Maximum: 4 sprays/day; 8 sprays/wk.
Rectal
Adults, Elderly. 1 suppository at onset of headache; may repeat dose in 1 hr. Maximum: 2 suppositories/episode; 5 suppositories/wk.

CONTRAINDICATIONS

Coronary artery disease, hypertension, impaired hepatic or renal function, malnutrition, peripheral vascular diseases (such as thromboangiitis obliterans, syphilitic arteritis, severe arteriosclerosis, thrombophlebitis, and Raynaud's disease), sepsis, severe pruritus

INTERACTIONS

Drug

Beta blockers, erythromycin: May increase the risk of vasospasm.
Ergot alkaloids, systemic vasoconstrictors: May increase pressor effect.
Nitroglycerin: May decrease the effects of nitroglycerin.

Herbal

None known.

Food

None known.

DIAGNOSTIC TEST EFFECTS

None known.

SIDE EFFECTS

Occasional (5%–2%)

Cough, dizziness

Rare (less than 2%)

Myalgia, fatigue, diarrhea, upper respiratory tract infection, dyspepsia

SERIOUS REACTIONS

! Prolonged administration or excessive dosage may produce ergotamine poisoning, manifested as nausea and vomiting; paresthesia, muscle pain or weakness; precordial pain; tachycardia or bradycardia; and hypertension or hypotension. Vasoconstriction of peripheral arteries and arterioles may result in localized edema and pruritus. Muscle pain will occur when walking and later, even at rest. Other rare effects include confusion, depression, drowsiness, seizures, and gangrene.

NURSING CONSIDERATIONS

Baseline Assessment

- Determine if the patient has a history of peripheral vascular disease or renal or hepatic impairment.
- Perform a careful assessment of the patient's peripheral circulation, including the temperature, color, and strength of pulses in the extremities.
- Determine if the patient is pregnant before beginning therapy.
- Determine the onset, location, and duration of the patient's vascular headaches and possible precipitating factors.

Lifespan Considerations

- Ergotamine use is contraindicated in pregnancy because it may result in fetal harm and even death.
- Ergotamine is distributed in breast milk and may inhibit lactation.
- Ergotamine use may produce diarrhea or vomiting in neonates.
- Ergotamine may be used safely in children 6 years and older, but only use when the patient has been unresponsive to other drugs.
- In the elderly, age-related occlusive peripheral vascular disease increases the risk of peripheral vasoconstriction; in addition, age-related renal impairment may require cautious use.

Administration and Handling

IV
- Administer dihydroergotamine undiluted over 1 minute.

Sublingual
- Have the patient place the sublingual tablet under the tongue, let it dissolve, and then swallow it. Don't administer it with water.

Nasal
- Before administration, prime the pump by squeezing it four times. Discard the drug within 8 hours of opening the container.
- Don't refrigerate the nasal form.

Intervention and Evaluation

- Monitor the patient closely for evidence of ergotamine overdose from prolonged administration or excessive dosage.

Patient Teaching

- Instruct the patient to begin taking ergotamine at the first sign of a vascular headache.
- Advise the patient to notify the physician if the drug does not relieve the headache or if he or she experiences an irregular heartbeat, nausea or vomiting, numbness or tingling of the fingers and toes, and pain or weakness of the extremities.
- Warn the female patient to avoid pregnancy during therapy and to notify the physician immediately if she becomes pregnant. Teach the patient methods of contraception if needed.

frovatriptan

fro-va-**trip**-tan
(Frovan)

CATEGORY AND SCHEDULE

Pregnancy Risk Category: C

MECHANISM OF ACTION

A serotonin receptor agonist that binds selectively to vascular receptors, producing a vasoconstrictive effect on cranial blood vessels. **Therapeutic Effect:** Relieves migraine headache.

PHARMACOKINETICS

Well absorbed after PO administration. Metabolized by the liver to inactive metabolite. Eliminated in urine. ***Half-life:*** 26 hr (increased in hepatic impairment).

AVAILABILITY

Tablets: 2.5 mg.

INDICATIONS AND DOSAGES

▸ **Acute migraine attack**

PO

Adults, Elderly. Initially 2.5 mg. If headache improves but then returns, dose may be repeated after 2 hr. Maximum: 7.5 mg/day.

CONTRAINDICATIONS

Basilar or hemiplegic migraine, cerebrovascular or peripheral vascular disease, coronary artery disease, ischemic heart disease (including angina pectoris, history of MI, silent ischemia, and Prinzmetal's angina), severe hepatic impairment (Child-Pugh grade C), uncontrolled hypertension, use within 24 hours of ergotamine-containing preparations or another serotonin receptor agonist, use within 14 days of MAOIs

INTERACTIONS

Drug

Ergotamine-containing medications: May produce a vasospastic reaction.
Fluoxetine, fluvoxamine, paroxetine, sertraline: May produce a vasospastic reaction.
Oral contraceptives: Decrease frovatriptan clearance and volume of distribution.
Propranolol: May dramatically increase frovatriptan plasma concentration.

Herbal

None known.

Food

None known.

DIAGNOSTIC TEST EFFECTS

None known.

SIDE EFFECTS

Occasional (8%–4%)

Dizziness, paresthesia, fatigue, flushing

Rare (3%–2%)
Hot or cold sensation, dry mouth, dyspepsia

SERIOUS REACTIONS

! Cardiac reactions (including ischemia, coronary artery vasospasm, and MI) and noncardiac vasospasm-related reactions (such as hemorrhage and CVA) occur rarely, particularly in patients with hypertension, diabetes, or a strong family history of coronary artery disease; obese patients; smokers; males older than 40 years; and postmenopausal women.

NURSING CONSIDERATIONS

Baseline Assessment

• Determine if the patient has a history of hepatic or renal impairment or peripheral vascular disease.
• Determine if the patient is pregnant or planning to become pregnant.
• Determine the onset, location, and duration of the patient's migraines and possible precipitating factors.

Lifespan Considerations

• It is unknown if frovatriptan is excreted in breast milk.
• The safety and efficacy of this drug have not been established in children.
• Frovatriptan use is not recommended for the elderly; however, the drug may be prescribed for patients for whom the benefits outweigh the risk.

Precautions

• Use frovatriptan cautiously in patients with mild to moderate hepatic impairment or cardiovascular risk factors.

Administration and Handling

PO
• Administer film-coated tablets whole; don't crush them.

Intervention and Evaluation

• Assess the patient for relief of migraines and associated symptoms, including nausea and vomiting, photophobia, and phonophobia (sound sensitivity).

Patient Teaching

• Instruct the patient not to crush or chew film-coated tablets.
• Instruct the patient to take a single dose of frovatriptan as soon as migraine symptoms appear. Explain that if the headache improves but then recurs, he or she may take a second dose at least 2 hours after the first dose.
• Inform the patient that frovatriptan is intended to relieve migraine headaches, not to prevent them or reduce the number of attacks.
• Instruct the patient to avoid tasks that require mental alertness or motor skills until his or her response to the drug has been established.
• Caution the patient to notify the physician immediately if he or she experiences palpitations, pain or weakness in the extremities, pain or tightness in the chest or throat, or sudden or severe abdominal pain.
• Urge the female patient of childbearing age to use contraceptives during therapy and to inform the physician if she suspects she is pregnant.
• Encourage the patient to lie down in a dark, quiet room for additional benefit after taking frovatriptan.

naratriptan

nare-a-**trip**-tan
(Amerge, Naramig[AUS])
Do not confuse Amerge with Amaryl.

CATEGORY AND SCHEDULE

Pregnancy Risk Category: C

MECHANISM OF ACTION

A serotonin receptor agonist that binds selectively to vascular receptors producing a vasoconstrictive effect on cranial blood vessels. **Therapeutic Effect:** Relieves migraine headache.

PHARMACOKINETICS

Well absorbed after PO administration. Protein binding: 28%–31%. Metabolized by the liver to inactive metabolite. Eliminated primarily in urine and, to a lesser extent, in feces. ***Half-life:*** 6 hr (increased in hepatic or renal impairment).

AVAILABILITY

Tablets: 1 mg, 2.5 mg.

INDICATIONS AND DOSAGES

▸ **Acute migraine attack**

PO

Adults. 1 mg or 2.5 mg. If headache improves but then returns, dose may be repeated after 4 hr. Maximum: 5 mg/24 hr.

▸ **Dosage in mild to moderate hepatic or renal impairment**

A lower starting dose is recommended. Don't exceed 2.5 mg/24 hr.

CONTRAINDICATIONS

Basilar or hemiplegic migraine, cerebrovascular or peripheral vascular disease, coronary artery disease, ischemic heart disease (including angina pectoris, history of MI, silent ischemia, and Prinzmetal's angina), severe hepatic impairment (Child-Pugh grade C), severe renal impairment (serum creatinine less than 15 ml/min), uncontrolled hypertension, use within 24 hours of ergotamine-containing preparations or another serotonin receptor agonist, use within 14 days of MAOIs

INTERACTIONS

Drug

Ergotamine-containing medications: May produce a vasospastic reaction.
Fluoxetine, fluvoxamine, paroxetine, sertraline: May produce hyperreflexia, incoordination, and weakness.
Oral contraceptives: Decrease naratriptan clearance and volume of distribution.

Herbal

None known.

Food

None known.

DIAGNOSTIC TEST EFFECTS

None known.

SIDE EFFECTS

Occasional (5%)
Nausea
Rare (2%)
Paresthesia; dizziness; fatigue; somnolence; jaw, neck, or throat pressure

SERIOUS REACTIONS

! Corneal opacities and other ocular defects may occur.
! Cardiac reactions (including ischemia, coronary artery vasospasm, and MI) and noncardiac vasospasm-related reactions (such as hemorrhage and CVA) occur rarely, particularly in patients with hypertension, diabetes, or a strong family history of coronary artery disease;

obese patients; smokers; males older than 40 years; and postmenopausal women.

NURSING CONSIDERATIONS

Baseline Assessment

• Determine if the patient has a history of peripheral vascular disease or hepatic or renal impairment.
• Determine if the patient is pregnant before starting therapy.
• Determine the onset, location, and duration of the patient's migraines and possible precipitating factors.

Lifespan Considerations

• It is unknown if naratriptan is excreted in breast milk.
• The safety and efficacy of naratriptan have not been established in children.
• Naratriptan is not recommended for the elderly.

Precautions

• Use naratriptan cautiously in patients with mild to moderate hepatic or renal impairment or cardiovascular risk factors.

Administration and Handling

PO
• Give naratriptan without regard to food.

Intervention and Evaluation

• Assess the patient for relief of migraines and associated symptoms, including nausea and vomiting, photophobia, and phonophobia (sound sensitivity).

Patient Teaching

• Teach the patient to swallow tablets whole with water—not to crush or chew them.
• Inform the patient that he or she may take another dose of naratriptan, if needed, 4 hours after the first dose for a maximum of 5 mg/24 hours.
• Advise the patient that naratriptan use may cause dizziness, drowsiness, and fatigue.
• Warn the patient to avoid tasks that require mental alertness or motor skills until his or her response to the drug has been established.
• Instruct the patient to notify the physician if he or she experiences anxiety, chest pain, palpitations, or tightness in the throat.
• Instruct the female patient of childbearing age to use contraceptives during therapy and to notify the physician immediately if she suspects she is pregnant.
• Encourage the patient to lie down in a dark, quiet room for additional benefit after taking naratriptan.

rizatriptan benzoate

rize-a-**trip**-tan
(Maxalt, Maxalt-MLT)

CATEGORY AND SCHEDULE

Pregnancy Risk Category: C

MECHANISM OF ACTION

A serotonin receptor agonist that binds selectively to vascular receptors, producing a vasoconstrictive effect on cranial blood vessels. **Therapeutic Effect:** Relieves migraine headache.

PHARMACOKINETICS

Well absorbed after PO administration. Protein binding: 14%. Crosses the blood-brain barrier. Metabolized by the liver to inactive metabolite. Eliminated primarily in urine and, to a lesser extent, in feces. ***Half-life:*** 2–3 hr.

AVAILABILITY

Tablets (Maxalt): 5 mg, 10 mg.
Tablets (Oral-Disintegrating [Maxalt-MLT]): 5 mg, 10 mg.

INDICATIONS AND DOSAGES

▸ Acute migraine attack

PO

Adults older than 18 yr, Elderly. 5–10 mg. If headache improves, but then returns, dose may be repeated after 2 hr. Maximum: 30 mg/24 hr.

CONTRAINDICATIONS

Basilar or hemiplegic migraine, coronary artery disease, ischemic heart disease (including angina pectoris, history of MI, silent ischemia, and Prinzmetal's angina), uncontrolled hypertension, use within 24 hours of ergotamine-containing preparations or another serotonin receptor agonist, use within 14 days of MAOIs

INTERACTIONS

Drug

Ergotamine-containing medications: May produce a vasospastic reaction.

Fluoxetine, fluvoxamine, paroxetine, sertraline: May produce hyperreflexia, incoordination, and weakness.

MAOIs, propranolol: May dramatically increase plasma concentration of rizatriptan.

Herbal

None known.

Food

All foods: Delay peak drug concentration by 1 hour.

DIAGNOSTIC TEST EFFECTS

None known.

SIDE EFFECTS

Frequent (9%–7%)

Dizziness, somnolence, paraesthesia, fatigue

Occasional (6%–3%)

Nausea, chest pressure, dry mouth

Rare (2%)

Headache; neck, throat, or jaw pressure; photosensitivity

SERIOUS REACTIONS

! Cardiac reactions (such as ischemia, coronary artery vasospasm, and MI) and noncardiac vasospasm-related reactions (including hemorrhage and CVA) occur rarely, particularly in patients with hypertension, diabetes, or a strong family history of coronary artery disease; obese patients; smokers; males older than 40 years; and postmenopausal women.

NURSING CONSIDERATIONS

Baseline Assessment

- Determine if the patient has a history peripheral vascular disease or hepatic or renal impairment.
- Obtain BUN level and serum alkaline phosphatase, bilirubin, creatinine AST (SGOT), and ALT (SGPT) levels to assess renal and hepatic function.
- Determine the onset, location, and duration of the patient's migraines and possible precipitating factors.
- Obtain a baseline EKG.

Lifespan Considerations

- It is unknown if rizatriptan is distributed in breast milk.
- The safety and efficacy of rizatriptan have not been established in children.
- No age-related precautions have been noted in the elderly.

Precautions

- Use rizatriptan cautiously in patients with mild to moderate hepatic or renal impairment or cardiovascular risk factors.

Administration and Handling

PO

- The orally disintegrating tablets come packaged in individual aluminum blister packs. Open packet with dry hands, and place tablet on the patient's tongue to dissolve. Then have the patient swallow it. Don't administer the orally disintegrating tablets with water.

Intervention and Evaluation

- Monitor the patient for dizziness.
- Assess the patient for relief of migraines and associated symptoms, including nausea and vomiting, photophobia, and phonophobia (sound sensitivity).

Patient Teaching

- Instruct the patient to take a single dose of rizatriptan as soon as migraine symptoms appear.
- Teach the patient not to remove the orally disintegrating tablet from the blister pack until just before he or she intends to take it.
- Explain that rizatriptan is intended to relieve migraines, not to prevent them or reduce the number of attacks.
- Caution the patient to avoid tasks that require mental alertness or motor skills until his or her response to the drug has been established.
- Warn the patient to notify the physician immediately if he or she experiences palpitations, pain or tightness in the chest or throat, or pain or weakness in the extremities.
- Instruct the patient to protect against exposure to sunlight and ultraviolet rays by using sunscreen and wearing protective clothing.
- Urge the patient not to smoke during rizatriptan therapy.
- Encourage the patient to lie down in a dark, quiet room for additional benefit after taking the drug.

sumatriptan

soo-ma-**trip**-tan
(Imigran[AUS], Imitrex, Suvalan[AUS])

Do not confuse sumatriptan with somatropin.

CATEGORY AND SCHEDULE

Pregnancy Risk Category: C

MECHANISM OF ACTION

A serotonin receptor agonist that binds selectively to vascular receptors, producing a vasoconstrictive effect on cranial blood vessels. **Therapeutic Effect:** Relieves migraine headache.

PHARMACOKINETICS

Route	Onset	Peak	Duration
Nasal	15 min	N/A	24–48hr
PO	30 min	2 hr	24–48hr
Subcutaneous	10 min	1 hr	24–48hr

Rapidly absorbed after subcutaneous administration. Absorption after PO administration is incomplete, with significant amounts undergoing hepatic metabolism, resulting in low bioavailability (about 14%). Protein binding: 10%–21%. Widely distributed. Undergoes first-pass metabolism in the liver. Excreted in urine. ***Half-life:*** 2 hr.

AVAILABILITY

Tablets: 25 mg, 50 mg, 100 mg.
Injection: 6 mg/0.5 ml.
Nasal Spray: 5 mg, 20 mg.

INDICATIONS AND DOSAGES

▸ **Acute migraine attack**

PO

Adults, Elderly. 25–50 mg. Dose may be repeated after at least 2 hr.

Maximum: 100 mg/single dose; 200 mg/24 hr.
Subcutaneous
Adults, Elderly. 6 mg. Maximum: Two 6-mg injections/24 hr (separated by at least 1 hr).
Intranasal
Adults, Elderly. 5–20 mg; may repeat in 2 hr. Maximum: 40 mg/24 hr.

CONTRAINDICATIONS

CVA, ischemic heart disease (including angina pectoris, history of MI, silent ischemia, and Prinzmetal's angina), severe hepatic impairment, transient ischemic attack, uncontrolled hypertension, use within 14 days of MAOIs, use within 24 hr of ergotamine preparations

INTERACTIONS

Drug

Ergotamine-containing medications: May produce vasospastic reaction.
MAOIs: May increase sumatriptan blood concentration and half-life.

Herbal

None known.

Food

None known.

DIAGNOSTIC TEST EFFECTS

None known.

SIDE EFFECTS

Frequent

Oral (10%–5%): Tingling, nasal discomfort
Subcutaneous (greater than 10%): Injection site reactions, tingling, warm or hot sensation, dizziness, vertigo
Nasal (greater than 10%): Bad or unusual taste, nausea, vomiting

Occasional

Oral (5%–1%): Flushing, asthenia, visual disturbances
Subcutaneous (10%–2%): Burning sensation, numbness, chest discomfort, drowsiness, asthenia
Nasal (5%–1%): Nasopharyngeal discomfort, dizziness

Rare

Oral (less than 1%): Agitation, eye irritation, dysuria
Subcutaneous (less than 2%): Anxiety, fatigue, diaphoresis, muscle cramps, myalgia
Nasal (less than 1%): Burning sensation

SERIOUS REACTIONS

! Excessive dosage may produce tremor, red extremities, reduced respirations, cyanosis, seizures, and paralysis.
! Serious arrhythmias occur rarely, especially in patients with hypertension, diabetes, or a strong family history of coronary artery disease; obese patients; and smokers.

NURSING CONSIDERATIONS

Baseline Assessment

- Determine if the patient has a history of peripheral vascular disease or hepatic or renal impairment.
- Determine if the patient is pregnant or planning to become pregnant.
- Determine the onset, location, and duration of the patient's migraines and possible precipitating factors.
- Obtain a baseline EKG.

Lifespan Considerations

- It is unknown if sumatriptan is distributed in breast milk.
- The safety and efficacy of sumatriptan have not been established in children.
- No age-related precautions have been noted in the elderly.

Precautions

- Use sumatriptan cautiously in patients with epilepsy, a hypersensitivity to sulfonamides, or hepatic or renal impairment.

Administration and Handling

PO

• Have the patient swallow tablets whole with a full glass of water.

Subcutaneous

• Follow the manufacturer's instructions for using the autoinjection device.

Nasal

• Each unit contains only one spray, so don't test the spray before use.
• Have the patient blow the nose gently to clear nasal passages.
• With the patient's head upright, close one of the patient's nostrils with an index finger and have him or her breathe gently through the mouth.
• Insert the nozzle about 1/2 inch into the patient's open nostril.
• Instruct the patient to close his or her mouth, then breathe through the nose while depressing the blue plunger and releasing the spray.
• Remove the nozzle from the patient's nose, and instruct the patient to gently breathe in through the nose and out through the mouth for 10–20 seconds. Tell the patient not to breathe in deeply.

Intervention and Evaluation

• Evaluate the patient for relief of migraines and associated symptoms, including nausea and vomiting, photophobia, and phonophobia (sound sensitivity).

Patient Teaching

• Teach the patient how to properly load the autoinjector, inject the medication, and discard the syringe.
• Instruct the patient to inject the drug into an area with adequate subcutaneous tissue because the needle will penetrate the skin and adipose tissue as deeply as 6 mm.
• Tell the patient not to administer more than two subcutaneous injections during any 24-hour period and to allow at least 1 hour between injections.
• Warn the patient to notify the physician immediately if he or she experiences palpitations, a rash, wheezing, pain or tightness in the chest or throat, or facial edema.
• Advise the patient to lie down in a dark, quiet room for additional benefit after taking sumatriptan.

zolmitriptan

zohl-mih-**trip**-tan
(Zomig, Zomig Rapimelt[CAN], Zomig-ZMT)

CATEGORY AND SCHEDULE

Pregnancy Risk Category: C

MECHANISM OF ACTION

A serotonin receptor agonist that binds selectively to vascular receptors, producing a vasoconstrictive effect on cranial blood vessels. **Therapeutic Effect:** Relieves migraine headache.

PHARMACOKINETICS

Rapidly but incompletely absorbed after PO administration. Protein binding: 15%. Undergoes first-pass metabolism in the liver to active metabolite. Eliminated primarily in urine (60%) and, to a lesser extent, in feces (30%). ***Half-life:*** 3 hr.

AVAILABILITY

Tablets (Zomig): 2.5 mg, 5 mg.
Tablets (Orally-Disintegrating [Zomig-ZMT]): 2.5 mg, 5 mg.
Nasal Spray (Zomig): 5 mg/0.1 ml.

INDICATIONS AND DOSAGES

▸ Acute migraine attack

PO

Adults, Elderly, Children older than 18 yr. Initially, 2.5 mg or less. If headache returns, may repeat dose in 2 hr. Maximum: 10 mg/24 hr.

Intranasal

Adults, Elderly. 5 mg. May repeat in 2 hr. Maximum: 10 mg/24hr.

CONTRAINDICATIONS

Arrhythmias associated with conduction disorders, basilar or hemiplegic migraine, coronary artery disease, ischemic heart disease (including angina pectoris, history of MI, silent ischemia, and Prinzmetal's angina), uncontrolled hypertension, use within 24 hr of ergotamine-containing preparations or another serotonin receptor agonist, use within 14 days of MAOIs, Wolff-Parkinson-White syndrome

INTERACTIONS

Drug

Ergotamine-containing medications: May produce a vasospastic reaction.

Fluoxetine, fluvoxamine, paroxetine, sertraline: May produce hyperreflexia, incoordination, and weakness.

MAOIs: May dramatically increase plasma concentration of zolmitriptan.

Oral contraceptives: Decrease zolmitriptan clearance and volume of distribution.

Herbal

None known.

Food

None known.

DIAGNOSTIC TEST EFFECTS

None known.

SIDE EFFECTS

Frequent (8%–6%)

Oral: Dizziness; tingling; neck, throat, or jaw pressure; somnolence

Nasal: Altered taste, paraesthesia

Occasional (5%–3%)

Oral: Warm or hot sensation, asthenia, chest pressure

Nasal: Nausea, somnolence, nasal discomfort, dizziness, asthenia, dry mouth

Rare (2%–1%)

Diaphoresis, myalgia, paresthesia

SERIOUS REACTIONS

! Cardiac reactions (including ischemia, coronary artery vasospasm, and MI) and noncardiac vasospasm-related reactions (such as hemorrhage and CVA) occur rarely, particularly in patients with hypertension, diabetes, or a strong family history of coronary artery disease; obese patients; smokers; males older than 40 years; and postmenopausal women.

NURSING CONSIDERATIONS

Baseline Assessment

- Determine if the patient has a history of hepatic or renal impairment, MAOI use, and peripheral vascular or coronary artery disease.
- Determine the onset, location, and duration of the patient's migraines and possible precipitating factors.

Lifespan Considerations

- It is unknown if zolmitriptan is distributed in breast milk.
- The safety and efficacy of zolmitriptan have not been established in children younger than 12 years.
- No age-related precautions have been noted in the elderly.

Precautions

- Use zolmitriptan cautiously in patients with controlled hypertension, a history of CVA, mild to moderate hepatic or renal impairment, or cardiovascular risk factors.

Administration and Handling

PO

- Give zolmitriptan without regard to food.

Nasal

- Instruct the patient to blow his or her nose gently to clear nasal passages.
- With the patient's head upright, close one of the patient's nostrils with an index finger and have the patient breathe gently through the mouth.
- Insert the nozzle about 1/2 inch into the patient's open nostril.
- Instruct the patient to close his or her mouth, then take a breath through the nose while depressing the plunger and releasing the spray.
- Remove the nozzle from the patient's nose, and instruct the patient to gently breathe in through the nose and out through the mouth for 15–20 seconds. Tell the patient not to breathe in deeply.

Intervention and Evaluation

- Monitor the patient for dizziness.
- Monitor BP, especially in patients with hepatic impairment.
- Assess the patient for relief of migraines and associated symptoms, including nausea and vomiting, photophobia, and phonophobia (sound sensitivity).

Patient Teaching

- Instruct the patient to take a single dose of zolmitriptan as soon as migraine symptoms appear.
- Explain to the patient that zolmitriptan is intended to relieve migraines, not to prevent them or reduce the number of attacks.
- Advise the patient to avoid tasks that require mental alertness or motor skills until his or her response to the drug has been established.
- Warn the patient to notify the physician if he or she experiences blood in urine or stool, chest pain, palpitations, easy bruising, numbness or pain in the arms or legs, throat tightness, or swelling of the eyelids, face, or lips.
- Advise the patient to lie down in a dark, quiet room for additional benefit after taking zolmitriptan.

37 Antiparkinson Agents

amantadine hydrochloride
apomorphine
benztropine mesylate
bromocriptine mesylate
carbidopa and levodopa
entacapone
pergolide mesylate
pramipexole
ropinirole hydrochloride
selegiline hydrochloride
tolcapone

Uses: Antiparkinson agents are used to treat Parkinson's disease. They're prescribed to reduce parkinsonian signs and symptoms, to correct the disease-induced dopamine deficit, or both. In addition, some drugs in this class have other indications. For example, bromocriptine is also used to treat hyperprolactemia and acromegaly.

Action: Because antiparkinson agents belong to four distinct subclasses, they work by different mechanisms. *Dopaminergics,* such as carbidopa and levodopa, increase dopamine synthesis. *Dopamine agonists,* such as pramipexole, directly activate dopamine receptors and promote the release of dopamine. *Monoamine oxidase (MAO)-B inhibitors,* such as selegiline, are used with levodopa or carbidopa and levodopa; by inhibiting the enzymes that break down dopamine, they extend levodopa's antiparkinsonian effect. *Catechol-*O*-methyltransferase (COMT) inhibitors,* such as entacapone, are given with carbidopa and levodopa; they inhibit the enzyme COMT, which increases the levodopa concentration. (See the illustration *Mechanisms of Action: Antiparkinson Agents,* page 768.)

COMBINATION PRODUCTS

STALEVO: entacapone/carbidopa and levodopa 200 mg/12.5 mg/50 mg; 200 mg/ 25 mg/100 mg; 200 mg/37.5 mg/150 mg.

amantadine hydrochloride

(Symmetrel)
See Antiviral Agents

apomorphine

aye-poe-**more**-feen
(Apokyn)

CATEGORY AND SCHEDULE

Pregnancy Risk Category: C

MECHANISM OF ACTION

An antiparkinson agent that stimulates postsynaptic dopamine receptors in the brain. **Therapeutic Effect:** Relieves signs and symptoms of Parkinson's disease and improves motor function.

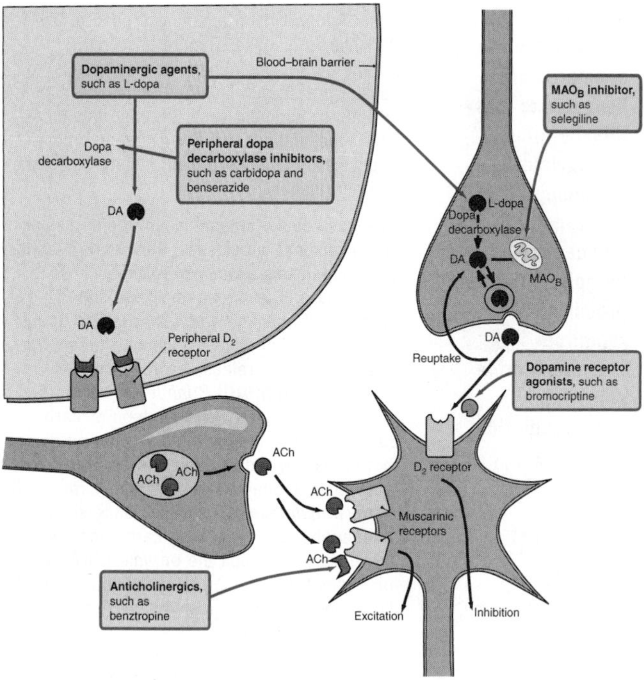

Mechanisms of Action: Antiparkinson Agents

In Parkinson's disease, voluntary movement is hampered because of reduced levels of dopamine (DA) in the brain, especially the corpus striatum and substantia nigra, along with a loss of dopaminergic neurons in the basal ganglia. The goal of treatment is to increase dopaminergic activity and reduce cholinergic activity.

Antiparkinson agents treat Parkinson's disease in several ways. Dopaminergic agents, such as the dopamine precursor, levodopa (L-dopa), cross the blood-brain barrier and convert to dopamine, restoring the brain's content of the neurotransmitter. Consequently, hyperactive cholinergic activity is reduced. To prevent the breakdown of levodopa, the drug carbidopa inhibits the enzyme dopa decarboxylase. As a result, more levodopa is available to move into the brain. Similarly, the monoamine oxidase B (MAO$_B$) inhibitor, selegiline, helps to prevent the breakdown of dopamine. Normally MAO$_B$ degrades dopamine.

Peripheral dopamine receptor agonists, such as bromocriptine, work directly on dopamine 2 (D$_2$) receptors in the corpus striatum. These drugs are often used as adjunctive therapy with levodopa.

Anticholinergic agents, such as benztropine, reduce cholinergic activity by blocking the action of acetylcholine (ACh) on muscarinic receptors responsible for striatal cholinergic excitation.

PHARMACOKINETICS

Rapidly absorbed after subcutaneous administration. Protein binding: 99.9%. Widely distributed. Rapidly eliminated from plasma. Not detected in urine or secretions. ***Half-life:*** 41–45 min.

AVAILABILITY

Injection: 10 mg/ml.

INDICATIONS AND DOSAGES

▸ **Acute, intermittent treatment of hypomobility ("off" episodes) associated with advanced Parkinson's disease**

Subcutaneous

Adults, Elderly. Initially, 0.2 ml (2 mg); may be increased in 0.1-ml (1-mg) increments every few days. Maximum: 0.6 ml (6 mg).

CONTRAINDICATIONS

Concurrent use of alosetron, dolasetron, granisetron, ondansetron, or palonosetron

INTERACTIONS

Drug

Alosetron, dolasetron, granisetron, ondansetron, palonosetron: May produce profound hypotension and loss of consciousness.

Butyrophenones, metoclopramide, phenothiazines, thioxanthenes: Decrease the effectiveness of apomorphine.

CNS depressants: May increase CNS depressant effects.

Herbal

None known.

Food

None known.

DIAGNOSTIC TEST EFFECTS

May increase serum alkaline phosphatase level.

SIDE EFFECTS

Occasional (4%–3%)

Injection site discomfort, arthralgia, somnolence, hypersalivation, pallor, yawning, headache, dizziness, diaphoresis, vomiting, orthostatic hypotension

Rare (less than 2%)

Psychosis, stomatitis, altered taste, hallucinations

SERIOUS REACTIONS

! Respiratory depression or CNS stimulation (characterized by tachypnea, bradycardia or persistent vomiting) may occur.

! Apomorphine use may cause or exacerbate preexisting dyskinesia.

NURSING CONSIDERATIONS

Baseline Assessment

- Assess the patient for symptoms of Parkinson's disease to establish a baseline. Also document vital signs, including BP.

Lifespan Considerations

- It is unknown if apomorphine is distributed in breast milk.
- The safety and efficacy of apomorphine have not been established in children.
- No age-related precautions have been noted in the elderly; however, they may be more prone to develop hallucinations.

Precautions

- Use apomorphine cautiously in patients with cardiac decompensation or impaired hepatic or renal function.

Administration and Handling

◂**ALERT**▸ Don't give apomorphine without also administering an antiemetic other than a 5-HT3 antagonist. Antiemetic therapy should begin 3 days before the initial dose of apomorphine and continue for at least the first 3 months of therapy.

Subcutaneous

- Store apomorphine at room temperature.
- Apomorphine should appear clear and colorless. Discard the solution if it's cloudy or green or contains particles.

Intervention and Evaluation

- Assist the patient with ambulation if he or she experiences dizziness.
- Assess the patient for clinical improvement of symptoms, including mask-like facial expression, muscle rigidity, shuffling gait, and tremors of the head or hands at rest.

Patient Teaching

- Inform the patient that dizziness and drowsiness may be the initial response to the drug.
- Instruct the patient to change positions slowly to prevent orthostatic hypotension.
- Warn the patient to avoid performing tasks that require mental alertness or motor skills until his or her response to the drug has been established.
- Inform the patient, especially if elderly, that he or she may experience hallucinations during apomorphine therapy.

benztropine mesylate

benz-troe-peen

(Apo-Benztropine[CAN], Bentrop [AUS], Cogentin)

Do not confuse benztropine with bromocriptine.

CATEGORY AND SCHEDULE

Pregnancy Risk Category: C

MECHANISM OF ACTION

An antiparkinson agent that selectively blocks central cholinergic receptors, helping to balance cholinergic and dopaminergic activity.
Therapeutic Effect: Reduces the incidence and severity of akinesia, rigidity, and tremor.

AVAILABILITY

Tablets: 0.5 mg, 1 mg, 2 mg.
Injection: 1 mg/ml.

INDICATIONS AND DOSAGES

▸ **Parkinsonism**

PO

Adults. 0.5–6 mg/day as a single dose or in 2 divided doses. Titrate by 0.5 mg at 5–6 day intervals.
Elderly. Initially, 0.5 mg once or twice a day. Titrate by 0.5 mg at 5–6 day intervals. Maximum: 4 mg/day.

▸ **Drug-induced extrapyramidal symptoms**

PO, IM

Adults. 1–4 mg once or twice a day.
Children older than 3 yr. 0.02–0.05 mg/kg/dose once or twice a day.

▸ **Acute dystonic reactions**

IV, IM

Adults. Initially, 1–2 mg; then 1–2 mg PO twice a day to prevent recurrence.

CONTRAINDICATIONS

Angle-closure glaucoma, benign prostatic hyperplasia, children younger than 3 years, GI obstruction, intestinal atony, megacolon, myasthenia gravis, paralytic ileus, severe ulcerative colitis

INTERACTIONS

Drug

Alcohol, other CNS depressants: May increase sedation.
Amantadine, anticholinergics, MAOIs: May increase the effects of benztropine.
Antacids, antidiarrheals: May decrease the absorption and effects of benztropine.

Herbal
None known.
Food
None known.

DIAGNOSTIC TEST EFFECTS
None known.

SIDE EFFECTS
Frequent
Somnolence, dry mouth, blurred vision, constipation, decreased sweating or urination, GI upset, photosensitivity
Occasional
Headache, memory loss, muscle cramps, anxiety, peripheral paresthesia, orthostatic hypotension, abdominal cramps
Rare
Rash, confusion, eye pain

SERIOUS REACTIONS
! Overdose may produce severe anticholinergic effects, such as unsteadiness, somnolence, tachycardia, dyspnea, skin flushing, and severe dryness of the mouth, nose, or throat.
! Severe paradoxical reactions, marked by hallucinations, tremor, seizures, and toxic psychosis, may occur.

NURSING CONSIDERATIONS
Baseline Assessment
- Assess the patient's mental status for agitation, confusion, disorientation, and psychotic-like symptoms because benztropine frequently produces such side effects in patients older than 60 years.
Precautions
◀ALERT▶ Patients older than 60 years are more likely to develop agitation, disorientation, confusion, and psychotic-like symptoms.
- Use benztropine cautiously in patients with arrhythmias, heart disease, hypertension, hepatic or renal impairment, obstructive diseases of the GI or GU tracts, urine retention, benign prostatic hyperplasia, tachycardia, or treated open-angle glaucoma.
Intervention and Evaluation
- Be alert for neurologic effects, including agitation, headache, somnolence, and confusion.
- Assess the patient for relief of symptoms, such as an improvement of masklike facial expression, muscular rigidity, shuffling gait, and resting tremors of the hands and head.
Patient Teaching
- Inform the patient that dizziness, drowsiness, and dry mouth are expected responses to the drug. Explain that drowsiness tends to diminish or disappear with continued therapy.
- Warn the patient to avoid tasks that require mental alertness or motor skills until his or her response to the drug has been established.
- Urge the patient to avoid alcoholic beverages during benztropine therapy.

bromocriptine mesylate
broe-moe-**krip**-teen
(Apo-Bromocriptine[CAN], Bromohexal[AUS], Kripton[AUS], Parlodel)
Do not confuse bromocriptine with benztropine, or Parlodel with pindolol.

CATEGORY AND SCHEDULE
Pregnancy Risk Category: C

MECHANISM OF ACTION

A dopamine agonist that directly stimulates dopamine receptors in the corpus striatum and inhibits prolactin secretion. Also suppresses secretion of growth hormone. **Therapeutic Effect:** Improves symptoms of parkinsonism, suppresses galactorrhea, and reduces serum growth hormone concentrations in acromegaly.

PHARMACOKINETICS

Indication	Onset	Peak	Duration
Prolactin lowering	2 hr	8 hr	24 hr
Antiparkinson	0.5–1.5 hr	2 hr	N/A
Growth hormone suppressant	1–2 hr	4–8 wk	4–8 hr

Minimally absorbed from the GI tract. Protein binding: 90%–96%. Metabolized in the liver. Excreted in feces by biliary secretion. ***Half-life:*** 15 hr.

AVAILABILITY

Capsules: 5 mg.
Tablets: 2.5 mg.

INDICATIONS AND DOSAGES

▸ Hyperprolactinemia

PO

Adults, Elderly. Initially, 1.25–2.5 mg/day. May increase by 2.5 mg/day at 3- to 7-day intervals. Range: 2.5 mg 2–3 times a day.

▸ Parkinson's disease

PO

Adults, Elderly. Initially, 1.25 mg twice a day. May increase by 2.5 mg/day every 14–28 days. Range: 30–90 mg/day.

▸ Acromegaly

PO

Adults, Elderly. Initially, 1.25–2.5 mg. May increase at 3- to 7-day intervals. Usual dose 20–30 mg/day.

OFF-LABEL USES

Treatment of cocaine addiction, hyperprolactinemia associated with pituitary adenomas, neuroleptic malignant syndrome

CONTRAINDICATIONS

Hypersensitivity to ergot alkaloids, peripheral vascular disease, pregnancy, severe ischemic heart disease, uncontrolled hypertension

INTERACTIONS

Drug

Alcohol: May produce a disulfiram-like reaction (chest pain, confusion, flushed face, nausea, vomiting).
Erythromycin, ritonavir: May increase bromocriptine blood concentration and risk of toxicity.
Estrogens, progestins: May decrease the effects of bromocriptine.
Haloperidol, MAOIs, phenothiazines, risperidone: May decrease bromocriptine's prolactin-lowering effect.
Hypotension-producing medications: May increase hypotension.
Levodopa: May increase the effects of bromocriptine.

Herbal

None known.

Food

None known.

DIAGNOSTIC TEST EFFECTS

May increase plasma growth hormone concentration.

SIDE EFFECTS

Frequent

Nausea (49%), headache (19%), dizziness (17%)

Occasional (7%–3%)

Fatigue, light-headedness, vomiting, abdominal cramps, diarrhea, constipation, nasal congestion, somnolence, dry mouth

Rare

Muscle cramps, urinary hesitancy

SERIOUS REACTIONS

! Visual or auditory hallucinations have been noted in patients with Parkinson's disease.

! Long-term, high-dose therapy may produce continuing rhinorrhea, syncope, GI hemorrhage, peptic ulcer, and severe abdominal pain.

NURSING CONSIDERATIONS

Baseline Assessment

• Expect to rule out a pituitary gland tumor before beginning treatment for hyperprolactinemia with amenorrhea or galactorrhea and infertility.

• Plan to obtain a pregnancy test to rule out pregnancy.

Lifespan Considerations

• Bromocriptine use is not recommended during pregnancy or breast-feeding.

• The safety and efficacy of bromocriptine have not been established in children.

• Elderly patients are more prone to CNS adverse effects.

Precautions

◀ALERT▶ The incidence of side effects is high, especially at the beginning of therapy and with high dosages.

• Use bromocriptine cautiously in patients with cardiac or hepatic function impairment, hypertension, or psychiatric disorders.

Administration and Handling

PO

• Make sure the patient is lying down before administering the first dose to avoid light-headedness.

• Give bromocriptine after food to decrease the incidence of nausea.

Intervention and Evaluation

• Assist the patient with ambulation if dizziness occurs after drug administration.

• Assess the patient for a therapeutic response, such as a decrease in breast engorgement or parkinsonian symptoms.

• Monitor the patient for constipation.

Patient Teaching

• Instruct the patient change positions slowly and to dangle the legs momentarily before standing to avoid light-headedness.

• Warn the patient to avoid tasks that require mental alertness or motor skills until his or her response to the drug has been established.

• Urge the patient to use nonhormonal contraceptives during treatment.

• Instruct the patient to notify the physician if he or she experiences watery nasal discharge.

carbidopa and levodopa

kar-bee-**doe**-pa; lee-voe-**doe**-pa

(Apo-Levocarb[CAN], Kinson[AUS], Parcopa, Sinemet, Sinemet CR)

CATEGORY AND SCHEDULE

Pregnancy Risk Category: C

MECHANISM OF ACTION

Levodopa is converted to dopamine in the basal ganglia thus increasing dopamine concentration in brain and inhibiting hyperactive cholinergic activity. Carbidopa prevents peripheral breakdown of levodopa, allowing more levodopa to be available for transport into the brain. **Therapeutic Effect:** Reduces tremor.

PHARMACOKINETICS
Carbidopa is rapidly and completely absorbed from the GI tract. Widely distributed. Excreted primarily in urine. Levodopa is converted to dopamine. Excreted primarily in urine. ***Half-life:*** 1–2 hr (carbidopa); 1–3 hr (levodopa).

AVAILABILITY
Tablets: 10 mg carbidopa/100 mg levodopa, 25 mg carbidopa/100 mg levodopa, 25 mg carbidopa/250 mg levodopa.
Tablets (Orally-Disintegrating [Parcopa]): 10 mg carbidopa/100 mg levodopa, 25 mg carbidopa/100 mg levodopa, 25 mg carbidopa/250 mg levodopa.
Tablets (Extended-Release): 25 mg carbidopa/100 mg levodopa, 50 mg carbidopa/200 mg levodopa.

INDICATIONS AND DOSAGES
▸ Parkinsonism
PO
Adults. Initially, 25/100 mg 2–4 times a day. May increase up 200/2,000 mg daily.
Elderly. Initially, 25/100 mg twice a day. May increase as necessary.
When converting a patient from Sinemet to Sinemet CR (50 mg/200 mg), dosage is based on the total daily dose of levodopa, as follows:

Sinemet	Sinemet CR
300–400 mg	1 tablet twice a day
500–600 mg	1.5 tablets twice a day or 1 tab 3 times a day
700–800 mg	4 tablets in 3 or more divided doses
900–1,000 mg	5 tablets in 3 or more divided doses

Intervals between doses of Sinemet CR should be 4–8 hr while awake.

CONTRAINDICATIONS
Angle-closure glaucoma, use within 14 days of MAOIs

INTERACTIONS
Drug
Anticonvulsants, benzodiazepines, haloperidol, phenothiazines: May decrease the effects of carbidopa and levodopa.
MAOIs: May increase the risk of hypertensive crisis.
Selegiline: May increase levodopa-induced dyskinesias, nausea, orthostatic hypotension, confusion, and hallucinations.
Herbal
None known.
Food
None known.

DIAGNOSTIC TEST EFFECTS
May increase BUN level and serum LDH, alkaline phosphatase, bilirubin, AST (SGOT), and ALT (SGPT) levels.

SIDE EFFECTS
Frequent (90%–10%)
Uncontrolled movements of face, tongue, arms, or upper body; nausea and vomiting (80%); anorexia (50%)
Occasional
Depression, anxiety, confusion, nervousness, urine retention, palpitations, dizziness, light-headedness, decreased appetite, blurred vision, constipation, dry mouth, flushed skin, headache, insomnia, diarrhea, unusual fatigue, darkening of urine and sweat
Rare
Hypertension, ulcer, hemolytic anemia (marked by fatigue)

SERIOUS REACTIONS

! Patients on long-term therapy have a high incidence of involuntary choreiform, dystonic, and dyskinetic movements.

! Numerous mild to severe CNS and psychiatric disturbances may occur, including reduced attention span, anxiety, nightmares, daytime somnolence, euphoria, fatigue, paranoia, psychotic episodes, depression, and hallucinations.

NURSING CONSIDERATIONS

Baseline Assessment

• Assess the patient's mental status, including affect, mood, and evidence of CNS depression, before and at regular intervals throughout drug therapy.

Lifespan Considerations

• It is unknown if carbidopa and levodopa crosses the placenta or is distributed in breast milk. However, this drug may inhibit lactation. Women should not breast-feed while taking this drug.

• The safety and efficacy of carbidopa and levodopa have not been established in children younger than 18 years.

• The elderly are more sensitive to levodopa's effects. Elderly patients receiving anticholinergics are at increased risk for adverse CNS effects, such as anxiety, confusion, and nervousness.

Precautions

• Use carbidopa and levodopa cautiously in patients with active peptic ulcer; severe cardiac, endocrine, hepatic, pulmonary, or renal impairment; treated open-angle glaucoma; or a history of MI, bronchial asthma (because of tartrazine sensitivity), or emphysema.

Administration and Handling

◀ **ALERT** ▶ Plan to discontinue levodopa at least 12 hours before giving carbidopa and levodopa. Expect the initial dose to provide at least 25% of the previous levodopa dose. Instruct the patient to void before giving carbidopa and levodopa to reduce the risk of urine retention.

PO

• Give carbidopa and levodopa without regard to food.

• Scored tablets may be crushed as needed. Extended-release tablets may be cut in half but not crushed.

Intervention and Evaluation

• Be alert for dyskinesia and neurologic effects, including agitation, headache, lethargy, and confusion.

• Assess the patient for relief of symptoms, such as improvement of masklike facial expression, muscular rigidity, shuffling gait, and resting tremors of the hands and head.

Patient Teaching

• Instruct the patient to take carbidopa and levodopa with food to minimize GI upset.

• Inform the patient that the drug's therapeutic effects may be delayed from several weeks to months.

• Warn the patient to avoid tasks that require mental alertness or motor skills until his or her response to the drug has been established.

• Caution the patient to avoid alcoholic beverages during therapy.

• Suggest that the patient take sips of tepid water and chew sugarless gum to relieve dry mouth.

• Inform the patient that carbidopa and levodopa may darken sweat and urine, but that this is not harmful.

• Warn the patient to notify the physician if he or she experiences difficulty urinating, irregular heartbeats, mental changes, severe nausea or vomiting, or uncontrolled movement of the hands, arms, legs, eyelids, face, mouth, or tongue.

entacapone

en-**tak**-a-pone
(Comtan)

CATEGORY AND SCHEDULE

Pregnancy Risk Category: C

MECHANISM OF ACTION

An antiparkinson agent that inhibits the enzyme catechol-*O*-methyltransferase (COMT), potentiating dopamine activity and increasing the duration of action of levodopa. **Therapeutic Effect:** Decreases signs and symptoms of Parkinson's disease.

PHARMACOKINETICS

Rapidly absorbed after PO administration. Protein binding: 98%. Metabolized in the liver. Primarily eliminated by biliary excretion. Not removed by hemodialysis. ***Half-life:*** 2.4 hr.

AVAILABILITY

Tablets: 200 mg.

INDICATIONS AND DOSAGES

▸ **Adjunctive treatment of Parkinson's disease**

PO

Adults, Elderly. 200 mg concomitantly with each dose of carbidopa and levodopa up to a maximum of 8 times a day (1,600 mg).

CONTRAINDICATIONS

Hypersensitivity, use within 14 days of MAOIs

INTERACTIONS

Drug

Ampicillin, cholestyramine, erythromycin, probenecid: May decrease the excretion of entacapone.

Bitolterol, dobutamine, dopamine, epinephrine, isoetharine, isoproterenol, epinephrine, methyldopa, norepinephrine: May increase the risk of arrhythmias and changes in BP.

Nonselective MAOIs (including phenelzine): May inhibit catecholamine metabolism.

Other CNS depressants: May increase CNS depression.

Herbal

None known.

Food

None known.

DIAGNOSTIC TEST EFFECTS

None known.

SIDE EFFECTS

Frequent (greater than 10%)

Dyskinesia, nausea, dark yellow or orange urine and sweat, diarrhea

Occasional (9%–3%)

Abdominal pain, vomiting, constipation, dry mouth, fatigue, back pain

Rare (less than 2%)

Anxiety, somnolence, agitation, dyspepsia, flatulence, diaphoresis, asthenia, dyspnea

SERIOUS REACTIONS

! None known.

NURSING CONSIDERATIONS

Baseline Assessment

- Obtain baseline vital signs, including BP.

Lifespan Considerations

- It is unknown if entacapone is distributed in breast milk.
- This drug is not indicated for use in children.
- No age-related precautions have been noted in the elderly.

Precautions

- Use entacapone cautiously in patients with hepatic or renal impairment, dyskinesia, orthostatic hypotension, or syncope.

Administration and Handling

◀ALERT▶ Always administer entacapone with carbidopa and levodopa.

PO

• Give entacapone without regard to food.

Intervention and Evaluation

• Monitor the patient for dyskinesia, diarrhea, and orthostatic hypotension.
• Assess the patient for relief of symptoms, including improvement of masklike facial expression, muscular rigidity, shuffling gait, and resting tremors of the hands and head.
• Monitor the patient's BP.

Patient Teaching

• Instruct the patient to take entacapone with carbidopa and levodopa for best results.
• Caution the patient to avoid tasks that require mental alertness or motor skills until his or her response to the drug has been established.
• Inform the patient that entacapone may cause sweat or urine to turn dark yellow or orange.
• Advise the patient to notify the physician if he or she experiences uncontrolled movement of the hands, arms, legs, eyelids, face, mouth, or tongue.

pergolide mesylate

per-go-lide

(Permax)

Do not confuse Permax with Pentrax or Pernox.

CATEGORY AND SCHEDULE

Pregnancy Risk Category: B

MECHANISM OF ACTION

A centrally active dopamine agonist that directly stimulates dopamine receptors. **Therapeutic Effect:** Decreases signs and symptoms of Parkinson's disease.

PHARMACOKINETICS

Well absorbed from the GI tract. Protein binding: 90%. Undergoes extensive first-pass metabolism in the liver. Primarily excreted in urine. Unknown if removed by hemodialysis.

AVAILABILITY

Tablets: 0.05 mg, 0.25 mg, 1 mg.

INDICATIONS AND DOSAGES

▸ **Parkinsonism**

PO

Adults, Elderly. Initially, 0.05 mg/day for 2 days. May increase by 0.1–0.15 mg/day every 3 days over the next 12 days; afterward may increase by 0.25 mg/day every 3 days. Range: 2–3 mg/day in 3 divided doses. Maximum: 5 mg/day.

CONTRAINDICATIONS

Hypersensitivity to pergolide or other ergot derivatives

INTERACTIONS

Drug

Haloperidol, loxapine, methyldopa, metoclopramide, phenothiazines: May decrease the effectiveness of pergolide.

Hypotension-producing medications: May increase the hypotensive effect.

Herbal

None known.

Food

None known.

DIAGNOSTIC TEST EFFECTS

May increase the serum growth hormone level.

SIDE EFFECTS

Frequent (24%–10%)
Nausea, dizziness, hallucinations, constipation, rhinitis, dystonia, confusion, somnolence
Occasional (9%–3%)
Orthostatic hypotension, insomnia, dry mouth, peripheral edema, anxiety, diarrhea, dyspepsia, abdominal pain, headache, abnormal vision, anorexia, tremor, depression, rash
Rare (less than 2%)
Urinary frequency, vivid dreams, neck pain, hypotension, vomiting

SERIOUS REACTIONS

! Symptoms of overdose may vary from CNS depression, characterized by sedation, apnea, cardiovascular collapse, and death, to severe paradoxical reactions, such as hallucinations, tremor, and seizures.

NURSING CONSIDERATIONS

Baseline Assessment

- Obtain a baseline EKG for patients with a history of cardiac disease.
- Monitor the patient's BP and pulse rate to detect hypotension and irregularities that could indicate an arrhythmia.

Lifespan Considerations

- It is unknown if pergolide crosses the placenta or is distributed in breast milk. However, pergolide may interfere with lactation.
- The safety and efficacy of this drug have not been established in children.
- No age-related precautions have been noted in the elderly.

Precautions

- Use pergolide cautiously in patients with pre-existing cardiac arrhythmias, confusion, or hallucinations.

Administration and Handling

PO
◀ **ALERT** ▶ Pergolide is usually given in 3 divided doses daily.
- Crush scored tablets as needed.
- Give pergolide without regard to food.

Intervention and Evaluation

- Be alert for the drug's neurologic effects, including agitation, headache, lethargy, and confusion.
- Monitor the patient for dyskinesia.
- Monitor the patient's BP and EKG.
- Assess the patient for relief of parkinsonian symptoms, such as improvement of masklike facial expression, muscular rigidity, shuffling gait, and resting tremors of the hands and head.
- Overdose may require supportive measures to maintain BP. Plan to monitor cardiac function, obtain vital signs, and check ABG and serum electrolyte levels.
- Activated charcoal may be more effective than emesis or lavage for overdose.

Patient Teaching

- Inform the patient that dizziness, drowsiness, and dry mouth are expected side effects of pergolide.
- Warn the patient to avoid tasks that require mental alertness or motor skills until his or her response to the drug has been established.
- Urge the patient to avoid alcoholic beverages during therapy.

pramipexole

pram-eh-**pex**-ol
(Mirapex)
Do not confuse Mirapex with Mifeprex or MiraLax.

CATEGORY AND SCHEDULE

Pregnancy Risk Category: C

MECHANISM OF ACTION

An antiparkinson agent that stimulates dopamine receptors in the striatum. **Therapeutic Effect:** Relieves signs and symptoms of Parkinson's disease.

PHARMACOKINETICS

Rapidly and extensively absorbed after PO administration. Protein binding: 15%. Widely distributed. Steady-state concentrations achieved within 2 days. Primarily eliminated in urine. Not removed by hemodialysis. ***Half-life:*** 8 hr (12 hr in patients older than 65 yr).

AVAILABILITY

Tablets: 0.125 mg, 0.25 mg, 0.5 mg, 1 mg, 1.5 mg.

INDICATIONS AND DOSAGES

▸ **Parkinson's disease**

PO

Adults, Elderly. Initially, 0.375 mg/day in 3 divided doses. Don't increase dosage more frequently than every 5–7 days. Maintenance: 1.5–4.5 mg/day in 3 equally divided doses.

▸ **Dosage in renal impairment**

Dosage and frequency are modified based on creatinine clearance.

Creatinine clearance	Initial Dose	Maximum Dose
Greater than 60 ml/min	0.125 mg 3 times a day	1.5 mg 3 times a day
35–59 ml/min	0.125 mg twice a day	1.5 mg twice a day
15–34 ml/min	0.125 mg once a day	1.5 mg once a day

CONTRAINDICATIONS

History of hypersensitivity to pramipexole

INTERACTIONS

Drug

Carbidopa and levodopa, levodopa: May increase plasma level of levodopa.

Cimetidine: Increases pramipexole plasma concentration and half-life.

Cimetidine, diltiazem, quinidine, quinine, ranitidine, triamterene, verapamil: May decrease pramipexole clearance.

Herbal

None known.

Food

All foods: Delay peak drug plasma levels by 1 hour but don't affect drug absorption.

DIAGNOSTIC TEST EFFECTS

None known.

SIDE EFFECTS

Frequent

Early Parkinson's disease (28%–10%): Nausea, asthenia, dizziness, somnolence, insomnia, constipation

Advanced Parkinson's disease (53%–17%): Orthostatic hypotension, extrapyramidal reactions, insomnia, dizziness, hallucinations

Occasional

Early Parkinson's disease (5%–2%): Edema, malaise, confusion, amnesia, akathisia, anorexia, dysphagia, peripheral edema, vision changes, impotence

Advanced Parkinson's disease (10%–7%): Asthenia, somnolence, confusion, constipation, abnormal gait, dry mouth

Rare

Advanced Parkinson's disease (6%–2%): General edema, malaise, chest pain, amnesia, tremor, urinary frequency or incontinence, dyspnea, rhinitis, vision changes

SERIOUS REACTIONS

! None known.

NURSING CONSIDERATIONS

Baseline Assessment

- Expect to perform renal function studies to guide drug dosage.
- Obtain baseline vital signs, including BP.

Lifespan Considerations

- It is unknown if pramipexole is distributed in breast milk.
- The safety and efficacy of pramipexole have not been established in children.
- Elderly patients are at increased risk for hallucinations.

Precautions

- Use pramipexole cautiously in patients with hallucinations, syncope, renal impairment, or a history of orthostatic hypotension and in those using CNS depressants concurrently.

Administration and Handling

PO

- Give pramipexole without regard to food.

Intervention and Evaluation

- Instruct the patient to change positions slowly to prevent orthostatic hypotension.
- Assist the patient with ambulation if he or she experiences dizziness.
- Assess the patient for constipation, a common side effect of the drug.
- Assess the patient for relief of symptoms, such as improvement of masklike facial expression, muscular rigidity, shuffling gait, and resting tremors of the hands and head.

Patient Teaching

- Instruct the patient to take pramipexole with food if nausea is a problem.
- Caution the patient against abruptly discontinuing pramipexole.
- Inform the patient (especially if elderly) that the drug may cause hallucinations.
- Tell the patient that orthostatic hypotension occurs more commonly during initial therapy.
- Warn the patient to avoid tasks that require mental alertness or motor skills until his or her response to the drug has been established.

ropinirole hydrochloride

ro-**pin**-i-role
(Requip)

CATEGORY AND SCHEDULE

Pregnancy Risk Category: C

MECHANISM OF ACTION

An antiparkinson agent that stimulates dopamine receptors in the striatum. **Therapeutic Effect:** Relieves signs and symptoms of Parkinson's disease.

PHARMACOKINETICS

Rapidly absorbed after PO administration. Protein binding: 40%. Extensively distributed throughout the body. Extensively metabolized. Steady-state concentrations achieved within 2 days. Eliminated in urine. Unknown if removed by hemodialysis. ***Half-life:*** 6 hr.

AVAILABILITY

Tablets: 0.25 mg, 0.5 mg, 1 mg, 2 mg, 3 mg, 4 mg, 5 mg.

INDICATIONS AND DOSAGES

▸ **Parkinson's disease**

PO

Adults, Elderly. Initially, 0.25 mg 3 times a day. May increase dosage every 7 days.

CONTRAINDICATIONS

None known.

INTERACTIONS

Drug

Butyrophenones, metoclopramide, phenothiazines, thioxanthenes: Decrease the effectiveness of ropinirole.
Cimetidine, diltiazem, enoxacin, erythromycin, fluvoxamine, mexiletine, norfloxacin, tacrine: Alter ropinirole blood concentration.
Ciprofloxacin: Increases ropinirole blood concentration.
CNS depressants: May increase CNS depressant effects.
Estrogens: Reduce the clearance of ropinirole.
Levodopa: Increases the blood concentration of levodopa.

Herbal

None known.

Food

All foods: Delay peak plasma levels by 1 hour but don't affect drug absorption.

DIAGNOSTIC TEST EFFECTS

May increase serum alkaline phosphatase level.

SIDE EFFECTS

Frequent (60%–40%)

Nausea, dizziness, somnolence

Occasional (12%–5%)

Syncope, vomiting, fatigue, viral infection, dyspepsia, diaphoresis, asthenia, orthostatic hypotension, abdominal discomfort, pharyngitis, abnormal vision, dry mouth, hypertension, hallucinations, confusion

Rare (less than 4%)

Anorexia, peripheral edema, memory loss, rhinitis, sinusitis, palpitations, impotence

SERIOUS REACTIONS

! None known.

NURSING CONSIDERATIONS

Baseline Assessment

- Obtain baseline vital signs, especially BP and serum alkaline phosphatase levels.

Lifespan Considerations

- Because ropinirole is distributed in breast milk, it may cause drug-related effects in the breast-feeding infant.
- The safety and efficacy of ropinirole have not been established in children.
- No age-related precautions have been noted in the elderly, but they are more likely than other age-groups to experience hallucinations.

Precautions

- Use ropinirole cautiously in patients with hallucinations (especially the elderly), syncope, or a history of orthostatic hypotension, and in patients who take CNS depressants concurrently.

Administration and Handling

PO

- Expect the dosage schedule to increase very gradually, as follow: Week 1, 0.25 mg 3 times a day to total daily dose of 0.75 mg; Week 2, 0.5 mg 3 times a day to total daily dose of 1.5 mg; Week 3, 0.75 mg 3 times a day to total daily dose of 2.25 mg; Week 4, 1 mg 3 times a day to total daily dose of 3 mg, as prescribed. After week 4, dosage may be increased every week, if needed, by 1.5–3 mg/day to a total dose of 24 mg/day.
- Plan to discontinue the drug gradually at 7-day intervals, as follows: first decrease the frequency from 3 times a day to twice a day for 4 days; for the remaining 3 days, decrease the frequency to once a day before complete withdrawal, as prescribed.

Intervention and Evaluation

- Assess the patient for relief of

symptoms, such as improvement of masklike facial expression, muscular rigidity, shuffling gait, and resting tremors of the hands and head.
• Assist the patient with ambulation if he or she experiences dizziness.

Patient Teaching

• Instruct the patient to take ropinirole with food if nausea is a problem.
• Inform the patient that dizziness, drowsiness, and orthostatic hypotension are common initial responses to the drug. Advise the patient to change positions slowly to help prevent orthostatic hypotension.
• Warn the patient to avoid tasks that require mental alertness or motor skills until his or her response to the drug has been established.
• Inform the patient (especially if elderly) that the drug may cause hallucinations.

selegiline hydrochloride

seh-**leg**-ill-ene
(Apo-Selegiline[CAN], Eldepryl, Novo-Selegiline[CAN], Selgene[AUS])
Do not confuse selegiline with Stelazine, or Eldepryl with enalapril.

CATEGORY AND SCHEDULE

Pregnancy Risk Category: C

MECHANISM OF ACTION

An antiparkinson agent that irreversibly inhibits the activity of monoamine oxidase type B, the enzyme that breaks down dopamine, thereby increasing dopaminergic action.
Therapeutic Effect: Relieves signs and symptoms of Parkinson's disease.

PHARMACOKINETICS

Rapidly absorbed from the GI tract. Crosses the blood-brain barrier. Metabolized in the liver to the active metabolites. Primarily excreted in urine. ***Half-life:*** 17 hr (amphetamine), 20 hr (methamphetamine).

AVAILABILITY

Capsules: 5 mg.
Tablets: 5 mg.

INDICATIONS AND DOSAGES

▸ **Adjunctive treatment for parkinsonism**

PO

Adults. 10 mg/day in divided doses, such as 5 mg at breakfast and lunch, given concomitantly with each dose of carbidopa and levodopa.
Elderly. Initially, 5 mg in the morning. May increase up to 10 mg/day.

CONTRAINDICATIONS

None known.

INTERACTIONS

Drug

Fluoxetine: May cause serotonin syndrome.
Meperidine: May cause diaphoresis, excitation, hypertension or hypotension, coma, and even death.

Herbal

None known.

Food

Caffeine, tyramine-rich foods: Large amounts of these substances may produce a severe hypertensive reaction.

DIAGNOSTIC TEST EFFECTS

None known.

SIDE EFFECTS

Frequent (10%–4%)

Nausea, dizziness, light-headedness, syncope, abdominal discomfort

Occasional (3%–2%)
Confusion, hallucinations, dry mouth, vivid dreams, dyskinesia
Rare (1%)
Headache, myalgia, anxiety, diarrhea, insomnia

SERIOUS REACTIONS

! Symptoms of overdose may vary from CNS depression, characterized by sedation, apnea, cardiovascular collapse, and death, to severe paradoxical reactions, such as hallucinations, tremor, and seizures.
! Other serious effects may include involuntary movements, impaired motor coordination, loss of balance, blepharospasm, facial grimaces, feeling of heaviness in the lower extremities, depression, nightmares, delusions, overstimulation, sleep disturbance, and anger.

NURSING CONSIDERATIONS

Baseline Assessment

- Obtain baseline vital signs, especially BP.

Lifespan Considerations

- It is unknown if selegiline crosses the placenta or is distributed in breast milk.
- The safety and efficacy of selegiline have not been established in children.
- No age-related precautions have been noted in the elderly.

Precautions

- Use selegiline cautiously in patients with cardiac arrhythmias, dementia, history of peptic ulcer disease, profound tremor, psychosis, or tardive dyskinesia.

Administration and Handling

PO
- Expect to administer selegiline with carbidopa and levodopa therapy.

◀ALERT▶ Keep in mind that therapy should begin with the lowest dosage, then increase gradually over 3 to 4 weeks.

Intervention and Evaluation

- Be alert for neurologic effects, including agitation, headache, lethargy, and confusion.
- Monitor the patient for dyskinetic effects.
- Assess the patient for clinical reversal of symptoms, including improvement of masklike facial expression, muscular rigidity, shuffling gait, and resting tremor of the hands and head.

Patient Teaching

- Inform the patient that dizziness, drowsiness, light-headedness, and dry mouth are common side effects of the drug but will diminish or disappear with continued treatment.
- Instruct the patient change positions slowly and to let legs dangle momentarily before standing to reduce the drug's hypotensive effect.
- Warn the patient to avoid tasks that require mental alertness or motor skills until his or her response to the drug has been established.
- Urge the patient to avoid alcoholic beverages during therapy.
- Instruct the patient to avoid ingesting large amounts of caffeine or tyramine-rich foods, such as wine and aged cheese, to prevent a hypertensive reaction.

tolcapone

toll-ka-pone
(Tasmar)

CATEGORY AND SCHEDULE

Pregnancy Risk Category: C

MECHANISM OF ACTION

An antiparkinson agent that inhibits the enzyme catechol-*O*-methyltransferase (COMT), potentiating dopamine activity and increasing the duration of action of levodopa. **Therapeutic Effect:** Relieves signs and symptoms of Parkinson's disease.

PHARMACOKINETICS
Rapidly absorbed after PO administration. Protein binding: 99%. Metabolized in the liver. Eliminated primarily in urine (60%) and, to a lesser extent, in feces (40%). Unknown if removed by hemodialysis. ***Half-life:*** 2–3 hr.

AVAILABILITY
Tablets: 100 mg, 200 mg.

INDICATIONS AND DOSAGES
▸ Adjunctive treatment of Parkinson's disease
PO
Adults, Elderly. Initially, 100–200 mg 3 times a day concomitantly with each dose of carbidopa and levodopa. Maximum: 600 mg/day.
▸ Dosage in hepatic impairment
Patients with moderate to severe cirrhosis should not receive more than 200 mg tolcapone 3 times a day.

CONTRAINDICATIONS
None known.

INTERACTIONS
Drug
Levodopa: Increases the duration of action of this drug.
Herbal
None known.
Food
All foods: Decrease tolcapone bioavailability by 10%–20% if given within 1 hour before or 2 hour after drug administration.

DIAGNOSTIC TEST EFFECTS
May increase AST (SGOT) and ALT (SGPT) levels.

SIDE EFFECTS
◂ALERT▸ Frequency of side effects increases with dosage. The following effects are based on a 200-mg dose.
Frequent (35%–16%)
Nausea, insomnia, somnolence, anorexia, diarrhea, muscle cramps, orthostatic hypotension, excessive dreaming
Occasional (11%–4%)
Headache, vomiting, confusion, hallucinations, constipation, diaphoresis, bright yellow urine, dry eyes, abdominal pain, dizziness, flatulence
Rare (3%–2%)
Dyspepsia, neck pain, hypotension, fatigue, chest discomfort

SERIOUS REACTIONS
! Upper respiratory tract infection and UTI occur in 7%–5% of patients.
! Too-rapid withdrawal from therapy may produce withdrawal-emergent hyperpyrexia, characterized by fever, muscular rigidity, and altered LOC.
! Dyskinesia and dystonia occur frequently.

NURSING CONSIDERATIONS
Baseline Assessment
• Monitor the patient's AST (SGOT) and ALT (SGPT) levels every 2 weeks for the first year, every 4 weeks for the next 6 months, and every 8 weeks thereafter.
Lifespan Considerations
• It is unknown if tolcapone is distributed in breast milk.
• Tolcapone is not used in children.
• Elderly patients are at increased risk for hallucinations.
Precautions
• Use tolcapone cautiously in pa-

tients with baseline hypotension, severe hepatic or renal impairment, or a history of hallucinations or orthostatic hypotension.

Administration and Handling

◀ALERT▶ Always administer tolcapone with carbidopa and levodopa.

◀ALERT▶ Expect to discontinue tolcapone if the patient's ALT and AST levels exceed the upper limits of normal or the patient develops signs and symptoms of hepatic failure.

PO

- Give tolcapone without regard to food.

Intervention and Evaluation

- Plan to reduce the levodopa dosage if the patient experiences hallucinations. Keep in mind that hallucinations are usually accompanied by confusion and, to a lesser extent, insomnia.
- Assist the patient with ambulation if he or she experiences dizziness.
- Assess the patient for relief of symptoms, such as improvement of masklike facial expression, muscular rigidity, shuffling gait, and resting tremors of the hands and head.

Patient Teaching

- Advise the patient to take tolcapone with food if he or she experiences nausea.
- Inform the patient that dizziness, drowsiness, and nausea may occur initially but will diminish or disappear with continued treatment.
- Inform the patient that orthostatic hypotension commonly occurs during initial therapy but that changing positions slowly can help prevent or minimize this effect.
- Warn the patient to avoid tasks that require mental alertness or motor skills until his or her response to the drug has been established.
- Inform the patient that hallucinations occur more often in elderly patients, typically within the first 2 weeks of therapy.
- Tell the patient that urine may turn bright yellow.
- Instruct the patient to notify the physician if he or she experiences dark urine, falls, fatigue, itching, loss of appetite, persistent nausea, yellowing of the skin and sclera of the eyes, or abnormal contractions of the head, neck, or trunk.
- Caution the female patient to notify the physician if she is or plans to become pregnant.
- Instruct the patient to report to the physician if he or she experiences frequent falls.

38 Antipsychotics

aripiprazole
chlorpromazine
clozapine
fluphenazine hydrochloride
haloperidol
mesoridazine besylate
olanzapine
perphenazine
quetiapine
risperidone
thioridazine
thiothixene
trifluoperazine hydrochloride
ziprasidone

Uses: Antipsychotics are used primarily to manage psychotic illness, especially in patients with increased psychomotor activity. They're also used to treat the manic phase of bipolar disorder, behavioral problems in children, nausea and vomiting, intractable hiccups, anxiety, and agitation. In addition, these agents are used to potentiate the effects of narcotics and, as adjuncts, to treat tetanus.

Action: Antipsychotic agents produce effects at all levels of the CNS. Although their exact mechanism of action is unknown, they may antagonize the action of dopamine as a neurotransmitter in the basal ganglia and limbic system by blocking postsynaptic dopamine receptors, inhibiting dopamine release, or increaseing dopamine turnover. This class of drugs is divided into phenothiazines, such as chlorpromazine, mesoridazine, and thioridazine, and nonphenothiazines, such as aripiprazole and haloperidol.

COMBINATION PRODUCTS

ETRAFON: perphenazine/amitriptyline (an antidepressant) 2 mg/10 mg; 2 mg/25 mg; 4 mg/10mg; 4 mg/25 mg; 4 mg/50 mg.
SYMBYAX: olanzapine/fluoxetine (an antidepressant) 6 mg/25mg; 6 mg/50 mg; 12 mg/25 mg; 12 mg/50 mg.
TRIAVIL: perphenazine/amitriptyline (an antidepressant) 2 mg/10 mg; 2 mg/25 mg; 4 mg/10 mg; 4 mg/25 mg; 4 mg/50 mg.

aripiprazole

ara-**pip**-rah-zole
(Abilify)

CATEGORY AND SCHEDULE

Pregnancy Risk Category: C

MECHANISM OF ACTION

An antipsychotic agent that provides partial agonist activity at dopamine and serotonin (5-HT_{1A}) receptors and antagonist activity at serotonin (5-HT_{2A}) receptors. **Therapeutic Effect:** Diminishes schizophrenic behavior.

PHARMACOKINETICS

Well absorbed through the GI tract. Protein binding: 99% (primarily albumin). Reaches steady levels in 2 wk. Metabolized in the liver. Eliminated primarily in feces and, to a lesser extent, in urine. Not removed by hemodialysis. ***Half-life:*** 75 hr.

AVAILABILITY

Tablets: 5 mg, 10 mg, 15 mg, 20 mg, 30 mg.

INDICATIONS AND DOSAGES

▸ **Schizophrenia, bipolar disorder**

PO

Adults, Elderly. Initially, 10–15 mg once a day. May increase up to 30 mg/day.

OFF-LABEL USES

Schizoaffective disorder

CONTRAINDICATIONS

None known.

INTERACTIONS

Drug

Carbamazepine: May decrease the aripiprazole blood concentration.

Fluoxetine, ketoconazole, quinidine, paroxetine: May increase the aripiprazole blood concentration.

Herbal

None known.

Food

None known.

DIAGNOSTIC TEST EFFECTS

None known.

SIDE EFFECTS

Frequent (11%–5%)

Weight gain, headache, insomnia, vomiting

Occasional (4%–3%)

Light-headedness, nausea, akathisia, somnolence

Rare (2% or less)

Blurred vision, constipation, asthenia or loss of energy and strength, anxiety, fever, rash, cough, rhinitis, orthostatic hypotension

SERIOUS REACTIONS

! Extrapyramidal symptoms and neuroleptic malignant syndrome occur rarely.

NURSING CONSIDERATIONS

Baseline Assessment

- Assess the patient's appearance, behavior, emotional status, response to environment, speech pattern, and thought content.
- Correct dehydration and hypovolemia, if present, before beginning therapy.

Lifespan Considerations

- It is unknown if aripiprazole crosses the placenta. Because this drug may be distributed in breast milk, female patients should avoid breast-feeding during therapy.
- The safety and efficacy of aripiprazole have not been established in children.
- No age-related precautions have been noted in the elderly.

Precautions

- Use aripiprazole cautiously in patients concurrently using CNS depressants, including alcohol.
- Use aripiprazole cautiously in patients with cardiovascular or cerebrovascular diseases (because it may induce hypotension), history of seizures or conditions that may lower the seizure threshold (such as Alzheimer's disease), hepatic or renal impairment, or Parkinson's disease (because of potential for exacerbation).

Administration and Handling

◂ALERT▸ Keep in mind that at least 2 weeks should elapse between dosage adjustments.

PO

- Give aripiprazole without regard to food.

Intervention and Evaluation

- Monitor the patient for extrapyramidal symptoms and tardive dyskinesia, manifested as chewing or puckering of the mouth, puffing of the cheeks, or tongue protrusion.
- Periodically monitor the patient's

BP and pulse rate, particularly in patients with pre-existing cardiovascular disease.
- Check the patient's weight periodically.
- Assess the patient for evidence of a therapeutic response, such as increased interest in surroundings and ability to concentrate, improvement in self-care, and relaxed facial expression.

Patient Teaching
- Urge the patient to avoid alcohol during aripiprazole therapy.
- Warn the patient to avoid tasks that require mental alertness or motor skills until his or her response to aripiprazole has been established.

chlorpromazine
(Thorazine)
See Antiemetics

clozapine
klo-za-peen
(Clopine[AUS], Clozaril, FazaClo)
Do not confuse clozapine with Cloxapen or clofazimine, or Clozaril with Clinoril or Colazal.

CATEGORY AND SCHEDULE
Pregnancy Risk Category: B

MECHANISM OF ACTION
A dibenzodiazepine derivative that interferes with the binding of dopamine at dopamine receptor sites; binds primarily at nondopamine receptor sites. **Therapeutic Effect:** Diminishes schizophrenic behavior.

AVAILABILITY
Tablets (Clozaril): 12.5 mg, 25 mg, 100 mg.
Tablets (Oral-Disintegrating [FazaClo]): 25 mg, 100 mg.

INDICATIONS AND DOSAGES
▸ **Schizophrenic disorders, reduce suicidal behavior**
PO
Adults. Initially, 25 mg once or twice a day. May increase by 25–50 mg/day over 2 wk until dosage of 300–450 mg/day is achieved. May further increase by 50–100 mg/day no more than once or twice a week, Range: 200–600 mg/day. Maximum: 900 mg/day.
Elderly. Initially, 25 mg/day. May increase by 25 mg/day. Maximum: 450 mg/day.

CONTRAINDICATIONS
Coma, concurrent use of other drugs that may suppress bone marrow function, history of clozapine-induced agranulocytosis or severe granulocytopenia, myeloproliferative disorders, severe CNS depression

INTERACTIONS
Drug
Alcohol, other CNS depressants: May increase CNS depressant effects.
Bone marrow depressants: May increase myelosuppression.
Lithium: May increase the risk of confusion, dyskinesia, and seizures.
Phenobarbital: Decreases clozapine blood concentration.
Herbal
None known.
Food
None known.

DIAGNOSTIC TEST EFFECTS
May increase serum glucose levels.

SIDE EFFECTS

Frequent

Somnolence (39%), salivation (31%), tachycardia (25%), dizziness (19%), constipation (14%)

Occasional

Hypotension (9%); headache (7%); tremor, syncope, diaphoresis, dry mouth (6%); nausea, visual disturbances (5%); nightmares, restlessness, akinesia, agitation, hypertension, abdominal discomfort or heartburn, weight gain (4%)

Rare

Rigidity, confusion, fatigue, insomnia, diarrhea, rash

SERIOUS REACTIONS

! Seizures occur in about 3% of patients.

! Overdose produces CNS depression (including sedation, coma, and delirium), respiratory depression, and hypersalivation.

! Blood dyscrasias, particularly agranulocytosis; and mild leukopenia, may occur.

NURSING CONSIDERATIONS

Baseline Assessment

- Obtain the patient's baseline WBC count before beginning treatment.
- Assess the patient's appearance, behavior, emotional status, response to environment, speech pattern, and thought content.

Precautions

- Use clozapine cautiously in patients undergoing alcohol withdrawal and in those with cardiovascular disease, glaucoma, history of seizures, benign prostatic hyperplasia, myocarditis, urine retention, or impaired hepatic, renal, or respiratory function.

Administration and Handling

PO

- Give clozapine without regard to food.

Intervention and Evaluation

- Monitor the patient's BP for hypertension or hypotension.
- Assess the patient's heart rate for tachycardia, a common side effect.
- Monitor the patient's CBC for blood dyscrasias, particularly agranulocytosis and mild leukopenia.
- Obtain the patient's WBC count every week for the first 6 months of continuous therapy, then biweekly for patients with acceptable WBC counts.
- Closely supervise suicidal patients during early therapy. As depression lessens, the patient's energy level improves, which increases the suicide potential.
- Assess the patient for evidence of a therapeutic response, such as increased interest in surroundings and ability to concentrate, improvement in self-care, and relaxed facial expression.

Patient Teaching

- Caution the patient against abruptly discontinuing clozapine.
- Inform the patient that drowsiness generally subsides with continued therapy.
- Warn the patient to avoid tasks that require mental alertness or motor skills until his or her response to the drug has been established.
- Urge the patient to avoid alcohol during clozapine therapy.

fluphenazine hydrochloride

floo-**fen**-a-zeen
(Anatensol[AUS], Modecate[AUS], Moditen[CAN], Permitil, Prolixin, Prolixin Decanoate)
Do not confuse Moditen with Modane or Mobidin.

CATEGORY AND SCHEDULE

Pregnancy Risk Category: C

MECHANISM OF ACTION

A phenothiazine that antagonizes dopamine neurotransmission at synapses by blocking postsynaptic dopaminergic receptors in the brain. **Therapeutic Effect:** Decreases psychotic behavior. Also produces weak anticholinergic, sedative, and antiemetic effects and strong extrapyramidal effects.

AVAILABILITY

Elixir (Prolixin): 2.5 mg/5 ml.
Tablets (Prolixin): 1 mg, 2.5 mg, 5 mg, 10 mg.
Injection (Prolixin): 2.5 mg/ml.
Injection (Prolixin Decanoate): 25 mg/ml.

INDICATIONS AND DOSAGES

▸ **Psychosis**

PO

Adults, Elderly. 0.5–10 mg/day in divided doses q6–8h.

IM

Adults, Elderly. 2.5–10 mg/day in divided doses q6–8h or 12.5 mg (decanoate) q2wk.

OFF-LABEL USES

Treatment of neurogenic pain (adjunct to tricyclic antidepressants)

CONTRAINDICATIONS

Angle-closure glaucoma, myelosuppression, severe cardiac or hepatic disease, severe hypertension or hypotension, subcortical brain damage

INTERACTIONS

Drug

Alcohol, other CNS depressants: May increase hypotensive and CNS and respiratory depressant effects.
Antithyroid agents: May increase the risk of agranulocytosis.
Extrapyramidal symptom–producing medications: May increase extrapyramidal symptoms.
Hypotension-producing medications: May increase hypotension.
Levodopa: May decrease the effects of this drug.
Lithium: May decrease the absorption of fluphenazine and produce adverse neurologic effects.
MAOIs, tricyclic antidepressants: May increase anticholinergic and sedative effects.

Herbal

None known.

Food

None known.

DIAGNOSTIC TEST EFFECTS

May produce false-positive pregnancy and phenylketonuria test results. May cause EKG changes, including Q- and T-wave disturbances.

SIDE EFFECTS

Frequent

Hypotension, dizziness, and syncope (occur frequently after first injection, occasionally after subsequent injections, and rarely with oral doses)

Occasional

Somnolence (during early therapy), dry mouth, blurred vision, lethargy, constipation or diarrhea, nasal congestion, peripheral edema, urine retention

Rare
Ocular changes, altered skin pigmentation (with prolonged use of high doses)

SERIOUS REACTIONS

! Extrapyramidal symptoms appear to be related to high dosages and are divided into 3 categories: akathisia (inability to sit still, tapping of feet), parkinsonian symptoms (such as hypersalivation, masklike facial expression, shuffling gait, and tremors), and acute dystonias (such as torticollis, opisthotonos, and oculogyric crisis).
! Tardive dyskinesia, manifested as tongue protrusion, puffing of the cheeks, and chewing or puckering of the mouth occurs rarely but may be irreversible.
! Abrupt withdrawal after long-term therapy may precipitate dizziness, gastritis, nausea and vomiting, and tremors.
! Blood dyscrasias, particularly agranulocytosis and mild leukopenia, may occur.
! Fluphenzine use may lower the seizure threshold.

NURSING CONSIDERATIONS

- Assess the patient's appearance, behavior, emotional status, response to environment, speech pattern, and thought content.

Precautions
- Use fluphenazine cautiously in patients with Parkinson's disease or seizures.

Administration and Handling
- Avoid skin contact with the fluphenazine solution to prevent contact dermatitis.

Intervention and Evaluation
- Monitor the patient's BP for hypotension and CBC for blood dyscrasias.
- Evaluate the patient's fine tongue movement for signs of tardive dyskinesia.
- Closely supervise suicidal patients during early therapy. As depression lessens, the patient's energy level generally improves, which increases the suicide potential.
- Assess the patient for a therapeutic response, such as improvement in self-care, increased ability to concentrate and interest in surroundings, and relaxed facial expression.

Patient Teaching
- Inform the patient that the drug's full therapeutic effect may take up to 6 weeks to appear.
- Caution the patient against abruptly discontinuing fluphenazine.
- Explain to the patient that drowsiness generally subsides during continued therapy.
- Warn the patient to avoid tasks that require mental alertness or motor skills until his or her response to the drug has been established.

haloperidol

ha-loe-**per**-idole
(Apo-Haloperidol[CAN], Haldol, Haldol Decanoate, Novoperidol[CAN], Peridol[CAN], Serenace[AUS])
Do not confuse Haldol with Halcion, Halog, or Stadol.

CATEGORY AND SCHEDULE

Pregnancy Risk Category: C

MECHANISM OF ACTION

An antipsychotic, antiemetic, and antidyskinetic agent that competitively blocks postsynaptic dopamine receptors, interrupts nerve impulse movement, and increases turnover of dopamine in the brain. Has strong extrapyramidal and antiemetic effects; weak anticholinergic and sedative effects. **Therapeutic Effect:** Produces tranquilizing effect.

PHARMACOKINETICS

Readily absorbed from the GI tract. Protein binding: 92%. Extensively metabolized in the liver. Primarily excreted in urine. Not removed by hemodialysis. ***Half-life:*** 12–37 hr PO; 10–19 hr IV; 17–25 hr IM.

AVAILABILITY

Oral Concentrate: 2 mg/ml.
Tablets: 0.5 mg, 1 mg, 2 mg, 5 mg, 10 mg, 20 mg.
Injection (Lactate): 5 mg/ml.
Injection (Decanoate): 50 mg/ml, 100 mg/ml.

INDICATIONS AND DOSAGES

▸ Treatment of psychotic disorders
PO
Adults, Children 12 yr and older. Initially, 0.5–5 mg 2–3 times/day. Dosage gradually adjusted as needed.
Elderly. 0.5–2 mg 2–3 times/day. Dosage gradually adjusted as needed.
Children 3–12 yr or weighing 15–40 kg. Initially, 0.05 mg/kg/day in 2–3 divided doses. May increase by 0.5 mg increments at 5- to 7-day intervals. Maximum: 0.15 mg/kg/day in divided doses.
IM
Adults, Elderly, Children 12 yr and older. Initially, 2–5 mg. May repeat at 1-hour intervals as needed. Maximum: 100 mg/day.
IM (Decanoate)
Adults, Elderly, Children 12 yr and older. Initially, 10–15 times previous daily oral dose up to maximum initial dose of 100 mg. Maximum: 300 mg/month.

▸ Treatment of non-psychotic disorders, Tourette's syndrome
PO
Children 3–12 yr or weighing 15–40 kg. Initially, 0.05 mg/kg/day in 2–3 divided doses. May increase by 0.5 mg at 5- to 7-day intervals. Maximum: 0.075 mg/kg/day.

OFF-LABEL USES

Treatment of Huntington's chorea, infantile autism, nausea or vomiting associated with cancer chemotherapy

CONTRAINDICATIONS

Angle-closure glaucoma, CNS depression, myelosuppression, Parkinson's disease, severe cardiac or hepatic disease

INTERACTIONS

Drug

Alcohol, other CNS depressants: May increase CNS depression.
Epinephrine: May block alpha-adrenergic effects.
Extrapyramidal symptom-producing medications: May increase extrapyramidal symptoms.
Lithium: May increase neurologic toxicity.

Herbal

None known.

Food

None known.

DIAGNOSTIC TEST EFFECTS

None known. Therapeutic serum drug level is 0.2–1 mcg/ml; toxic serum drug level is greater than 1 mcg/ml.

IV INCOMPATIBILITIES

Allopurinol (Aloprim), amphotericin B complex (Abelcet, AmBisome, Amphotec), cefepime (Maxipime), fluconazole (Diflucan), foscarnet (Foscavir), heparin, nitroprusside

(Nipride), piperacillin and tazobactam (Zosyn)

IV COMPATIBILITIES

Dobutamine (Dobutrex), dopamine (Intropin), fentanyl (Sublimaze), hydromorphone (Dilaudid), lidocaine, lorazepam (Ativan), midazolam (Versed), morphine, nitroglycerin, norepinephrine (Levophed), propofol (Diprivan)

SIDE EFFECTS

Frequent

Blurred vision, constipation, orthostatic hypotension, dry mouth, swelling or soreness of female breasts, peripheral edema

Occasional

Allergic reaction, difficulty urinating, decreased thirst, dizziness, decreased sexual function, drowsiness, nausea, vomiting, photosensitivity, lethargy

SERIOUS REACTIONS

! Extrapyramidal symptoms appear to be dose-related and typically occur in the first few days of therapy. Marked drowsiness and lethargy, excessive salivation, and fixed stare occur frequently. Less common reactions include severe akathisia (motor restlessness) and acute dystonias (such as torticollis, opisthotonos, and oculogyric crisis).

! Tardive dyskinesia (tongue protrusion, puffing of the cheeks, chewing or puckering of the mouth) may occur during long-term therapy or after discontinuing the drug and may be irreversible. Elderly female patients have a greater risk of developing this reaction.

NURSING CONSIDERATIONS

Baseline Assessment

- Assess the patient's appearance, behavior, emotional status, response to environment, speech pattern, and thought content.

Lifespan Considerations

- Haloperidol crosses the placenta and is distributed in breast milk.
- Children are more susceptible to dystonias. Haloperidol use is not recommended for children younger than 3 years.
- A decreased dosage is recommended for the elderly, who are more susceptible to extrapyramidal and anticholinergic effects, orthostatic hypotension, and sedation.

Precautions

- Use haloperidol cautiously in patients with cardiovascular disease, hepatic or renal dysfunction, or a history of seizures.

Administration and Handling

PO

- Give haloperidol without regard to food.
- Crush scored tablets as needed.

IV

◀ALERT▶ Only haloperidol lactate is given IV.

- Store vials at room temperature. Protect them from freezing and light.
- Discard the solution if it becomes discolored or contains precipitate.
- Haloperidol may be given undiluted by IV push.
- Flush with at least 2 ml 0.9% NaCl before and after administration.
- To dilute, add the drug to 30 to 50 ml of most solutions; D_5W is preferred.
- Give IV push at a rate of 5 mg/minute.
- Infuse IV piggyback over 30 minutes.
- For IV infusion, administer up to 25 mg/hour, titrating dosage to patient response.

IM

- Prepare haloperidol decanoate IM injection using a 21-gauge needle.

• Don't exceed a volume of 3 ml per IM injection site.
• Slowly inject the drug deep into the upper outer quadrant of the gluteus maximus.
• Keep the patient recumbent (head low and legs raised) for 30 to 60 minutes after administration to minimize hypotensive effects.

Intervention and Evaluation

• Closely supervise suicidal patients during early therapy. As depression lessens, the patient's energy level improves, which increases the suicide potential.
• Monitor the patient for fine tongue movement, masklike facial expression, rigidity, and tremor.
• Assess the patient for evidence of a therapeutic response, including improvement in self-care, increased interest in surroundings and ability to concentrate, and relaxed facial expression.
• Know that the therapeutic serum level for haloperidol is 0.2 to 1 mcg/ml, and the toxic serum level is greater than 1 mcg/ml.

Patient Teaching

• Inform the patient that the drug's full therapeutic effect may take up to 6 weeks to appear.
• Caution the patient against abruptly discontinuing haloperidol after long-term use.
• Inform the patient that drowsiness generally subsides with continued therapy.
• Warn the patient to avoid tasks that require mental alertness or motor skills until his or her response to the drug has been established.
• Urge the patient to avoid alcohol during haloperidol therapy.
• Instruct the patient to notify the physician if muscle stiffness occurs.
• Urge the patient to avoid exposure to sunlight and any conditions that may cause dehydration or overheating because they may increase the risk of heat stroke.
• Suggest taking sips of tepid water or chewing sugarless gum to help relieve dry mouth.

mesoridazine besylate

mez-oh-**rid**-a-zeen

(Serentil)

Do not confuse Serentil with Proventil, Serevent, or sertraline.

CATEGORY AND SCHEDULE

Pregnancy Risk Category: C

MECHANISM OF ACTION

A phenothiazine that blocks dopamine at postsynaptic receptor sites in the brain. **Therapeutic Effect:** Diminishes schizophrenic behavior. Also has anticholinergic and sedative effects.

AVAILABILITY

Oral Solution: 25 mg/ml.
Tablets: 10 mg, 25 mg, 50 mg, 100 mg.
Injection: 25 mg/ml.

INDICATIONS AND DOSAGES

▸ Schizophrenia

PO

Adults, Elderly. 25–50 mg 3 times a day. Maximum: 400 mg/day.

IM

Adults, Elderly. Initially, 25 mg. May repeat in 30–60 min. Range: 25–200 mg.

▸ Severe behavioral problems (combativeness or explosive, hyperexcitable behavior) associated with neurologic diseases

PO

Elderly. Initially, 10 mg once or

twice a day. May increase at 4- to 7-day intervals. Maximum: 250 mg.
IM
Adults, Elderly. Initially, 25 mg. May repeat in 30–60 min. Range: 25–200 mg.

CONTRAINDICATIONS

Coma, myelosuppression, severe cardiovascular disease, severe CNS depression, subcortical brain damage

INTERACTIONS

Drug

Alcohol, other CNS depressants: May increase CNS and respiratory depression and the hypotensive effects of mesoridazine.
Antithyroid agents: May increase the risk of agranulocytosis.
Extrapyramidal symptom producing medications: May increase extrapyramidal symptoms.
Hypotension-producing medications: May increase hypotension.
Levodopa: May decrease the effects of levodopa.
Lithium: May decrease mesoridazine absorption and produce adverse neurologic effects.
MAOIs, tricyclic antidepressants: May increase the anticholinergic and sedative effects of mesoridazine.

Herbal

None known.

Food

None known.

DIAGNOSTIC TEST EFFECTS

May produce false-positive pregnancy and phenylketonuria test results. May produce EKG changes, including prolonged QT and QTc intervals and T-wave depression or inversion.

SIDE EFFECTS

Frequent

Orthostatic hypotension, dizziness, syncope (occur frequently after first injection, occasionally after subsequent injections, and rarely with oral form)

Occasional

Somnolence (during early therapy), dry mouth, blurred vision, lethargy, constipation or diarrhea, nasal congestion, peripheral edema, urine retention

Rare

Ocular changes, altered skin pigmentation (in those taking high doses for prolonged periods), darkening of urine

SERIOUS REACTIONS

! Abrupt withdrawal after long-term therapy may precipitate nausea, vomiting, gastritis, dizziness, and tremors.
! Blood dyscrasias, particularly agranulocytosis and mild leukopenia may occur.
! Mesoridazine use may lower the seizure threshold.

NURSING CONSIDERATIONS

Baseline Assessment

- Assess the patient's appearance, behavior, emotional status, response to environment, speech pattern, and thought content.
- Expect to perform a baseline EKG and measure the QT and QTc intervals.

Precautions

- Use mesoridazine cautiously in patients undergoing alcohol withdrawal and in those with glaucoma, history of seizures, benign prostatic hyperplasia, myocarditis, urine retention, or impaired cardiac, hepatic, renal, or respiratory function.

Administration and Handling

• Avoid skin contact with the oral solution because it may cause contact dermatitis.

Intervention and Evaluation

• Assess the patient for orthostatic hypotension.
• Assess the patient's pattern of daily bowel activity and stool consistency.
• Closely supervise suicidal patients during early therapy. As depression lessens, the patient's energy level improves, which increases the suicide potential.
• Assess the patient for evidence of a therapeutic response, such as improvement in self-care, increased interest in surroundings and ability to concentrate, and relaxed facial expression.

Patient Teaching

• Inform the patient that the drug's full therapeutic effect may take up to 6 weeks to appear.
• Caution the patient against abruptly discontinuing the drug after long-term use.
• Explain that drowsiness generally subsides with continued therapy.
• Inform the patient that the drug may darken the urine.
• Advise the patient to notify the physician if visual disturbances occur.
• Urge the patient to avoid alcohol and other CNS depressants during mesoridazine therapy.

olanzapine

oh-**lan**-za-peen
(Zyprexa, Zyprexa Intramuscular, Zyprexa Zydis)
Do not confuse olanzapine with olsalazine, or Zyprexa with Zyrtec.

CATEGORY AND SCHEDULE

Pregnancy Risk Category: C

MECHANISM OF ACTION

A dibenzepin derivative that antagonizes $alpha_1$-adrenergic, dopamine, histamine, muscarinic, and serotonin receptors. Produces anticholinergic, histaminic, and CNS depressant effects. **Therapeutic Effect:** Diminishes manifestations of psychotic symptoms.

PHARMACOKINETICS

Well absorbed after PO administration. Protein binding: 93%. Extensively distributed throughout the body. Undergoes extensive first-pass metabolism in the liver. Excreted primarily in urine and, to a lesser extent, in feces. Not removed by dialysis. ***Half-life:*** 21–54 hr.

AVAILABILITY

Tablets (Zyprexa): 2.5 mg, 5 mg, 7.5 mg, 10 mg, 15 mg, 20 mg).
Tablets (Orally-Disintegrating [Zyprexa Zydis]): 5 mg, 10 mg, 15 mg, 20 mg.
Injection (Zyprexa Intramuscular): 10 mg.

INDICATIONS AND DOSAGES

▸ Schizophrenia

PO

Adults. Initially, 5–10 mg once daily. May increase by 10 mg/day at 5- to 7-day intervals. If further adjustments are indicated, may

increase by 5–10 mg/day at 7-day intervals. Range: 10–30 mg/day.
Elderly. Initially, 2.5 mg/day. May increase as indicated. Range: 2.5–10 mg/day.
Children. Initially, 2.5 mg/day. Titrate as necessary up to 20 mg/day.

▸ **Bipolar mania**

PO
Adults. Initially, 10–15 mg/day. May increase by 5 mg/day at intervals of at least 24 hr. Maximum: 20 mg/day.
Children. Initially, 2.5 mg/day. Titrate as necessary up to 20 mg/day.

▸ **Dosage for elderly or debilitated patients and those predisposed to hypotensive reactions**

The initial dosage for these patients is 5 mg/day.

▸ **Control agitation in schizophrenic or bipolar patients**

IM
Adults, Elderly. 2.5–10 mg. May repeat 2 hr after first dose and 4 hr after second dose. Maximum: 30 mg/day.

OFF-LABEL USES

Treatment of anorexia, maintenance of long-term treatment response in schizophrenic patients, nausea, vomiting

CONTRAINDICATIONS

None known.

INTERACTIONS

Drug

Alcohol, other CNS depressants: May increase CNS depressant effects.
Antihypertensives: May increase the hypotensive effects of these drugs.
Carbamazepine: Increases olanzapine clearance.
Ciprofloxacin, fluvoxamine: May increase the olanzapine blood concentration.
Dopamine agonists, levodopa: May antagonize the effects of these drugs.
Imipramine, theophylline: May inhibit the metabolism of these drugs.

Herbal

None known.

Food

None known.

DIAGNOSTIC TEST EFFECTS

May significantly increase serum GGT, prolactin, AST (SGOT), and ALT (SGPT) levels.

SIDE EFFECTS

Frequent

Somnolence (26%), agitation (23%), insomnia (20%), headache (17%), nervousness (16%), hostility (15%), dizziness (11%), rhinitis (10%)

Occasional

Anxiety, constipation (9%); nonaggressive atypical behavior (8%); dry mouth (7%); weight gain (6%); orthostatic hypotension, fever, arthralgia, restlessness, cough, pharyngitis, visual changes (dim vision) (5%)

Rare

Tachycardia; back, chest, abdominal, or extremity pain; tremor

SERIOUS REACTIONS

! Rare reactions include seizures and neuroleptic malignant syndrome, a potentially fatal syndrome characterized by hyperpyrexia, muscle rigidity, irregular pulse or BP, tachycardia, diaphoresis, and cardiac arrhythmias.
! Extrapyramidal symptoms and dysphagia may also occur.
! Overdose (300 mg) produces drowsiness and slurred speech.

NURSING CONSIDERATIONS

Baseline Assessment

- Obtain liver function test results, as ordered, before beginning olanzapine treatment.
- Assess the patient's appearance, behavior, emotional status, response to environment, speech pattern, and thought content.

Lifespan Considerations

- It is unknown if olanzapine crosses the placenta or is distributed in breast milk.
- The safety and efficacy of olanzapine have not been established in children.
- No age-related precautions have been noted in the elderly.

Precautions

- Use olanzapine cautiously in patients with a hypersensitivity to clozapine, hepatic impairment, cerebrovascular disease, cardiovascular disease (such as conduction abnormalities, heart failure, or history of MI or ischemia), history of seizures or conditions that lower the seizure threshold (such as Alzheimer's disease), and conditions predisposing patients to hypotension (such as dehydration, hypovolemia, and use of antihypertensives).
- Use the drug cautiously in elderly patients, patients at risk for aspiration pneumonia, patients concurrently taking hepatotoxic drugs, and those who should avoid anticholinergics (such as patients with benign prostatic hyperplasia).
- Use caution with each dosage increase.

Administration and Handling

PO

- Give olanzapine without regard to food.

Intervention and Evaluation

- Monitor the patient's BP.
- Assess the patient for tremors, changes in gait, and abnormal muscular movements.
- Closely supervise suicidal patients during early therapy. As depression lessens, the patient's energy level improves, which increases the suicide potential.
- Assess the patient for evidence of a therapeutic response, such as improvement in self-care increased interest in surroundings and ability to concentrate, and relaxed facial expression.
- Assist the patient with ambulation if he or she experiences dizziness.
- Assess the patient's sleep pattern.
- Monitor the patient for extrapyramidal symptoms, and notify the physician if they occur.

Patient Teaching

- Instruct the patient to take olanzapine as ordered. Caution the patient against abruptly discontinuing the drug or increasing the dosage.
- Inform the patient that drowsiness generally subsides with continued therapy.
- Warn the patient to avoid tasks requiring mental alertness or motor skills until his or her response to the drug has been established.
- Caution the patient to notify the physician if she becomes pregnant or intends to become pregnant during olanzapine therapy.
- Advise the patient to avoid dehydration, particularly during exercise; exposure to extreme heat; and concurrent use of medications that cause dry mouth or other drying effects.
- Suggest taking sips of tepid water and chewing sugarless gum to help relieve dry mouth.
- Instruct the patient to maintain a healthy diet and exercise program to prevent weight gain.

perphenazine

per-**fen**-ah-zeen
(Trilafon)
Do not confuse perphenazine with promazine.

CATEGORY AND SCHEDULE

Pregnancy Risk Category: C

MECHANISM OF ACTION

An antipsychotic agent and antiemetic that blocks postsynaptic dopamine receptor sites in the brain. **Therapeutic Effect:** Suppresses behavioral response in psychosis, and relieves nausea and vomiting.

AVAILABILITY

Oral Concentrate: 15 mg/5 ml.
Tablets: 2 mg, 4 mg, 8 mg, 16 mg.

INDICATIONS AND DOSAGES

▸ **Severe schizophrenia**

PO

Adults. 4–16 mg 2–4 times/day. Maximum: 64 mg/day.
Elderly. Initially, 2–4 mg/day. May increase at 4- to 7-day intervals by 2–4 mg/day up to 32 mg/day.

▸ **Severe nausea and vomiting**

PO

Adults. 8–16 mg/day in divided doses up to 24 mg/day.

CONTRAINDICATIONS

Coma, myelosuppression, severe cardiovascular disease, severe CNS depression, subcortical brain damage

INTERACTIONS

Drug

Alcohol, other CNS depressants: May increase hypotensive effects and CNS and respiratory depression.
Antihypotensives: May increase the risk of hypotension.
Antithyroid agents: May increase the risk of agranulocytosis.
Extrapyramidal symptom–producing medications: May increase the severity and frequency of extrapyramidal symptoms.
Levodopa: May decrease the effects of this drug.
Lithium: May decrease perphenazine absorption and produce adverse neurologic effects.
MAOIs, tricyclic antidepressants: May increase anticholinergic and sedative effects.

Herbal

None known.

Food

Apple juice, caffeine- or tannic-containing beverages (such as tea): Don't mix oral concentrate with these beverages.

DIAGNOSTIC TEST EFFECTS

May produce false-positive pregnancy and phenylketonuria test results. May produce EKG changes, including prolonged QT and QTc intervals and T-wave depression or inversion.

IV INCOMPATIBILITIES

Aminophylline, cefoperazone (Cefobid), midazolam (Versed), opium alkaloids, oxytocin, pentobarbital (Nembutal), secobarbital (Seconal), thiopental (Pentothal)

IV COMPATIBILITIES

Atropine, chlorpromazine (Librium), dimenhydrinate (Dramamine), diphenhydramine (Benadryl), droperidol (Inapsine), fentanyl (Sublimaze), hydroxyzine (Vistaril), meperidine (Demerol), morphine, pentazocine (Talwin), prochlorperazine (Compazine), promethazine (Phenergan), ranitidine (Zantac), scopolamine (Transderm)

SIDE EFFECTS

Occasional

Marked photosensitivity, somnolence, dry mouth, blurred vision, lethargy, constipation or diarrhea, nasal congestion, peripheral edema, urine retention

Rare

Ocular changes, altered skin pigmentation, hypotension, dizziness, syncope

SERIOUS REACTIONS

! Extrapyramidal symptoms appear to be dose-related and are divided into 3 categories: akathisia (characterized by inability to sit still, tapping of feet), parkinsonian symptoms (including masklike face, tremors, shuffling gait, hypersalivation), and acute dystonias (such as torticollis, opisthotonos, and oculogyric crisis).

! Tardive dyskinesia occurs rarely.

! Abrupt withdrawal after long-term therapy may precipitate nausea, vomiting, gastritis, dizziness, and tremors.

NURSING CONSIDERATIONS

Baseline Assessment

• When perphenzine is given as an antiemetic, assess the patient for signs and symptoms of dehydration, such as dry mucous membranes, longitudinal furrows in the tongue, and poor skin turgor.

• When perphenzine is given as an antipsychotic, assess the patient's appearance, behavior, emotional status, response to environment, speech pattern, and thought content.

Precautions

• Use perphenzine cautiously in patients experiencing alcohol withdrawal and in patients with glaucoma; history of seizures; hypocalcemia; cardiac, hepatic, renal, or respiratory impairment; benign prostatic hyperplasia; or urine retention.

Administration and Handling

◀ ALERT ▶

• Decrease the dose gradually to optimum response. Decrease to lowest effective level for maintenance. Replace parenteral therapy with oral therapy as soon as possible.

• Avoid skin contact with perphenazine solutions because they may cause contact dermatitis.

PO

• Store tablets at room temperature.

• Refrigerate the oral concentrate. Shake it well before using.

• Give perphenazine without regard to food.

• Crush tablets if needed.

• Dilute the oral concentrate with clear carbonated beverages, carbonated orange drink, milk, tomato or vegetable juice, apricot, grapefruit, pineapple, prune, or orange juice. Mix each 5 ml of oral concentrate with 2 fluid ounces of diluent.

Intervention and Evaluation

• Monitor the patient's BP for hypotension.

• When perphenazine is given as an antiemetic, maintain a quiet and supportive atmosphere and assess the patient for extrapyramidal symptoms and early signs of tardive dyskinesia, including fine tongue movement. Assess the patient for relief from nausea and vomiting.

• When perphenazine is given as an antipsychotic, closely supervise the suicidal patient during early therapy. As depression lessens, the patient's energy level improves, increasing the likelihood of a suicide attempt.

• Assess the patient taking perphenazine as an antipsychotic for evidence of a therapeutic response, such as increased ability to concentrate and interest in surroundings, improvement in self-care, and a relaxed facial expression.

Patient Teaching

- Warn the patient not to abruptly discontinue the drug after long-term use.
- Tell the patient that drowsiness generally subsides during continued therapy.
- Inform the patient that urine may turn pink or reddish brown during perphenazine therapy.
- Advise the patient to wear protective clothing and sunscreen outdoors to prevent a photosensitivity reaction.

quetiapine

kwe-**tye**-a-peen
(Seroquel)

CATEGORY AND SCHEDULE

Pregnancy Risk Category: C

MECHANISM OF ACTION

A dibenzepin derivative that antagonizes dopamine, serotonin, histamine, and alpha$_1$-adrenergic receptors. **Therapeutic Effect:** Diminishes manifestations of psychotic disorders. Produces moderate sedation, few extrapyramidal effects, and no anticholinergic effects.

PHARMACOKINETICS

Well absorbed after PO administration. Protein binding: 83%. Widely distributed in tissues; CNS concentration exceeds plasma concentration. Undergoes extensive first-pass metabolism in the liver. Primarily excreted in urine. ***Half-life:*** 6 hr.

AVAILABILITY

Tablets: 25 mg, 100 mg, 200 mg, 300 mg.

INDICATIONS AND DOSAGES

▸ To manage manifestations of psychotic disorders, Bipolar disorder

PO

Adults, Elderly. Initially, 25 mg twice a day, then 25–50 mg 2–3 times a day on the second and third days, up to 300–400 mg/day in divided doses 2–3 times a day by the fourth day. Further adjustments of 25–50 mg twice a day may be made at intervals of 2 days or longer. Maintenance: 300–800 mg/day (adults); 50–200 mg/day (elderly).

▸ Dosage in hepatic impairment, elderly or debilitated patients, and those predisposed to hypotensive reactions

These patients should receive a lower initial dose and lower dosage increases.

CONTRAINDICATIONS

None known.

INTERACTIONS

Drug

Alcohol, other CNS depressants: May increase CNS depression.
Antihypertensives: May increase the hypotensive effects of these drugs.
Hepatic enzyme inducers (such as phenytoin): May increase quetiapine clearance.

Herbal

None known.

Food

None known.

DIAGNOSTIC TEST EFFECTS

May decrease serum total and free thyroxine (T_4) serum levels. May increase serum cholesterol, triglyceride, AST (SGOT), and ALT (SGPT) levels. May produce a false-positive pregnancy test result.

SIDE EFFECTS

Frequent (19%–10%)
Headache, somnolence, dizziness
Occasional (9%–3%)
Constipation, orthostatic hypotension, tachycardia, dry mouth, dyspepsia, rash, asthenia, abdominal pain, rhinitis
Rare (2%)
Back pain, fever, weight gain

SERIOUS REACTIONS

! Overdose may produce heart block hypotension, hypokalemia, and tachycardia.

NURSING CONSIDERATIONS

Baseline Assessment

- Assess the patient's appearance, behavior, emotional status, response to environment, speech pattern, and thought content.
- Obtain the patient's CBC and blood chemistry values to assess hepatic enzyme levels before and periodically during treatment, as ordered.

Lifespan Considerations

- It is unknown if quetiapine is distributed in breast milk. However, this drug is not recommended for breast-feeding women.
- The safety and efficacy of quetiapine have not been established in children.
- Although no age-related precautions have been noted in the elderly, lower initial and target dosages may be necessary for this age-group.

Precautions

- Use quetiapine cautiously in patients with Alzheimer's disease, cardiovascular disease (such as CHF or history of MI), cerebrovascular disease, seizures, hepatic impairment, dehydration, hypothyroidism, hypovolemia, a history of breast cancer, or a history of drug abuse or dependence.

Administration and Handling

PO
- Give quetiapine without regard to food.
- Know that dosage adjustments should occur at 2-day intervals.
- When restarting therapy for patients who have been off quetiapine for longer than 1 week, follow the initial titration schedule, as prescribed. When restarting therapy for patients who have been off quetiapine for less than 1 week, titration is not required and the maintenance dose can be reinstituted.

Intervention and Evaluation

- Assist the patient with ambulation if he or she experiences dizziness.
- Closely supervise suicidal patients during early therapy. As depression lessens, the patient's energy level improves, which increases the suicide potential.
- Monitor the patient's BP for hypotension and pulse rate for tachycardia, especially if the drug dosage has been increased rapidly.
- Assess the patient's pattern of daily bowel activity and stool consistency.
- Assess the patient for evidence of a therapeutic response, such as improvement in self-care, increased interest in surroundings and ability to concentrate, and relaxed facial expression.

Patient Teaching

- Instruct the patient to take quetiapine as ordered. Caution the patient against abruptly discontinuing the drug or increasing the dosage.
- Inform the patient that drowsiness generally subsides during continued therapy.
- Warn the patient to avoid tasks that require mental alertness or motor skills until his or her response to the drug has been established.

• Instruct the patient to change positions slowly to reduce the hypotensive effect of quetiapine.
• Urge the patient to avoid alcohol and exposure to extreme heat.
• Advise the patient to drink lots of fluids, especially during physical activity.

risperidone

ris-**per**-i-done
(Risperdal, Risperdal Consta, Risperdol M-Tabs)
Do not confuse risperidone with reserpine.

CATEGORY AND SCHEDULE

Pregnancy Risk Category: C

MECHANISM OF ACTION

A benzisoxazole derivative that may antagonize dopamine and serotonin receptors. **Therapeutic Effect:** Suppresses psychotic behavior.

PHARMACOKINETICS

Well absorbed from the GI tract; unaffected by food. Protein binding: 90%. Extensively metabolized in the liver to active metabolite. Primarily excreted in urine. ***Half-life:*** 3–20 hr; metabolite: 21–30 hr (increased in elderly).

AVAILABILITY

Oral Solution (Risperdal): 1 mg/ml.
Tablets (Risperdal): 0.25 mg, 0.5 mg, 1 mg, 2 mg, 3 mg, 4 mg.
Tablets (Orally-Disintegrating [Risperdal M-Tabs]): 0.5 mg, 1 mg, 2 mg.
Injection (Risperdal Consta): 25 mg, 37.5 mg, 50 mg.

INDICATIONS AND DOSAGES

▸ **Psychotic disorder**

PO

Adults. 0.5–1 mg twice a day. May increase dosage slowly. Range: 2–6 mg/day.
Elderly. Initially, 0.25–2 mg/day in 2 divided doses. May increase dosage slowly. Range: 2–6 mg/day.

IM

Adults, Elderly. 25 mg q2wk. Maximum: 50 mg q2wk.

▸ **Mania**

PO

Adults, Elderly. Initially, 2–3 mg as a single daily dose. May increase at 24-hour intervals of 1 mg/day. Range: 2–6 mg/day.

▸ **Dosage in renal impairment**

Initial dosage for adults and elderly patients is 0.25–0.5 mg twice a day. Dosage is titrated slowly to desired effect.

OFF-LABEL USES

Autism in children, behavioral symptoms associated with dementia, Tourette's disorder

CONTRAINDICATIONS

None known.

INTERACTIONS

Drug

Alcohol, other CNS depressants: May increase CNS depression.
Carbamazepine: May decrease the risperidone blood concentration.
Clozapine: May increase the risperidone blood concentration.
Dopamine agonists, levodopa: May decrease the effects of these drugs.
Paroxetine: May increase the risperidone blood concentration and the risk of extrapyramidal symptoms.

Herbal

None known.

Food
None known.

DIAGNOSTIC TEST EFFECTS
May increase serum prolactin, creatinine, alkaline phosphatase, uric acid, AST (SGOT), ALT (SGPT), and triglyceride levels. May decrease blood glucose and serum potassium, protein, and sodium levels. May cause EKG changes.

SIDE EFFECTS
Frequent (26%–13%)
Agitation, anxiety, insomnia, headache, constipation
Occasional (10%–4%)
Dyspepsia, rhinitis, somnolence, dizziness, nausea, vomiting, rash, abdominal pain, dry skin, tachycardia
Rare (3%–2%)
Visual disturbances, fever, back pain, pharyngitis, cough, arthralgia, angina, aggressive behavior, orthostatic hypotension, breast swelling

SERIOUS REACTIONS
! Rare reactions include tardive dyskinesia (characterized by tongue protrusion, puffing of the cheeks, and chewing or puckering of the mouth) and neuroleptic malignant syndrome (marked by hyperpyrexia, muscle rigidity, change in mental status, irregular pulse or BP, tachycardia, diaphoresis, cardiac arrhythmias, rhabdomyolysis, and acute renal failure).

NURSING CONSIDERATIONS
Baseline Assessment
- Expect to obtain blood chemistry values, including BUN level and serum alkaline phosphatase, bilirubin, creatinine, AST (SGOT), and ALT (SGPT) levels, to assess hepatic and renal function before beginning risperidone therapy, as ordered.
- Assess the patient's appearance, behavior, emotional status, response to environment, speech pattern, and thought content.

Lifespan Considerations
- It is unknown if risperidone crosses the placenta or is excreted in breast milk. Breast-feeding is not recommended for patients taking this drug.
- The safety and efficacy of this drug have not been established in children.
- The elderly are more susceptible to orthostatic hypotension. They may require a dosage adjustment because of age-related renal or hepatic impairment.

Precautions
- Use risperidone cautiously in suicidal patients; patients with cardiac disease, breast cancer, hepatic or renal impairment, seizure disorders, or recent MI; and in those at risk for aspiration pneumonia.
- Use risperidone cautiously in patients with dementia because the drug may increase the risk of CVA in these patients.
- Risperidone use may increase the risk of hyperglycemia.

Administration and Handling
PO
- Give risperidone without regard to food.
- Mix the oral solution with water, orange juice, coffee, or low-fat milk, but not with cola or tea.

IM
- Use only the diluent and needle supplied in the dose pack. You'll require all the components in the dose pack for administration. Don't substitute any components. Prepare the suspension according to the manufacturer's directions.
- The drug may be given up to 6 hours after reconstitution, but imme-

diate administration is recommended. If 2 minutes pass before the injection, reconstitute the solution by shaking the upright vial vigorously back and forth for as long as it takes to resuspend the microspheres.
- Store the drug below 77° F (25° C) once it's in suspension.
- Inject the drug IM into the upper outer quadrant of the gluteus maximus.
- Do not administer the drug by the IV route.

Intervention and Evaluation
- Monitor the patient's BP, heart rate, liver function test results, EKG, and weight.
- Observe the patient for fine tongue movement, which may be the first sign of irreversible tardive dyskinesia.
- Closely supervise suicidal patients during early therapy. As depression lessens, the patient's energy level improves, which increases the suicide potential.
- Assess the patient for evidence of a therapeutic response, such as increased ability to concentrate and interest in surroundings, improvement in self-care, and relaxed facial expression.
- Monitor the patient for signs of neuroleptic malignant syndrome, such as altered mental status, fever, irregular BP or pulse, and muscle rigidity.

Patient Teaching
- Inform the patient that risperidone may cause dizziness or drowsiness. Warn the patient to avoid tasks that require mental alertness or motor skills until his or her response to the drug has been established.
- Urge the patient to notify the physician if he or she experiences altered gait, difficulty breathing, palpitations, pain or swelling in breasts, severe dizziness or fainting, trembling fingers, unusual movements, rash, or visual changes.
- Instruct the patient to change positions slowly to minimize the drug's hypotensive effects.
- Urge the patient to avoid alcohol during risperidone therapy.

thioridazine

thye-or-**rid**-a-zeen
(Aldazine[AUS], Apo-Thioridazine[CAN], Mellaril, Melleril[AUS], Thioridazine Intensol)

Do not confuse thioridazine with thiothixene or Thorazine, or Mellaril with Mebaral.

CATEGORY AND SCHEDULE

Pregnancy Risk Category: C

MECHANISM OF ACTION

A phenothiazine that blocks dopamine at postsynaptic receptor sites. Possesses strong anticholinergic and sedative effects. **Therapeutic Effect:** Suppresses behavioral response in psychosis; reduces locomotor activity and aggressiveness.

AVAILABILITY

Oral Solution (Concentrate [Thioridazine Intensol]): 30 mg/ml.
Tablets (Melleril): 10 mg, 15 mg, 25 mg, 50 mg, 100 mg, 150 mg, 200 mg.

INDICATIONS AND DOSAGES

▸ Psychosis

PO

Adults, Elderly, Children 12 yr and older. Initially, 25–100 mg 3 times a day; dosage increased gradually. Maximum: 800 mg/day.
Children 2–11 yr. Initially, 0.5 mg/kg/day in 2–3 divided doses. Maximum: 3 mg/kg/day.

OFF-LABEL USES
Treatment of behavioral problems in children, dementia, depressive neurosis

CONTRAINDICATIONS
Angle-closure glaucoma, blood dyscrasias, cardiac arrhythmias, cardiac or hepatic impairment, concurrent use of drugs that prolong QT interval, severe CNS depression

INTERACTIONS
Drug
Alcohol, other CNS depressants: May increase respiratory depression and the hypotensive effects of thioridazine.
Antithyroid agents: May increase the risk of agranulocytosis.
Extrapyramidal symptom–producing medications: May increase the risk of extrapyramidal symptoms.
Hypotension-producing agents: May increase hypotension.
Levodopa: May decrease the effects of levodopa.
Lithium: May decrease the absorption of thioridazine and produce adverse neurologic effects.
MAOIs, tricyclic antidepressants: May increase the anticholinergic and sedative effects of thioridazine.
Herbal
None known.
Food
None known.

DIAGNOSTIC TEST EFFECTS
May cause EKG changes. Therapeutic serum level is 0.2–2.6 mcg/ml; toxic serum level is not established.

SIDE EFFECTS
Occasional
Drowsiness during early therapy, dry mouth, blurred vision, lethargy, constipation or diarrhea, nasal congestion, peripheral edema, urine retention
Rare
Ocular changes, altered skin pigmentation (in those taking high doses for prolonged periods), photosensitivity, darkening of urine

SERIOUS REACTIONS
! Prolonged QT interval may produce torsades de pointes, a form of ventricular tachycardia, and sudden death.

NURSING CONSIDERATIONS
Baseline Assessment
- Assess the patient's appearance, behavior, emotional status, response to environment, speech pattern, and thought content.
- Plan to obtain a baseline EKG and to measure the QT and QTc intervals.
Precautions
- Use thioridazine cautiously in patients with benign prostatic hypertrophy, decreased GI motility, seizures, urinary retention, and visual problems.
Administration and Handling
- Avoid skin contact with the oral solution because it can cause contact dermatitis.
Intervention and Evaluation
- Assess the patient for extrapyramidal symptoms.
- Monitor the patient's BP, CBC, EKG, serum potassium level, and liver function test results, including serum alkaline phosphatase, bilirubin, AST (SGOT), and ALT (SGPT) levels.
- Observe the patient for fine tongue movement, which may be an early sign of tardive dyskinesia.
- Closely supervise suicidal patients during early therapy. As depression lessens, the patient's energy level

improves, which increases the suicide potential.

• Assess the patient for evidence of a therapeutic response, such as improvement in self-care and ability to concentrate, increased interest in surroundings, and relaxed facial expression.

• Know that the therapeutic serum level for thioridazine is 0.2 to 2.6 mcg/ml, and the toxic serum level is not established.

Patient Teaching

• Inform the patient that the drug's full therapeutic effect may take up to 6 weeks to appear.

• Caution the patient against abruptly discontinuing the drug after long-term use.

• Inform the patient that the drug may darken urine.

• Warn the patient to avoid tasks that require mental alertness or motor skills until his or her response to the drug has been established. Explain that drowsiness generally subsides during continued therapy.

• Advise the patient to notify the physician if he or she experiences visual disturbances.

• Urge the patient to avoid alcohol and exposure to artificial light and sunlight during thioridazine therapy.

• Suggest taking sips of tepid water or chewing sugarless gum to relieve dry mouth.

thiothixene

thye-oh-**thix**-een

(Navane)

Do not confuse thiothixene with thioridazine.

CATEGORY AND SCHEDULE

Pregnancy Risk Category: C

MECHANISM OF ACTION

An antipsychotic that blocks postsynaptic dopamine receptor sites in brain. Has alpha-adrenergic blocking effects, and depresses the release of hypothalamic and hypophyseal hormones. **Therapeutic Effect:** Suppresses psychotic behavior.

PHARMACOKINETICS

Well absorbed from the GI tract after IM administration. Widely distributed. Metabolized in the liver. Primarily excreted in urine. Unknown if removed by hemodialysis. ***Half-life:*** 34 hr.

AVAILABILITY

Capsules: 1 mg, 2 mg, 5 mg, 10 mg, 20 mg.

Oral Concentrate: 5 mg/ml.

Injection: 5 mg of thiothixene and 59.6 mg of mannitol per ml when reconstituted with 2.2 ml of sterile water for injection.

INDICATIONS AND DOSAGES

▸ Psychosis

PO

Adults, Elderly, Children older than 12 yr. Initially, 2 mg 3 times a day. Maximum: 60 mg/day.

IM

Adults, Elderly, Children older than 12 yr. Initially, 4 mg 2–4 times a day. Maximum: 30 mg/day.

CONTRAINDICATIONS

Blood dyscrasias, circulatory collapse, CNS depression, coma, history of seizures

INTERACTIONS

Drug

Alcohol, other CNS depressants: May increase CNS and respiratory depression and the hypotensive effects of thiothixene.

Extrapyramidal symptom–producing medications: May increase the risk of extrapyramidal symptoms.
Levodopa: May inhibit the effects of levodopa.
Quinidine: May increase cardiac effects.

Herbal

Kava kava, St. John's wort, valerian:
May increase CNS depression.

Food

None known.

DIAGNOSTIC TEST EFFECTS

May decrease serum uric acid level.

SIDE EFFECTS

Expected

Hypotension, dizziness, syncope (occur frequently after first injection, occasionally after subsequent injections, and rarely with oral form)

Frequent

Transient drowsiness, dry mouth, constipation, blurred vision, nasal congestion

Occasional

Diarrhea, peripheral edema, urine retention, nausea

Rare

Ocular changes, altered skin pigmentation (in those taking high doses for prolonged periods), photosensitivity

SERIOUS REACTIONS

! The most common extrapyramidal reaction is akathisia, characterized by motor restlessness and anxiety. Akinesia, marked by rigidity, tremor, increased salivation, masklike facial expression, and reduced voluntary movements, occurs less frequently. Dystonias, including torticollis, opisthotonos, and oculogyric crisis, occur rarely.

! Tardive dyskinesia, characterized by tongue protrusion, puffing of the cheeks, and chewing or puckering of the mouth, occurs rarely but may be irreversible. Elderly female patients have a greater risk of developing this reaction.

! Grand mal seizures may occur in epileptic patients, especially those receiving the drug by IM administration.

! Neuroleptic malignant syndrome occurs rarely.

NURSING CONSIDERATIONS

Baseline Assessment

- Assess the patient's appearance, behavior, emotional status, response to environment, speech pattern, and thought content.

Lifespan Considerations

- Thiothixene crosses the placenta and is distributed in breast milk.
- Children are more prone to develop extrapyramidal and neuromuscular symptoms, especially dystonias.
- The elderly are more prone to anticholinergic effects (such as dry mouth), extrapyramidal symptoms, orthostatic hypotension, and increased sedation.

Precautions

- Use thiothixene cautiously in patients undergoing alcohol withdrawal; in those with severe cardiovascular disorders, glaucoma, or benign prostatic hyperplasia; and in those who may be exposed to extreme heat.

Administration and Handling

PO

- Give thiothixene without regard to food.
- Avoid skin contact with the oral solution because it can cause contact dermatitis.

IM

- Reconstitute drug with 2.2 ml of sterile water.

Intervention and Evaluation

- Closely supervise suicidal patients during early therapy. As depression lessens, the patient's energy level improves, which increases the suicide potential.
- Monitor the patient's BP for hypotension.
- Assess the patient for peripheral edema.
- Assess the patient's pattern of daily bowel activity and stool consistency.
- Monitor the patient for extrapyramidal reactions and early signs of tardive dyskinesia and potentially fatal neuroleptic malignant syndrome (such as altered mental status, fever, irregular pulse or BP, and muscle rigidity).
- Assess the patient for evidence of a therapeutic response, such as improvement in self-care and ability to concentrate, increased interest in surroundings, and relaxed facial expression.

Patient Teaching

- Inform the patient that the drug's full therapeutic effect may take up to 6 weeks to appear.
- Warn the patient to avoid tasks that require mental alertness or motor skills until his or her response to the drug has been established. Explain that drowsiness generally subsides during continued therapy.
- Advise the patient to notify the physician if visual disturbances occur.
- Urge the patient to avoid alcohol, exposure to artificial light or direct sunlight, and other CNS depressants during thiothixene therapy.
- Suggest taking sips of tepid water and chewing sugarless gum to relieve dry mouth.

trifluoperazine hydrochloride

trye-floo-oh-**per**-a-zeen
(Apo-Trifluoperazine[CAN], Nono-Trifluzine[CAN], PMS-Trifluoperazine[CAN], Stelazine)
Do not confuse trifluoperazine with triflupromazine, or Stelazine with selegiline.

CATEGORY AND SCHEDULE

Pregnancy Risk Category: C

MECHANISM OF ACTION

A phenothiazine derivative that blocks dopamine at postsynaptic receptor sites. Possess strong extrapyramidal and antiemetic effects and weak anticholinergic and sedative effects. **Therapeutic Effect:** Suppresses behavioral response in psychosis; reduces locomotor activity and aggressiveness.

AVAILABILITY

Tablets: 1 mg, 2 mg, 5 mg, 10 mg.
Injection: 2 mg/ml.

INDICATIONS AND DOSAGES

▸ Psychotic disorders

PO

Adults, Elderly, Children 12 yr and older. Initially, 2–5 mg once or twice a day. Range: 15–20 mg/day. Maximum: 40 mg/day.
Children 6–11 yr. Initially, 1 mg once or twice a day. Maintenance: Up to 15 mg/day.

IM

Adults. 1–2 mg q4–6h. Maximum: 10 mg/24h.
Elderly. 1 mg q4–6h. Maximum: 6 mg/24h.
Children. 1 mg 2 times/day.

CONTRAINDICATIONS

Angle-closure glaucoma, circulatory

collapse, myelosuppression, severe cardiac or hepatic disease, severe hypertension or hypotension

INTERACTIONS

Drug

Alcohol, other CNS depressants: May increase CNS and respiratory depression and the hypotensive effects of trifluoperazine.
Antacids: May inhibit absorption of trifluoperzine if given within 1 hour of drug.
Antithyroid agents: May increase the risk of agranulocytosis.
Extrapyramidal symptom–producing medications: May increase extrapyramidal symptoms.
Hypotension-producing agents: May increase hypotension.
Levodopa: May decrease the effects of levodopa.
Lithium: May decrease the absorption of trifluoperazine and produce adverse neurologic effects.
MAOIs, tricyclic antidepressants: May increase the anticholinergic and sedative effects of trifluoperazine.

Herbal

None known.

Food

None known.

DIAGNOSTIC TEST EFFECTS

May cause EKG changes.

SIDE EFFECTS

Frequent

Hypotension, dizziness, and syncope (occur frequently after first injection, occasionally after subsequent injections, and rarely with oral form)

Occasional

Drowsiness during early therapy, dry mouth, blurred vision, lethargy, constipation or diarrhea, nasal congestion, peripheral edema, urine retention

Rare

Ocular changes, altered skin pigmentation (in those taking high doses for prolonged periods), photosensitivity

SERIOUS REACTIONS

! Extrapyramidal symptoms appear to be dose-related (particularly high doses) and are divided into 3 categories: akathisia (inability to sit still, tapping of feet), parkinsonian symptoms (such as masklike face, tremors, shuffling gait, and hypersalivation), and acute dystonias (such as torticollis, opisthotonos, and oculogyric crisis). Dystonic reactions may also produce diaphoresis and pallor.
! Tardive dyskinesia, marked by tongue protrusion, puffing of the cheeks, and chewing or puckering of the mouth, occurs rarely but may be irreversible.
! Abrupt withdrawal after long-term therapy may precipitate nausea, vomiting, gastritis, dizziness, and tremors.
! Blood dyscrasias, particularly agranulocytosis, and mild leukopenia may occur.
! Trifluoperazine may lower the seizure threshold.

NURSING CONSIDERATIONS

Baseline Assessment

- Assess the patient's appearance, behavior, emotional status, response to environment, speech pattern, and thought content.

Precautions

- Use trifluoperazine cautiously in patients with Parkinson's disease or seizure disorders.

Administration and Handling

PO

- May give with food to decrease GI effects.

IM

- Administer deep injection in large muscle mass.

Intervention and Evaluation
- Monitor the patient's BP for hypotension.
- Observe the patient for extrapyramidal symptoms, such as gait changes, tremors, and abnormal movement in the trunk, neck, or extremities.
- Monitor the patient's WBC count for blood dyscrasias, such as anemia, neutropenia, pancytopenia, and thrombocytopenia.
- Monitor the patient for fine tongue movement, an early sign of tardive dyskinesia.
- Closely supervise suicidal patients during early therapy. As depression lessens, the patient's energy level improves, increasing the suicide potential.
- Assess the patient for signs of a therapeutic response, such as improvement in self-care and ability to concentrate, increased interest in surroundings, and relaxed facial expression.

Patient Teaching
- Inform the patient that trifluoperazine may cause drowsiness. Warn the patient to avoid tasks requiring mental alertness or motor skills until his or her response to the drug has been established.
- Instruct the patient not to take antacids within 1 hour of trifluoperazine.
- Urge the patient to avoid alcohol and excessive exposure to artificial light and sunlight during trifluoperazine therapy.
- Instruct the patient to rise slowly from a lying or sitting position to prevent hypotension.

ziprasidone
zye-**pray**-za-done
(Geodon)

CATEGORY AND SCHEDULE
Pregnancy Risk Category: C

MECHANISM OF ACTION
A piperazine derivative that antagonizes alpha-adrenergic, dopamine, histamine, and serotonin receptors; also inhibits reuptake of serotonin and norepinephrine. **Therapeutic Effect:** Diminishes symptoms of schizophrenia and depression.

PHARMACOKINETICS
Well absorbed after PO administration. Food increases bioavailability. Protein binding: 99%. Extensively metabolized in the liver. Not removed by hemodialysis. ***Half-life:*** 7 hr.

AVAILABILITY
Capsules: 20 mg, 40 mg, 60 mg, 80 mg.
Injection: 20 mg/ml.

INDICATIONS AND DOSAGES
▸ Schizophrenia
PO
Adults, Elderly. Initially, 20 mg twice a day with food. Titrate at intervals of no less than 2 days. Maximum: 80 mg twice a day.
IM
Adults, Elderly. 10 mg q2h or 20 mg q4h. Maximum: 40 mg/day.
▸ Bipolar Mania
PO
Adults, Elderly. 40 mg 2 times/day.

CONTRAINDICATIONS
Conditions that prolong the QT interval, such as congenital long QT syndrome

INTERACTIONS

Drug

Alcohol, other CNS depressants: May increase CNS depression.
Carbamazepine: May decrease ziprasidone blood concentration.
Ketoconazole: May increase ziprasidone blood concentration.

Herbal

None known.

Food

All foods: Enhance the bioavailability of ziprasidone.

DIAGNOSTIC TEST EFFECTS

May prolong the QT interval.

SIDE EFFECTS

Frequent (30%–16%)
Headache, somnolence, dizziness
Occasional
Rash, orthostatic hypotension, weight gain, restlessness, constipation, dyspepsia

SERIOUS REACTIONS

! Prolongation of QT interval may produce torsades de pointes, a form of ventricular tachycardia. Patients with bradycardia, hypokalemia, or hypomagnesemia are at increased risk.

NURSING CONSIDERATIONS

Baseline Assessment

- Assess the patient's appearance, behavior, emotional status, response to environment, speech pattern, and thought content.
- Obtain an EKG, as ordered, to assess for prolonged QT interval before beginning treatment.
- Plan to obtain blood chemistry tests to check magnesium and potassium levels before beginning therapy and routinely thereafter.

Lifespan Considerations

- It is unknown if ziprasidone crosses the placenta or is distributed in breast milk.
- The safety and efficacy of ziprasidone have not been established in children.
- No age-related precautions have been noted in the elderly.

Precautions

- Use ziprasidone cautiously in patients with bradycardia, hypokalemia, or hypomagnesemia because they may be at greater risk for developing torsades de pointes or atypical ventricular tachycardia.

Administration and Handling

PO

- Give ziprasidone with food to increase its bioavailability.

IM

- Store vials at room temperature, and protect them from light.
- Reconstitute each vial with 1.2 ml sterile water for injection to provide a concentration of 20 mg/ml.
- The reconstituted solution is stable for 24 hours at room temperature or 7 days refrigerated.

Intervention and Evaluation

- Closely supervise suicidal patients during early therapy. As depression lessens, the patient's energy level improves, which increases the suicide potential.
- Assess the patient for evidence of a therapeutic response, such as a greater interest in surroundings, improved self-care and ability to concentrate, and relaxed facial expression.
- Monitor the patient's weight.

Patient Teaching

- Instruct the patient to take ziprasidone with food to increase its effectiveness.
- Warn the patient to avoid tasks requiring mental alertness or motor skills until his or her response to the drug has been established.

39 Cholinesterase Inhibitors

donepezil hydrochloride
galantamine
memantine hydrochloride
rivastigmine tartrate
tacrine hydrochloride

Uses: Cholinesterase inhibitors are used to treat mild to moderate dementia of Alzheimer's disease and to slow the progression of the disease.

Action: Most agents in this class inhibit acetyl cholinesterase, which normally hydrolyzes acetylcholine. By preventing acetylcholine breakdown, these agents increase the acetylcholine level at cholinergic synapses, which enhances cholinergic transmission in the CNS. This is helpful in Alzheimer's disease, which is thought to involve degeneration of cholinergic neuronal pathways. Memantine decreases the effects of glutamate, which is the main excitatory neurotransmitter in the brain and which may contribute to symptoms of Alzheimer's disease.

donepezil hydrochloride

dah-**nep**-eh-zil
(Aricept)
Do not confuse Aricept with Aciphex or Ascriptin.

CATEGORY AND SCHEDULE

Pregnancy Risk Category: C

MECHANISM OF ACTION

A cholinesterase inhibitor that inhibits the enzyme acetylcholinesterase, thus increasing the concentration of acetylcholine at cholinergic synapses and enhancing cholinergic function in the CNS. **Therapeutic Effect:** Slows the progression of Alzheimer's disease.

PHARMACOKINETICS

Well absorbed after PO administration. Protein binding: 96%. Extensively metabolized. Eliminated in urine and feces. ***Half-life:*** 70 hr.

AVAILABILITY

Tablets: 5 mg, 10 mg.
Tablets (Orally-Disintegrating): 5 mg, 10 mg.

INDICATIONS AND DOSAGES

▸ **Alzheimer's disease**

PO

Adults, Elderly. 5–10 mg/day as a single dose. If initial dose is 5 mg, do not increase to 10 mg for 4–6 wk.

OFF-LABEL USES

Treatment of autism

CONTRAINDICATIONS

History of hypersensitivity to donepezil or piperidine derivatives

INTERACTIONS

Drug

Anticholinergics: May decrease the effect of anticholinergics.
Cholinergic agonists, neuromuscular blockers, succinylcholine: May increase the synergistic effects of these drugs.

Ketoconazole, quinidine: May inhibit the metabolism of donepezil.
NSAIDs: May increase gastric acid secretion of NSAIDs.
Paroxetine: May decrease the metabolism and increase the blood concentration of donepezil.

Herbal

None known.

Food

None known.

DIAGNOSTIC TEST EFFECTS

May increase blood glucose and serum creatine kinase and LDH concentrations. May decrease the serum potassium level.

SIDE EFFECTS

Frequent (11%–8%)

Nausea, diarrhea, headache, insomnia, nonspecific pain, dizziness

Occasional (6%–3%)

Mild muscle cramps, fatigue, vomiting, anorexia, ecchymosis

Rare (3%–2%)

Depression, abnormal dreams, weight loss, arthritis, somnolence, syncope, frequent urination

SERIOUS REACTIONS

! Overdose may result in cholinergic crisis, characterized by severe nausea, increased salivation, diaphoresis, bradycardia, hypotension, flushed skin, abdominal pain, respiratory depression, seizures, and cardiorespiratory collapse. Increasing muscle weakness may result in death if respiratory muscles are involved. The antidote is 1–2 mg IV atropine sulfate with subsequent doses based on therapeutic response.

NURSING CONSIDERATIONS

Baseline Assessment

- Obtain the patient's baseline vital signs.
- Determine if the patient has a history of asthma, cardiac conduction disturbances, COPD, peptic ulcer disease, seizure disorder, or urinary obstruction.
- Assess the patient's behavioral, cognitive, and functional deficits.

Lifespan Considerations

- It is unknown if donepezil is distributed in breast milk.
- Donepezil is not prescribed for children.
- No age-related precautions have been noted in the elderly.

Precautions

- Use donepezil cautiously in patients with asthma, bladder outflow obstruction, COPD, peptic ulcer disease, history of seizures, or sick sinus syndrome or other supraventricular conduction disturbances.
- Use the drug cautiously in patients taking NSAIDs concurrently.

Administration and Handling

PO

- Give donepezil without regard to food. The drug may be given in the morning or evening; however, best results may be achieved if it's given at bedtime.

Intervention and Evaluation

- Monitor the patient's behavioral, cognitive, and functional status.
- Monitor the patient for cholinergic reactions, such as diaphoresis, dizziness, excessive salivation, facial warmth, abdominal cramps or discomfort, lacrimation, pallor, and urinary urgency.
- Monitor the patient for diarrhea, headache, insomnia, and nausea.

Patient Teaching

- Inform the patient that donepezil may be taken with or without food.
- Instruct the patient to notify the physician if he or she experiences abdominal pain, diarrhea, excessive sweating or salivation, dizziness, or nausea and vomiting.

- Inform the patient and family that donepezil is not a cure for Alzheimer's disease but may slow the progression of its symptoms.
- Refer the patient's family to the local chapter of the Alzheimer's Disease Association for a guide to available services.

galantamine

ga-**lan**-ta-mene
(Reminyl)
Do not confuse Reminyl with Remeron, Remicade, or Robinul.

CATEGORY AND SCHEDULE

Pregnancy Risk Category: B

MECHANISM OF ACTION

A cholinesterase inhibitor that inhibits the enzyme acetylcholinesterase, thus increasing the concentration of acetylcholine at cholinergic synapses and enhancing cholinergic function in the CNS. **Therapeutic Effect:** Slows the progression of Alzheimer's disease.

PHARMACOKINETICS

Rapidly absorbed from the GI tract. Protein binding: 18%. Distributed to blood cells; binds to plasma proteins, mainly albumin. Metabolized in the liver. Excreted in urine. ***Half-life:*** 7 hr.

AVAILABILITY

Oral Solution: 4 mg/ml.
Tablets: 4 mg, 8 mg, 12 mg.

INDICATIONS AND DOSAGES

▸ **Alzheimer's disease**

PO

Adults, Elderly. Initially, 4 mg twice a day (8 mg/day). After a minimum of 4 wk (if well tolerated), may increase to 8 mg twice a day (16 mg/day). After another 4 wk, may increase to 12 mg twice daily (24 mg/day). Range: 16–24 mg/day in 2 divided doses.

▸ **Dosage in renal impairment**

For moderate impairment, maximum dosage is 16 mg/day. Drug is not recommended for patients with severe impairment.

CONTRAINDICATIONS

Severe hepatic or renal impairment

INTERACTIONS

Drug

Bethanechol, succinylcholine: May interfere with the effects of these drugs.
Cimetidine, erythromycin, ketoconazole, paroxetine: May increase the galantamine blood concentration.

Herbal

None known.

Food

None known.

DIAGNOSTIC TEST EFFECTS

None known.

SIDE EFFECTS

Frequent (17%–5%)
Nausea, vomiting, diarrhea, anorexia, weight loss
Occasional (9%–4%)
Abdominal pain, insomnia, depression, headache, dizziness, fatigue, rhinitis
Rare (less than 3%)
Tremors, constipation, confusion, cough, anxiety, urinary incontinence

SERIOUS REACTIONS

! Overdose may cause cholinergic crisis, characterized by increased salivation, lacrimation, severe nausea and vomiting, bradycardia, respiratory depression, hypotension, and increased muscle weakness. Treatment usually consists of supportive measures and an anticholinergic such as atropine.

NURSING CONSIDERATIONS

Baseline Assessment

• Assess the patient's behavioral, cognitive, and functional deficits.
• Obtain the patient's liver and renal function test results.

Lifespan Considerations

• It is unknown if galantamine crosses the placenta or is distributed in breast milk.
• Galantamine is not prescribed for children.
• No age-related precautions have been noted in the elderly, but galantamine is not recommended for those with severe hepatic or renal impairment (creatinine clearance of less than 9 ml/minute).

Precautions

• Use galantamine cautiously in patients with asthma, bladder outflow obstruction, COPD, peptic ulcer disease, history of seizures, moderate hepatic or renal impairment, or supraventricular conduction disturbances.
• Use the drug cautiously in patients taking NSAIDs concurrently.

Administration and Handling

◀**ALERT**▶ If galantamine therapy is interrupted for several days or longer, reinstitute therapy as prescribed.

PO

• Give galantamine with morning and evening meals.

Intervention and Evaluation

• Monitor the patient's behavioral, cognitive, and functional status.
• Periodically assess the 12-lead EKG and rhythm strips of patients with underlying arrhythmias.
• Assess the patient for signs of GI distress, including nausea, vomiting, diarrhea, anorexia, and weight loss.

Patient Teaching

• Instruct the patient to take galantamine with morning and evening meals to reduce the risk of nausea.
• Warn the patient to avoid tasks that require mental alertness or motor skills until his or her response to the drug has been established.
• Advise the patient to notify the physician if he or she experiences excessive sweating, tearing, or salivation; depression; dizziness; excessive fatigue; muscle weakness; insomnia; or persistent GI disturbances.
• Inform the patient and family that galantamine is not a cure for Alzheimer's disease but may slow the progression of its symptoms.
• Refer the patient's family to the local chapter of the Alzheimer's Disease Association for a guide to available services.

memantine hydrochloride

meh-**man**-teen

(Ebixa[AUS], Namenda)

CATEGORY AND SCHEDULE

Pregnancy Risk Category: B

MECHANISM OF ACTION

A neurotransmitter inhibitor that decreases the effects of glutamate, the principle excitatory neurotransmitter in the brain. Persistent CNS excitation by glutamate is thought to cause the symptoms of Alzheimer's disease. **Therapeutic Effect:** May reduce clinical deterioration in moderate to severe Alzheimer's disease.

PHARMACOKINETICS

Rapidly and completely absorbed after PO administration. Protein binding: 45%. Undergoes little metabolism; most of the dose is excreted unchanged in urine. ***Half-life:*** 60–80 hr.

AVAILABILITY

Tablets: 5 mg, 10 mg.

INDICATIONS AND DOSAGES

▸ Alzheimer's disease

PO

Adults, Elderly. Initially, 5 mg once a day. May increase dosage at intervals of at least 1 wk in 5-mg increments to 10 mg/day (5 mg twice a day), then 15 mg/day (5 mg and 10 mg as separate doses), and finally 20 mg/day (10 mg twice a day). Target dose: 20 mg/day.

CONTRAINDICATIONS

Severe renal impairment

INTERACTIONS

Drug

Carbonic anhydrase inhibitors, sodium bicarbonate: May decrease the renal elimination of memantine.

Herbal

None known.

Food

None known.

DIAGNOSTIC TEST EFFECTS

None known.

SIDE EFFECTS

Occasional (7%–4%)

Dizziness, headache, confusion, constipation, hypertension, cough

Rare (3%–2%)

Back pain, nausea, fatigue, anxiety, peripheral edema, arthralgia, insomnia

SERIOUS REACTIONS

! None known.

NURSING CONSIDERATIONS

Baseline Assessment

- Evaluate the patient's behavioral, cognitive, and functional deficits.
- Expect to obtain baseline renal function tests, including BUN and serum creatinine levels.

Lifespan Considerations

- It is unknown if memantine crosses the placenta or is distributed in breast milk.
- Memantine is not prescribed for use in children.
- No age-related precautions have been noted in the elderly, but memantine is not recommended for elderly patients with severe renal impairment (creatinine clearance less than 9 ml/minute).

Precautions

- Use memantine cautiously in patients with moderate renal impairment.

Administration and Handling

PO

- Give memantine without regard to food.

Intervention and Evaluation

- Monitor the patient's behavioral, cognitive, and functional status.
- Monitor the patient's urine pH because alkaline urine may lead to an accumulation of the drug and a possible increase in side effects.
- Monitor the patient's renal function.

Patient Teaching

- Caution the patient against abruptly discontinuing memantine or adjusting the drug dosage.
- If therapy is interrupted for several days, instruct the patient to restart the drug at the lowest dose and increase the dosage at intervals of at

least 1 week to the most recent dose, as prescribed.

- Urge the patient to maintain adequate fluid intake.
- Inform the patient and family that memantine is not a cure for Alzheimer's disease but may slow the progression of its symptoms.
- Refer the patient's family to the local chapter of the Alzheimer's Disease Association for a guide to available services.

rivastigmine tartrate

riv-a-**stig**-meen
(Exelon)

CATEGORY AND SCHEDULE

Pregnancy Risk Category: B

MECHANISM OF ACTION

A cholinesterase inhibitor that inhibits the enzyme acetylcholinesterase, thus increasing the concentration of acetylcholine at cholinergic synapses and enhancing cholinergic function in the CNS. **Therapeutic Effect:** Slows the progression of symptoms of Alzheimer's disease.

PHARMACOKINETICS

Rapidly and completely absorbed. Protein binding: 60%. Widely distributed throughout the body. Rapidly and extensively metabolized. Primarily excreted in urine. ***Half-life:*** 1.5 hr.

AVAILABILITY

Capsules: 1.5 mg, 3 mg, 4.5 mg, 6 mg.
Oral Solution: 2 mg/ml.

INDICATIONS AND DOSAGES

▸ Alzheimer's disease

PO

Adults, Elderly. Initially, 1.5 mg twice a day. May increase at intervals of least 2 wk to 3 mg twice a day, then 4.5 mg twice a day, and finally 6 mg twice a day. Maximum: 6 mg twice a day.

CONTRAINDICATIONS

None known.

INTERACTIONS

Drug

Anticholinergics: May decrease the effects of rivastigmine or anticholinergics.
Bethanecol: May increase the effects of rivastigmine or bethanecol.

Herbal

None known.

Food

None known.

DIAGNOSTIC TEST EFFECTS

None known.

SIDE EFFECTS

Frequent (47%–17%)
Nausea, vomiting, dizziness, diarrhea, headache, anorexia
Occasional (13%–6%)
Abdominal pain, insomnia, dyspepsia (heartburn, indigestion, epigastric pain), confusion, UTI, depression
Rare (5%–3%)
Anxiety, somnolence, constipation, malaise, hallucinations, tremor, flatulence, rhinitis, hypertension, flulike symptoms, weight loss, syncope

SERIOUS REACTIONS

! Overdose may result in cholinergic crisis, characterized by severe nausea and vomiting, increased salivation, diaphoresis, bradycardia, hypotension, respiratory depression, and seizures.

NURSING CONSIDERATIONS

Baseline Assessment

- Obtain the patient's baseline vital signs.
- Determine if the patient has a history of asthma, COPD, peptic ulcer disease, or urinary obstruction.
- Assess the patient's behavioral, cognitive, and functional deficits.

Lifespan Considerations

- It is unknown if rivastigmine is distributed in breast milk.
- Rivastigmine is not prescribed for children.
- No age-related precautions have been noted in the elderly.

Precautions

- Use rivastigmine cautiously in patients with asthma, bradycardia, COPD, peptic ulcer disease, history of seizures, sick sinus syndrome, or urinary obstruction.
- Use the drug cautiously in patients taking NSAIDs concurrently.

Administration and Handling

PO

- Give rivastigmine with morning and evening meals.
- When administering the oral solution, withdraw the prescribed amount of rivastigmine from the container, using the oral syringe provided by the manufacturer.
- The drug may be slowly placed in the patient's mouth directly from the syringe or mixed in a small glass of water, cold fruit juice, or soda. Use the solution within 4 hours of mixing it.

Intervention and Evaluation

- Monitor the patient for a cholinergic reaction, including diaphoresis, dizziness, excessive salivation, facial warmth, abdominal cramps or discomfort, lacrimation, pallor, and urinary urgency.
- Monitor for the patient for diarrhea, nausea, headache, and insomnia.

Patient Teaching

- Instruct the patient to take rivastigmine with morning and evening meals.
- Teach the patient to swallow the capsules whole, not to break, chew, or crush them.
- If the patient is using the oral solution, explain that he or she should withdraw the prescribed amount of drug into the syringe and either sip it directly from the syringe or first mix it with a small glass of water, cold fruit juice, or soda and then stir and drink the mixture.
- Advise the patient to notify the physician if he or she experiences diarrhea, excessive sweating or salivation, dizziness, nausea and vomiting, or severe abdominal pain.
- Inform the patient and family that rivastigmine is not a cure for Alzheimer's disease but may slow the progression of its symptoms.
- Refer the patient's family to the local chapter of the Alzheimer's Disease Association for a guide to available services.

tacrine hydrochloride

tack-rin
(Cognex)

CATEGORY AND SCHEDULE

Pregnancy Risk Category: C

MECHANISM OF ACTION

A cholinesterase inhibitor that inhibits the enzyme acetylcholinesterase, thus increasing the concentration of acetylcholine at cholinergic synapses and enhancing cholinergic function in the CNS. **Therapeutic Effect:** Slows the progression of Alzheimer's disease.

AVAILABILITY

Capsules: 10 mg, 20 mg, 30 mg, 40 mg.

INDICATIONS AND DOSAGES

▸ Alzheimer's disease

PO

Adults, Elderly. Initially, 10 mg 4 times a day for 6 wk, followed by 20 mg 4 times a day for 6 wk, 30 mg 4 times a day for 12 wk, then 40 mg 4 times a day if needed.

▸ Dosage in hepatic impairment

For patients with ALT (SGPT) greater than 3–5 times normal, decrease the dose by 40 mg/day and resume the normal dose when ALT (SGPT) returns to normal. For patients with ALT (SGPT) greater than 5 times normal, stop treatment and resume it when ALT (SGPT) returns to normal.

CONTRAINDICATIONS

Active, severe hepatic disease; active and untreated duodenal or gastric ulcers; breast-feeding women; concurrent use of other cholinesterase inhibitors; hypersensitivity to cholinergics; mechanical obstruction of intestine or urinary tract; pregnancy; women with childbearing potential

INTERACTIONS

Drug

Anticholinergics: May decrease the effects of tacrine oranticholinergics.
Cimetidine: May increase the tacrine blood concentration.
NSAIDs: May increase the adverse effects of NSAIDs.
Theophylline: May increase the theophylline blood concentration.

Herbal

None known.

Food

None known.

DIAGNOSTIC TEST EFFECTS

Increases AST (SGOT) and ALT (SGPT) levels. Alters blood Hgb, Hct, and serum electrolyte levels.

SIDE EFFECTS

Frequent (28%–11%)

Headache, nausea, vomiting, diarrhea, dizziness

Occasional (9%–4%)

Fatigue, chest pain, dyspepsia, anorexia, abdominal pain, flatulence, constipation, confusion, agitation, rash, depression, ataxia, insomnia, rhinitis, myalgia

Rare (less than 3%)

Weight loss, anxiety, cough, facial flushing, urinary frequency, back pain, tremor

SERIOUS REACTIONS

! Overdose can cause cholinergic crisis, marked by increased salivation, lacrimation, bradycardia, respiratory depression, hypotension, and increased muscle weakness. Treatment usually consists of supportive measures and an anticholinergic such as atropine.

NURSING CONSIDERATIONS

Baseline Assessment

- Assess the patient's behavioral, cognitive, and functional deficits.
- Expect to obtain liver function test results.

Precautions

- Use tacrine cautiously in patients with alcohol abuse, asthma, bradycardia, cardiac arrhythmias, COPD, peptic ulcer disease, hyperthyroidism, hepatic dysfunction, or a history of seizures.

Administration and Handling

◀ **ALERT** ▶ If tacrine therapy is stopped for longer than 14 days, reinstitute therapy as prescribed.

PO
- Give tacrine without regard to food.

Intervention and Evaluation
- Monitor the patient's behavioral, cognitive, and functional status.
- Monitor the patient's AST (SGOT) and ALT (SGPT) levels.
- Periodically monitor the EKG and rhythm strips of patients with underlying arrhythmias.
- Assess the patient for signs of GI distress.

Patient Teaching
- Instruct the patient to take tacrine at regular intervals, between meals. However, inform the patient that he or she may take the drug with meals if GI upset occurs.
- Caution the patient against abruptly discontinuing tacrine or adjusting the drug dosage.
- Urge the patient to avoid smoking during tacrine therapy because smoking reduces the drug's blood level.
- Inform the patient and family that tacrine is not a cure for Alzheimer's disease but may slow the progression of its symptoms.
- Refer the patient's family to the local chapter of the Alzheimer's Disease Association for a guide to available services.

40 CNS Stimulants

atomoxetine
dexmethylphenidate hydrochloride
dextroamphetamine sulfate
methylphenidate hydrochloride
modafinil
pemoline

Uses: Most CNS stimulants are used to treat attention deficit hyperactivity disorder, primarily in children age 6 and younger. In adults, several of these agents are used to treat narcolepsy. In addition, dextroamphetamine is used for short-term treatment of obesity.

Action: In this classification, specific subgroups and individual agents act by different mechanisms. *Amphetamines,* such as dextroamphetamine, promote the release and action of norepinephrine and dopamine by blocking reuptake from synapses; they also inhibit the action of monoamine oxidase. *Atomoxetine* selectively blocks presynaptic norepinephrine release. *Dexmethylphenidate* and *methylphenidate* block the reuptake of norepinephrine and dopamine into presynaptic neurons. *Modafinil's* exact mechanism of action is unknown, but the drug may bind to dopamine reuptake carrier sites, increasing alpha activity and decreasing delta, theta, and beta brain wave activity. *Pemoline* blocks the reuptake of dopamine at neurons in the cerebral cortex and subcortical structures.

atomoxetine

auto-**mox**-eh-teen
(Strattera)

CATEGORY AND SCHEDULE

Pregnancy Risk Category: C

MECHANISM OF ACTION

A norepinephrine reuptake inhibitor that enhances noradrenergic function by selective inhibition of the presynaptic norepinephrine transporter. **Therapeutic Effect:** Improves symptoms of attention-deficit hyperactivity disorder (ADHD).

PHARMACOKINETICS

Rapidly absorbed after PO administration. Protein binding: 98% (primarily to albumin). Eliminated primarily in urine and, to a lesser extent, in feces. Not removed by hemodialysis. ***Half-life:*** 4–5 hr in general population, 22 hr in 7% of Caucasians and 2% of African-Americans (increased in moderate to severe hepatic insufficiency).

AVAILABILITY

Capsules: 10 mg, 18 mg, 25 mg, 40 mg, 60 mg.

INDICATIONS AND DOSAGES

▸ **ADHD**

PO

Adults, Children weighing 70 kg and more. 40 mg once a day. May in-

crease after at least 3 days to 80 mg as a single daily dose or in divided doses. Maximum: 100 mg.
Children weighing less than 70 kg. Initially, 0.5 mg/kg/day. May increase after at least 3 days to 1.2 mg/kg/day. Maximum: 1.4 mg/kg/day or 100 mg.

▸ **Dosage in hepatic impairment**
Expect to administer 50% of normal atomoxetine dosage to patients with moderate hepatic impairment and 25% of normal dosage to those with severe hepatic impairment.

OFF-LABEL USES
Treatment of depression

CONTRAINDICATIONS
Angle-closure glaucoma, use within 14 days of MAOIs

INTERACTIONS
Drug
Fluoxetine, paroxetine, quinidine: May increase atomoxetine blood concentration.
MAOIs: May increase the risk of toxic effects.
Herbal
None known.
Food
None known.

DIAGNOSTIC TEST EFFECTS
None known.

SIDE EFFECTS
Frequent
Headache, dyspepsia, nausea, vomiting, fatigue, decreased appetite, dizziness, altered mood
Occasional
Tachycardia, hypertension, weight loss, delayed growth in children, irritability
Rare
Insomnia, sexual dysfunction in adults, fever

SERIOUS REACTIONS
! Urine retention or urinary hesitance may occur.
! In overdose, gastric emptying and repeated use of activated charcoal may prevent systemic absorption.

NURSING CONSIDERATIONS
Baseline Assessment
- Assess the patient's BP and pulse rate before beginning atomoxetine therapy, after dosage increases, and periodically during therapy.
Lifespan Considerations
- It is unknown if atomoxetine is excreted in breast milk.
- The safety and efficacy of atomoxetine have not been established in children younger than 6 years.
- Age-related cardiovascular or cerebrovascular disease and hepatic or renal impairment may increase the risk of side effects in the elderly.
Precautions
◂**ALERT**▸ Avoid concurrent use of medications that can increase heart rate or blood pressure.
- Use atomoxetine cautiously in patients with cardiovascular disease, tachycardia, hypertension, moderate or severe hepatic impairment, or a risk of urine retention.
Administration and Handling
PO
- Give atomoxetine without regard to food.
Intervention and Evaluation
- Monitor the patient's urine output. Inability to urinate or urinary hesitancy may be an adverse reaction.
- Assist the patient with ambulation if he or she experiences dizziness.
- Be alert for mood changes.
- Monitor the fluid and electrolyte status of patients who experience significant vomiting.
Patient Teaching
- Instruct the patient to take the last

daily dose of atomoxetine early in the evening to avoid insomnia.

- Advise the patient to avoid tasks that require mental alertness and motor skills until his or her response to the drug has been established.
- Instruct the patient to notify the physician if he or she experiences fever, irritability, palpitations, or vomiting.

dexmethylphenidate hydrochloride

dex-meth-ill-**fen**-i-date
(Focalin)

CATEGORY AND SCHEDULE

Pregnancy Risk Category: C
Controlled Substance: Schedule II

MECHANISM OF ACTION

A CNS stimulant that blocks the reuptake of norepinephrine and dopamine into presynaptic neurons, increasing the release of these neurotransmitters into the synaptic cleft. **Therapeutic Effect:** Decreases motor restlessness and fatigue; increases motor activity, mental alertness, and attention span; elevates mood.

PHARMACOKINETICS

Route	Onset	Peak	Duration
PO	N/A	N/A	4–5 hr

Readily absorbed from the GI tract. Plasma concentrations increase rapidly. Metabolized in the liver. Excreted unchanged in urine. ***Half-life:*** 2.2 hr.

AVAILABILITY

Tablets: 2.5 mg, 5 mg, 10 mg.

INDICATIONS AND DOSAGES

▸ **Attention deficit hyperactivity disorder (ADHD)**

PO

Patients new to dexmethylphenidate or methylphenidate. 2.5 mg twice a day (5 mg/day). May adjust dosage in 2.5- to 5-mg increments. Maximum: 20 mg/day.

Patients currently taking methylphenidate. Half the methylphenidate dosage. Maximum: 20 mg/day.

CONTRAINDICATIONS

Diagnosis or family history of Tourette syndrome; glaucoma; history of marked agitation, anxiety, or tension; motor tics; use within 14 days of MAOIs

INTERACTIONS

Drug

Amitriptyline, phenobarbital, phenytoin, primidone: Dosage of these drugs may need to be decreased.

MAOIs: May increase the effects of dexmethylphenidate.

Other CNS stimulants: May have an additive effect.

Warfarin: May inhibit the metabolism of warfarin.

Herbal

None known.

Food

None known.

DIAGNOSTIC TEST EFFECTS

None known.

SIDE EFFECTS

Frequent

Abdominal pain, nausea, anorexia, fever

Occasional

Tachycardia, arrhythmias, palpitations, insomnia, twitching

Rare
Blurred vision, rash, arthralgia.

SERIOUS REACTIONS

! Withdrawal after prolonged therapy may unmask symptoms of the underlying disorder.
! Dexmethylphenidate may lower the seizure threshold in those with a history of seizures.
! Overdose produces excessive sympathomimetic effects, including vomiting, tremor, hyperreflexia, seizures, confusion, hallucinations, and diaphoresis.
! Prolonged administration to children may delay growth.

NURSING CONSIDERATIONS

Baseline Assessment

- Obtain baseline height and weight, and weigh the patient regularly to detect delayed growth in children.

Lifespan Considerations

- It is unknown if dexmethylphenidate is excreted in breast milk.
- Children are more prone to develop abdominal pain, insomnia, anorexia, and weight loss.
- Long-term dexmethylphenidate use may inhibit growth in children.
- In psychotic children, dexmethylphenidate use may exacerbate behavior disturbances and abnormal thoughts.
- No age-related precautions have been noted in the elderly.

Precautions

- Use dexmethylphenidate cautiously in patients with cardiovascular disease, psychosis, or seizure disorders.
- Avoid dexmethylphenidate use in patients with a history of substance abuse.

Administration and Handling

PO
- Give dexmethylphenidate without regard to food. Crush tablets as needed.
- Administer the last dose of the day several hours before bedtime to prevent insomnia.

Intervention and Evaluation

- Plan to obtain CBC, WBC count with differential, and platelet count routinely during therapy.
- Expect to discontinue the drug or reduce the dosage if symptoms of ADHD return.

Patient Teaching

- Instruct the patient to take the last dose of the day several hours before bedtime to prevent insomnia.
- Warn the patient to avoid tasks that require mental alertness or motor skills until his or her response to the drug has been established.

dextroamphetamine sulfate

dex-troe-am-**fet**-a-meen
(Dexamphetamine[AUS], Dexedrine, Dexedrine Spansule, Dextrostat)
Do not confuse dextroamphetamine with dextromethorphan, or Dexedrine with Dextran or Excedrin.

CATEGORY AND SCHEDULE

Pregnancy Risk Category: C
Controlled Substance: Schedule II

MECHANISM OF ACTION

An amphetamine that enhances the action of dopamine and norepinephrine by blocking their reuptake from synapses; also inhibits monoamine oxidase and facilitates the release of catecholamines. **Therapeutic Effect:** Increases motor activity and mental alertness; decreases motor restlessness, drowsiness, and fatigue; suppresses appetite.

AVAILABILITY

Capsules (Sustained-Release [Dexedrine Spansule]): 5 mg, 10 mg, 15 mg.
Tablets (Dexedrine): 5 mg.
Tablets (Dextrostat): 5 mg, 10 mg.

INDICATIONS AND DOSAGES

▸ Narcolepsy

PO

Adults, Children older than 12 yr. Initially, 10 mg/day. Increase by 10 mg/day at weekly intervals until therapeutic response is achieved.
Children 6–12 yr. Initially, 5 mg/day. Increase by 5 mg/day at weekly intervals until therapeutic response is achieved. Maximum: 60 mg/day.

▸ Attention deficit hyperactivity disorder (ADHD)

PO

Children 6 yr and older. Initially, 5 mg once or twice a day. Increase by 5 mg/day at weekly intervals until therapeutic response is achieved.
Children 3–5 yr. Initially, 2.5 mg/day. Increase by 2.5 mg/day at weekly intervals until therapeutic response is achieved. Maximum: 40 mg/day.

▸ Appetite suppressant

PO

Adults. 5–30 mg daily in divided doses of 5–10 mg each, given 30–60 min before meals; or 1 extended-release capsule in the morning.

CONTRAINDICATIONS

Advanced arteriosclerosis, agitated states, glaucoma, history of drug abuse, hypersensitivity to sympathomimetic amines, hyperthyroidism, moderate to severe hypertension, symptomatic cardiovascular disease, use within 14 days of MAOIs

INTERACTIONS

Drug

Beta blockers: May increase the risk of bradycardia, heart block, and hypertension.
Digoxin: May increase the risk of arrhythmias.
MAOIs: May prolong and intensify the effects of dextroamphetamine.
Meperidine: May increase the risk of hypotension, respiratory depression, seizures, and vascular collapse.
Other CNS stimulants: May increase the effects of dextroamphetamine.
Thyroid hormones: May increase the effects of either drug.
Tricyclic antidepressants: May increase cardiovascular effects.

Herbal

None known.

Food

None known.

DIAGNOSTIC TEST EFFECTS

May increase plasma corticosteroid concentrations.

SIDE EFFECTS

Frequent

Irregular pulse, increased motor activity, talkativeness, nervousness, mild euphoria, insomnia

Occasional

Headache, chills, dry mouth, GI distress, worsening depression in patients who are clinically depressed, tachycardia, palpitations, chest pain, dizziness, decreased appetite

SERIOUS REACTIONS

! Overdose may produce skin pallor or flushing, arrhythmias, and psychosis.
! Abrupt withdrawal after prolonged use of high doses may produce lethargy lasting for weeks.
! Prolonged administration to

children with ADHD may inhibit growth.

NURSING CONSIDERATIONS

Precautions

- Use dextroamphetamine cautiously in debilitated, elderly, or tartrazine-sensitive patients.

Intervention and Evaluation

- Monitor the patient for CNS overstimulation, hypertension, and weight loss.

Patient Teaching

- Instruct the patient to take dextroamphetamine early in the day.
- Inform the patient that he or she may develop a tolerance to the drug's appetite-suppressant and mood-elevating effects within a few weeks.
- Warn the patient to avoid performing tasks that require mental alertness or motor skills until his or her response to the drug has been established.
- Caution the patient that this drug may mask signs and symptoms of extreme fatigue.
- Instruct the patient to notify the physician if he or she experiences decreased appetite, dizziness, dry mouth, or pronounced nervousness.
- Suggest taking sips of tepid water and chewing sugarless gum to relieve dry mouth.

methylphenidate hydrochloride

meth-ill-**fen**-i-date
(Attenta[AUS], Concerta, Metadate CD, Metadate ER, Methylin, Methylin ER, PMS-Methylphenidate[CAN], Riphenidate[CAN], Ritalin, Ritalin LA, Ritalin SR)

Do not confuse Ritalin with Rifadin.

CATEGORY AND SCHEDULE

Pregnancy Risk Category: C
Controlled Substance: Schedule II

MECHANISM OF ACTION

A CNS stimulant that blocks the reuptake of norepinephrine and dopamine into presynaptic neurons. **Therapeutic Effect:** Decreases motor restlessness and fatigue; increases motor activity, attention span, and mental alertness; produces mild euphoria.

PHARMACOKINETICS

Onset	Peak	Duration
Immediate-release	2 hr	3–5 hr
Sustained-release	4–7 hr	3–8 hr
Extended-release	N/A	8–12 hr

Slowly and incompletely absorbed from the GI tract. Protein binding: 15%. Metabolized in the liver. Eliminated in urine and in feces by biliary system. Unknown if removed by hemodialysis. ***Half-life:*** 2–4 hr.

AVAILABILITY

Capsules (Extended-Release [Metadate CD]): 10 mg, 20 mg, 30 mg.
Capsules (Extended-Release [Ritalin LA]): 20 mg, 30 mg, 40 mg.

Tablets (Ritalin): 5 mg, 10 mg, 20 mg.
Tablets (Extended-Release [Metadate ER, Mehtylin ER]): 10 mg, 20 mg.
Tablets (Extended-Release [Concerta]): 18 mg, 27 mg, 36 mg, 54 mg, 72 mg.
Tablets (Sustained-Release [Ritalin SR]): 20 mg.
Tablets (Chewable [Methylin]): 2.5 mg, 5 mg, 10 mg.
Oral Solution (Methylin): 5 mg/5 ml, 10 mg/5 ml.

INDICATIONS AND DOSAGES

▸ Attention deficit hyperactivity disorder (ADHD)

PO
Children 6 yr and older. Immediate release: Initially, 2.5–5 mg before breakfast and lunch. May increase by 5–10 mg/day at weekly intervals. Maximum: 60 mg/day.
PO (Concerta)
Children 6 yr and older. Initially, 18 mg once a day; may increase by 18 mg/day at weekly intervals. Maximum: 72 mg/day.
PO (Metadate CD)
Children 6 yr and older. Initially, 20 mg/day. May increase by 20 mg/day at weekly intervals. Maximum: 60 mg/day.
PO (Ritalin LA)
Children 6 yr and older. Initially, 20 mg/day. May increase by 10 mg/day at weekly intervals. Maximum: 60 mg/day.

▸ Narcolepsy

PO
Adults, Elderly. 10 mg 2–3 times a day. Range: 10–60 mg/day.

OFF-LABEL USES

Treatment of secondary mental depression

CONTRAINDICATIONS

Use within 14 days of MAOIs

INTERACTIONS

Drug

MAOIs: May increase the effects of methylphenidate.
Other CNS stimulants: May have an additive effect.

Herbal

None known.

Food

None known.

DIAGNOSTIC TEST EFFECTS

None known.

SIDE EFFECTS

Frequent

Anxiety, insomnia, anorexia

Occasional

Dizziness, drowsiness, headache, nausea, abdominal pain, fever, rash, arthralgia, vomiting

Rare

Blurred vision, Tourette syndrome (marked by uncontrolled vocal outbursts, repetitive body movements, and tics), palpitations

SERIOUS REACTIONS

! Prolonged administration to children with ADHD may delay growth.
! Overdose may produce tachycardia, palpitations, arrhythmias, chest pain, psychotic episode, seizures, and coma.
! Hypersensitivity reactions and blood dyscrasias occur rarely.

NURSING CONSIDERATIONS

Baseline Assessment

- Obtain baseline height and weight, and weigh the patient regularly to detect delayed growth in children.

Lifespan Considerations

- It is unknown if methylphenidate crosses the placenta or is distributed in breast milk.
- Children are more prone to develop abdominal pain, anorexia, weight loss, and insomnia.
- Long-term methylphenidate use may inhibit growth in children. Monitor the growth of pediatric patients.
- No age-related precautions have been noted in the elderly.

Precautions

- Use methylphenidate cautiously in patients with heart failure, hypertension, hyperthyroidism, recent MI, seizures, acute stress reaction, emotional instability, or a history of drug dependence.

Administration and Handling

◀ **ALERT** ▶ Sustained- and extended-release tablets may be given in place of regular tablets once the daily dose is titrated using regular tablets and if the titrated dosage corresponds to the sustained- or extended-release tablet strength.

- Give methylphenidate 30 to 45 minutes before meals (usually before breakfast and lunch). Give last dose before 6 p.m. to help prevent insomnia.
- Crush tablets as needed, but don't crush or break extended-release capsules.
- Open the Metadate CD capsule and sprinkle the pellets on applesauce, if desired.

Intervention and Evaluation

- Perform a CBC, WBC count with differential, and platelet count routinely during therapy.
- Expect to discontinue methylphenidate or reduce the dosage if symptoms of ADHD return.

Patient Teaching

- Instruct the patient to take the last dose of methylphenidate before 6 p.m. to avoid insomnia.
- Caution the patient against discontinuing the drug abruptly after prolonged use.
- Warn the patient to avoid tasks that require mental alertness or motor skills until his or her response to the drug has been established.
- Advise the patient to notify the physician if he or she experiences fever, anxiety, palpitations, a rash, vomiting or, for those with a seizure disorder, an increase in the number of seizures.
- Urge the patient to avoid consuming caffeinated beverages during methylphenidate therapy.
- Inform the patient that taking sips of tepid water and chewing sugarless gum may relieve dry mouth.

modafinil

mode-ah-**feen**-awl
(Alertec[CAN], Modavigil[AUS], Provigil)

CATEGORY AND SCHEDULE

Pregnancy Risk Category: C

MECHANISM OF ACTION

An alpha$_1$-agonist that may bind to dopamine reuptake carrier sites, increasing alpha activity and decreasing delta, theta, and beta brain wave activity. **Therapeutic Effect:** Reduces the number of sleep episodes and total daytime sleep.

PHARMACOKINETICS

Well absorbed. Protein binding: 60%. Widely distributed. Metabolized in the liver. Excreted by the kidneys. Unknown if removed by hemodialysis. ***Half-life:*** 8–10 hr.

AVAILABILITY

Tablets: 100 mg, 200 mg.

INDICATIONS AND DOSAGES

▸ **Narcolepsy, other sleep disorders**

PO

Adults, Elderly. 200–400 mg/day.

OFF-LABEL USES

Treatment of depression

CONTRAINDICATIONS

None known.

INTERACTIONS

Drug

Cyclosporine, oral contraceptives, theophylline: May decrease plasma concentrations of these drugs.

Diazepam, phenytoin, propranolol, tricyclic antidepressants, warfarin: May increase plasma concentrations of these drugs.

Other CNS stimulants: May increase CNS stimulation.

Herbal

None known.

Food

None known.

DIAGNOSTIC TEST EFFECTS

None known.

SIDE EFFECTS

Frequent

Anxiety, insomnia, nausea

Occasional

Anorexia, diarrhea, dizziness, dry mouth or skin, muscle stiffness, polydipsia, rhinitis, paraesthesia, tremor, headache, vomiting

SERIOUS REACTIONS

! Agitation, excitation, hypertension, and insomnia may occur.

NURSING CONSIDERATIONS

Baseline Assessment

- Obtain a history of the patient's narcolepsy or other sleep disorder, including the duration, pattern, frequency, and severity of sleep episodes and the environmental situations in which they occurred.
- Ask the patient if he or she has experienced a sudden loss of muscle tone (cataplexy) precipitated by strong emotional responses before a sleep episode.

Lifespan Considerations

- It is unknown if modafinil is excreted in breast milk. Use caution when giving modafinil to pregnant women.
- The safety and efficacy of this drug have not been established in children younger than 16 years.
- Age-related hepatic or renal impairment may require decreased dosage in the elderly.

Precautions

- Use modafinil cautiously in patients with hepatic impairment or a history of clinically significant mitral valve prolapse, left ventricular hypertrophy, or seizures.

Administration and Handling

- Give modafinil without regard to food.

Intervention and Evaluation

- Monitor the patient's sleep pattern, including restlessness during sleep and the duration of insomnia at night.
- Assess the patient for anxiety and dizziness. Institute safety precautions as needed.

Patient Teaching

- Instruct the patient not to increase the drug dose without physician approval.
- Warn the patient to avoid tasks that require mental alertness or motor

skills until his or her response to the drug has been established.
• Tell the patient to use a nonhormonal contraceptive method during modafinil therapy and for 1 month afterward. Explain that modafinil may decrease the effectiveness of hormonal contraceptives.
• Inform the patient that taking sips of tepid water and chewing sugarless gum may relieve dry mouth.

pemoline

pem-oh-leen
(Cylert, PemADD, PemADD CT)

CATEGORY AND SCHEDULE

Pregnancy Risk Category: B
Controlled Substance: Schedule IV

MECHANISM OF ACTION

A CNS stimulant that blocks the reuptake mechanism present in dopaminergic neurons in the cerebral cortex and subcortical structures. **Therapeutic Effect:** Reduces motor restlessness and fatigue, increases alertness, elevates mood.

AVAILABILITY

Tablets (Cylert, PemADD): 18.75 mg, 37.5 mg, 75 mg.
Tablets (Chewable [PemADD CT]): 37.5 mg.

INDICATIONS AND DOSAGES

▸ **ADHD**

PO

Children 6 yr and older. Initially, 37.5 mg/day as a single dose in morning. May increase by 18.75 mg at weekly intervals until therapeutic response is achieved. Range: 56.25–75 mg/day. Maximum: 112.5 mg/day.

CONTRAINDICATIONS

Family history of Tourette syndrome, hepatic impairment, motor tics

INTERACTIONS

Drug

Other CNS stimulants: May increase CNS stimulation.

Herbal

None known.

Food

None known.

DIAGNOSTIC TEST EFFECTS

May increase serum LDH, AST (SGOT), and ALT (SGPT) levels.

SIDE EFFECTS

Frequent

Anorexia, insomnia

Occasional

Nausea, abdominal discomfort, diarrhea, headache, dizziness, somnolence

SERIOUS REACTIONS

! Visual disturbances, rash, and dyskinetic movements of the tongue, lips, face, and extremities have occurred.
! Large doses of pemoline may produce extreme nervousness and tachycardia.
! Hepatic effects, such as hepatitis and jaundice, appear to be reversible when the drug is discontinued.
! Prolonged administration to children with ADHD may temporarily delay growth.

NURSING CONSIDERATIONS

Baseline Assessment

• Perform hepatic function tests before and periodically during pemoline therapy.

- Obtain baseline height and weight, and weigh the patient regularly to detect delayed growth in children.

Precautions

- Use pemoline cautiously in patients with hypertension, psychosis, renal impairment, seizures, or a history of drug abuse.

Patient Teaching

- Warn the patient to avoid tasks that require mental alertness or motor skills until his or her response to the drug has been established.
- Explain to the patient that pemoline may be habit forming. Caution the patient against abruptly discontinuing the drug.
- Advise the patient to notify the physician if he or she experiences dark urine, GI complaints, loss of appetite, or yellow skin.
- Urge the patient to avoid alcohol and caffeine during pemoline therapy.

41 Narcotic Agonist-Antagonist Analgesics

buprenorphine hydrochloride
butorphanol tartrate
nalbuphine hydrochloride

Uses: Narcotic agonist-antagonist analgesics are used to relieve mild to moderate pain.

Action: *Agonist-antagonists* primarily act as antagonists at mu receptors and as agonists at kappa receptors. Although these agents have less abuse potential and cause less respiratory depression than narcotic analgesics, they generally produce weaker analgesic effects. (See the illustration *Mechanism of Action: Narcotic Agonist-Antagonist Analgesics,* page 834.)

COMBINATION PRODUCTS

SUBOXONE**:** buprenorphine/naloxone (a narcotic antagonist) 2 mg/0.5 mg; 8 mg/2 mg.

buprenorphine hydrochloride

byoo-pre-**nor**-feen
(Buprenex, Subutex, Temgesic[CAN])

CATEGORY AND SCHEDULE

Pregnancy Risk Category: C
Controlled Substance: Schedule V (opioid agonist), III (tablet)

MECHANISM OF ACTION

An opioid agonist-antagonist that binds with opioid receptors in the CNS. **Therapeutic Effect:** Alters the perception of and emotional response to pain; blocks the effects of herion and produces minimal opioid withdrawal symptoms.

AVAILABILITY

Tablets (Sublingual): 2 mg, 8 mg.
Injection: 0.3 mg/ml.

INDICATIONS AND DOSAGES

▸ **Analgesia**

IV, IM

Adults, Children older than 12 yr. 0.3 mg q6–8h as needed. May repeat once in 30–60 min. Range: 0.15–0.6 mg q4–8h as needed.

Children 2–12 yr. 2–6 mcg/kg q4–6h as needed.

Elderly. 0.15 mg q6h as needed.

▸ **Opioid dependence**

Sublingual

Adults, Elderly, Children older than 16 yr. Initially, 12–16 mg/day, beginning at least 4 hr after last use of heroin or short-acting opioid. Maintenance: 16 mg/day. Range: 4–24 mg/day. Patients should be switched to buprenorphine and naloxone combination drug, which is preferred for maintenance treatment.

CONTRAINDICATIONS

Hypersensitivity to buprenorphine; hypersensitivity to naloxone for those receiving the fixed combination product containing naloxone (Suboxone)

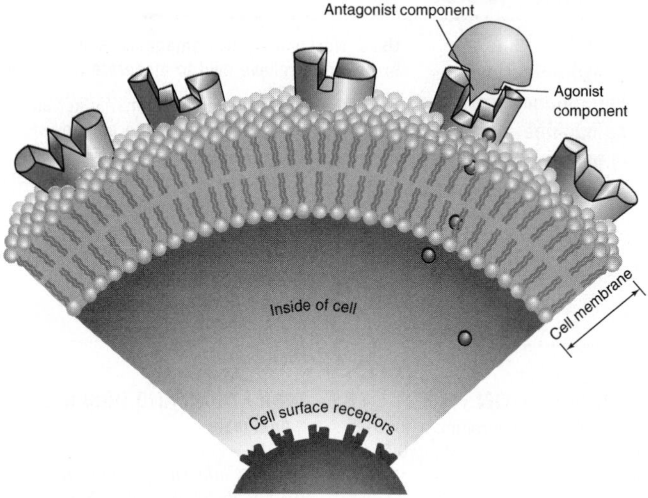

Mechanism of Action: Narcotic Agonist-Antagonist Analgesics

Cell membranes have different types of opioid receptors, such as mu, kappa, and delta receptors. Opioid agonist-antagonists work by stimulating one type of receptor while simultaneously blocking another type. As agonists, they work primarily by activating kappa receptors to produce analgesia and such other effects as CNS and respiratory depression, decreased GI motility, and euphoria. As antagonists, they compete with opioids at mu receptors, helping to reverse or block some of the other effects of agonists.

INTERACTIONS

Drug

CNS depressants, MAOIs: May increase CNS or respiratory depression and hypotension.

Other opioid analgesics: May decrease the effects of other opioid analgesics.

Herbal

Kava kava, St. John's wort, valerian: May increase CNS depression.

Food

None known.

DIAGNOSTIC TEST EFFECTS

May increase serum amylase and lipase levels.

SIDE EFFECTS

Frequent

Tablet: Headache, pain, insomnia, anxiety, depression, nausea, abdominal pain, constipation, back pain, weakness, rhinitis, withdrawal syndrome, infection, diaphoresis

Injection (more than 10%): Sedation

Occasional

Injection: Hypotension, respiratory depression, dizziness, headache, vomiting, nausea, vertigo

SERIOUS REACTIONS

! Overdose results in cold and clammy skin, weakness, confusion, severe respiratory depression, cyanosis, pinpoint pupils, and extreme somnolence progressing to seizures, stupor, and coma.

NURSING CONSIDERATIONS

Baseline Assessment

- Assess the duration, location, onset, and type of pain.

Precautions

- Use buprenorphine cautiously in patients with hepatic impairment or possible neurologic injury.

Administration and Handling

PO

- Place the tablet under the patient's tongue until dissolved. If two or more tablets are needed, all may be placed under the tongue at the same time.

IV

- Administer buprenorphine slowly, over at least 2 minutes.

Intervention and Evaluation

- Know that buprenorphine's analgesic effect is reduced if full pain response recurs before the next dose.
- Monitor the patient's BP, pulse rate, and respiratory status.
- Initiate deep-breathing and coughing exercises, particularly in patients with impaired pulmonary function.
- Assess the patient for clinical improvement, and record the onset of pain relief.

Patient Teaching

- Instruct the patient to change positions slowly to avoid dizziness.
- Warn the patient to avoid tasks requiring mental alertness or motor skills until his or her response to the drug has been established.

butorphanol tartrate

byoo-**tor**-fa-nole

(Stadol, Stadol NS)

Do not confuse butorphanol with butabarbital, or Stadol with Haldol.

CATEGORY AND SCHEDULE

Pregnancy Risk Category: C (D if used for prolonged periods or at high dosages at term)

Controlled Substance: Schedule IV

MECHANISM OF ACTION

An opioid that binds to opiate receptor sites in the CNS. Reduces intensity of pain stimuli incoming from sensory nerve endings. **Therapeutic Effect:** Alters pain perception and emotional response to pain.

PHARMACOKINETICS

Route	Onset	Peak	Duration
IM	10–30 min	30–60 min	3–4 hr
IV	less than 1 min	30 min	2–4 hr
Nasal	15 min	1–2 hr	4–5 hr

Rapidly absorbed after IM injection. Protein binding: 80%. Extensively metabolized in the liver. Primarily excreted in urine. ***Half-life:*** 2.5–4 hr.

AVAILABILITY

Injection: 1 mg/ml, 2 mg/ml.
Nasal Spray: 10 mg/ml.

INDICATIONS AND DOSAGES

▸ **Analgesia**

IV

Adults. 0.5–2 mg q3–4h as needed.
Elderly. 1 mg q4–6h as needed.

IM
Adults. 1–4 mg q3–4h as needed.
Elderly. 1 mg q4–6h as needed.

▸ **Migraine**

Nasal
Adults. 1 mg or 1 spray in one nostril. May repeat in 60–90 min. May repeat 2-dose sequence q3–4h as needed. Alternatively, 2 mg or 1 spray each nostril if patient remains recumbent, may repeat in 3–4 hr.

CONTRAINDICATIONS

CNS disease that affects respirations, physical dependence on other opioid analgesics, preexisting respiratory depression, pulmonary disease

INTERACTIONS

Drug

Alcohol, CNS depressants: May increase CNS or respiratory depression and hypotension.
Buprenorphine: Effects may be decreased with buprenorphine.
MAOIs: May produce severe, fatal reaction unless dose is reduced by one-fourth.

Herbal

None known.

Food

None known.

DIAGNOSTIC TEST EFFECTS

None known.

IV INCOMPATIBILITIES

Amphotericin B complex (Abelcet, AmBisome, Amphotec)

IV COMPATIBILITIES

Atropine, diphenhydramine (Benadryl), droperidol (Inapsine), hydroxyzine (Vistaril), morphine, promethazine (Phenergan), propofol (Diprivan)

SIDE EFFECTS

Frequent

Parenteral: Somnolence (43%), dizziness (19%)
Nasal: Nasal congestion (13%), insomnia (11%)

Occasional

Parenteral (3%–9%): Confusion, diaphoresis, clammy skin, lethargy, headache, nausea, vomiting, dry mouth
Nasal (3%–9%): Vasodilation, constipation, unpleasant taste, dyspnea, epistaxis, nasal irritation, upper respiratory tract infection, tinnitus

Rare

Parenteral: Hypotension, pruritus, blurred vision, sensation of heat, CNS stimulation, insomnia
Nasal: Hypertension, tremor, ear pain, paresthesia, depression, sinusitis

SERIOUS REACTIONS

! Abrupt withdrawal after prolonged use may produce symptoms of narcotic withdrawal, such as abdominal cramping, rhinorrhea, lacrimation, anxiety, increased temperature, and piloerection or goose bumps.
! Overdose results in severe respiratory depression, skeletal muscle flaccidity, cyanosis, and extreme somnolence progressing to seizures, stupor, and coma.
! Tolerance to analgesic effect and physical dependence may occur with chronic use.

NURSING CONSIDERATIONS

Baseline Assessment

- Obtain the patient's vital signs before giving butorphanol.
- Withhold the medication and notify the physician if the adult patient's respirations are 12/minute or less, or 20/minute or less in children.

• Assess duration, location, onset, and type of pain the patient is experiencing.
• Know that the effect of the medication is reduced if the patient experiences full pain before the next dose.
• Protect the patient from falls.
• During labor, assess fetal heart tones, and the patient's uterine contractions.

Lifespan Considerations

• During labor, assess fetal heart tones, and the patient's uterine contractions.
• Be aware that the safety and efficacy of butorphanol have not been established in children younger than 18 years of age.
• Be aware that the elderly may be more sensitive to effects. Adjust drug dose and interval in the elderly.

Precautions

• Use cautiously in patients who are debilitated or elderly.
• Use cautiously in patients with head injury, hypertension, impaired liver or renal function, myocardial infarction, and prior to biliary tract surgery, because the drug produces spasm of sphincter of Oddi.

Administration and Handling

◀**ALERT**▶ May be given by IM or IV push.

IV
• Store at room temperature.
• May be given undiluted.
• Administer over 3 to 5 minutes.

Intranasal
• Instruct patient to blow nose to clear nasal passages as much as possible.
• Spray into nostril while holding other nostril closed and instruct patient to concurrently inspire through nose to permit medication as high into nasal passages as possible.

Intervention and Evaluation

• Monitor the patient for a change in blood pressure (BP), pulse rate and quality, and respirations.
• Initiate deep-breathing and coughing exercises, particularly in patients with impaired pulmonary function.
• Help the patient change position every 2 to 4 hours.
• Assess the patient for clinical improvement, and record the onset of relief of pain.

Patient Teaching

• Instruct the patient to change positions slowly to avoid dizziness.
• Warn the patient to avoid tasks that require mental alertness or motor skills until his or her response to the drug is established.
• Teach the patient the proper use of nasal spray.
• Urge the patient to avoid alcohol or CNS depressants during butorphanol therapy.
• Instruct the patient to alert you to the onset of pain, and not to wait until the pain is unbearable. Butorphanol is more effective when given at the onset of pain.

nalbuphine hydrochloride

nal-byoo-feen
(Nubain)
Do not confuse Nubain with Navane.

CATEGORY AND SCHEDULE

Pregnancy Risk Category: B (D if used for prolonged periods or at high dosages at term)

MECHANISM OF ACTION

A narcotic agonist-antagonist that binds with opioid receptors in the CNS. May displace opioid agonists and competitively inhibit their action; may precipitate withdrawal symptoms. **Therapeutic Effect:** Alters the perception of and emotional response to pain.

PHARMACOKINETICS

Route	Onset	Peak	Duration
IV	2–3 min	30 min	3–6 hr
IM	less than 15 min	60 min	3–6 hr
Subcutaneous	less than 15 min	N/A	3–6 hr

Well absorbed after IM or subcutaneous administration. Protein binding: 50%. Metabolized in the liver. Primarily eliminated in feces by biliary secretion. ***Half-life:*** 3.5–5 hr.

AVAILABILITY

Injection: 10 mg/ml, 20 mg/ml.

INDICATIONS AND DOSAGES

▸ **Analgesia**

IV, IM, Subcutaneous

Adults, Elderly. 10 mg q3–6h as needed. Don't exceed maximum single dose of 20 mg or daily dose of 160 mg. For patients receiving long-term narcotic analgesics of similar duration of action, give 25% of usual dose.

Children. 0.1–0.15 mg/kg q3–6h as needed.

▸ **Supplement to anesthesia**

IV

Adults, Elderly. Induction: 0.3–3 mg/kg over 10–15 min. Maintenance: 0.25–0.5 mg/kg as needed.

CONTRAINDICATIONS

Respiratory rate less than 12 breaths/minute

INTERACTIONS

Drug

Alcohol, other CNS depressants: May increase CNS or respiratory depression and hypotension.

Buprenorphine: May decrease the effects of nalbuphine.

MAOIs: May produce a severe, possibly fatal reaction; plan to administer 25% of the usual nalbuphine dose.

Herbal

None known.

Food

None known.

DIAGNOSTIC TEST EFFECTS

May increase serum amylase and lipase levels.

IV INCOMPATIBILITIES

Amphotericin B complex (Abelcet, AmBisome, Amphotec), cefepime (Maxipime), docetaxel (Doxil), methotrexate, nafcillin (Nafcil), piperacillin and tazobactam (Zosyn), sargramostim (Leukine, Prokine), sodium bicarbonate

IV COMPATIBILITIES

Diphenhydramine (Benadryl), droperidol (Inapsine), glycopyrrolate (Robinul), hydroxyzine (Vistaril), ketorolac (Toradol), lidocaine, midazolam (Versed), propofol (Diprivan)

SIDE EFFECTS

Frequent (35%)

Sedation

Occasional (9%–3%)

Diaphoresis, cold and clammy skin, nausea, vomiting, dizziness, vertigo, dry mouth, headache

Rare (less than 1%)

Restlessness, emotional lability, paresthesia, flushing, paradoxical reaction

SERIOUS REACTIONS

! Abrupt withdrawal after prolonged use may produce symptoms of narcotic withdrawal, such as abdominal cramping, rhinorrhea, lacrimation, anxiety, fever, and piloerection (goose bumps).
! Overdose results in severe respiratory depression, skeletal muscle flaccidity, cyanosis, and extreme somnolence progressing to seizures, stupor, and coma.
! Repeated use may result in drug tolerance and physical dependence.

NURSING CONSIDERATIONS

Baseline Assessment

- Obtain the patient's vital signs before giving nalbuphine.
- Withhold the drug and notify the physician if the respiratory rate is 12 breaths/minute or less in an adult or 20 breaths/minute or less in a child.
- Assess the duration, location, onset, and type of pain.

Lifespan Considerations

- Nalbuphine readily crosses the placenta and is distributed in breast milk. Breast-feeding is not recommended for patients taking this drug.
- Children may experience paradoxical excitement.
- Children younger than 2 years and the elderly are more likely to develop respiratory depression.
- In the elderly, age-related renal impairment may increase the risk of urine retention.

Precautions

- Use nalbuphine cautiously in pregnant patients; opioid-dependent patients; patients with head trauma, increased intracranial pressure, hepatic or renal impairment, recent MI, or respiratory depression; and those about to undergo biliary tract surgery.

Administration and Handling

◀ **ALERT** ▶ Keep in mind that nalbuphine dosage is based on the patient's physical condition, the severity of pain, and concurrent use of other drugs.

IV

- Store vials at room temperature.
- Nalbuphine may be given undiluted.
- For IV push, administer each 10 mg over 3 to 5 minutes.

IM

- Rotate IM injection sites.

Intervention and Evaluation

- Know that the drug's analgesic effect is reduced if a full pain response recurs before the next dose.
- Be aware that nalbuphine has a low abuse potential.
- Monitor the patient's BP, pulse rate, and respiratory status.
- Assess the patient's pattern of daily bowel activity and stool consistency.
- Initiate deep-breathing and coughing exercises, particularly in patients with impaired pulmonary function.
- Assess the patient for clinical improvement, and record the onset of relief of pain. Notify the physician if pain relief is inadequate.

Patient Teaching

- Instruct the patient to alert you as soon as pain occurs and not to wait until the pain is unbearable because nalbuphine is more effective when given at the onset of pain.
- Inform the patient that nalbuphine may be habit-forming.
- Urge the patient to avoid alcohol and CNS depressants during nalbuphine therapy.
- Warn the patient to avoid tasks that require mental alertness or motor skills until his or her response to the drug has been established.
- Inform the patient that nalbuphine may cause dry mouth.

42 Narcotic (Opioid) Analgesics

codeine phosphate, codeine sulfate
fentanyl
hydrocodone bitartrate
hydromorphone hydrochloride
meperidine hydrochloride
methadone hydrochloride
morphine sulfate
oxycodone
propoxyphene hydrochloride, propoxyphene napsylate

Uses: Narcotic (opoid) analgesics are used to relieve moderate to severe pain related to surgery, MI, burns, cancer, and other conditions. These agents may be used as an adjunct to anesthesia, either as preoperative medication or as an intraoperative supplement to anesthesia. They're also used for obstetric analgesia. *Codeine* may be prescribed for its antitussive and antidiarrheal effects. Although *methadone* can relieve severe pain, it's used primarily as part of heroin detoxification.

Action: All narcotic analgesics bind to opioid receptors and have actions similar to morphine, which is why they're also referred to as *opioid analgesics*. (See the illustration *Mechanism of Action: Narcotic Analgesics,* page 842.) These agents produce major effects on the CNS (causing analgesia, drowsiness, mood changes, mental clouding, analgesia without loss of consciousness, nausea, and vomiting) and the GI tract (reducing hydrochloric acid secretion; biliary, pancreatic, and intestinal secretions; and propulsive peristalsis). They also depress respirations and cause such cardiovascular effects as peripheral vasodilation, decreased peripheral resistance, and inhibited baroreceptors reflexes.

COMBINATION PRODUCTS

ANEXSIA: hydrocodone/acetaminophen (a non-narcotic analgesic) 5 mg/500 mg; 7.5 mg/650 mg; 10 mg/650 mg.
CAPITAL WITH CODEINE: acetaminophen (a non-narcotic analgesic)/codeine 120 mg/12 mg per 5 ml.
COMBUNOX: oxycodone/ibuprofen (an NSAID) 5 mg/400 mg.
DARVOCET A 500: propoxyphene/acetaminophen (a non-narcotic analgesic) 100 mg/500 mg.
DARVOCET-N: propoxyphene/acetaminophen (a non-narcotic analgesic) 50 mg/325 mg; 100 mg/650 mg.
DUOCET: hydrocodone/acetaminophen (a non-narcotic analgesic) 5 mg/500 mg.
LORCET: hydrocodone/acetaminophen (a non-narcotic analgesic) 7.5 mg/650 mg; 10 mg/650 mg.
LORTAB: hydrocodone/acetaminophen (a non-narcotic analgesic) 2.5 mg/500 mg; 5 mg/500 mg; 7.5 mg/500 mg; 10 mg/500 mg.
LORTAB ELIXIR: hydrocodone/acetaminophen (a non-narcotic analgesic) 2.5 mg/167 mg per 5 ml.
LORTAB WITH ASA: hydrocodone/aspirin (a non-narcotic analgesic) 5 mg/500 mg.

NORCO: hydrocodone/acetaminophen (a non-narcotic analgesic) 10 mg/325 mg.
PERCOCET: oxycodone/acetaminophen (a non-narcotic analgesic) 2.5 mg/325 mg; 5 mg/325 mg; 5 mg/500 mg; 7.5 mg/325 mg; 7.5 mg/500 mg; 10 mg/325 mg; 10 mg/650 mg.
PERCODAN: oxycodone/aspirin (a non-narcotic analgesic) 2.25 mg/325 mg; 4.5 mg/325 mg.
PHENERGAN WITH CODEINE: codeine/promethazine (an antihistamine) 10 mg/6.25 mg.
PHENERGAN VC WITH CODEINE: codeine/promethazine (an antihistamine)/phenylephrine (a vasopressor) 10 mg/6.25 mg/5 mg.
REPREXAIN CIII: hydrocodone/ibuprofen (an NSAID) 5 mg/200 mg.
ROBITUSSIN AC: codeine/guaifenesin (an antitussive) 10 mg/100 mg.
ROXICET: oxycodone/acetaminophen (a non-narcotic analgesic) 5 mg/500 mg.
TYLENOL WITH CODEINE: acetaminophen (a non-narcotic analgesic)/codeine 120 mg/12 mg per 5 ml; 300 mg/15 mg; 300 mg/30 mg; 300 mg/60 mg.
TYLOX: oxycodone/acetaminophen (a non-narcotic analgesic) 5 mg/500 mg.
VICODIN: hydrocodone/acetaminophen (a non-narcotic analgesic) 5 mg/500 mg.
VICODIN ES: hydrocodone/acetaminophen (a non-narcotic analgesic) 7.5 mg/750 mg.
VICODIN HP: hydrocodone/acetaminophen (a non-narcotic analgesic) 10 mg/650 mg.
VICOPROFEN: hydrocodone/ibuprofen (an NSAID) 7.5 mg/200 mg.
ZYDONE: hydrocodone/acetaminophen (a non-narcotic analgesic) 5 mg/400 mg; 7.5 mg/400 mg; 10 mg/400 mg.

codeine phosphate

koe-deen
(Actacode[AUS], Codeine Phosphate Injection, Codeine Linctus[AUS])

codeine sulfate

(Contin[CAN])
Do not confuse codeine with Cardene or Lodine.

CATEGORY AND SCHEDULE

Pregnancy Risk Category: C (D if used for prolonged periods or at high dosages at term)
Controlled Substance: Schedule II (analgesic), III (fixed-combination form)

MECHANISM OF ACTION

An opioid agonist that binds to opioid receptors at many cites in the CNS, particularly in the medulla. This action inhibits the ascending pain pathways. **Therapeutic Effect:** Alters the perception of and emotional response to pain, suppresses cough reflex.

AVAILABILITY

Tablets: 15 mg, 30 mg, 60 mg.
Oral Solution: 15 mg/5 ml.
Injection: 15 mg/ml, 30 mg/ml.

INDICATIONS AND DOSAGES

▸ **Analgesia**
PO, IM, Subcutaneous
Adults, Elderly. 30 mg q4–6h. Range: 15–60 mg.
Children. 0.5–1 mg/kg q4–6h. Maximum: 60 mg/dose.

▸ **Cough**
PO
Adults, Elderly, Children 12 yr and older. 10–20 mg q4–6h.
Children 6–11 yr. 5–10 mg q4–6h.
Children 2–5 yr. 2.5–5 mg q4–6h.

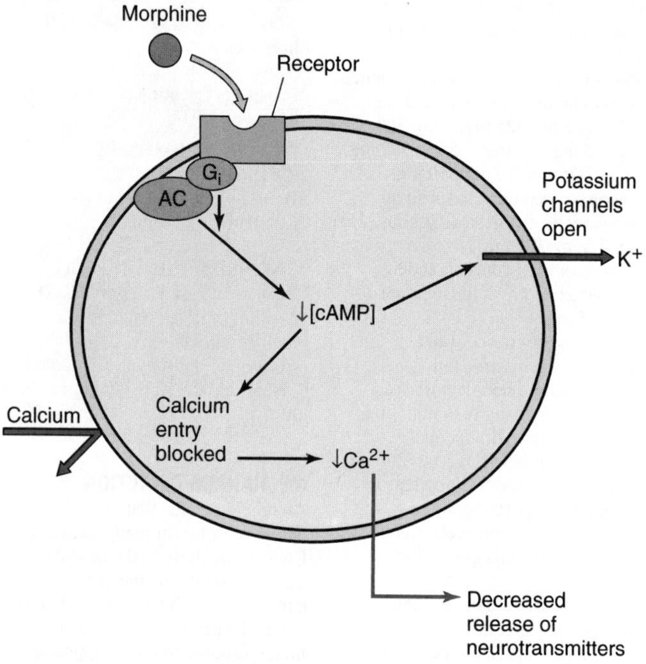

Mechanism of Action: Narcotic Analgesics

Narcotic analgesics bind to three types of opioid receptors: mu, kappa, and delta receptors. They produce analgesia primarily by activating mu receptors. However, they also engage with and activate kappa and delta receptors, producing other effects, such as sedation and vasomotor stimulation.

When morphine or another narcotic analgesic binds to opioid receptors, activation occurs. The receptors send signals to the enzyme adenyl cyclase (AC) to slow activity by way of G proteins (G_i). Decreased adenyl cyclase activity causes less cyclic adenosine monophosphate (cAMP) to be produced. A secondary messenger substance, cAMP, is important for regulating cell membrane channels. A reduced cAMP level allows fewer potassium ions to leave the cell and blocks calcium ions from entering the cell. This ion imbalance—especially the reduced intracellular calcium level—ultimately decreases the release of neurotransmitters from the cell, thereby blocking or reducing pain impulse transmission.

▸ **Dosage in renal impairment**

Dosage is modified based on creatinine clearance.

Creatinine Clearance	Dosage
10–50 ml/min	75% of usual dose
less than 10 ml/min	50% of usual dose

OFF-LABEL USES
Treatment of diarrhea

CONTRAINDICATIONS
None known.

INTERACTIONS
Drug
Alcohol, other CNS depressants: May increase CNS or respiratory depression, and hypotension.
MAOIs: May produce a severe, sometimes fatal reaction; plan to administer a test dose, which is one-quarter of usual codeine dose.
Herbal
None known.
Food
None known.

DIAGNOSTIC TEST EFFECTS
May increase serum amylase and lipase levels.

SIDE EFFECTS
Frequent
Constipation, somnolence, nausea, vomiting
Occasional
Paradoxical excitement, confusion, palpitations, facial flushing, decreased urination, blurred vision, dizziness, dry mouth, headache, hypotension (including orthostatic hypotension), decreased appetite, injection site redness, burning, or pain
Rare
Hallucinations, depression, abdominal pain, insomnia

SERIOUS REACTIONS
! Too-frequent use may result in paralytic ileus.
! Overdose may produce cold and clammy skin, confusion, seizures, decreased BP, restlessness, pinpoint pupils, bradycardia, respiratory depression, decreased LOC, and severe weakness.
! The patient who uses codeine repeatedly may develop a tolerance to the drug's analgesic effect as well as physical dependence.

NURSING CONSIDERATIONS
Baseline Assessment
- Assess the duration, location, onset, and type of pain.
- If the patient is being treated for cough, assess the frequency, severity, and type of cough, as well as sputum production.

Lifespan Considerations
- Codeine crosses the placenta and is distributed in breast milk.
- Regular use of opioids during pregnancy may produce withdrawal symptoms in the neonate, such as diarrhea, excessive crying, fever, hyperactive reflexes, irritability, seizures, sneezing, tremors, vomiting, and yawning.
- Codeine may prolong labor if administered in the latent phase of the first stage of labor or before the cervix is dilated 4 to 5 cm.
- The neonate may develop respiratory depression if the mother receives codeine during labor.
- Children and the elderly are more prone to experience paradoxical excitement.
- Children younger than 2 years and the elderly are more susceptible to the drug's respiratory depressant effects.
- In the elderly, age-related renal impairment may increase the risk of codeine-induced urine retention.

Precautions
- Use codeine extremely cautiously in patients with acute alcoholism, anoxia, CNS depression, hypercapnia, respiratory depression or

dysfunction, seizures, shock, or untreated myxedema.
• Use codeine cautiously in patients with acute abdominal conditions, Addison's disease, COPD, hypothyroidism, hepatic impairment, increased intracranial pressure, benign prostatic hyperplasia, or urethral stricture.

Administration and Handling

◀ALERT▶ Be aware that ambulatory patients and patients not in severe pain may be more prone to dizziness, hypotension, nausea, and vomiting than patients in the supine position and those in severe pain.

◀ALERT▶ Expect to reduce the initial dosage in elderly and debilitated patients; those with hypothyroidism, Addison's disease, or renal insufficiency; and those using other CNS depressants concurrently.

PO
• Give codeine with food or milk to minimize adverse GI effects.

IM, Subcutaneous
• Inspect drug for cloudiness or precipitate. If present, discard drug.

Intervention and Evaluation

• Keep in mind that the drug's effect is reduced if the full pain response recurs before the next dose.
• Assess the patient's daily pattern of bowel activity and stool consistency.
• Increase the patient's fluid intake and environmental humidity to help improve the viscosity of lung secretions.
• Encourage deep-breathing and coughing exercises.
• Assess the patient for clinical improvement and record the onset of pain or cough relief.

Patient Teaching

• Instruct the patient to alert you as soon as pain recurs because this drug is less effective if full pain response recurs before the next dose.
• Caution the patient that drug dependence or tolerance may occur with prolonged use of high doses.
• Instruct the patient to change positions slowly to avoid orthostatic hypotension.
• Warn the patient to avoid tasks that require mental alertness or motor skills until his or her response to the drug has been established.
• Urge the patient to avoid alcohol during codeine therapy.

fentanyl

fen-ta-nill
(Actig, Duragesic, Sublimaze)
Do not confuse fentanyl with alfentanil.

CATEGORY AND SCHEDULE

Pregnancy Risk Category: C (D if used for prolonged periods or at high dosages at term)
Controlled Substance: Schedule II

MECHANISM OF ACTION

An opioid agonist that binds to opioid receptors in the CNS, reducing stimuli from sensory nerve endings and inhibiting ascending pain pathways. **Therapeutic Effect:** Alters pain reception and increases the pain threshold.

PHARMACOKINETICS

Route	Onset	Peak	Duration
IV	1–2 min	3–5 min	0.5–1 hr
IM	7–15 min	20–30 min	1–2 hr
Transdermal	6–8 hr	24 hr	72 hr
Transmucosal	5–15 min	20–30 min	1–2 hr

Well absorbed after IM or topical administration. Transmucosal form absorbed through the buccal mucosa and GI tract. Protein binding: 80%–85%. Metabolized in the liver. Primarily eliminated by biliary system. ***Half-life:*** 2–4 hr IV; 17 hr transdermal; 6.6 hr transmucosal.

AVAILABILITY

Injection (Sublimaze): 50 mcg/ml.
Transdermal Patch (Duragesic): 25 mcg/hr, 50 mcg/hr, 75 mcg/hr, 100 mcg/hr.
Transmucosal Lozenges (Actig): 200 mcg, 400 mcg, 600 mcg, 800 mcg, 1,200 mcg, 1,600 mcg.

INDICATIONS AND DOSAGES

▸ Sedation in minor procedures, analgesia

IV, IM

Adults, Elderly, Children 12 yr and older. 0.5–1 mcg/kg/dose; may repeat in 30–60 min.
Children 1–11 yr. 1–2 mcg/kg/dose.
Children younger than 1 yr. 1–4 mcg/kg/dose.

▸ Preoperative sedation, postoperative pain, adjunct to regional anesthesia

IV, IM

Adults, Elderly, Children 12 yr and older. 50–100 mcg/dose.

▸ Adjunct to general anesthesia

IV

Adults, Elderly, Children 12 yr and older. 2–50 mcg/kg.

▸ Usual Transdermal Dose

Adults, Elderly, Children 12 yr and older. Initially, 25 mcg/hr. May increase after 3 days.

▸ Usual Transmucosal Dose

Adults, Children. 200–400 mcg for breakthrough cancer pain.

▸ Usual Epidural Dose

Adults, Elderly. Bolus dose of 100 mcg, followed by continuous infusion of 10 mcg/ml concentration at 4–12 ml/hr.

▸ Continuous analgesia

IV

Adults, Elderly, Children 1–12 yr. Bolus dose of 1–2 mcg/kg, followed by continuous infusion of 1 mcg/kg/hr. Range: 1–5 mcg/kg/hr.
Children younger than 1 yr. Bolus dose of 1–2 mcg/kg, followed by continuous infusion of 0.5–1 mcg/kg/hr.

▸ Dosage in renal impairment

Dosage is modified based on creatinine clearance.

Creatinine Clearance	Dosage
10–50 ml/min	75% of usual dose
less than 10 ml/min	50% of usual dose

CONTRAINDICATIONS

Increased intracranial pressure, severe hepatic or renal impairment, severe respiratory depression

INTERACTIONS

Drug

Benzodiazepines, CNS depressants: May increase the risk of hypotension and respiratory depression.
Buprenorphine: May decrease the effects of fentanyl.

Herbal

None known.

Food

None known.

DIAGNOSTIC TEST EFFECTS

May increase serum amylase and lipase concentrations.

IV INCOMPATIBILITIES

Phenytoin (Dilantin)

IV COMPATIBILITIES

Atropine, bupivacaine (Marcaine, Sensorcaine), clonidine (Duraclon), diltiazem (Cardizem), diphenhydramine (Benadryl), dobutamine (Dobutrex), dopamine (Intropin), droperidol (Inapsine), heparin, hydromorphone (Dilaudid), ketorolac (Toradol), lorazepam (Ativan), metoclopramide (Reglan), midazolam (Versed), milrinone (Primacor), morphine, nitroglycerin, norepinephrine (Levophed), ondansetron (Zofran), potassium chloride, propofol (Diprivan)

SIDE EFFECTS

Frequent

IV: Postoperative drowsiness, nausea, vomiting
Transdermal (10%–3%): Headache, pruritus, nausea, vomiting, diaphoresis, dyspnea, confusion, dizziness, somnolence, diarrhea, constipation, decreased appetite

Occasional

IV: Postoperative confusion, blurred vision, chills, orthostatic hypotension, constipation, difficulty urinating
Transdermal (3%–1%): Chest pain, arrhythmias, erythema, pruritus, swelling of skin, syncope, agitation, tingling or burning of skin

SERIOUS REACTIONS

! Overdose or too-rapid IV administration may produce severe respiratory depression and skeletal and thoracic muscle rigidity (which may lead to apnea), laryngospasm, bronchospasm, cold and clammy skin, cyanosis, and coma.
! The patient who uses fentanyl repeatedly may develop a tolerance to the drug's analgesic effect.

NURSING CONSIDERATIONS

Baseline Assessment

- Obtain the patient's baseline BP and respiratory rate.
- Assess the duration, intensity, location, and type of pain the patient is experiencing.

Lifespan Considerations

- Fentanyl readily crosses the placenta; it is unknown whether fentanyl is distributed in breast milk. Fentanyl may prolong labor if administered in the latent phase of the first stage of labor or before the cervix has dilated 4 to 5 cm.
- Fentanyl may cause respiratory depression in the neonate if it's given to the mother during labor.
- The transdermal form of fentanyl is not recommended for children younger than 12 years or children younger than 18 years who weigh less than 50 kg.
- Neonates and the elderly are more susceptible to the drug's respiratory depressant effects.
- Age-related renal impairment may require a dosage adjustment in the elderly.

Precautions

- Use fentanyl cautiously in patients with bradycardia, head injuries, altered LOC, and hepatic, renal, or respiratory disease.
- Use fentanyl cautiously in patients who use MAOIs within 14 days of fentanyl administration.

Administration and Handling

◀ALERT▶ Keep in mind that fentanyl may be combined with a local anesthetic, such as bupivacaine.

IV

- Store the parenteral form at room temperature.
- Make sure resuscitative equipment and an opiate antagonist (naloxone 0.5 mcg/kg) is readily available before administering the drug.
- For initial anesthesia induction, give a small amount by tuberculin syringe, as prescribed.
- Give by slow IV push, over 1 to 2 minutes.

• A too-rapid IV infusion increases the of severe adverse reactions, such as anaphylaxis, bronchospasm, laryngospasm, peripheral circulatory collapse, cardiac arrest, and skeletal and thoracic muscle rigidity (which may result in apnea).
Transdermal
• To clean the patch site before application, use only water because soap and oils may irritate the skin.
• Apply the patch to a flat, unirritated, non-hairy area of intact skin on the upper torso.
• Press the patch onto the patient's skin firmly and evenly for 10 to 20 seconds, ensuring that it comes in full contact with the skin, especially around the edges.
• Rotate application sites.
• Carefully fold used patches so that they adhere to themselves, and discard them in the toilet.
Transmucosal
• Have the patient suck the lozenge vigorously.

Intervention and Evaluation
• Monitor the patient's BP, heart rate, respiratory rate, and oxygen saturation.
• Encourage the patient to cough, turn, and breathe deeply every 2 hours.
• Assess the patient for relief of pain.
• Assist the patient with ambulation.

Patient Teaching
• Instruct the patient to use fentanyl as directed to avoid an overdosage. Explain that prolonged use of the drug may cause physical dependence.
• Teach the patient to properly apply the fentanyl transdermal patch.
• Instruct the patient to discontinue fentanyl slowly after long-term use.
• Urge the patient to avoid alcohol during fentanyl therapy and to consult the physician before taking any other drugs.
• Warn the patient to avoid tasks requiring mental alertness or motor skills until his or her response to the drug has been established.

hydrocodone bitartrate

high-drough-**koe**-doan
(Hycodan[CAN], Robidone[CAN])

CATEGORY AND SCHEDULE

Pregnancy Risk Category: C (D if used for prolonged periods or at high dosages at term)
Controlled Substance: Schedule III

MECHANISM OF ACTION

A narcotic analgesic and antitussive that binds with opioid receptors in the CNS. **Therapeutic Effect:** Alters the perception of and emotional response to pain; suppresses cough reflex.

PHARMACOKINETICS

Route	Onset	Peak	Duration
PO (analgesic)	10–20 min	30–60 min	4–6 hr
PO (antitussive)	N/A	N/A	4–6 hr

Well absorbed from the GI tract. Metabolized in the liver. Primarily excreted in urine. ***Half-life:*** 3.8 hr (increased in elderly).

INDICATIONS AND DOSAGES

▸ **Analgesia**
PO
Adults, Children older than 12 yr. 5–10 mg q4–6h.
Elderly. 2.5–5 mg q4–6h.

▸ **Cough**
PO
Adults. 5–10 mg q4–6h as needed. Maximum: 15 mg/dose.
Children. 0.6 mg/kg/day in 3–4 divided doses at intervals of at least 4 hr. Maximum single dose: 5 mg (children 2–12 yr), 1.25 mg (children younger than 2 yr).
PO (Extended-Release)
Adults. 10 mg q12h.
Children 6–12 yr. 5 mg q12h.

CONTRAINDICATIONS
None known.

INTERACTIONS
Drug
Alcohol, other CNS depressants: May increase CNS or respiratory depression and hypotension.
MAOIs: May produce a severe, sometimes fatal reaction; plan to administer one-quarter of usual hydrocodone dose.
Herbal
None known.
Food
None known.

DIAGNOSTIC TEST EFFECTS
May increase serum amylase and lipase levels.

SIDE EFFECTS
Frequent
Sedation, hypotension, diaphoresis, facial flushing, dizziness, somnolence
Occasional
Urine retention, blurred vision, constipation, dry mouth, headache, nausea, vomiting, difficult or painful urination, euphoria, dysphoria

SERIOUS REACTIONS
! Overdose results in respiratory depression, skeletal muscle flaccidity, cold or clammy skin, cyanosis, and extreme somnolence progressing to seizures, stupor, and coma.
! The patient who uses hydrocodone repeatedly may develop a tolerance to the drug's analgesic effect as well as physical dependence.
! The drug may have a prolonged duration of action and cumulative effect in patients with hepatic or renal impairment.

NURSING CONSIDERATIONS
Baseline Assessment
- Obtain the patient's vital signs before giving hydrocodone.
- Withhold the drug and notify the physician if the respiratory rate is 12 breaths/minute or less in an adult or 20 breaths/minute or less in a child.
- If hydrocodone is administered as an analgesic, assess the duration, location, onset, and type of pain the patient experiences.
- If hydrocodone is administered as an antitussive, assess the frequency, severity, and type of cough.

Lifespan Considerations
- Hydrocodone readily crosses the placenta and is distributed in breast milk.
- Regular use of hydrocodone during pregnancy may produce withdrawal symptoms in the neonate, including irritability, excessive crying, tremors, hyperactive reflexes, fever, vomiting, diarrhea, yawning, sneezing, and seizures.
- Hydrocodone use may prolong labor if administered in the latent phase of the first stage of labor or before the cervix has dilated 4 to 5 cm.
- The neonate may develop respiratory depression if the mother receives hydrocodone during labor.
- Children younger than 2 years may

be more susceptible to respiratory depression.
- Elderly patients may be more susceptible to respiration depression and paradoxical excitement.
- In the elderly, age-related renal impairment, benign prostatic hyperplasia, or obstruction may increase the risk of urine retention. A dosage adjustment is recommended.

Precautions
- Use hydrocodone extremely cautiously in patients with acute alcoholism, anoxia, CNS depression, hypercapnia, respiratory depression or dysfunction, seizures, shock, or untreated myxedema.
- Use hydrocodone cautiously in patients with acute abdominal conditions, Addison's disease, COPD, hypothyroidism, hepatic impairment, increased intracranial pressure, benign prostatic hyperplasia, or urethral stricture.

Administration and Handling

◀ALERT▶ Although side effects depend on the dosage and administration route, they occur infrequently when hydromorphone is administered orally as an antitussive.
- Ambulatory patients and those not in severe pain may be more prone to dizziness, hypotension, nausea, and vomiting than patients in the supine position and those in severe pain.

PO
- Give hydrocodone without regard to food.
- Crush tablets if needed.

Intervention and Evaluation
- Keep in mind that hydrocodone's effect is reduced if the full pain response recurs before the next dose.
- Palpate the patient's bladder for urine retention.
- Assess the patient's pattern of daily bowel activity and stool consistency.
- Initiate deep-breathing and coughing exercises, particularly in patients with impaired pulmonary function.
- Assess the patient for clinical improvement of symptoms, and record the onset of pain or cough relief.

Patient Teaching
- Inform the patient that he or she may take hydrocodone with food.
- Instruct the patient to change positions slowly to help prevent orthostatic hypotension. Warn the patient to avoid tasks that require mental alertness or motor skills until his or her response to hydrocodone has been established.
- Explain to the patient that drug dependence and tolerance may occur with prolonged use of high doses.
- Urge the patient to avoid consuming alcohol during hydrocodone treatment.
- Caution the patient to notify the health care provider if he or she experiences constipation, difficulty breathing, nausea, and vomiting during hydrocodone therapy.

hydromorphone hydrochloride

hye-droe-**mor**-fone
(Dilaudid, Dilaudid HP, Hydromorph Contin[CAN], Palladone)
Do not confuse hydromorphone with morphine, or Dilaudid with Dilantin.

CATEGORY AND SCHEDULE

Pregnancy Risk Category: B (D if used for prolonged periods or at high dosages at term)
Controlled Substance: Schedule II

MECHANISM OF ACTION

An opioid agonist that binds to

opioid receptors in the CNS, reducing the intensity of pain stimuli from sensory nerve endings. **Therapeutic Effect:** Alters the perception of and emotional response to pain; suppresses cough reflex.

PHARMACOKINETICS

Route	Onset	Peak	Duration
PO	30 min	90–120 min	4 hr
IV	10–15 min	15–30 min	2–3 hr
IM	15 min	30–60 min	4–5 hr
Subcutaneous	15 min	30–90 min	4 hr
Rectal	15–30 min	N/A	N/A

Well absorbed from the GI tract after IM administration. Widely distributed. Metabolized in the liver. Excreted in urine. ***Half-life:*** 1–3 hr.

AVAILABILITY

Liquid (Dilaudid): 5 mg/5 ml.
Capsules (Extended-Release [Palladone]): 12 mg, 16 mg, 24 mg, 32 mg.
Tablets (Dilaudid): 2 mg, 3 mg, 4 mg, 8 mg.
Injection (Dilaudid): 1 mg/ml, 2 mg/ml, 4 mg/ml.
Injection (Dilaudid HP): 10 mg/ml.
Suppository (Dilaudid): 3 mg.

INDICATIONS AND DOSAGES

▸ **Analgesia**

PO

Adults, Elderly, Children weighing 50 kg and more. 2–4 mg q3–4h. Range: 2–8 mg/dose.
Children older than 6 mo and weighing less than 50 kg. 0.03-0.08 mg/kg/dose q3–4h.

PO (Extended-Release)

Adults, Elderly. 12–32 mg once a day.

IV

Adults, Elderly, Children weighing more than 50 kg. 0.2–0.6 mg q2–3h.
Children weighing 50 kg or less. 0.015 mg/kg/dose q3–6h as needed.

Rectal

Adults, Elderly. 3 mg q4–8h.

▸ **Patient-controlled analgesia (PCA)**

IV

Adults, Elderly. 0.05–0.5 mg at 5–15 min lockout. Maximum (4-hr): 4–6 mg.

Epidural

Adults, Elderly. Bolus dose of 1–1.5 mg at rate of 0.04–0.4 mg/hr. Demand dose of 0.15 mg at 30 min lockout.

▸ **Cough**

PO

Adults, Elderly, Children older than 12 yr. 1 mg q3–4h.
Children 6–12 yr. 0.5 mg q3–4h.

CONTRAINDICATIONS

None known.

INTERACTIONS

Drug

Alcohol, other CNS depressants: May increase CNS or respiratory depression and hypotension.
MAOIs: May produce a severe, sometimes fatal reaction; plan to administer one-quarter of usual hydromorphone dose.

Herbal

None known.

Food

None known.

DIAGNOSTIC TEST EFFECTS

May increase serum amylase and lipase concentrations.

IV INCOMPATIBILITIES

Amphotericin B complex (Abelcet, AmBisome, Amphotec), cefazolin

(Ancef, Kefzol), diazepam (Valium), phenobarbital, phenytoin (Dilantin)

IV COMPATIBILITIES

Diltiazem (Cardizem), diphenhydramine (Benadryl), dobutamine (Dobutrex), dopamine (Intropin), fentanyl (Sublimaze), furosemide (Lasix), heparin, lorazepam (Ativan), magnesium sulfate, metoclopramide (Reglan), midazolam (Versed), milrinone (Primacor), morphine, propofol (Diprivan)

SIDE EFFECTS

Frequent
Somnolence, dizziness, hypotension (including orthostatic hypotension), decreased appetite
Occasional
Confusion, diaphoresis, facial flushing, urine retention, constipation, dry mouth, nausea, vomiting, headache, pain at injection site
Rare
Allergic reaction, depression

SERIOUS REACTIONS

! Overdose results in respiratory depression, skeletal muscle flaccidity, cold or clammy skin, cyanosis, and extreme somnolence progressing to seizures, stupor, and coma.
! The patient who uses hydromorphone repeatedly may develop a tolerance to the drug's analgesic effect as well as physical dependence.
! This drug may have a prolonged duration of action and cumulative effect in patients with hepatic or renal impairment.

NURSING CONSIDERATIONS

Baseline Assessment

- Obtain the patient's vital signs before administering hydromorphone.
- Withhold the drug, and notify the physician if the respiratory rate is 12 breaths/minute or less in an adult, or 20 breaths/minute or less in a child.
- Assess the duration, location, onset, and type of pain.
- If the patient is being treated for cough, assess the frequency, severity, and type of cough.

Lifespan Considerations

- Hydromorphone readily crosses the placenta; it is unknown if it is distributed in breast milk.
- Regular use of opioids during pregnancy may produce withdrawal symptoms in the neonate, including diarrhea, excessive crying, fever, hyperactive reflexes, irritability, seizures, sneezing, tremors, vomiting, and yawning.
- Hydromorphone use may prolong labor if administered in the latent phase of the first stage of labor or before cervical dilation of 4 to 5 cm.
- The neonate may develop respiratory depression if the mother receives hydromorphone during labor.
- Children younger than 2 years may be more susceptible to respiratory depression.
- Elderly patients may be more susceptible to respiratory depression and paradoxical excitement.
- In the elderly, age-related benign prostatic hyperplasia, obstruction, or renal impairment may increase the risk of urine retention; a dosage adjustment is recommended.

Precautions

- Use hydromorphone extremely cautiously in patients with acute alcoholism, anoxia, CNS depression, hypercapnia, respiratory depression or dysfunction, seizures, shock, or untreated myxedema.
- Use hydromorphone cautiously in patients with acute abdominal conditions, Addison's disease, COPD, hypothyroidism, hepatic impairment,

increased intracranial pressure, benign prostatic hyperplasia, or urethral stricture.

Administration and Handling

◀ALERT▶ Although side effects depend on the dosage and administration route, they occur infrequently when hydromorpone is administered orally as an antitussive.

• Ambulatory patients and those not in severe pain may be more prone to dizziness, hypotension, nausea, and vomiting than patients in the supine position and those in severe pain.

PO

• Give hydromorphone without regard to food.

• Crush tablets, as needed.

IV

◀ALERT▶ Be aware that a high concentration (10 mg/ml) should be used only in patients currently receiving high doses of another opioid agonist for severe, chronic pain caused by cancer or those who have developed a tolerance to high doses of other opioids.

• Store vials at room temperature; protect from light.

• A slight yellow discoloration of the parenteral form does not indicate a loss of potency.

• Hydromorphone may be given undiluted as IV push over 2 to 5 minutes, or it may be further diluted with 5 ml sterile water for injection or 0.9% NaCl.

• Be aware that rapid IV administration increases the risk of a severe anaphylactic reaction, marked by apnea, cardiac arrest, and circulatory collapse.

IM, Subcutaneous

• Use a short 25- to 30-gauge needle for subcutaneous injection.

• Administer the drug slowly; rotate injection sites.

• Know that patients with circulatory impairment are at increased risk for overdose because of delayed absorption of repeated injections.

Rectal

• Refrigerate suppositories.

• Moisten the suppository with cold water before inserting it well into the rectum.

Intervention and Evaluation

• Keep in mind that the drug's effect is reduced if the full pain response recurs before the next dose

• Monitor the patient's vital signs.

• For patients being treated for a cough, auscultate the lungs for adventitious breath sounds and increase fluid intake and environmental humidity to decrease the viscosity of lung secretions.

• Initiate deep-breathing and coughing exercises, particularly in patients with impaired respiratory function.

• Assess the patient's pattern of daily bowel activity and stool consistency, especially with long-term use.

• Assess the patient for clinical improvement and record the onset of pain or cough relief.

Patient Teaching

• Instruct the patient to alert you as soon as pain occurs because the drug is less effective if a full pain response recurs before the next dose.

• Explain to the patient that drug dependence and tolerance may occur with prolonged use of high dosages.

• Urge the patient to avoid alcohol during hydromorphone therapy.

• Warn the patient to avoid tasks that require mental alertness and motor skills until his or her response to the drug has been established.

• Instruct the patient to change positions slowly to avoid orthostatic hypotension.

meperidine hydrochloride

me-**per**-i-deen
(Demerol, Pethidine Injection[AUS])
Do not confuse Demerol with Demulen or Dymelor.

CATEGORY AND SCHEDULE

Pregnancy Risk Category: B (D if used for prolonged periods or at high dosages at term)
Controlled Substance: Schedule II

MECHANISM OF ACTION

An opioid agonist that binds to opioid receptors in the CNS. **Therapeutic Effect:** Alters the perception of and emotional response to pain.

PHARMACOKINETICS

Route	Onset	Peak	Duration
PO	15 min	60 min	2–4 hr
IV	less than 5 min	5–7 min	2–3 hr
IM	10–15 min	30–50 min	2–4 hr
Subcutaneous	10–15 min	30–50 min	2–4 hr

Variably absorbed from the GI tract; well absorbed after IM administration. Protein binding: 60%–80%. Widely distributed. Metabolized in the liver to active metabolite. Primarily excreted in urine. Not removed by hemodialysis. ***Half-life:*** 2.4–4 hr; metabolite 8-16 hr (increased in hepatic impairment and disease).

AVAILABILITY

Syrup: 50 mg/5 ml.
Tablets: 50 mg, 100 mg.
Injection: 25 mg/ml, 50 mg/ml, 75 mg/ml, 100 mg/ml.

INDICATIONS AND DOSAGES

▸ **Analgesia**
PO, IM, Subcutaneous
Adults, Elderly. 50–150 mg q3–4h.
Children. 1.1–1.5 mg/kg q3–4h. Don't exceed single dose of 100 mg.

▸ **Patient-controlled analgesia (PCA)**
IV
Adults. Loading dose: 50–100 mg. Intermittent bolus: 5–30 mg. Lockout interval: 10–20 min. Continuous infusion: 5–40 mg/hr. Maximum (4-hr): 200–300 mg.

▸ **Dosage in renal impairment**
Dosage is based on creatinine clearance.

Creatinine Clearance	Dosage
10–50 ml/min	75% of usual dose
less than 10 ml/min	50% of usual dose

CONTRAINDICATIONS

Delivery of premature infant, diarrhea due to poisoning, use within 14 days of MAOIs

INTERACTIONS

Drug

Alcohol, other CNS depressants: May increase CNS or respiratory depression and hypotension.
MAOIs: May produce a severe, sometimes fatal reaction. Meperidine use is contraindicated.

Herbal

Valerian: May increase CNS depression.

Food

None known.

DIAGNOSTIC TEST EFFECTS

May increase serum amylase and lipase levels. Therapeutic serum level is 100–550 ng/ml; toxic serum level is greater than 1,000 ng/ml.

IV INCOMPATIBILITIES

Allopurinol (Aloprim), amphotericin B complex (Abelcet, AmBisome, Amphotec), cefepime (Maxipime), cefoperazone (Cefobid), doxorubicin liposomal (Doxil), furosemide (Lasix), idarubicin (Idamycin), nafcillin (Nafcil)

IV COMPATIBILITIES

Atropine, bumetanide (Bumex), diltiazem (Cardizem), diphenhydramine (Benadryl), dobutamine (Dobutrex), dopamine (Intropin), glycopyrrolate (Robinul), heparin, hydroxyzine (Vistaril), insulin, lidocaine, magnesium, midazolam (Versed), oxytocin (Pitocin), potassium

SIDE EFFECTS

Frequent

Sedation, hypotension (including orthostatic hypotension), diaphoresis, facial flushing, dizziness, nausea, vomiting, constipation

Occasional

Confusion, arrhythmias, tremors, urine retention, abdominal pain, dry mouth, headache, irritation at injection site, euphoria, dysphoria

Rare

Allergic reaction (rash, pruritus), insomnia

SERIOUS REACTIONS

! Overdose results in respiratory depression, skeletal muscle flaccidity, cold or clammy skin, cyanosis, and extreme somnolence progressing to seizures, stupor, and coma. The antidote is 0.4 mg naloxone.

! The patient who uses meperidine repeatedly may develop a tolerance to the drug's analgesic effect and physical dependence.

NURSING CONSIDERATIONS

Baseline Assessment

- Assess the duration, location, onset, and type of pain the patient.
- Obtain the patient's vital signs before giving meperidine.
- Withhold the drug and notify the physician if the respiratory rate is 12 breaths/minute or less in an adult or 20 breaths/minute or less in a child.

Lifespan Considerations

- Meperidine crosses the placenta and is distributed in breast milk.
- Regular use of opiates during pregnancy may produce withdrawal symptoms in the neonate, such as diarrhea, excessive crying, fever, hyperactive reflexes, irritability, seizures, sneezing, tremors, vomiting, and yawning.
- The neonate may develop respiratory depression if the mother receives meperidine during labor.
- Children are more prone to develop paradoxical excitement.
- Children younger than 2 years and the elderly are more susceptible to the drug's respiratory depressant effects.
- In the elderly, age-related renal impairment may increase the risk of urine retention.

Precautions

- Use meperidine cautiously in elderly or debilitated patients and in patients with acute abdominal conditions, cor pulmonale, history of seizures, increased intracranial pressure, hepatic or renal impairment, respiratory abnormalities, or supraventricular tachycardia.
- Use cautiously in patients with renal impairment as meperidine's metabolite may increase and cause seizures, tremors, and twitching.

Administration and Handling

◀ **ALERT** ▶ Be aware that meperidine's side effects are dependent on the dosage and route of administration.

• Know that ambulatory patients and those not in severe pain may be more prone to dizziness, nausea, and vomiting than those in the supine position and those in severe pain.

◀ **ALERT** ▶ Meperidine's metabolite may increase in patients with renal impairment and cause seizures, tremors, and twitching.

PO

• Give meperidine without regard to food.

• Dilute the syrup in a glass of water to prevent an anesthetic effect on mucous membranes.

IV

◀ **ALERT** ▶ Give meperidine by slow IV push or IV infusion.

• Store vials at room temperature.

• Meperidine may be given undiluted or may be diluted in D_5W, Ringer's solution, lactated Ringer's solution, a dextrose-saline combination (such as 2.5%, 5%, or 10% dextrose and 0.45% or 0.9% NaCl), or Molar (M/6) Sodium Lactate Injection for IV injection or infusion.

• Place the patient in a recumbent position before administering parenteral meperidine.

• Administer IV push very slowly, over 2 to 3 minutes.

• Rapid IV administration increases the risk of a severe anaphylactic reaction, marked by apnea, cardiac arrest, and circulatory collapse.

IM, Subcutaneous

◀ **ALERT** ▶ The IM route is preferred over the subcutaneous route because subcutaneous injection can produce induration, local irritation, and pain.

• Inject the drug slowly.

• Know that patients with circulatory impairment are at increased risk for overdose because of delayed absorption of repeated injections.

Intervention and Evaluation

• Know that meperidine's effects are reduced if a full pain response recurs before the next dose.

• Monitor the patient's vital signs for 15 to 30 minutes after an IM or subcutaneous dose and for 5 to 10 minutes after an IV dose. Be alert for decreased BP, as well as a change in quality and rate of pulse.

• Monitor the patient's level of pain and sedation.

• Assess the patient's pattern of daily bowel activity and stool consistency.

• Evaluate the patient for adequate urination.

• Initiate deep-breathing and coughing exercises, particularly in patients with impaired respiratory function. Therapeutic serum drug level is 100 to 550 ng/ml; toxic serum drug level is greater than 1,000 ng/ml.

Patient Teaching

• Instruct the patient to take meperidine before pain fully returns, within prescribed intervals.

• Inform the the patient that injection may cause discomfort.

• Caution the patient that drug dependence and tolerance may occur with prolonged use of high doses.

• Warn the patient to avoid tasks that require mental alertness or motor skills until his or her response to the drug has been established.

• Instruct the patient to change positions slowly to avoid orthostatic hypotension.

• Advise the patient to increase fluid intake and consumption of high-fiber foods to prevent constipation.

• Urge the patient to avoid alcohol and other CNS depressants while taking meperidine.

methadone hydrochloride

meth-a-done
(Dolophine, Metadol[CAN], Methadone Intensol, Methadose, Physeptone[AUS])

CATEGORY AND SCHEDULE

Pregnancy Risk Category: B (D if used for prolonged periods or at high dosages at term)
Controlled Substance: Schedule II

MECHANISM OF ACTION

An opioid agonist that binds with opioid receptors in the CNS. **Therapeutic Effect:** Alters the perception of and emotional response to pain; reduces withdrawal symptoms from other opioid drugs.

PHARMACOKINETICS

Route	Onset	Peak	Duration
Oral	0.5-1 hr	1.5-2 hr	6–8 hr
IM	10–20 min	1–2 hr	4–5 hr
IV	N/A	15-30 min	3-4 hr

Well absorbed after IM injection. Protein binding: 80%–85%. Metabolized in the liver. Primarily excreted in urine. Not removed by hemodialysis. ***Half-life:*** 15–25 hr.

AVAILABILITY

Oral Concentrate (Methadone Intensol, Methadose): 10 mg/ml.
Oral Solution: 5 mg/5 ml, 10 mg/5 ml.
Tablets (Dolophine, Methadose): 5 mg, 10 mg.
Tablets (Dispersible [Methadose]): 40 mg.
Injection (Dolophine): 10 mg/ml.

INDICATIONS AND DOSAGES

▸ **Analgesia**
PO, IV, IM, Subcutaneous
Adults. 2.5–10 mg q3–8h as needed up to 5–20 mg q6–8h.
Elderly. 2.5 mg q8–12h.
Children. Initially, 0.1 mg/kg/dose q4h for 2–3 doses, then q6–12h. Maximum: 10 mg/dose.

▸ **Detoxification**
PO
Adults, Elderly. 15–40 mg/day.

▸ **Temporary maintenance treatment of narcotic abstinence syndrome**
PO
Adults, Elderly. 20–120 mg/day.

CONTRAINDICATIONS

Delivery of premature infant, diarrhea due to poisoning, hypersensitivity to narcotics, labor

INTERACTIONS

Drug

Alcohol, other CNS depressants: May increase CNS or respiratory depression and hypotension.
MAOIs: May produce a severe, sometimes fatal reaction; plan to administer one-quarter of usual methadone dose.

Herbal

Valerian: May increase CNS depression.

Food

None known.

DIAGNOSTIC TEST EFFECTS

May increase serum amylase and lipase levels.

SIDE EFFECTS

Frequent

Sedation, decreased BP (including orthostatic hypotension), diaphoresis, facial flushing, constipation, dizziness, nausea, vomiting

Occasional
Confusion, urine retention, palpitations, abdominal cramps, visual changes, dry mouth, headache, decreased appetite, anxiety, insomnia
Rare
Allergic reaction (rash, pruritus)

SERIOUS REACTIONS

! Overdose results in respiratory depression, skeletal muscle flaccidity, cold or clammy skin, cyanosis, and extreme somnolence progressing to seizures, stupor, and coma. The antidote is 0.4 mg naloxone.
! The patient who uses methadone long term may develop a tolerance to the drug's analgesic effect and physical dependence.

NURSING CONSIDERATIONS

Baseline Assessment

• Obtain the patient's vital signs before giving methadone.
• Withhold the drug, and notify the physician if the respiratory rate is 12 breaths/minute or less in an adult or 20 breaths/minute or less in a child.

Lifespan Considerations

• Methadone crosses the placenta and is distributed in breast milk.
• Regular use of opioids during pregnancy may produce withdrawal symptoms in the neonate, such as diarrhea, excessive crying, fever, hyperactive reflexes, irritability, seizures, sneezing, tremors, vomiting, and yawning.
• The neonate may develop respiratory depression if the mother receives methadone during labor.
• Children are more prone to experience paradoxical excitement.
• Children younger than 2 years and the elderly are more susceptible to the drug's respiratory depressant effects.
• Age-related renal impairment may increase the risk of urine retention in the elderly.

Precautions

• Use methadone extremely cautiously in patients with acute abdominal conditions, cor pulmonale, history of seizures, impaired hepatic or renal function, increased intracranial pressure, respiratory abnormalities, or supraventricular tachycardia.
• Use methadone cautiously in debilitated or elderly patients.

Administration and Handling

PO
• Know that oral methadone is one-half as potent as parenteral methadone.
• Give methadone without regard to food.
• Dilute the syrup in a glass of water to prevent an anesthetic effect on mucous membranes.
IM, Subcutaneous
◀ALERT▶ Be aware that the IM route is preferred over the subcutaneous route because the subcutaneous route may produce induration, local irritation, and pain.
• Don't use the solution if it appears cloudy or contains a precipitate.
• Place the patient in the recumbent position before giving parenteral methadone.
• Inject the drug slowly.
• Know that patients with circulatory impairment are at increased risk for overdose because of delayed absorption of repeated injections.

Intervention and Evaluation

• Monitor the patient's vital signs for 15 to 30 minutes after an IM or subcutaneous dose and for 5 to 10 minutes after an IV dose.
• Assess the patient for adequate urination.
• Assess the patient for clinical improvement, and record the onset of pain relief.
• Provide support to the patient in a

detoxification program. Monitor the patient for withdrawal symptoms.

Patient Teaching

- Caution the patient against abruptly discontinuing methadone after prolonged use.
- Inform the patient that methadone may cause dizziness and dry mouth.
- Warn the patient to avoid tasks that require mental alertness or motor skills until his or her reponse to the drug has been established.
- Urge the patient to avoid alcohol and CNS depressants during methadone therapy.

morphine sulfate

mor-feen

(Anamorph[AUS], Astramorph, Avinza, DepoDur, Duramorph, Infumorph, Kadian, Kapanol[AUS], M-Eslon, Morphine Mixtures[AUS], MS Contin, MSIR, MS Mono[AUS], Oramorph SR, RMS, Roxanol, Statex[CAN])

Do not confuse morphine with hydromorphone, or Roxanol with Roxicet.

CATEGORY AND SCHEDULE

Pregnancy Risk Category: C (D if used for prolonged periods or at high dosages at term)

Controlled Substance: Schedule II

MECHANISM OF ACTION

An opioid agonist that binds with opioid receptors in the CNS. **Therapeutic Effect:** Alters the perception of and emotional response to pain; produces generalized CNS depression.

PHARMACOKINETICS

Route	Onset	Peak	Duration
Oral Solution	N/A	1 hr	3–5 hr
Tablets	N/A	1 hr	3–5 hr
Tablets (ER)	N/A	3–4 hr	8–12 hr
IV	Rapid	0.3 hr	3–5 hr
IM	5–30 min	0.5–1 hr	3–5 hr
Epidural	N/A	1 hr	12–20 hr
Subcutaneous	N/A	1.1–5 hr	3–5 hr
Rectal	N/A	0.5–1 hr	3–7 hr

Variably absorbed from the GI tract. Readily absorbed after IM or subcutaneous administration. Protein binding: 20%–35%. Widely distributed. Metabolized in the liver. Primarily excreted in urine. Removed by hemodialysis. ***Half-life:*** 2–3 hr. (increased in patients with hepatic disease)

AVAILABILITY

Capsules (Extended-Release [Kadian]): 20 mg, 30 mg, 50 mg, 60 mg, 100 mg.
Capsules (Extended-Release [Avinza]): 30 mg, 60 mg, 90 mg, 120 mg.
Capsules (MSIR): 15 mg, 30 mg.
Solution for Injection: 2 mg/ml, 4 mg/ml, 5 mg/ml, 8 mg/ml, 10 mg/ml, 15 mg/ml, 25 mg/ml.
Solution for Injection (Preservative-Free): 10 mg/ml, 15 mg/ml, 25 mg/ml, 50 mg/ml.
Epidural and Intrathecal via Infusion Device (Infumorph): 10 mg/ml, 25 mg/ml.
Epidural, Intrathecal, IV Infusion (Astramorph, Duramorph): 0.5 mg/ml, 1 mg/ml.

Oral Solution (MSIR): 10 mg/ml, 20 mg/ml.
Oral Solution (Roxanol): 20 mg/ml, 100 mg/ml.
Suppositories (RMS): 5 mg, 10 mg, 20 mg, 30 mg.
Tablets (MSIR): 15 mg, 30 mg.
Tablets (Extended-Release [MS Contin]): 15 mg, 30 mg, 60 mg, 100 mg, 200 mg.
Tablets (Extended-Release [Oramorph SR]): 15 mg, 30 mg, 60 mg, 100 mg.
Liposomal Injection (DepoDur): 10 mg/ml, 15 mg/1.5 ml, 20 mg/2 ml.

INDICATIONS AND DOSAGES

◀ALERT▶ Dosage should be titrated to desired effect.

▸ **Analgesia**

PO (Prompt-release)
Adults, Elderly. 10–30 mg q3–4h as needed.
Children. 0.2–0.5 mg/kg q3–4h as needed.

◀ALERT▶ For the Avinza dosage below, be aware that this drug is to be administered once a day only.

◀ALERT▶ For the Kadian dosage information below, be aware that this drug is to be administered q12h or once a day only.

◀ALERT▶ Be aware that pediatric dosages of extended-release preparations Kadian and Avinza have not been established.

◀ALERT▶ For the MS Contin and Oramorph SR dosage information below, be aware that the daily dosage is divided and given q8h or q12h.

PO (Extended-Release [Avinza])
Adults, Elderly. Dosage requirment should be established using prompt-release formulations and is based on total daily dose. Avinza is given once a day only.

PO (Extended-Release [Kadian])
Adults, Elderly. Dosage requirment should be established using prompt-release formulations and is based on total daily dose. Dose is given once a day or divided and given q12h.

PO (Extended-Release [MS Contin, Oramorph SR])
Adults, Elderly. Dosage requirment should be established using prompt-release formulations and is based on total daily dose. Daily dose is divided and given q8h or q12h.
Children. 0.3-0.6 mg/kg/dose q12h.

IM
Adults, Elderly. 5–10 mg q3–4h as needed.
Children. 0.1 mg/kg q3–4h as needed.

IV
Adults, Elderly. 2.5–5 mg q3–4h as needed. Note: Repeated doses (e.g. 1–2 mg) may be given more frequently (e.g., every hour) if needed.
Children. 0.05–0.1 mg/kg q3–4h as needed.

IV Continuous Infusion
Adults, Elderly. 0.8–10 mg/h. Range: Up to 80 mg/h.
Children. 10–30 mcg/kg/hr.

Epidural
Adults, Elderly. Initially, 1–6 mg bolus, infusion rate: 0.1–1 mg/hr. Maximum: 10 mg/24 hr.

Intrathecal
Adults, Elderly. One-tenth of the epidural dose: 0.2–1 mg/dose.

▸ **PCA**

IV
Adults, Elderly. Loading dose: 5–10 mg. Intermittent bolus: 0.5–3 mg. Lockout interval: 5–12 min. Continuous infusion: 1–10 mg/hr. 4-hr limit: 20–30 mg.

CONTRAINDICATIONS

Acute or severe asthma, GI obstruction, severe hepatic or renal impairment, severe respiratory depression, asthma, severe liver or renal impairment

INTERACTIONS

Drug

Alcohol, other CNS depressants: May increase CNS or respiratory depression and hypotension.
MAOIs: May produce a severe, sometimes fatal reaction; expect to administer one-quarter of usual morphine dose.

Herbal

None known.

Food

None known.

DIAGNOSTIC TEST EFFECTS

May increase serum amylase and lipase levels.

IV INCOMPATIBILITIES

Amphotericin B complex (Abelcet, AmBisome, Amphotec), cefepime (Maxipime), doxorubicin liposomal (Doxil), thiopental

IV COMPATIBILITIES

Amiodarone (Cordarone), atropine, bumetanide (Bumex), bupivacaine (Marcaine, Sensorcaine), diltiazem (Cardizem), diphenhydramine (Benadryl), dobutamine (Dobutrex), dopamine (Intropin), glycopyrrolate (Robinul), heparin, hydroxyzine (Vistaril), lidocaine, lorazepam (Ativan), magnesium, midazolam (Versed), milrinone (Primacor), nitroglycerin, potassium, propofol (Diprivan)

SIDE EFFECTS

Frequent

Sedation, decreased BP (including orthostatic hypotension), diaphoresis, facial flushing, constipation, dizziness, somnolence, nausea, vomiting

Occasional

Allergic reaction (rash, pruritus), dyspnea, confusion, palpitations, tremors, urine retention, abdominal cramps, vision changes, dry mouth, headache, decreased appetite, pain or burning at injection site

Rare

Paralytic ileus

SERIOUS REACTIONS

! Overdose results in respiratory depression, skeletal muscle flaccidity, cold or clammy skin, cyanosis, and extreme somnolence progressing to seizures, stupor, and coma.
! The patient who uses morphine repeatedly may develop a tolerance to the drug's analgesic effect and physical dependence.
! The drug may have a prolonged duration of action and cumulative effect in those with hepatic and renal impairment.

NURSING CONSIDERATIONS

Baseline Assessment

- Assess the duration, location, onset, and type of pain.
- Obtain the patient's vital signs before giving morphine.
- Withhold the drug and notify the physician if the respiratory rate is 12 breaths/minute or less in an adult or 20 breaths/minute or less in a child.

Lifespan Considerations

- Morphine crosses the placenta and is distributed in breast milk.
- Regular use of opioids during pregnancy may produce withdrawal symptoms in the neonate, such as diarrhea, excessive crying, fever, hyperactive reflexes, irritability, seizures, sneezing, tremors, vomiting, and yawning.
- Morphine may prolong labor if administered in the latent phase of the first stage of labor or before the cervix is dilated 4 to 5 cm.
- The neonate may develop respiratory depression if the mother receives morphine during labor.

• Children and the elderly are more prone to experience paradoxical excitement.
• Children younger than 2 years and the elderly are more susceptible to the drug's respiratory depressant effects.
• Age-related renal impairment may increase the risk of urine retention in the elderly.

Precautions

• Use morphine extremely cautiously in patients with COPD, cor pulmonale, head injury, hypoxia, hypercapnia, increased intracranial pressure, preexisting respiratory depression, or severe hypotension.
• Use morphine cautiously in debilitated patients and in those with Addison's disease, alcoholism, biliary tract disease, CNS depression, hypothyroidism, pancreatitis, benign prostatic hyperplasia, seizure disorders, toxic psychosis, or urethral stricture.

Administration and Handling

◀ALERT▶ Expect to reduce morphine dosage for debilitated and elderly patients and those using CNS depressants concurrently. Titrate dosage to desired effect, as prescribed.

◀ALERT▶ Morphine's side effects are dependent on the dosage and route of administration.

• Ambulatory patients and those not in severe pain are more prone to experience dizziness, nausea, and vomiting than those in the supine position and those in severe pain.

PO

• Mix the liquid form with fruit juice to improve the taste.
• Don't crush, open, or break extended-release capsules.
• Kadian (extended-release capsules) may be mixed with applesauce just before administration.

IV

• Store vials at room temperature.
• Morphine may be given undiluted as IV push.
• For IV injection, 2.5 to 15 mg morphine may be diluted in 4 to 5 ml sterile water for injection.
• For continuous IV infusion, dilute to a concentration of 0.1 to 1 mg/ml in D_5W and administer through a controlled infusion device.
• Place the patient in the recumbent position before giving parenteral morphine.
• Always administer IV morphine very slowly because rapid IV administration increases the risk of a severe anaphylactic reaction, marked by apnea, cardiac arrest, and circulatory collapse.

IM, Subcutaneous

• Inject the drug slowly; rotate injection sites.
• Know that patients with circulatory impairment are at increased risk for overdose because of delayed absorption of repeated injections.

Rectal

• If the suppository is too soft, refrigerate it for 30 minutes or run cold water over the foil wrapper.
• Moisten the suppository with cold water before inserting it well into the rectum.

Intervention and Evaluation

• Keep in mind that morphine's effect is reduced if a full pain response recurs before the next dose.
• Monitor the patient's vital signs for 5 to 10 minutes after IV administration and 15 to 30 minutes after IM or subcutaneous injection.
• Be alert for bradycardia and hypotension.
• Assess the patient's pattern of daily bowel activity and stool consistency, and determine if the patient has difficulty urinating.
• Initiate deep-breathing and coughing exercises, particularly in patients with impaired respiratory function.

• Assess the patient for clinical improvement, and record the onset of pain relief. Consult the physician if pain relief is not adequate.

Patient Teaching

• Inform the patient that injection of morphine may cause discomfort.
• Explain that drug dependence and tolerance may occur with prolonged use of high morphine doses.
• Instruct the patient to change positions slowly to avoid orthostatic hypotension.
• Warn the patient to avoid tasks that require mental alertness or motor skills until his or her response to the drug has been established.
• Urge the patient to avoid alcohol and CNS depressants during morphine therapy.

oxycodone

ox-ee-**koe**-done
(Endone[AUS], OxyContin, Oxydose, OxyFast, OxyIR, Oxynorm[AUS], Roxicodone, Roxicodone Intensol)
Do not confuse oxycodone with oxybutynin.

CATEGORY AND SCHEDULE

Pregnancy Risk Category: B (D if used for prolonged periods or at high dosages at term)
Controlled Substance: Schedule II

MECHANISM OF ACTION

An opioid analgesic that binds with opioid receptors in the CNS. **Therapeutic Effect:** Alters the perception of and emotional response to pain.

PHARMACOKINETICS

Route	Onset	Peak	Duration
PO, Immediate-release	N/A	N/A	4–5 hr
PO, Controlled-release	N/A	N/A	12 hr

Moderately absorbed from the GI tract. Protein binding: 38%–45%. Widely distributed. Metabolized in the liver. Excreted in urine. Unknown if removed by hemodialysis. ***Half-life:*** 2–3 hr (3.2 hr controlled-release).

AVAILABILITY

Capsules (Immediate-Release [OxyIR]): 5 mg.
Oral Concentrate (Oxydose, OxyFast, Roxicodone Intensol): 20 mg/ml.
Oral Solution (Roxicodone): 5 mg/5 ml.
Tablets (Roxicodone): 5 mg, 15 mg, 30 mg.
Tablets (Extended-Release [OxyContin]): 10 mg, 20 mg, 40 mg, 80 mg, 160 mg.

INDICATIONS AND DOSAGES

▸ **Analgesia**

PO (Controlled-Release)
Adults, Elderly. Initially, 10 mg q12h. May increase every 1–2 days by 25%–50%. Usual: 40 mg/day (100 mg/day for cancer pain).
PO (Immediate-Release)
Adults, Elderly. Initially, 5 mg q6h as needed. May increase up to 30 mg q4h. Usual: 10–30 mg q4h as needed.
Children. 0.05–0.15 mg/kg/dose q4–6h.

CONTRAINDICATIONS

None known.

INTERACTIONS

Drug

Alcohol, other CNS depressants: May increase CNS or respiratory depression and hypotension.
MAOIs: May produce a severe, sometimes fatal reaction; expect to administer one-quarter of usual oxycodone dose.

Herbal

None known.

Food

None known.

DIAGNOSTIC TEST EFFECTS

May increase serum amylase and lipase levels.

SIDE EFFECTS

Frequent

Somnolence, dizziness, hypotension (including orthostatic hypotension), anorexia

Occasional

Confusion, diaphoresis, facial flushing, urine retention, constipation, dry mouth, nausea, vomiting, headache

Rare

Allergic reaction, depression, paradoxical CNS hyperactivity or nervousness in children, paradoxical excitement and restlessness in elderly or debilitated patients

SERIOUS REACTIONS

! Overdose results in respiratory depression, skeletal muscle flaccidity, cold or clammy skin, cyanosis, and extreme somnolence progressing to seizures, stupor, and coma.
! Hepatotoxicity may occur with overdose of the acetaminophen component of fixed-combination products.
! The patient who uses oxycodone repeatedly may develop a tolerance to the drug's analgesic effect and physical dependence.

NURSING CONSIDERATIONS

Baseline Assessment

- Assess the duration, location, onset, and type of pain.
- Obtain the patient's vital signs before giving oxycodone.
- Withhold the drug and notify the physician if the respiratory rate is 12 breaths/minute or less in an adult or 20 breaths/minute or less in a child.

Lifespan Considerations

- Oxycodone readily crosses the placenta and is distributed in breast milk.
- Regular use of opioids during pregnancy may produce withdrawal symptoms in the neonate, including irritability, diarrhea, excessive crying, fever, hyperactive reflexes, irritability, seizures, sneezing, tremors, vomiting, and yawning.
- The neonate may develop respiratory depression if the mother receives oxycodone during labor.
- Children are more prone to experience paradoxical excitement.
- Children younger than 2 years and the elderly are more susceptible to the drug's respiratory depressant effects.
- Age-related renal impairment may increase the risk of urine retention in the elderly.

Precautions

- Use oxycodone extremely cautiously in patients with acute alcoholism, anoxia, CNS depression, hypercapnia, respiratory depression or dysfunction, seizures, shock, or untreated myxedema.
- Use oxycodone cautiously in patients with acute abdominal conditions, Addison's disease, chronic obstructive pulmonary disease (COPD), hypothyroidism, hepatic impairment, increased intracranial pressure, prostatic hypertrophy, or urethral stricture.

Administration and Handling

◀ALERT▶ Be aware that oxycodone's side effects are dependent on the dosage.

• Know that ambulatory patients and patients not in severe pain are more likely to experience dizziness, hypotension, nausea, and vomiting than those in the supine position or those in severe pain.

PO

• Give oxycodone without regard to food.

• Crush immediate-release tablets as needed.

◀ALERT▶ Have the patient swallow controlled-release tablets (OxyContin) whole because crushing, breaking, or chewing them may lead to the rapid release and absorption of a potentially fatal dose.

Intervention and Evaluation

• Know that oxycodone's effect is reduced if the patient experiences a full pain response before the next dose.

• Monitor the patient's pattern of daily bowel activity and stool consistency, and palpate the patient's bladder for urine retention.

• Monitor the patient's BP, respiratory rate, and mental status.

• Assess the patient for clinical improvement, and record the onset of pain relief.

• Initiate deep-breathing and coughing exercises, particularly in patients with impaired respiratory function.

Patient Teaching

• Instruct the patient not to break, chew, or crush controlled-release tablets (OxyContin).

• Advise the patient to take oxycodone before the pain fully returns, within prescribed intervals.

• Caution the patient that oxycodone may be habit-forming.

◀ALERT▶ Strongly warn the patient that OxyContin has a potential for abuse and that accidental overdose may result in death.

• Inform the patient that oxycodone may cause drowsiness, dizziness, and dry mouth.

• Warn the patient to avoid performing tasks that require mental alertness or motor skills until his or her response to the drug has been established.

• Urge the patient to avoid alcohol while taking oxycodone.

propoxyphene hydrochloride 🏴

pro-**pox**-ih-feen

(Darvon)

propoxyphene napsylate

(Darvon-N[CAN], Doloxene[AUS])

Do not confuse Darvon with Diovan.

CATEGORY AND SCHEDULE

Pregnancy Risk Category: C (D if used for prolonged periods)

Controlled Substance: Schedule IV

MECHANISM OF ACTION

An opioid agonist that binds with opioid receptors in the CNS. **Therapeutic Effect:** Alters the perception of and emotional response to pain.

PHARMACOKINETICS

Route	Onset	Peak	Duration
PO	15–60 min	N/A	4–6 hr

Well absorbed from the GI tract. Protein binding: High. Widely distributed. Metabolized in the liver. Primarily excreted in urine. Not removed by hemodialysis. ***Half-life:*** 6–12 hr; metabolite: 30–36 hr.

AVAILABILITY

Capsules (Hydrochloride): 65 mg.
Tablets (Napsylate): 100 mg.

INDICATIONS AND DOSAGES

Mild to moderate pain

PO (propoxyphene hydrochloride)
Adults, Elderly. 65 mg q4h as needed. Maximum: 390 mg/day.
PO (propoxyphene napsylate)
Adults, Elderly. 100 mg q4h as needed. Maximum: 600 mg/day.

CONTRAINDICATIONS

None known.

INTERACTIONS

Drug

Alcohol, other CNS depressants: May increase CNS or respiratory depression and risk of hypotension.
Buprenorphine: May decrease the effects of propoxyphene.
Carbamazepine: May increase the blood concentration and risk of toxicity of carbamazepine.
MAOIs: May produce a severe, sometimes fatal reaction; plan to administer 25% of usual propoxyphene dose.

Herbal

None known.

Food

None known.

DIAGNOSTIC TEST EFFECTS

May increase serum alkaline phosphatase, lipase, amylase, bilirubin, LDH, AST (SGOT), and ALT (SGPT) levels. Therapeutic serum drug level is 100–400 ng/ml; toxic serum drug level is greater than 500 ng/ml.

SIDE EFFECTS

Frequent

Dizziness, somnolence, dry mouth, euphoria, hypotension (including orthostatic hypotension), nausea, vomiting, fatigue

Occasional

Allergic reaction (including decreased BP), diaphoresis, flushing, and wheezing), trembling, urine retention, vision changes, constipation, headache

Rare

Confusion, increased BP, depression, abdominal cramps, anorexia

SERIOUS REACTIONS

! Overdose results in respiratory depression, skeletal muscle flaccidity, cold or clammy skin, cyanosis, and extreme somnolence progressing to seizures, stupor, and coma.
! Hepatotoxicity may occur with overdose of the acetaminophen component of fixed-combination products.
! The patient who uses propoxyphene repeatedly may develop a tolerance to the drug's analgesic effect and physical dependence.

NURSING CONSIDERATIONS

Baseline Assessment

- Obtain the patient's vital signs before administering propoxyphene.
- Withhold the drug and notify the physician if the respiratory rate is 12 breaths/minute or less in an adult or 20 breaths/minute or less in a child.
- Expect to obtain baseline blood chemistry tests to assess hepatic function.
- Assess the duration, location, onset, and type of pain.

Lifespan Considerations

- Propoxyphene crosses the placenta and a minimal amount of the drug is distributed in breast milk.

• Be aware that regular use of opioids during pregnancy may produce withdrawal symptoms in the neonate, including diarrhea, excessive crying, fever, hyperactive reflexes, irritability, seizures, sneezing, tremors, vomiting, and yawning.
• The neonate may develop respiratory depression if the mother receives propoxyphene during labor.
• The pediatric dosage of this drug has not been established.
• Avoid use in the elderly, if possible. They may be more susceptible to propoxyphene's CNS effects and constipation.

Precautions

• Use propoxyphene cautiously in patients with hepatic or renal impairment and those who are narcotic-dependent.

Administration and Handling

◀ALERT▶ Be aware that propoxyphene's side effects are dependent on the dosage.
• Know that ambulatory patients and patients not in severe pain are more likely to experience dizziness, hypotension, nausea, and vomiting than patients in the supine position and those in severe pain.
◀ALERT▶ Expect to reduce the initial dosage for patients with Addison's disease, hypothyroidism, and renal insufficiency; for debilitated or elderly patients; and for patients concurrently taking CNS depressants.

PO

• Give propoxyphene without regard to food.
• Empty capsules and mix with food as needed.
• Do not crush or break film-coated tablets.

Intervention and Evaluation

• Know that the drug's effect is reduced if the patient experiences a full pain response before the next dose.
• Monitor the patients' pattern of daily bowel activity and stool consistency. Palpate the bladder for urine retention.
• Initiate deep-breathing and coughing exercises, particularly in patients with impaired respiratory function.
• Assess the patient for clinical improvement and record the onset of pain relief. Contact the physician if pain relief is inadequate.
• Know that the therapeutic serum level of propoxyphene is 100 to 400 ng/ml, and the toxic serum level is over 500 ng/ml.

Patient Teaching

• Instruct the patient to take propoxyphene before the pain fully returns, within prescribed intervals.
• Caution the patient not to abruptly discontinue the drug.
• Inform the patient that propoxyphene may be habit-forming.
• Warn the patient to avoid performing tasks that require mental alertness or motor skills until his or her response to the drug has been established.
• Urge the patient to avoid alcohol during propoxyphene therapy.

43 Narcotic Antagonists

naloxone hydrochloride
naltrexone hydrochloride

Uses: Narcotic antagonists are primarily used to reverse the respiratory depression caused by a narcotic overdose. Naloxone is the drug of choice for reversal of respiratory depression. In patients with severe respiratory depression, treatment requires additional measures, including oxygen administration and mechanical ventilation. Naltrexone is used as an adjunct with other interventions to treat alcohol dependence.

Action: By displacing narcotics (opioid agonists) at receptor sites in the CNS, narcotic antagonists prevent or reverse the effects of narcotics on mu receptors. For example, they increase respiration and reverse sedative effects.

COMBINATION PRODUCTS

SUBOXONE: naloxone/buprenorphine (a non-narcotic analgesic) 0.5 mg/2 mg; 2 mg/8 mg.

naloxone hydrochloride

nal-**oks**-one
(Narcan)
Do not confuse naloxone with naltrexone, or Narcan with Norcuron.

CATEGORY AND SCHEDULE

Pregnancy Risk Category: B

MECHANISM OF ACTION

A narcotic antagonist that displaces opioids at opioid-occupied receptor sites in the CNS. **Therapeutic Effect:** Reverses opioid-induced sleep or sedation, increases respiratory rate, raises BP to normal range.

PHARMACOKINETICS

Route	Onset	Peak	Duration
IV	1–2 min	N/A	20–60 min
IM	2–5 min	N/A	20–60 min
Subcutaneous	2–5 min	N/A	20–60 min

Well absorbed after IM or subcutaneous administration. Metabolized in the liver. Primarily excreted in urine. ***Half-life:*** 60-100 min.

AVAILABILITY

Injection: 0.02 mg/ml, 0.4 mg/ml, 1 mg/ml.

INDICATIONS AND DOSAGES

▸ **Opioid toxicity**

IV, IM, Subcutaneous

Adults, Elderly. 0.4–2 mg q2–3min as needed. May repeat q20–60min.

Children 5 yr and older and weighing 22 kg or more. 2 mg/dose; if no response, may repeat q2–3min. May need to repeat q20–60min.

Children younger than 5 yr and weighing less than 22 kg. 0.1 mg/kg;

if no response, repeat q2–3min. May need to repeat q20–60min.

▸ **Postanesthesia narcotic reversal**

IV

Children. 0.01 mg/kg; may repeat q2–3min.

▸ **Neonatal opioid-induced depression**

IV

Neonates. May repeat q2–3min as needed. May need to repeat q1–2h.

OFF-LABEL USES

Treatment of PCP, ethanol ingestion

CONTRAINDICATIONS

Respiratory depression due to non-opioid drugs

INTERACTIONS

Drug

Butorphanol, nalbuphine, opioid agonist analgesics, pentazocine: Reverses the analgesic and adverse effects of these drugs and may precipitate withdrawal symptoms.

Herbal

None known.

Food

None known.

DIAGNOSTIC TEST EFFECTS

None known.

IV INCOMPATIBILITIES

Amphotericin B complex (Abelcet, AmBisome, Amphotec)

IV COMPATIBILITIES

Heparin, ondansetron (Zofran), propofol (Diprivan)

SIDE EFFECTS

None known; little or no pharmacologic effect in absence of narcotics.

SERIOUS REACTIONS

! Too-rapid reversal of narcotic-induced respiratory depression may result in nausea, vomiting, tremors, increased BP, and tachycardia.

! Excessive dosage in postoperative patients may produce significant excitement, tremors, and reversal of analgesia.

! Patients with cardiovascular disease may experience hypotension or hypertension, ventricular tachycardia and fibrillation, and pulmonary edema.

NURSING CONSIDERATIONS

Baseline Assessment

- Establish and maintain the patient's airway.
- Obtain the body weight of pediatric patients to calculate the drug dosage.

Lifespan Considerations

- It is unknown if naloxone crosses the placenta or is distributed in breast milk.
- No age-related precautions have been noted in children or the elderly.

Precautions

- Use naloxone cautiously in patients with chronic cardiovascular or pulmonary disease, postoperative patients (to avoid cardiovascular complications), and patients suspected of being opioid dependent.

Administration and Handling

◂ **ALERT** ▸ The American Academy of Pediatrics recommends an initial dose of 0.1 mg/kg for infants and children younger than 5 years and weighing less than 20 kg, and an initial dose of 2 mg for children 5 years and older and weighing more than 20 kg.

IV

- Store the parenteral form at room temperature, and protect it from light.
- The reconstituted solution remains stable in D_5W or 0.9% NaCl at 4 mcg/ml for 24 hours. Discard any unused solution.

• For IV injection, dilute 1 mg/ml with 50 ml sterile water for injection to provide a concentration of 0.02 mg/ml.
• For continuous IV infusion, dilute each 2 mg of naloxone with 500 ml D_5W or 0.9% NaCl to provide a concentration of 0.004 mg/ml.
• Naloxone may also be administered undiluted.
• Give each 0.4 mg as IV push over 15 seconds.
• Use the 0.4-mg/ml and 1-mg/ml vials for adults and the 0.02-mg/ml concentration for neonates.
IM
• Inject naloxone in a large muscle mass.

Intervention and Evaluation

• Monitor the patient's vital signs, especially respiratory rate, depth, and rhythm, during and frequently after administration.
• Continue to monitor the patient even after a satisfactory response has been achieved. If the duration of action of the opioid exceeds that of naloxone, respiratory depression may recur.
• Assess the patient for increased pain with reversal of the opioid.

Patient Teaching

• Instruct the patient to let you know if he or she experiences pain or increased sedation.

naltrexone hydrochloride

nal-**trex**-one
(Revia)

CATEGORY AND SCHEDULE

Pregnancy Risk Category: C

MECHANISM OF ACTION

A narcotic antagonist that displaces opioids at opioid-occupied receptor sites in the CNS. **Therapeutic Effect:** Blocks physical effects of opioid analgesics; decreases craving for alcohol and relapse rate in alcoholism.

AVAILABILITY

Tablets: 50 mg.

INDICATIONS AND DOSAGES

▸ **Naloxone challenge test to determine if patient is opioid dependent**

◂**ALERT**▸ Expect to perform the naloxone challenge test if there is any question that the patient is opioid dependent. Don't administer naltrexone until the naloxone challenge test is negative.

IV

Adults, Elderly. Draw 2 ml (0.8 mg) of naloxone into syringe. Inject 0.5 ml (0.2 mg); while needle is still in vein, observe patient for 30 sec for withdrawal signs or symptoms. If no evidence of withdrawal, inject remaining 1.5 ml (0.6 mg); observe patient for additional 20 min for withdrawal signs or symptoms.

Subcutaneous

Adults, Elderly. Inject 2 ml (0.8 mg) of naloxone; observe patient for 45 min for withdrawal signs or symptoms.

▸ **Treatment of opioid dependence in patients who have been opioid free for at least 7-10 days**

PO

Adults, Elderly. Initially, 25 mg. Observe patient for 1 hr. If no withdrawal signs or symptoms appear, give another 25 mg. May be given as 100 mg every other day or 150 mg every 3 days.

▸ Adjunctive treatment of alcohol dependence
PO
Adults, Elderly. 50 mg once a day.

OFF-LABEL USES
Treatment of eating disorders, post-concussional syndrome unresponsive to other treatments

CONTRAINDICATIONS
Acute hepatitis, acute opioid withdrawal, failed naloxone challenge test, hepatic failure, history of hypersensitivity to naltrexone, opioid dependence, positive urine screen for opioids

INTERACTIONS
Drug
Opioid-containing products (including analgesics, antidiarrheals, and antitussives): Blocks the therapeutic effects of these drugs.
Thioridazine: May produce lethargy and somnolence.
Herbal
None known.
Food
None known.

DIAGNOSTIC TEST EFFECTS
May increase AST (SGOT) and ALT (SGPT) levels.

SIDE EFFECTS
Frequent
Alcoholism (10%–7%): Nausea, headache, depression
Narcotic addiction (10%–5%): Insomnia, anxiety, nervousness, headache, low energy, abdominal cramps, nausea, vomiting, arthralgia, myalgia
Occasional
Alcoholism (4%–2%): Dizziness, nervousness, fatigue, insomnia, vomiting, anxiety, suicidal ideation
Narcotic addiction (5%–2%): Irritability, increased energy, dizziness, anorexia, diarrhea or constipation, rash, chills, increased thirst

SERIOUS REACTIONS
! Signs and symptoms of opioid withdrawal include stuffy or runny nose, tearing, yawning, diaphoresis, tremor, vomiting, piloerection, feeling of temperature change, bone pain, arthralgia, myalgia, abdominal cramps, and feeling of skin crawling.
! Accidental naltrexone overdose produces withdrawal symptoms within 5 minutes of ingestion that may last for up to 48 hours. Symptoms include confusion, visual hallucinations, somnolence, and significant vomiting and diarrhea.
! Hepatocellular injury may occur with large doses.

NURSING CONSIDERATIONS
Baseline Assessment
- Perform a naloxone challenge test on the patient if there is any question of opioid dependence.
- Establish the patient's medication history, especially opioid use, and other medical conditions, including hepatitis or other hepatic disease.
- Plan to perform baseline laboratory tests, including creatinine clearance, serum bilirubin, AST (SGOT), and ALT (SGPT) levels.

Precautions
- Use naltrexone cautiously in patients with active hepatic disease.

Administration and Handling
PO
- Give naltrexone with antacids, after meals, or with food to avoid adverse GI effects.

Intervention and Evaluation
- Assess liver function test results and monitor the patient closely for evidence of hepatotoxicity.
- Monitor the patient's creatinine

clearance, serum bilirubin, AST (SGOT), and ALT (SGPT) levels.

Patient Teaching

• Instruct the patient to take naltrexone tablets with antacids, after meals, or with food to avoid GI upset.

• Inform the patient that any opioid-containing drugs used during naltrexone therapy will have no effect. Stress that any attempt to overcome naltrexone's prolonged 24- to 72-hour blockade of opioid effects by taking large amount of opioids may result in coma, serious injury, or death.

• Warn the patient to notify the physician if he or she experiences abdominal pain that lasts longer than 3 days, dark urine, white stools, or yellowing of the whites of the eyes.

• Refer the patient to an alcohol or drug rehab center.

44 Non-Narcotic Analgesics

acetaminophen
aspirin (acetylsalicylic acid, ASA)
diflunisal
salsalate
tramadol hydrochloride

Uses: Non-narcotic analgesics are used to relieve mild to moderate pain. Acetaminophen and salicylates, such as aspirin, also have anti-inflammatory and antipyretic effects. By virtue of its action on platelet function, aspirin is also used to prevent and treat diseases associated with hypercoagulability and to reduce the risk of stroke and MI.

Actions: Different nonnarcotic analgesics act in distinct ways. For example, *acetaminophen* may act by inhibiting prostaglandin synthesis in the CNS; *salicylates*, such as aspirin, inhibit cyclooxygenase, thereby inhibiting prostaglandin synthesis in the CNS and periphery.

COMBINATION PRODUCTS

AGGRENOX: aspirin/dipyridamole (an antiplatelet agent) 25 mg/200 mg.
ANEXSIA: acetaminophen/hydrocodone (a narcotic analgesic) 500 mg/5 mg; 650 mg/7.5 mg; 650 mg/10 mg.
CAPITAL WITH CODEINE: acetaminophen/codeine (a narcotic analgesic) 120 mg/12 mg per 5 ml.
DARVOCET A 500: acetaminophen/propoxyphene (a narcotic analgesic) 500 mg/100 mg.
DARVOCET-N: acetaminophen/propoxyphene (a narcotic analgesic) 325 mg/50 mg; 650 mg/100 mg.
DUOCET: acetaminophen/hydrocodone (a narcotic analgesic) 500 mg/5 mg.
FIORICET: acetaminophen/caffeine (a CNS stimulant)/butabarbital (a sedative-hypnotic) 325 mg/40 mg/50 mg.
FIORINAL: aspirin/butabarbital (a sedative-hypnotic)/caffeine (a CNS stimulant) 325 mg/50 mg/40 mg.
LORCET: acetaminophen/hydrocodone (a narcotic analgesic) 650 mg/7.5 mg, 650 mg/10 mg.
LORTAB: acetaminophen/hydrocodone (a narcotic analgesic) 500 mg/2.5 mg; 500 mg/5 mg; 500 mg/7.5 mg, 500 mg/10 mg.
LORTAB/ASA: aspirin/hydrocodone (a narcotic analgesic) 500 mg/5 mg.
LORTAB ELIXIR: acetaminophen/hydrocodone (a narcotic analgesic) 167 mg/2.5 mg per 5 ml.
NORCO: acetaminophen/hydrocodone (a narcotic analgesic) 325 mg/10 mg.
PERCOCET: acetaminophen/oxycodone (a narcotic analgesic) 325 mg/5 mg.
PERCODAN: aspirin/oxycodone (a narcotic analgesic) 325 mg/2.25 mg; 325 mg/4.5 mg.
PRAVIGARD: aspirin/pravastatin (an antihyperlipidemic) 81 mg/20 mg; 325 mg/20 mg; 81 mg/40 mg; 325 mg/40 mg; 81 mg/80 mg; 325 mg/80 mg.
ROXICET: acetaminophen/oxycodone (a narcotic analgesic) 325 mg/5 mg.
TYLENOL WITH CODEINE: acetaminophen/codeine (a narcotic analgesic) 120 mg/12 mg per 5 ml; 300 mg/15 mg; 300 mg/30 mg; 300 mg/60 mg.
TYLOX: acetaminophen/oxycodone (a narcotic analgesic) 500 mg/5 mg.

ULTRACET: acetaminophen/tramadol (a nonnarcotic analgesic) 325 mg/ 37.5 mg.
VICODIN: acetaminophen/ hydrocodone (a narcotic analgesic) 500 mg/5 mg.
VICODIN ES: acetaminophen/ hydrocodone (a narcotic analgesic) 750 mg/7.5 mg.
VICODIN HP: acetaminophen/ hydrocodone (a narcotic analgesic) 650 mg/10 mg.
ZYDONE: acetaminophen/hydrocodone (a narcotic analgesic) 400 mg/5 mg; 400 mg/7.5 mg; 400 mg/10 mg.

acetaminophen

ah-**seet**-ah-min-oh-fen
(Abenol[CAN], Apo-Acetaminophen[CAN], Atasol[CAN], Dymadon[AUS], Feverall, Panadol[AUS], Panamax[AUS], Paralgin [AUS], Setamol[AUS], Tempra, Tylenol)
Do not confuse Feverall with Fiorinal, Hycodan, Indocin, Percodan, or Tuinal.

CATEGORY AND SCHEDULE

Pregnancy Risk Category: B
OTC

MECHANISM OF ACTION

A central analgesic whose exact mechanism is unknown, but appears to inhibit prostaglandin synthesis in the CNS and, to a lesser extent, block pain impulses through peripheral action. Acetaminophen acts centrally on hypothalamic heat-regulating center, producing peripheral vasodilation (heat loss, skin erythema, sweating). **Therapeutic Effect:** Results in antipyresis. Produces analgesic effect. Results in antipyresis.

PHARMACOKINETICS

Route	Onset	Peak	Duration
PO	15–30 min	1–1.5 hr	4–6 hr

Rapidly, completely absorbed from the GI tract; rectal absorption variable. Protein binding: 20%–50%. Widely distributed to most body tissues. Metabolized in the liver; excreted in urine. Removed by hemodialysis. ***Half-life:*** 1–4 hr (half-life is increased in those with liver disease, elderly, neonates; decreased in children).

AVAILABILITY

Caplets (Genapap, Tylenol): 500 mg.
Caplets (Extended-Release [Mapap, Tylenol Arthritis Pain]): 650 mg.
Capsules (Mapap): 500 mg.
Elixir: 160 mg/5 ml.
Oral Liquid (Tylenol Extra Strength): 500 mg/15 ml.
Solution (Oral Drops [Tylenol]): 80 mg/0.8 ml.
Suppositories, Rectal (Feverall): 80 mg
Suppositories (Acephen, Feverall): 120 mg, 325 mg, 650 mg.
Tablets (Genapap, Mapap, Tylenol): 325 mg, 500 mg.
Tablets (Chewable [Genapap, Mapap, Tylenol]): 80 mg.

INDICATIONS AND DOSAGES

▸ **Analgesia and antipyresis**

PO

Adults, Elderly. 325-650 mg q4–6h or 1 g 3–4 times a day. Maximum: 4 g/day.
Children. 10–15 mg/kg/dose q4–6h as needed. Maximum: 5 doses/24 hr.
Neonates. 10–15 mg/kg/dose q6–8h as needed.

Rectal

Adults. 650 mg q4–6h. Maximum: 6 doses/24 hr.

Children. 10–20 mg/kg/dose q4–6h as needed.
Neonates. 10–15 mg/kg/dose q6–8h as needed.

▸ **Dosage in renal impairment**

Creatinine Clearance	Frequency
10–50 ml/min	q6h
less than 10 ml/min	q8h

CONTRAINDICATIONS

Active alcoholism, liver disease, or viral hepatitis, all of which increase the risk of hepatotoxicity

INTERACTIONS

Drug

Alcohol (chronic use), hepatotoxic medications (e.g., phenytoin), liver enzyme inducers (e.g., cimetidine): May increase risk of hepatotoxicity with prolonged high dose or single toxic dose.
Warfarin: May increase the risk of bleeding with regular use.

Herbal

None known.

Food

None known.

DIAGNOSTIC TEST EFFECTS

May increase serum bilirubin, prothrombin time (may indicate hepatotoxicity), AST (SGOT), and ALT (SGPT). Therapeutic serum level: 10–30 mcg/ml; toxic serum level: greater than 200 mcg/ml.

SIDE EFFECTS

Rare

Hypersensitivity reaction

SERIOUS REACTIONS

! Acetaminophen toxicity is the primary serious reaction.
! Early signs and symptoms of acetaminophen toxicity include anorexia, nausea, diaphoresis, and generalized weakness within the first 12 to 24 hr.
! Later signs of acetaminophen toxicity include vomiting, right upper quadrant tenderness, and elevated liver function tests within 48 to 72 hr after ingestion.
! The antidote to acetaminophen toxicity is acetylcysteine.

NURSING CONSIDERATIONS

Baseline Assessment

- Assess onset, type, location, and duration of pain before acetaminophen is given for analgesia. The effect of the medication is reduced if full pain response recurs before the next dose.
- Expect to obtain the patient's vital signs before giving any of acetaminophen's fixed combinations. If respirations are 12 per minute or lower (20 per minute or lower in children), withhold the medication and contact the physician.

Lifespan Considerations

- Acetaminophen crosses the placenta and is distributed in breast milk.
- Acetaminophen is routinely used in all stages of pregnancy and appears safe for short-term use.
- There are no age-related precautions noted in children or the elderly.

◂ **ALERT** ▸ Children may receive repeat doses 4 to 5 times a day to a maximum of 5 doses in 24 hours.

Precautions

- Use cautiously in patients with G6PD deficiency, phenylketonuria, sensitivity to acetaminophen, or severe impaired renal function.

Administration and Handling

PO

- Give without regard to meals.
- Tablets may be crushed.

Rectal
- Moisten suppository with cold water before inserting well up into the rectum.

Intervention and Evaluation
- Assess for clinical improvement and relief of pain or fever.
- Monitor serum levels. A therapeutic serum level is 10 to 30 mcg/ml and a toxic serum level is greater than 200 mcg/ml.

Patient Teaching
- Caution the patient to consult with the physician before using acetaminophen in children under 2 years of age; oral use for more than 5 days in children, more than 10 days in adults, or fever lasting more than 3 days. Monitor patient for severe or recurrent pain or high, continuous fever, which may indicate a serious illness.

aspirin (acetylsalicylic acid, ASA)

as-pir-in
(Ascriptin, Aspro[AUS], Bayer, Bex[AUS], Bufferin, Disprin[AUS], Ecotrin, Entrophen[CAN], Halfprin, Novasen[CAN], Solprin[AUS], Spren[AUS])
Do not confuse aspirin or Ascriptin with Aricept, Afrin, or Asendin; or Ecotrin with Edecrin.

CATEGORY AND SCHEDULE

Pregnancy Risk Category: C (D if full dose used in third trimester of pregnancy)
OTC

MECHANISM OF ACTION

A nonsteroidal salicylate that inhibits prostaglandin synthesis, acts on the hypothalamus heat-regulating center, and interferes with the production of thromboxane A, a substance that stimulates platelet aggregation. **Therapeutic Effect:** Reduces inflammatory response and intensity of pain; decreases fever; inhibits platelet aggregation.

PHARMACOKINETICS

Route	Onset	Peak	Duration
PO	1 hr	2–4 hr	24 hr

Rapidly and completely absorbed from GI tract; enteric-coated absorption delayed; rectal absorption delayed and incomplete. Protein binding: High. Widely distributed. Rapidly hydrolyzed to salicylate. ***Half-life:*** 15–20 min (aspirin); 2–3 hr (salicylate at low dose); more than 20 hr (salicylate at high dose).

AVAILABILITY

Tablets (Bayer): 325 mg, 500 mg.
Tablets (Chewable [Bayer and St. Joseph]): 81 mg.
Tablets (Enteric-Coated [Bayer, Ecotrin, St. Joseph]): 81 mg, 325 mg, 500 mg, 650 mg.
Tablets (Hafprin): 162 mg.
Caplets (Bayer): 81 mg, 325 mg, 500 mg.
Gelcap (Bayer): 325 mg, 500 mg.
Suppositories: 60 mg, 120 mg, 125 mg, 200 mg, 325 mg, 600 mg, 650 mg.

INDICATIONS AND DOSAGES

▸ **Analgesia, fever**

PO, Rectal
Adults, Elderly. 325–1,000 mg q4–6h
Children. 10–15 mg/kg/dose q4–6h. Maximum: 4 g/day.

Anti-inflammatory
PO
Adults, Elderly. Initially, 2.4–3.6 g/day in divided doses; then 3.6–5.4 g/day.
Children. Initially, 60–90 mg/kg/day in divided doses; then 80–100 mg/kg/day.

Suspected MI
PO
Adults, Elderly. 162 mg as soon as the MI is suspected, then daily for 30 days after the MI.

Prevention of MI
PO
Adults, Elderly. 75–325 mg/day.

Prevention of stroke after transient ischemic attack
PO
Adults, Elderly. 50–325 mg/day.

Kawasaki disease
PO
Children. 80–100 mg/kg/day in divided doses.

OFF-LABEL USES

Prevention of thromboembolism, treatment of Kawasaki disease

CONTRAINDICATIONS

Allergy to tartrazine dye, bleeding disorders, chickenpox or flu in children and teenagers, GI bleeding or ulceration, hepatic impairment, history of hypersensitivity to aspirin or NSAIDs

INTERACTIONS

Drug

Alcohol, NSAIDs: May increase the risk of adverse GI effects, including ulceration.
Antacids, urinary alkalinizers: Increase the excretion of aspirin.
Anticoagulants, heparin, thrombolytics: Increase the risk of bleeding.
Insulin, oral antidiabetics: May increase the effects of these drugs (with large doses of aspirin).
Methotrexate, zidovudine: May increase the risk of toxicity of these drugs.
Ototoxic medications, vancomycin: May increase the risk of ototoxicity.
Platelet aggregation inhibitors, valproic acid: May increase the risk of bleeding.
Probenecid, sulfinpyrazone: May decrease the effects of these drugs.

Herbal

None known.

Food

None known.

DIAGNOSTIC TEST EFFECTS

May alter serum alkaline phosphatase, uric acid, AST (SGOT), and ALT (SGPT) levels. May prolong PT and bleeding time. May decrease serum cholesterol, serum potassium, and T_3 and T_4 levels.

SIDE EFFECTS

Occasional

GI distress (including abdominal distention, cramping, heartburn, and mild nausea); allergic reaction (including bronchospasm, pruritus, and urticaria)

SERIOUS REACTIONS

! High doses of aspirin may produce GI bleeding and gastric mucosal lesions.
! Dehydrated, febrile children may experience aspirin toxicity quickly. Reye's syndrome may occur in children with the chickenpox or the flu.
! Low-grade toxicity characterized is by tinnitus, generalized pruritus (possibly severe), headache, dizziness, flushing, tachycardia, hyperventilation, diaphoresis, and thirst.

! Market toxicity is characterized by hyperthermia, restlessness, seizures, abnormal breathing patterns, respiratory failure, and coma.

NURSING CONSIDERATIONS

Baseline Assessment

- Assess the duration, location, and type of inflammation or pain.
- Inspect the arthritic patient's affected joints for deformities, immobility, and skin condition.
- The therapeutic serum aspirin level for antiarthritic effect is 20 to 30 mg/dl. The toxic serum level is over 30 mg/dl.

Lifespan Considerations

- Aspirin readily crosses the placenta and is distributed in breast milk.
- Pregnant women should not take aspirin during the last trimester of pregnancy because the drug may prolong gestation and labor and cause adverse effects in the fetus such as premature closure of the ductus arteriosus, low birth weight, hemorrhage, stillbirth, and death.
- Use caution in giving aspirin to children with acute febrile illness. Don't give aspirin to children with chickenpox or the flu because this increases their risk of developing Reye's syndrome.
- Lower aspirin dosages are recommended for the elderly because they're more susceptible to aspirin toxicity.

Precautions

- Use aspirin cautiously in patients with chronic renal insufficiency, vitamin K deficiency, or the "aspirin triad" of asthma, nasal polyps, and rhinitis.

Administration and Handling

PO

- Don't give aspirin to children or teenagers with chickenpox or the flu because this increases their risk of developing Reye's syndrome.
- Do not use aspirin that smells of vinegar because this odor indicates chemical breakdown of the drug.
- Don't crush or break enteric-coated tablets.
- Give aspirin with water, milk, or meals if GI distress occurs.

Rectal

- Refrigerate suppositories.
- If the suppository is too soft, refrigerate it for 30 minutes or run cold water over the foil wrapper.
- Moisten the suppository with cold water before inserting it well into the rectum.

Intervention and Evaluation

- Monitor the patient's urine pH for signs of sudden acidification, indicated by a pH of 6.5 to 5.5. Sudden acidification may cause the serum salicylate level to greatly increase, leading to toxicity.
- Assess the patient's skin for evidence of ecchymosis.
- If aspirin is given as an antipyretic, take the patient's temperature just before and 1 hour after giving the drug.
- Evaluate the arthritic patient for a therapeutic response to the drug such as improved grip strength, increased joint mobility, reduced joint tenderness, and relief of pain, stiffness, and swelling.

Patient Teaching

◀ **ALERT** ▶ Explain to the patient and family that behavioral changes and vomiting may be early signs of Reye's syndrome. If these occur, urge them to contact the physician at once.

- Instruct the patient not to crush or chew enteric-coated tablets.
- Caution the patient to report ringing in the ears (tinnitus) or persistent abdominal or GI pain to the physician.

• Inform the patient that aspirin's anti-inflammatory effect should occur within 1 to 3 weeks.
• Because of the increased risk of GI bleeding, advise the patient to avoid taking NSAIDs and drinking alcohol while taking aspirin.

diflunisal

dye-**floo**-ni-sal
(Apo-Diflunisal[CAN], Dolobid, Novo-Diflunisal[CAN])
Do not confuse diflunisal with Dicarbosil, or Dolobid with Slo-bid.

CATEGORY AND SCHEDULE

Pregnancy Risk Category: C (D if used in third trimester or near delivery)

MECHANISM OF ACTION

A nonsteroidal anti-inflammatory that inhibits prostaglandin synthesis, reducing inflammatory response and intensity of pain stimulus reaching sensory nerve endings. **Therapeutic Effect:** Produces analgesic and anti-inflammatory effect.

PHARMACOKINETICS

Route	Onset	Peak	Duration
PO	1 hr	2–3 hr	8–12 hr

Completely absorbed from the GI tract. Widely distributed. Protein binding: greater than 99%. Metabolized in liver. Primarily excreted in urine. Not removed by hemodialysis. ***Half-life:*** 8–12 hr.

AVAILABILITY

Tablets: 250 mg, 500 mg.

INDICATIONS AND DOSAGES

▸ **Mild to moderate pain**
PO
Adults, Elderly. Initially, 0.5–1 g, then 250–500 mg q8-12h. Maximum: 1.5 g/day.

▸ **Rheumatoid arthritis, osteoarthritis**
PO
Adults, Elderly. 0.5–1 g/day in 2 divided doses. Maximum: 1.5 g/day.

OFF-LABEL USES

Treatment of psoriatic arthritis, vascular headache

CONTRAINDICATIONS

Active GI bleeding, factor VII or factor IX deficiencies, hypersensitivity to aspirin or NSAIDs

INTERACTIONS

Drug

Antihypertensives, diuretics: May decrease the effects of these drugs.
Aspirin, salicylates: May increase the risk of GI bleeding and side effects.
Bone marrow depressants: May increase the risk of hematologic reactions.
Heparin, oral anticoagulants, thrombolytics: May increase the effects of these drugs.
Lithium: May increase the blood concentration and risk of toxicity of lithium.
Methotrexate: May increase the risk of toxicity of methotrexate.
Probenecid: May increase diflunisal blood concentration.

Herbal

Ginkgo biloba: May increase the risk of bleeding.

Food

None known.

DIAGNOSTIC TEST EFFECTS

May increase serum AST (SGOT) and ALT (SGPT) levels. May decrease serum uric acid levels.

SIDE EFFECTS

Side effects are less common with short-term treatment.

Occasional (9%–3%)

Nausea, dyspepsia (heartburn, indigestion, epigastric pain), diarrhea, headache, rash

Rare (3%–1%)

Vomiting, constipation, flatulence, dizziness, somnolence, insomnia, fatigue, tinnitus

SERIOUS REACTIONS

! Overdosage may produce drowsiness, vomiting, nausea, diarrhea, hyperventilation, tachycardia, diaphoresis, stupor, and coma.

! Peptic ulcer, GI bleeding, gastritis, and severe hepatic reaction, including cholestasis and jaundice, occur rarely.

! Nephrotoxicity, including dysuria, hematuria, proteinuria, and nephrotic syndrome, and severe hypersensitivity reaction, marked by bronchospasm and angioedema, occur rarely.

NURSING CONSIDERATIONS

Baseline Assessment

- Assess the duration, location, onset, and type of inflammation or pain.
- Inspect the arthritic patient's affected joints for deformities, immobility, and skin condition.
- Plan to obtain baseline laboratory tests, including PT, aPTT, renal and liver function studies, and CBC.

Lifespan Considerations

- Be aware that diflunisal crosses the placenta and is distributed in breast milk. Avoid diflunisal use during the last trimester of pregnancy as the drug may adversely affect the fetal cardiovascular system, causing premature closure of ductus arteriosus.
- Be aware that the safety and efficacy of this drug have not been established in children.
- In the elderly, GI bleeding or ulceration is more likely to cause serious adverse effects.
- In the elderly, age-related renal impairment may increase risk of liver or renal toxicity; a decreased drug dosage is recommended.

Precautions

- Use cautiously in patients with edema, elevated liver function tests, erosive gastritis, impaired renal or liver function, peptic ulcer disease, platelet and bleeding disorders, and vitamin K deficiency.

Administration and Handling

PO

- May give diflunisal with meals, milk, or water.
- Don't crush or break film-coated tablets.

Intervention and Evaluation

- Monitor the patient for dyspepsia and nausea.
- Assess the patient's skin for evidence of rash.
- Assess the patient's pattern of daily bowel activity and stool consistency.
- Evaluate the patient for therapeutic response, improved grip strength, increased joint mobility, reduced joint tenderness, and relief of pain, stiffness, and swelling.

Patient Teaching

- Instruct the patient to swallow tablets whole; do not chew or crush.
- Teach the patient that if he or she experiences GI upset, he or she may take diflunisal with food or milk.
- Warn the patient to notify the physician if he or she experiences GI distress, headache, or rash.

• Tell the patient to inform the physician if she suspects pregnancy, or plans to become pregnant.

salsalate

sal-sa-late
(Amigesic, Disalcid, Mono-Gesic, Salflex)

CATEGORY AND SCHEDULE

Pregnancy Risk Category: C

MECHANISM OF ACTION

An NSAID that inhibits prostaglandin synthesis, reducing the inflammatory response and the intensity of pain stimuli reaching the sensory nerve endings. **Therapeutic Effect:** Produces analgesic and anti-inflammatory effects.

AVAILABILITY

Tablets (Amigesic, Disalcid): 500 mg, 750 mg.
Tablets (Mono-Gesic, Slaflex): 750 mg.

INDICATIONS AND DOSAGES

▸ **Rheumatoid arthritis, osteoarthritis pain**

PO

Adults, Elderly. Initially, 3 g/day in 2–3 divided doses. Maintenance: 2–4 g/day.

CONTRAINDICATIONS

Bleeding disorders, hypersensitivity to salicylates or NSAIDs

INTERACTIONS

Drug

Alcohol, NSAIDs: May increase the risk of GI effects, such as ulceration.
Antacids, urinary alkalinizers: Increase the excretion of salsalate.
Anticoagulants, heparin, thrombolytics: Increase the risk of bleeding.
Insulin, oral antidiabetics: May increase the effects of these drugs (with large doses of salsalate).
Methotrexate, zidovudine: May increase the toxicity of these drugs.
Ototoxic medications, vancomycin: May increase the risk of ototoxicity.
Platelet aggregation inhibitors, valproic acid: May increase the risk of bleeding.
Probenecid, sulfinpyrazone: May decrease the effects of these drugs.

Herbal

Ginkgo biloba: May increase the risk of bleeding.

Food

None known.

DIAGNOSTIC TEST EFFECTS

May alter serum alkaline phosphatase, uric acid, AST (SGOT), and ALT (SGPT) levels. May prolong PT and bleeding time. May decrease serum cholesterol, potassium, T_3, and T_4 levels.

SIDE EFFECTS

Occasional

Nausea, dyspepsia (including heartburn, indigestion, and epigastric pain)

SERIOUS REACTIONS

! Tinnitus may be the first indication that the serum salicylic acid concentration is reaching or exceeding the upper therapeutic range.
! Salsalate use may also produce vertigo, headache, confusion, drowsiness, diaphoresis, hyperventilation, vomiting, and diarrhea.
! Reye's syndrome may occur in children with chickenpox or the flu.
! Severe overdose may result in electrolyte imbalance, hyperthermia,

dehydration, and blood pH imbalance.

! GI bleeding, peptic ulcer, and Reye's syndrome rarely occur.

NURSING CONSIDERATIONS

Baseline Assessment

- Assess the duration, location, onset, and type of inflammation or pain.
- Inspect the arthritic patient's affected joints for deformities, immobility, and skin condition.
- Expect to obtain baseline liver function and coagulation studies.

Precautions

- Use salsalate cautiously in patients with asthma, bleeding disorders, gastritis, history of gastric irritation, hepatic or renal impairment, peptic ulcer disease, or platelet disorders.

Administration and Handling

- Don't give salsalate to children or teenagers with chickenpox or the flu because this increases their risk of developing Reye's syndrome.

PO

- To minimize GI discomfort, administer the drug with food.

Intervention and Evaluation

- Assess the patient for dyspepsia and nausea.
- Evaluate the arthritic patient for evidence of a therapeutic response, such as improved grip strength, increased joint mobility, reduced joint tenderness, and relief of pain, stiffness, and swelling.

Patient Teaching

- Instruct the patient to take salsalate with food and to use antacids to relieve stomach upset.
- Urge the patient to notify the physician if he or she experiences persistent GI pain or ringing in the ears.
- Urge the patient to avoid alcohol and and NSAIDs during salsalate therapy.
- Instruct the patient to report if he or she experiences behavioral changes or vomiting as these symptoms may be early signs of developing Reye's syndrome.

tramadol hydrochloride

tray-mah-doal

(Tramal[AUS], Tramal SR[AUS], Ultram, Zydol[AUS])

Do not confuse tramadol with Toradol, or Ultram with Ultane.

CATEGORY AND SCHEDULE

Pregnancy Risk Category: C

MECHANISM OF ACTION

An analgesic that binds to mu-opioid receptors and inhibits reuptake of norepinephrine and serotonin. Reduces the intensity of pain stimuli reaching sensory nerve endings. **Therapeutic Effect:** Alters the perception of and emotional response to pain.

PHARMACOKINETICS

Route	Onset	Peak	Duration
PO	less than 1 hr	2–3 hr	4–6 hr

Rapidly and almost completely absorbed after PO administration. Protein binding: 20%. Extensively metabolized in the liver to active metabolite (reduced in patients with advanced cirrhosis). Primarily excreted in urine. Minimally removed by hemodialysis. ***Half-life:*** 6–7 hr.

AVAILABILITY

Tablets: 50 mg.

INDICATIONS AND DOSAGES

▸ **Moderate to moderately severe pain**

PO

Adults, Elderly. 50–100 mg q4–6h. Maximum: 400 mg/day for patients 75 yr and younger; 300 mg/day for patients older than 75 yr.

▸ **Dosage in renal impairment**

For patients with creatinine clearance of less than 30 ml/min, increase dosing interval to q12h. Maximum: 200 mg/day.

▸ **Dosage in hepatic impairment**

Dosage is decreased to 50 mg q12h.

CONTRAINDICATIONS

Acute alcohol intoxication; concurrent use of centrally acting analgesics, hypnotics, opioids, or psychotropic drugs

INTERACTIONS

Drug

Alcohol, other CNS depressants: May increase CNS or respiratory depression and hypotension.

Carbamazepine: Decreases tramadol blood concentration.

MAOIs: Increase tramadol blood concentration.

Herbal

None known.

Food

None known.

DIAGNOSTIC TEST EFFECTS

May increase serum creatinine, AST (SGOT), and ALT (SGPT) hepatic levels. May decrease blood Hgb level. May cause proteinuria.

SIDE EFFECTS

Frequent (25%–15%)

Dizziness or vertigo, nausea, constipation, headache, somnolence

Occasional (10%–5%)

Vomiting, pruritus, CNS stimulation (such as nervousness, anxiety, agitation, tremor, euphoria, mood swings, and hallucinations), asthenia, diaphoresis, dyspepsia, dry mouth, diarrhea

Rare (less than 5%)

Malaise, vasodilation, anorexia, flatulence, rash, blurred vision, urine retention or urinary frequency, menopausal symptoms

SERIOUS REACTIONS

! Overdose results in respiratory depression and seizures.

! Tramadol may have a prolonged duration of action and cumulative effect in patients with hepatic or renal impairment.

NURSING CONSIDERATIONS

Baseline Assessment

• Assess the duration, location, onset, and type of pain.

• Determine the patient's medication history, especially the use of carbamazepine, CNS depressants, and MAOIs. Review the patient's medical history, especially for seizures.

• Obtain a CBC and liver and renal function studies.

Lifespan Considerations

• Tramadol crosses the placenta and is distributed in breast milk.

• The safety and efficacy of tramadol have not been established in children.

• Age-related renal impairment may require a dosage adjustment in the elderly.

Precautions

• Use tramadol extremely cautiously in patients with acute alcoholism, advanced cirrhosis, anoxia, CNS depression, epilepsy, respiratory depression, or shock.

• Use the drug cautiously in patients with acute abdominal conditions, hepatic or renal impairment, increased intracranial pressure, opioid dependence, or a sensitivity to opioids.

Administration and Handling

◀ALERT▶ Be aware that dialysis patients can receive their regular dose on the day of dialysis.

PO

• Give tramadol without regard to food.

Intervention and Evaluation

• Know that tramadol's analgesic effect is reduced if the patient experiences full pain before the next dose.
• Monitor the patient's BP and pulse rate.
• Assist the patient with ambulation if he or she experiences dizziness or vertigo.
• Offer the patient cola and dry crackers to relieve nausea and sips of tepid water to relieve dry mouth.
• Assess the patient's pattern of daily bowel activity and stool consistency.
• Palpate the patient's bladder for urine retention.
• Assess the patient for clinical improvement, and record the onset of pain relief.

Patient Teaching

• Caution the patient that tramadol use may cause dependence.
• Urge the patient to avoid alcohol and OTC drugs such as analgesics and sedatives during tramadol therapy.
• Inform the patient that tramadol may cause blurred vision, dizziness, and drowsiness. Warn the patient to avoid tasks requiring mental alertness or motor skills until his or her reaction to the drug has been established.
• Instruct the patient to notify the physician about chest pain, difficulty breathing, excessive sedation, muscle weakness, palpitations, seizures, severe constipation, or tremors.

45 Nonsteroidal Anti-inflammatory Drugs (NSAIDs)

celecoxib
diclofenac
etodolac
fenoprofen calcium
flurbiprofen
ibuprofen
indomethacin
ketoprofen
ketorolac tromethamine
meloxicam
nabumetone
naproxen, naproxen sodium
oxaprozin
piroxicam
sulindac
valdecoxib

Uses: NSAIDs relieve the pain and inflammation of musculoskeletal disorders, such as rheumatoid arthritis, osteoarthritis, and ankylosing spondylitis. They're also used to provide analgesia for mild to moderate pain and to reduce fever. However, many of these agents aren't suited for long-term therapy because of toxicity.

Action: The NSAIDs' exact mechanism of action in relieving inflammation, pain, and fever is unknown. They may work by inhibiting cyclooxygenase, the enzyme responsible for prostaglandin synthesis, and other mediators of inflammation, such as leukotrienes. In addition, they may produce their antipyretic effects by acting centrally on the heat-regulating center of the hypothalamus.

COMBINATION PRODUCTS

ADVIL COLD: ibuprofen/pseudoephedrine (a nasal decongestant) 200 mg/30 mg; 100 mg/15 mg per 5 ml.
ARTHROTEC: diclofenac/misoprostol (an antisecretory gastric protectant) 50 mg/200 mcg; 75 mg/200 mcg.
CHILDREN'S ADVIL COLD: ibuprofen/pseudoephedrine (a nasal decongestant) 100 mg/15 mg per 5 ml.
COMBUNOX: ibuprofen/oxycodone (a narcotic analgesic) 400 mg/5 mg.
MOTRIN COLD: ibuprofen/pseudoephedrine (a nasal decongestant) 200 mg/30 mg; 100 mg/15 mg per 5 ml.
PREVACID NAPRAPAC: naproxen/lansoprazole (a proton pump inhibitor) 375 mg/15 mg; 500 mg/15 mg.
REPREXIAN CIII: ibuprofen/hydrocodone (a narcotic analgesic) 200 mg/5 mg.
VICOPROFEN: ibuprofen/hydrocodone (a narcotic analgesic) 200 mg/7.5 mg.

celecoxib

sel-eh-**cox**-ib
(Celebrex, DisperDose, Panixine)
Do not confuse Celebrex with Cerebyx or Celexa.

CATEGORY AND SCHEDULE

Pregnancy Risk Category: C (D if used in third trimester or near delivery)

MECHANISM OF ACTION

An NSAID that inhibits cyclo-oxygenase-2, the enzyme responsible for prostaglandin synthesis. Mechanism of action in treating familial adenomatous polyposis is unknown. **Therapeutic Effect:** Reduces inflammation and relieves pain.

PHARMACOKINETICS

Widely distributed. Protein binding: 97%. Metabolized in the liver. Primarily eliminated in feces. ***Half-life:*** 11.2 hr.

AVAILABILITY

Capsules: 100 mg, 200 mg, 400 mg.

INDICATIONS AND DOSAGES

▸ **Osteoarthritis**

PO

Adults, Elderly. 200 mg/day as a single dose or 100 mg twice a day.

▸ **Rheumatoid arthritis**

PO

Adults, Elderly. 100–200 mg twice a day.

▸ **Acute pain**

PO

Adults, Elderly. Initially, 400 mg with additional 200 mg on day 1, if needed. Maintenance: 200 mg twice a day as needed.

▸ **Familial adenomatous polyposis**

PO

Adults, Elderly. 400 mg twice daily (with food).

CONTRAINDICATIONS

Hypersensitivity to aspirin, NSAIDs, or sulfonamides

INTERACTIONS

Drug

Fluconazole: May increase celecoxib blood level.

Lithium: May increase lithium blood levels.

Warfarin: May increase the risk of bleeding.

Herbal

None known.

Food

None known.

DIAGNOSTIC TEST EFFECTS

May increase AST (SGOT) and ALT (SGPT) levels.

SIDE EFFECTS

Frequent (greater than 5%)

Diarrhea, dyspepsia, headache, upper respiratory tract infection

Occasional (5%–1%)

Abdominal pain, flatulence, nausea, back pain, peripheral edema, dizziness, rash

SERIOUS REACTIONS

! None known.

NURSING CONSIDERATIONS

Baseline Assessment

- Assess the duration, location, onset, and type of inflammation or pain.
- Inspect the patient's affected joints for deformity, immobility, and skin condition.

Lifespan Considerations

- It is unknown if celecoxib crosses the placenta or is distributed in breast milk.
- Celecoxib should not be used during the third trimester of pregnancy because it may cause adverse effects in the fetus, such as premature closure of the ductus arteriosus.
- The safety and efficacy of celecoxib have not been established in children younger than 18 years.
- No age-related precautions have been noted in the elderly.

Precautions

◂ALERT▸ When high doses of celecoxib are given to prevent colon

cancer the risk of adverse cardiovascular effects increases.
• Use celecoxib cautiously in patients older than 60 years, smokers, those with active alcoholism, or history of peptic ulcer disease, and those receiving anticoagulant or steroid therapy.

Administration and Handling

PO
• Give celecoxib without regard to food.
• Don't crush or break capsules.

Intervention and Evaluation

• Evaluate the patient for evidence of a therapeutic response, such as decreased pain, stiffness, swelling, and tenderness; improved grip strength, and increased joint mobility.

Patient Teaching

• Advise the patient to take celecoxib with food if GI upset occurs.
• Warn the patient to avoid alcohol and aspirin during celecoxib therapy because these substances increase the risk of GI bleeding.

diclofenac

dye-**kloe**-fen-ak
(Cataflam, Diclohexal[AUS], Diclotek[CAN], Fenac[AUS], Novo-Difenac[CAN], Solaraze, Voltaren, Voltaren Emulgel[AUS], Voltaren Ophthalmic, Voltaren Rapid[AUS], Voltaren XR)
Do not confuse diclofenac with Diflucan or Duphalac, or Voltaren with Verelan.

CATEGORY AND SCHEDULE

Pregnancy Risk Category: B (D if used in third trimester or near delivery; C for ophthalmic solution)

MECHANISM OF ACTION

An NSAID that inhibits prostaglandin synthesis, reducing the intensity of pain. Also constricts the iris sphincter. May inhibit angiogenesis (the formation of blood vessels) by inhibiting substance P or blocking the angiogenic effects of prostaglandin E. **Therapeutic Effect:** Produces analgesic and anti-inflammatory effects. Prevents miosis during cataract surgery. May reduce angiogenesis in inflammed tissue.

PHARMACOKINETICS

Route	Onset	Peak	Duration
PO	30 min	2–3 hr	Up to 8 hr

Completely absorbed from the GI tract; penetrates cornea after ophthalmic administration (may be systemically absorbed). Protein binding: greater than 99%. Widely distributed. Metabolized in the liver. Primarily excreted in urine. Minimally removed by hemodialysis. ***Half-life:*** 1.2–2 hr.

AVAILABILITY

Topical Gel (Solaraze): 3%.
Tablets (Cataflam): 50 mg.
Tablets (Enteric-Coated [Voltaren]): 25 mg, 50 mg, 75 mg.
Tablets (Extended-Release [Voltaren XR]): 100 mg.
Ophthalmic Solution (Voltaren Ophthalmic): 0.1%.

INDICATIONS AND DOSAGES

▸ **Osteoarthritis**

PO (Cataflam, Voltaren)
Adults, Elderly. 50 mg 2–3 times a day.
PO (Voltaren XR)
Adults, Elderly. 100 mg/day as a single dose.

▸ **Rheumatoid arthritis**
PO (Cataflam, Voltaren)
Adults, Elderly. 50 mg 2–4 times a day. Maximum: 225 mg/day.
PO (Voltaren XR)
Adults, Elderly. 100 mg once a day. Maximum: 100 mg twice a day.

▸ **Ankylosing spondylitis**
PO (Voltaren)
Adults, Elderly. 100–125 mg/day in 4–5 divided doses.

▸ **Analgesia, primary dysmenorrhea**
PO (Cataflam)
Adults, Elderly. 30 mg 3 times a day.

▸ **Usual pediatric dosage**
Children. 2–3 mg/kg/day in 2-4 divided doses.

▸ **Actinic keratoses**
Topical
Adults, Adolescents. Apply twice a day to lesion for 60–90 days.

▸ **Cataract surgery**
Ophthalmic
Adults, Elderly. Apply 1 drop to eye 4 times a day commencing 24 hr after cataract surgery. Continue for 2 wk afterward.

▸ **Pain, relief of photophobia in patients undergoing corneal refractive surgery**
Ophthalmic
Adults, Elderly. Apply 1 drop to affected eye 1 hr before surgery, within 15 min after surgery, then 4 times a day for 3 days.

OFF-LABEL USES

Treatment of vascular headaches (oral); to reduce the occurrence and severity of cystoid macular edema after cataract surgery (ophthalmic form)

CONTRAINDICATIONS

Hypersensitivity to aspirin, diclofenac, and other NSAIDs; porphyria

INTERACTIONS

Drug

Acetylcholine, carbachol: May decrease the effects of these drugs (with ophthalmic diclofenac).
Antihypertensives, diuretics: May decrease the effects of these drugs.
Aspirin, other salicylates: May increase the risk of GI side effects such as bleeding.
Bone marrow depressants: May increase the risk of hematologic reactions.
Epinephrine, other antiglaucoma medications: May decrease the antiglaucoma effect of these drugs.
Heparin, oral anticoagulants, thrombolytics: May increase the effects of these drugs.
Lithium: May increase the blood concentration and risk of toxicity of lithium.
Methotrexate: May increase the risk of methotrexate toxicity.
Probenecid: May increase diclofenac blood concentration.

Herbal

Ginkgo biloba: May increase the risk of bleeding.

Food

None known.

DIAGNOSTIC TEST EFFECTS

May increase BUN level; urine protein level; and serum LDH, potassium, alkaline phosphatase, creatinine, AST (SGOT), and ALT (SGPT) levels. May decrease serum uric acid level.

SIDE EFFECTS

Frequent (9%–4%)
PO: Headache, abdominal cramps, constipation, diarrhea, nausea, dyspepsia
Ophthalmic: Burning or stinging on instillation, ocular discomfort

Occasional (3%–1%)
PO: Flatulence, dizziness, epigastric pain
Ophthalmic: Ocular itching or tearing
Rare (less than 1%)
PO: Rash, peripheral edema or fluid retention, visual disturbances, vomiting, drowsiness

SERIOUS REACTIONS

! Overdose may result in acute renal failure.
! Rare reactions with long-term use include peptic ulcer disease, GI bleeding, gastritis, a severe hepatic reaction (jaundice), nephrotoxicity (hematuria, dysuria, proteinuria), and a severe hypersensitivity reaction (bronchospasm or angioedema).

NURSING CONSIDERATIONS

Baseline Assessment
- Assess the duration, location, onset, and type of inflammation or pain.
- Inspect the arthritic patient's affected joints for deformity, immobility, and skin condition.
- Plan to obtain baseline BUN level; urinary protein levels; as well as serum potassium, LDH, alkaline phosphatase, creatinine, AST (SGOT), and ALT (SGPT) levels.

Lifespan Considerations
- Diclofenac crosses the placenta; it is unknown if the drug is distributed in breast milk.
- Diclofenac should not be used during the last trimester of pregnancy because it may casue adverse effects in the fetus, such as premature closure of the ductus arteriosus.
- The safety and efficacy of diclofenac have not been established in children.
- In elderly patients, GI bleeding or ulceration is more likely to cause serious complications and age-related renal impairment may increase the risk of hepatotoxicity or renal toxicity; a decreased drug dosage is recommended.

Precautions
- Use diclofenac cautiously in patients with CHF, hypertension, hepatic or renal impairment, or a history of GI disease.
- Don't use diclofenac topical gel on children, infants, or neonates. Avoid applying the gel around eyes or on open skin wounds, infected areas, or areas affected by exfoliative dermatitis.

Administration and Handling
PO
- Don't crush or break enteric-coated tablets.
- Give diclofenac with food, milk, or antacids if the patient experiences GI distress.

Ophthalmic
- Place a gloved finger on the patient's lower eyelid, and pull it out until a pocket is formed between the eye and lower lid.
- Hold the dropper above the pocket, and place the prescribed number of drops in the pocket.
- Gently close the patient's eye, and apply digital pressure to the lacrimal sac for 1 to 2 minutes to minimize drainage into the nose and throat, reducing the risk of systemic effects.
- Remove excess solution with a tissue.

Intervention and Evaluation
- Monitor the patient for dyspepsia and headache.
- Assess the patient's pattern of daily bowel activity and stool consistency.
- Evaluate the patient for evidence of a therapeutic response, such as improved grip strength, increased joint mobility, and decreased joint pain, tenderness, stiffness, and swelling.

Patient Teaching

- Instruct the patient to swallow diclofenac tablets whole and not to crush or chew them.
- Advise the patient to take diclofenac with food or milk if he or she experiences GI upset
- Warn the patient to avoid alcohol and aspirin during diclofenac therapy because these substances increase the risk of GI bleeding.
- Warn the patient to notify the physician if he or she experiences a persistent headache, black stools, changes in vision, pruritus, rash, or weight gain.
- Instruct the patient not to use hydrogel soft contact lenses during ophthalmic diclofenac therapy.
- Advise the patient using topical diclofenac to notify the physician if he or she experiences a rash.
- Instruct the female patient to notify the physician if she is or plans to become pregnant.

etodolac

e-toe-**doe**-lak
(Apo-Etodolac[CAN], Lodine, Lodine XL, Ultradol[CAN])
Do not confuse Lodine with codeine or iodine.

CATEGORY AND SCHEDULE

Pregnancy Risk Category: C (D if used in third trimester or near delivery)

MECHANISM OF ACTION

An NSAID that produces analgesic and anti-inflammatory effects by inhibiting prostaglandin synthesis. **Therapeutic Effect:** Reduces the inflammatory response and intensity of pain.

PHARMACOKINETICS

Route	Onset	Peak	Duration
PO (analgesic)	30 min	N/A	4–12 hr

Completely absorbed from the GI tract. Protein binding: greater than 99%. Widely distributed. Metabolized in the liver. Primarily excreted in urine. Not removed by hemodialysis. ***Half-life:*** 6–7 hr.

AVAILABILITY

Capsules (Lodine): 200 mg, 300 mg.
Tablets (Lodine): 400 mg, 500 mg.
Tablets (Extended-Release [Lodine XL]): 400 mg, 500 mg, 600 mg.

INDICATIONS AND DOSAGES

▸ **Osteoarthritis**

PO

Adults, Elderly. Initially, 800–1,200 mg/day in 2–4 divided doses. Maintenance: 600–1,200 mg/day.

▸ **Rheumatoid arthritis**

PO

Adults, Elderly. Initially, 300 mg 2–3 times a day or 400–500 mg twice a day. Maintenance: 600–1,200 mg/day.

▸ **Analgesia**

PO

Adults, Elderly. 200–400 mg q6–8h as needed. Maximum: 1,200 mg/day.

OFF-LABEL USES

Treatment of acute gouty arthritis, vascular headache

CONTRAINDICATIONS

Active peptic ulcer disease, chronic inflammation of GI tract, GI bleeding or ulceration, history of hypersensitivity to aspirin or NSAIDs

INTERACTIONS

Drug

Antihypertensives, diuretics: May decrease the effects of these drugs.

Aspirin, other salicylates: May increase the risk of GI side effects such as bleeding.
Bone marrow depressants: May increase the risk of hematologic reactions.
Heparin, oral anticoagulants, thrombolytics: May increase the effects of these drugs.
Lithium: May increase the blood concentration and risk of toxicity of lithium.
Methotrexate: May increase the risk of methotrexate toxicity.
Probenecid: May increase etodolac blood concentration.

Herbal

Feverfew, ginkgo biloba: May increase the risk of bleeding.

Food

None known.

DIAGNOSTIC TEST EFFECTS

May increase bleeding time, liver function test results, and serum creatinine level. May decrease serum uric acid level.

SIDE EFFECTS

Occasional (9%–4%)

Dizziness, headache, abdominal pain or cramps, bloated feeling, diarrhea, nausea, indigestion

Rare (3%–1%)

Constipation, rash, pruritus, visual disturbances, tinnitus

SERIOUS REACTIONS

! Overdose may result in acute renal failure.

! Rare reactions with long-term use include peptic ulcer disease, GI bleeding, gastritis, severe hepatic reactions (jaundice), nephrotoxicity (hematuria, dysuria, proteinuria), and a severe hypersensitivity reaction (bronchospasm, angioedema).

NURSING CONSIDERATIONS

Baseline Assessment

- Assess the duration, location, onset, and type of inflammation or pain.
- Inspect the affected joints for deformity, immobility, and skin condition.

Lifespan Considerations

- It is unknown if etodolac crosses the placenta or is distributed in breast milk.
- Etodolac should not be used during the last trimester of pregnancy because it may cause adverse effects in the fetus, such as premature closure of the ductus arteriosus.
- The safety and efficacy of etodolac have not been established in children.
- In elderly patients, GI bleeding or ulceration is more likely to cause serious complications and age-related renal impairment may increase the risk of hepatotoxicity or renal toxicity; a decreased dosage is recommended.

Precautions

- Use etodolac cautiously in patients with a hepatic or renal impairment, a predisposition to fluid retention, or a history of GI tract disease.

Administration and Handling

◀ **ALERT** ▶ Expect to reduce etodolac dosage for elderly patients. Know that the maximum dose for patients weighing 60 kg or less is 20 mg/kg.

PO

- Do not crush, open, or break capsules or extended-release tablets.
- Give etodolac with food, milk, or antacids if the patient experiences GI distress.

Intervention and Evaluation

- Monitor the patient's CBC and blood chemistry studies to assess hepatic and renal function.
- Evaluate the patient for bleeding and ecchymosis.

• Assess the patient for evidence of a therapeutic response, such as improved grip strength, increased joint mobility, and decreased pain, tenderness, stiffness, and swelling.

Patient Teaching

• Instruct the patient to swallow etodolac capsules whole and not to open, chew, or crush them.
• Advise the patient to take etodolac with food, milk, or antacids if GI distress occurs.
• Instruct the patient to notify the physician if he or she experiences edema, GI distress, headache, rash, signs of bleeding, or visual disturbances.
• Instruct the patient to avoid alcohol and aspirin during etodolac therapy because these substances increase the risk of GI bleeding.
• Warn the patient to avoid performing tasks that require mental alertness or motor skills until his or her response to the drug has been established.
• Advise the patient to notify the physician if she is or plans to become pregnant.

fenoprofen calcium

fen-oh-**proe**-fen
(Nalfon)
Do not confuse Nalfon with Naldecon.

CATEGORY AND SCHEDULE

Pregnancy Risk Category: B (D if used in third trimester or near delivery)

MECHANISM OF ACTION

An NSAID that produces analgesic and anti-inflammatory effects by inhibiting prostaglandin synthesis. **Therapeutic Effect:** Reduces the inflammatory response and intensity of pain.

AVAILABILITY

Capsules: 200 mg, 300 mg.
Tablets: 600 mg.

INDICATIONS AND DOSAGES

▸ **Mild to moderate pain**
PO
Adults, Elderly. 200 mg q4–6h as needed.

▸ **Rheumatoid arthritis, osteoarthritis**
PO
Adults, Elderly. 300–600 mg 3–4 times a day.

OFF-LABEL USES

Treatment of ankylosing spondylitis, psoriatic arthritis, vascular headaches

CONTRAINDICATIONS

Active peptic ulcer disease, chronic inflammation of GI tract, GI bleeding or ulceration, history of hypersensitivity to aspirin or NSAIDs, significant renal impairment

INTERACTIONS

Drug

Antihypertensives, diuretics: May decrease the effects of these drugs.
Aspirin, other salicylates: May increase the risk of GI side effects such as bleeding.
Bone marrow depressants: May increase the risk of hematologic reactions.
Heparin, oral anticoagulants, thrombolytics: May increase the effects of these drugs.
Lithium: May increase the blood concentration and risk of toxicity of lithium.
Methotrexate: May increase the risk of methotrexate toxicity.
Probenecid: May increase fenoprofen blood concentration.

Herbal
None known.
Food
None known.

DIAGNOSTIC TEST EFFECTS
May increase bleeding time, BUN and blood glucose levels, and serum protein, alkaline phosphatase, LDH, creatinine, AST (SGOT), and ALT (SGPT) levels.

SIDE EFFECTS
Frequent (9%–3%)
Headache, somnolence, dyspepsia, nausea, vomiting, constipation
Occasional (2%–1%)
Dizziness, pruritus, nervousness, asthenia, diarrhea, abdominal cramps, flatulence, tinnitus, blurred vision, peripheral edema and fluid retention

SERIOUS REACTIONS
! Overdose may result in acute hypotension and tachycardia.
! Rare reactions with long-term use include peptic ulcer disease, GI bleeding, gastritis, severe hepatic reaction (jaundice), nephrotoxicity (hematuria, dysuria, proteinuria), and a severe hypersensitivity reaction (bronchospasm, angioedema).

NURSING CONSIDERATIONS
Baseline Assessment
• Assess the duration, location, onset, and type of inflammation or pain.
• Inspect the arthritic patient's affected joints for deformity, immobility, and skin condition.
• Plan to check baseline bleeding time; BUN and blood glucose levels; serum alkaline phosphatase, LDH, creatinine, AST (SGOT), and ALT (SGPT) levels; and urinary protein levels.
Lifespan Considerations
• Fenoprofen crosses the placenta and is distributed in breast milk.
• Fenoprofen should not be used during the last trimester of pregnancy because it may cause adverse effects in the fetus, such as premature closure of the ductus arteriosus.
• The safety and efficacy of fenoprofen have not been established in children.
• In elderly patients, GI bleeding or ulceration is more likely to cause serious complications and age-related renal impairment may increase the risk of hepatotoxicity or renal toxicity; a decreased drug dosage is recommended.
Precautions
• Use fenoprofen cautiously in patients with hepatic or renal impairment, a predisposition to fluid retention, or a history of GI tract disease.
Administration and Handling
PO
◀ALERT▶ Don't exceed a fenoprofen dosage of 3.2 g/day, as prescribed.
• Do not crush, open, or break capsules.
Intervention and Evaluation
• Assist the patient with ambulation if he or she experiences dizziness or somnolence.
• Monitor the patient for dyspepsia.
• Assess the patient's pattern of daily bowel activity and stool consistency.
• Examine the area behind the medial malleolus for fluid.
• Evaluate the patient for evidence of a therapeutic response, such as improved grip strength, increased joint mobility, and decreased pain, stiffness, and swelling.
Patient Teaching
• Instruct the patient to swallow fenoprofen capsules whole and not to chew or crush them.
• Advise the patient to take fenopro-

fen with food or milk if GI upset occurs.
• Warn the patient to avoid tasks that require mental alertness or motor skills until his or her response to the drug has been established.
• Warn the patient to avoid alcohol and aspirin during fenoprofen therapy because these substances increase the risk of GI bleeding.

flurbiprofen

flure-**bi**-proe-fen
(Ansaid, Froben[CAN], Ocufen, Strepfen[AUS])
Do not confuse Ocufen with Ocuflox.

CATEGORY AND SCHEDULE

Pregnancy Risk Category: B (D if used in third trimester or near delivery; C for ophthalmic solution)

MECHANISM OF ACTION

A phenylalkanoic acid that produces analgesic and anti-inflammatory effect by inhibiting prostaglandin synthesis. Also relaxes the iris sphincter. **Therapeutic Effect:** Reduces the inflammatory response and intensity of pain. Prevents or decreases miosis during cataract surgery.

PHARMACOKINETICS

Well absorbed from the GI tract; ophthalmic solution penetrates cornea after administration, and may be systemically absorbed. Protein binding: 99%. Widely distributed. Metabolized in the liver. Primarily excreted in urine. ***Half-life:*** 3–4 hr.

AVAILABILITY

Tablets (Ansaid): 50 mg, 100 mg.
Ophthalmic Solution (Ocufen): 0.03%.

INDICATIONS AND DOSAGES

▸ **Rheumatoid arthritis, osteoarthritis**
PO
Adults, Elderly. 200–300 mg/day in 2–4 divided doses. Maximum: 100 mg/dose or 300 mg/day.
▸ **Dysmenorrhea, pain**
PO
Adults. 50 mg 4 times a day
▸ **Usual Ophthalmic Dosage**
Adults, Elderly, Children. Apply 1 drop q30min starting 2 hr before surgery for total of 4 doses.

CONTRAINDICATIONS

Active peptic ulcer, chronic inflammation of GI tract, GI bleeding or ulceration, history of hypersensitivity to aspirin or NSAIDs

INTERACTIONS

Drug

Acetylcholine, carbachol: May decrease the effects of these drugs (with ophthalmic flurbiprofen).
Antihypertensives, diuretics: May decrease the effects of these drugs.
Aspirin, other salicylates: May increase the risk of GI side effects such as bleeding.
Bone marrow depressants: May increase the risk of hematologic reactions.
Epinephrine, other antiglaucoma medications: May decrease the antiglaucoma effect of these drugs.
Heparin, oral anticoagulants, thrombolytics: May increase the effects of these drugs.
Lithium: May increase the blood concentration and risk of toxicity of lithium.
Methotrexate: May increase the risk of methotrexate toxicity.

Probenecid: May increase the flurbiprofen blood concentration.

Herbal

Feverfew: May decrease the effects of feverfew.

Ginkgo biloba: May increase the risk of bleeding.

Food

None known.

DIAGNOSTIC TEST EFFECTS

May increase bleeding time and serum LDH, alkaline phosphatase, AST (SGOT), and ALT (SGPT) levels.

SIDE EFFECTS

Occasional

PO (9%–3%): Headache, abdominal pain, diarrhea, indigestion, nausea, fluid retention

Ophthalmic: Burning or stinging on instillation, keratitis, elevated intraocular pressure

Rare (less than 3%)

PO: Blurred vision, flushed skin, dizziness, somnolence, nervousness, insomnia, unusual fatigue, constipation, decreased appetite, vomiting, confusion

SERIOUS REACTIONS

! Overdose may result in acute renal failure.

! Rare reactions with long-term use include peptic ulcer disease, GI bleeding, gastritis, severe hepatic reaction (jaundice), nephrotoxicity (hematuria, dysuria, proteinuria), a severe hypersensitivity reaction (angioedema, bronchospasm), and cardiac arrhythmias.

NURSING CONSIDERATIONS

Baseline Assessment

- Assess the duration, location, onset, and type of inflammation or pain.
- Inspect the arthritic patient's affected joints for deformity, immobility, and skin condition.

Lifespan Considerations

- Flurbiprofen crosses the placenta; it is unknown whether the drug is distributed in breast milk.
- Flurbiprofen should not be used during the last trimester of pregnancy because it may cause adverse effects in the fetus, such as premature closure of the ductus arteriosus.
- The safety and efficacy of flurbiprofen have not been established in children.
- In the elderly, GI bleeding or ulceration is more likely to cause serious complications and age-related renal impairment may increase the risk of hepatotoxicity or renal toxicity; a decreased dosage is recommended.

Precautions

- Use flurbiprofen cautiously in patients who wear soft contact lens; those with hepatic or renal impairment, a predisposition to fluid retention, or a history of GI tract disease; and surgical patients with a bleeding tendency.

Administration and Handling

PO

- Don't crush or break enteric-coated tablets.
- Give with food, milk, or antacids if the patient experiences GI distress.

Ophthalmic

- Place a gloved finger on the patient's lower eyelid, and pull it out until a pocket is formed between the eye and lower lid.
- Hold the dropper above the pocket, and place the prescribed number of drops into the pocket.
- Gently close the patient's eye and apply digital pressure to the lacrimal sac for 1 to 2 minutes to minimize drainage into the nose and throat, reducing the risk of systemic effects.

• Remove excess solution with a tissue.

Intervention and Evaluation

• Monitor the patient for dizziness, dyspepsia, and headache.

• Assess the patient's pattern of daily bowel activity and stool consistency.

• For patients taking oral flurbiprofen, monitor the BUN level, CBC, and serum alkaline phosphatase, bilirubin, creatinine, AST (SGOT), and ALT (SGPT) levels. Check stools for occult blood.

• Perform periodic eye exams on patients using ophthalmic flurbiprofen.

• Evaluate the patient for evidence of a therapeutic response, such as improved grip strength, increased joint mobility, and decreased pain, stiffness, and swelling.

Patient Teaching

• Instruct the patient to swallow flurbiprofen tablets whole and not to chew or crush them.

• Advise the patient to take flurbiprofen with food or milk if GI upset occurs.

• Urge the patient to avoid alcohol and aspirin during flurbiprofen therapy because these substances increase the risk of GI bleeding.

• Warn the patient to notify the physician if he or she experiences edema, GI distress, headache, rash, or visual disturbances.

• Inform patients using ophthalmic flurbiprofen that the eyes may sting momentarily during drug instillation.

• Instruct the patient to notify the physician if she is or plans to become pregnant.

ibuprofen

eye-**byoo**-pro-fen

(Act-3[AUS], Advil, Apo-Ibuprofen, Brufen[AUS], Codral Period Pain[AUS], Motrin, Novoprofen[CAN], Nurofen[AUS], Rafen[AUS])

CATEGORY AND SCHEDULE

Pregnancy Risk Category: B (D if used in third trimester or near delivery)

OTC (Tablets: 200 mg, Oral Suspension: 100 mg/5 ml)

MECHANISM OF ACTION

An NSAID that inhibits prostaglandin synthesis. Also produces vasodilation by acting centrally on the heat-regulating center of the hypothalamus. **Therapeutic Effect:** Produces analgesic and anti-inflammatory effects and decreases fever.

PHARMACOKINETICS

Route	Onset	Peak	Duration
PO (analgesic)	0.5 hr	N/A	4–6 hr
PO (antirheumatic)	2 days	1–2 wk	N/A

Rapidly absorbed from the GI tract. Protein binding: greater than 90%. Metabolized in the liver. Primarily excreted in urine. Not removed by hemodialysis. ***Half-life:*** 2–4 hr.

AVAILABILITY

Caplets (Advil, Menadol, Motrin): 200 mg.

Capsules (Advil, Advil Migraine): 200 mg.

Gelcaps (Advil, Motrin IB): 200 mg.

Tablets (Advil, Motrin IB): 200 mg.

Tablets (Motin): 400 mg, 600 mg, 800 mg.
Tablets (Chewable [Children's Advil, Children's Motrin]): 50 mg.
Tablets (Chewable [Junior Advil, Junior Strength Motrin]): 100 mg.
Oral Suspension (Children's Advil, Children's Motrin): 100 mg/5 ml.
Oral Drops (Infant Advil, Infant Motrin): 40 mg/ml.

INDICATIONS AND DOSAGES

▸ Acute or chronic rheumatoid arthritis, osteoarthritis, migraine pain, gouty arthritis
PO
Adults, Elderly. 400–800 mg 3–4 times a day. Maximum: 3.2 g/day.

▸ Mild to moderate pain, primary dysmenorrhea
PO
Adults, Elderly. 200–400 mg q4–6h as needed. Maximum: 1.6 g/day.

▸ Fever, minor aches or pain
PO
Adults, Elderly. 200–400 mg q4–6h. Maximum: 1.6 g/day.
Children. 5–10 mg/kg/dose q6–8h. Maximum: 40 mg/kg/day. OTC: 7.5 mg/kg/dose q6–8h. Maximum: 30 mg/kg/day.

▸ Juvenile arthritis
PO
Children. 30–70 mg/kg/day in 3–4 divided doses. Maximum: 400 mg/day in children weighing less than 20 kg, 600 mg/day in children weighing 20–30 kg, 800 mg/day in children weighing greater than 30–40 kg.

OFF-LABEL USES

Treatment of psoriatic arthritis, vascular headaches

CONTRAINDICATIONS

Active peptic ulcer, chronic inflammation of GI tract, GI bleeding disorders or ulceration, history of hypersensitivity to aspirin or NSAIDs

INTERACTIONS

Drug

Antihypertensives, diuretics: May decrease the effects of these drugs.
Aspirin, other salicylates: May increase the risk of GI side effects such as bleeding.
Bone marrow depressants: May increase the risk of hematologic reactions.
Heparin, oral anticoagulants, thrombolytics: May increase the effects of these drugs.
Lithium: May increase the blood concentration and risk of toxicity of lithium.
Methotrexate: May increase the risk of methotrexate toxicity.
Probenecid: May increase the ibuprofen blood concentration.

Herbal

Feverfew: May decrease the effects of feverfew.
Ginkgo biloba: May increase the risk of bleeding.

Food

None known.

DIAGNOSTIC TEST EFFECTS

May prolong bleeding time. May alter blood glucose level. May increase BUN level, and serum creatinine, potassium, AST (SGOT), and ALT (SGPT) levels. May decrease blood Hgb and Hct.

SIDE EFFECTS

Occasional (9%–3%)
Nausea with or without vomiting, dyspepsia, dizziness, rash
Rare (less than 3%)
Diarrhea or constipation, flatulence, abdominal cramps or pain, pruritus

SERIOUS REACTIONS

! Acute overdose may result in metabolic acidosis.

! Rare reactions with long-term use include peptic ulcer disease, GI bleeding, gastritis, a severe hepatic reaction (cholestasis, jaundice), nephrotoxicity (dysuria, hematuria, proteinuria, nephrotic syndrome), and a severe hypersensitivity reaction (particularly in patients with systemic lupus erythematosus or other collagen diseases).

NURSING CONSIDERATIONS

Baseline Assessment

- Assess the duration, location, onset, and type of inflammation or pain.
- Inspect the arthritic patient's affected joints for deformity, immobility, and skin condition.

Lifespan Considerations

- It is unknown if ibuprofen crosses the placenta or is distributed in breast milk.
- Ibuprofen should not be used during the third trimester of pregnancy because it may cause adverse effects in the fetus, such as premature closure of the ductus arteriosus.
- The safety and efficacy of this drug have not been established in children younger than 6 months.
- In the elderly, GI bleeding or ulceration is more likely to cause serious complications, and age-related renal impairment may increase the risk of hepatotoxicity or renal toxicity; a reduced dosage is recommended.

Precautions

- Use ibuprofen cautiously in patients with CHF, hypertension, dehydration, GI disease (such as GI bleeding or ulcers), or hepatic or renal impairment and in those using anticoagulants concurrently.

Administration and Handling

PO

- Don't crush or break enteric-coated tablets.
- Give ibuprofen with food, milk, or antacids if the patient experiences GI distress.

Intervention and Evaluation

- Monitor the patient's body temperature for fever.
- Assess the patient for dyspepsia and nausea.
- Monitor the patient's CBC, platelet count, and serum alkaline phosphatase, bilirubin, creatinine, AST (SGOT), and ALT (SGPT) levels.
- Assess the patient's pattern of daily bowel activity and stool consistency.
- Examine the patient's skin for rash.
- Evaluate the patient for evidence of a therapeutic response, such as improved grip strength, increased joint mobility, and decreased pain, tenderness, stiffness, and swelling.

Patient Teaching

- Teach the patient not to chew or crush enteric-coated ibuprofen tablets.
- Instruct the patient to take ibuprofen with food, milk, or antacids if GI upset occurs.
- Inform the patient that ibuprofen use may cause dizziness.
- Urge the patient to avoid alcohol and aspirin during ibuprofen therapy because these substances increase the risk of GI bleeding.
- Warn the patient to avoid performing tasks that require mental alertness or motor skills until his or her response to the drug has been established.

indomethacin

in-doe-**meth**-a-sin
(Apo-Indomethacin[CAN], Arthrexin[AUS], Indocid[CAN], Indocin, Indocin-IV, Indocin-SR, Novomethacin[CAN])
Do not confuse Indocin with Imodium or Vicodin.

CATEGORY AND SCHEDULE

Pregnancy Risk Category: B (D if used after 34 weeks' gestation, close to delivery, or for longer than 48 hours)

MECHANISM OF ACTION

An NSAID that produces analgesic and anti-inflammatory effects by inhibiting prostaglandin synthesis. Also increases the sensitivity of the premature ductus to the dilating effects of prostaglandins. **Therapeutic Effect:** Reduces the inflammatory response and intensity of pain. Closure of the patent ductus arteriosus.

AVAILABILITY

Capsules (Indocin): 25 mg, 50 mg.
Capsules (Sustained-Release [Indocin SR]): 75 mg.
Oral Suspension (Indocin): 25 mg/5 ml.
Powder for Injection (Indocin IV): 1 mg.
Suppositories: 50 mg.

INDICATIONS AND DOSAGES

▸ **Moderate to severe rheumatoid arthritis, osteoarthritis, ankylosing spondylitis**
PO
Adults, Elderly. Initially, 25 mg 2–3 times a day; increased by 25–50 mg/wk up to 150–200 mg/day. Or 75 mg/day (extended-release) up to 75 mg twice a day.
Children. 1–2 mg/kg/day. Maximum: 150–200 mg/day.

▸ **Acute gouty arthritis**
PO
Adults, Elderly. Initially, 100 mg, then 50 mg 3 times a day.

▸ **Acute shoulder pain**
PO
Adults, Elderly. 75–150 mg/day in 3–4 divided doses.

▸ **Usual rectal dosage**
Adults, Elderly. 50 mg 4 times a day.
Children. Initially, 1.5–2.5 mg/kg/day, increased up to 4 mg/kg/day. Maximum: 150–200 mg/day.

▸ **Patent ductus arteriosus**
IV
Neonates. Initially, 0.2 mg/kg. Subsquent doses are based on age, as follows:
Neonates older than 7 days. 0.25 mg/kg for 2nd and 3rd doses.
Neonates 2–7 days. 0.2 mg/kg for 2nd and 3rd doses.
Neonates less than 48 hr. 0.1 mg/kg for 2nd and 3rd doses.

OFF-LABEL USES

Treatment of fever due to malignancy, pericarditis, psoriatic arthritis, rheumatic complications associated with Paget's disease of bone, vascular headache

CONTRAINDICATIONS

Active GI bleeding or ulcerations; hypersensitivity to aspirin, indomethacin, or other NSAIDs; renal impairment, thrombocytopenia

INTERACTIONS

Drug

Aminoglycosides: May increase the blood concentration of these drugs in neonates.
Antihypertensives, diuretics: May decrease the effects of these drugs.

Aspirin, other salicylates: May increase the risk of GI side effects such as bleeding.
Bone marrow depressants: May increase the risk of hematologic reactions.
Heparin, oral anticoagulants, thrombolytics: May increase the effects of these drugs.
Lithium: May increase the blood concentration and risk of toxicity of lithium.
Methotrexate: May increase the risk of methotrexate toxicity.
Probenecid: May increase the indomethacin blood concentration.
Triamterene: May potentiate acute renal failure. Don't give concurrently.

Herbal

Feverfew: May decrease the effects of feverfew.
Ginkgo biloba: May increase the risk of bleeding.

Food

None known.

DIAGNOSTIC TEST EFFECTS

May prolong bleeding time. May alter blood glucose level. May increase BUN level, and serum creatinine, potassium, AST (SGOT), and ALT (SGPT) levels. May decrease serum sodium level and platelet count.

IV INCOMPATIBILITIES

Amino acid injection, calcium gluconate, cimetidine (Tagamet), dobutamine (Dobutrex), dopamine (Intropin), gentamicin (Garamycin), tobramycin (Nebcin)

IV COMPATIBILITIES

Insulin, potassium

SIDE EFFECTS

Frequent (11%–3%)

Headache, nausea, vomiting, dyspepsia, dizziness

Occasional (less than 3%)

Depression, tinnitus, diaphoresis, somnolence, constipation, diarrhea, bleeding disturbances in patent ductus arteriosus

Rare

Hypertension, confusion, urticaria, pruritus, rash, blurred vision

SERIOUS REACTIONS

! Paralytic ileus and ulceration of the esophagus, stomach, duodenum, or small intestine may occur.
! Patients with impaired renal function may develop hyperkalemia and worsening of renal impairment.
! Indomethacin use may aggravate epilepsy, parkinsonism, and depression or other psychiatric disturbances.
! Nephrotoxicity, including dysuria, hematuria, proteinuria, and nephrotic syndrome, occurs rarely.
! Metabolic acidosis or alkalosis, apnea, and bradycardia occur rarely in patients with patent ductus arteriosus.

NURSING CONSIDERATIONS

Baseline Assessment

- Assess the duration, location, onset, and type of fever, inflammation, or pain.
- Inspect the arthritic patient's affected joints for deformity, immobility, and skin condition.
- Expect to obtain baseline CBC, blood chemistry studies, PT, aPTT, and liver and renal function tests.
- Assess baseline heart sounds in neonates with patent ductus arteriosus. Note the location, intensity, quality, and timing of murmurs.

Precautions

- Use indomethacin cautiously in patients with cardiac dysfunction, hypertension, epilepsy, or hepatic or renal impairment and in those receiving anticoagulant therapy concurrently.

Administration and Handling

PO

- Give indomethacin after meals or with food or antacids.
- Don't crush extended-release capsules.

IV

◀ALERT▶ IV injection is the preferred route for neonatal patients with patent ductus arteriosus. The drug may also be given orally, by NG tube, or rectally. Administer no more than 3 doses at 12- to 24-hour intervals.

- To reconstitute, add 1 or 2 ml preservative-free sterile water for injection or 0.9% NaCl to the 1-mg vial to provide a concentration of 1 mg or 0.5 mg/ml, respectively. Don't dilute the solution any further.
- Administer the IV immediately after reconstitution. The solution normally appears clear, discard if it becomes cloudy or contains precipitate. Discard any unused portion.
- Administer the drug over 5 to 10 seconds.
- Restrict the patient's fluid intake, as ordered.

Rectal

- If suppository is too soft, refrigerate it for 30 minutes or run cold water over the foil wrapper.
- Moisten the suppository with cold water before inserting it into the rectum.

Intervention and Evaluation

- Know that indomethacin use may mask signs of infection.
- Monitor the patient for dyspepsia and nausea.
- Monitor the patient's BUN level and serum alkaline phosphatase, bilirubin, creatinine, potassium, AST (SGOT), and ALT (SGPT) levels.
- In neonatal patients, monitor the BP, EKG, heart rate, platelet count, serum sodium and blood glucose levels, and urine output. Also auscultate heart sounds to detect the presence of changes in a murmur.
- Assist the patient with ambulation if he or she experiences dizziness.
- Evaluate the patient for evidence of therapeutic response, such as improved grip strength, increased joint mobility, and reduced pain, tenderness, stiffness, and swelling.

Patient Teaching

- Instruct the patient to swallow capsules whole and not to chew, open, or crush them.
- Advise the patient to take indomethacin with food or milk if GI upset occurs.
- Warn the patient to avoid tasks that require mental alertness or motor skills until his or her response to the drug has been established.
- Urge the patient to avoid alcohol and aspirin during indomethacin therapy because these substances increase the risk of GI bleeding.

ketoprofen

kee-toe-**proe**-fen
(Apo-Keto[CAN], Novo-Keto-EC, Orudis[AUS], Orudis KT[CAN], Orudis SR[AUS], Oruvail, Oruvail SR[AUS], Rhodis[CAN])

CATEGORY AND SCHEDULE

Pregnancy Risk Category: B (D if used in third trimester or near delivery)
OTC (tablets)

MECHANISM OF ACTION

An NSAID that produces analgesic and anti-inflammatory effects by inhibiting prostaglandin synthesis. **Therapeutic Effect:** Reduces the inflammatory response and intensity of pain.

AVAILABILITY

Capsules: 50 mg, 75 mg.
Capsules (Extended-Release [Oruvail]): 100 mg, 150 mg, 200 mg.
Tablets (Orudis KT): 12.5 mg (OTC).

INDICATIONS AND DOSAGES

‣ Acute or chronic rheumatoid arthritis and osteoarthritis

PO

Adults. Initially, 75 mg 3 times a day or 50 mg 4 times a day.
Elderly. Initially, 25–50 mg 3–4 times a day. Maintenance: 150–300 mg/day in 3–4 divided doses.

PO (Extended-Release)

Adults, Elderly. 100–200 mg once a day.

‣ Mild to moderate pain, dysmenorrhea

PO

Adults, Elderly. 25–50 mg q6–8h. Maximum: 300 mg/day.

‣ Over-the-counter (OTC) dosage

PO

Adults, Elderly. 12.5 mg q4-6h. Maximum: 6 tabs/day.

‣ Dosage in renal impairment

Mild. 150 mg/day maximum.
Severe. 100 mg/day maximum.

OFF-LABEL USES

Treatment of acute gouty arthritis, psoriatic arthritis, ankylosing spondylitis, vascular headache

CONTRAINDICATIONS

Active peptic ulcer disease, chronic inflammation of the GI tract, GI bleeding or ulceration, history of hypersensitivity to aspirin or NSAIDs

INTERACTIONS

Drug

Antihypertensives, diuretics: May decrease the effects of these drugs.
Aspirin, other salicylates: May increase the risk of GI side effects such as bleeding.
Bone marrow depressants: May increase the risk of hematologic reactions.
Heparin, oral anticoagulants, thrombolytics: May increase the effects of these drugs.
Lithium: May increase the blood concentration and risk of toxicity of lithium.
Methotrexate: May increase the risk of methotrexate toxicity.
Probenecid: May increase the ketoprofen blood concentration.

Herbal

Feverfew: May decrease the effects of feverfew.
Ginkgo biloba: May increase the risk of bleeding.

Food

None known.

DIAGNOSTIC TEST EFFECTS

May prolong bleeding time. May increase serum alkaline phosphatase and levels and liver function test results. May decrease Hct, blood Hgb, and serum sodium levels.

SIDE EFFECTS

Frequent (11%)

Dyspepsia

Occasional (more than 3%)

Nausea, diarrhea or constipation, flatulence, abdominal cramps, headache

Rare (less than 2%)

Anorexia, vomiting, visual disturbances, fluid retention

SERIOUS REACTIONS

! Rare reactions with long-term use include peptic ulcer disease, GI bleeding, gastritis, and severe hepatic reactions (cholestasis, jaundice), nephrotoxicity (dysuria, hematuria, proteinuria, nephrotic syndrome), and severe hypersensitivity reaction (bronchospasm, angioedema).

NURSING CONSIDERATIONS

Baseline Assessment

- Assess the duration, location, onset, and type of inflammation or pain.
- Inspect the arthritic patient's affected joints for deformity, immobility, and skin condition.
- Plan to obtain baseline CBC, blood chemistry studies, PT, aPTT, and renal and liver function tests.

Precautions

- Use ketoprofen cautiously in patients with a history of GI tract disease, hepatic or renal impairment, or a predisposition to fluid retention.

Administration and Handling

◀ALERT▶ Don't exceed a ketoprofen dosage of 300 mg/day. Oruvail is not recommended as initial therapy for small patients, those older than 75 years, or those with renal impairment.

PO

- Give ketoprofen with food, a full glass (8 oz) of water, or milk to minimize GI distress.
- Don't break, open, or chew extended-release capsules.

Intervention and Evaluation

- Monitor the patient for dyspepsia and nausea.
- Monitor the patient's liver and renal function test results and mental function.
- Evaluate the patient for evidence of a therapeutic response, such as improved grip strength, increased mobility, improved range of motion, and decreased pain, tenderness, stiffness, and swelling.

Patient Teaching

- Instruct the patient to swallow capsules whole and not to chew or crush them.
- Advise the patient to take the drug with food or milk if he or she experiences GI upset.
- Warn the patient to avoid alcohol and aspirin during ketoprofen therapy because these substances increase the risk of GI bleeding.
- Instruct the patient to inform the physician if she is or plans to become pregnant.

ketorolac tromethamine

kee-**toe**-role-ak

(Acular, Acular LS, Acular PF, Toradol)

Do not confuse Acular with Acthar or Ocular.

CATEGORY AND SCHEDULE

Pregnancy Risk Category: C (D if used in third trimester)

MECHANISM OF ACTION

An NSAID that inhibits prostaglandin synthesis and reduces prostaglandin levels in the aqueous humor. **Therapeutic Effect:** Relieves pain stimulus and reduces intraocular inflammation.

PHARMACOKINETICS

Route	Onset	Peak	Duration
PO	30–60 min	1.5–4 hr	4–6 hr
IV/IM	30 min	1–2 hr	4–6 hr

Readily absorbed from the GI tract, after IM administration. Protein binding: 99%. Largely metabolized in the liver. Primarily excreted in urine. Not removed by hemodialysis. ***Half-life:*** 3.8–6.3 hr (increased with impaired renal function and in the elderly).

AVAILABILITY

Tablets (Toradol): 10 mg.
Injection (Toradol): 15 mg/ml, 30 mg/ml.
Ophthalmic Solution (Acular): 0.5%.
Ophthalmic Solution (Acular LS): 0.4%.
Ophthalmic Solution (Acular PF): 0.5%.

INDICATIONS AND DOSAGES

▸ **Short-term relief of mild to moderate pain (multiple doses)**
PO
Adults, Elderly. 10 mg q4–6h. Maximum: 40 mg/24 hr.
IV/IM
Adults younger than 65 yr. 30 mg q6h. Maximum: 120 mg/24 hr.
Adults 65 yr and older, those with renal impairment, those weighing less than 50 kg. 15 mg q6h. Maximum: 60 mg/24 hr.
Children 2–16 yr. 0.5 mg/kg q6h.

▸ **Short-term relief of mild to moderate pain (single dose)**
IV
Adults younger than 65 yr, Children 17 yr and older weighing more than 50 kg. 30 mg.
Adults 65 yr and older, with renal impairment, weighing less than 50 kg. 15 mg.
Children 2-16 yr. 0.5 mg/kg. Maximum: 15 mg.
IM
Adults younger than 65 yr, Children 17 yr and older, weighing more than 50 kg. 60 mg.
Adults 65 yrs and older, with renal impairment, weighing less than 50 kg. 30 mg.
Children 2–16 yr. 1 mg/kg. Maximum: 15 kg.

▸ **Allergic conjunctivitis**
Ophthalmic
Adults, Elderly, Children 3 yr and older. 1 drop 4 times a day.

▸ **Cataract extraction**
Ophthalmic
Adults, Elderly. 1 drop 4 times a day. Begin 24 hr after surgery and continue for 2 wk.

▸ **Refractive surgery**
Ophthalmic
Adults, Elderly. 1 drop 4 times a day for 3 days.

OFF-LABEL USES

Prevention or treatment of ocular inflammation (ophthalmic form)

CONTRAINDICATIONS

Active peptic ulcer disease, chronic inflammation of GI tract, GI bleeding or ulceration, history of hypersensitivity to aspirin or NSAIDs

INTERACTIONS

Drug

Antihypertensives, diuretics: May decrease the effects of these drugs.
Aspirin, other salicylates: May increase the risk of GI side effects such as bleeding.
Bone marrow depressants: May increase the risk of hematologic reactions.
Heparin, oral anticoagulants, thrombolytics: May increase the effects of these drugs.
Lithium: May increase the blood concentration and risk of toxicity of lithium.
Methotrexate: May increase the risk of methotrexate toxicity.
Probenecid: May increase ketorolac blood concentration.

Herbal

Feverfew: May decrease the effects of feverfew.

Ginkgo biloba: May increase the risk of bleeding.

Food

None known.

DIAGNOSTIC TEST EFFECTS

May prolong bleeding time. May increase liver function test results.

IV INCOMPATIBILITIES

Promethazine (Phenergan)

IV COMPATIBILITIES

Fentanyl (Sublimaze), hydromorphone (Dilaudid), morphine, nalbuphine (Nubain)

SIDE EFFECTS

Frequent (17%–12%)

Headache, nausea, abdominal cramps or pain, dyspepsia

Occasional (9%–3%)

Diarrhea

Ophthalmic: Transient stinging and burning

Rare (3%–1%)

Constipation, vomiting, flatulence, stomatitis, dizziness

Ophthalmic: Ocular irritation, allergic reactions, superficial ocular infection, keratitis

SERIOUS REACTIONS

! Rare reactions with long-term use include peptic ulcer disease, GI bleeding, gastritis, severe hepatic reactions (cholestasis, jaundice), nephrotoxicity (glomerular nephritis, interstitial nephritis, nephrotic syndrome), and an acute hypersensitivity reaction (including fever, chills, and joint pain).

NURSING CONSIDERATIONS

Baseline Assessment

- Assess the duration, location, onset, and type of pain.

Lifespan Considerations

- It is unknown if ketorolac is excreted in breast milk.
- Ketorolac should not be used during the third trimester of pregnancy because it may cause adverse effects in the fetus, such as premature closure of the ductus arteriosus.
- Although the safety and efficacy of ketorolac have not been established in children, doses of 0.5 mg/kg have been used.
- In the elderly, GI bleeding or ulceration is more likely to cause serious complications and age-related renal impairment may increase the risk of hepatotoxicity or renal toxicity; a decreased dosage is recommended.

Precautions

- Use ketorolac cautiously in patients with a history of GI tract disease, hepatic or renal impairment, or a predisposition to fluid retention.

Administration and Handling

◀ALERT▶ Ketorolac should not be administered by any route or combination of routes for more than 5 days. This drug may be given as a single dose, on a schedule, or on an as-needed basis, as prescribed.

PO

- Give ketorolac with food, milk, or antacids if the patient experiences GI distress.

IV

- Administer ketorolac undiluted by IV push over at least 15 seconds.

IM

- Slowly inject the drug deeply and into a large muscle mass.

Ophthalmic

- Place a gloved finger on the patient's lower eyelid, and pull it out until a pocket is formed between the eye and lower lid.
- Hold the dropper above the pocket, and place the prescribed number of drops in the pocket.

• Gently close the patient's eye and apply digital pressure to the lacrimal sac for 1 to 2 minutes to minimize drainage into the nose and throat, reducing the risk of systemic effects.
• Remove excess solution with a tissue.

Intervention and Evaluation

• Monitor the patient's CBC, liver and renal function test results, urine output, BUN level, and serum alkaline phosphatase, bilirubin, and creatinine levels.
• Be alert for signs of bleeding, which may also occur with ophthalmic use if systemic absorption occurs.
• Evaluate the patient for evidence of a therapeutic response, such as improved grip strength, increased joint mobility, and decreased pain, tenderness, stiffness, and swelling.

Patient Teaching

• Instruct the patient to take ketorolac with food or milk GI upset occurs.
• Instruct the patients not to administer ketorolac ophthalmic solution while wearing soft contact lenses. Inform the patient that transient burning and stinging may occur after instillation.
• Warn the patient to avoid alcohol and aspirin during ketorolac therapy with oral or ophthalmic ketorolac, which increase the tendency to bleed.
• Warn the patient to avoid tasks that require mental alertness or motor skills until his or her response to the drug has been established.
• Urge the female patient to inform the physician if she is or plans to become pregnant.

meloxicam

mel-**oks**-i-kam
(Mobic)

CATEGORY AND SCHEDULE

Pregnancy Risk Category: C (D if used in third trimester or near delivery)

MECHANISM OF ACTION

An NSAID that produces analgesic and anti-inflammatory effects by inhibiting prostaglandin synthesis. **Therapeutic Effect:** Reduces the inflammatory response and intensity of pain.

PHARMACOKINETICS

Route	Onset	Peak	Duration
PO (analgesic)	30 min	4–5 hr	N/A

Well absorbed after PO administration. Protein binding: 99%. Metabolized in the liver. Eliminated in urine and feces. Not removed by hemodialysis. ***Half-life:*** 15–20 hr.

AVAILABILITY

Tablets: 7.5 mg, 15 mg.

INDICATIONS AND DOSAGES

▸ **Osteoarthritis, Rheumatoid arthritis**

PO

Adults. Initially, 7.5 mg/day. Maximum: 15 mg/day.

CONTRAINDICATIONS

Aspirin-induced nasal polyps associated with bronchospasm

INTERACTIONS

Drug

Aspirin: May increase the risk of

epigastric distress, such as heartburn and indigestion.

Lithium: May increase the plasma concentration and risk of toxicity of lithium.

Herbal

Ginkgo biloba: May increase the risk of bleeding.

Food

None known.

DIAGNOSTIC TEST EFFECTS

May increase serum creatinine, AST (SGOT), and ALT (SGPT) levels.

SIDE EFFECTS

Frequent (9%–7%)

Dyspepsia, headache, diarrhea, nausea

Occasional (4%–3%)

Dizziness, insomnia, rash, pruritus, flatulence, constipation, vomiting

Rare (less than 2%)

Somnolence, urticaria, photosensitivity, tinnitus

SERIOUS REACTIONS

! Rare reactions with long-term use include peptic ulcer disease, GI bleeding, gastritis, severe hepatic reaction (jaundice), nephrotoxicity (hematuria, dysuria, proteinuria), and a severe hypersensitivity reaction (bronchospasm, angioedema).

NURSING CONSIDERATIONS

Baseline Assessment

- Assess the duration, location, onset, and type of inflammation or pain.
- Inspect the arthritic patient's affected joints for deformity, immobility, and skin condition.

Lifespan Considerations

- Meloxicam should not be used during pregnancy because it may cause fetal harm.
- Meloxicam is excreted in breast milk.
- The safety and efficacy of meloxicam have not been established in children.
- Elderly patients require a dosage adjustment because of age-related renal impairment and increased susceptibility to GI toxicity.

Precautions

- Use meloxicam cautiously in patients with asthma, CHF, hypertension, dehydration, hemostatic disease, hepatic or renal impairment, or a history of GI disorders (such as ulcers) and in those using anticoagulants concurrently.

Administration and Handling

PO

- Give meloxicam without regard to food.

Intervention and Evaluation

- Monitor the patient's CBC, BUN level, and serum alkaline phosphatase, bilirubin, creatinine, AST (SGOT), and ALT (SGPT) levels.
- Evaluate the patient for evidence of a therapeutic response, such as improved grip strength, increased joint mobility, and decreased pain, tenderness, stiffness, and swelling.

Patient Teaching

- Instruct the patient to take meloxicam with food or milk to reduce GI upset.
- Urge the patient to notify the physician if he or she experiences chest pain, difficulty breathing, palpitations, peripheral edema, persistent abdominal cramps or pain, a rash, ringing in the ears, severe nausea or vomiting, or unusual bleeding or ecchymosis.
- Tell the patient to inform the physician if she suspects pregnancy or plans to become pregnant.
- Warn the patient to avoid tasks that require mental alertness or motor skills until his or her response to the drug has been established.

nabumetone

na-**byu**-me-tone
(Apo-Nabumetone, Relafen)

CATEGORY AND SCHEDULE

Pregnancy Risk Category: C (D if used in third trimester or near delivery)

MECHANISM OF ACTION

An NSAID that produces analgesic and anti-inflammatory effects by inhibiting prostaglandin synthesis.
Therapeutic Effect: Reduces the inflammatory response and intensity of pain.

PHARMACOKINETICS

Readily absorbed from the GI tract. Protein binding: 99%. Widely distributed. Metabolized in the liver to active metabolite. Primarily excreted in urine. Not removed by hemodialysis. ***Half-life:*** 22–30 hr.

AVAILABILITY

Tablets: 500 mg, 750 mg.

INDICATIONS AND DOSAGES

▸ **Acute or chronic rheumatoid arthritis and osteoarthritis**

PO

Adults, Elderly. Initially, 1,000 mg as a single dose or in 2 divided doses. May increase up to 2,000 mg/day as a single or in 2 divided doses.

CONTRAINDICATIONS

Active peptic ulcer disease, chronic inflammation of GI tract, GI bleeding or ulceration, history of hypersensitivity to aspirin or NSAIDs, history of significant renal impairment

INTERACTIONS

Drug

Antihypertensives, diuretics: May decrease the effects of these drugs.
Aspirin, other salicylates: May increase the risk of GI side effects such as bleeding.
Bone marrow depressants: May increase the risk of hematologic reactions.
Heparin, oral anticoagulants, thrombolytics: May increase the effects of these drugs.
Lithium: May increase the blood concentration and risk of toxicity of lithium.
Methotrexate: May increase the risk of methotrexate toxicity.
Probenecid: May increase the nabumetone blood concentration.

Herbal

Feverfew: May decrease the effects of feverfew.
Ginkgo biloba: May increase the risk of bleeding.

Food

None known.

DIAGNOSTIC TEST EFFECTS

May increase BUN level; urine protein levels; and serum LDH, alkaline phosphatase, creatinine, potassium, AST (SGOT), and ALT (SGPT) levels. May decrease serum uric acid level.

SIDE EFFECTS

Frequent (14%–12%)
Diarrhea, abdominal cramps or pain, dyspepsia
Occasional (9%–4%)
Nausea, constipation, flatulence, dizziness, headache
Rare (3%–1%)
Vomiting, stomatitis, confusion

SERIOUS REACTIONS

! Overdose may result in acute hypotension and tachycardia.

! Rare reactions with long-term use include peptic ulcer disease, GI bleeding, gastritis, nephrotoxicity (dysuria, cystitis, hematuria, proteinuria, nephrotic syndrome), severe hepatic reactions (cholestasis, jaundice), and severe hypersensitivity reactions (bronchospasm, angioedema).

NURSING CONSIDERATIONS

Baseline Assessment

- Assess the duration, location, onset, and type of inflammation or pain.
- Inspect the arthritic patient's affected joints for deformity, immobility, and skin condition.
- Plan to obtain baseline blood chemistry studies, renal and liver function studies, and CBC.

Lifespan Considerations

- Nabumetone is distributed in low concentrations in breast milk.
- Nabumetone should not be used during the last trimester of pregnancy because it may cause adverse effects in the fetus, such as premature closing of the ductus arteriosus.
- The safety and efficacy of this drug have not been established in children.
- In the elderly, GI bleeding or ulceration is more likely to cause serious complications and age-related renal impairment may increase the risk of hepatotoxicity or renal toxicity; a reduced drug dosage is recommended.

Precautions

- Use nabumetone cautiously in patients with CHF, hypertension, or hepatic or renal impairment and in those using anticoagulants concurrently.

Administration and Handling

PO

- Have the patient swallow tablets whole.
- Give nabumetone with food, milk, or antacids if the patient experiences GI distress.

Intervention and Evaluation

- Assist the patient with ambulation if he or she experiences dizziness or drowsiness.
- Monitor the patient for dyspepsia.
- Assess the patient's pattern of daily bowel activity and stool consistency.
- Evaluate the patient for evidence of a therapeutic response, such as improved grip strength, increased joint mobility, and decreased pain, tenderness, stiffness, and swelling.

Patient Teaching

- Instruct the patient to take nabumetone with food if GI upset occurs.
- Caution the patient that nabumetone may cause serious GI bleeding with or without pain. Warn the patient to avoid aspirin during nabumetone therapy because it increases the risk of GI bleeding.
- Inform the patient that nabumetone may cause confusion or dizziness. Warn the patient to avoid performing tasks that require mental alertness or motor skills until his or her response to the drug has been established.
- Advise the female pateint to inform the physician if she is or plans to become pregnant.

naproxen

na-**prox**-en
(Crysanal[AUS], EC-Naprosyn, Inza[AUS], Naprelan, Naprosyn)

naproxen sodium

(Aleve, Anaprox, Anaprox DS, Apo-Naprosyn[CAN], Naprogesic[AUS], Novo-Naprox[CAN], Nu-Naprox[CAN], Pamprin)
Do not confuse Aleve with Allese, or Anaprox with Anaspaz.

CATEGORY AND SCHEDULE

Pregnancy Risk Category: B (D if used in third trimester or near delivery)
OTC (220-mg gelcaps, 220-mg tablets)

MECHANISM OF ACTION

An NSAID that produces analgesic and anti-inflammatory effects by inhibiting prostaglandin synthesis. **Therapeutic Effect:** Reduces the inflammatory response and intensity of pain.

PHARMACOKINETICS

Route	Onset	Peak	Duration
PO (analgesic)	less than 1 hr	N/A	7 hr or less
PO (antirheumatic)	less than 14 days	2–4 wk	N/A

Completely absorbed from the GI) tract. Protein binding: 99%. Metabolized in the liver. Primarily excreted in urine. Not removed by hemodialysis. ***Half-life:*** 13 hr.

AVAILABILITY

Gelcaps (Aleve): 220 mg naproxen sodium (equivalent to 200 mg naproxen).
Oral Suspension (Naprosyn): 125 mg/5 ml naproxen.
Tablets (Aleve): 220 mg naproxen.
Tablets (Anaprox): 275 mg naproxen sodium (equivalent to 250 mg naproxen).
Tablets (Anaprox DS): 550 mg naproxen sodium (equivalent to 500 mg naproxen).
Tablets (Controlled-Release [EC-Naprosyn]): 375 mg naproxen, 500 mg naproxen.
Tablets (Controlled-Release [Naprelan]): 421 mg naproxen, 550 mg naproxen sodium (equivalent to 500 mg naproxen).

INDICATIONS AND DOSAGES

▸ **Rheumatoid arthritis, osteoarthritis, ankylosing spondylitis**
PO
Adults, Elderly. 250–500 mg naproxen (275–550 mg naproxen sodium) twice a day or 250 mg naproxen (275 mg naproxen sodium) in morning and 500 mg naproxen (550 mg naproxen sodium) in evening. Naprelan: 750–1,000 mg once a day.

▸ **Acute gouty arthritis**
PO
Adults, Elderly. Initially, 750 mg naproxen (825 mg naproxen sodium), then 250 mg naproxen (275 mg naproxen sodium) q8h until attack subsides. Naprelan: Initially, 1,000–1,500 mg, then 1,000 mg once a day until attack subsides.

▸ **Mild to moderate pain, dysmenorrhea, bursitis, tendinitis**
PO
Adults, Elderly. Initially, 500 mg naproxen (550 mg naproxen sodium), then 250 mg naparoxen (275 mg naproxen sodium) q6–8h as needed. Maximum: 1.25 g/day naproxen (1.375 g/day naproxen

sodium). Naprelan: 1,000 mg once a day.

▸ **Juvenile rheumatoid arthritis**
PO (naproxen only)
Children. 10–15 mg/kg/day in 2 divided doses. Maximum: 1,000 mg/day.

OFF-LABEL USES

Treatment of vascular headaches

CONTRAINDICATIONS

Hypersensitivity to aspirin, naproxen, or other NSAIDs

INTERACTIONS

Drug

Antihypertensives, diuretics: May decrease the effects of these drugs.
Aspirin, other salicylates: May increase the risk of GI side effects such as bleeding.
Bone marrow depressants: May increase the risk of hematologic reactions.
Heparin, oral anticoagulants, thrombolytics: May increase the effects of these drugs.
Lithium: May increase the blood concentration and risk of toxicity of lithium.
Methotrexate: May increase the risk of methotrexate toxicity.
Probenecid: May increase the naproxen blood concentration.

Herbal

Feverfew: May decrease the effects of feverfew.
Ginkgo biloba: May increase the risk of bleeding.

Food

None known.

DIAGNOSTIC TEST EFFECTS

May prolong bleeding time and alter blood glucose level. May increase serum hepatic function test results. May decrease serum sodium and uric acid levels.

SIDE EFFECTS

Frequent (9%–4%)
Nausea, constipation, abdominal cramps or pain, heartburn, dizziness, headache, somnolence
Occasional (3%–1%)
Stomatitis, diarrhea, indigestion
Rare (less than 1%)
Vomiting, confusion

SERIOUS REACTIONS

! Rare reactions with long-term use include peptic ulcer disease, GI bleeding, gastritis, severe hepatic reactions (cholestasis, jaundice), nephrotoxicity (dysuria, hematuria, proteinuria, nephrotic syndrome), and a severe hypersensitivity reaction (fever, chills, bronchospasm).

NURSING CONSIDERATIONS

Baseline Assessment

- Assess the duration, location, onset, and type of inflammation or pain.
- Inspect the arthritic patient's affected joints for deformity, immobility, and skin condition.

Lifespan Considerations

- Naproxen crosses the placenta and is distributed in breast milk.
- Naproxen should not be used during the third trimester of pregnancy because it may cause adverse effects in the fetus, such as premature closing of the ductus arteriosus.
- The safety and efficacy of naproxen have not been established in children younger than 2 years.
- Children older than 2 years are at an increased risk for developing a rash during naproxen therapy.
- In the elderly, GI bleeding or ulceration is more likely to cause serious complications and age-related renal impairment may increase the risk of hepatotoxicity and

renal toxicity; a reduced dosage is recommended.

Precautions

• Use naproxen cautiously in patients with cardiac disease or GI disease, or impaired hepatic or renal function and in patients using anticoagulants concurrently.

Administration and Handling

PO

◀ **ALERT** ▶ Be aware that each 275- or 550-mg tablet of naproxen sodium equals 250 or 500 mg of naproxen, respectively.

• Have the patient swallow enteric-coated tablets whole; scored tablets may be broken or crushed.

• Give naproxen with food, milk, or antacids if the patient experiences GI distress.

Intervention and Evaluation

• Monitor the patient's CBC (particularly Hgb, Hct, and platelet count), BUN level, and serum alkaline phosphatase, bilirubin, creatinine, AST (SGOT), and ALT (SGPT) levels to assess hepatic and renal function.

• Assess the patient's pattern of daily bowel activity and stool consistency.

• Assist the patient with ambulation if he or she experiences dizziness.

• Evaluate the patient for evidence of a therapeutic response, such as improved grip strength, increased joint mobility, and decreased pain, tenderness, stiffness, and swelling.

Patient Teaching

• Instruct the patient to take naproxen with food or milk if GI upset occurs.

• Advise the patient to notify the physician if he or she experiences black or tarry stools, persistent headache, rash, visual disturbances, or weight gain.

• Warn the patient to avoid tasks that require mental alertness or motor skills until his or her response to the drug has been established.

• Caution the patient to avoid alcohol and aspirin during naproxen therapy because these substances increase the risk of GI bleeding.

• Advise the female patient to inform the physician if she is or plans to become pregnant.

oxaprozin

ox-a-**pro**-zin

(Daypro)

Do not confuse oxaprozin with oxazepam.

CATEGORY AND SCHEDULE

Pregnancy Risk Category: C (D if used in third trimester or near delivery)

MECHANISM OF ACTION

An NSAID that produces analgesic and anti-inflammatory effects by inhibiting prostaglandin synthesis. **Therapeutic Effect:** Reduces the inflammatory response and intensity of pain.

PHARMACOKINETICS

Well absorbed from the GI tract. Protein binding: 99%. Widely distributed. Metabolized in the liver. Primarily excreted in urine; partially eliminated in feces. Not removed by hemodialysis. ***Half-life:*** 42–50 hr.

AVAILABILITY

Tablets: 600 mg.

INDICATIONS AND DOSAGES

▸ **Osteoarthritis**

PO

Adults, Elderly. 1,200 mg once a day (600 mg in patients with low body weight or mild disease). Maximum: 1,800 mg/day.

▸ **Rheumatoid arthritis**

PO

Adults, Elderly. 1,200 mg once a day. Range: 600–1,800 mg/day.

▸ **Juvenile rheumatoid arthritis**

Children weighing more than 54 kg. 1,200 mg/day.

Children weighing 32-54 kg. 900 mg/day.

Children weighing 22-31 kg. 600 mg/day.

▸ **Dosage in renal impairment**

For adults and elderly patients with renal impairment, the recommended initial dose is 600 mg/day; may be increased up to 1,200 mg/day.

CONTRAINDICATIONS

Active peptic ulcer disease, chronic inflammation of GI tract, GI bleeding or ulceration, history of hypersensitivity to aspirin or NSAIDs

INTERACTIONS

Drug

Antihypertensives, diuretics: May decrease the effects of these drugs.

Aspirin, other salicylates: May increase the risk of GI side effects such as bleeding.

Bone marrow depressants: May increase the risk of hematologic reactions.

Heparin, oral anticoagulants, thrombolytics: May increase the effects of these drugs.

Lithium: May increase the blood concentration and risk of toxicity of lithium.

Methotrexate: May increase the risk of methotrexate toxicity.

Probenecid: May increase the oxaprozin blood concentration.

Herbal

Feverfew: May decrease the effects of feverfew.

Ginkgo biloba: May increase the risk of bleeding.

Food

None known.

DIAGNOSTIC TEST EFFECTS

May increase BUN, serum creatinine, AST (SGOT), and ALT (SGPT) levels.

SIDE EFFECTS

Occasional (9%–3%)

Nausea, diarrhea, constipation, dyspepsia, edema

Rare (less than 3%)

Vomiting, abdominal cramps or pain, flatulence, anorexia, confusion, tinnitus, insomnia, somnolence

SERIOUS REACTIONS

! Hypertension, acute renal failure, respiratory depression, GI bleeding, and coma occur rarely.

NURSING CONSIDERATIONS

Baseline Assessment

• Assess the duration, location, onset, and type of inflammation or pain.

Lifespan Considerations

• It is unknown if oxaprozin is excreted in breast milk.

• Oxaprozin should not be used during the third trimester of pregnancy because it may cause adverse effects in the fetus, such as premature closure of the ductus arteriosus.

• The safety and efficacy of oxaprozin have not been established in children.

• In the elderly, GI bleeding or ulceration is more likely to cause serious complications and age-related renal impairment may increase the risk of hepatotoxicity or renal toxicity; a decreased dosage is recommended.

Precautions
• Use oxaprozin cautiously in patients with a history of GI tract disease, hepatic or renal impairment, or a predisposition to fluid retention.
Administration and Handling
PO
• Give oxaprozin with food, milk, or antacids if the patient experiences GI distress.
Intervention and Evaluation
• Assess the patient for bleeding, ecchymosis, edema, confusion and weight gain.
• Monitor the patient's BUN and serum alkaline phosphatase, bilirubin, creatinine, AST (SGOT), and ALT (SGPT) levels to assess hepatic and renal function.
• Evaluate the patient for evidence of a therapeutic response, such as improved grip strength, increased joint mobility, and decreased pain, tenderness, stiffness, and swelling.
Patient Teaching
• Instruct the patient to take oxaprozin with food or milk if GI upset occurs.
• Caution the patient to avoid alcohol and aspirin, which increase the risk of GI bleeding, during oxaprozin therapy.
• Warn the patient to avoid performing tasks that require mental alertness or motor skills until his or her response to the drug has been established.
• Instruct the patient to notify the physician if he or she experiences persistent GI effects, especially black, tarry stools.
• Tell the female patient to inform the physician if she is or plans to become pregnant.

piroxicam
peer-**ox**-i-kam
(Apo-Piroxicam[CAN], Candyl-D[AUS], Feldene, Fexicam[CAN], Mobilis[AUS], Novopirocam[CAN], Pirohexal-D[AUS], Rosig[AUS], Rosig-D[AUS])
Do not confuse Feldene with Seldane.

CATEGORY AND SCHEDULE
Pregnancy Risk Category: C (D if used in third trimester or near delivery)

MECHANISM OF ACTION
An NSAID that produces analgesic and anti-inflammatory effects by inhibiting prostaglandin synthesis. **Therapeutic Effect:** Reduces inflammatory response and intensity of pain.

AVAILABILITY
Capsules: 10 mg, 20 mg.

INDICATIONS AND DOSAGES
▸ **Acute or chronic rheumatoid arthritis and osteoarthritis**
PO
Adults, Elderly. Initially, 10–20 mg/day as a single dose or in divided doses. Some patients may require up to 30–40 mg/day.
Children. 0.2–0.3 mg/kg/day. Maximum: 15 mg/day.

OFF-LABEL USES
Treatment of acute gouty arthritis, ankylosing spondylitis, dysmenorrhea

CONTRAINDICATIONS
Active peptic ulcer disease, chronic inflammation of the GI tract, GI bleeding or ulceration, history of hypersensitivity to aspirin or NSAIDs

INTERACTIONS

Drug

Antihypertensives, diuretics: May decrease the effects of these drugs.
Aspirin, other salicylates: May increase the risk of GI side effects such as bleeding.
Bone marrow depressants: May increase the risk of hematologic reactions.
Heparin, oral anticoagulants, thrombolytics: May increase the effects of these drugs.
Lithium: May increase the blood concentration and risk of toxicity of lithium.
Methotrexate: May increase the risk of methotrexate toxicity.
Probenecid: May increase the piroxicam blood concentration.

Herbal

Feverfew: May decrease the effects of feverfew.
Ginkgo biloba: May increase the risk of bleeding.
St. John's wort: May increase the risk of phototoxicity.

Food

None known.

DIAGNOSTIC TEST EFFECTS

May increase AST (SGOT) and ALT (SGPT) levels. May decrease serum uric acid levels.

SIDE EFFECTS

Frequent (9%–4%)
Dyspepsia, nausea, dizziness
Occasional (3%–1%)
Diarrhea, constipation, abdominal cramps or pain, flatulence, stomatitis
Rare (less than 1%)
Hypertension, urticaria, dysuria, ecchymosis, blurred vision, insomnia, phototoxicity

SERIOUS REACTIONS

! Rare reactions with long-term use include peptic ulcer disease, GI bleeding, gastritis, severe hepatic reaction (cholestasis, jaundice), nephrotoxicity (dysuria, hematuria, proteinuria, nephrotic syndrome), hematologic sensitivity (anemia, leukopenia, eosinophilia, thrombocytopenia), and a severe hypersensitivity reaction (fever, chills, bronchospasm).

NURSING CONSIDERATIONS

Baseline Assessment

• Assess the duration, location, onset, and type of inflammation or pain.
• Inspect the arthritic patient's affected joints for deformity, immobility, and skin condition.
• Expect to obtain baseline CBC and serum chemistry tests, especially BUN and serum alkaline phosphatase, bilirubin, creatinine, AST (SGOT), and ALT (SGPT) levels to assess hepatic and renal function.

Precautions

• Use piroxicam cautiously in patients with GI disease, hypertension, or impaired cardiac or hepatic function and in patients using anticoagulants concurrently.

Administration and Handling

PO
• Don't crush or break capsules.
• Give piroxicam with food, milk, or antacids if the patient experiences GI distress.

Intervention and Evaluation

• Monitor the patient for GI distress and nausea.
• Monitor the patient's CBC and hepatic and renal function test results.
• Assess the patient's pattern of daily bowel activity and stool consistency.
• Evaluate the patient for evidence of a therapeutic response, such as improved grip strength, increased

joint mobility, and decreased pain, tenderness, stiffness, and swelling.

Patient Teaching

- Instruct the patient to take piroxicam with food, milk, or antacids if GI upset occurs.
- Warn the patient to avoid tasks that require mental alertness or motor skills until his or her response to the drug has been established.
- Caution the patient to avoid alcohol and aspirin during piroxicam therapy because these substances increase the risk of GI bleeding.
- Advise the female patient to inform the physician if she is or plans to become pregnant.

sulindac

sul-**in**-dak

(Aclin[AUS], Apo-Sulin[CAN], Clinoril, Novo Sundac[CAN])

Do not confuse Clinoril with Clozaril.

CATEGORY AND SCHEDULE

Pregnancy Risk Category: B (D if used in third trimester or near delivery)

MECHANISM OF ACTION

An NSAID that produces analgesic and anti-inflammatory effects by inhibiting prostaglandin synthesis. **Therapeutic Effect:** Reduces inflammatory response and intensity of pain.

PHARMACOKINETICS

Route	Onset	Peak	Duration
PO (Antirheumatic)	7 days	2–3 wk	N/A

Well absorbed from the GI tract. Metabolized in liver to active metabolite. Primarily excreted in urine. Not removed by hemodialysis. ***Half-life:*** 7.8 hr; metabolite: 16.4 hr.

AVAILABILITY

Tablets: 150 mg, 200 mg.

INDICATIONS AND DOSAGES

▸ Rheumatoid arthritis, osteoarthritis, ankylosing spondylitis

PO

Adults, Elderly. Initially, 150 mg twice a day; may increase up to 400 mg/day.

▸ Acute shoulder pain, gouty arthritis, bursitis, tendinitis

PO

Adults, Elderly. 200 mg twice a day.

CONTRAINDICATIONS

Active peptic ulcer disease, chronic inflammation of GI tract, GI bleeding or ulceration, history of hypersensitivity to aspirin or NSAIDs

INTERACTIONS

Drug

Antacids: May decrease the sulindac blood concentration.
Antihypertensives, diuretics: May decrease the effects of these drugs.
Aspirin, other salicylates: May increase the risk of GI side effects such as bleeding.
Bone marrow depressants: May increase the risk of hematologic reactions.
Heparin, oral anticoagulants, thrombolytics: May increase the effects of these drugs.
Lithium: May increase the blood concentration and risk of toxicity of lithium.
Methotrexate: May increase the risk of methotrexate toxicity.
Probenecid: May increase the sulindac blood concentration.

Herbal

Feverfew: May decrease the effects of feverfew.
Ginkgo biloba: May increase the risk of bleeding.

Food

None known.

DIAGNOSTIC TEST EFFECTS

May increase liver function test results and serum alkaline phosphatase level.

SIDE EFFECTS

Frequent (9%–4%)

Diarrhea or constipation, indigestion, nausea, maculopapular rash, dermatitis, dizziness, headache

Occasional (3%–1%)

Anorexia, abdominal cramps, flatulence

SERIOUS REACTIONS

! Rare reactions with long-term use include peptic ulcer disease GI bleeding, gastritis, nephrotoxicity (glomerular nephritis, interstitial nephritis, nephrotic syndrome), severe hepatic reactions (cholestasis, jaundice), and severe hypersensitivity reactions (fever, chills, and joint pain).

NURSING CONSIDERATIONS

Baseline Assessment

- Assess the duration, location, onset, and type of inflammation or pain.
- Inspect the arthritic patient's affected joints for deformity, immobility, and skin condition.
- Expect to obtain baseline CBC, particularly platelet count, and baseline blood chemistry values, especially BUN and serum alkaline phosphatase, bilirubin, creatinine, AST (SGOT), ALT (SGPT) levels to assess hepatic and renal function.

Lifespan Considerations

- It is unknown if sulindac is excreted in breast milk.
- Sulindac should not be used during the third trimester of pregnancy because it may cause adverse effects in the fetus, such as premature closure of the ductus arteriosus.
- The safety and efficacy of naproxen have not been established in children.
- In the elderly, GI bleeding or ulceration is more likely to cause serious complications and age-related renal impairment may increase the risk of hepatotoxicity and renal toxicity; a reduced drug dosage is recommended.

Precautions

- Use sulindac cautiously in patients with history of GI tract disease, hepatic or renal impairment, or a predisposition to fluid retention. Also use cautiously in patients receiving concurrent anticoagulant therapy.

Administration and Handling

PO

- Give sulindac with food, milk, or antacids if the patient experiences GI distress.

Intervention and Evaluation

- Monitor the patient's CBC, especially platelet count, and liver and renal function test results.
- Assess the patient's pattern of daily bowel activity and stool consistency.
- Examine the patient's skin for a rash.
- Assist the patient with ambulation if he or she experiences dizziness.
- Evaluate the patient for evidence of a therapeutic response, such as improved grip strength, increased joint mobility, and decreased pain, tenderness, stiffness, and swelling.

Patient Teaching

- Instruct the patient to take sulindac with food or milk if GI upset occurs.
- Inform the patient that sulindac's

therapeutic antiarthritic effect will occur 1 to 3 weeks after therapy begins.
- Caution the patient to avoid alcohol and aspirin during naproxen therapy because these substances increase the risk of GI bleeding.
- Advise the female patient to inform the physician if she is or plans to become pregnant.
- Warn the patient not to perform tasks that require mental alertness or motor skills until his or her response to the drug has been established.

valdecoxib

val-de-**cocks**-ib
(Bextra)

CATEGORY AND SCHEDULE

Pregnancy Risk Category: C (D if used in third trimester or near delivery)

MECHANISM OF ACTION

An NSAID that inhibits cyclooxygenase-2, the enzyme responsible for producing prostaglandins, which cause pain and inflammation. **Therapeutic Effect:** Reduces inflammatory response and intensity of pain.

PHARMACOKINETICS

Rapidly and almost completely absorbed from the GI tract. Widely distributed. Extensively metabolized in the liver. Primarily eliminated in urine. ***Half-life:*** 8-11 hr.

AVAILABILITY

Tablets: 10 mg, 20 mg.

INDICATIONS AND DOSAGES

▸ Osteoarthritis, rheumatoid arthritis

PO

Adults, Elderly. 10 mg once a day.

▸ Primary dysmenorrhea

PO

Adults, Elderly. 20 mg twice a day.

CONTRAINDICATIONS

Hypersensitivity to aspirin or NSAIDs, severe hepatic or renal impairment

INTERACTIONS

Drug

Anticoagulants: May increase the effects of anticoagulants.
Aspirin, other salicylates: May increase the risk of GI side effects such as bleeding.
Dextromethorphan: May increase the plasma level of dextromethorphan.
Fluconazole, ketoconazole: May increase the plasma concentration of valdecoxib.

Herbal

None known.

Food

None known.

DIAGNOSTIC TEST EFFECTS

May increase BUN and serum creatinine levels and liver function test results.

SIDE EFFECTS

Frequent (8%-4%)
Headache

Occasional (3%-2%)
Dizziness

Rare (less than 2%)
Dyspepsia, nausea, diarrhea, sinusitis, peripheral edema

SERIOUS REACTIONS

! None known.

NURSING CONSIDERATIONS

Baseline Assessment
- Assess the duration, location,

onset, and type of inflammation or pain.
- Inspect the arthritic patient's affected joints for deformity, immobility, and skin condition.

Lifespan Considerations
- Valdecoxib is excreted in breast milk.
- Valdecoxib should not be used during the third trimester of pregnancy because it may cause adverse effects in the fetus, such as premature closure of the ductus arteriosus.
- The safety and efficacy of valdecoxib have not been established in children younger than 18 years.
- Elderly patients are more likely to experience adverse reactions than younger patients.

Precautions
- Use valdecoxib cautiously in patients 65 years and older, smokers, and patients with alcoholism or moderate hepatic impairment, and those who use anticoagulants or steroids concurrently.

Administration and Handling
- Do not crush or break film-coated tablets.
- Give valdecoxib without regard to food.

Intervention and Evaluation
- Monitor the patient's BUN and serum creatinine levels and liver function test results.
- Assess the patient's pattern of daily bowel activity and stool consistency.
- Monitor the patient for headache.
- Assist the patient with ambulation if he or she experiences dizziness.
- Assess the patient with dysmenorrhea for relief of abdominal cramps.
- Evaluate the arthritis patient for evidence of a therapeutic response, such as improved grip strength, increased joint mobility, and decreased joint tenderness, pain, stiffness, and swelling.

Patient Teaching
- Instruct the patient to take valdecoxib with food or milk if he or she experiences GI upset.
- Caution the patient to avoid alcohol and aspirin during valdecoxib therapy. These substances increase the risk of GI bleeding.
- Advise the patient to inform the physician if she is or plans to become pregnant.

46 Sedative-Hypnotics

chloral hydrate
dexmedetomidine hydrochloride
eszopiclone
flurazepam hydrochloride
temazepam
triazolam
zaleplon
zolpidem tartrate

Uses: Sedative-hypnotics are used to treat insomnia, which includes difficulty falling asleep initially, frequent awakenings, and awakening too early. Benzodiazepines, such as flurazepam and triazolam, are the most widely used agents. They have largely replaced barbiturates as sedative-hypnotics because they offer greater safety and a lower risk of drug dependence. Nonbenzodiazepines, including zaleplon and zolpidem, have a rapid onset and short duration of action and are used to treat short-term insomnia. In addition, some sedative-hypnotics, such as chloral hydrate, are used to premedicate patients before a dental or medical procedure.

Action: Sedatives decrease motor activity, moderate excitement, and have calming effects. Hypnotics produce drowsiness and enhance the onset and maintenance of sleep, resembling natural sleep. *Benzodiazepines* potentiate gamma-aminobutyric acid (GABA), which inhibits impulse transmission in the reticular formation in the brain. They increase the total sleep time by decreasing sleep latency (time before the onset of sleep), the number of awakenings, and the time spent in the awake stage of sleep (light sleep). *Nonbenzodiazepines* bind selectively to a subunit of GABA to enhance its action.

chloral hydrate

klor-al **hye**-drate
(Aquachloral Supprettes, PMS-Chloral Hydrate[CAN], Somnote)

CATEGORY AND SCHEDULE

Pregnancy Risk Category: C

MECHANISM OF ACTION

A nonbarbiturate chloral derivative that produces CNS depression. **Therapeutic Effect:** Induces quiet, deep sleep, with only a slight decrease in respiratory rate and BP.

AVAILABILITY

Capsules (Somnote): 500 mg.
Syrup: 500 mg/5 ml.
Suppositories (Aquachloral Supprettes): 324 mg, 648 mg.

INDICATIONS AND DOSAGES

▸ **Premedication for dental or medical procedures**

PO, Rectal

Adults. 0.5–1 g.

Children. 75 mg/kg up to 1 g total.

▸ **Premedication for EEG**

PO, Rectal

Adults. 0.5–1.5 g.

Children. 25–50 mg/kg/dose 30–60 min prior to EEG. May repeat in 30 min. Maximum: 1 g for infants, 2 g for children.

CONTRAINDICATIONS

Gastritis, marked hepatic or renal impairment, severe cardiac disease

INTERACTIONS

Drug

Alcohol, other CNS depressants: May increase the effects of chloral hydrate.

Furosemide (IV): May alter BP and cause diaphoresis if given within 24 hours after chloral hydrate.

Warfarin: May increase the effect of warfarin.

Herbal

None known.

Food

None known.

DIAGNOSTIC TEST EFFECTS

None known.

SIDE EFFECTS

Occasional

Gastric irritation (nausea, vomiting, flatulence, diarrhea), rash, sleepwalking

Rare

Headache, paradoxical CNS hyperactivity or nervousness in children, excitement or restlessness in the elderly (particularly in patients with pain).

SERIOUS REACTIONS

! Overdose may produce somnolence, confusion, slurred speech, severe incoordination, respiratory depression, and coma.

NURSING CONSIDERATIONS

Baseline Assessment

- Assess the patient's BP, pulse rate, and respiratory rate, rhythm, and depth immediately before administering chloral hydrate.
- Institute safety measures including raising the patient's bed rails and providing a call bell.
- Provide the patient with an environment conducive to sleep. For example, offer a back rub, a quiet environment, and low lighting.
- Expect to obtain baseline blood chemistry studies to assess renal and hepatic function.

Precautions

- Use chloral hydrate cautiously in patients with clinical depression or a history of drug abuse.

Administration and Handling

PO

- Administer chloral hydrate capsules with a full glass of water or fruit juice.
- Have the patient swallow the capsules whole and not chew them.
- Dilute the dose of syrup in water to minimize gastric irritation.

Rectal

- Store suppositories at room temperature; don't refrigerate them.

Intervention and Evaluation

- Monitor the patient's mental status and vital signs.
- Assess pediatric and elderly patients for paradoxical reactions, such as excitability.

Patient Teaching

- Urge the patient not to drive if he or she will take chloral hydrate before a procedure.

dexmedetomidine hydrochloride

decks-meh-deh-**tome**-ih-deen
(Precedex)
Do not confuse Precedex with Peridex or Percocet.

CATEGORY AND SCHEDULE

Pregnancy Risk Category: C

MECHANISM OF ACTION

A selective $alpha_2$-adrenergic agonist. **Therapeutic Effect:** Produces analgesic, hypnotic, and sedative effects.

AVAILABILITY

Injection: 100 mcg/ml.

INDICATIONS AND DOSAGES

▸ **Sedation before, during, and after intubation and mechanical ventilation while in ICU**

IV

Adults. Loading dose of 1 mcg/kg over 10 min followed by maintenance infusion of 0.2–0.7 mcg/kg/hr.
Elderly. May require decreased dosage. No guidelines available.

CONTRAINDICATIONS

None known.

INTERACTIONS

Drug

Anesthetics, opioids, other sedative-hypnotics: May enhance the effects of dexmedetomidine.

Herbal

None known.

Food

None known.

DIAGNOSTIC TEST EFFECTS

May increase serum potassium, alkaline phosphatase, AST (SGOT), and ALT (SGPT) levels.

IV INCOMPATIBILITIES

Do not mix dexmedetomidine with any other medications.

SIDE EFFECTS

Frequent

Hypotension (30%), nausea (11%)

Occasional (3%–2%)

Pain, fever, oliguria, thirst

SERIOUS REACTIONS

! Bradycardia, atrial fibrillation, hypoxia, anemia, pain, and pleural effusion may occur with too-rapid IV infusion.

NURSING CONSIDERATIONS

Baseline Assessment

- Obtain baseline vital signs, including BP and heart rate.
- Expect to obtain baseline liver function test results as well as serum electrolyte levels.
- Expect to perform a baseline EKG to help rule out underlying cardiac disease.

Precautions

- Use dexmedetomidine cautiously in patients with CHF, advanced heart block, hypovolemia, or hepatic or renal impairment.
- Make sure that the patient is on a continuous cardiac monitor and pulse oximeter to assess for arrhythmias and hypoxemia before administering the drug.

Administration and Handling

◂**ALERT**▸ Dilute dexmedetomidine with 48 ml 0.9% NaCl before use. Don't infuse the drug for longer than 24 hours.

IV

- Store vials at room temperature.
- Dilute 2 ml of dexmedetomidine with 48 ml of 0.9% NaCl.
- Administer the drug as a maintenance infusion, as prescribed.

Intervention and Evaluation
- Monitor the patient's EKG for atrial fibrillation, BP for hypotension and level of sedation, and pulse rate for bradycardia. Also assess respiratory rate and rhythm.
- Monitor the patient's ventilator settings.

Patient Teaching
- Explain to the patient that dexmedetomidine will provide relaxation and sedation before, during, and after insertion of the endotracheal tube, and during mechanical ventilation.
- Provide comfort measures, such as mouth care and repositioning while the patient is sedated. Inform the patient that his or her hands and arms will be restrained during mechanical ventilation.

eszopiclone

es-zoe-**pick**-lone
(Lunesta)

CATEGORY AND SCHEDULE

Pregnancy Risk Category: C

MECHANISM OF ACTION

A nonbenzodiazepine that may interact with GABA-receptor complexes at binding domains located close to or allosterically coupled to benzodiazepine receptors. **Therapeutic Effect:** Induces sleep and helps maintain sleep at night.

AVAILABILITY

Tablets (Film-Coated): 1 mg, 2 mg, 3 mg.

INDICATIONS AND DOSAGES

▸ Insomnia

PO

Adults. 2 mg before bedtime. Maximum: 3 mg.

Adults using CYP3A4 inhibitors concurrently. 1 mg before bedtime; may be increased to 2 mg if needed.

Elderly. Initially, 1 mg before bedtime. Maximum: 2 mg.

▸ Difficulty Maintaining Sleep

PO

Adults, Elderly. 2 mg before bedtime.

CONTRAINDICATIONS

None known.

INTERACTIONS

Drug

Alcohol, olanzapine: May lead to decreased psychomotor function.

Aminoglutethimide, carbamazepine, nafcillin, nevirapine, phenobarbital, phenytoin, rifampicin: May decrease the blood level and effects of eszopiclone.

Clarithromycin, ketoconazole, nefazodone, nelfinavir, ritonavir, traconazole, troleandomycin: May increase the blood level and effects of eszopiclone.

Herbal

Gotu kola, kava kava, St. John's wort, valerian: May increase CNS depression.

Food

Heavy meals: May reduce onset of eszopiclone action if taken with or immediately after a heavy meal.

DIAGNOSTIC TEST EFFECTS

None known.

SIDE EFFECTS

Frequent (34%–21%)
Unpleasant taste, headache

Occasional (10%–4%)
Somnolence, dry mouth, dyspepsia, dizziness, nervousness, nausea, rash, pruritus, depression, diarrhea

Rare (3%–2%)
Hallucinations, anxiety, confusion,

abnormal dreams, decreased libido, neuralgia.

SERIOUS REACTIONS

! Chest pain and peripheral edema occur occasionally.

NURSING CONSIDERATIONS

Precautions

• Use eszopiclone cautiously in patients with clinical depression and hepatic impairment compromised respiratory function.

Administration and Handling

PO

• Give immediately before bedtime. Don't give with, or immediately following, a high-fat meal.
• Don't crush or break tablets.

flurazepam hydrochloride

flure-**az**-e-pam
(Apo-Flurazepam[CAN], Dalmane)
Do not confuse Dalmane with Dialume.

CATEGORY AND SCHEDULE

Pregnancy Risk Category: X
Controlled Substance: Schedule IV

MECHANISM OF ACTION

A benzodiazepine that enhances action of inhibitory neurotransmitter gamma-aminobutyric acid (GABA). **Therapeutic Effect:** Produces hypnotic effect due to CNS depression.

PHARMACOKINETICS

Route	Onset	Peak	Duration
PO	15–20 min	3–6 hr	7–8 hr

Well absorbed from the GI tract. Protein binding: 97%. Crosses the blood-brain barrier. Widely distributed. Metabolized in liver to active metabolite. Primarily excreted in urine. Not removed by hemodialysis. ***Half-life:*** 2.3 hr; metabolite: 40–114 hr.

AVAILABILITY

Capsules: 15 mg, 30 mg.

INDICATIONS AND DOSAGES

▸ **Insomnia**

PO

Adults. 15–30 mg at bedtime.
Elderly, debilitated, liver disease, low serum albumin, Children 15 yr and older. 15 mg at bedtime.

CONTRAINDICATIONS

Acute alcohol intoxication, acute angle-closure glaucoma, pregnancy or breast-feeding

INTERACTIONS

Drug

Alcohol, CNS depressants: May increase CNS depression.

Herbal

Kava kava, valerian: May increase CNS depression.

Food

None known.

DIAGNOSTIC TEST EFFECTS

None known.

SIDE EFFECTS

Frequent

Drowsiness, dizziness, ataxia, sedation

Morning drowsiness may occur initially.

Occasional

GI disturbances, nervousness, blurred vision, dry mouth, headache, confusion, skin rash, irritability, slurred speech

Rare

Paradoxical CNS excitement or restlessness, particularly noted in elderly or debilitated

SERIOUS REACTIONS

! Abrupt or too-rapid withdrawal after long-term use may result in pronounced restlessness and irritability, insomnia, hand tremors, abdominal or muscle cramps, vomiting, diaphoresis, and seizures.

! Overdose results in somnolence, confusion, diminished reflexes, and coma.

NURSING CONSIDERATIONS

Baseline Assessment

- Assess the patient's BP, pulse, and respirations immediately before beginning flurazepam administration.
- Raise the patient's bed rails and place the call bell within reach.
- Provide the patient with an environment conducive to sleep. For example, offer a back rub, quiet environment, and low lighting.

Lifespan Considerations

- Be aware that flurazepam crosses the placenta and may be distributed in breast milk.
- Be aware that chronic flurazepam ingestion during pregnancy may produce withdrawal symptoms and CNS depression in neonates.
- Be aware that the safety and efficacy of flurazepam have not been established in children younger than 15 years of age.
- Use small initial doses with gradual dose increases to avoid ataxia or excessive sedation in the elderly.

Precautions

- Use cautiously in patients with impaired liver or renal function.

Administration and Handling

PO

- Give flurazepam without regard to meals.
- If desired, empty capsules and mix with food.

Intervention and Evaluation

- Assess patients for paradoxical reaction, such as excitability, particularly during early therapy.
- Evaluate the patient for therapeutic response to insomnia, a decrease in number of nocturnal awakenings and an increase in length of sleep.

Patient Teaching

- Tell the patient that smoking reduces the drug's effectiveness.
- Caution the patient against abruptly withdrawing the medication after long-term use.
- Explain to the patient that he or she may have disturbed sleep 1 to 2 nights after discontinuing the drug.
- Instruct the patient to notify the physician if she becomes pregnant or plans to become pregnant. Explain to the patient that flurazepam is pregnancy risk category X and that the drug cannot be taken due to its risk factor.
- Urge the patient to avoid alcohol and other CNS depressants during flurazepam therapy.
- Advise the patient that flurazepam may be habit-forming.

temazepam

te-**maz**-e-pam
(Apo-Temazepam[CAN], Novo-Temazepam[CAN], PMS-Temazepam[CAN], Restoril)
Do not confuse Restoril with Vistaril or Zestril.

CATEGORY AND SCHEDULE
Pregnancy Risk Category: X
Controlled Substance: Schedule IV

MECHANISM OF ACTION
A benzodiazepine that enhances the action of the inhibitory neurotransmitter gamma-aminobutyric acid, resulting in CNS depression. **Therapeutic Effect:** Induces sleep.

PHARMACOKINETICS
Well absorbed from the GI tract. Protein binding: 96%. Widely distributed. Crosses the blood-brain barrier. Metabolized in the liver. Primarily excreted in urine. Not removed by hemodialysis. ***Half-life:*** 4–18 hr.

AVAILABILITY
Capsules: 7.5 mg, 15 mg, 22.5 mg, 30 mg.

INDICATIONS AND DOSAGES
Insomnia
PO
Adults, Children 18 yr and older. 15-30 mg at bedtime.
Elderly, Debilitated. 7.5–15 mg at bedtime.

CONTRAINDICATIONS
Angle-closure glaucoma; CNS depression; pregnancy or breast-feeding; severe, uncontrolled pain; sleep apnea

INTERACTIONS
Drug
Alcohol, other CNS depressants: May increase CNS depression.
Herbal
Kava kava, valerian: May increase CNS depression.
Food
None known.

DIAGNOSTIC TEST EFFECTS
None known.

SIDE EFFECTS
Frequent
Somnolence, sedation, rebound insomnia (may occur for 1–2 nights after drug is discontinued), dizziness, confusion, euphoria
Occasional
Asthenia, anorexia, diarrhea
Rare
Paradoxical CNS excitement or restlessness (particularly in elderly or debilitated patients)

SERIOUS REACTIONS
! Abrupt or too-rapid withdrawal may result in pronounced restlessness, irritability, insomnia, hand tremor, abdominal or muscle cramps, vomiting, diaphoresis, and seizures.
! Overdose results in somnolence, confusion, diminished reflexes, respiratory depression, and coma.

NURSING CONSIDERATIONS

Baseline Assessment
- Determine if the patient is pregnant before beginning temazepam therapy.
- Assess the patient's BP, pulse rate, and respiratory rate, rhythm, and depth before administering temazepam.
- Provide the patient with an environment conducive to sleep. For

example, offer a back rub, low lighting, and a quiet environment.
- Assess the patient's baseline sleep pattern, including time needed to fall asleep and number of nocturnal awakenings.

Lifespan Considerations
- Temazepam crosses the placenta and may be distributed in breast milk.
- Long-term use of flurazepam during pregnancy may produce withdrawal symptoms and CNS depression in neonates. Keep in mind that the drug is FDA pregnancy risk category X and should not be used during pregnancy.
- Temazepam use is not recommended for children younger than 18 years.
- To avoid ataxia or excessive sedation in the elderly, plan to administer small doses initially and to increase dosage gradually.

Precautions
- Use temazepam cautiously in patients with mental impairment or the potential for drug dependence.

Administration and Handling
PO
- If desired, open temazepam capsules and mix the contents with food.

Intervention and Evaluation
- Monitor the patient's cardiovascular, mental, and respiratory status.
- Assess elderly or debilitated patients for paradoxical reactions, particularly during early therapy.
- Evaluate the patient for a therapeutic response, such as a decrease in the number of nocturnal awakenings and a longer duration of sleep.

Patient Teaching
- Instruct the patient to take temazepam about 30 minutes before bedtime.
- Inform the patient that temazepam may cause daytime drowsiness. Warn the patient to avoid activities requiring mental alertness or motor skills until his or her response to the drug has been established.
- Urge the patient to avoid alcohol and other CNS depressants during therapy.
- Instruct the patient to notify the physician if she is or plans to become pregnant during temazepam therapy.

triazolam

trye-**ay**-zoe-lam
(Apo-Triazo[CAN], Halcion)
Do not confuse Halcion with Haldol or Healon.

CATEGORY AND SCHEDULE

Pregnancy Risk Category: X
Controlled Substance: Schedule IV

MECHANISM OF ACTION

A benzodiazepine that enhances the action of the inhibitory neurotransmitter gamma-aminobutyric acid, resulting in CNS depression. **Therapeutic Effect:** Induces sleep.

AVAILABILITY

Tablets: 0.125 mg, 0.25 mg.

INDICATIONS AND DOSAGES

▸ **Insomnia**

PO

Adults, Children 18 yr and older. 0.125–0.5 mg at bedtime.
Elderly. 0.0625–0.125 mg at bedtime.

CONTRAINDICATIONS

Angle-closure glaucoma; CNS depression; pregnancy or breast-feeding; severe, uncontrolled pain; sleep apnea

INTERACTIONS

Drug

Alcohol, other CNS depressants: May increase CNS depression.

Herbal

Kava kava, valerian: May increase CNS depression.

Food

Grapefruit, grapefruit juice: May alter the absorption of triazolam.

DIAGNOSTIC TEST EFFECTS

None known.

SIDE EFFECTS

Frequent

Somnolence, sedation, dry mouth, headache, dizziness, nervousness, light-headedness, incoordination, nausea, rebound insomnia (may occur for 1–2 nights after drug is discontinued)

Occasional

Euphoria, tachycardia, abdominal cramps, visual disturbances

Rare

Paradoxical CNS excitement or restlessness (particularly in elderly or debilitated patients)

SERIOUS REACTIONS

! Abrupt or too-rapid withdrawal may result in pronounced restlessness, irritability, insomnia, hand tremors, abdominal or muscle cramps, vomiting, diaphoresis, and seizures.

! Overdose results in somnolence, confusion, diminished reflexes, respiratory depression, and coma.

NURSING CONSIDERATIONS

Baseline Assessment

- Determine if the patient is pregnant before beginning triazolam therapy.
- Assess the patient's vital signs immediately before administering triazolam.
- Raise the patient's bed rails and provide a call bell.
- Provide the patient with an environment conducive to sleep. For example, offer a back rub, a quiet environment, and low lighting.

Precautions

- Use triazolam cautiously in patients with a potential for drug abuse.

Administration and Handling

PO

- Give triazolam without regard to food. Crush tablets as needed.
- Don't administer the drug with grapefruit juice.

Intervention and Evaluation

- Assess the patient's sleep pattern.
- Monitor the patient's cardiovascular, mental, and respiratory status. Also monitor hepatic function of patients on long-term therapy.
- Assess elderly or debilitated patients for a paradoxical reaction, particularly during early therapy.
- Evaluate the patient for a therapeutic response, such as a decrease in the number of nocturnal awakenings and a longer duration of sleep.

Patient Teaching

- Inform the patient that triazolam may cause drowsiness. Warn the patient to avoid activities requiring mental alertness or motor skills until his or her response to the drug has been established.
- Urge the patient to avoid alcohol and other CNS depressants during therapy.
- Inform the patient that triazolam may cause dry mouth and physical or psychological dependence.
- Inform the patient that he or she may experience disturbed sleep patterns for 1 or 2 nights after discontinuing triazolam.
- Urge the patient to avoid consuming grapefruit or grapefruit juice during triazolam therapy because

grapefruit decreases the drug's absorption.
- Inform the patient that smoking reduces the drug's effectiveness. Provide the patient with information about smoking cessation.
- Caution the patient to notify the physician if she is or plans to become pregnant during triazolam therapy.

zaleplon

zal-e-plon
(Sonata, Stamoc[CAN])

CATEGORY AND SCHEDULE

Pregnancy Risk Category: C

MECHANISM OF ACTION

A nonbenzodiazepine that enhances the action of the inhibitory neurotransmitter gamma-aminobutyric acid. **Therapeutic Effect:** Induces sleep.

AVAILABILITY

Capsules: 5 mg, 10 mg.

INDICATIONS AND DOSAGES

▸ Insomnia

PO
Adults. 10 mg at bedtime. Range: 5-20 mg.
Elderly. 5 mg at bedtime.

CONTRAINDICATIONS

Severe hepatic impairment

INTERACTIONS

Drug

Alcohol, other CNS depressants: May increase CNS depression.
Cimetidine: May increase the effect of zaleplon.
Rifampin: Decreases the zaleplon blood concentration.

Herbal

None known.

Food

High-fat, heavy meals: May delay onset of sleep by approximately 2 hours.

DIAGNOSTIC TEST EFFECTS

None known.

SIDE EFFECTS

Expected
Somnolence, sedation, mild rebound insomnia (on first night after drug is discontinued)
Frequent (28%–7%)
Nausea, headache, myalgia, dizziness
Occasional (5%–3%)
Abdominal pain, asthenia, dyspepsia, eye pain, paresthesia
Rare (2%)
Tremors, amnesia, hyperacusis (acute sense of hearing), fever, dysmenorrhea

SERIOUS REACTIONS

! Zaleplon may produce altered concentration, behavior changes, and impaired memory.
! Taking the drug while up and about may result in adverse CNS effects, such as hallucinations, impaired coordination, dizziness, and light-headedness.
! Overdose results in somnolence, confusion, diminished reflexes, and coma.

NURSING CONSIDERATIONS

Baseline Assessment

- Raise the patient's bed rails and provide a call light immediately after drug administration.
- Provide the patient with an environment conducive to sleep. For example, offer a back rub, a quiet environment, and low lighting.

Precautions
• Use zaleplon cautiously in patients with mild to moderate hepatic impairment, signs or symptoms of depression, or a hypersensitivity to aspirin (may cause an allergic-type reaction).

Administration and Handling
PO
• If desired, open zaleplon capsules and mix the contents with food.
• Avoid giving this drug with or immediately after a high-fat meal to avoid delayed absorption.

Intervention and Evaluation
• Assess the patient's sleep pattern, including the time needed to fall asleep and the number of nocturnal awakenings.

Patient Teaching
• Instruct the patient to take zaleplon right before bedtime, but not immediately after a high-fat or heavy meal.
• Caution the patient not to exceed the prescribed drug dosage.
• Urge the patient to avoid alcohol and other CNS depressants during therapy.
• Warn the patient to avoid activities requiring mental alertness or motor skills until his or her response to the drug has been established.
• Inform the patient that sleep may be disturbed for 1 or 2 nights after discontinuing the drug.

zolpidem tartrate
zole-**pi**-dem
(Ambien, Stilnox[AUS])
Do not confuse Ambien with Amen.

CATEGORY AND SCHEDULE
Pregnancy Risk Category: B
Controlled Substance: Schedule IV

MECHANISM OF ACTION
A nonbenzodiazepine that enhances the action of the inhibitory neurotransmitter gamma-aminobutyric acid. **Therapeutic Effect:** Induces sleep and improves sleep quality.

PHARMACOKINETICS

Route	Onset	Peak	Duration
PO	30 min	N/A	6–8 hr

Rapidly absorbed from the GI tract. Protein binding: 92%. Metabolized in the liver; excreted in urine. Not removed by hemodialysis. ***Half-life:*** 1.4–4.5 hr (increased in hepatic impairment).

AVAILABILITY
Tablets: 5 mg, 10 mg.

INDICATIONS AND DOSAGES
▸ **Insomnia**
PO
Adults. 10 mg at bedtime.
Elderly, Debilitated. 5 mg at bedtime.

CONTRAINDICATIONS

None known.

INTERACTIONS

Drug

Alcohol, other CNS depressants: May increase CNS depression.

Herbal

None known.

Food

None known.

DIAGNOSTIC TEST EFFECTS

None known.

SIDE EFFECTS

Occasional (7%)

Headache

Rare (less than 2%)

Dizziness, nausea, diarrhea, muscle pain

SERIOUS REACTIONS

! Overdose may produce severe ataxia, bradycardia, altered vision (such as diplopia), severe drowsiness, nausea and vomiting, difficulty breathing, and unconsciousness.
! Abrupt withdrawal of the drug after long-term use may produce asthenia, facial flushing, diaphoresis, vomiting, and tremor.
! Drug tolerance or dependence may occur with prolonged, high-dose therapy.

NURSING CONSIDERATIONS

Baseline Assessment

- Assess the patient's BP, pulse rate, and respiratory rate, rhythm, and depth immediately before administering zolpidem.
- Raise the patient's bed rails and provide a call light.
- Provide the patient with an environment conducive to sleep. For example, offer a back rub, a quiet environment, and low lighting.

Lifespan Considerations

- It is unknown if zolpidem crosses the placenta or is distributed in breast milk.
- The safety and efficacy of zolpidem have not been established in children.
- In the elderly, age-related hepatic impairment and an increased susceptibilty to falls or confusion may require a dosage adjustment.

Precautions

- Use zolpidem cautiously in patients with depression, hepatic impairment, or a history of drug dependence.

Administration and Handling

PO

- For faster sleep onset, give zolpidem on an empty stomach.

Intervention and Evaluation

- Assess the patient's sleep pattern, including time needed to fall asleep and number of nocturnal awakenings.
- Evaluate the patient for a therapeutic response, such as a decrease in the number of nocturnal awakenings and an increased duration of sleep.

Patient Teaching

- Caution the patient against abruptly stopping zolpidem after long-term use.
- Inform the patient that drug dependence or tolerance may occur with prolonged use of high doses.
- Urge the patient to avoid alcohol during zolpidem therapy.
- Warn the patient to avoid activities requiring mental alertness or motor skills until his or her response to the drug has been established.

47 Skeletal Muscle Relaxants

baclofen
carisoprodol
cyclobenzaprine hydrochloride
dantrolene sodium
tizanidine

Uses: As adjuncts to rest and physical therapy, skeletal muscle relaxants are used to relieve discomfort in acute, painful musculoskeletal disorders, such as local spasms from muscle injury. Baclofen (a direct-acting skeletal muscle relaxant) and dantrolene are used to treat spasticity—characterized by heightened muscle tone, spasm, and loss of dexterity—caused by multiple sclerosis, cerebral palsy, spinal cord lesions, or CVA.

Action: Skeletal muscle relaxants work by a mechanism that's not fully understood. They may act at various levels of the CNS to depress polysynaptic reflexes, and their sedative effect may be responsible for their ability to relax muscles. Baclofen may mimic the actions of gamma-aminobutyric acid on spinal neurons; it doesn't directly affect skeletal muscles. Dantrolene acts directly on skeletal muscles, relieving spasticity.

baclofen

bak-loe-fen
(Apo-Baclofen[CAN], Baclo[AUS], Clofen[AUS], Lioresal, Liotec[CAN], Stelax[AUS])
Do not confuse baclofen with Bactroban or Beclovent.

CATEGORY AND SCHEDULE

Pregnancy Risk Category: C

MECHANISM OF ACTION

A direct-acting skeletal muscle relaxant that inhibits transmission of reflexes at the spinal cord level. **Therapeutic Effect:** Relieves muscle spasticity.

PHARMACOKINETICS

Well absorbed from the GI tract. Protein binding: 30%. Partially metabolized in the liver. Primarily excreted in urine. ***Half-life:*** 2.5–4 hr; intrathecal: 1.5 hr.

AVAILABILITY

Tablets: 10 mg, 20 mg.
Intrathecal Injection: 500 mcg/ml.

INDICATIONS AND DOSAGES

▸ **Spasticity**

PO

Adults. Initially, 5 mg 3 times a day. May increase by 15 mg/day at 3-day intervals. Range: 40–80 mg/day. Maximum: 80 mg/day.
Elderly. Initially, 5 mg 2–3 times a day. May gradually increase dosage.
Children. Initially, 10–15 mg/day in divided doses q8h. May increase by 5–15 mg/day at 3-day intervals. Maximum: 40 mg/day (children 2–7 yr); 60 mg/day (children 8 yr and older).

▸ **Usual Intrathecal Dosage**

Adults, Elderly, Children older than 12 yr. 300–800 mcg/day.
Children 12 yr and younger. 100–300 mcg/day.

OFF-LABEL USES

Treatment of trigeminal neuralgia

CONTRAINDICATIONS

Skeletal muscle spasm due to cerebral palsy, Parkinson's disease, rheumatic disorders, CVA

INTERACTIONS

Drug

Alcohol, other CNS depressants: May increase CNS depression.

Herbal

None known.

Food

None known.

DIAGNOSTIC TEST EFFECTS

May increase blood glucose level and serum alkaline phosphatase, AST (SGOT), and ALT (SGPT) levels.

SIDE EFFECTS

Frequent (greater than 10%)

Transient somnolence, asthenia, dizziness, light-headedness, nausea, vomiting

Occasional (10%–2%)

Headache, paresthesia, constipation, anorexia, hypotension, confusion, nasal congestion

Rare (less than 1%)

Paradoxical CNS excitement or restlessness, slurred speech, tremor, dry mouth, diarrhea, nocturia, impotence

SERIOUS REACTIONS

! Abrupt discontinuation of baclofen may produce hallucinations and seizures.

! Overdose results in blurred vision, seizures, myosis, mydriasis, severe muscle weakness, strabismus, respiratory depression, and vomiting.

NURSING CONSIDERATIONS

Baseline Assessment

- Record the duration, location, onset, and type of muscle spasm.
- Evaluate the patient for signs and symptoms of immobility, stiffness, or swelling.

Lifespan Considerations

- It is unknown if baclofen crosses the placenta or is distributed in breast milk.
- The safety and efficacy of baclofen have not been established in children younger than 12 years.
- Elderly patients may require decreased dosage because of age-related renal impairment. They're also at increased risk for CNS toxicity, manifested as confusion, hallucinations, depression, and sedation.

Precautions

- Use baclofen cautiously in patients with diabetes mellitus, epilepsy, impaired renal function, pre-existing psychiatric disorders, or a history of CVA.

Administration and Handling

PO

- Give baclofen without regard to food.
- Crush tablets as needed.

Intervention and Evaluation

- Assess the patient for paradoxical reactions.
- Assist the patient with ambulation at all times.
- Expect to obtain blood counts and liver and renal function tests periodically for those on long-term therapy.
- Evaluate the patient for evidence of a therapeutic response, such as decreased intensity of skeletal muscle pain.

Patient Teaching

- Inform the patient that drowsiness usually diminishes with continued therapy.
- Caution the patient against discontinuing baclofen abruptly after long-term therapy.
- Warn the patient to avoid tasks that require mental alertness or motor skills until his or her response to baclofen has been established.
- Urge the patient to avoid alcohol and CNS depressants during therapy.

carisoprodol

kar-i-so-**pro**-dol
(Soma)

CATEGORY AND SCHEDULE

Pregnancy Risk Category: C

MECHANISM OF ACTION

A centrally-acting skeletal muscle relaxant whose exact mechanism is unknown. Effects may be due to its CNS depressant actions. **Therapeutic Effect:** Relieves muscle spasms and pain.

AVAILABILITY

Tablets: 350 mg.

INDICATIONS AND DOSAGES

▸ Adjunct to rest, physical therapy, analgesics, and other measures for relief of discomfort from acute, painful musculoskeletal conditions

PO

Adults, Elderly. 350 mg 4 times a day.

CONTRAINDICATIONS

Acute intermittent porphyria, sensitivity to meprobamate

INTERACTIONS

Drug

Alcohol, other CNS depressants: May increase CNS depression.

Herbal

None known.

Food

None known.

DIAGNOSTIC TEST EFFECTS

None known.

SIDE EFFECTS

Frequent (greater than 10%)

Somnolence

Occasional (10%–1%)

Tachycardia, facial flushing, dizziness, headache, lightheadedness, dermatitis, nausea, vomiting, abdominal cramps, dyspnea

SERIOUS REACTIONS

! Overdose may cause CNS and respiratory depression, shock, and coma.

NURSING CONSIDERATIONS

Baseline Assessment

- Assess the patient's use of other medications, especially other CNS depressants.
- Expect to obtain baseline liver and renal function test results.

Precautions

- Use carisoprodol cautiously in patients with hepatic or renal impairment.

Administration and Handling

PO

- Give carisoprodol without regard to food.
- Give the last dose at bedtime.

Intervention and Evaluation

- Assess the patient for relief of muscle spasm and pain.
- Institute safety measures.
- Assist the patient with ambulation.

Patient Teaching

- Inform the patient that carisoprodol may cause dizziness or drowsiness.
- Urge the patient to avoid alcohol and other CNS depressants during carisoprodol therapy.

cyclobenzaprine hydrochloride

sye-kloe-**ben**-za-preen
(Flexeril, Flexitec[CAN], Novo-Cycloprine[CAN])
Do not confuse cyclobenzaprine with cycloserine or cyproheptadine, or Flexeril with Floxin.

CATEGORY AND SCHEDULE

Pregnancy Risk Category: B

MECHANISM OF ACTION

A centrally acting skeletal muscle relaxant that reduces tonic somatic muscle activity at the level of the brainstem. **Therapeutic Effect:** Relieves local skeletal muscle spasm.

PHARMACOKINETICS

Route	Onset	Peak	Duration
PO	1 hr	3–4 hr	12–24 hr

Well but slowly absorbed from the GI tract. Protein binding: 93%. Metabolized in the GI tract and the liver. Primarily excreted in urine. ***Half-life:*** 1–3 days.

AVAILABILITY

Tablets: 5 mg, 10 mg.

INDICATIONS AND DOSAGES

▸ Acute, painful musculoskeletal conditions

PO

Adults. Initially, 5 mg 3 times a day. May increase to 10 mg 3 times a day.
Elderly. 5 mg 3 times a day.

▸ Dosage in hepatic impairment

Mild: 5 mg 3 times a day.
Moderate and severe: Not recommended.

OFF-LABEL USES

Treatment of fibromyalgia

CONTRAINDICATIONS

Acute recovery phase of MI, arrhythmias, CHF, heart block, conduction disturbances, hyperthyroidism, use within 14 days of MAOIs

INTERACTIONS

Drug

Alcohol, other CNS depression-producing medications (such as tricyclic antidepressants): May increase CNS depression.
MAOIs: May increase the risk of hypertensive crisis and severe seizures.

Herbal

None known.

Food

None known.

DIAGNOSTIC TEST EFFECTS

None known.

SIDE EFFECTS

Frequent

Somnolence (39%), dry mouth (27%), dizziness (11%)

Rare (3%–1%)

Fatigue, asthenia, blurred vision, headache, nervousness, confusion, nausea, constipation, dyspepsia, unpleasant taste

SERIOUS REACTIONS

! Overdose may result in visual hallucinations, hyperactive reflexes, muscle rigidity, vomiting, and hyperpyrexia.

NURSING CONSIDERATIONS

Baseline Assessment

• Record the duration, location, onset, and type of muscle spasm.
• Examine the patient for immobility, stiffness, and swelling.

Lifespan Considerations

• It is unknown if cyclobenzaprine crosses the placenta or is distributed in breast milk.
• The safety and efficacy of cyclobenzaprine have not been established in children.
• The elderly have an increased sensitivity to the drug's anticholinergic effects, such as confusion and urine retention.

Precautions

• Use cyclobenzaprine cautiously in patients with angle-closure glaucoma, impaired hepatic or renal function, increased intraocular pressure, or a history of urine retention.

Administration and Handling

◀ **ALERT** ▶ Don't administer cyclobenzaprine for longer than 2 to 3 weeks.
PO
• Give cyclobenzaprine without regard to food.

Intervention and Evaluation

• Assist the patient with ambulation at all times.
• Evaluate the patient for evidence of a therapeutic response, such as decreased skeletal muscle pain, stiffness, and tenderness and improved mobility.

Patient Teaching

• Inform the patient that drowsiness usually diminishes with continued therapy.
• Warn the patient to avoid tasks that require mental alertness or motor skills until his or her response to the drug has been established.
• Urge the patient to avoid alcohol and other CNS depressants while taking cyclobenzaprine.
• Instruct the patient to change positions slowly to help avoid the drug's hypotensive effects.
• Suggest that the patient sip tepid water and chew sugarless gum to relieve dry mouth.

dantrolene sodium

dan-troe-leen
(Dantrium)
Do not confuse Dantrium with Daraprim.

CATEGORY AND SCHEDULE

Pregnancy Risk Category: C

MECHANISM OF ACTION

A skeletal muscle relaxant that reduces muscle contraction by interfering with release of calcium ion. Reduces calcium ion concentration. **Therapeutic Effect:** Dissociates excitation-contraction coupling. Interferes with catabolic process associated with malignant hyperthermic crisis.

PHARMACOKINETICS

Poorly absorbed from the GI tract. Protein binding: High. Metabolized in the liver. Primarily excreted in urine. ***Half-life:*** IV: 4–8 hr; PO: 8.7 hr.

AVAILABILITY

Capsules: 25 mg, 50 mg, 100 mg.
Powder for Injection: 20-mg vial.

INDICATIONS AND DOSAGES

▸ Spasticity

PO

Adults, Elderly. Initially, 25 mg/day. Increase to 25 mg 2–4 times a day, then by 25-mg increments up to 100 mg 2–4 times a day.

Children. Initially, 0.5 mg/kg twice a day. Increase to 0.5 mg/kg 3–4 times a day, then in increments of 0.5 mg/kg/day up to 3 mg/kg 2–4 times a day. Maximum: 400 mg/day.

▸ Prevention of malignant hyperthermic crisis

PO

Adults, Elderly, Children. 4–8 mg/kg/day in 3–4 divided doses 1–2 days before surgery; give last dose 3–4 hr before surgery.

IV

Adults, Elderly, Children. 2.5 mg/kg about 1.25 hr before surgery.

▸ Management of malignant hyperthermic crisis

IV

Adults, Elderly, Children. Initially a minimum of 1 mg/kg rapid IV; may repeat up to total cumulative dose of 10 mg/kg. May follow with 4–8 mg/kg/day PO in 4 divided doses up to 3 days after crisis.

OFF-LABEL USES

Relief of exercise-induced pain in patients with muscular dystrophy, treatment of flexor spasms and neuroleptic malignant syndrome

CONTRAINDICATIONS

Active hepatic disease

INTERACTIONS

Drug

Central nervous system (CNS) depressants: May increase CNS depression with short-term use.

Liver toxic medications: May increase the risk of liver toxicity with chronic use.

Herbal

None known.

Food

None known.

DIAGNOSTIC TEST EFFECTS

May alter liver function test results.

IV INCOMPATIBILITIES

None known.

SIDE EFFECTS

Frequent

Drowsiness, dizziness, weakness, general malaise, diarrhea (mild)

Occasional

Confusion, diarrhea (may be severe), headache, insomnia, constipation, urinary frequency

Rare

Paradoxical CNS excitement or restlessness, paresthesia, tinnitus, slurred speech, tremor, blurred vision, dry mouth, nocturia, impotence, rash, pruritus

SERIOUS REACTIONS

! There is a risk of liver toxicity, most notably in females, those 35 years of age and older, and those taking other medications concurrently.

! Overt hepatitis noted most frequently between 3rd and 12th month of therapy.

! Overdosage results in vomiting, muscular hypotonia, muscle twitching, respiratory depression, and seizures.

NURSING CONSIDERATIONS

Baseline Assessment

- Plan to obtain the patient's baseline liver function test results, including serum alkaline phosphatase, AST (SGOT), ALT (SGPT), and total bilirubin levels.

• Record the duration, location, onset, and type of muscle spasm.
• Examine the patient for immobility, stiffness, and swelling.

Lifespan Considerations

• Be aware that dantrolene readily crosses the placenta and should not be used in breast-feeding mothers.
• There are no age-related precautions noted in children 5 years and older.
• There is no information available on dantrolene use in the elderly.

Precautions

• Use cautiously in patients with a history of previous liver disease and impaired cardiac or pulmonary function.

Administration and Handling

◀ **ALERT** ▶ Begin with low-dose therapy, as prescribed, then increase gradually at 4- to 7-day intervals to reduces incidence of side effects.

PO

• Give dantrolene without regard to meals.

IV

• Store at room temperature.
• Use within 6 hours after reconstitution.
• Solution normally appears clear, colorless.
• Discard if cloudy or precipitate is present.
• Reconstitute 20-mg vial with 60 ml sterile water for injection to provide a concentration of 0.33 mg/ml.
• For IV infusion, administer over 1 hour.
• Diligently monitor for extravasation because of high pH of IV preparation. May produce severe complications.

Intervention and Evaluation

• Assist the patient with ambulation.
• Perform periodic blood tests, such as liver and renal function tests, as ordered, for patients on long-term therapy.
• Evaluate the patient for a therapeutic response, such as decreased intensity of skeletal muscle pain or spasm.

Patient Teaching

• Explain to the patient that drowsiness usually diminishes with continued therapy.
• Caution the patient to avoid tasks that require mental alertness or motor skills until his or her response to the drug is established.
• Urge the patient to avoid alcohol or other depressants while taking dantrolene.
• Warn the patient to notify the physician if he or she experiences bloody or tarry stools, continued weakness, diarrhea, fatigue, itching, nausea, or skin rash.

tizanidine

tye-**zan**-i-deen
(Zanaflex)

CATEGORY AND SCHEDULE

Pregnancy Risk Category: C

MECHANISM OF ACTION

A skeletal muscle relaxant that increases presynaptic inhibition of spinal motor neurons mediated by $alpha_2$-adrenergic agonists, reducing facilitation to postsynaptic motor neurons. **Therapeutic Effect:** Reduces muscle spasticity.

PHARMACOKINETICS

Route	Onset	Peak	Duration
PO	N/A	1–2 hr	3–6 hr

Metabolized in the liver. ***Half-life:*** 4–8 hr.

AVAILABILITY

Tablets: 2 mg, 4 mg.

INDICATIONS AND DOSAGES

Muscle spasticity

PO

Adults, Elderly. Initially 2–4 mg, gradually increased in 2- to 4-mg increments and repeated q6–8h. Maximum: 3 doses/day or 36 mg/24 hr.

OFF-LABEL USES

Spasticity associated with multiple sclerosis or spinal cord injury

CONTRAINDICATIONS

None known.

INTERACTIONS

Drug

Alcohol, other CNS depressants: May increase CNS depressant effects.

Antihypertensives: May increase tizanidine's hypotensive potential.

Oral contraceptives: May reduce tizanidine clearance.

Phenytoin: May increase serum levels and risk of toxicity of phenytoin.

Herbal

None known.

Food

None known.

DIAGNOSTIC TEST EFFECTS

May increase serum alkaline phosphatase, AST (SGOT), and ALT (SGPT) levels.

SIDE EFFECTS

Frequent (49%–41%)

Dry mouth, somnolence, asthenia

Occasional (16%–4%)

Dizziness, UTI, constipation

Rare (3%)

Nervousness, amblyopia, pharyngitis, rhinitis, vomiting, urinary frequency

SERIOUS REACTIONS

! Hypotension (a reduction in either diastolic or systolic BP) may be associated with bradycardia, orthostatic hypotension and, rarely, syncope. The risk of hypotension increases as dosage increases; BP may decrease within 1 hour after administration.

NURSING CONSIDERATIONS

Baseline Assessment

- Record the duration, location, onset, and type of muscle spasm.
- Examine the patient for immobility, stiffness, and swelling.
- Obtain the patient's baseline serum alkaline phosphatase and total bilirubin levels.

Lifespan Considerations

- The safety and efficacy of tizanidine have not been established in children.
- In the elderly, age-related renal impairment may warrant cautious use.

Precautions

- Use tizanidine cautiously in patients with hypotension or cardiac, hepatic, or renal disease.

Intervention and Evaluation

- Assist the patient with ambulation at all times.
- Evaluate the patient for a therapeutic response, such as decreased stiffness, tenderness, and intensity of skeletal muscle pain and improved mobility.
- Perform periodic liver and renal function tests for patients on long-term therapy, as ordered.

Patient Teaching

- Inform the patient that tizanidine may cause low blood pressure, impaired coordination, and sedation.

- Warn the patient to avoid tasks that require mental alertness or motor skills until his or her response to the drug has been established.
- Instruct the patient to change positions slowly to help prevent dizziness.

48 Miscellaneous CNS Agents

acamprosate
alosetron
botulinum toxin type a
botulinum toxin type b
flumazenil
fluvoxamine maleate
ketamine
lithium carbonate, lithium citrate
nicotine
poly-L-lactic acid
propofol
riluzole
ziconotide

Uses: Miscellaneous CNS agents have a wide variety of uses. *Acamprosate* is used to maintain abstinence in patients who are alcohol-dependent. *Alosetron* is prescribed to treat severe diarrhea, especially in women with irritable bowel syndrome who don't respond to conventional therapy. Both types of *botulinum toxin* are used to block the neuromuscular effects of cervical dystonia; in addition, botulinum type A can reduce brow furrow lines. *Flumazenil* is used as an antidote for benzodiazepine overdose. *Fluvoxamine* is used to treat obsessive-compulsive disorder. *Ketamine* is a rapidly-acting anesthetic that has several uses and is the sole anesthetic for short diagnostic and surgical procedures that don't require skeletal muscle relaxation. *Lithium* is used to prevent and treat acute mania and the manic phase of bipolar disorder. *Nicotine* is helpful as a smoking deterrent. *Poly-L-lactic acid* is used to treat facial lipoatrophy. *Propofol* is a rapidly-acting general anesthetic used as a sedative in intensive care units and as an anesthetic. *Riluzole* is ordered to treat amyotrophic lateral sclerosis. *Ziconotide,* an intrathecal agent, is used for pain control.

Action: Most of these miscellaneous agents act on receptors in the CNS. *Acamprosate* interacts with glutamate and gamma-aminobutyric acid neurotransmitters, restoring their balance. *Alosetron* is a serotonin subtype 3 (5-HT_3) receptor antagonist that affects enteric neurons in the GI tract. Both types of *botulinum toxin* inhibit acetylcholine release to produce neuromuscular blockade. *Flumazenil* antagonizes the effect of benzodiazepines on gamma-aminobutyric acid receptors in the CNS. *Fluvoxamine* selectively inhibits serotonin reuptake by neurons in the CNS. *Ketamine* blocks afferent impulses and interacts with CNS neurotransmitters. *Lithium* affects the storage, release, and reuptake of neurotransmitters, including norepinephrine and serotonin. *Nicotine* produces autonomic effects by binding with acetylcholine receptors, which causes stimulation followed by depression of the peripheral and central nervous systems.

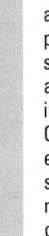

Poly-L-lactic acid works through the implantable injection of microparticles of a synthetic polymer. *Propofol* works by inhibiting sympathetic vasoconstrictor nerve activity and decreasing vascular resistance. *Riluzole* inhibits presynaptic glutamate release in the CNS and interferes postsynaptically with the effects of excitatory amino acids. *Ziconotide* selectively binds to calcium channels on affect nerve fibers in the spinal cord, blocking N-type calcium channels.

acamprosate

ah-**camp**-ro-sate
(Campral)

CATEGORY AND SCHEDULE

Pregnancy Risk Category: C

MECHANISM OF ACTION

An alcohol abuse deterrent that appears to interact with glutamate and gamma-aminobutyric acid neurotransmitter systems centrally, restoring their balance. **Therapeutic Effect:** Reduces alcohol dependence.

PHARMACOKINETICS

Slowly absorbed from the GI tract. Steady-state plasma concentrations are reached within 5 days. Does not undergo metabolism. Excreted in urine. ***Half-life:*** 20–33 hr.

AVAILABILITY

Tablets: 333 mg.

INDICATIONS AND DOSAGES

▸ Maintenance of alcohol abstinence in alcohol-dependent patients who are abstinent at initiation of treatment.

PO

Adults, Elderly: Two tablets 3 times a day.

▸ Dosage in renal impairment

For patients with creatinine clearance of 30–49 ml/min, dosage is decreased to one tablet 3 times a day.

CONTRAINDICATIONS

Severe renal impairment (creatinine clearance of 30 ml/min or less)

INTERACTIONS

Drug

Antidepressants: May cause weight gain or loss.

Naltrexone: May increase acamprosate blood concentration.

Herbal

None known.

Food

None known.

DIAGNOSTIC TEST EFFECTS

None known.

SIDE EFFECTS

Frequent (17%)

Diarrhea

Occasional (6%–4%)
Insomnia, asthenia, fatigue, anxiety, flatulence, nausea, depression, pruritus
Rare (3%–1%)
Dizziness, anorexia, paresthesia, diaphoresis, dry mouth

SERIOUS REACTIONS

! None known.

NURSING CONSIDERATIONS

Baseline Assessment

- Obtain the patient's BUN and serum creatinine levels before beginning treatment.
- Assess the patient for agitation, tension, trembling, cold or clammy hands, and diaphoresis.

Lifespan Considerations

- It is unknown if acamprosate is distributed in breast milk.
- The safety and efficacy of acamprosate have not been established in children.
- Age-related renal impairment may require a dosage adjustment in the elderly.

Administration and Handling

◀ALERT▶ Expect to decrease the dosage for patients with moderate renal impairment (creatinine clearance of 30–50 ml/minute).

PO

- Don't crush or break enteric-coated tablets.
- Give acamprosate without regard to food. However, patients who regularly eat three meals a day may be more compliant with the drug regimen if instructed to take acamprosate with food.

Intervention and Evaluation

- Assess the patient's pattern of daily bowel activity and stool consistency.
- Assess the patient's sleep pattern and provide an environment conducive to sleep, such as a quiet room with low lighting.
- Offer emotional support to the anxious patient.
- Assist the patient with ambulation if he or she experiences dizziness.

Patient Teaching

- Explain to the patient that acamprosate does not eliminate or diminish withdrawal symptoms.
- Inform the patient that acamprosate helps maintain abstinence only when used as part of a treatment program that includes counseling and support.
- Warn the patient to avoid tasks that require mental alertness or motor skills until his or her response to the drug has been established.

alosetron

al-**ohs**-eh-tron
(Lotronex)
Do not confuse Lotronex with Lovenox.

CATEGORY AND SCHEDULE

Pregnancy Risk Category: B

MECHANISM OF ACTION

A serotonin (5-HT_3) receptor antagonist that mediates abdominal pain, bloating, nausea, vomiting, peristalsis, and secretory reflexes.
Therapeutic Effect: Alleviates diarrhea, reduces gastric pain.

PHARMACOKINETICS

Rapidly absorbed after PO administration. Extensively metabolized in liver. Excreted primarily in urine and, to a lesser extent, in feces. ***Half-life:*** 1.5 hr.

AVAILABILITY

Tablets: 1 mg.

INDICATIONS AND DOSAGES

▸ Irritable bowel syndrome

PO

Adults (Women older than 18 yr). 1 mg twice a day. Maximum: 2 mg/day.

OFF-LABEL USES

Treatment of carcinoid diarrhea, irritable bowel syndrome in men

CONTRAINDICATIONS

Breast-feeding; constipation; diverticulitis (active or history of); GI bleeding, obstruction, or perforation; history ischemic colitis, ulcerative colitis, or Crohn's disease; thrombophlebitis

INTERACTIONS

Drug

Hydralazine, isoniazid, procainamide: May alter the effects of these drugs.

Herbal

St. John's wort: May increase alosetron blood concentration.

Food

All foods: May decrease the absorption or delay the peak blood concentration of alosetron.

DIAGNOSTIC TEST EFFECTS

May increase serum alkaline phosphatase, bilirubin, ALT (SGPT) and AST (SGOT) levels.

SIDE EFFECTS

Frequent (28%)

Constipation

Occasional (10%–2%)

Nausea, GI or abdominal discomfort or pain, dyspepsia, flatulence, hypertension, clinical depression

Rare

Sedation, abnormal dreams, anxiety

SERIOUS REACTIONS

! Acute ischemic colitis and serious complications of constipation have resulted in the need for blood transfusions and surgery.

NURSING CONSIDERATIONS

Baseline Assessment

- Determine the patient's history of abdominal distress, abdominal pain or discomfort, bloating, blood in stools, and diarrhea.
- Assess the patient's skin turgor, urinary status, and mucous membranes for dryness to determine baseline hydration status.

Lifespan Considerations

◂ALERT▸ Alosetron is indicated for use in women only. The safety and efficacy of this drug have not been established in men.

- It is unknown if alosetron is excreted in breast milk.
- The safety and efficacy of alosetron have not been established in children.
- No age-related precautions have been noted in the elderly.

Precautions

- Use alosetron cautiously in patients with hepatic function impairment.

Administration and Handling

PO

- Give alosetron without regard to food.

Intervention and Evaluation

- Encourage the patient to maintain adequate fluid intake.
- Monitor the patient's pattern of daily bowel activity and stool consistency. Auscultate the patient's bowel sounds for peristalsis.
- Evaluate the patient for a decrease in signs and symptoms.

Patient Teaching

- Inform the patient that urgency and diarrhea may be reduced within 1 week of treatment but that the drug's full therapeutic effects may not occur for up to 4 weeks.

• Inform the patient that persistent constipation may require interruption of treatment or drug management.
• Advise the patient to notify the physician or nurse if bloody diarrhea, severe constipation, or a sudden worsening of stomach pain occurs.

botulinum toxin type a

botch-you-lin-em
(Botox, Dysport[AUS])

CATEGORY AND SCHEDULE
Pregnancy Risk Category: C

MECHANISM OF ACTION

A neurotoxin that blocks neuromuscular conduction by binding to receptor sites on motor nerve endings, and inhibiting the release of acetylcholine, resulting in muscle denervation. **Therapeutic Effect:** Reduces muscle activity.

AVAILABILITY

Injection: 100 units/vial.

INDICATIONS AND DOSAGES

▸ **Cervical dystonia in patients who have previously tolerated botulinum toxin type A**
IM
Adults, Elderly. Mean dose of 236 units (range: 198–300 units) divided among the affected muscles, based on patient's head and neck position, localization of pain, muscle hypertrophy, patient response, and adverse reaction history.

▸ **Cervical dystonia in patients who have not previously been treated with botulinum toxin type A**
IM
Adults, Elderly. Administer at lower dosage than for patients who have previously tolerated the drug.

▸ **Strabismus**
IM
Adults, Children older then 12 yr. 1.25–2.5 units into any one muscle.
Children 2 mo–12 yr. 1–2.5 units into any one muscle.

▸ **Blepharospasm**
IM
Adults. Initially, 1.25–2.5 units. May increase up to 2.5–5.0 units at repeat treatments. Maximum: 5 units per injection or cumulative dose of 200 units over a 30-day period.

▸ **Cerebral palsy spasticity**
IM
Children older than 18 mo. 1–6 units/kg. Maximum: 50 units per injection site. No more than 400 units per visit or during a 3-month period.

▸ **Improvement of brow furrow**
IM
Adults 65 yr and younger. Individualized.

OFF-LABEL USES

Treatment of dynamic muscle contracture in children with cerebral palsy, focal task-specific dystonia, head and neck tremor unresponsive to drug therapy, hemifacial spasms, laryngeal dystonia, oromandibular dystonia, spasmoditic torticollis, writer's cramp

CONTRAINDICATIONS

Infection at proposed injection sites

INTERACTIONS

Drug

Aminoglycoside antibiotics, other drugs that interfere with neuromuscular transmission (such as curare-like compounds): May potentiate the effects of botulinum toxin type A.

Herbal
None known.
Food
None known.

DIAGNOSTIC TEST EFFECTS
None known.

SIDE EFFECTS
◀ALERT▶ Side effects usually occur within the first week after injection.
Frequent (15%–11%)
Localized pain, tenderness, or bruising at injection site; localized weakness in injected muscle; upper respiratory tract infection; neck pain; headache
Occasional (10%–2%)
Increased cough, flulike symptoms, back pain, rhinitis, dizziness, hypertonia, soreness at injection site, asthenia, dry mouth, nausea, somnolence
Rare
Stiffness, numbness, diplopia, ptosis

SERIOUS REACTIONS
! Mild to moderate dysphagia occurs in approximately 20% of patients.
! Arrhythmias and severe dysphagia (manifested as aspiration, pneumonia, and dyspnea) occur rarely.
! Overdose produces systemic weakness and muscle paralysis.

NURSING CONSIDERATIONS
Baseline Assessment
- Assess the onset, location, duration, and type of dystonia the patient is experiencing.
- Examine the proposed injection site for signs of infection, such as erythema or swelling.

Precautions
- Use botulinum toxin type A cautiously in patients with neuromuscular junctional disorders, such as amyotrophic lateral sclerosis, Lambert-Eaton syndrome, motor neuropathy, and myasthenia gravis, because they may experience significant systemic effects, including respiratory compromise, and severe dysphagia.

Administration and Handling
IM
◀ALERT▶ Plan to have a physician inject the drug into the affected muscle.
- Expect to administer the drug at the lowest effective dosage, and at the longest effective dosing interval to avoid formation of neutralizing antibodies.
- Store drug vials in the freezer. The reconstituted solution may be refrigerated for up to 4 hours.
- Administer the drug within 4 hours after reconstitution.
- The solution normally appears as a clear and colorless. Discard the solution if particulate matter is present.
- Dilute drug with 0.9% NaCl. For a resulting dose of units/0.1 ml draw up 1 ml of diluent to provide 10 units, 2 ml to provide 5 units, 4 ml to provide 2.5 units, or 8 ml to provide 1.25 units.
- Slowly and gently inject the diluent into the vial to avoid producing bubbles. Then, rotate the vial gently to mix the drug. If a vacuum doesn't pull the diluent into the vial, discard it.
- Assist the physician, as necessary, while he or she injects the drug into the affected muscles using a 25-, 27-, or 30-gauge needle for superficial muscles, and a 22-gauge needle for deeper muscles.

Intervention and Evaluation
- Assess for signs of dysphagia and aspiration pneumonia, including fever, sputum production, and adventitious breath sounds.

Patient Teaching

- Inform the patient that clinical improvement should begin within 2 weeks of the injection but that the drug's maximum benefit will appear approximately 6 weeks after the injection.
- Advise the patient to resume normal activity slowly and carefully.
- Urge the patient to seek medical attention immediately if respiratory, speech, or swallowing difficulties occur.

botulinum toxin type b

botch-you-lin-em
(Myobloc)

CATEGORY AND SCHEDULE

Pregnancy Risk Category: C

MECHANISM OF ACTION

A neurotoxin that inhibits acetylcholine release at the neuromuscular junction. **Therapeutic Effect:** Produces flaccid paralysis.

AVAILABILITY

Injection: 2,500 units, 5,000 units, 10,000 units.

INDICATIONS AND DOSAGES

▸ **To reduce the severity of symptoms in patients with cervical dystonia who have previously tolerated botulinum toxin type B**

IM

Adults, Elderly. 2,500–5,000 units divided among the affected muscles.

▸ **To reduce the severity of symptoms in patients with cervical dystonia who have not previously been treated with botulinum toxin type B**

IM

Adults, Elderly. Administer at lower dosage than for patients who have previously tolerated the drug.

CONTRAINDICATIONS

None known.

INTERACTIONS

Drug

Aminoglycoside antibiotics, other drugs that interfere with neuromuscular transmission (such as curare-like compounds): May potentiate the effects of botulinum toxin type B.

Herbal

None known.

Food

None known.

DIAGNOSTIC TEST EFFECTS

None known.

SIDE EFFECTS

◀ **ALERT** ▶ Side effects usually occur within the first week after the injection.

Frequent (19%–12%)

Infection, neck pain, headache, injection site pain, dry mouth

Occasional (10%–4%)

Flulike symptoms, generalized pain, increased cough, back pain, myasthenia

Rare

Dizziness, nausea, rhinitis, headache, vomiting, edema, allergic reaction

SERIOUS REACTIONS

! Mild to moderate dysphagia occurs in approximately 10% of patients.

! Arrhythmias and severe dysphagia (manifested as aspiration, pneumonia, and dyspnea) occur rarely.

! Overdose produces systemic weakness and muscle paralysis.

NURSING CONSIDERATIONS

Baseline Assessment

• Assess the onset, location, duration, and type of dystonia the patient is experiencing.
• Examine the proposed injection site for signs of infection, such as erythema or swelling.

Precautions

• Use botulinum toxin type B cautiously in patients with neuromuscular junctional disorders, such as amyotrophic lateral sclerosis, Lambert-Eaton syndrome, motor neuropathy, and myasthenia gravis, because they may experience significant systemic effects, including respiratory compromise, and severe dysphagia.

Administration and Handling

IM

◀ **ALERT** ▶ Plan to have a physician inject the drug into the affected muscle.
• Unreconstituted vials may be refrigerated for up to 21 months. Do not freeze them. The reconstituted solution may be stored in the refrigerator for up to 4 hours.
• Administer the drug within 4 hours after reconstitution.
• The solution normally appears clear and colorless. Discard it if particulate matter is present.
• Dilute drug with 0.9% NaCl. Slowly and gently inject the diluent into the vial to avoid producing bubbles. Then rotate the vial gently to mix the drug. If a vacuum doesn't pull the diluent into the vial, discard it.
• Assist the physician as necessary, while he or she injects the drug into the affected muscles using a 25-, 27-, or 30-gauge needle for superficial muscles, and a 22-gauge needle for deeper muscles.

Intervention and Evaluation

• Know that drug's effect lasts for 12 to 16 weeks at doses of 5,000 or 10,000 units.
• Assess for signs of dysphagia and aspiration pneumonia, including fever, sputum production, and adventitious breath sounds.

Patient Teaching

• Tell the patient to resume normal activity slowly and carefully.
• Urge the patient to seek medical attention immediately if respiratory, speech, or swallowing difficulties occur.

flumazenil

flew-**maz**-ah-nil
(Anexate[CAN], Romazicon)

CATEGORY AND SCHEDULE

Pregnancy Risk Category: C

MECHANISM OF ACTION

An antidote that antagonizes the effect of benzodiazepines on the gamma-aminobutyric acid receptor complex in the CNS. **Therapeutic Effect:** Reverses sedative effect of benzodiazepines.

PHARMACOKINETICS

Route	Onset	Peak	Duration
IV	1–2 min	6–10 min	less than 1 hr

Duration and degree of benzodiazepine reversal depend on dosage and plasma concentration. Protein binding: 50%. Metabolized by the liver; excreted in urine.

AVAILABILITY

Injection: 0.1 mg/ml.

INDICATIONS AND DOSAGES

▸ Reversal of conscious sedation or general anesthesia

IV

Adults, Elderly. Initially, 0.2 mg (2 ml) over 15 sec; may repeat dose in 45 sec; then at 60-sec intervals. Maximum: 1 mg (10 ml) total dose.

Children, Neonates. Initially, 0.01 mg/kg; may repeat in 45 sec, then at 60-sec intervals. Maximum: 0.2 mg single dose; 0.05 mg/kg or 1 mg cumulative dose.

▸ Benzodiazepine overdose

IV

Adults, Elderly. Initially, 0.2 mg (2 ml) over 30 sec; if desired LOC is not achieved after 30 sec, 0.3 mg (3 ml) may be given over 30 sec. Further doses of 0.5 mg (5 ml) may be administered over 30 sec at 60-sec intervals. Maximum: 3 mg (30 ml) total dose.

Children, Neonates. Initially, 0.01 mg/kg; may repeat in 45 sec, then at 60-sec intervals. Maximum: 0.2 mg single dose; 1 mg cumulative dose.

CONTRAINDICATIONS

Anticholinergic signs (such as mydriasis, dry mucosa, and hypoperistalsis), arrhythmias, cardiovascular collapse, history of hypersensitivity to benzodiazepines, patients with signs of serious cyclic antidepressant overdose (such as motor abnormalities), patients who have been given a benzodiazepine for control of a potentially life-threatening condition (such as control of status epilepticus or increased intracranial pressure)

INTERACTIONS

Drug

Tricyclic antidepressants: May produce seizures and arrhythmias as flumazenil reverses the sedative effects of tricyclic antidepressants.

Herbal

None known.

Food

None known.

DIAGNOSTIC TEST EFFECTS

None known.

IV INCOMPATIBILITIES

No information available for Y-site administration.

IV COMPATIBILITIES

Aminophylline, cimetidine (Tagamet), dobutamine (Dobutrex), dopamine (Intropin), famotidine (Pepcid), heparin, lidocaine, procainamide (Pronestyl), ranitidine (Zantac)

SIDE EFFECTS

Frequent (11%–4%)

Agitation, anxiety, dry mouth, dyspnea, insomnia, palpitations, tremors, headache, blurred vision, dizziness, ataxia, nausea, vomiting, pain at injection site, diaphoresis

Occasional (3%–1%)

Fatigue, flushing, auditory disturbances, thrombophlebitis, rash

Rare (less than 1%)

Urticaria, pruritus, hallucinations

SERIOUS REACTIONS

! Toxic effects, such as seizures and arrhythmias, of other drugs taken in overdose, especially tricyclic antidepressants, may emerge with reversal of sedative effect of benzodiazepines.

! Flumazenil may provoke a panic attack in those with a history of panic disorder.

NURSING CONSIDERATIONS

Baseline Assessment

- Obtain ABG levels before and every 30 minutes during IV flumazenil administration.

Lifespan Considerations

- It is unknown if flumazenil crosses the placenta or is distributed in breast milk. Flumazenil use is not recommended during labor and delivery.
- No age-related precautions have been noted in children.
- In the elderly, benzodiazepine-induced sedation tends to be deeper and more prolonged, requiring careful monitoring.

Precautions

- Use flumazenil cautiously in patients with alcoholism, drug dependence, head injury, or hepatic impairment.

Administration and Handling

IV

◀ ALERT ▶ If sedation recurs, give up to 1 mg (as 0.2 mg/minute) as a single dose or up to 3 mg in 1 hour.

- Flumazenil is compatible with D_5W, lactated Ringer's solution, or 0.9% NaCl.
- Store the parenteral form at room temperature.
- Discard the injection 24 hours after it has been drawn into a syringe or mixed with any other IV solutions; also discard it if it becomes discolored or contains particulate.
- Rinse any spilled solution from the skin with cool water.
- Administer flumazenil over 15 seconds, as prescribed, for reversal of conscious sedation or general anesthesia or over 30 seconds, as prescribed, for benzodiazepine overdose.
- Inject the drug into a large vein through a free-flowing IV infusion because local injection produces pain and inflammation at injection site.

Intervention and Evaluation

- Monitor and maintain a patent airway and prepare to assist with ventilation if flumazenil does not fully reverse the respiratory depressant effects of the benzodiazepine.
- Know that the effects of flumazenil may wear off before the effects of the benzodiazepine wear off.
- Frequently monitor the patient's heart rate and rhythm and BP.
- For benzodiazepine overdose, administer activated charcoal, if ordered, and perform gastric lavage as ordered.
- Monitor the patient for benzodiazepine's effect.
- Assess the patient for hypoventilation, resedation, and respiratory depression.
- Closely monitor the patient for return of unconsciousness or narcosis for at least 1 hour after he or she is fully alert.

Patient Teaching

- Advise the patient to avoid tasks requiring mental alertness or motor skills until for least 24 hours after discharge.
- Instruct the patient to avoid taking OTC drugs for 18 to 24 hours after discharge.

fluvoxamine maleate

floo-**vox**-a-meen

(Faverin[AUS], Luvox)

CATEGORY AND SCHEDULE

Pregnancy Risk Category: C

MECHANISM OF ACTION

An antidepressant and antiobsessive agent that selectively inhibits neuronal reuptake of serotonin. **Therapeutic Effect:** Relieves depression and symptoms of obsessive-compulsive disorder.

AVAILABILITY

Tablets: 25 mg, 50 mg, 100 mg.

INDICATIONS AND DOSAGES

Obsessive-compulsive disorder

PO

Adults. 50 mg at bedtime; may increase by 50 mg every 4–7 days. Dosages greater than 100 mg/day given in 2 divided doses. Maximum: 300 mg/day.

Children 8–17 yr. 25 mg at bedtime; may increase by 25 mg every 4–7 days. Dosages greater than 50 mg/day given in 2 divided doses. Maximum: 200 mg/day.

OFF-LABEL USES

Treatment of depression, panic disorder, anxiety disorders in children

CONTRAINDICATIONS

Use within 14 days of MAOIs

INTERACTIONS

Drug

Benzodiazepines, carbamazepine, clozapine, theophylline: May increase the blood concentration and risk of toxicity of these drugs.

Lithium, tryptophan: May enhance fluvoxamine's serotonergic effects.

MAOIs: May produce serious reactions, including hyperthermia, rigidity, and myoclonus.

Tricyclic antidepressants: May increase the fluvoxamine blood concentration.

Warfarin: May increase the effects of warfarin.

Herbal

St. John's wort: May increase fluvoxamine's pharmacologic effects and risk of toxicity.

Food

None known.

DIAGNOSTIC TEST EFFECTS

None known.

SIDE EFFECTS

Frequent

Nausea (40%), headache, somnolence, insomnia (21%–22%)

Occasional (14%–8%)

Dizziness, diarrhea, dry mouth, asthenia, weakness, dyspepsia, constipation, abnormal ejaculation

Rare (6%–3%)

Anorexia, anxiety, tremor, vomiting, flatulence, urinary frequency, sexual dysfunction, altered taste

SERIOUS REACTIONS

! Overdose may produce seizures, nausea, vomiting, and extreme agitation and restlessness.

NURSING CONSIDERATIONS

Baseline Assessment

- Perform baseline blood chemistry tests to assess hepatic function.

Precautions

- Use fluvoxamine cautiously in elderly patients and patients with impaired hepatic or renal function.

Administration and Handling

PO

◀ALERT▶ Expect to decrease the dosage or dosing frequency for elderly patients and those with impaired hepatic function.

Intervention and Evaluation

- Closely supervise suicidal patients during early therapy. As depression lessens, the patient's energy level improves, which increases the suicide potential.
- Assess the patient's appearance, behavior, level of interest, mood, and sleep pattern.
- Assist the patient with ambulation if he or she experiences dizziness or somnolence.
- Assess the patient's pattern of daily bowel activity and stool consistency.

Patient Teaching

- Tell the patient that fluvoxamine's

maximum therapeutic response may require 4 weeks or more to appear.
- Caution the patient not to discontinue the drug abruptly.
- Warn the patient to avoid tasks that require mental alertness or motor skills until his or her response to the drug has been established.
- Suggest that the patient that take sips of tepid water and chew sugarless gum to relieve dry mouth.

ketamine

key-tah-meen
(Ketalar)

CATEGORY AND SCHEDULE

Pregnancy Risk Category: B

MECHANISM OF ACTION

A rapidly acting general anesthetic that selectively blocks afferent impulses and interacts with CNS transmitter systems. **Therapeutic Effect:** Produces an anesthetic state characterized by profound analgesia and normal pharyngeal-laryngeal reflexes.

PHARMACOKINETICS

Route	Onset	Peak	Duration
IM (anesthetic)	3–4 min	N/A	12–25 min
IM (analgesic)	30 min	N/A	15–30 min
IV (anesthetic)	30 sec	N/A	5–10 min
IV (analgesic)	10–15 min	N/A	N/A

Rapidly distributed. Metabolized in the liver. Primarily excreted in urine. ***Half-life:*** Distribution: 10–15 min, elimination: 2–3 hr.

AVAILABILITY

Injection: 10 mg/ml, 50 mg/ml, 100 mg/ml.

INDICATIONS AND DOSAGES

▸ **Sole anesthetic for short diagnostic and surgical procedures that don't require skeletal muscle relaxation, induction of anesthesia before administering other general anesthetics, supplement to low-potency agents**

IV

Adults, Elderly. 1–4.5 mg/kg.
Children. 0.5–2 mg/kg.

IM

Adults, Elderly. 3–8 mg/kg.
Children. 3–7 mg/kg.

CONTRAINDICATIONS

Aneurysms, angina, CHF, elevated ICP, hypertension, psychotic disorders, thyrotoxicosis

INTERACTIONS

Drug

Antihypertensives, CNS depressants: May increase the risk of hypotension and respiratory depression.

Herbal

None known.

Food

None known.

DIAGNOSTIC TEST EFFECTS

May increase IOP.

IV INCOMPATIBILITIES

No information available for Y-site administration.

IV COMPATIBILITIES

Bupivacaine (Marcaine), clonidine (Duraclon), fentanyl (Sublimaze), lidocaine, morphine, propofol (Diprivan)

SIDE EFFECTS

Frequent
Increased BP and pulse rate; emergence reaction (marked by dreamlike state, delirium, hallucinations, and vivid imagery and occasionally accompanied by confusion, excitement, and irrational behavior; lasts from few hours to 24 hours after ketamine administration)

Occasional
Pain at injection site

Rare
Rash

SERIOUS REACTIONS

! Continuous or repeated intermittent infusion may result in extreme somnolence and circulatory or respiratory depression.

! Too-rapid IV administration of ketamine may produce severe hypotension, respiratory depression, and irregular muscle movements.

NURSING CONSIDERATIONS

Baseline Assessment

- Obtain the patient's vital signs before giving ketamine.
- Have resuscitative equipment and oxygen available.

Lifespan Considerations

- Ketamine is not recommended for pregnant or breast-feeding women.
- No age-related precautions have been noted in children or the elderly.

Precautions

- Use ketamine cautiously in intoxicated or chronic alcoholic patients and in patients with a full stomach, gastroesophageal reflux disease, or hepatic impairment.

Administration and Handling

IV

- Give ketamine by IV push when it's used to induce anesthesia.
- Dilute the 100 mg/ml vial of ketamine with an equal volume of sterile water for injection, D_5W, or 0.9% NaCl.
- For a maintenance IV infusion, dilute the 50-mg/ml vial (10 ml) or 100-mg/ml vial (5 ml) of ketamine with 250–500 ml D_5W or 0.9% NaCl to provide a concentration of 1–2 mg/ml.
- Administer maintenance dose by IV push slowly at a rate of 0.5 mg/kg/minute over 60 seconds. A too-rapid IV administration may result in severe hypotension and respiratory depression.

IM

- Use the 10-mg/ml vial of ketamine. Do not dilute the 10-mg/ml vial.

Intervention and Evaluation

- Monitor vital signs every 3 to 5 minutes during and after ketamine administration until the patient has recovered.
- Assess the patient for an emergence reaction. Be prepared to administer a barbituate or hypnotic in case this reaction occurs.
- Minimize verbal, tactile, and visual stimulation during the recovery period.

Patient Teaching

- Warn the patient to avoid performing tasks that require mental alertness or motor skills for 24 hours after anesthesia has been discontinued.

lithium carbonate

lith-ee-um
(Duralith[CAN], Eskalith, Lithicarb[AUS], Lithobid, Quilonum SR[AUS])

lithium citrate

(Cibalith-S)

Do not confuse Lithobid with Levbid, Lithostat, or Lithotabs.

CATEGORY AND SCHEDULE

Pregnancy Risk Category: D

MECHANISM OF ACTION

A psychotherapeutic agent that affects the storage, release, and reuptake of neurotransmitters. Antimanic effect may result from increased norepinephrine reuptake and serotonin receptor sensitivity.
Therapeutic Effect: Produces antimanic and antidepressant effects.

PHARMACOKINETICS

Rapidly and completely absorbed from the GI tract. Primarily excreted unchanged in urine. Removed by hemodialysis. ***Half-life:*** 18–24 hr (increased in elderly).

AVAILABILITY

Capsules: 150 mg, 300 mg, 600 mg.
Syrup: 300 mg/ml.
Tablets: 300 mg.
Tablets (Controlled-Release): 450 mg.
Tablets (Slow-Release): 300 mg.

INDICATIONS AND DOSAGES

◀ALERT▶ During acute phase, a therapeutic serum lithium concentration of 1–1.4 mEq/L is required. For long-term control, the desired level is 0.5–1.3 mEq/L. Monitor serum drug concentration and clinical response to determine proper dosage.

▸ Prevention or treatment of acute mania, manic phase of bipolar disorder (manic-depressive illness)
PO
Adults. 300 mg 3–4 times a day or 450–900 mg slow-release form twice a day. Maximum: 2.4 g/day.
Elderly. 300 mg twice a day. May increase by 300 mg/day q1wk. Maintenance: 900–1,200 mg/day.
Children 12 yr and older. 600–1,800 mg/day in 3–4 divided doses (2 doses/day for slow-release).
Children younger than 12 yr. 15–60 mg/kg/day in 3–4 divided doses.

OFF-LABEL USES

Prevention of vascular headache; treatment of depression, neutropenia

CONTRAINDICATIONS

Debilitated patients, severe cardiovascular disease, severe dehydration, severe renal disease, severe sodium depletion

INTERACTIONS

Drug

Antithyroid medications, iodinated glycerol, potassium iodide: May increase the effects of these drugs.
Diuretics, NSAIDs: May increase lithium serum concentration and risk of toxicity.
Haloperidol: May increase extrapyramidal symptoms and the risk of neurologic toxicity.
Molindone: May increase the risk of neurotoxicity.
Phenothiazines: May decrease the absorption of phenothiazines, increase the intracellular concentration and renal excretion of lithium, and increase delirium and extrapyramidal symptoms. Antiemetic effect of some phenothiazines may mask early signs of lithium toxicity.

Herbal

None known.

Food

None known.

DIAGNOSTIC TEST EFFECTS

May increase blood glucose, immunoreactive parathyroid hormone, and serum calcium levels. Therapeutic lithium serum level is 0.6–1.2 mEq/L; toxic serum level is greater than 1.5 mEq/L.

SIDE EFFECTS

◀ALERT▶ Side effects are dose related and seldom occur at lithium serum levels less than 1.5 mEq/L.

Occasional
Fine hand tremor, polydipsia, polyuria, mild nausea
Rare
Weight gain, bradycardia or tachycardia, acne, rash, muscle twitching, cold and cyanotic extremities, pseudotumor cerebri (eye pain, headache, tinnitus, vision disturbances)

SERIOUS REACTIONS

! A lithium serum concentration of 1.5–2.0 mEq/L may produce vomiting, diarrhea, drowsiness, confusion, incoordination, coarse hand tremor, muscle twitching, and T-wave depression on EKG.
! A lithium serum concentration of 2.0–2.5 mEq/L may result in ataxia, giddiness, tinnitus, blurred vision, clonic movements, and severe hypotension.
! Acute toxicity may be characterized by seizures, oliguria, circulatory failure, coma, and death.

NURSING CONSIDERATIONS

Baseline Assessment

- Assess the patient's appearance, behavior, emotional status, response to environment, speech pattern, and thought content.
- Obtain lithium serum level every 3 to 4 days during the initial phase of lithium therapy, every 1 to 2 months thereafter, and weekly if symptoms fail to improve or adverse reactions occur.

Lifespan Considerations

- Lithium freely crosses the placenta and is distributed in breast milk. Warn the patient of the potential risks to the fetus if she uses lithium during pregnancy.
- Lithium use may decrease bone formation or density in children by altering parathyroid hormone concentrations.
- A lower lithium dosage is recommended for elderly patients, who are more likely to develop lithium-induced goiter, clinical hypothyroidism, CNS toxicity, increased thirst, and urinary frequency.

Precautions

- Use lithium cautiously in elderly patients and patients with cardiovascular or thyroid disease.

Administration and Handling

PO
- Lithium may be given on an empty stomach, but administration with meals or milk is preferred.
- Don't break, chew, or crush slow-release or film-coated tablets.

Intervention and Evaluation

- Monitor the patient's lithium serum level every 3 to 4 days at the beginning of therapy, then every 1 to 2 months. Obtain the serum level as close as possible to 12 hours after the patient's last dose. Lithium's therapeutic serum level is 0.6 to 1.2 mEq/L; its toxic serum level is greater than 1.5 mEq/L. Monitoring the drug level and assessing lithium's therapeutic effect is necessary for maintaining the correct dosage.
- Monitor the patient's cardiac, hepatic, renal, and thyroid function; CBC with differential; creatinine clearance; serum electrolyte levels; and urinalysis results.
- Observe the patient for signs and symptoms of lithium toxicity.
- Assess the patient for increased urine output and persistent thirst.
- Notify the physician if the patient experiences diarrhea, fever, polyuria, or prolonged vomiting.
- These side effects may indicate the need for a temporary dosage reduction or discontinuation of lithium therapy.
- Assess the patient for therapeutic response to the drug, as characterized by increased ability to concentrate,

improvement in self-care, interest in his or her surroundings, and a relaxed facial expression.

Patient Teaching

- Inform the patient that regular monitoring of the lithium blood level is necessary to determine the proper dosage.
- Inform the patient that lithium may cause excessive thirst and increased urination.
- Advise the patient to drink plenty of fluids and maintain a steady salt intake to avoid dehydration.
- Urge the patient to limit consumption of alcohol and caffeine.
- Warn the patient to avoid tasks that require mental alertness or motor skills until his or her response to the drug has been established.
- Instruct the patient to contact the physician if he or she experiences incoordination, diarrhea, vomiting, drowsiness, muscle weakness, or tremor.

nicotine

nik-o-teen

(Commit, Habitrol[CAN], Nicabate[AUS], Nicabate CQ Clear[AUS], Nicabate CQ Lozenges[AUS], NicoDerm[CAN], NicoDerm CQ, Nicorette, Nicorette Plus[CAN], Nicotinell [AUS], Nicotrol, Nicotrol NS, Nicotrol Patch[CAN])

Do not confuse Nicoderm with Nitroderm.

CATEGORY AND SCHEDULE

Pregnancy Risk Category: D (transdermal)

OTC (Nicoderm transdermal patch, Nicotrol transdermal patch, Nicorette chewing gum)

MECHANISM OF ACTION

A cholinergic-receptor agonist binds to acetylcholine receptors, producing both stimulating and depressant effects on the peripheral and central nervous systems. **Therapeutic Effect:** Provides a source of nicotine during nicotine withdrawal and reduces withdrawal symptoms.

PHARMACOKINETICS

Absorbed slowly after transdermal administration. Protein binding: 5%. Metabolized in the liver. Excreted primarily in urine. ***Half-life:*** 4 hr.

AVAILABILITY

Chewing Gum (Nicorette): 2 mg, 4 mg.
Lozenge (Commit): 2 mg, 4 mg.
Transdermal patch (NicoDerm CQ, Nicotrol): 7 mg, 14 mg, 21 mg.
Nasal Spray (Nicotrol NS): 0.5 mg/spray.
Inhalation (Nicotrol Inhaler): 10 mg cartridge.

INDICATIONS AND DOSAGES

▸ **Smoking cessation aid to relieve nicotine withdrawal symptoms**

PO (Chewing gum)

Adults, Elderly. Usually, 10–12 pieces/day. Maximum: 30 pieces/day.

PO (Lozenge)

◀ **ALERT** ▶ For those who smoke the first cigarette within 30 min of waking, administer the 4-mg lozenge; otherwise administer the 2-mg lozenge.

Adults, Elderly. One 4-mg or 2-mg lozenge q1–2h for the first 6 weeks; one lozenge q2–4h for wk 7–9; and one lozenge q4–8h for wk 10–12. Maximum: one lozenge at a time, 5 lozenges/6 hr, 20 lozenges/day.

Transdermal

Adults, Elderly who smoke 10

cigarettes or more per day. Follow the guidelines below.
Step 1: 21 mg/day for 4–6 wk.
Step 2: 14 mg/day for 2 wk.
Step 3: 7 mg/day for 2 wk.
Adults, Elderly who smoke less than 10 cigarettes per day. Follow the guidelines below.
Step 1: 14 mg/day for 6 wk.
Step 2: 7 mg/day for 2 wk.
Patients weighing less than 100 lb, patients with a history of cardiovascular disease. Initially, 14 mg/day for 4–6 wk, then 7 mg/day for 2–4wk.
Transdermal (Nicotrol)
Adults, Elderly. One patch a day for 6 wk.
Nasal
Adults, Elderly. 1–2 doses/hr (1 dose = 2 sprays [1 in each nostril] = 1 mg). Maximum: 5 doses (5 mg)/hr; 40 doses (40 mg) /day.
Inhaler (Nicotrol)
Adults, Elderly. Puff on nicotine cartridge mouthpiece for about 20 min as needed.

CONTRAINDICATIONS

Immediate post-MI period, life-threatening arrhythmias, severe or worsening angina

INTERACTIONS

Drug

Beta-adrenergic blockers, bronchodilators (such as theophylline), insulin, propoxyphene: May increase the effects of these drugs.

Herbal

None known.

Food

None known.

DIAGNOSTIC TEST EFFECTS

None known.

SIDE EFFECTS

Frequent

All forms: Hiccups, nausea
Gum: Mouth or throat soreness, nausea, hiccups
Transdermal: Erythema, pruritus, or burning at application site

Occasional

All forms: Eructation, GI upset, dry mouth, insomnia, diaphoresis, irritability
Gum: Hiccups, hoarseness
Inhaler: Mouth or throat irritation, cough

Rare

All forms: Dizziness, myalgia, arthralgia

SERIOUS REACTIONS

! Overdose produces palpitations, tachyarrhythmias, seizures, depression, confusion, diaphoresis, hypotension, rapid or weak pulse, and dyspnea. Lethal dose for adults is 40–60 mg. Death results from respiratory paralysis.

NURSING CONSIDERATIONS

Baseline Assessment

- Screen and evaluate patients with Buerger's disease, coronary artery disease (including angina pectoris and history of MI), Prinzmetal's variant angina, and serious cardiac arrhythmias.
- Plan to perform a baseline EKG.

Lifespan Considerations

- Nicotine passes freely into breast milk and smoking or nicotine gum are associated with a decrease in fetal breathing movements. The use of nicotine is not recommended for breast-feeding women.
- Nicotine use is not recommended for children.
- In the elderly, an age-related decrease in cardiac function may require cautious use.

Precautions

- Use nicotine cautiously in patients with eczematous dermatitis, esophagitis, hyperthyroidism, insulin-dependent diabetes mellitus, oral or pharyngeal inflammation, peptic ulcer disease, pheochromocytoma, or severe renal impairment.

Administration and Handling

◀ALERT▶ Expect to individualize nicotine dosage and to administer the drug when the patient plans to stop smoking.

Gum

• Instruct the pateint to chew 1 piece slowly and intermittently for 30 minutes when he or she feels the urge to smoke. The patient should chew until the distinctive, peppery nicotine taste or slight tingling in mouth occurs. When the tingling is almost gone, after approximately 1 minute, the patient should repeat the chewing procedure to allow constant, slow buccal absorption.
• Advise the patient not to chew too rapidly because this may cause excessive release of nicotine, resulting in adverse effects similar to those of oversmoking, such as nausea and throat irritation.
• Tell the patient not to swallow the gum.

Transdermal

◀ALERT▶ Decrease the dosage, as prescribed, for patients taking more than 600 mg cimetidine (Tagamet) daily.

• Apply the patch as soon as it has been removed from the protective pouch. This wrapping prevents evaporation and loss of nicotine. Use only an intact pouch. Do not cut the patch.
• Apply the patch only once daily to a hairless, clean, dry area on the upper body or outer arm.
• Rotate application sites; don't use the same site for 7 days or the same patch for longer than 24 hours.
• Wash hands with water alone after applying the patch because soap may increase nicotine absorption.
• To discard a used patch, fold it in half with the sticky sides together, place it in the empty pouch of the new patch, and discard it in a receptacle that is not accessible to children or pets.

Inhaler

• Insert the cartridge into mouthpiece, and have the patient puff vigorously for 20 minutes.

Intervention and Evaluation

• If the transdermal system is used, monitor the application site for burning, erythema, and pruritus.
• Obtain baseline vital signs, including BP and pulse rate.
• Assess smoking habits in relation to sleep patterns.

Patient Teaching

• Instruct the patient using nicotine gum to chew slowly to avoid jaw ache, nausea, and throat irritation and to maximize therapeutic benefits. Tell the patient not to swallow the gum.
• Teach the patient how to properly apply and discard the nicotine patches. Instruct the patient not to cut patches.
• Advise the patient to notify the physician if he or she experiences itching or a persistent rash during treatment with the transdermal patch.
• Urge the patient not to smoke while wearing nicotine transdermal patches.

poly-L-lactic acid

polly-el-**lack**-tic
(Sculptra)

CATEGORY AND SCHEDULE

Pregnancy Risk Category: Not established

MECHANISM OF ACTION

A lipoatrophy agent containing microparticles of a synthetic polymer that is used as an injectable implant. **Therapeutic Effect:** Restores facial fat.

PHARMACOKINETICS

Biodegradable, biocompatible synthetic polymer.

AVAILABILITY

Powder for Injection (freeze-dried).

INDICATIONS AND DOSAGES

▸ **Facial lipoatrophy**

Subcutaneous

Adults, Elderly. For severe facial fat loss, one vial usually injected into multiple points of each cheek during each injection session. Volume of drug for each injection and number of injection sessions depend on severity of condition. Typically, 3–6 injection sessions, separated by intervals of at least 2 weeks, are required.

CONTRAINDICATIONS

None known.

INTERACTIONS

Drug

None known.

Herbal

None known.

Food

None known.

DIAGNOSTIC TEST EFFECTS

None known.

SIDE EFFECTS

Frequent

Ecchymosis

Occasional

Discomfort, edema

Rare

Erythema

SERIOUS REACTIONS

! Subcutaneous papules at injection sites and hematoma occur occasionally.

NURSING CONSIDERATIONS

Baseline Assessment

- If the skin in or near the treatment area is inflamed or infected, defer use of poly-L-lactic acid until the inflammatory or infectious process has been controlled.

Lifespan Considerations

- The safety and efficacy of poly-L-lactic acid have not been established in patients younger than 18 years.
- No age-related precautions have been noted in the elderly.

Precautions

- Use poly-L-lactic acid cautiously in patients with a tendency to develop keloid formations.

Administration and Handling

Subcutaneous

- Store unopened vials at room temperature. Reconstituted product is stable for up to 72 hours at room temperature.
- Draw 3 to 5 ml sterile water for injection into a 5-ml sterile syringe.
- Slowly add all of the sterile water for injection into the vial, using an 18-gauge sterile needle.
- Let the vial stand for at least 2 hours. Don't shake it during this period.
- After 2 hours, agitate the vial until a uniform translucent suspension is obtained.
- Withdraw the dose (usually 1 ml) into a syringe, using a new 18-gauge needle.
- Replace the 18-gauge needle with a 26-gauge needle before injecting the product into the deep dermis or subcutaneous layer.

Intervention and Evaluation

- Apply ice packs to the treated area to reduce inflammation.

• Massage the treatment area daily for several days after each injection session.

Patient Teaching

• Inform the patient that pain, bruising, redness, and swelling typically resolve within 1 week after injection.
• Tell the patient that it may take weeks or months for the drug's full therapeutic effect to appear.
• Instruct the patient to avoid exposure to excessive sunlight and UV lamps until the initial redness and swelling resolve.

propofol

pro-poe-**fall**
(Diprivan, Recofol[AUS])

CATEGORY AND SCHEDULE

Pregnancy Risk Category: B

MECHANISM OF ACTION

A rapidly acting general anesthetic that inhibits sympathetic vasoconstrictor nerve activity and decreases vascular resistance. **Therapeutic Effect:** Produces hypnosis rapidly.

PHARMACOKINETICS

Route	Onset	Peak	Duration
IV	40 sec	N/A	3–10 min

Rapidly and extensively distributed. Protein binding: 97%–99%. Metabolized in the liver. Primarily excreted in urine. Unknown if removed by hemodialysis. ***Half-life:*** 3–12 hr.

AVAILABILITY

Injection: 10 mg/ml.

INDICATIONS AND DOSAGES

▸ **Intensive care unit sedation**

IV

Adults, Elderly. Initially, 0.3 mg/kg/hr. May increase by 0.3–0.6 mg/kg/hr q5–10min until desired effect is obtained. Maintenance: 0.3–3 mg/kg/h.

▸ **Anesthesia**

IV

Adults, American Society of Anesthesiologists (ASA) I and II patients. 2–2.5 mg/kg (about 40 mg q10sec until onset of anesthesia). Maintenance: 0.1–0.2 mg/kg/min.
Elderly, Debilitated, Hypovolemic, ASA III or IV patients. 1–1.5 mg/kg (about 20 mg q10sec until onset of anesthesia). Maintenance: 0.05–0.1 mg/kg/min.
Children 3 yr and older, ASA I or II patients. 2.5–3.5 mg/kg (lower dosage for ASA III or IV patients).
Children 2 mo–16 yr. Maintenance dose: 0.125–0.15 mg/kg/min.

CONTRAINDICATIONS

Impaired cerebral circulation, increased ICP

INTERACTIONS

Drug

Alcohol, other CNS depressants: May increase hypotensive and CNS and respiratory depressant effects of propofol.

Herbal

None known.

Food

None known.

DIAGNOSTIC TEST EFFECTS

None known.

IV INCOMPATIBILITIES

Amikacin (Amikin), amphotericin B complex (Abelcet, AmBisome, Amphotec), bretylium (Bretylol), calcium chloride, ciprofloxacin

(Cipro), diazepam (Valium), digoxin (Lanoxin), doxorubicin (Adriamycin), gentamicin (Garamycin), methylprednisolone (Solu-Medrol), minocycline (Minocin), phenytoin (Dilantin), tobramycin (Nebcin), verapamil (Isoptin)

IV COMPATIBILITIES

Acyclovir (Zovirax), bumetanide (Bumex), calcium gluconate, ceftazidime (Fortaz), dobutamine (Dobutrex), dopamine (Intropin), enalapril (Vasotec), fentanyl, heparin, insulin, labetalol (Normodyne, Trandate), lidocaine, lorazepam (Ativan), magnesium, milrinone (Primacor), nitroglycerin, norepinephrine (Levophed), potassium chloride, vancomycin (Vancocin)

SIDE EFFECTS

Frequent

Involuntary muscle movements, apnea (common during induction; lasts longer than 60 seconds), hypotension, nausea, vomiting, IV site burning or stinging

Occasional

Twitching, bucking, jerking, thrashing, headache, dizziness, bradycardia, hypertension, fever, abdominal cramps, paresthesia, coldness, cough, hiccups, facial flushing, greenish-colored urine

Rare

Rash, dry mouth, agitation, confusion, myalgia, thrombophlebitis

SERIOUS REACTIONS

! A continuous infusion or repeated intermittent infusions of propofol may result in extreme somnolence, respiratory depression, and circulatory depression.

! Too-rapid IV administration may produce severe hypotension, respiratory depression, and involuntary muscle movements.

! The patient may experience an acute allergic reaction, characterized by abdominal pain, anxiety, restlessness, dyspnea, erythema, hypotension, pruritus, rhinitis, and urticaria.

NURSING CONSIDERATIONS

Baseline Assessment

- Have resuscitative equipment, suction equipment, and oxygen available.
- Obtain the patient's vital signs before giving propofol.

Lifespan Considerations

- Propofol crosses the placenta and is not recommended for obstetric use.
- Propofol is distributed in breast milk and is not recommended for breast-feeding women.
- The safety and efficacy of propofol have not been established in children. However, the Food and Drug Administration has approved the drug for use in children 2 months and older.
- Lower propofol dosages are recommended for the elderly.

Precautions

- Use propofol cautiously in debilitated patients; patients with circulatory, hepatic, lipid metabolism, renal, or respiratory disorders; and those with a history of epilepsy.

Administration and Handling

◀ALERT▶ Don't give propofol through the same IV line as blood or plasma.

IV

- Store propofol at room temperature.
- Don't use propofol if the emulsion separates.
- Shake well before using.
- Propofol may be given undiluted, or it may be diluted only with D_5W to a concentration of no less than 2

mg/ml (4 ml D_5W to 1 ml propofol yields 2 mg/ml).

- Discard any unused portions of drug.
- Too-rapid IV administration of propofol may produce irregular muscle movements, respiratory depression, and severe hypotension.
- Observe the patient for signs of inadvertent intra-arterial injection, such as delayed onset of drug action, pain or discolored skin near the injection site, or blue or white discoloration of the hand if a hand or arm IV site is used.

Intervention and Evaluation

- Monitor the patient's ABG levels, BP, heart and respiratory rates, oxygen saturation, depth of sedation, and lipid and triglyceride levels if propofol is given for longer than 24 hours.

Patient Teaching

- Inform the patient that propofol may turn urine green.

riluzole

rye-loo-zole
(Rilutek)

CATEGORY AND SCHEDULE

Pregnancy Risk Category: C

MECHANISM OF ACTION

An amyotrophic lateral sclerosis (ALS) agent that inhibits presynaptic glutamate release in the CNS and intereferes postsynaptically with the effects of excitatory amino acids.
Therapeutic Effect: Extends survival of ALS patients.

AVAILABILITY

Tablets: 50 mg.

INDICATIONS AND DOSAGES

ALS

PO
Adults, Elderly. 50 mg q12h.

CONTRAINDICATIONS

None significant.

INTERACTIONS

Drug

Alcohol: May increase CNS depression.
Amitriptyline, quinolones, theophylline: May increase the effects and risk of toxicity of riluzole.
Omeprazole, rifampin: May decrease the effects of riluzole.

Herbal

None known.

Food

Caffeine: May increase the effects and risk of toxicity of riluzole.
High-fat meals: May decrease the absorption and effects of riluzole.

DIAGNOSTIC TEST EFFECTS

May increase liver function test results.

SIDE EFFECTS

Frequent (greater than 10%)
Nausea, asthenia, reduced respiratory function
Occasional (10%–1%)
Edema, tachycardia, headache, dizziness, somnolence, depression, vertigo, tremor, pruritus, alopecia, abdominal pain, diarrhea, anorexia, dyspepsia, vomiting, stomatitis, increased cough

SERIOUS REACTIONS

! None known.

NURSING CONSIDERATIONS

Baseline Assessment

- Obtain baseline blood chemisty tests to evaluate hepatic function.

Precautions

• Use riluzole cautiously in patients with a renal or hepatic impairment.

Administration and Handling

PO

• Administer riluzole at least 1 hour before or 2 hours after a meal.

Intervention and Evaluation

• Monitor the patient's liver function test results. Expect to discontinue the drug if the ALT level exceeds 10 times the upper normal limit.

Patient Teaching

• Instruct the patient to take riluzole at least 1 hour before or 2 hours after a meal and at the same times each day.

• Inform the patient that riluzole may cause drowsiness, dizziness, or vertigo.

• Warn the patient to avoid tasks requiring mental alertness or motor skills until his or her response to the medication has been established.

• Urge the patient to avoid alcohol during therapy.

• Caution the patient to notify the physician if he or she develops a fever.

ziconotide

zi-**koe**-no-tide

(Prialt)

CATEGORY AND SCHEDULE

Pregnancy Risk Category: C

MECHANISM OF ACTION

A synthetic peptide that selectively binds to N-type voltage-sensitive calcium channels located on afferent nerves in the spinal cord. This binding is thought to block N-type calcium channels. **Therapeutic Effect:** Blocks excitatory neurotransmitter release, reducing sensitivity to painful stimuli.

AVAILABILITY

Solution: 25-mcg/ml (20-ml), 100-mcg/ml (1-ml, 2-ml, 5-ml) vials.

INDICATIONS AND DOSAGES

‣ Pain control

Intrathecal

Adults, Elderly. Initially, 2.4 mcg/day (0.1 mcg/hour). May titrate to maximum of 19.2 mcg/day (0.8 mcg/hr).

CONTRAINDICATIONS

History of psychosis, presence of infection at the injection site, uncontrolled bleeding, or spinal canal obstruction that impairs CSF circulation, IV administration

INTERACTIONS

Drug

Other CNS depressants: May enhance the adverse and toxic effects of these drugs.

Herbal

None known.

Food

None known.

DIAGNOSTIC TEST EFFECTS

May increase serum kinase levels.

SIDE EFFECTS

Frequent (47%–11%)

Dizziness, nausea, somnolence, weakness, diarrhea, confusion, ataxia, headache, vomiting, gait disturbance, memory impairment, hypertonia

Occasional (10%–7%)

Anorexia, visual disturbances, anxiety, urinary retention, speech disorder, aphasia, nystagmus, paresthesia, fever, hallucinations, nervousness, vertigo

Rare
Insomnia, dry skin, constipation, arthralgia, myalgia, tremor

SERIOUS REACTIONS

! Atrial fibrillation, cerebral vascular accident, seizures, kidney failure (acute), myoclonus, and psychosis occurs rarely.

NURSING CONSIDERATIONS

Precautions

- Use ziconotide cautiously in elderly patients because they are at increased risk of developing confusion.

Administration and Handling

Intrathecal

- Administer ziconotide only with a Medtronic SynchroMed EL or SynchroMed II Infusion System, or the Simms Deltec Cadd Micro External Microinfusion Device and Catheter. Refer to the manufacturer's manuals for instructions for initial filling and refilling of the reservoir.

49 Anticholinergics and Antispasmodics

atropine sulfate
dicyclomine hydrochloride
glycopyrrolate
hyoscyamine
scopolamine

Uses: Anticholinergic and antispasmodic agents are used to treat a wide variety of GI conditions that involve bowel irritability and increased tone (spasticity) or motility of the GI tract.

Action: Also known as parasympatholytics, antimuscarinics, and muscarinic blockers, anticholinergics and antispasmodics competitively block the actions of acetylcholine at muscarinic receptors. Through this action, they reduce GI tone and motility and suppress gastric acid secretion.

COMBINATION PRODUCTS

DONNATAL: hyoscyamine/atropine/phenobarbital (a sedative)/scopolamine 0.1037 mg/0.0194 mg/16.2 mg/0.0065 mg.
LOMOTIL: atropine sulfate/diphenoxylate hydrochloride (an antidiarrheal) 0.025 mg/2.5 mg.
ATROPINE SULFATE: See antiarrhythmic agents
SCOPOLAMINE: See antiemetics

atropine sulfate

See Antiarrhythmic Agents

dicyclomine hydrochloride

dye-**sye**-kloe-meen
(Bentyl, Bentylol[CAN], Formulex[CAN], Lomine[CAN], Merbentyl[AUS])
Do not confuse dicyclomine with doxycycline or dyclonime, or Bentyl with Aventyl or Benadryl.

CATEGORY AND SCHEDULE

Pregnancy Risk Category: B

MECHANISM OF ACTION

A GI antispasmodic and anticholinergic agent that directly acts as a relaxant on smooth muscle. **Therapeutic Effect:** Reduces tone and motility of GI tract.

PHARMACOKINETICS

Route	Onset	Peak	Duration
PO	1–2 hr	N/A	4 hr

Readily absorbed from the GI tract. Widely distributed. Metabolized in the liver. ***Half-life:*** 9–10 hr.

AVAILABILITY

Capsules: 10 mg.
Tablets: 20 mg.
Syrup: 10 mg/5 ml.
Injection: 10 mg/ml.

INDICATIONS AND DOSAGES

▸ **Functional disturbances of GI motility**

PO

Adults. 10–20 mg 3–4 times a day up to 40 mg 4 times/day.
Children older than 2 yr. 10 mg 3–4 times a day.

Children 6 mo–2 yr. 5 mg 3–4 times a day.
Elderly. 10–20 mg 4 times a day. May increase up to 160 mg/day.
IM
Adults. 20 mg q4–6h.

CONTRAINDICATIONS

Bladder neck obstruction due to prostatic hyperplasia, coronary vasospasm, intestinal atony, myasthenia gravis in patients not treated with neostigmine, narrow-angle glaucoma, obstructive disease of the GI tract, paralytic ileus, severe ulcerative colitis, tachycardia secondary to cardiac insufficiency or thyrotoxicosis, toxic megacolon, unstable cardiovascular status in acute hemorrhage

INTERACTIONS

Drug

Antacids, antidiarrheals: May decrease the absorption of dicyclomine.
Ketoconazole: May decrease the absorption of ketoconazole.
Other anticholinergics: May increase the effects of dicyclomine.
Potassium chloride: May increase the severity of GI lesions with the wax matrix formulation of potassium chloride.

Herbal

None known.

Food

None known.

DIAGNOSTIC TEST EFFECTS

None known.

SIDE EFFECTS

Frequent

Dry mouth (sometimes severe), constipation, diminished sweating ability

Occasional

Blurred vision; photophobia; urinary hesitancy; somnolence (with high dosage); agitation, excitement, confusion, or somnolence noted in elderly (even with low dosages); transient light-headedness (with IM route), irritation at injection site (with IM route)

Rare

Confusion, hypersensitivity reaction, increased IOP, nausea, vomiting, unusual fatigue

SERIOUS REACTIONS

! Overdose may produce temporary paralysis of ciliary muscle; pupillary dilation; tachycardia; palpitations; hot, dry, or flushed skin; absence of bowel sounds; hyperthermia; increased respiratory rate; EKG abnormalities; nausea; vomiting; rash over face or upper trunk; CNS stimulation; and psychosis (marked by agitation, restlessness, rambling speech, visual hallucinations, paranoid behavior, and delusions, followed by depression).

NURSING CONSIDERATIONS

Baseline Assessment

- Instruct the patient to void before giving dicyclomine to reduce the risk of urine retention.

Lifespan Considerations

- It is unknown if dicyclomine crosses the placenta or is distributed in breast milk.
- Infants and young children are more susceptible to the drug's toxic effects.
- Dicyclomine use in the elderly may cause agitation, confusion, somnolence, or excitement.

Precautions

- Use dicyclomine extremely cautiously in patients with autonomic neuropathy, diarrhea, known or suspected GI infections, or mild to moderate ulcerative colitis.

• Use cautiously in patients with CHF, COPD, coronary artery disease, esophageal reflux or hiatal hernia associated with reflux esophagitis, gastric ulcer, hyperthyroidism, hypertension, hepatic or renal disease, or tachyarrhythmias.
• Use cautiously in infants and elderly patients.

Administration and Handling

• Store capsules, tablets, syrup, and parenteral form at room temperature.

PO

• Dilute syrup with an equal volume of water just before administration.
• May give dicyclomine without regard to meals because food may slightly decrease absorption.

IM

• Injection normally appears colorless.
• Do not administer IV or subcutaneously.
• Inject IM deep in large muscle mass.
• Do not give for longer than 2 days, as prescribed.

Intervention and Evaluation

• Evaluate the patient for urine retention.
• Monitor changes in the patient's BP and body temperature.
• Be alert for fever because it increases the risk of hyperthermia.
• Assess the patient's bowel sounds for peristalsis, and mucous membranes and skin turgor for hydration status.
• Encourage adequate fluid intake.
• Assess the patient's pattern of daily bowel activity and stool consistency.

Patient Teaching

• Tell the patient not to become overheated while exercising in hot weather because this may cause heat stroke.
• Urge the patient to avoid hot baths and saunas.
• Warn the patient to avoid tasks that require mental alertness or motor skills until his or her response to the drug has been established.
• Instruct the patient not to take antacids or antidiarrheals within 1 hour of taking dicyclomine because these drugs decrease dicyclomine's effectiveness.

glycopyrrolate

glye-koe-**pye**-roe-late
(Robinul, Robinul Forte, Robinul Injection[AUS])
Do not confuse Robinul with Reminyl.

CATEGORY AND SCHEDULE

Pregnancy Risk Category: B

MECHANISM OF ACTION

A quaternary anticholinergic that inhibits action of acetylcholine at postganglionic parasympathetic sites in smooth muscle, secretory glands, and CNS. **Therapeutic Effect:** Reduces salivation and excessive secretions of respiratory tract; reduces gastric secretions and acidity.

AVAILABILITY

Injection: 0.2 mg/ml.

INDICATIONS AND DOSAGES

▸ **Preoperative inhibition of salivation and excessive respiratory tract secretions**

IM

Adults, Elderly. 4.4 mcg/kg 30–60 min before procedure.
Children 2 yr and older. 4.4 mcg/kg.
Children younger than 2 yr. 4.4–8.8 mcg/kg.

▸ **To block effects of anticholinesterase agents**

IV

Adults, Elderly. 0.2 mg for each 1

mg neostigmine or 5 mg pyridostigmine.

CONTRAINDICATIONS

Acute hemorrhage, myasthenia gravis, narrow-angle glaucoma, obstructive uropathy, paralytic ileus, tachycardia, ulcerative colitis

INTERACTIONS

Drug

Antacids, antidiarrheals: May decrease the absorption of glycopyrrolate.
Ketoconazole: May decrease the absorption of ketoconazole.
Other anticholinergics: May increase the effects of glycopyrrolate.
Potassium chloride: May increase the severity of GI lesions with the wax matrix formulation of potassium chloride.

Herbal

None known.

Food

None known.

DIAGNOSTIC TEST EFFECTS

May decrease serum uric acid levels.

IV INCOMPATIBILITIES

None known.

IV COMPATIBILITIES

Diphenhydramine (Benadryl), droperidol (Inapsine), hydromorphone (Dilaudid), hydroxyzine (Vistaril), lidocaine, midazolam (Versed), morphine, promethazine (Phenergan)

SIDE EFFECTS

Frequent

Dry mouth, decreased sweating, constipation

Occasional

Blurred vision, gastric bloating, urinary hesitancy, somnolence (with high dosage), headache, intolerance to light, loss of taste, nervousness, flushing, insomnia, impotence, mental confusion or excitement (particularly in the elderly and children), temporary light-headedness (with parenteral form), local irritation (with parenteral form)

Rare

Dizziness, faintness

SERIOUS REACTIONS

! Overdose may produce temporary paralysis of ciliary muscle; pupillary dilation; tachycardia; palpitations; hot, dry, or flushed skin; absence of bowel sounds; hyperthermia; increased respiratory rate; EKG abnormalities; nausea; vomiting; rash over face or upper trunk; CNS stimulation; and psychosis (marked by agitation, restlessness, rambling speech, visual hallucinations, paranoid behavior, and delusions, followed by depression).

NURSING CONSIDERATIONS

Baseline Assessment

- Instruct the patient to void before giving glycopyrrolate to reduce the risk of urine retention.
- Perform a careful health history that screens for the presence of myasthenia gravis, narrow-angle glaucoma, obstructive uropathy, tachyarrhythmias, and ulcerative colitis.

Precautions

- Use glycopyrrolate cautiously in patients with CHF, diarrhea, fever, GI infections, hepatic or renal disease, hypothyroidism, or reflux esophagitis.

Administration and Handling

IV

- For direct injection, administer undiluted through the tubing of a free-flowing compatible IV solution.

IM
• Administer undiluted or diluted with D_5W, $D_{10}W$, or 0.9% NaCl.

Intervention and Evaluation
• Palpate the patient's bladder for signs of urine retention, and monitor urine output.
• Monitor the patient's BP, body temperature, and heart rate.
• Assess the patient's bowel sounds for peristalsis and mucous membranes and skin turgor for hydration status.
• Encourage adequate fluid intake.
• Be alert for fever because it increases the risk of hyperthermia.
• Assess the patient's pattern of daily bowel activity and stool consistency.

Patient Teaching
• Inform the patient that glycopyrrolate use may cause dry mouth.
• Instruct the patient not to become overheated while exercising in hot weather becauses this may cause heat stroke.
• Urge the patient to avoid hot baths and saunas.
• Warn the patient to avoid tasks that require mental alertness or motor skills until his or her response to the drug has been established.
• Instruct the patient not to take antacids or antidiarrheals within 1 hour of taking glycopyrrolate because these drugs decrease glycopyrrolate's effectiveness.

hyoscyamine

hye-oh-**sye**-a-meen
(Anaspaz, Buscopan[CAN], Cystospaz, Cystospaz-M, Hyosine, Levbid, Levsin, Levsinex, Levin S/L, NuLev, Spacol, Spacol T/S, Symax SL, Symax SR)
Do not confuse Anaspaz with Anaprox.

CATEGORY AND SCHEDULE

Pregnancy Risk Category: C

MECHANISM OF ACTION

A GI antispasmodic and anticholinergic agent that inhibits the action of acetylcholine at post-ganglionic (muscarinic) receptor sites. **Therapeutic Effect:** Decreases secretions (bronchial, salivary, sweat gland) and gastric juices and reduces motility of GI and urinary tract.

AVAILABILITY

Tablets (Anaspaz, Cystospaz, Levsin, Spacol): 0.125 mg.
Tablets (Oral-Disintegrating [NuLev]): 0.125 mg.
Tablets (Sublingual [Levsin S/L, Symax SL]): 0.125 mg.
Tablets (Extended-Release [Levbid, Spacol T/S, Symax SR]): 0.375 mg.
Capsules (Extended-Release [Cystospaz-M, Levsinex]): 0.375 mg.
Liquid (Hyosine, Spacol): 0.125 mg/5 ml.
Oral Solution (Hyosine, Levsin): 0.125 mg/5 ml

INDICATIONS AND DOSAGES

▸ **GI tract disorders**

PO
Adults, Elderly, Children 12 yr and older. 0.125–0.25 mg q4h as needed. Extended-release: 0.375–

0.75 mg q12h. Maximum: 1.5 mg/day.
Children 2–11 yr. 0.0625–0.125 mg q4h as needed. Extended-release: 0.375 mg q12h. Maximum: 0.75 mg/day.
IV, IM
Adults, Elderly, Children 12 yr and older. 0.25–0.5 mg q4h for 1–4 doses.

▸ **Hypermotility of lower urinary tract**
PO, Sublingual
Adults, Elderly. 0.15–0.3 mg 4 times a day; or extended-release 0.375 mg q12h.

▸ **Infant colic**
PO
Infants. Individualized drops dosed q4h as needed.

CONTRAINDICATIONS

GI or GU obstruction, myasthenia gravis, narrow-angle glaucoma, paralytic ileus, severe ulcerative colitis

INTERACTIONS

Drug

Antacids, antidiarrheals: May decrease the absorption of hyoscyamine.
Ketoconazole: May decrease the absorption of this drug.
Other anticholinergics: May increase the effects of hyoscyamine.
Potassium chloride: May increase the severity of GI lesions with the matrix formulation of potassium chloride.

Herbal

None known.

Food

None known.

DIAGNOSTIC TEST EFFECTS

None known.

SIDE EFFECTS

Frequent

Dry mouth (sometimes severe), decreased sweating, constipation

Occasional

Blurred vision; bloated feeling; urinary hesitancy; somnolence (with high dosage); headache; intolerance to light; loss of taste; nervousness; flushing; insomnia; impotence; mental confusion or excitement (particularly in the elderly and children); temporary light-headedness (with parenteral form); local irritation (with parenteral form)

Rare

Dizziness, faintness

SERIOUS REACTIONS

! Overdose may produce temporary paralysis of ciliary muscle; pupillary dilation; tachycardia; palpitations; hot, dry, or flushed skin; absence of bowel sounds; hyperthermia; increased respiratory rate; EKG abnormalities; nausea; vomiting; rash over face or upper trunk; CNS stimulation; and psychosis (marked by agitation, restlessness, rambling speech, visual hallucinations, paranoid behavior, and delusions, followed by depression).

NURSING CONSIDERATIONS

Baseline Assessment

- Instruct the patient to void before giving hyoscyamine to reduce the risk of urine retention.

Precautions

- Use hyoscyamine cautiously in patients with cardiac arrhythmias, CHF, chronic lung disease, hyperthyroidism, neuropathy, or prostatic hyperplasia.

Administration and Handling

PO

- Give hyoscyamine without regard to meals.

- Crush or have patient chew tablets.
- Extended-release capsule should be swallowed whole.

Parenteral

- May give undiluted.

Intervention and Evaluation

- Assess the patient's pattern of daily bowel activity and stool consistency.
- Palpate the patient's bladder for signs of urine retention, and monitor urine output.
- Monitor changes in the patient's BP and body temperature.
- Be alert for fever because it increases the risk of hyperthermia.
- Assess the patient's bowel sounds for peristalsis and mucous membranes and skin turgor for hydration status.
- Encourage adequate fluid intake.

Patient Teaching

- Advise the patient that dry mouth may occur during hyoscyamine therapy. Urge the patient to maintain good oral hygiene because the lack of saliva may increase the risk of cavities.
- Warn the patient to notify the physician if constipation, difficulty urinating, eye pain, or rash occurs.
- Urge the patient to avoid hot baths and saunas.
- Caution the patient to avoid tasks that require mental alertness or motor skills until his or her response to the drug has been established.

scopolamine

See Antiemetics

50 Antidiarrheals

bismuth subsalicylate
diphenoxylate hydrochloride with atropine sulfate
loperamide hydrochloride
nitazoxanide

Uses: Antidiarrheals are used to treat acute diarrhea and chronic diarrhea of inflammatory bowel disease. The goal of antidiarrheal therapy is to determine and treat the underlying cause of diarrhea, replenish fluids and electrolytes, relieve GI cramping, and reduce the passage of unformed stools. Some antidiarrheals are also used to reduce fluid from ileostomies.

Action: Systemic and local antidiarrheals act in different ways. *Systemic agents,* such as diphenoxylate, act at receptors in enteric smooth muscles, disrupting peristaltic movements, decreasing GI motility, and decreasing the transit time of intestinal contents. *Local agents,* such as bismuth subsalicylate, adsorb toxic substances and fluids to large surface areas of particles in the preparation. Some of these agents coat and protect irritated intestinal walls. They may also have local anti-inflammatory action. Nitazoxanide interferes with an enzyme-dependent reaction that's essential for anaerobic metabolism in *Cryptosporidium parvum* and *Giardia lamblia,* two organisms responsible for diarrhea.

COMBINATION PRODUCTS

HELIDAC: bismuth/metronidazole (an anti-infective)/tetracycline (an anti-infective) 262 mg/250 mg/500 mg.
IMODIUM ADVANCED: loperamide/simethicone (an antiflatulent) 2 mg/125 mg.
LOMOTIL: diphenoxylate/atropine (an anticholinergic and antispasmodic) 2.5 mg/0.025 mg.

bismuth subsalicylate

bis-muth sub-sal-**ih**-sah-late
(Bismed[CAN], Colo-Fresh, Devrom, Kaopectate, Pepto-Bismol)

CATEGORY AND SCHEDULE

Pregnancy Risk Category: C
OTC

MECHANISM OF ACTION

An antinauseant and antiulcer agent that absorbs water and toxins in the large intestine and forms a protective coating in the intestinal mucosa. Also possesses antisecretory and antimicrobial effects. **Therapeutic Effect:** Prevents diarrhea. Helps treat *Helicobacter pylori*–associated peptic ulcer disease.

AVAILABILITY

Caplet (Devrom): 200 mg.
Liquid (Kaopectate, Pepto-Bismol): 262 mg/15 ml, 525 mg/15 ml.
Tablet (Colo-Fresh): 324 mg.
Tablets (Chewable [Devrom]): (Devrom): 200 mg.
Tablets (Chewable [Pepto-Bismol]): 262 mg.

INDICATIONS AND DOSAGES

▸ **Diarrhea, gastric distress**
PO
Adults, Elderly. 2 tablets (30 ml) q30–60min. Maximum: 8 doses in 24 hr.
Children 9–12 yr. 1 tablet or 15 ml q30–60min. Maximum: 8 doses in 24 hr.
Children 6–8 yr. Two-thirds of a tablet or 10 ml q30–60min. Maximum: 8 doses in 24 hr.
Children 3–5 yr. One-third of a tablet or 5 ml q30–60min. Maximum: 8 doses in 24 hr.

▸ ***H. pylori*–associated duodenal ulcer, gastritis**
PO
Adults, Elderly. 525 mg 4 times a day, with 500 mg amoxicillin and 500 mg metronidazole, 3 times a day after meals, for 7–14 days.

▸ **Chronic infant diarrhea**
PO
Children 2–24 mo. 2.5 ml q4h.

OFF-LABEL USES

Prevention of traveler's diarrhea

CONTRAINDICATIONS

Bleeding ulcers, gout, hemophilia, hemorrhagic states, renal impairment

INTERACTIONS

Drug

Anticoagulants, heparin, thrombolytics: May increase the risk of bleeding.
Aspirin, other salicylates: May increase the risk of salicylate toxicity.
Insulin, oral antidiabetics: Large dose may increase the effects of insulin and oral antidiabetics.
Tetracyclines: May decrease the absorption of tetracyclines.

Herbal

None known.

Food

None known.

DIAGNOSTIC TEST EFFECTS

May alter serum alkaline phosphatase, AST (SGOT), ALT (SGPT), and uric acid levels. May decrease serum potassium level. May prolong PT.

SIDE EFFECTS

Frequent

Grayish black stools

Rare

Constipation

SERIOUS REACTIONS

! Debilitated patients and infants may develop impaction.

NURSING CONSIDERATIONS

Baseline Assessment

• Before administering, assess the patient's abdomen for signs of tenderness, rigidity, and the presence of bowel sounds.
• Determine when the patient last had a bowel movement, and find out the amount and consistency.

Precautions

• Use bismuth cautiously in diabetic and elderly patients.

Administration and Handling

- Shake the suspension well before administration.
- Have the patient chew the chewable tablet before swallowing. Alternatively, have the patient allow the chewable tablet to dissolve before swallowing.

Intervention and Evaluation

- Encourage the patient to drink and maintain adequate fluid intake.
- Assess the patient's bowel sounds for peristaltic activity.
- Monitor the patient's pattern of daily bowel activity and stool consistency.

Patient Teaching

- Explain to the patient that his or her stool may appear black or gray.
- Instruct the patient to chew tablets thoroughly before swallowing.
- Warn the patient to avoid bismuth if he or she is taking aspirin or other salicylates because of the increased risk of toxicity.
- Instruct the patient taking anticoagulants to ask the physician about using bismuth because this drug combination can dangerously prolong bleeding time.

diphenoxylate hydrochloride with atropine sulfate

dye-fen-**ox**-i-late
(Lomotil, Lonox)
Do not confuse Lomotil with Lamictal; or Lofenoxal or Lonox with Lanoxin, Loprox, or Lovenox.

CATEGORY AND SCHEDULE

Pregnancy Risk Category: C

MECHANISM OF ACTION

A meperidine derivative that acts locally and centrally on gastric mucosa. **Therapeutic Effect:** Reduces intestinal motility.

PHARMACOKINETICS

Well absorbed from the GI tract. Metabolized in the liver to active metabolite. Primarily eliminated in feces. ***Half-life:*** 2.5 hr; metabolite, 12–24 hr.

AVAILABILITY

Tablets (Lomotil, Lonox): 2.5 mg.
Liquid (Lomotil): 2.5 mg/5 ml.

INDICATIONS AND DOSAGES

▸ Diarrhea

PO

Adults, Elderly. Initially, 15–20 mg/day in 3–4 divided doses; then 5–15 mg/day in 2–3 divided doses.
Children 9–12 yr. 2 mg 5 times a day.
Children 6–8 yr. 2 mg 4 times a day.
Children 2–5 yr. 2 mg 3 times a day.

CONTRAINDICATIONS

Children younger than 2 years, dehydration, jaundice, narrow-angle glaucoma, severe hepatic disease

INTERACTIONS

Drug

Alcohol, other CNS depressants: May increase CNS depressant effects.
Anticholinergics: May increase the effects of atropine.
MAOIs: May precipitate hypertensive crisis.

Herbal

None known.

Food

None known.

DIAGNOSTIC TEST EFFECTS

May increase serum amylase level.

SIDE EFFECTS

Frequent
Somnolence, light-headedness, dizziness, nausea

Occasional
Headache, dry mouth

Rare
Flushing, tachycardia, urine retention, constipation, paradoxical reaction (marked by restlessness and agitation), blurred vision

SERIOUS REACTIONS

! Dehydration may predispose to diphenoxylate toxicity.

! Paralytic ileus and toxic megacolon (marked by constipation, decreased appetite, and stomach pain with nausea or vomiting) occur rarely.

! Severe anticholinergic reaction, manifested by severe lethargy, hypotonic reflexes, and hyperthermia, may result in severe respiratory depression and coma.

NURSING CONSIDERATIONS

Baseline Assessment

- Check the patient's hydration status. Assess the mucous membranes, skin turgor, and urine output.
- Perform an abdominal assessment, checking for tenderness, distention, and guarding, as well as the presence and activity of bowel sounds.

Lifespan Considerations

- It is unknown if diphenoxylate crosses the placenta or is distributed in breast milk.
- Diphenoxylate is not recommended for use in children because of the increased risk of toxicity, which can lead to respiratory depression.
- The elderly are more susceptible to the anticholinergic effects of diphenoxylate, and they may experience confusion and respiratory depression.

Precautions

- Use diphenoxylate cautiously in patients with acute ulcerative colitis, cirrhosis, hepatic or renal disease, or renal impairment.

Administration and Handling

PO

- Give without regard to meals. If GI irritation occurs, give with food.
- Administer the liquid form to children 2 to 12 years of age, using a graduated dropper for accurate measurement.

Intervention and Evaluation

- Encourage the patient to maintain adequate fluid intake.
- Assess the patient's bowel sounds for peristalsis.
- Assess the patient's pattern of daily bowel activity and stool consistency and record time of evacuation.
- Evaluate the patient for abdominal disturbances.
- Discontinue the medication if the patient experiences abdominal distention.

Patient Teaching

- Warn the patient to avoid tasks that require mental alertness or motor skills until his or her response to the drug has been established.
- Urge the patient to avoid alcohol and barbiturates during drug therapy.
- Tell the patient to notify the physician if abdominal distention, fever, palpitations, or persistent diarrhea occurs.

loperamide hydrochloride

loe-**per**-a-mide
(Apo-Loperamide[CAN], Gastro-Stop[AUS], Imodium, Imodium A-D, Loperacap[CAN], Novo-Loperamide[CAN])
Do not confuse Imodium with Indocin or Ionamin.

CATEGORY AND SCHEDULE

Pregnancy Risk Category: B
OTC liquid, tablets

MECHANISM OF ACTION

An antidiarrheal that directly affects the intestinal wall muscles. **Therapeutic Effect:** Slows intestinal motility and prolongs transit time of intestinal contents by reducing fecal volume, diminishing loss of fluid and electrolytes, and increasing viscosity and bulk of stool.

PHARMACOKINETICS

Poorly absorbed from the GI tract. Protein binding: 97%. Metabolized in the liver. Eliminated in feces and excreted in urine. Not removed by hemodialysis. ***Half-life:*** 9.1–14.4 hr.

AVAILABILITY

Capsules: 2 mg.
Liquid: 1 mg/5 ml.
Tablets: 2 mg.

INDICATIONS AND DOSAGES

▸ Acute diarrhea

PO (Capsules)
Adults, Elderly. Initially, 4 mg; then 2 mg after each unformed stool. Maximum: 16 mg/day.
Children 9–12 yr, weighing more than 30 kg. Initially, 2 mg 3 times a day for 24 hr.
Children 6–8 yr, weighing 20–30 kg. Initially, 2 mg twice a day for 24 hr.
Children 2–5 yr, weighing 13–20 kg. Initially, 1 mg 3 times/day for 24 hr. Maintenance: 1 mg/10 kg only after loose stool.

▸ Chronic diarrhea

PO
Adults, Elderly. Initially, 4 mg; then 2 mg after each unformed stool until diarrhea is controlled.
Children. 0.08–0.24 mg/kg/day in 2–3 divided doses. Maximum: 2 mg/dose.

▸ Traveler's diarrhea

PO
Adults, Elderly. Initially, 4 mg; then 2 mg after each loose bowel movement (LBM). Maximum: 8 mg/day for 2 days.
Children 9–11 yr. Initially, 2 mg; then 1 mg after each LBM. Maximum: 6 mg/day for 2 days.
Children 6–8 yr. Initially, 1 mg; then 1 mg after each LBM. Maximum: 4 mg/day for 2 days.

CONTRAINDICATIONS

Acute ulcerative colitis (may produce toxic megacolon), diarrhea associated with pseudomembranous enterocolitis due to broad-spectrum antibiotics or to organisms that invade intestinal mucosa (such as *Escherichia coli*, shigella, and salmonella), patients who must avoid constipation

INTERACTIONS

Drug

Opioid (narcotic) analgesics: May increase the risk of constipation.

Herbal

None known.

Food

None known.

DIAGNOSTIC TEST EFFECTS

None known.

SIDE EFFECTS

Rare

Dry mouth, somnolence, abdominal discomfort, allergic reaction (such as rash and itching)

SERIOUS REACTIONS

! Toxicity results in constipation, GI irritation, including nausea and vomiting, and CNS depression. Activated charcoal is used to treat loperamide toxicity.

NURSING CONSIDERATIONS

Baseline Assessment

- Do not administer to the patient who has bloody diarrhea or a temperature greater than 101°F.
- Determine if the patient has a history of ulcerative colitis.
- Expect to obtain stool specimens for culture and sensitivity and for ova and parasites, if infectious diarrhea is suspected.

Lifespan Considerations

- It is unknown if loperamide crosses the placenta or is distributed in breast milk.
- Loperamide use is not recommended in children younger than 6 years of age. Infants younger than 3 months of age are more susceptible to CNS effects.
- Loperamide use in the elderly may mask dehydration and electrolyte depletion.

Precautions

- Use loperamide cautiously in patients with fluid and electrolyte depletion or hepatic impairment.

Administration and Handling

Oral Liquid

- When administering the drug to children, use the accompanying plastic dropper to measure the liquid.

Intervention and Evaluation

- Encourage the patient to maintain adequate fluid intake.
- Assess the patient's bowel sounds for peristalsis.
- Monitor the patient's pattern of daily bowel activity and stool consistency.
- Withhold the drug and notify the physician promptly if abdominal distention, pain, or fever occurs.

Patient Teaching

- Caution the patient not to exceed the prescribed dosage.
- Tell the patient that loperamide may cause dry mouth.
- Urge the patient to avoid alcohol during loperamide therapy.
- Instruct the patient to avoid tasks that require mental alertness or motor skills until his or her response to the drug has been established.
- Warn the patient to notify the physician if abdominal distention and pain, diarrhea that does not stop within 3 days, or fever occurs.

nitazoxanide

nigh-tazz-**oks**-ah-nide

(Alinia)

CATEGORY AND SCHEDULE

Pregnancy Risk Category: B

MECHANISM OF ACTION

An antiparasitic that interferes with the body's reaction to pyruvate ferredoxin oxidoreductase, an enzyme essential for anaerobic energy metabolism. **Therapeutic Effect:** Produces antiprotozoal activity, reducing or terminating diarrheal episodes.

PHARMACOKINETICS

Rapidly hydrolyzed to an active metabolite. Protein binding: 99%. Excreted in the urine, bile, and feces. ***Half-life:*** 2–4 hr.

AVAILABILITY

Powder for Oral Suspension: 100 mg/5 ml.

INDICATIONS AND DOSAGES

▸ Diarrhea

PO

Children 12 yr and older. 200 mg q12h.

Children 4–11 yr. 200 mg (10 ml) q12h for 3 days.

Children 12–47 mo. 100 mg (5 ml) q12h for 3 days.

CONTRAINDICATIONS

History of sensitivity to aspirin and salicylates

INTERACTIONS

Drug

None known.

Herbal

None known.

Food

None known.

DIAGNOSTIC TEST EFFECTS

May increase serum creatinine and ALT (SGPT) levels.

SIDE EFFECTS

Occasional (8%)

Abdominal pain

Rare (2%–1%)

Diarrhea, vomiting, headache

SERIOUS REACTIONS

! None known.

NURSING CONSIDERATIONS

Baseline Assessment

- Establish the patient's blood glucose and electrolyte levels, BP, and weight.
- Assess the patient for dehydration.

Lifespan Considerations

- It is unknown if nitazoxanide is distributed in breast milk.
- The safety and efficacy of nitazoxanide have not been established in children older than 11 years of age.
- Nitazoxanide is not indicated for use in the elderly.

Precautions

- Use nitazoxanide cautiously in patients with biliary or hepatic disease, GI disorders, or renal impairment.

Administration and Handling

PO

- Store unreconstituted powder at room temperature.
- Reconstitute oral suspension with 48 ml water to provide a concentration of 100 mg/5 ml.
- Shake vigorously to suspend powder.
- Reconstituted solution is stable for 7 days at room temperature.
- Give with food.

Intervention and Evaluation

- Evaluate the blood glucose level in the patient with diabetes.
- Assess the patient's electrolyte levels for abnormalities that may have been caused by diarrhea.
- Weigh the patient each day and encourage him or her to maintain adequate fluid intake.
- Assess the patient's bowel sounds for peristalsis.
- Assess the patient's pattern of daily bowel activity and stool consistency.

Patient Teaching

- Tell parents of children with diabetes mellitus that the oral suspension of nitazoxanide contains 1.48 g of sucrose per 5 ml.
- Explain to the patient that nitazoxanide therapy should significantly improve his or her diarrhea.
- Instruct the patient and his or her parents to make sure the drug is taken with food.

51 Histamine (H_2) Antagonists

cimetidine
famotidine
nizatidine
ranitidine hydrochloride, ranitidine bismuth citrate

Uses: Histamine (H_2) antagonists are used for short-term treatment of duodenal ulcer and active benign gastric ulcer and for maintenance therapy of duodenal ulcer. They're also used to treat pathologic hypersecretory conditions, such as Zollinger-Ellison syndrome, and gastroesophageal reflux disease (GERD). In addition, these agents are used to prevent upper GI bleeding in critically ill patients.

Action: H_2 antagonists inhibit gastric acid secretion by interfering with histamine at H_2 receptors in parietal cells. (See the illustration *Sites of Action: Drugs Used to Treat GERD,* page 980.) They also inhibit acid secretion, which is regulated by the hormone gastrin, whether the secretion is basal (fasting), nocturnal, or stimulated by food or fundic distention. H_2 antagonists decrease the volume and H_2 concentration of gastric juices.

COMBINATION PRODUCTS

PEPCID COMPLETE: famotidine/calcium chloride (an antacid)/magnesium hydroxide (an antacid) 10 mg/800 mg/165 mg.

cimetidine

sye-**met**-i-deen
(Apo-Cimetidine[CAN], Cimehexal[AUS], Magicul[AUS], Novocimetine[CAN], Peptol[CAN], Sigmetadine[AUS], Tagamet, Tagamet HB)
Do not confuse cimetidine with simethicone.

CATEGORY AND SCHEDULE

Pregnancy Risk Category: B
OTC (100 mg tablets)

MECHANISM OF ACTION

An antiulcer agent and gastric acid secretion inhibitor that inhibits histamine action at histamine 2 receptor sites of parietal cells. **Therapeutic Effect:** Inhibits gastric acid secretion during fasting, at night, or when stimulated by food, caffeine, or insulin.

PHARMACOKINETICS

Well absorbed from the GI tract. Protein binding: 15%–20%. Widely distributed. Metabolized in the liver. Primarily excreted in urine. Not removed by hemodialysis. ***Half-life:*** 2 hr; increased with impaired renal function.

AVAILABILITY

Tablets: (Tagamet HB): 200 mg.
Tablets (Tagamet): 300 mg, 400 mg.
Liquid: 300 mg/5 ml.
Liquid (Tagamet HB): 200 mg/20 ml.
Injection: 150 mg/ml.

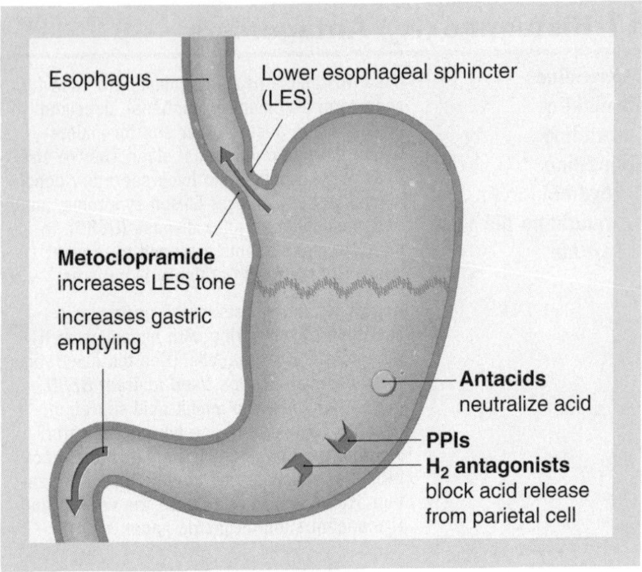

Sites of Action: Drugs Used to Treat GERD

Gastroesophageal reflux disease (GERD) occurs when acidic stomach contents regurgitate into the esophagus, causing heartburn. The disorder may result from a weakness or incompetence of the lower esophageal sphincter (LES). Because the malfunctioning LES makes the reflux leave the esophagus and re-enter the stomach slowly, the esophageal mucosa is exposed to the acid for a long time. Because the enzymatic action of parietal cells in the stomach makes the reflux highly acidic, GERD causes irritation and possible erosion of the esophageal mucosa.

Treatment of GERD can employ drugs from several classes: histamine (H_2) antagonists, proton pump inhibitors (PPIs), the miscellaneous GI agent metoclopramide, and antacids. H_2 antagonists, such as cimetidine, act in parietal cells of the stomach. Normally, H_2-receptor stimulation results in gastric acid secretion. By blocking these receptors, H_2 antagonists decrease the amount and acidity of gastric secretion, including secretion that occurs with fasting, food consumption at night, and abdominal distension.

PPIs, such as esomeprazole, also suppress gastric acid secretion. However, they do it by inhibiting the hydrogen-potassium-adenosine triphosphatase enzyme system, which is located on the surface of parietal cells and controls their gastric acid secretion. PPIs block acid secretion that results from fasting or abdominal distension caused by food ingestion.

Metoclopramide increases the tone and motility of the upper GI tract. It works by stimulating the release of acetylcholine from GI nerve endings, which improves LES tone and leads to decreased reflux. The drug also stimulates gastric emptying, which reduces gastric contents.

Antacids, such as aluminum hydroxide, act primarily in the stomach by chemically combining with the hydrogen ions (H^+) in gastric acid and raising the pH of gastric contents. They don't prevent reflux. However, they make the reflux less acidic, so it causes less damage to the esophageal mucosa.

INDICATIONS AND DOSAGES

▸ **Active ulcer**

PO

Adults, Elderly. 300 mg 4 times a day or 400 mg twice a day or 800 mg at bedtime.

IV, IM

Adults, Elderly. 300 mg q6h or 150 mg as single dose followed by 37.5 mg/hr continuous infusion.

▸ **Prevention of duodenal ulcer**

PO

Adults, Elderly. 400–800 mg at bedtime.

▸ **Gastric hypersecretory secretions**

PO, IV, IM

Adults, Elderly. 300–600 mg q6h. Maximum: 2,400 mg/day.

Children. 20–40 mg/kg/day in divided doses q6h.

Infants. 10–20 mg/kg/day in divided doses q6–12h.

Neonates. 5–10 mg/kg/day in divided doses q8–12h.

▸ **Gastrointestinal reflux disease**

PO

Adults, Elderly. 800 mg twice a day or 400 mg 4 times a day for 12 wk.

▸ **OTC use**

PO

Adults, Elderly. 100 mg up to 30 min before meals. Maximum: 2 doses/day.

▸ **Prevention of upper GI bleeding**

IV Infusion

Adults, Elderly. 50 mg/hr.

▸ **Dosage in renal impairment**

Dosage is based on a 300-mg dose in adults. Dosage interval is modified based on creatinine clearance.

Creatinine Clearance	Dosage Interval
greater than 40 ml/min	q6h
20–40 ml/min	q8h or decrease dose by 25%
less than 20 ml/min	q12h or decrease dose by 50%

Give after hemodialysis and q12h between dialysis sessions.

OFF-LABEL USES

Prevention of aspiration pneumonia; treatment of acute urticaria, chronic warts, upper GI bleeding

CONTRAINDICATIONS

None known.

INTERACTIONS

Drug

Antacids: May decrease the absorption of cimetidine.

Calcium channel blockers, cyclosporine, lidocaine, metoprolol, metronidazole, oral anticoagulants, oral antidiabetics, phenytoin, propranolol, theophylline, tricyclic antidepressants: May decrease the metabolism and increase the blood concentrations of these drugs.

Ketoconazole: May decrease the absorption of ketoconazole.

Herbal

None known.

Food

None known.

DIAGNOSTIC TEST EFFECTS

Interferes with skin tests using allergen extracts. May increase prolactin, serum creatinine, and transaminase levels. May decrease parathyroid hormone concentration.

IV INCOMPATIBILITIES

Allopurinol (Aloprim), amphotericin B complex (AmBisome, Amphotec, Abelcet), cefepime (Maxipime)

IV COMPATIBILITIES

Aminophylline, diltiazem (Cardizem), furosemide (Lasix), heparin, hydromorphone (Dilaudid), insulin (regular), lidocaine, lorazepam (Ativan), midazolam (Versed), morphine, potassium chloride, propofol (Diprivan)

SIDE EFFECTS

Occasional (4%–2%)
Headache
Elderly and severely ill patients, patients with impaired renal function: Confusion, agitation, psychosis, depression, anxiety, disorientation, hallucinations. Effects reverse 3 to 4 days after discontinuance.
Rare (less than 2%)
Diarrhea, dizziness, somnolence, nausea, vomiting, gynecomastia, rash, impotence

SERIOUS REACTIONS

! Rapid IV administration may produce cardiac arrhythmias and hypotension.

NURSING CONSIDERATIONS

Baseline Assessment

- Assess the patient for the presence of abdominal pain and occult or frank blood in stool, gastric aspirate, or emesis.

Lifespan Considerations

- Cimetidine crosses the placenta and is distributed in breast milk.
- Cimetidine use in infants cimetidine use may suppress gastric acidity, inhibit drug metabolism, and produce CNS stimulation.
- Long-term use in children may induce cerebral toxicity and affect the hormonal system.
- The elderly are more likely to experience confusion, especially those with impaired renal function.

Precautions

- Use cimetidine cautiously in elderly patients and in those with impaired hepatic and renal function.

Administration and Handling

PO
- Give cimetidine without regard to meals; however, it is best given with meals and at bedtime.
- Do not administer within 1 hour of antacids. Give at least 2 hours after ketoconazole administration.

IV
- Store at room temperature.
- Reconstituted IV solution is stable for 48 hours at room temperature.
- Dilute each 300 mg (2 ml) with 18 ml 0.9% NaCl, 0.45% NaCl, 0.2% NaCl, D_5W, $D_{10}W$, Ringer's solution, or lactated Ringer's solution to a total volume of 20 ml.
- For IV push, administer over not less than 2 minutes to prevent arrhythmias and hypotension.
- For intermittent IV (piggyback) administration, infuse over 15 to 20 minutes.
- For IV infusion, dilute with 100 to 1,000 ml 0.9% NaCl, D_5W, or other compatible solution, and infuse over 24 hours.

IM
- Administer undiluted.
- Inject deep into large muscle mass, such as the gluteus maximus muscle.

Intervention and Evaluation

- Monitor the patient's BP for hypotension during IV infusion.
- Assess the patient for GI bleeding manifested by blood in stool and hematemesis.
- Check the mental status in elderly and severely ill patients and in those with impaired renal function.

Patient Teaching

- Warn the patient that IM administration may produce transient discomfort at the injection site.
- Instruct the patient not to take antacids within 1 hour of oral cimetidine administration.
- Warn the patient to avoid tasks that require mental alertness or motor

skills until his or her response to the drug has been established.
- Urge the patient to avoid smoking.
- Caution the patient to notify the physician if he or she experiences blood in emesis or stool, or dark, tarry stool.
- Urge the patient to avoid alcohol and aspirin, both of which may cause GI distress, during cimetidine therapy.

famotidine

fam-**o**-tah-deen
(Amfamox [AUS], Novo-Famotidine[CAN] Pepcid, Pepcid AC, Pepcidine[AUS], Ulcidine[CAN])

CATEGORY AND SCHEDULE

Pregnancy Risk Category: B
OTC (10 mg tablets)

MECHANISM OF ACTION

An antiulcer agent and gastric acid secretion inhibitor that inhibits histamine action at histamine 2 receptors of parietal cells. **Therapeutic Effect:** Inhibits gastric acid secretion when fasting, at night, or when stimulated by food, caffeine, or insulin.

PHARMACOKINETICS

Route	Onset	Peak	Duration
PO	1 hr	1–4 hr	10–12 hr
IV	1 hr	0.5–3 hr	10–12 hr

Rapidly, incompletely absorbed from the GI tract. Protein binding: 15%–20%. Partially metabolized in the liver. Primarily excreted in urine. Not removed by hemodialysis. ***Half-life:*** 2.5–3.5 hr (increased with impaired renal function).

AVAILABILITY

Oral Suspension (Pepcid): 40 mg/5 ml.
Tablets (Pepcid): 20 mg, 40 mg.
Tablets (Pepcid AC): 10 mg, 20 mg.
Tablets (Chewable [Pepcid AC]): 10 mg.
Capsules (Pepcid AC): 10 mg.
Injection (Pepcid): 10 mg/ml.

INDICATIONS AND DOSAGES

▸ **Acute treatment of duodenal and gastric ulcers**
PO
Adults, Elderly, Children 12 yr and older. 40 mg/day at bedtime.
Children 1–11 yr. 0.5 mg/kg/day at bedtime. Maximum: 40 mg/day.

▸ **Duodenal ulcer maintenance**
PO
Adults, Elderly. 20 mg/day at bedtime.

▸ **Gastroesophageal reflux disease**
PO
Adults, Elderly, Children 12 yr and older. 20 mg twice a day.
Children 1–11 yr. 1 mg/kg/day in 2 divided doses.
Children 3 mo to 11 mo. 0.5 mg/kg/dose twice a day.
Children younger than 3 mo. 0.5 mg/kg/dose once a day.

▸ **Esophagitis**
PO
Adults, Elderly, Children 12 yr and older. 2-40 mg twice a day.

▸ **Hypersecretory conditions**
PO
Adults, Elderly, Children 12 yr and older. Initially, 20 mg q6h. May increase up to 160 mg q6h.

▸ **Acid indigestion, heartburn (OTC)**
PO
Adults, Elderly, Children 12 yr and older. 10–20 mg 15–60 min before eating. Maximum: 2 doses per day.

Usual Parenteral Dosage
IV
Adults, Elderly, Children 12 yr and older. 20 mg q12h.
Dosage in renal impairment
Dosing frequency is modified based on creatinine clearance.

Creatinine Clearance	Dosing Frequency
10–50 ml/min	q24h
less than 10 ml/min	q36–48h

OFF-LABEL USES
Autism, prevention of aspiration pneumonitis

CONTRAINDICATIONS
None known.

INTERACTIONS
Drug
Antacids: May decrease the absorption of famotidine.
Ketoconazole: May decrease the absorption of ketoconazole.
Herbal
None known.
Food
None known.

DIAGNOSTIC TEST EFFECTS
Interferes with skin tests using allergen extracts. May increase liver enzyme levels.

IV INCOMPATIBILITIES
Amphotericin B complex (Abelcet, Amphotec, AmBisome), cefepime (Maxipime), furosemide (Lasix), piperacillin/tazobactam (Zosyn)

IV COMPATIBILITIES
Calcium gluconate, dobutamine (Dobutrex), dopamine (Intropin), heparin, hydromorphone (Dilaudid), insulin (regular), lidocaine, lorazepam (Ativan), magnesium sulfate, midazolam (Versed), morphine, nitroglycerin, norepinephrine (Levophed), potassium chloride, potassium phosphate, propofol (Diprivan)

SIDE EFFECTS
Occasional (5%)
Headache
Rare (2% or less)
Constipation, diarrhea, dizziness

SERIOUS REACTIONS
! None known.

NURSING CONSIDERATIONS
Baseline Assessment
- Assess patient for the presence of abdominal pain and occult or frank blood in stool, gastric aspirate, or emesis.

Lifespan Considerations
- It is unknown if famotidine crosses the placenta or is distributed in breast milk.
- No age-related precautions have been noted in children.
- The elderly are more likely to experience confusion, especially those with impaired hepatic or renal function.

Precautions
- Use famotidine cautiously in patients with impaired hepatic or renal function.

Administration and Handling
PO
- Store tablets and suspension at room temperature.
- After reconstitution, oral suspension is stable for 30 days at room temperature.
- Shake suspension well before use.
- Give famotidine without regard to meals; however it's best given after meals or at bedtime.
- Do not administer within 30 minutes to 1 hour of antacids. Give at

least 2 hours after ketoconazole administration.

IV

- Refrigerate unreconstituted vials.
- IV solution normally appears clear and is colorless.
- After dilution, IV solution is stable for 48 hours at room temperature.
- For IV push, dilute 20 mg with 5 to 10 ml 0.9% NaCl, D_5W, $D_{10}W$, lactated Ringer's solution, or 5% sodium bicarbonate. Give push over 2 minutes.
- For intermittent IV piggyback infusion, dilute with 50 to 100 ml D_5W, or 0.9% NaCl. Administer over 15 to 30 minutes.

Intervention and Evaluation

- Monitor the patient's pattern of bowel activity and stool consistency.
- Assess the patient for constipation, diarrhea, and headache.

Patient Teaching

- Tell the patient that he or she may take famotidine without regard to meals but that it's best taken after meals or at bedtime.
- Warn the patient to notify the physician if headache occurs.
- Urge the patient to avoid alcohol, aspirin, and coffee, all of which may cause GI distress, during famotidine therapy.
- Instruct the patient to contact the physician if persistent acid indigestion, heartburn, or sour stomach persists despite the medication.

nizatidine

ni-**za**-ti-deen

(Axid, Axid AR, Tazac[AUS])

CATEGORY AND SCHEDULE

Pregnancy Risk Category: B

OTC (75 mg capsules)

MECHANISM OF ACTION

An antiulcer agent and gastric acid secretion inhibitor that inhibits histamine action at histamine 2 receptors of parietal cells. **Therapeutic Effect:** Inhibits basal and nocturnal gastric acid secretion.

PHARMACOKINETICS

Rapidly, well absorbed from the GI tract. Protein binding: 35%. Metabolized in the liver. Primarily excreted in urine. Not removed by hemodialysis. ***Half-life:*** 1–2 hr (increased with impaired renal function).

AVAILABILITY

Capsules: 75 mg, 150 mg, 300 mg.
Oral Solution.

INDICATIONS AND DOSAGES

▸ **Active duodenal ulcer**

PO

Adults, Elderly. 300 mg at bedtime or 150 mg twice a day.

▸ **Prevention of duodenal ulcer recurrence**

PO

Adults, Elderly. 150 mg at bedtime.

▸ **Gastroesophageal reflux disease**

PO

Adults, Elderly. 150 mg twice a day.

▸ **Active benign gastric ulcer**

PO

Adults, Elderly. 150 mg twice a day or 300 mg at bedtime.

▸ **Dyspepsia**

PO

Adults, Elderly. 75 mg 30–60 min before meals; no more than 2 tablets a day.

▸ **Dosage in renal impairment**

Dosage adjustment is based on creatinine clearance.

Creatinine Clearance	Active Ulcer	Maintenance Therapy
20–50 ml/min	150 mg at bedtime	150 mg every other day
less than 20 ml/min	150 mg every other day	150 mg q3 days

OFF-LABEL USES
Gastric hypersecretory conditions, multiple endocrine adenoma, Zollinger-Ellison syndrome, weight gain reduction in patients taking Zyprexa

CONTRAINDICATIONS
None known.

INTERACTIONS
Drug
Antacids: May decrease the absorption of nizatidine.
Ketoconazole: May decrease the absorption of ketoconazole.
Herbal
None known.
Food
None known.

DIAGNOSTIC TEST EFFECTS
Interferes with skin tests using allergen extracts. May increase serum alkaline phosphatase, AST (SGOT), and ALT (SGPT) levels.

SIDE EFFECTS
Occasional (2%)
Somnolence, fatigue
Rare (1%)
Diaphoresis, rash

SERIOUS REACTIONS
! Asymptomatic ventricular tachycardia, hyperuricemia not associated with gout, and nephrolithiasis occur rarely.

NURSING CONSIDERATIONS
Baseline Assessment
• Expect to obtain blood chemistry laboratory test results, including BUN, serum alkaline phosphatase, bilirubin, creatinine, AST (SGOT), and ALT (SGPT) levels to assess hepatic and renal function.
Lifespan Considerations
• It is unknown if nizatidine crosses the placenta or is distributed in breast milk.
• The safety and efficacy of nizatidine have not been established in children younger than 16 years of age.
• No age-related precautions have been noted in the elderly.
Precautions
• Use nizatidine cautiously in patients with hepatic or renal impairment.
Administration and Handling
PO
• Give nizatidine without regard to meals; however, it's best given after meals or at bedtime.
• Give right before eating for heartburn prevention.
• Do not administer within 1 hour of magnesium- or aluminum-containing antacids because it can decrease the absorption of nizatidine.
Intervention and Evaluation
• Assess the patient for abdominal pain and GI bleeding. Observe for overt blood in emesis or stool and for tarry stools.
• Monitor the patient's serum alkaline phosphatase, bilirubin, AST (SGOT), and ALT (SGPT) levels.
Patient Teaching
• Warn the patient to avoid tasks that require mental alertness or motor skills until his or her response to the drug has been established.
• Urge the patient to avoid alcohol,

aspirin, and smoking during nizatidine therapy.
• Instruct the patient to notify the physician if acid indigestion, gastric distress, or heartburn occur after 2 weeks of continuous nizatidine therapy.

ranitidine hydrochloride

ra-**ni**-ti-deen
(Apo-Ranitidine[CAN], Ausran[AUS], Novo-Ranidine[CAN], Rani-2[AUS], Ranihexal[AUS], Zantac, Zantac-75, Zantac EFFERdose)
Do not confuse Zantac with Xanax, Ziac, or Zyrtec.

ranitidine bismuth citrate

(Pylorid[AUS], Tritec)

CATEGORY AND SCHEDULE

Pregnancy Risk Category: B
OTC (Tablets, 75 mg)

MECHANISM OF ACTION

An antiulcer agent that inhibits histamine action at histamine 2 receptors of gastric parietal cells. **Therapeutic Effect:** Inhibits gastric acid secretion when fasting, at night, or when stimulated by food, caffeine, or insulin. Reduces volume and hydrogen ion concentration of gastric juice.

PHARMACOKINETICS

Rapidly absorbed from the GI tract. Protein binding: 15%. Widely distributed. Metabolized in the liver. Primarily excreted in urine. Not removed by hemodialysis. ***Half-life:*** PO, 2.5 hr; IV, 2–2.5 hr (increased with impaired renal function).

AVAILABILITY

Tablets (Effervescent [Zantac EFFERdose]): 25 mg, 150 mg.
Capsules: 150 mg, 300 mg.
Granules (Zantac EFFERdose): 150 mg.
Syrup (Zantac): 15 mg/ml.
Tablets (Zantac 75): 75 mg.
Tablets (Zantac): 150 mg, 300 mg.
Injection (Zantac): 25 mg/ml.

INDICATIONS AND DOSAGES

▸ **Duodenal ulcers, gastric ulcers, gastroesophageal reflux disease**
PO
Adults, Elderly. 150 mg twice a day or 300 mg at bedtime. Maintenance: 150 mg at bedtime.
Children. 2–4 mg/kg/day in divided doses twice a day. Maximum: 300 mg/day.
▸ **Erosive esophagitis**
PO
Adults, Elderly. 150 mg 4 times a day. Maintenance: 150 mg 2 times/day or 300 mg at bedtime.
Children. 4–10 mg/kg/day in 2 divided doses. Maximum: 600 mg/day.
▸ **Hypersecretory conditions**
PO
Adults, Elderly. 150 mg twice a day. May increase up to 6 g/day.
▸ **Usual parenteral dosage**
IV, IM
Adults, Elderly. 50 mg/dose q6–8h. Maximum: 400 mg/day.
Children. 2–4 mg/kg/day in divided doses q6–8h. Maximum: 200 mg/day.
▸ **Usual neonatal dosage**
PO
Neonates. 2 mg/kg/day in divided doses q12h.
IV
Neonates. Initially, 1.5 mg/kg/dose; then 1.5–2 mg/kg/day in divided doses q12h.

Dosage in renal impairment

For patients with creatinine clearance less than 50 ml/min, give 150 mg PO q24h or 50 mg IV or IM q18–24h.

OFF-LABEL USES

Prevention of aspiration pneumonia

CONTRAINDICATIONS

History of acute porphyria

INTERACTIONS

Drug

Antacids: May decrease the absorption of ranitidine.
Ketoconazole: May decrease the absorption of ketoconazole.

Herbal

None known.

Food

None known.

DIAGNOSTIC TEST EFFECTS

Interferes with skin tests using allergen extracts. May increase hepatic function enzyme, gamma-glutamyl transpeptidase, and serum creatinine levels.

IV INCOMPATIBILITIES

Amphotericin B complex (Abelcet, AmBisome, Amphotec)

IV COMPATIBILITIES

Diltiazem (Cardizem), dobutamine (Dobutrex), dopamine (Intropin), heparin, hydromorphone (Dilaudid), insulin, lidocaine, lorazepam (Ativan), morphine, norepinephrine (Levophed), potassium chloride, propofol (Diprivan)

SIDE EFFECTS

Occasional (2%)
Diarrhea
Rare (1%)
Constipation, headache (may be severe)

SERIOUS REACTIONS

! Reversible hepatitis and blood dyscrasias occur rarely.

NURSING CONSIDERATIONS

Baseline Assessment

- Expect to obtain blood chemistry test results including BUN, serum alkaline phosphatase, bilirubin, creatinine, AST (SGOT), and ALT (SGPT) levels to assess hepatic and renal function.

Lifespan Considerations

- It is unknown if ranitidine crosses the placenta or is distributed in breast milk.
- No age-related precautions have been noted in children.
- The elderly are more likely to experience confusion, especially those with hepatic or renal impairment.

Precautions

- Use ranitidine cautiously in elderly patients and those with impaired hepatic and renal function.

Administration and Handling

PO

- Give ranitidine without regard to meals; however it's best given after meals or at bedtime.
- Do not administer within 1 hour of magnesium- or aluminum-containing antacids because they decrease ranitidine absorption by 33%.
- Give 2 hours after ketoconazole administration.

IV

- IV solutions normally appear clear and are colorless to yellow; slight darkening does not affect potency.
- IV infusion (piggyback) is stable for 48 hours at room temperature. Discard if discolored or precipitate forms.
- For IV push, dilute each 50 mg with 20 ml 0.9% NaCl or D_5W.
- For intermittent IV infusion (pig-

gyback), dilute each 50 mg with 50 ml 0.9% NaCl or D_5W.
- For IV infusion, dilute with 250 to 1,000 ml 0.9% NaCl or D_5W.
- Administer IV push over minimum of 5 minutes to prevent arrhythmias and hypotension.
- Infuse IV piggyback over 15 to 20 minutes.
- Infuse IV infusion over 24 hours.

IM
- May be given undiluted.
- Give deep IM into large muscle mass, such as the gluteus maximus.

Intervention and Evaluation
- Monitor the patient's serum alkaline phosphatase, bilirubin, AST and ALT levels.
- Assess the elderly patient's mental status.

Patient Teaching
- Tell the patient that smoking decreases the effectiveness of ranitidine.
- Instruct the patient not to take ranitidine within 1 hour of magnesium- or aluminum-containing antacids.
- Warn the patient that transient burning or itching may occur with IV administration.
- Instruct the patient to notify the physician if headache occurs during ranitidine therapy.
- Urge the patient to avoid alcohol and aspirin, both of which may cause GI distress, during ranitidine therapy.

52 Laxatives

bisacodyl
cascara sagrada
docusate
lactulose
magnesium chloride, magnesium citrate, magnesium hydroxide, magnesium oxide, magnesium protein complex, magnesium sulfate
methylcellulose
polycarbophil
polyethylene glycol-electrolyte solution (PEG-ES)
psyllium
senna

Uses: Laxatives are used for short-term treatment of constipation and for colon evacuation before rectal or bowel examinations. They're also used to prevent straining, such as after anorectal surgery or MI; to prevent fecal impaction; and to reduce painful elimination, such as in patients with recent episiotomy, hemorrhoids, or anorectal lesions. In addition, these agents are helpful in modifying ileostomy effluent and in removing ingested poisons.

Action: Laxatives ease or stimulate defecation by three basic mechanisms. They attract and retain fluid in the colonic contents through their hydrophilic or osmotic properties. They act directly or indirectly on the mucosa to decrease water and sodium absorption. Or they increase intestinal motility and decrease water and sodium absorption. (See the illustration *Mechanisms of Action: Laxatives,* page 992.)

—*Bulk-forming laxatives,* such as psyllium and polycarbophil, act primarily in the small and large intestines. They retain water in stool and may bind with water and ions in the colonic lumen to soften feces and increase stool bulk. They may also increase colonic bacteria growth, which increases fecal mass. Typically, they produce soft stool in 1 to 3 days.

—*Osmotic laxatives,* including lactulose, act in the colon like saline laxatives. Their osmotic action may be enhanced in the distal ileum and colon by bacterial metabolism to lactate and other organic acids. This decreases the pH and increases the osmotic pressure, which in turn increases the stool water content and softens the stool. They produce soft stool in 1 to 3 days.

—*Stimulant laxatives,* such as bisacodyl and senna, act in the colon. They enhance water and electrolyte accumulation in the colonic lumen, which enhances intestinal motility, and may also act directly on the intestinal mucosa. Most of them produce semifluid stool in 6 to 12 hours. However, bisacodyl suppositories act in 15 to 60 minutes.

—*Surfactant laxatives,* such as docusate, act in the small and large intestines. By their surfactant action, they hydrate and soften stool, helping fat and water penetrate it. They produce soft stool in 1 to 3 days.

COMBINATION PRODUCTS

FERRO-SEQUELS: docusate/ferrous fumarate (a hematinic) 100 mg/150 mg.
GELUSIL: magnesium hydroxide/aluminum hydroxide (an antacid)/simethicone (an antiflatulent) 200 mg/200 mg/25 mg.
GENTLAX-S: senna/docusate (a laxative) 8.6 mg/50 mg.
HALEY'S MO: magnesium/mineral oil (a lubricant laxative) 300 mg/1.25 ml.
PEPCID COMPLETE: magnesium hydroxide/famotidine (a histamine [H_2] antagonist)/calcium chloride (an antacid) 165 mg/10 mg/800 mg.
SENOKOT-S: senna/docusate (a laxative) 8.6 mg/50 mg.

bisacodyl

bis-a-**koe**-dill
(Alophen, Apo-Bisacodyl[CAN], Bisalax[AUS], Dulcolax, Femilax, Gentlax, Modane, Veracolate)
Do not confuse Veracolate with Accolate, or Modane with Mudrane.

CATEGORY AND SCHEDULE

Pregnancy Risk Category: C
OTC

MECHANISM OF ACTION

A GI stimulant that has a direct effect on colonic smooth musculature by stimulating the intramural nerve plexi. **Therapeutic Effect:** Promotes fluid and ion accumulation in the colon increasing peristalsis and producing a laxative effect.

PHARMACOKINETICS

Route	Onset	Peak	Duration
PO	6–12 hr	N/A	N/A
Rectal	15–60 min	N/A	N/A

Minimal absorption following oral and rectal administration. Absorbed drug is excreted in urine; remainder is eliminated in feces.

AVAILABILITY

Tablets (Enteric-Coated): 5 mg.
Suppositories: 10 mg.

INDICATIONS AND DOSAGES

▸ **Treatment of constipation**
PO
Adults, Children older than 12 yr. 5–15 mg as needed. Maximum: 30 mg.
Children 3–12 yr. 5–10 mg or 0.3 mg/kg at bedtime or after breakfast.
Elderly. Initially, 5 mg/day.
Rectal
Adults, Children 12 yr and older. 10 mg to induce bowel movement.
Children 2–11 yr. 5–10 mg as a single dose.
Children younger than 2 yr. 5 mg.
Elderly. 5–10 mg/day.

CONTRAINDICATIONS

Abdominal pain, appendicitis, intes-

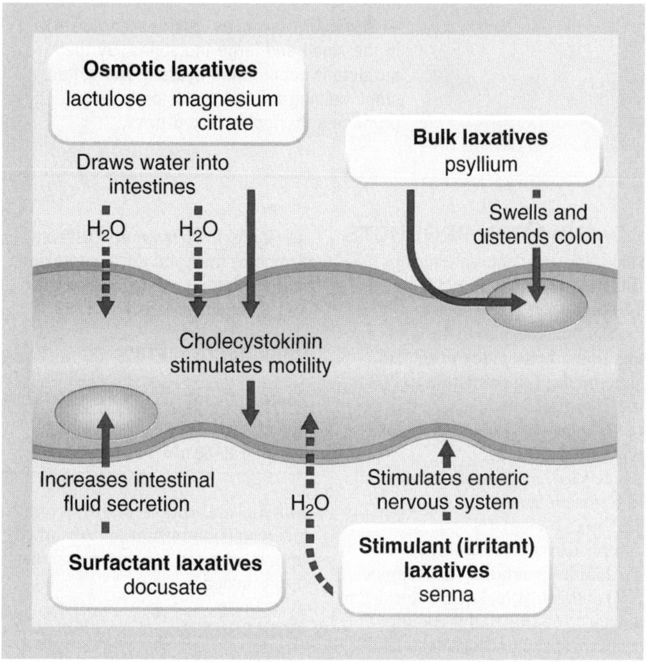

Mechanisms of Action: Laxatives

Laxatives ease or stimulate defecation. Typically, they're classified by their mechanism of action as bulk-forming, osmotic, stimulant, or surfactant laxatives.

Bulk-forming laxatives, such as psyllium, act in the small and large bowel. Because ingredients in these laxatives are undigestible, they remain within the stool and increase the fecal mass by drawing in water. These agents also enhance bacterial growth in the colon, further adding to the fecal mass.

Osmotic laxatives, such as lactulose, draw water into the intestinal lumen, causing the fecal mass to soften and swell. This osmotic action may be enhanced by the metabolism of colonic bacteria to lactate and other organic acids. These acids decrease colonic pH and increase colonic motility.

Stimulant (or irritant) laxatives, such as senna, act on the intestinal wall to increase water and electrolytes in the intestinal lumen. In addition, they directly irritate the colon, increasing motility.

Surfactant laxatives (or fecal softeners), such as docusate, reduce the surface tension of the stool, allowing water to enter it. These laxatives may also help to increase water and electrolyte excretion into the intestinal lumen, softening and increasing the fecal mass.

tinal obstruction, nausea, undiagnosed rectal bleeding, vomiting

INTERACTIONS

Drug

Antacids, cimetidine, famotidine, ranitidine: May cause rapid dissolution of bisacodyl, producing abdominal cramping, and vomiting.
Oral medications: May decrease transit time of concurrently administered oral medications, decreasing absorption of bisacodyl.

Herbal

None known.

Food

Milk: May cause rapid dissolution of bisacodyl.

DIAGNOSTIC TEST EFFECTS

None known.

SIDE EFFECTS

Frequent

Some degree of abdominal discomfort, nausea, mild cramps, faintness

Occasional

Rectal administration: burning of rectal mucosa, mild proctitis

SERIOUS REACTIONS

! Long-term use may result in laxative dependence, chronic constipation, and loss of normal bowel function.
! Prolonged use or overdose may result in electrolyte or metabolic disturbances (such as hypokalemia, hypocalcemia, and metabolic acidosis or alkalosis), as well as persistent diarrhea, vomiting, muscle weakness, malabsorption, and weight loss.

NURSING CONSIDERATIONS

Baseline Assessment

- Before bisacodyl administration, assess the patient's abdomen for signs of tenderness, rigidity, and the presence of bowel sounds.
- Try to determine when the patient last had a bowel movement, and find out the amount and consistency.

Lifespan Considerations

- It is unknown if bisacodyl crosses the placenta or is distributed in breast milk.
- Avoid bisacodyl use in children younger than 6 years of age because this patient population is usually unable to describe symptoms or more severe side effects.
- Repeated use of bisacodyl in the elderly may cause orthostatic hypotension and weakness due to electrolyte loss.

Precautions

- Excessive use of bisacodyl may lead to fluid and electrolyte imbalance.

Administration and Handling

PO

- Give bisacodyl on an empty stomach for faster action.
- Offer 6 to 8 glasses of water a day to aid in stool softening.
- Administer tablets whole; make sure the patient does not chew or crush them.
- Avoid giving within 1 hour of antacids, milk, or other oral medications.

Rectal

- If suppository is too soft, chill for 30 minutes in refrigerator or run cold water over foil wrapper.
- Moisten suppository with cold water before inserting deep into rectum.

Intervention and Evaluation

- Encourage the patient to maintain adequate fluid intake.
- Assess the patient's bowel sounds for peristalsis.
- Assess the patient's pattern of daily bowel activity and stool consistency and record time of evacuation.

- Monitor the patient for abdominal disturbances.
- Monitor serum electrolyte levels in patients with excessive, frequent, or prolonged use of bisacodyl.

Patient Teaching

- Tell the patient to institute measures to promote defecation, such as increasing his or her fluid intake, exercising, and eating a high-fiber diet.
- Instruct the patient not to take antacids, milk, or other medications within 1 hour of taking bisacodyl because these substances may decrease the effectiveness of bisacodyl.
- Warn the patient to notify the physician if unrelieved constipation, dizziness, muscle cramps or pain, rectal bleeding, or weakness occurs.

cascara sagrada

cass-**care**-ah sah-**graud**-ah
(Cascara Sagrada)

CATEGORY AND SCHEDULE

Pregnancy Risk Category: C

MECHANISM OF ACTION

A GI stimulant that has a direct effect on colonic smooth musculature, by stimulating intramural nerve plexi. **Therapeutic Effect:** Promotes fluid and ion accumulation in the colon, increasing peristalsis and promoting a laxative effect.

AVAILABILITY

Liquid: (18% alcohol) 1 g/ml.

INDICATIONS AND DOSAGES

▸ Treatment of constipation

PO

Adults, Elderly. 5 ml at bedtime.
Children 2–11 yr. 2.5 ml, 1–3 ml as a single dose.
Infants. 1.25 ml, 0.5–2 ml as a single dose.

CONTRAINDICATIONS

Abdominal pain, appendicitis, intestinal obstruction, nausea, vomiting

INTERACTIONS

Drug

Oral medications: May decrease transit time of concurrently administered oral medications, decreasing the absorption of cascara sagrada.

Herbal

None known.

Food

None known.

DIAGNOSTIC TEST EFFECTS

May increase blood glucose level. May decrease serum calcium and potassium levels.

SIDE EFFECTS

Frequent

Pink-red, red-violet, red-brown, or yellow-brown discoloration of urine

Occasional

Some degree of abdominal discomfort, nausea, mild cramps, faintness

SERIOUS REACTIONS

! Long-term use may result in laxative dependence, chronic constipation, and loss of normal bowel function.

! Prolonged use or overdose may result in electrolyte or metabolic disturbances (such as hypokalemia, hypocalcemia, and metabolic acidosis or alkalosis), as well as persistent diarrhea, vomiting, muscle weakness, malabsorption, and weight loss.

NURSING CONSIDERATIONS

Baseline Assessment

- Before cascara sagrada administra-

tion, assess the patient's abdomen for signs of tenderness, rigidity, and the presence of bowel sounds.
• Try to determine when the patient last had a bowel movement, and find out the amount and consistency.

Lifespan Considerations
• Because cascara sagrada is a strong stimulant, use cautiously in pregnant patients.

Precautions
• Excessive use of cascara sagrada may lead to fluid and electrolyte imbalance.

Administration and Handling
PO
• Give cascara sagrada on an empty stomach for faster action.
• Avoid giving within 1 hour of antacids, milk, or other oral medications.

Intervention and Evaluation
• Encourage the patient to maintain adequate fluid intake.
• Assess the patient's bowel sounds for peristalsis.
• Assess the patient's pattern of daily bowel activity and stool consistency and record time of evacuation.
• Monitor the patient for abdominal disturbances.
• Monitor serum electrolyte levels in patients with excessive, frequent, or prolonged use of cascara sagrada.

Patient Teaching
• Explain to the patient that his or her urine may temporarily turn pink-red, red-violet, red-brown, or yellow-brown.
• Tell the patient to institute measures to promote defecation, such as increasing his or her fluid intake, exercising, and eating a high-fiber diet.
• Instruct the patient not to take other oral medications within 1 hour of taking cascara sagrada because these substances may decrease the effectiveness of cascara sagrada.
• Warn the patient not to use cascara sagrada if abdominal pain, nausea, or vomiting lasting longer than 1 week occurs.
• Tell the patient that the liquid form contains alcohol.

docusate

dok-yoo-sate
(Apo-Docusate[CAN], Colace, Colax-C[CAN], Coloxyl[AUS], Diocto, Docusoft-S, Novo-Ducosate[CAN], PMS-Docusate[CAN], Pro-Cal-Sof, Regulex[CAN], Selax[CAN], Soflax[CAN], Surfak)

CATEGORY AND SCHEDULE
Pregnancy Risk Category: C
OTC

MECHANISM OF ACTION
A bulk-producing laxative that decreases surface film tension by mixing liquid and bowel contents. **Therapeutic Effect:** Increases infiltration of liquid to form a softer stool.

PHARMACOKINETICS
Minimal absorption from the GI tract. Acts in small and large intestines. Results usually occur 1–2 days after first dose, but may take 3–5 days.

AVAILABILITY
Capsules (Colace): 50 mg, 100 mg.
Capsules (Docusoft-S): 100 mg.
Capsules (Surfak): 240 mg.
Liquid (Colace): 50 mg/5 ml (sodium).
Syrup (Colace, Diocto): 60 mg/15 ml.

INDICATIONS AND DOSAGES

▸ **Stool softener**

PO

Adults, Elderly, Children 12 yr and older. 50–500 mg/day in 1–4 divided doses.
Children 6–11 yr. 40–150 mg/day in 1–4 divided doses.
Children 3–5 yr. 20–60 mg/day in 1–4 divided doses.
Children younger than 3 yr. 10–40 mg in 1–4 divided doses.

CONTRAINDICATIONS

Acute abdominal pain, concomitant use of mineral oil, intestinal obstruction, nausea, vomiting

INTERACTIONS

Drug

Danthron, mineral oil: May increase the absorption of danthron or mineral oil.

Herbal

None known.

Food

None known.

DIAGNOSTIC TEST EFFECTS

None known.

SIDE EFFECTS

Occasional

Mild GI cramping, throat irritation (with liquid preparation)

Rare

Rash

SERIOUS REACTIONS

! None known.

NURSING CONSIDERATIONS

Baseline Assessment

- Before docusate administration, assess the patient's abdomen for signs of tenderness, rigidity, and the presence of bowel sounds.
- Try to determine when the patient last had a bowel movement, and find out the amount and consistency.

Lifespan Considerations

- It is unknown if docusate is distributed in breast milk.
- Docusate use is not recommended in children younger than 6 years of age.
- No age-related precautions have been noted in the elderly.

Administration and Handling

PO

- Have the patient drink 6 to 8 glasses of water a day to aid in stool softening.
- Give each dose with full glass of water or fruit juice.
- Administer docusate liquid with infant formula, fruit juice, or milk to mask the bitter taste.

Intervention and Evaluation

- Encourage the patient to maintain adequate fluid intake.
- Assess the patient's bowel sounds for peristalsis.
- Assess the patient's pattern of daily bowel activity and stool consistency and record time of evacuation.
- Monitor the patient for abdominal disturbances.

Patient Teaching

- Advise the patient to institute measures to promote defecation, such as increasing his or her fluid intake, exercising, and eating a high-fiber diet.
- Warn the patient to notify the physician if unrelieved constipation, dizziness, muscle cramps or pain, rectal bleeding, or weakness occurs.

lactulose

lak-tyoo-lose
(Acilac[CAN], Actilax[AUS], Cholac, Constilac, Constulose, Duphalac[CAN], Enulose, Generlac, Genlac[AUS], Kristalose, Laxilose[CAN])
Do not confuse Cholac with diclofenac, or lactulose with lactose.

CATEGORY AND SCHEDULE
Pregnancy Risk Category: B

MECHANISM OF ACTION
A lactose derivative that retains ammonia in colon and decreases serum ammonia concentration, producing osmotic effect. **Therapeutic Effect:** Promotes increased peristalsis and bowel evacuation, which expels ammonia from the colon.

PHARMACOKINETICS

Route	Onset	Peak	Duration
PO	24–48 hr	N/A	N/A
Rectal	30–60 min	N/A	N/A

Poorly absorbed from the GI tract. Acts in the colon. Primarily excreted in feces.

AVAILABILITY
Syrup: 10 g/15 ml.
Packets: 10 g, 20 g.

INDICATIONS AND DOSAGES
▸ Constipation
PO
Adults, Elderly. 15–30 ml (10-20 g)/day, up to 60 ml (40 g)/day.
Children. 7.5 ml (5 g)/day after breakfast.

▸ Portal-systemic encephalopathy
PO
Adults, Elderly. Initially, 30–45 ml every hr. Then, 30–45 ml (20-30 g) 3–4 times a day. Adjust dose q1–2 days to produce 2–3 soft stools a day.
Children. 40–90 ml/day in divided doses.
Infants. 2.5–10 ml/day in divided doses.
Rectal (as retention enema)
Adults, Elderly, 300 ml with 700 ml water or saline solution; patient should retain 30–60 min. Repeat q4–6h. If evacuation occurs too promptly, repeat immediately.

CONTRAINDICATIONS
Abdominal pain, appendicitis, nausea, patients on a galactose-free diet, vomiting

INTERACTIONS
Drug
Oral medication: May decrease transit time of concurrently administered oral medications, decreasing lactulose absorption.
Herbal
None known.
Food
None known.

DIAGNOSTIC TEST EFFECTS
May decrease serum potassium level.

SIDE EFFECTS
Occasional
Abdominal cramping, flatulence, increased thirst, abdominal discomfort
Rare
Nausea, vomiting

SERIOUS REACTIONS
! Diarrhea indicates overdose.
! Long-term use may result in laxative dependence, chronic

constipation, and loss of normal bowel function.

NURSING CONSIDERATIONS

Baseline Assessment

- Before lactulose administration, assess the patient's abdomen for signs of tenderness, rigidity, and the presence of bowel sounds.
- Try to determine when the patient last had a bowel movement, and find out the amount and consistency.
- Plan to obtain the patient's serum ammonia levels.
- Assess the patient's mental status, and look for signs and symptoms of a high ammonia level, such as asterixis.

Lifespan Considerations

- It is unknown if lactulose crosses the placenta or is distributed in breast milk.
- Lactulose use should be avoided in children younger than 6 years of age because this patient population is usually unable to describe symptoms.
- No age-related precautions have been noted in the elderly.

Precautions

- Use lactulose cautiously in patients with diabetes mellitus.

Administration and Handling

PO

- Store solution at room temperature.
- Solution normally appears pale yellow to yellow in color and viscous in consistency. However, cloudy, darkened solution does not indicate potency loss.
- Have patient drink juice, milk, or water with each dose to aid in stool softening and increase palatability.

Rectal

- Lubricate anus with petroleum jelly before applicator insertion.
- Insert applicator carefully, to prevent damage to the rectal wall, with nozzle toward navel.
- Squeeze container until entire dose has been expelled.
- Have patient retain liquid until definite lower abdominal cramping is felt.

Intervention and Evaluation

- Encourage the patient to maintain adequate fluid intake.
- Assess the patient's bowel sounds for peristalsis.
- Assess the patient's pattern of daily bowel activity and stool consistency and record time of evacuation.
- Monitor the patient for abdominal disturbances.
- Monitor serum electrolyte levels in patients with excessive, frequent, or prolonged use of lactulose.
- Obtain periodic serum ammonia levels, looking for a reduction.
- Assess the patient's mental status, and watch for signs of reduced ammonia level, such as lessening of asterixis.

Patient Teaching

- Instruct the patient receiving lactulose rectally to retain the liquid until cramping is felt. Tell him or her that evacuation occurs in 24 to 48 hours of the initial drug dose.
- Advise the patient to institute measures to promote defecation, such as increasing his or her fluid intake, exercising, and eating a high-fiber diet.

magnesium chloride

mag-**knee**-see-um
(Mag-Delay SR, Slow-Mag)

magnesium citrate

(Citrate of Magnesia, Citro-Mag[CAN])

magnesium hydroxide

(Phillips Milk of Magnesia)

magnesium oxide

(Mag-Ox 400, Uro-Mag)

magnesium protein complex

(Mg-PLUS)

magnesium sulfate

(Epsom salt, magnesium sulfate injection)
Do not confuse magnesium sulfate with manganese sulfate.

CATEGORY AND SCHEDULE

Pregnancy Risk Category: B

MECHANISM OF ACTION

An antacid, laxative, electrolyte, and anticonvulsant. As an antacid acts in the stomach to neutralize gastric acid. **Therapeutic Effect:** Increases pH. As a laxative has an osmotic effect, primarily in the small intestine, and draws water into the intestinal lumen. **Therapeutic Effect:** Produces distention and promotes peristalsis and bowel evacuation. As a systemic dietary supplement and electrolyte replacement, is found primarily in intracellular fluids and is essential for enzyme activity, nerve conduction, and muscle contraction. As an anticonvulsant, blocks neuromuscular transmission and the amount of acetylcholine released at the motor end plate. **Therapeutic Effect:** Controls seizure. Maintains and restores magnesium levels.

PHARMACOKINETICS

Antacid, laxative: Minimal absorption through the intestine. Absorbed dose primarily excreted in urine. Systemic: Widely distributed. Primarily excreted in urine.

AVAILABILITY

Magnesium chloride
Tablets (Mag Delay SR, Slo-Mag): 64 mg.
Magnesium citrate
Oral Solution (Citrate of Magnesia): 290 mg/5 ml.
Magnesium hydroxide
Oral Liquid (Phillips Milk of Magnesia): 400 mg/5 ml, 800 mg/5 ml.
Tablets (Chewable [Phillips Milk of Magnesia]): 311 mg.
Magnesium oxide
Tablets (Mag-Ox 400): 400 mg.
Capsules (Uro-Mag): 140 mg.
Magnesium sulfate
Premix Infusion Solution: 10 mg/ml, 20 mg/ml, 40 mg/ml, 80 mg/ml.
Injection: 125 mg/ml, 500 mg/ml.

INDICATIONS AND DOSAGES

▸ **Hypomagnesemia**

PO (magnesium sulfate)
Adults, Elderly. 3 g q6h for 4 doses as needed.
IV, IM
Adults, Elderly. 1–12 g/day in divided doses.
Children. 25–50 mg/kg/dose q4–6h for 3–4 doses. Maintenance: 30–60 mg/kg/day.

▸ **Hypertension, seizures**

IV, IM (magnesium sulfate)
Children. 20–100 mg/kg/dose q4–6h as needed.
IV (magnesium sulfate)
Adults. Initially, 4 g then 1–4 g/hr by continuous infusion.

Arrhythmias
IV (magnesium sulfate)
Adults, Elderly. Initially, 1–2 g then infusion of 1–2 g/hr.
Treat constipation
PO (magnesium sulfate)
Adults, Elderly, Children 12 yr and older. 10–30 g/day in divided doses.
Children 6–11 yr. 5–10 g/day in divided doses.
Children 2–5 yr. 2.5–5 g/kg/day in divided doses.
Treat constipation
PO (magnesium hydroxide)
Adults, Elderly, Children 12 yr and older. 6–8 tablets or 30–60 ml/day.
Children 6–11 yr. 3–4 tablets or 7.5–15 ml/day.
Children 2–5 yr. 1–2 tablets or 2.5–7.5 ml/day.
Treatment of hyperacidity
PO (magnesium hydroxide)
Adults, Elderly. 2–4 tablets or 5–15 ml as needed up to 4 times a day.
Children 7–14 yr. 1 tablet or 2.5–5 ml as needed up to 4 times a day.
Magnesium deficiency
PO (magnesium oxide)
Adults, Elderly. 1–2 tablets 2–3 times/day.
Dietary supplement
PO (magnesium chloride)
Adults, Elderly. 54–483 mg/day in 2–4 divided doses.
Cathartic
PO (magnesium citrate)
Adults, Elderly, Children 12 yr and older. 120–300 ml.
Children 6–11 yr. 100–150 ml.
Children younger than 6 yr. 0.5 ml/kg up to maximum of 200 ml.

CONTRAINDICATIONS

Antacid: Appendicitis or symptoms of appendicitis, ileostomy, intestinal obstruction, severe renal impairment
Laxative: Appendicitis, CHF, colostomy, hypersensitivity, ileostomy, intestinal obstruction, undiagnosed rectal bleeding
Systemic: Heart block, myocardial damage, renal failure

INTERACTIONS

Drug

Antacid
Ketoconazole, tetracyclines: May decrease the absorption of ketoconazole and tetracyclines.
Methenamine: May decrease the effects of methenamine.
Antacid, laxative
Digoxin, oral anticoagulants, phenothiazines: May decrease the effects of these drugs.
Tetracyclines: May form nonabsorbable complex with tetracyclines.
Systemic (dietary supplement, electrolyte replacement)
Calcium: May neutralize the effects of magnesium.
CNS depression-producing medications: May increase CNS depression.
Digoxin: May cause changes in cardiac conduction or heart block with digoxin.

Herbal

None known.

Food

None known.

DIAGNOSTIC TEST EFFECTS

Antacid: May increase gastrin production and pH.
Laxative: May decrease serum potassium level.
Systemic (dietary supplement, electrolyte replacement): None known.

IV INCOMPATIBILITIES

Amphotericin B complex (Abelcet, AmBisome, Amphotec), cefepime (Maxipime)

IV COMPATIBILITIES

Amikacin (Amikin), cefazolin

(Ancef), ciprofloxacin (Cipro), dobutamine (Dobutrex), enalapril (Vasotec), gentamicin, heparin, hydromorphone (Dilaudid), insulin, milrinone (Primacor), morphine, piperacillin/tazobactam (Zosyn), potassium chloride, propofol (Diprivan), tobramycin (Nebcin), vancomycin (Vancocin)

SIDE EFFECTS

Frequent

Antacid: Chalky taste, diarrhea, laxative effect

Occasional

Antacid: Nausea, vomiting, stomach cramps

Antacid, laxative: With prolonged use or large doses in renal impairment, possible hypermagnesemia, marked by dizziness, irregular heartbeat, mental changes, fatigue, and weakness

Laxative: Cramping, diarrhea, increased thirst, flatulence

Systemic (dietary supplement, electrolyte replacement): Reduced respiratory rate, decreased reflexes, flushing, hypotension, decreased heart rate

SERIOUS REACTIONS

! Magnesium as an antacid or laxative has no known serious reactions.

! Systemic use of magnesium may produce prolonged PR interval and widening of QRS interval.

! Magnesium toxicity may cause loss of deep tendon reflexes, heart block, respiratory paralysis, and cardiac arrest. The antidote for toxicity is 10–20 ml 10% calcium gluconate (5–10 mEq of calcium).

NURSING CONSIDERATIONS

Baseline Assessment

- Determine if the patient is sensitive to magnesium.
- Assess for the presence of GI pain. Note its duration, quality, location, and causative and exacerbative factors.
- If the patient will be taking magnesium as a laxative, assess the amount, color, and consistency of the stool. Also assess the pattern of daily bowel activity and evaluate the bowel sounds for peristalsis.
- Assess the patient for history of recent abdominal surgery, nausea, vomiting, and weight loss.
- Obtain the BUN and serum creatinine and magnesium levels of the patient taking magnesium for systemic use.

Lifespan Considerations

- It is unknown if antacid forms of magnesium are distributed in breast milk.
- Parenteral magnesium readily crosses the placenta and is distributed in breast milk for 24 hours after therapy has been discontinued.
- Continuous IV infusion of magnesium increases the risk of magnesium toxicity in the neonate.
- Magnesium should not be administered IV during the 2 hours preceding delivery.
- The elderly are at increased risk for developing magnesium deficiency, because of decreased magnesium absorption, other medications they may be taking, and poor diet.

Precautions

- Use magnesium cautiously in children younger than 6 years of age. Safety is unknown.
- Use magnesium antacids cautiously in patients with chronic diarrhea, colostomy, diverticulitis,

ulcerative colitis, or undiagnosed GI or rectal bleeding.
• Use laxative form cautiously in patients with diabetes mellitus and in those on a low-salt diet because some magnesium supplements contain sugar or sodium.
• When magnesium is given for systemic use, use cautiously in patients with severe renal impairment.

Administration and Handling

PO (Antacid)

◀ALERT▶ Keep in mind that antacids may be given up to 4 times a day.
• Shake suspension well before use.
• Make sure that chewable tablets are chewed thoroughly before swallowing and are followed by a full glass of water.

PO (Laxative)
• Have patient drink a full glass of liquid (8 oz) with each dose to prevent dehydration.
• Follow dose with citrus carbonated beverage or fruit juice to improve flavor.
• Refrigerate citrate of magnesia to retain potency and improve palatability.

IV
• Store at room temperature.
• The solution must be diluted to avoid exceeding 20 mg/ml concentration.
• For infusion, do not exceed magnesium sulfate concentration of 200 mg/ml (20%).
• Do not exceed infusion rate of 150 mg/minute.

IM
• For adults and elderly patients, use 250 mg/ml (25%) or 500 mg/ml (50%) magnesium sulfate concentration, as prescribed.
• For children and infants, do not exceed 200 mg/ml (20%) as prescribed.

Intervention and Evaluation
• Assess the patient taking magnesium antacids for relief of gastric distress.
• Monitor renal function in the patient taking magnesium antacids, especially if dosing is long-term or frequent.
• Monitor the patient taking the laxative form for constipation or diarrhea.
• Ensure that the patient taking the laxative form maintains adequate fluid intake.
• Monitor EKG and BUN, serum creatinine and magnesium levels in the patient taking systemic form.
• Test the patellar reflexes before giving repeat parenteral doses of systemic magnesium to assess for CNS depression. Know that suppressed reflexes may indicate impending respiratory arrest. Make sure that patellar reflexes are present and that the patient has a respiratory rate greater than 16 breaths/minute, before giving each parenteral dose.
• Provide seizure precautions for the patient taking systemic magnesium.

Patient Teaching
• Instruct the patient to take magnesium antacids at least 2 hours before or 2 hours after other medications.
• Tell the patient not to take magnesium antacids for longer than 2 weeks, unless directed by the physician.
• Instruct the patient with peptic ulcer disease to take magnesium antacids 1 and 3 hours after meals and at bedtime for 4 to 6 weeks.
• Teach the patient to chew tablets thoroughly followed by a glass of water and to shake suspensions well.
• Warn the patient that repeat dosing or taking large doses of magnesium antacids may have a laxative effect.
• Instruct the patient taking magne-

sium laxatives to drink a full glass (8 oz) of liquid to aid stool softening.
- Tell the patient taking magnesium laxatives that these drugs are for short-term use only.
- Warn the patient taking a magnesium laxative to stop the drug if abdominal pain, nausea, or vomiting occurs.
- Warn the patient taking systemic magnesium to notify the physician if signs and symptoms of hypermagnesemia occur, including confusion, cramping, dizziness, irregular heartbeat, light-headedness, or unusual fatigue or weakness.

methylcellulose

meth-ill-**cell**-you-los
(Citrucel, Cologel)
Do not confuse Citrucel with Citracal.

CATEGORY AND SCHEDULE

Pregnancy Risk Category: C
OTC

MECHANISM OF ACTION

A bulk-forming laxative that dissolves and expands in water. **Therapeutic Effect:** Provides increased bulk and moisture content in stool, increasing peristalsis and bowel motility.

PHARMACOKINETICS

Route	Onset	Peak	Duration
PO	12–24 hr	N/A	N/A

Acts in small and large intestines. Full effect may not be evident for 2–3 days.

AVAILABILITY

Powder.

INDICATIONS AND DOSAGES

▸ Constipation

PO

Adults, Elderly. 1 tbsp (15 ml) in 8 oz water 1–3 times a day.
Children 6–12 yr. 1 tsp (5 ml) in 4 oz water 3–4 times a day.

CONTRAINDICATIONS

Abdominal pain, dysphagia, nausea, partial bowel obstruction, symptoms of appendicitis, vomiting

INTERACTIONS

Drug

Digoxin, oral anticoagulants, salicylates: May decrease the effects of digoxin, oral anticoagulants, and salicylates by decreasing absorption of these drugs.
Potassium-sparing diuretics, potassium supplements: May interfere with the effects of potassium-sparing diuretics and potassium supplements.

Herbal

None known.

Food

None known.

DIAGNOSTIC TEST EFFECTS

May increase blood glucose level. May decrease serum potassium level.

SIDE EFFECTS

Rare

Some degree of abdominal discomfort, nausea, mild cramps, griping, faintness

SERIOUS REACTIONS

! Esophageal or bowel obstruction may occur if administered with less than 250 ml or 1 full glass of liquid.

NURSING CONSIDERATIONS

Baseline Assessment

• Before methylcellulose administration, assess the patient's abdomen for signs of tenderness, rigidity, and the presence of bowel sounds.
• Try to determine when the patient last had a bowel movement, and find out the amount and consistency.

Lifespan Considerations

• Methylcellulose may be used safely in pregnancy.
• Safety and efficacy of methylcellulose have not been established in children younger than 6 years of age. Methylcellulose use is not recommended in this age-group.
• No age-related precautions have been noted in the elderly.

Administration and Handling

PO
• Instruct the patient to drink 6 to 8 glasses of water a day to aid in stool softening.
• Drug should not be swallowed in dry form but should be mixed with at least 1 full glass (8 oz) of liquid.

Intervention and Evaluation

• Encourage the patient to maintain adequate fluid intake.
• Assess the patient's bowel sounds for peristalsis.
• Assess the patient's pattern of daily bowel activity and stool consistency and record time of evacuation.
• Monitor serum electrolyte levels in patients with excessive, frequent, or prolonged use of methylcellulose.

Patient Teaching

• Tell the patient to institute measures to promote defecation such as increasing fluid intake, exercising, and eating a high-fiber diet.
• Instruct the patient to take each dose with a full glass of water.
• Warn the patient that taking methylcellulose with an inadequate amount of fluid may cause choking or swelling in the throat.

polycarbophil

polly-**car**-bow-fill
(Fibercon, Replens[CAN])

CATEGORY AND SCHEDULE

Pregnancy Risk Category: C
OTC

MECHANISM OF ACTION

A bulk-forming laxative and antidiarrheal. As a laxative, retains water in the intestine and opposes dehydrating forces of the bowel. **Therapeutic Effect:** Promotes well-formed stools. As an antidiarrheal, absorbs fecal-free water, restores normal moisture level, and provides bulk. **Therapeutic Effect:** Forms gel and produces formed stool.

PHARMACOKINETICS

Route	Onset	Peak	Duration
PO	12–72 hr	N/A	N/A

Acts in small and large intestines.

AVAILABILITY

Tablets: 500 mg, 625 mg.
Tablets (Chewable): 500 mg.

INDICATIONS AND DOSAGES

▸ Constipation, diarrhea

PO
Adults, Elderly, Children 12 yr and older. 1 g 1–4 times a day, or as needed. Maximum: 4 g/24 hr.
Children 6–11 yr. 500 mg 1–4 times a day, or as needed. Maximum: 2 g/24 hr.
Children younger than 6 yr. Consult product labeling.

CONTRAINDICATIONS

Abdominal pain, dysphagia, nausea, partial bowel obstruction, symptoms of appendicitis, vomiting

INTERACTIONS

Drug

Digoxin, oral anticoagulants, salicylates, tetracyclines: May decrease the effects of digoxin, salicylates, and tetracyclines.
Potassium-sparing diuretics, potassium supplements: May interfere with the effects of potassium-sparing diuretics and potassium supplements.

Herbal

None known.

Food

None known.

DIAGNOSTIC TEST EFFECTS

May increase blood glucose level. May decrease serum potassium levels.

SIDE EFFECTS

Rare

Some degree of abdominal discomfort, nausea, mild cramps, griping, syncope/near syncope

SERIOUS REACTIONS

! Esophageal or bowel obstruction may occur if administered with less than 250 ml or 1 full glass of liquid.

NURSING CONSIDERATIONS

Baseline Assessment

- Before polycarbophil administration, assess the patient's abdomen for signs of tenderness, rigidity, and the presence of bowel sounds.
- Try to determine when the patient last had a bowel movement, and find out the amount and consistency.

Lifespan Considerations

- This drug may be used safely in pregnancy.
- Polycarbophil use is not recommended in children younger than 6 years of age.
- No age-related precautions have been noted in the elderly.

Administration and Handling

◀ALERT▶ For severe diarrhea, give every half hour up to maximum daily dosage; for constipation, give with 8 oz liquid, as prescribed.

Intervention and Evaluation

- Encourage the patient to maintain adequate fluid intake.
- Assess the patient's bowel sounds for peristalsis.
- Assess the patient's pattern of daily bowel activity and stool consistency and record time of evacuation.
- Monitor serum electrolyte levels in patients with excessive, frequent, or prolonged use of polycarbophil.

Patient Teaching

- Tell the patient to institute measures to promote defecation such as increasing fluid intake, exercising, and eating a high-fiber diet.
- Instruct the patient to drink 6 to 8 glasses of water a day when using polycarbophil as a laxative to aid in stool softening.

polyethylene glycol-electrolyte solution (PEG-ES)

poly-**eth**-ah-leen
(CoLyte, GoLYTELY, Klean-Prep[CAN], MiraLax, NuLytely, Peglyte[CAN], Pro-Lax[CAN], TriLyte)

CATEGORY AND SCHEDULE

Pregnancy Risk Category: C

MECHANISM OF ACTION

A laxative that has an osmotic effect. **Therapeutic Effect:** Induces diarrhea and cleanses bowel without depleting electrolytes.

PHARMACOKINETICS

Route	Onset	Peak	Duration
PO (Bowel cleansing)	1–2 hr	N/A	N/A
PO (Constipation)	2–4 days	N/A	N/A

AVAILABILITY

Powder for Oral Solution.
Oral Solution.

INDICATIONS AND DOSAGES

▸ Bowel cleansing

PO

Adults, Elderly. Before GI examination: 240 ml (8 oz) q10min until 4 liters consumed or rectal effluent clear. NG tube: 20–30 ml/min until 4 liters given.
Children. 25–40 ml/kg/hr until rectal effluent clear.

▸ Constipation

PO (MiraLax)

Adults. 17 g or 1 heaping tbsp a day.

CONTRAINDICATIONS

Bowel perforation, gastric retention, GI obstruction, megacolon, toxic colitis, toxic ileus

INTERACTIONS

Drug

Oral medications: May decrease the absorption of oral medications if given within 1 hour because they may be flushed from GI tract.

Herbal

None known.

Food

None known.

DIAGNOSTIC TEST EFFECTS

None known.

SIDE EFFECTS

Frequent (50%)
Some degree of abdominal fullness, nausea, bloating
Occasional (10%–1%)
Abdominal cramping, vomiting, anal irritation
Rare (less than 1%)
Urticaria, rhinorrhea, dermatitis

SERIOUS REACTIONS

! None known.

NURSING CONSIDERATIONS

Baseline Assessment

- Do not give oral medication within 1 hour of the initiation of polyethylene therapy because the oral medication may not be adequately absorbed before GI cleansing.

Lifespan Considerations

- It is unknown if polyethylene crosses the placenta or is distributed in breast milk.
- No age-related precautions have been noted in children or the elderly.

Precautions

- Use polyethylene cautiously in patients with ulcerative colitis.

Administration and Handling

PO

- Refrigerate reconstituted solutions; use within 48 hours.
- May use tap water to prepare solution. Shake vigorously for several minutes to ensure complete dissolution of powder.
- Give the patient nothing by mouth 3 hours or more before ingestion of solution. Give only clear liquids after administration.
- May give via NG tube.
- Rapid drinking preferred. Chilled solution is more palatable.

Intervention and Evaluation

- Assess the patient's bowel sounds for peristalsis.
- Assess the patient's pattern of daily bowel activity and stool consistency and record time of evacuation.
- Monitor the patient for abdominal disturbances.
- Monitor the patient's blood glucose, BUN, and serum electrolyte levels, and urine osmolality.

Patient Teaching

- Tell the patient to chill the solution to make it more palatable; encourage fast ingestion.
- Instruct the patient to fast for 3 hours before taking the drug, and to ingest only clear liquids afterward, as prescribed.
- Warn the patient to notify the physician if severe abdominal pain or bloating occurs.

psyllium

sill-ee-yum
(Fiberall, Hydrocil, Konsyl, Metamucil, Novo-Mucilax [CAN], Perdiem)

CATEGORY AND SCHEDULE

Pregnancy Risk Category: B
OTC

MECHANISM OF ACTION

A bulk-forming laxative that dissolves and swells in water providing increased bulk and moisture content in stool. **Therapeutic Effect:** Promotes peristalsis and bowel motility.

PHARMACOKINETICS

Route	Onset	Peak	Duration
PO	12–24 hr	2–3 days	N/A

Acts in small and large intestines.

AVAILABILITY

Powder (Fiberall, Hydrocil, Konsyl, Metamucil).
Wafer (Metamucil): 3.4 g/dose
Capsules (Metamucil): 0.52 g.
Granules (Perdiem): 4 g/5 ml.

INDICATIONS AND DOSAGES

▸ Constipation, irritable bowel syndrome

PO

◂ALERT▸ 3.4 g powder equals 1 rounded tsp, 1 packet, or 1 wafer.
Adults, Elderly. 2–5 capsules/dose 1–3 times a day. 1–2 tsp granules 1–2 times a day. 1 rounded tsp or 1 tbsp of powder 1–3 times a day. 2 wafers 1–3 times a day.
Children 6–11 yr. One half (1/2)–1 tsp powder in water 1–3 times a day.

CONTRAINDICATIONS

Fecal impaction, GI obstruction

INTERACTIONS

Drug

Digoxin, oral anticoagulants, salicylates: May decrease the effects of digoxin, oral anticoagulants, and salicylates by decreasing absorption.
Potassium-sparing diuretics, potassium supplements: May interfere with the effects of potassium-sparing diuretics and potassium supplements.

Herbal

None known.

Food

None known.

DIAGNOSTIC TEST EFFECTS

May increase blood glucose level.
May decrease serum potassium level.

SIDE EFFECTS

Rare

Some degree of abdominal discomfort, nausea, mild abdominal cramps, griping, faintness

SERIOUS REACTIONS

! Esophageal or bowel obstruction may occur if administered with less than 250 ml of liquid.

NURSING CONSIDERATIONS

Baseline Assessment

- Before psyllium administration, assess the patient's abdomen for signs of tenderness, rigidity, and the presence of bowel sounds.
- Try to determine when the patient last had a bowel movement, and find out the amount and consistency.

Lifespan Considerations

- This drug may be used safely in pregnancy.
- Safety and efficacy of psyllium has not been established in children younger than 6 years of age.
- No age-related precautions have been noted in the elderly.

Precautions

- Use psyllium cautiously in patients with esophageal strictures, intestinal adhesions, stenosis, or ulcers.

Administration and Handling

PO

- Administer at least 2 hours before or after other medication administration.
- Have patient drink 6 to 8 glasses of water a day to aid in stool softening.
- Drugs should not be swallowed in dry form but should be mixed with at least 1 full glass (8 oz) of liquid and then followed by 8 ounces of liquid.

Intervention and Evaluation

- Encourage the patient to maintain adequate fluid intake.
- Assess the patient's bowel sounds for peristalsis.
- Assess the patient's pattern of daily bowel activity and stool consistency and record time of evacuation.
- Monitor the patient for abdominal disturbances.
- Monitor serum electrolyte levels in patients with excessive, frequent, or prolonged use of psyllium.

Patient Teaching

- Tell the patient to institute measures to promote defecation such as increasing fluid intake, exercising, and eating a high-fiber diet.
- Instruct the patient to take each dose with a full glass, at least 250 ml, of water.
- Warn the patient that taking psyllium with an inadequate amount of fluid may cause GI obstruction.

senna

sen-na

(Ex-lax, Senexon, Senna-Glen, Sennatural, Senokot, X-Prep)

CATEGORY AND SCHEDULE

Pregnancy Risk Category: C

OTC

MECHANISM OF ACTION

A GI stimulant that has a direct effect on intestinal smooth musculature by stimulating the intramural nerve plexi. **Therapeutic Effect:** Increases peristalsis and promotes laxative effect.

PHARMACOKINETICS

Route	Onset	Peak	Duration
PO	6–12 hr	N/A	N/A
Rectal	0.5–2 hr	N/A	N/A

Minimal absorption after oral administration. Hydrolyzed to active form by enzymes of colonic flora. Absorbed drug metabolized in the liver. Eliminated in feces via biliary system.

AVAILABILITY

Granules (Senokot): 15 mg/tsp.
Liquid (X-Prep): 8.8 mg/5 ml.
Syrup (Senokot): 8.8 mg/5 ml.
Tablets (Sennatural, Senokot, Senexon, Senna-Gen): 8.6 mg, 15 mg.
Tablets (Ex-Lax).

INDICATIONS AND DOSAGES

▸ **Constipation**

PO (Tablets)

Adults, Elderly, Children 12 yr and older. 2 tablets at bedtime. Maximum: 4 tablets twice a day.
Children 6–11 yr. 1 tablet at bedtime. Maximum: 2 tablets twice a day.
Children 2–5 yr. 1/2 tablet at bedtime. Maximum: 1 tablet twice a day.

PO (Syrup)

Adults, Elderly, Children 12 yr and older. 10–15 ml at bedtime. Maximum: 15 ml twice a day.
Children 6–11 yr. 5–7.5 ml at bedtime. Maximum: 7.5 ml twice a day.
Children 2–5 yr. 2.5–3.75 ml at bedtime. Maximum: 3.75 ml twice a day.

PO (Granules)

Adults, Elderly, Children 12 yr and older. 1 tsp at bedtime. Maximum: 2 tsp twice a day.
Children 6–11 yr. One half (1/2) teaspoon at bedtime up to 1 teaspoon 2 times/day.
Children 2–5 yr. One quarter (1/4) teaspoon at bedtime up to one half (1/2) teaspoon 2 times/day.

▸ **Bowel evacuation**

PO

Adults, Elderly, Children older than 1 yr. 75 ml between 2 p.m. and 4 p.m. on day prior to procedure.

CONTRAINDICATIONS

Abdominal pain, appendicitis, intestinal obstruction, nausea, vomiting

INTERACTIONS

Drug

Oral medications: May decrease transit time of concurrently administered oral medications, decreasing absorption of senna.

Herbal

None known.

Food

None known.

DIAGNOSTIC TEST EFFECTS

May increase blood glucose level. May decrease serum potassium level.

SIDE EFFECTS

Frequent

Pink-red, red-violet, red-brown, or yellow-brown discoloration of urine

Occasional

Some degree of abdominal discomfort, nausea, mild cramps, griping, faintness

SERIOUS REACTIONS

! Long-term use may result in laxative dependence, chronic constipation, and loss of normal bowel function.

! Prolonged use or overdose may result in electrolyte and metabolic disturbances (such as hypokalemia, hypocalcemia, and metabolic acidosis or alkalosis), vomiting, muscle weakness, persistent diarrhea, malabsorption, and weight loss.

NURSING CONSIDERATIONS

Baseline Assessment

- Before senna administration, assess the patient's abdomen for signs of tenderness, rigidity, and the presence of bowel sounds.
- Try to determine when the patient last had a bowel movement, and find out the amount and consistency.

Lifespan Considerations

- It is unknown if senna is distributed in breast milk.
- Safety and efficacy of senna have not been established in children younger than 6 years of age.
- No age-related precautions have been noted in the elderly, but this patient population should be monitored for signs and symptoms of dehydration and electrolyte loss.

Precautions

- Use senna cautiously for extended periods (greater than 1 week).

Administration and Handling

PO

- Give senna on an empty stomach for faster results.
- Offer the patient at least 6 to 8 glasses of water a day to aid in stool softening.
- Avoid giving within 1 hour of other oral medications because drug absorption is decreased.

Intervention and Evaluation

- Encourage the patient to maintain adequate fluid intake.
- Assess the patient's bowel sounds for peristalsis.
- Assess the patient's pattern of daily bowel activity and stool consistency and record time of evacuation.
- Monitor the patient for GI disturbances.
- Monitor serum electrolyte levels in patients with excessive, frequent, or prolonged use of senna.

Patient Teaching

- Explain to the patient that his or her urine may turn pink-red, red-violet, red-brown, or yellow-brown.
- Instruct the patient to institute measures to promote defecation, such as increasing fluid intake, exercising, and eating a high-fiber diet.
- Instruct the patient not to take other oral medications within 1 hour of taking senna because these substances may decrease the effectiveness of senna.
- Tell the patient that oral senna generally produces a laxative effect in 6 to 12 hours but that it may take 24 hours.

53 Proton Pump Inhibitors

esomeprazole
lansoprazole
omeprazole
pantoprazole
rabeprazole sodium

Uses: Proton pump inhibitors are used to treat various gastric disorders, including gastric and duodenal ulcers, gastroesophageal reflux disease (GERD), and pathologic hypersecretory conditions.

Action: Proton pump inhibitors suppress gastric acid secretion by specifically inhibiting the hydrogen-potassium-adenosine triphosphatase enzyme system found at the secretory surface of gastric parietal cells. This enzyme system is considered the acid pump of the gastric mucosa. (See the illustration *Sites of Action: Drugs Used to Treat GERD,* page 980.) Proton pump inhibitors don't have anticholinergic or histamine-receptor antagonistic properties.

COMBINATION PRODUCTS

PREVACID NAPRAPAC: lansoprazole/narpoxen (a NSAID) 15 mg/375 mg; 15 mg/500 mg.

esomeprazole

es-om-eh-**pray**-zole
(Nexium)

CATEGORY AND SCHEDULE

Pregnancy Risk Category: B

MECHANISM OF ACTION

A proton pump inhibitor that is converted to active metabolites that irreversibly bind to and inhibit hydrogen-potassium adenosine triphosphates, an enzyme on the surface of gastric parietal cells. Inhibits hydrogen ion transport into gastric lumen. **Therapeutic Effect:** Increases gastric pH, reducing gastric acid production.

PHARMACOKINETICS

Well absorbed after oral administration. Protein binding: 97%. Extensively metabolized by the liver. Primarily excreted in urine. ***Half-life:*** 1–1.5 hr.

AVAILABILITY

Capsules (Delayed-Release): 20 mg, 40 mg.

INDICATIONS AND DOSAGES

▸ **Erosive esophagitis**
PO
Adults, Elderly. 20–40 mg once daily for 4–8 wk.

▸ **To maintain healing of erosive esophagitis**
PO
Adults, Elderly. 20 mg/day.

▸ **Gastroesophageal reflux disease, to reduce the risk of NSAID-induced gastric ulcer**
PO
Adults, Elderly. 20 mg once a day for 4 wk.

▸ **Duodenal ulcer caused by *Helicobacter pylori***
PO
Adults, Elderly. 40 mg (esomeprazole) once a day, with amoxicillin 1,000 mg and clarithromycin 500 mg twice a day for 10 days.

CONTRAINDICATIONS

None known.

INTERACTIONS

Drug

Digoxin, iron, ketoconazole: May decrease the concentration of digoxin, iron, and ketoconazole.

Herbal

None known.

Food

None known.

DIAGNOSTIC TEST EFFECTS

None known.

SIDE EFFECTS

Frequent (7%)
Headache
Occasional (3%–2%)
Diarrhea, abdominal pain, nausea
Rare (less than 2%)
Dizziness, asthenia or loss of strength, vomiting, constipation, rash, cough

SERIOUS REACTIONS

! None known.

NURSING CONSIDERATIONS

Baseline Assessment

- Before giving esomeprazole, determine if the patient can swallow capsules whole.

Lifespan Considerations

- It is unknown if esomeprazole crosses the placenta or is distributed in breast milk.
- Safety and efficacy of esomeprazole have not been established in children.
- No age-related precautions have been noted in the elderly.

Administration and Handling

PO

- Give 1 hour or more before eating.
- Do not crush or open capsule. Instruct the patient to swallow the capsule whole. If the patient has difficulty swallowing a capsule, open the capsule and mix pellets with 1 tablespoon of applesauce. Instruct the patient to swallow the spoonful without chewing.

Intervention and Evaluation

- Evaluate the patient for therapeutic response (relief of GI symptoms).
- Assess the patient for diarrhea, discomfort, or nausea.

Patient Teaching

- Warn the patient to notify the physician if headache occurs during esomeprazole therapy.
- Instruct the patient to take esomeprazole 1 hour or more before eating.
- Teach the patient who has difficulty swallowing to open the capsule, mix the pellets with 1 tablespoon of applesauce, and swallow the spoonful without chewing.

lansoprazole

lan-soe-**pray**-zole
(Prevacid, Prevacid IV, Prevacid Solu-Tab, Zoton[AUS])
Do not confuse Prevacid with Pepcid, Pravachol, or Prevpac.

CATEGORY AND SCHEDULE

Pregnancy Risk Category: B

MECHANISM OF ACTION

A proton pump inhibitor that selectively inhibits the parietal cell membrane enzyme system (hydrogen-potassium adenosine triphosphatase) or proton pump. **Therapeutic Effect:** Suppresses gastric acid secretion.

PHARMACOKINETICS

Route	Onset	Peak	Duration
PO (15 mg)	2–3 hr	N/A	24 hr
PO (30 mg)	1–2 hr	N/A	longer than 24 hr

Rapid and complete absorption (food may decrease absorption) once drug has left stomach. Protein binding: 97%. Distributed primarily to gastric parietal cells and converted to two active metabolites. Extensively metabolized in the liver. Eliminated in bile and urine. Not removed by hemodialysis. ***Half-life:*** 1.5 hr (increased in the elderly and in those with hepatic impairment).

AVAILABILITY

Capsules (Delayed-Release [Prevacid]): 15 mg, 30 mg.
Granules for Oral Suspension (Prevacid): 15 mg/pack; 30 mg/pack.
Injection Powder for Reconstitution (Prevacid IV): 30 mg.
Oral-Disintegrating Tablets (Prevacid Solu-Tab): 15 mg, 30 mg.

INDICATIONS AND DOSAGES

▸ **Duodenal ulcer**
PO
Adults, Elderly. 15 mg/day, before eating, preferably in the morning, for up to 4 wk.

▸ **Erosive esophagitis**
PO
Adults, Elderly. 30 mg/day, before eating, for up to 8 wks. If healing does not occur within 8 wk (in 5%–10% of cases), may give for additional 8 wk. Maintenance: 15 mg/day.
IV
Adults, Elderly. 30 mg once a day for up to 7 days. Switch to oral lansoprazole therapy as soon as patient can tolerate oral route.

▸ **Gastric ulcer**
PO
Adults. 30 mg/day for up to 8 wk.

▸ **NSAID gastric ulcer**
PO
Adults, Elderly. (Healing): 30 mg/day for up to 8 wk. (Prevention): 15 mg/day for up to 12 wk.

▸ **Healed duodenal ulcer, gastroesophageal reflux disease**
PO
Adults. 15 mg/day.

▸ **Usual pediatric dosage**
Children 3 mo–14 yr, weighing more than 20 kg. 30 mg once daily.
Children 3 mo–14 yr, weighing 10–20 kg. 15 mg once daily.
Children 3 mo–14 yr, weighing less than 10 kg. 7.5 mg once daily.

▸ ***Helicobacter pylori* infection**
PO
Adults. 30 mg twice a day for 10 days (with amoxicillin and clarithromycin).

▸ **Pathologic hypersecretory conditions (including Zollinger-Ellison syndrome)**
PO
Adults, Elderly. 60 mg/day. Individualize dosage according to patient needs and for as long as clinically indicated. Administer up to 120 mg/day in divided doses.

CONTRAINDICATIONS

None known.

INTERACTIONS

Drug

Ampicillin, digoxin, iron salts, ketoconazole: May interfere with the absorption of ampicillin, digoxin, iron salts, and ketoconazole.
Sucralfate: May delay the absorption of lansoprazole.

Herbal

None known.

Food

None known.

DIAGNOSTIC TEST EFFECTS

May increase LDH, serum alkaline phosphatase, bilirubin, cholesterol, creatinine, AST (SGOT), ALT (SGPT), triglyceride, and uric acid levels. May produce abnormal albumin/globulin ratio, electrolyte balance, and platelet, RBC, and WBC counts. May increase Hgb and Hct.

SIDE EFFECTS

Occasional (3%–2%)

Diarrhea, abdominal pain, rash, pruritus, altered appetite

Rare (1%)

Nausea, headache

SERIOUS REACTIONS

! Bilirubinemia, eosinophilia, and hyperlipemia occur rarely.

NURSING CONSIDERATIONS

Baseline Assessment

- Obtain the patient's laboratory values, including CBC and blood chemistry.
- Assess the patient's medication history, especially for the use of sucralfate.

Lifespan Considerations

- It is unknown if lansoprazole is distributed in breast milk.
- Safety and efficacy of lansoprazole have not been established in children.
- No age-related precautions have been noted in the elderly, but doses larger than 30 mg are not recommended in this patient population.

Precautions

- Use lansoprazole cautiously in patients with impaired hepatic function.

Administration and Handling

PO

- Give lansoprazole while the patient is fasting or before meals because food diminishes absorption.
- Instruct the patient not to chew or crush delayed-release capsules.
- If the patient has difficulty swallowing capsules, open capsules and sprinkle granules on 1 tablespoon of applesauce. Instruct the patient to swallow immediately.
- Give lansoprazole 30 minutes before sucralfate because sucralfate may delay lansoprazole absorption.

PO (Solu-Tab)

- May give with oral syringe or NG tube.
- May dissolve in 4 ml water (15 mg) or 10 ml water (30 mg).

IV

- Store drug at room temperature.
- Infuse over 30 minutes.

Intervention and Evaluation

- Monitor the patient's ongoing laboratory results.
- Assess the patient for abdominal pain, diarrhea, and nausea and watch for therapeutic response (relief of GI symptoms).

Patient Teaching

- Instruct the patient not to chew or crush delayed-release capsules.
- Teach the patient who has difficulty swallowing capsules to open the capsule, sprinkle the granules on 1 tablespoon of applesauce, and swallow immediately.
- Instruct the patient to take lansoprazole 30 minutes before sucralfate.

omeprazole

oh-**mep**-rah-zole
(Losec[CAN], Maxor[AUS], Prilosec, Prilosec OTC, Probitor [AUS], Zegerid)
Do not confuse Prilosec with prilocaine, Prinivil, or Prozac.

CATEGORY AND SCHEDULE

Pregnancy Risk Category: C

MECHANISM OF ACTION

A benzimidazole that is converted to active metabolites that irreversibly bind to and inhibit hydrogen-potassium adenosine triphosphatase, an enzyme on the surface of gastric parietal cells. Inhibits hydrogen ion transport into gastric lumen. **Therapeutic Effect:** Increases gastric pH, reduces gastric acid production.

PHARMACOKINETICS

Route	Onset	Peak	Duration
PO	1 hr	2 hr	72 hr

Rapidly absorbed from the GI tract. Protein binding: 99%. Primarily distributed into gastric parietal cells. Metabolized extensively in the liver. Primarily excreted in urine. Unknown if removed by hemodialysis. ***Half-life:*** 0.5–1 hr (increased in patients with hepatic impairment).

AVAILABILITY

Capsules (Delayed-Release [Prilosec]): 10 mg, 20 mg, 40 mg.
Oral Suspension (Zegerid): 20 mg.

INDICATIONS AND DOSAGES

▸ **Erosive esophagitis, poorly responsive gastroesophageal reflux disease, active duodenal ulcer, prevention and treatment of NSAID-induced ulcers**
PO
Adults, Elderly. 20 mg/day.

▸ **To maintain healing of erosive esophagitis**
PO
Adults, Elderly. 20 mg/day.

▸ **Pathologic hypersecretory conditions**
PO
Adults, Elderly. Initially, 60 mg/day up to 120 mg 3 times a day.

▸ **Duodenal ulcer caused by *Helibacter pylori***
PO
Adults, Elderly. 20 mg twice a day for 10 days.

▸ **Active benign gastric ulcer**
PO
Adults, Elderly. 40 mg/day for 4–8 wk.

▸ **Usual pediatric dosage**
Children older than 2 yr, weighing 20 kg and more. 20 mg/day.
Children older than 2 yr, weighing less than 20 kg. 10 mg/day.

OFF-LABEL USES

H. pylori–associated duodenal ulcer (with amoxicillin and clarithromycin), prevention and treatment of NSAID-induced ulcers, treatment of active benign gastric ulcers

CONTRAINDICATIONS

None known.

INTERACTIONS

Drug

Diazepam, oral anticoagulants, phenytoin: May increase the blood concentration of diazepam, oral anticoagulants, and phenytoin.

Herbal
None known.
Food
None known.

DIAGNOSTIC TEST EFFECTS
May increase serum alkaline phosphatase, AST (SGOT), and ALT (SGPT) levels.

SIDE EFFECTS
Frequent (7%)
Headache
Occasional (3%–2%)
Diarrhea, abdominal pain, nausea
Rare (2%)
Dizziness, asthenia or loss of strength, vomiting, constipation, upper respiratory tract infection, back pain, rash, cough

SERIOUS REACTIONS
! None known.

NURSING CONSIDERATIONS
Baseline Assessment
- Expect to obtain serum chemistry laboratory values, particularly serum alkaline phosphatase, AST and ALT levels, to assess liver function.

Lifespan Considerations
- It is unknown if omeprazole crosses the placenta or is distributed in breast milk.
- Safety and efficacy of omeprazole have not been established in children.
- No age-related precautions have been noted in the elderly.

Administration and Handling
PO
- Give omeprazole before meals.
- Do not crush or open capsules; have the patient swallow capsules whole.

Intervention and Evaluation
- Assess the patient for diarrhea, discomfort, and nausea.
- Evaluate the patient for therapeutic response (relief of GI symptoms).

Patient Teaching
- Warn the patient to notify the physician if headache occurs during omeprazole therapy.
- Instruct the patient to swallow omeprazole capsules whole and not to open or crush them.
- Teach the patient to take omeprazole capsules before eating.

pantoprazole
pan-toe-**pra**-zole
(Protonix, Pantoloc, Somac[AUS])
Do not confuse Protonix with Lotronex.

CATEGORY AND SCHEDULE
Pregnancy Risk Category: B

MECHANISM OF ACTION
A benzimidazole that is converted to active metabolites that irreversibly bind to and inhibit hydrogen-potassium adenosine triphosphate, an enzyme on the surface of gastric parietal cells. Inhibits hydrogen ion transport into gastric lumen. **Therapeutic Effect:** Increases gastric pH and reduces gastric acid production.

PHARMACOKINETICS

Route	Onset	Peak	Duration
PO	N/A	N/A	24 hr

Rapidly absorbed from the GI tract. Protein binding: 98%. Primarily distributed into gastric parietal cells. Metabolized extensively in the liver. Primarily excreted in urine. Not removed by hemodialysis. ***Half-life:*** 1 hr.

AVAILABILITY

Tablets (Delayed-Release): 20 mg, 40 mg.
Powder for Injection: 40 mg.

INDICATIONS AND DOSAGES

▸ Erosive esophagitis

PO

Adults, Elderly. 40 mg/day for up to 8 wk. If not healed after 8 wk, may continue an additional 8 wk.

IV

Adults, Elderly. 40 mg/day for 7–10 days.

▸ Hypersecretory conditions

PO

Adults, Elderly. Initially, 40 mg twice a day. May increase to 240 mg/day.

IV

Adults, Elderly. 80 mg twice a day. May increase to 80 mg q8h.

CONTRAINDICATIONS

None known.

INTERACTIONS

Drug

None known.

Herbal

None known.

Food

None known.

DIAGNOSTIC TEST EFFECTS

May increase serum creatinine, cholesterol, and uric acid levels.

IV INCOMPATIBILITIES

Do not mix with other medications. Flush IV with D_5W, 0.9% NaCl, or lactated Ringer's solution before and after administration.

SIDE EFFECTS

Rare (less than 2%)

Diarrhea, headache, dizziness, pruritus, rash

SERIOUS REACTIONS

! None known.

NURSING CONSIDERATIONS

Baseline Assessment

- Obtain the patient's serum chemistry laboratory values, including serum creatinine and cholesterol levels.

Lifespan Considerations

- It is unknown if pantoprazole crosses the placenta or is distributed in breast milk.
- Safety and efficacy of pantoprazole have not been established in children.
- No age-related precautions have been noted in the elderly.

Precautions

- Use pantoprazole cautiously in patients with a chronic or current hepatic disease.

Administration and Handling

PO

- Give pantoprazole without regard to meals.
- Do not crush or split tablet; have patient swallow tablet whole.

IV

- Refrigerate vials and protect from light; do not freeze reconstituted vials.
- Mix 40-mg vial with 10 ml 0.9% NaCl injection. May be further diluted with 100 ml D_5W, 0.9% NaCl, or lactated Ringer's solution.
- Once diluted with 10 ml 0.9% NaCl the solution is stable for 2 hours at room temperature. When further diluted with 100 ml, the solution is stable at room temperature for 22 hours.
- Infuse 10 ml solution over at least 2 minutes. Infuse 100 ml solution over at least 15 min.

Intervention and Evaluation

- Assess the patient for GI discomfort and nausea.

• Evaluate the patient for therapeutic response (relief of GI symptoms).

Patient Teaching

• Warn the patient to notify the physician if headache occurs during pantoprazole therapy.
• Instruct the patient to swallow tablets whole, and not to open, chew, or crush them.
• Teach the patient to take tablets before eating.

rabeprazole sodium

rah-**bep**-rah-zole
(Aciphex, Pariet[CAN])
Do not confuse Aciphex with Accupril or Aricept.

CATEGORY AND SCHEDULE

Pregnancy Risk Category: B

MECHANISM OF ACTION

A proton pump inhibitor that converts to active metabolites that irreversibly binds to and inhibit hydrogen-potassium adenosine triphosphate, an enzyme on the surface of gastric parietal cells. Actively secretes hydrogen ions for potassium ions, resulting in an accumulation of hydrogen ions in gastric lumen. **Therapeutic Effect:** Increases gastric pH, reducing gastric acid production.

PHARMACOKINETICS

Rapidly absorbed from the GI tract after passing through the stomach relatively intact. Protein binding: 96%. Metabolized extensively in the liver. Primarily excreted in urine. Unknown if removed by hemodialysis. ***Half-life:*** 1–2 hr (increased with hepatic impairment).

AVAILABILITY

Tablets (Delayed-Release): 20 mg.

INDICATIONS AND DOSAGES

▸ **Gastroesophageal reflux disease**
PO
Adults, Elderly. 20 mg/day for 4–8 wk. Maintenance: 20 mg/day.

▸ **Duodenal ulcer**
PO
Adults, Elderly. 20 mg/day after morning meal for 4 wk.

▸ **Non-steroidal antiinflammatory drug (NSAID)-induced ulcer**
PO
Adults, Elderly. 20 mg/day.

▸ **Pathologic hypersecretory conditions**
PO
Adults, Elderly. Initially, 60 mg once a day. May increase to 60 mg twice a day.

▸ ***Helibacter pylori* infection**
PO
Adults, Elderly. 20 mg 2 times a day for 7 days (given with amoxicillin 1,000 mg and clarithromycin 500 mg)

CONTRAINDICATIONS

None known.

INTERACTIONS

Drug

Digoxin: May increase the plasma concentration of digoxin.
Ketoconazole: May decrease the blood concentration of ketoconazole.

Herbal

None known.

Food

None known.

DIAGNOSTIC TEST EFFECTS

May increase serum alkaline phosphatase, AST (SGOT), and ALT (SGPT) levels.

SIDE EFFECTS

Rare (less than 2%)
Headache, nausea, dizziness, rash, diarrhea, malaise

SERIOUS REACTIONS

! Hyperglycemia, hypokalemia, hyponatremia, and hyperlipemia occur rarely.

NURSING CONSIDERATIONS

Baseline Assessment

- Obtain the patient's laboratory values, especially serum chemistries and liver function test results.

Lifespan Considerations

- It is unknown if rabeprazole crosses the placenta or is distributed in breast milk.
- Safety and efficacy of rabeprazole have not been established in children.
- No age-related precautions have been noted in the elderly.

Precautions

- Use rabeprazole cautiously in patients with impaired hepatic function.

Administration and Handling

PO

- Give rabeprazole before meals.
- Do not allow patient to crush, chew, or split tablet; have him or her swallow it whole.

Intervention and Evaluation

- Monitor the patient's ongoing laboratory results.
- Assess the patient for diarrhea, GI discomfort, headache, nausea, and skin rash.
- Evaluate the patient for therapeutic response (relief of GI symptoms).
- Observe the patient for dizziness and utilize appropriate safety precautions.

Patient Teaching

- Instruct the patient to swallow tablets whole, and not to chew, crush, or split them.
- Tell the patient to notify the physician if headache occurs during rabeprazole therapy.

54 Miscellaneous Gastrointestinal Agents

balsalazide
infliximab
mesalamine (5-aminosalicylic acid, 5-ASA)
metoclopramide
olsalazine sodium
orlistat
pancreatin, pancrelipase
simethicone
sucralfate
sulfasalazine
tegaserod
ursodiol

Uses: Because miscellaneous GI agents come from different classes, their uses vary greatly. *Balsalazide* is used to treat ulcerative colitis. *Infliximab* may be used alone to treat Crohn's disease or with other drugs to treat rheumatoid arthritis. As GI anti-inflammatory agents, *mesalamine, olsalazine, and sulfasalazine* are prescribed to manage ulcerative colitis; other indications include proctosigmoiditis and proctitis (mesalamine) and inflammatory bowel disease and rheumatoid arthritis (sulfasalazine). *Orlistat* is used to manage obesity as an adjunct to calorie reduction. *Metoclopramide* is used to stimulate gastric emptying and intestinal transit, which is helpful in facilitating small-bowel intubation and in relieving symptoms of gastroparesis, reflux esophagitis, and gastroesophageal reflux disease (GERD). *Pancreatin* and *pancrelipase* are used to replace or supplement pancreatic enzymes in chronic pancreatitis and other disorders; they can also treat steatorrhea caused by certain conditions. The antiflatulent *simethicone* is used to treat flatulence, gastric bloating, postoperative gas pain, and other conditions that may cause gas retention. *Sucralfate* is used to treat and prevent duodenal ulcers. *Tegaserod* may be used in short-term treatment of irritable bowel syndrome that features constipation. *Ursodiol* is used primarily to treat gallstone disease and prevent gallstone development.

Action: Miscellaneous GI agents act in different ways. *Balsalazide* diminishes colon inflammation by changing intestinal microflora, altering prostaglandin production, and inhibiting the function of mast cells, neutrophils, and macrophages. *Infliximab* binds to and inhibits tumor necrosis factor, producing GI anti-inflammatory effects. Among the other GI anti-inflammatory drugs, *mesalamine* acts locally to inhibit the production of arachidonic acid metabolites; *olsalazine* is converted to mesalamine by colonic bacteria; and *sulfasalazine* acts locally in the colon to inhibit prostaglandin synthesis. *Metoclopramide* stimulates upper GI motility, decreases esophageal reflux, and raises the threshold activity of the chemoreceptor trigger zone. (See the illustration *Sites of Action: Drugs Used to Treat GERD,* page 980.) *Orlistat* inhibits dietary fat absorption by inactivating gastric and pancreatic enzymes. *Pancreatin* and *pancrelipase* act by replacing endogenous pancreatic enzymes. The antiflatulent *simethicone* changes the surface tension of gas bubbles, allowing easier gas elimination. *Sucralfate* forms an ulcer-adherent complex at ulcer sites and an adhesive barrier on intact gastric and duodenal mucosa. *Tegaserod* binds to 5-HT_4 receptors in the GI tract, which increases bowel motility. *Ursodiol* may suppress cholesterol synthesis and inhibit intestinal absorption, which promotes cholesterol dissolution in gallstones.

COMBINATION PRODUCTS

EXTRA STRENGTH MAALOX: simethicone/magnesium hydroxide (an antacid)/aluminum hydroxide (an antacid) 20 mg/200 mg/200 mg; 40 mg/400 mg/400 mg.
GELUSIL: simethicone/aluminum hydroxide (an antacid)/magnesium hydroxide (an antacid) 25 mg/200 mg/200 mg.
IMODIUM ADVANCED: simethicone/loperamide (an antidiarrheal) 125 mg/2 mg.
MAALOX PLUS: simethicone/aluminum hydroxide (an antacid)/magnesium hydroxide (an antacid) 25 mg/200 mg/200 mg.
MYLANTA: simethicone/magnesium hydroxide (an antacid)/aluminum hydroxide (an antacid) 20 mg/200 mg/200 mg; 40 mg/400 mg/400 mg.
SILAIN-GEL: simethicone/magnesium hydroxide (an antacid)/aluminum hydroxide (an antacid).
METOCLOPRAMIDE: See antiemetics.
SULFASALAZINE: See miscellaneous anti-infectives.

balsalazide

ball-**sal**-a-zide
(Colazal)

CATEGORY AND SCHEDULE

Pregnancy Risk Category: B

MECHANISM OF ACTION

A 5-aminosalicylic acid derivative that changes intestinal microflora, altering prostaglandin production and inhibiting function of natural killer cells, mast cells, neutrophils, and macrophages. **Therapeutic Effect:** Diminishes inflammatory effect in colon.

AVAILABILITY

Capsules: 750 mg.

INDICATIONS AND DOSAGES

▸ **Ulcerative colitis**

PO

Adults, Elderly. Three 750-mg capsules 3 times a day for 8 wk.

CONTRAINDICATIONS
Hypersensitivity to salicylates

SIDE EFFECTS
Frequent (8%–6%)
Headache, abdominal pain, nausea, diarrhea
Occasional (4%–2%)
Vomiting, arthralgia, rhinitis, insomnia, fatigue, flatulence, coughing, dyspepsia

SERIOUS REACTIONS
! Liver toxicity occurs rarely.

NURSING CONSIDERATIONS

Baseline Assessment
- Assess the patient's serum chemistry laboratory values including BUN, alkaline phosphatase, bilirubin, creatinine, AST (SGOT), and ALT (SGPT) levels.

Precautions
- Use balsalazide cautiously in patients with hepatic or renal impairment.

Administration and Handling
- Administer capsules whole; don't open or crush them.

Intervention and Evaluation
- Monitor the patient's bowel sounds for peristalsis.
- Assess the patient's pattern of daily bowel activity and stool consistency.
- Evaluate the patient for abdominal discomfort.
- Monitor the patient's liver function test results for abnormalities.

Patient Teaching
- Instruct the patient to take balsalazide as directed.
- Teach the patient not to chew or open balsalazide capsules.
- Warn the patient to notify the physician if abdominal pain, severe headache or chest pain, or unresolved diarrhea occurs.

infliximab
in-**flicks**-ih-mab
(Remicade)
Do not confuse Remicade with Reminyl.

CATEGORY AND SCHEDULE
Pregnancy Risk Category: C

MECHANISM OF ACTION
A monoclonal antibody that binds to tumor necrosis factor (TNF), inhibiting functional activity of TNF. Reduces infiltration of inflammatory cells. **Therapeutic Effect:** Decreases inflamed areas of the intestine.

PHARMACOKINETICS

Route	Onset	Peak	Duration
IV (Crohn's disease)	1–2 wk	N/A	8–48 wk
IV (Rheumatoid arthritis [RA])	3–7 days	N/A	6–12 wk

Absorbed into the GI tissue; primarily distributed in the vascular compartment. ***Half-life:*** 9.5 days.

AVAILABILITY
Powder for Injection: 100 mg.

INDICATIONS AND DOSAGES
▸ **Moderate to severe Crohn's disease**
IV Infusion
Adults, Elderly. 5 mg/kg as a single IV infusion.
▸ **Fistulizing Crohn's disease**
IV Infusion
Adults, Elderly. Initially, 5 mg/kg followed by additional 5-mg/kg doses at 2 and 6 wk after first infusion.

▸ **RA**

IV Infusion

Adults, Elderly. 3 mg/kg; followed by additional doses at 2 and 6 wk after first infusion: Then q8wk.

OFF-LABEL USES

Sciatica

CONTRAINDICATIONS

Sensitivity to infliximab or murine proteins, sepsis, serious active infection

INTERACTIONS

Drug

Immunosuppressants: May reduce frequency of infusion reactions and antibodies to infliximab.

Live vaccines: May decrease immune response.

Herbal

None known.

Food

None known.

DIAGNOSTIC TEST EFFECTS

None known.

IV INCOMPATIBILITIES

Do not infuse infliximab in the same IV line with other agents.

SIDE EFFECTS

Frequent (22%–10%)

Headache, nausea, fatigue, fever

Occasional (9%–5%)

Fever or chills during infusion, pharyngitis, vomiting, pain, dizziness, bronchitis, rash, rhinitis, cough, pruritus, sinusitis, myalgia, back pain

Rare (4%–1%)

Hypotension or hypertension, paresthesia, anxiety, depression, insomnia, diarrhea, urinary tract infection

SERIOUS REACTIONS

! Hypersensitivity reaction, lupus-like syndrome, and severe hepatic reactions may occur.

NURSING CONSIDERATIONS

Baseline Assessment

- Assess the patient's pattern of daily bowel activity and stool consistency.
- Establish the patient's hydration status by examining the mucous membranes for dryness and assessing skin turgor and urinary status.

Lifespan Considerations

- It is unknown if infliximab is distributed in breast milk.
- Safety and efficacy of infliximab have not been established in children.
- Use infliximab cautiously in the elderly because of a higher rate of infection in this patient population.

Precautions

- Use infliximab cautiously in patients with a history of recurrent infections.

Administration and Handling

IV

- Refrigerate vials.
- Reconstitute each vial with 10 ml sterile water for injection, using 21-gauge or smaller needle. Direct the stream of sterile water to the glass wall of the vial.
- Swirl the vial gently to dissolve the contents. Do not shake. Allow the solution to stand for 5 minutes.
- Because infliximab is a protein, the solution may develop a few translucent particles; do not use if particles are opaque or foreign particles are present.
- The solution normally appears colorless to light yellow and opalescent; do not use if discolored.
- Withdraw and waste a volume of 0.9% NaCl from a 250-ml bag that is equal to the volume of reconstituted solution to be injected into the 250-ml bag (approximately 10 ml). Total dose to be infused should equal 250 ml.
- Slowly add the reconstituted infliximab solution to the 250-ml infusion bag. Gently mix. Infusion concentra-

tion should range between 0.4 and 4 mg/ml.
- Begin infusion within 3 hours of reconstitution.
- Administer IV infusion over 2 hours, using set with a low-protein-binding filter.

Intervention and Evaluation
- Monitor the patient's BP, erythrocyte sedimentation rate (ESR), and urinalysis.
- Assess the patient for signs of infection.
- Evaluate abdominal pain, C-reactive protein, and stool frequency in the patient with Crohn's disease.
- Evaluate the C-reactive protein and any decrease in pain, stiffness, and swollen joints in the patient with rheumatoid arthritis.

Patient Teaching
- Tell the patient to expect follow-up tests, such as ESR, C-reactive protein measurement, and urinalysis.
- Tell the patient to report signs of infection, such as fever.
- Instruct the patient with rheumatoid arthritis to report increase in pain, stiffness, or swelling of joints.
- Tell the patient with Crohn's disease to report changes in stool color, consistency, or elimination pattern.

mesalamine (5-aminosalicylic acid, 5-ASA)

mez-**al**-a-meen
(Asacol, Fiv-Canasa, Mesasal[CAN], Pentasa, Rowasa, Salofalk[CAN])
Do not confuse Asacol with Os-Cal.

CATEGORY AND SCHEDULE
Pregnancy Risk Category: B

MECHANISM OF ACTION
A salicylic acid derivative that locally inhibits arachidonic acid metabolite production, which is increased in patients with chronic inflammatory bowel disease. **Therapeutic Effect:** Blocks prostaglandin production and diminishes inflammation in the colon.

PHARMACOKINETICS
Poorly absorbed from the colon. Moderately absorbed from the GI tract. Metabolized in the liver to active metabolite. Unabsorbed portion eliminated in feces; absorbed portion excreted in urine. Unknown if removed by hemodialysis. ***Half-life:*** 0.5–1.5 hr; metabolite, 5–10 hr.

AVAILABILITY
Tablets (Delayed-Release [Asacol]): 400 mg.
Capsules (Controlled-Release [Pentasa]): 250 mg.
Rectal Suspension (Rowasa): 4 g/60 ml.
Suppositories (Canasa): 500 mg, 1 g.

INDICATIONS AND DOSAGES
▸ **Ulcerative colitis, proctosigmoiditis, proctitis**
PO (Asacol)
Adults, Elderly. 800 mg 3 times a day for 6 wk.
Children. 50 mg/kg/day q8–12h.
PO (Pentasa)
Adults, Elderly. 1 g 4 times a day for 8 wk.
Children. 50 mg/kg/day q6–12h.
Rectal (retention enema)
Adults, Elderly. 60 ml (4 g) at bedtime; retain overnight (about 8 hr) for 3–6 wk.
Rectal (suppository)
Adults, Elderly. 1 suppository (500 mg) twice a day, retain 1–3 hr for 3–6 wk.

▸ **To maintain remission in ulcerative colitis**
PO (Asacol)
Adults, Elderly. 1.6 g/day in divided doses.
PO (Pentasa)
Adults, Elderly. 1 g 4 times a day

CONTRAINDICATIONS
None known.

INTERACTIONS
Drug
None known.
Herbal
None known.
Food
None known.

DIAGNOSTIC TEST EFFECTS
May increase BUN, serum alkaline phosphatase, creatinine, AST (SGOT), and ALT (SGPT) levels.

SIDE EFFECTS
Mesalamine is generally well tolerated, with only mild and transient effects.
Frequent (greater than 6%)
PO: Abdominal cramps or pain, diarrhea, dizziness, headache, nausea, vomiting, rhinitis, unusual fatigue
Rectal: Abdominal or stomach cramps, flatulence, headache, nausea
Occasional (6%–2%)
PO: Hair loss, decreased appetite, back or joint pain, flatulence, acne
Rectal: Hair loss
Rare (less than 2%)
Rectal: Anal irritation

SERIOUS REACTIONS
! Sulfite sensitivity may occur in susceptible patients, manifested by cramping, headache, diarrhea, fever, rash, hives, itching, and wheezing. Discontinue drug immediately.
! Hepatitis, pancreatitis, and pericarditis occur rarely with oral forms.

NURSING CONSIDERATIONS
Baseline Assessment
• Expect to obtain BUN, serum alkaline phosphatase, creatinine, AST and ALT levels.
• Before administering mesalamine, ask the patient if he or she has an allergy to sulfa-based products.
Lifespan Considerations
• It is unknown if mesalamine crosses the placenta or is distributed in breast milk.
• Safety and efficacy of mesalamine have not been established in children.
• In the elderly, age-related renal impairment may require cautious use.
Precautions
• Use mesalamine cautiously in patients with preexisting renal disease or sulfasalazine sensitivity.
Administration and Handling
◂ **ALERT** ▸ Store rectal suspension, suppositories, and oral forms at room temperature.
PO
• Do not break outer coating of tablet. Have patient swallow whole.
• Give mesalamine without regard to food.
Rectal
• Shake bottle well.
• Instruct patient to lie on left side with lower leg extended, upper leg flexed forward, or to assume the knee-chest position.
• Insert applicator tip into rectum, pointing toward umbilicus. Squeeze bottle steadily until contents are emptied. Tell the patient to try to retain the enema for as long as tolerable, preferably for a minimum of 8 hours.

Intervention and Evaluation

- Encourage the patient to maintain adequate fluid intake.
- Assess the patient's bowel sounds for peristalsis.
- Assess the patient's pattern of daily bowel activity and stool consistency and record time of evacuation.
- Evaluate the patient for abdominal disturbances.
- Assess the patient's skin for rash and urticaria.
- Discontinue mesalamine if cramping, diarrhea, fever, or rash occurs.

Patient Teaching

- Warn the patient to avoid tasks that require mental alertness or motor skills until his or her response to the drug has been established.
- Tell the patient that mesalamine use may discolor urine yellow-brown.
- Explain to the patient that mesalamine suppositories will stain fabrics.

metoclopramide

See Antiemetics

olsalazine sodium

ohl-**sal**-ah-zeen
(Dipentum)
Do not confuse olsalazine with olanzapine.

CATEGORY AND SCHEDULE

Pregnancy Risk Category: C

MECHANISM OF ACTION

A salicylic acid derivative that is converted to mesalamine in the colon by bacterial action. Blocks prostaglandin production in bowel mucosa. **Therapeutic Effect:** Reduces colonic inflammation in inflammatory bowel disease.

AVAILABILITY

Capsules: 250 mg.

INDICATIONS AND DOSAGES

▸ **Maintenance of controlled ulcerative colitis**

PO

Adults, Elderly. 1 g/day in 2 divided doses, preferably q12h.

OFF-LABEL USES

Treatment of inflammatory bowel disease

CONTRAINDICATIONS

History of hypersensitivity to salicylates

INTERACTIONS

Drug

None known.

Herbal

None known.

Food

None known.

DIAGNOSTIC TEST EFFECTS

May increase AST (SGOT) and ALT (SGPT) levels.

SIDE EFFECTS

Frequent (10%–5%)

Headache, diarrhea, abdominal pain or cramps, nausea

Occasional (5%–1%)

Depression, fatigue, dyspepsia, upper respiratory tract infection, decreased appetite, rash, itching, arthralgia

Rare (1%)

Dizziness, vomiting, stomatitis

SERIOUS REACTIONS

! Sulfite sensitivity may occur in susceptible patients manifested by cramping, headache, diarrhea, fever, rash, hives, itching, and wheezing may occur. Discontinue drug immediately.

! Excessive diarrhea associated with extreme fatigue is noted rarely.

NURSING CONSIDERATIONS

Baseline Assessment

- Expect to obtain serum alkaline phosphatase, AST, and ALT levels.
- Before administering drug, determine if the patients has an allergy to sulfa-based products.

Precautions

- Use olsalazine cautiously in patients with pre-existing renal disease.

Administration and Handling

PO

- Give olsalazine with food in evenly divided doses.

Intervention and Evaluation

- Assess the patient's bowel sounds for peristalsis.
- Assess the patient's pattern of daily bowel activity and stool consistency and record time of evacuation.
- Evaluate the patient for abdominal disturbances.
- Assess the patient's skin for hives and rash.
- Discontinue olsalazine if the patient experiences cramping, diarrhea, fever, and rash.

Patient Teaching

- Warn the patient to notify physician if persistent or increasing cramping, diarrhea, fever, pruritus, and rash occur.
- Encourage the patient to maintain adequate fluid intake.

orlistat

ohr-lih-stat

(Xenical)

Do not confuse Xenical with Xeloda.

CATEGORY AND SCHEDULE

Pregnancy Risk Category: B

MECHANISM OF ACTION

A gastric and pancreatic lipase inhibitor that inhibits absorption of dietary fats by inactivating gastric and pancreatic enzymes. **Therapeutic Effect:** Resulting caloric deficit may positively affect weight control.

PHARMACOKINETICS

Minimal absorption after administration. Protein binding: 99%. Primarily eliminated unchanged in feces. Unknown if removed by hemodialysis. ***Half-life:*** 1–2 hr.

AVAILABILITY

Capsules: 120 mg.

INDICATIONS AND DOSAGES

▸ **Weight reduction**

PO

Adults, Elderly, Children 12–16 yr. 120 mg 3 times a day.

CONTRAINDICATIONS

Cholestasis, chronic malabsorption syndrome

INTERACTIONS

Drug

Pravastatin: May increase the blood concentration of pravastatin and risk of rhabdomyolysis.

Herbal

None known.

Food

None known.

DIAGNOSTIC TEST EFFECTS

Decreases blood glucose, total serum cholesterol, and serum LDL levels. Decreases absorption and levels of vitamins A and E.

SIDE EFFECTS

Frequent (30%–20%)

Headache, abdominal discomfort, flatulence, fecal urgency, fatty or oily stool

Occasional (14%–5%)
Back pain, menstrual irregularity, nausea, fatigue, diarrhea, dizziness
Rare (less than 4%)
Anxiety, rash, myalgia, dry skin, vomiting

SERIOUS REACTIONS

! None known.

NURSING CONSIDERATIONS

Baseline Assessment

• Expect to obtain laboratory studies, such as blood glucose levels and lipid profile.
• Obtain an accurate assessment of height and weight to help determine weight loss goals.
• Plan to consult a registered dietitian to review the patient's current diet, and to make dietary recommendations.

Lifespan Considerations

• It is unknown if orlistat is excreted in breast milk. Orlistat use is not recommended during pregnancy or in breast-feeding women.
• Safety and efficacy of orlistat have not been established in children.
• No age-related precautions have been noted in the elderly.

Administration and Handling

◀ALERT▶ Orlistat's side effects tend to be mild and transient in nature, gradually diminishing during treatment.
PO
• Give orlistat without regard to food.

Intervention and Evaluation

• Monitor the patient's blood glucose, cholesterol, and serum LDL levels.
• Monitor the patient for changes in coagulation parameters.

Patient Teaching

• Instruct the patient to maintain a nutritionally balanced, reduced-calorie diet. Teach the patient to distribute his or her daily intake of carbohydrates, fats, and protein over three main meals.
• Tell the patient that some of the unpleasant side effects, such as flatulence and urgency, should diminish with time.

pancreatin

pan-kree-**ah**-tin
(Ku-Zyme, Pancreatin)

pancrelipase

pan-kree-**lie**-pace
(Cotazym-S[AUS], Cotazym-S Forte[AUS], Creon, Pancrease[CAN], Pancrease MT, Ultrase, Viokase)

CATEGORY AND SCHEDULE

Pregnancy Risk Category: C

MECHANISM OF ACTION

Digestive enzymes that replace endogenous pancreatic enzymes. **Therapeutic Effect:** Assist in digestion of protein, starch, and fats.

AVAILABILITY

Capsules.
Tablets.

INDICATIONS AND DOSAGES

▸ **Pancreatic enzyme replacement or supplement when enzymes are absent or deficient, such as with chronic pancreatitis, cystic fibrosis, or ductal obstruction from cancer of the pancreas or common bile duct; to reduce malabsorption; treatment of steatorrhea associated with bowel resection or postgastrectomy syndrome**
PO
Adults, Elderly. 1–3 capsules or tablets before or with meals or

snacks. May increase to 8 tablets/dose.
Children. 1–2 tablets with meals or snacks.

CONTRAINDICATIONS

Acute pancreatitis, exacerbation of chronic pancreatitis, hypersensitivity to pork protein

INTERACTIONS

Drug

Antacids: May decrease the effects of pancreatin and pancrelipase.
Iron supplements: May decrease the absorption of iron supplements.

Herbal

None known.

Food

None known.

DIAGNOSTIC TEST EFFECTS

May increase serum uric acid level.

SIDE EFFECTS

Rare

Allergic reaction, mouth irritation, shortness of breath, wheezing

SERIOUS REACTIONS

! Excessive dosage may produce nausea, cramping, and diarrhea.
! Hyperuricosuria and hyperuricemia have occurred with extremely high dosages.

NURSING CONSIDERATIONS

Baseline Assessment

- Assess the patient's nutritional status before beginning and regularly throughout therapy.
- Determine if the patient is allergic to pork because hypersensitivity to pancreatin and pancrelipase may exist.

Lifespan Considerations

- It is unknown if pancreatin or pancrelipase cross the placenta or are distributed in breast milk.
- Information is not available on pancreatin or pancrelipase use in children.
- No age-related precautions have been noted in the elderly.

Precautions

- Use pancreatin and pancrelipase cautiously because inhalation of the powder form may precipitate an asthma attack.

Administration and Handling

PO

- Give pancreatin or pancrelipase before or with meals or snacks.
- Crush tablets as needed. Do not crush enteric-coated form.
- Spilling Viokase powder on the hands may irritate skin.
- Inhaling powder may irritate mucous membranes and produce bronchospasm.

Intervention and Evaluation

- Evaluate the patient for therapeutic response (relief from GI symptoms).
- Advise the patient not to change brands of the drug without first consulting the physician.

Patient Teaching

- Instruct the patient not to chew capsules or tablets, to minimize irritation to the mouth, lips, and tongue. If the patient cannot swallow capsules, instruct him or her to open capsules and spread contents over applesauce, mashed fruit, or rice cereal.
- Warn the patient not to spill Viokase powder on the hands because it may irritate the skin.
- Instruct the patient to avoid inhaling powder because it may irritate mucous membranes and produce bronchospasm.

simethicone

si-**meth**-i-kone
(Alka-Seltzer Gas Relief, Gas-X, Genasym, Infant Mylicon, Mylanta Gas, Ovol[CAN], Phazyme)

CATEGORY AND SCHEDULE

Pregnancy Risk Category: C
OTC

MECHANISM OF ACTION

An antiflatulent that changes surface tension of gas bubbles, allowing easier elimination of gas. **Therapeutic Effect:** Drug dispersal, prevents formation of gas pockets in the GI tract.

PHARMACOKINETICS

Does not appear to be absorbed from GI tract. Excreted unchanged in feces.

AVAILABILITY

Oral Drops (Infants Mylicon): 40 mg/0.6 ml.
Softgel (Alka-Seltzer Gas Relief, Gas-Z, Mylanta Gas): 125 mg.
Softgel (Phazyme): 180 mg.
Tablets (Chewable [Gas-X, Mylanta Gas]): 80 mg, 125 mg.

INDICATIONS AND DOSAGES

▸ **Antiflatulent**

PO

Adults, Elderly, Children 12 yr and older. 40–250 mg after meals and at bedtime. Maximum: 500 mg/day.
Children 2–11 yr. 40 mg 4 times a day.
Children younger than 2 yr. 20 mg 4 times a day.

OFF-LABEL USES

Adjunct to bowel radiography and gastroscopy

CONTRAINDICATIONS

None known.

INTERACTIONS

Drug

None known.

Herbal

None known.

Food

None known.

DIAGNOSTIC TEST EFFECTS

None known.

SIDE EFFECTS

None known.

SERIOUS REACTIONS

! None known.

NURSING CONSIDERATIONS

Baseline Assessment

- Before simethicone administration, assess the patient's abdomen for signs of tenderness, rigidity, and the presence of bowel sounds.
- Determine when the patient last had a bowel movement, and find out the amount and consistency.

Lifespan Considerations

- It is unknown if simethicone crosses the placenta or is distributed in breast milk.
- Simethicone may be used safely in children and the elderly.

Administration and Handling

PO

- Give simethicone after meals and at bedtime, as needed. Have the patient chew tablets thoroughly before swallowing.
- Shake suspension well before using.

Intervention and Evaluation

- Evaluate the patient for therapeutic response (relief of abdominal bloating and flatulence).

Patient Teaching

• Urge the patient to avoid carbonated beverages during simethicone therapy.
• Instruct the patient to chew tablets thoroughly before swallowing.

sucralfate

soo-**kral**-fate
(Apo-Sucralate[CAN], Carafate, Novo-Sucralate[CAN], Ulcyte[AUS])
Do not confuse Carafate with Cafergot.

CATEGORY AND SCHEDULE

Pregnancy Risk Category: B

MECHANISM OF ACTION

An antiulcer agent that forms an ulcer-adherent complex with proteinaceous exudate, such as albumin, at ulcer site. Also forms a viscous, adhesive barrier on the surface of intact mucosa of the stomach or duodenum. **Therapeutic Effect:** Protects damaged mucosa from further destruction by absorbing gastric acid, pepsin, and bile salts.

PHARMACOKINETICS

Minimally absorbed from the GI tract. Eliminated in feces, with small amount excreted in urine. Not removed by hemodialysis.

AVAILABILITY

Oral Suspension: 500 mg/ 5 ml.
Tablets: 1 g.

INDICATIONS AND DOSAGES

▸ **Active duodenal ulcers**
PO
Adults, Elderly. 1 g 4 times a day (before meals and at bedtime) for up to 8 wk.

▸ **Maintenance therapy after healing of acute duodenal ulcers**
PO
Adults, Elderly. 1 g twice a day.

OFF-LABEL USES

Prevention and treatment of stress-related mucosal damage, especially in acutely or critically ill patients; treatment of gastric ulcer and rheumatoid arthritis; relief of GI symptoms associated with NSAIDs; treatment of gastroesophageal reflux disease

CONTRAINDICATIONS

None known.

INTERACTIONS

Drug

Antacids: May interfere with binding of sucralfate.
Digoxin, phenytoin, quinolones, such as ciprofloxacin, theophylline: May decrease the absorption of these drugs.

Herbal

None known.

Food

None known.

DIAGNOSTIC TEST EFFECTS

None known.

SIDE EFFECTS

Frequent (2%)
Constipation
Occasional (less than 2%)
Dry mouth, backache, diarrhea, dizziness, somnolence, nausea, indigestion, rash, hives, itching, abdominal discomfort

SERIOUS REACTIONS

! None known.

NURSING CONSIDERATIONS

Baseline Assessment

• Before sucralfate administration, assess the patient's abdomen for signs of tenderness, rigidity, and the presence of bowel sounds.
• Determine when the patient last had a bowel movement, and find out the amount and consistency.

Lifespan Considerations

• It is unknown if sucralfate crosses the placenta or is distributed in breast milk.
• Safety and efficacy of sucralfate have not been established in children.
• No age-related precautions have been noted in the elderly.

Administration and Handling

◀ **ALERT** ▶ Know that 1 g equals 10 ml suspension.

PO

• Administer 1 hour before meals and at bedtime.
• Tablets may be crushed or dissolved in water.
• Do not give antacids within 30 minutes of sucralfate.
• Do not give digoxin, phenytoin, quinolones, or theophylline within 2 to 3 hours of sucralfate.

Intervention and Evaluation

• Assess the patient's pattern of daily bowel activity and stool consistency.

Patient Teaching

• Instruct the patient to take sucralfate on an empty stomach.
• Teach the patient that antacids should not be taken for 30 minutes before or after sucralfate because the formation of sucralfate gel is activated by stomach acid.
• Suggest that the patient take sips of tepid water or suck on sour hard candy to relieve dry mouth.

sulfasalazine

See Miscellaneous Anti-infective Agents

tegaserod

teh-**gas**-er-od
(Zelnorm)

CATEGORY AND SCHEDULE

Pregnancy Risk Category: B

MECHANISM OF ACTION

An anti-irritable bowel syndrome (IBS) agent that binds to 5-HT_4 receptors in the GI tract. **Therapeutic Effect:** Triggers a peristaltic reflex in the gut, increasing bowel motility.

PHARMACOKINETICS

Rapidly absorbed. Widely distributed. Protein binding: 98%. Metabolized by hydrolysis in the stomach and by oxidation and conjugation of the primary metabolite. Primarily excreted in feces. ***Half-life:*** 11 hr.

AVAILABILITY

Tablets: 2 mg, 6 mg.

INDICATIONS AND DOSAGES

▸ **IBS**

PO

Adults, Elderly women. 6 mg twice a day for 4–6 wk.

▸ **Chronic constipation**

PO

Adults. 6 mg twice a day.

CONTRAINDICATIONS

Abdominal adhesions, diarrhea, history of bowel obstruction, moderate to severe hepatic impairment, severe renal impairment, suspected sphincter of Oddi dysfunction, symptomatic gallbladder disease

INTERACTIONS

Drug

None known.

Herbal

None known.

Food

None known.

DIAGNOSTIC TEST EFFECTS

None known.

SIDE EFFECTS

Frequency (greater than 5%)

Headache, abdominal pain, diarrhea, nausea, flatulence

Occasional (5%–2%)

Dizziness, migraine, back pain, extremity pain

SERIOUS REACTIONS

! None known.

NURSING CONSIDERATIONS

Baseline Assessment

• Avoid tegaserod use if the patient has diarrhea.

Lifespan Considerations

• It is unknown if tegaserod is distributed in breast milk.

• Safety and efficacy of tegaserod have not been established in children.

• No age-related precautions have been noted in the elderly.

Administration and Handling

PO

• Give tegaserod before meals.

• Crush tablets as needed.

Intervention and Evaluation

• Evaluate the patient for therapeutic response (relief from abdominal discomfort, bloating, cramping, and urgency).

Patient Teaching

• Instruct the patient to take tegaserod before meals.

• Warn the patient to notify the physician if new or worsening episodes of abdominal pain or severe diarrhea occur.

ursodiol

your-**soo**-dee-ol

(Actigall, Urso)

CATEGORY AND SCHEDULE

Pregnancy Risk Category: B

MECHANISM OF ACTION

A gallstone solubilizing agent that suppresses hepatic synthesis and secretion of cholesterol; inhibits intestinal absorption of cholesterol. **Therapeutic Effect:** Changes the bile of patients with gallstones from precipitating (capable of forming crystals) to cholesterol solubilizing (capable of being dissolved).

AVAILABILITY

Capsules: 300 mg.
Tablets: 250 mg.

INDICATIONS AND DOSAGES

▸ **Dissolution of radiolucent, noncalcified gallstones when cholecystectomy is not recommended; treatment of biliary cirrhosis**

PO

Adults, Elderly. 8–10 mg/kg/day in 2–3 divided doses. Treatment may require months. Obtain ultrasound image of gallbladder at 6-mo intervals for first year. If gallstones have dissolved, continue therapy and repeat ultrasound within 1–3 mo.

▸ **Prevention of gallstones**

PO

Adults, Elderly. 300 mg twice a day.

OFF-LABEL USES

Treatment of alcoholic cirrhosis, biliary atresia, chronic hepatitis, gallstone formation, sclerosing cholangitis, prophylaxis of liver transplant rejection

CONTRAINDICATIONS

Allergy to bile acids, calcified cholesterol stones, chronic hepatic disease, radiolucent bile pigment stones, radiopaque stones

INTERACTIONS

Drug

Aluminum-containing antacids, cholestyramine: May decrease the absorption and effects of ursodiol.
Estrogens, oral contraceptives: May decrease the effects of ursodiol.

Herbal

None known.

Food

None known.

DIAGNOSTIC TEST EFFECTS

May alter liver functions test results.

SIDE EFFECTS

Occasional

Diarrhea

SERIOUS REACTIONS

! None significant.

NURSING CONSIDERATIONS

Baseline Assessment

- Obtain the patient's blood serum chemistry values including BUN, serum alkaline phosphatase, bilirubin, creatinine, AST (SGOT), and ALT (SGPT) levels before the start of ursodiol therapy, 1 and 3 months after therapy begins, and every 6 months thereafter, to assess hepatic function.

Administration and Handling

- Administer with meals or a snack because the drug dissolves more readily in the presence of bile acid and pancreatic juice.

Intervention and Evaluation

- Monitor the patient's liver function test results.
- Assess the patient for abdominal pain, especially right upper quadrant pain, nausea, and vomiting.

Patient Teaching

- Explain to the patient that ursodiol therapy requires months.
- Instruct the patient to avoid taking antacids within hours of taking ursodiol.

55 Anticoagulants

argatroban
bivalirudin
dalteparin sodium
desirudin
enoxaparin sodium
fondaparinux sodium
heparin sodium
lepirudin
tinzaparin sodium
warfarin sodium

Uses: Subclasses of anticoagulants have somewhat different indications. *Heparin* is used to treat pulmonary embolism, evolving stroke, and massive deep vein thrombosis (DVT). It's also used as an adjunct to thrombolytics to treat acute MI and in low doses to prevent postoperative venous thrombosis. *Low-molecular-weight (LMW) heparins* are used to prevent DVT after hip or knee replacement surgery and to treat DVT, ischemic stroke, pulmonary embolism, and non Q-wave MI. *Thrombin inhibitors* are prescribed for preventing and treating thrombosis in heparin-induced thrombocytopenia (HIT) and for preventing HIT during percutaneous coronary procedures. *Warfarin* is used to prevent venous thrombosis and associated pulmonary embolism.

Action: Each anticoagulant subclass acts by a different mechanism. *Heparin* combines with antithrombin III, accelerating the anticoagulant cascade that prevents thrombosis formation. (See the illustration *Mechanisms and Sites of Action: Hematologic Agents,* page 1036.) It inhibits the action of thrombin and factor Xa. By preventing the conversion of fibrinogen to fibrin, heparin prevents the formation of fibrin clots. *LMW heparins,* such as dalteparin and enoxaparin, are composed of shorter molecules than those in standard heparin. These agents preferentially inactivate factor Xa. *Thrombin inhibitors,* such as argatroban and bivalirudin, reversibly inhibit thrombin by binding to its receptor sites. *Warfarin* suppresses coagulation by acting as a vitamin K antagonist. It does this by blocking the synthesis of vitamin K–dependent factors (factors VII, IX, X, and prothrombin).

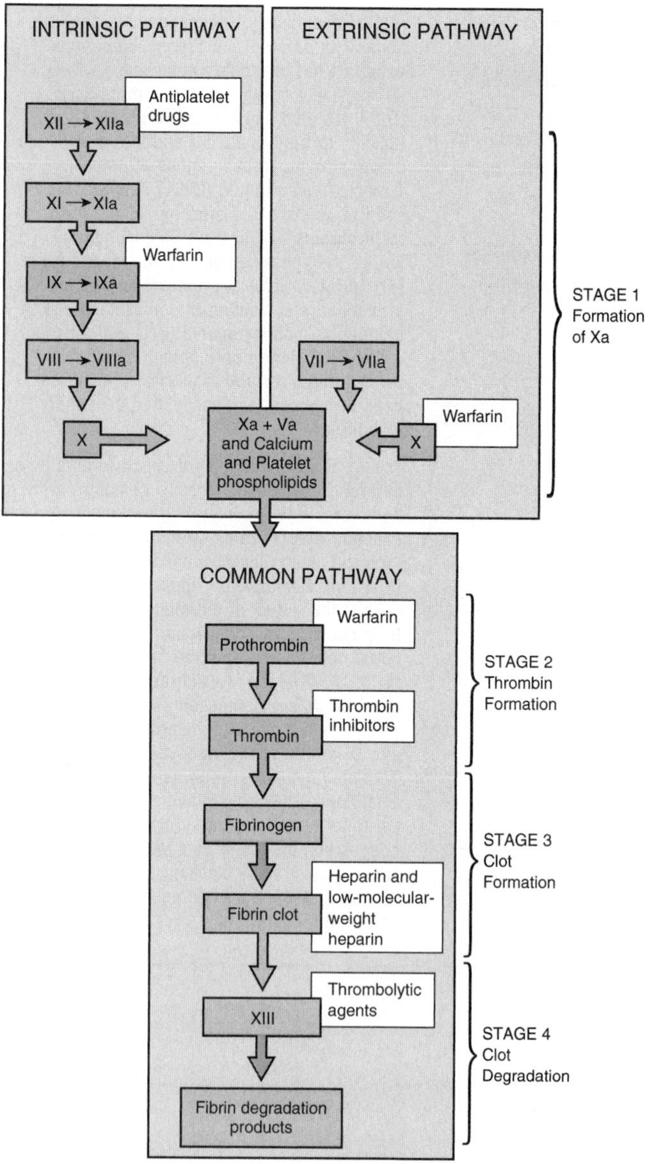
INTRINSIC PATHWAY
EXTRINSIC PATHWAY
Antiplatelet drugs
XII → XIIa
XI → XIa
Warfarin
IX → IXa
VIII → VIIIa
X
VII → VIIa
Warfarin
X
Xa + Va and Calcium and Platelet phospholipids
STAGE 1 Formation of Xa
COMMON PATHWAY
Warfarin
Prothrombin
Thrombin inhibitors
Thrombin
STAGE 2 Thrombin Formation
Fibrinogen
Heparin and low-molecular-weight heparin
Fibrin clot
STAGE 3 Clot Formation
Thrombolytic agents
XIII
Fibrin degradation products
STAGE 4 Clot Degradation

Mechanisms and Sites of Action: Hematologic Agents

Hemostasis causes the formation of a fibrin-platelet meshwork (clot) to stop bleeding. It results from activation of the coagulation cascade, which consists of intrinsic, extrinsic, and common pathways. Drugs that affect hemostasis include anticoagulants and antiplatelets (which prevent clot formation) and thrombolytics (which dissolve already-formed clots).

Different anticoagulants act at various points in the cascade. For example, heparin enhances antithrombin III in the plasma to inactivate factor Xa. As a result, prothrombin can't be converted to thrombin, which prevents fibrinogen from forming fibrin, a major clot component. Low-molecular-weight heparins, such as dalteparin, also inactivate factor Xa and thrombin by enhancing antithrombin III, ultimately preventing fibrinogen from forming fibrin. Thrombin inhibitors, such as argatroban, reversibly inhibit thrombin by binding to its receptor sites. This action prevents the conversion of fibrinogen to a fibrin clot. Warfarin depletes vitamin K–dependent factors X, IX, VII, and prothrombin. Consequently new clots can't form, and pre-existing clots can't extend.

Antiplatelet drugs inhibit platelet aggregation—and clotting—in different ways. Platelet aggregation and adhesion starts at the beginning of the clotting cascade that ultimately results in inactivated factor X. Aspirin inhibits cyclooxygenase and blocks the production of thromboxane A_2, a substance that causes vasoconstriction and platelet aggregation. Ticlopidine alters platelet membranes, preventing them from interacting. Dipyridamole stimulates prostacyclin release, which blocks thromboxane A_2 formation. Adenosine diphosphate (ADP) receptor antagonists, such as clopidogrel, block ADP receptors on platelets, inhibiting their aggregation. GP IIb/IIIa receptor inhibitors, such as abciximab, prevent fibrinogen from binding to GP IIb/IIIa receptors on platelets, rapidly inhibiting platelet aggregation.

Thrombolytic agents, such as streptokinase, break down clots that have already formed. They trigger the conversion of plasminogen to plasmin, an enzyme that dissolves fibrin clots into fibrin degradation products.

---

argatroban

ar-**gat**-tro-ban

(Acova)

Do not confuse argatroban with Aggrestat or Orgaran.

CATEGORY AND SCHEDULE

Pregnancy Risk Category: B

MECHANISM OF ACTION

A direct thrombin inhibitor that reversibly binds to thrombin-active sites. Inhibits thrombin-catalyzed or thrombin-induced reactions, including fibrin formation, activation of coagulant factors V, VIII, and XIII; also inhibits protein C formation; and platelet aggregation.

Therapeutic Effect: Produces anticoagulation.

PHARMACOKINETICS

Following IV administration, distributed primarily in extracellular fluid. Protein binding: 54%. Metabolized in the liver. Primarily excreted in the feces, presumably through biliary secretion. ***Half-life:*** 39–51 min.

AVAILABILITY

Injection: 100 mg/ml.

INDICATIONS AND DOSAGES

▸ **To prevent and treat heparin-induced thrombocytopenia**

IV Infusion

Adults, Elderly. Initially, 2 mcg/kg/min administered as a continuous infusion. After initial infusion, dose may be adjusted until steady state aPTT is 1.5–3 times initial baseline value, not to exceed 100 sec.

▸ **Percutaneous coronary intervention**

IV Infusion

Adults, Elderly. Initially, 25 mcg/kg/min and administer bolus of 350 mcg/kg over 3–5 min. ACT (activated clotting time) checked in 5–10 min following bolus. If ACT is less than 300 sec, give additional bolus 150 mcg/kg, increase infusion to 30 mcg/kg/min. If ACT is greater than 450 sec, decrease infusion to 15 mcg/kg/min. Once ACT of 300–450 sec achieved, proceed with procedure.

▸ **Dosage in hepatic impairment**

Adults, Elderly. Initially, 0.5 mcg/kg/min.

CONTRAINDICATIONS

Overt major bleeding

INTERACTIONS

Drug

Antiplatelet agents, thrombolytics, other anticoagulants: May increase the risk of bleeding.

Herbal

None known.

Food

None known.

DIAGNOSTIC TEST EFFECTS

Increases aPTT, international normalized ratio, and PT

IV INCOMPATIBILITIES

Do not mix with other medications or solutions.

SIDE EFFECTS

Frequent (8%–3%)

Dyspnea, hypotension, fever, diarrhea, nausea, pain, vomiting, infection, cough

SERIOUS REACTIONS

! Ventricular tachycardia and atrial fibrillation occur occasionally.

! Major bleeding and sepsis occur rarely.

NURSING CONSIDERATIONS

Baseline Assessment

- Evaluate the patient's CBC.
- Check the patient's PT and aPTT.
- Expect to obtain the patient's BP before therapy begins.
- Minimize procedures that involve puncturing the skin. Avoid numerous blood draws, catheter insertions, and injections.

Lifespan Considerations

- It is unknown if argatroban is excreted in breast milk.
- Safety and efficacy of argatroban have not been established in children younger than 18 years of age.
- No age-related precautions have been noted in the elderly.

Precautions

- Use argatroban cautiously in patients with congenital or acquired bleeding disorders, hepatic impairment, severe hypertension, or ulcerations.
- Use cautiously immediately following administration of spinal anesthesia, lumbar puncture, and major surgery.

Administration and Handling

IV

- Discard the solution if it appears cloudy or has an insoluble precipitate. Avoid exposing the solution to direct sunlight.
- Following reconstitution, the solution is stable for 24 hours at room temperature and for 48 hours if refrigerated.
- Before infusion, dilute the solution 100-fold in 0.9% NaCl, D_5W, or lactated Ringer's solution to provide a final concentration of 1 mg/ml.

• Mix the solution by repeatedly inverting the diluent bag for 1 minute.
• Following reconstitution, the solution may briefly appear hazy because of formation of microprecipitates. These rapidly dissolve when the solution is mixed.
• Rate of administration is based on body weight at 2 mcg/kg/min (for example, for a 50-kg patient, infuse at rate of 6 ml/hr).

Intervention and Evaluation

• Assess the patient for signs of bleeding, such as bleeding at a surgical site, or from the gums or injection sites; blood in the stool; ecchymosis; hematuria; and petechiae.
• Handle the patient carefully and as infrequently as possible to prevent bleeding. Do not obtain BP in the lower extremities, because a deep-vein thrombus may be present.
• Monitor the patient's activated coagulation time, aPTT, PT, and platelet count.
• Monitor the patient for any complaints of abdominal or back pain, a decrease in BP, increase in pulse rate, and severe headache, which indicates hemorrhage.
• Observe the patient for an increase in menstrual flow.
• Test the patient's urine for hematuria.
• Monitor the patient for hematomas.
• Gently remove the patient's dressings and tape.

Patient Teaching

• Instruct the patient to use an electric razor and soft toothbrush, to prevent bleeding.
• Warn the patient to report black or red stool, coffee-ground vomitus, red or dark urine, or blood-tinged mucus from cough.

bivalirudin

bye-va-**leer**-u-din
(Angiomax)

CATEGORY AND SCHEDULE

Pregnancy Risk Category: B

MECHANISM OF ACTION

An anticoagulant that specifically and reversibly inhibits thrombin by binding to its receptor sites. **Therapeutic Effect:** Decreases acute ischemic complications in patients with unstable angina pectoris.

PHARMACOKINETICS

Route	Onset	Peak	Duration
IV	Immediate	N/A	1 hr

Primarily eliminated by kidneys. Twenty-five percent removed by hemodialysis. ***Half-life:*** 25 min (increased in moderate to severe renal impairment).

AVAILABILITY

Injection, Powder for Reconstitution: 250 mg.

INDICATIONS AND DOSAGES

▸ Anticoagulant in patients with unstable angina who are undergoing percutaneous transluminal coronary angioplasty (PTCA) in conjunction with aspirin

IV

Adults, Elderly. 1 mg/kg as IV bolus followed by 4-hr IV infusion at rate of 2.5 mg/kg/hr. After initial 4-hr infusion is completed, give additional IV infusion at rate of 0.2 mg/kg/hr for 20 hr or less, if necessary.

▸ **Dosage in renal impairment**

GFR	Dosage Reduced by
30–59 ml/min	20%
10–29 ml/min	60%
Dialysis	90%

CONTRAINDICATIONS
Active major bleeding

INTERACTIONS
Drug

Platelet aggregation inhibitors other than aspirin, thrombolytics, warfarin: May increase the risk of bleeding complications.

Herbal

Ginkgo biloba: May increase the risk of bleeding.

Food

None known.

DIAGNOSTIC TEST EFFECTS
Prolongs aPTT and PT.

IV INCOMPATIBILITIES
Do not mix with other medications.

SIDE EFFECTS
Frequent (42%)

Back pain

Occasional (15%–12%)

Nausea, headache, hypotension, generalized pain

Rare (8%–4%)

Injection site pain, insomnia, hypertension, anxiety, vomiting, pelvic or abdominal pain, bradycardia, nervousness, dyspepsia, fever, urine retention

SERIOUS REACTIONS
! A hemorrhagic event occurs rarely and is characterized by a fall in BP or Hct.

NURSING CONSIDERATIONS
Baseline Assessment

- Establish the patient's baseline BP.
- Obtain the patient's bleeding time, CBC, and BUN and serum creatinine levels to assess renal function.

Lifespan Considerations

- It is unknown if bivalirudin is distributed in breast milk or crosses the placenta.
- Safety and efficacy of bivalirudin have not been established in children.
- In the elderly, age-related renal impairment may require dosage adjustment.

Precautions

- Use bivalirudin cautiously in patients with conditions associated with increased risk of bleeding, including bacterial endocarditis, cerebrovascular accident, hemorrhagic diathesis, intracerebral surgery, recent major bleeding, recent major surgery, stroke, severe hypertension, and severe hepatic or renal impairment.

Administration and Handling

◀ALERT▶ Bivalirudin is intended for use with aspirin, 300–325 mg daily.

◀ALERT▶ Treatment should be initiated immediately before angioplasty.

IV

- Store unreconstituted vials at room temperature. Reconstituted solution may be refrigerated for no more than 24 hours.
- Diluted drug with a concentration of 0.5 to 5 mg/ml is stable at room temperature for 24 hours or less.
- To each 250-mg vial add 5 ml sterile water for injection. Gently swirl until all material is dissolved.
- Further dilute each vial in 50 ml D_5W or 0.9% NaCl to yield final concentration of 5 mg/ml: 1 vial in 50 ml, 2 vials in 100 ml, 5 vials in 250 ml.
- If low-rate infusion is used after

the initial infusion, reconstitute the 250-mg vial with an additional 5 ml sterile water for injection. Gently swirl until all material is dissolved.
- Further dilute each vial in 500 ml D_5W or 0.9% NaCl to yield final concentration of 0.5 mg/ml.
- Diluting produces a clear, colorless solution; do not use solution if it is cloudy or contains a precipitate.
- Expect to adjust IV infusion based on aPTT or patient's body weight.

Intervention and Evaluation

- Monitor the patient's aPTT, Hct, BUN and serum creatinine levels, and stool or urine cultures for occult blood.
- Assess the patient for a decrease in BP and an increase in pulse rate.
- Determine the amount of female patient's menstrual discharge and monitor for any increase.
- Assess the patient's urine for hematuria.

Patient Teaching

- Warn female patient that her menstrual flow may be heavier than usual.
- Instruct the patient to report blood in the urine or stool.
- Urge the patient to report discomfort or pain, especially chest pain, after treatment.
- Instruct the patient to remain on bed rest and to keep the leg used during PTCA immobile, as ordered. Tell the patient to report bleeding from femoral vein site.

dalteparin sodium

doll-teh-pare-in
(Fragmin)

CATEGORY AND SCHEDULE

Pregnancy Risk Category: B

MECHANISM OF ACTION

An antithrombin that inhibits factor Xa and thrombin in the presence of low-molecular-weight heparin. Only slightly influences platelet aggregation, PT, and aPTT. **Therapeutic Effect:** Produces anticoagulation.

PHARMACOKINETICS

Route	Onset	Peak	Duration
Subcutaneous	N/A	4 hr	N/A

Protein binding: less than 10%. ***Half-life:*** 3–5 hr.

AVAILABILITY

Syringe: 2,500 international units/0.2 ml, 5,000 international units/0.2 ml, 7,500 international units/0.3 ml, 10,000 international units/ml.
Vial: 10,000 international units/ml, 25,000 international units/ml.

INDICATIONS AND DOSAGES

▸ Low- to moderate-risk abdominal surgery

Subcutaneous

Adults, Elderly. 2,500 international units 1–2 hr before surgery, then daily for 5–10 days.

▸ High-risk abdominal surgery

Subcutaneous

Adults, Elderly. 5,000 international units 1–2 hr before surgery, then daily for 5–10 days.

▸ Total hip surgery

Subcutaneous

Adults, Elderly. 2,500 international units 1–2 hr before surgery, then 2,500 units 6 hr after surgery, then 5,000 units/day for 7–10 days.

▸ Unstable angina, non–Q-wave MI

Subcutaneous

Adults, Elderly. 120 international units/kg q12h (maximum: 10,000 international units/dose) given with aspirin until clinically stable.

▸ **Prevention of DVT or PE in the acutely ill patient**

Subcutaneous

Adults, Elderly. 5,000 international units once a day.

CONTRAINDICATIONS

Active major bleeding; concurrent heparin therapy; hypersensitivity to dalteparin, heparin, or pork products; thrombocytopenia associated with positive in vitro test for antiplatelet antibody

INTERACTIONS

Drug

Anticoagulants, platelet inhibitors: May increase risk of bleeding.

Herbal

None known.

Food

None known.

DIAGNOSTIC TEST EFFECTS

Increases (reversible) LDH, serum alkaline phosphatase, AST (SGOT), and ALT (SGPT) levels.

SIDE EFFECTS

Occasional (7%–3%)

Hematoma at injection site

Rare (less than 1%)

Hypersensitivity reaction (chills, fever, pruritus, urticaria, asthma, rhinitis, lacrimation, headache); mild, local skin irritation

SERIOUS REACTIONS

! Overdose may lead to bleeding complications ranging from local ecchymoses to major hemorrhage.

! Thrombocytopenia occurs rarely.

NURSING CONSIDERATIONS

Baseline Assessment

- Assess the patient's CBC.
- Establish the patient's baseline BP.

Lifespan Considerations

- Dalteparin should be used with caution in pregnant women, particularly during the last trimester and immediately postpartum because it increases the risk of maternal hemorrhage.
- It is unknown if dalteparin is distributed in breast milk.
- Safety and efficacy of dalteparin have not been established in children.
- No age-related precautions have been noted in the elderly.

Precautions

- Use dalteparin cautiously in patients with bacterial endocarditis, conditions with increased risk of hemorrhage, history of heparin-induced thrombocytopenia, recent GI ulceration and hemorrhage, hypertensive or diabetic retinopathy, impaired hepatic or renal function, or uncontrolled arterial hypertension.

Administration and Handling

Subcutaneous

- Store drug at room temperature.
- Instruct the patient to sit or lie down before administering by deep subcutaneous injection.
- Inject into U-shaped area around the navel, upper outer side of thigh, or upper outer quadrangle of buttock.
- Use a fine needle (25- to 26-gauge) to minimize tissue trauma.
- Introduce the entire length of the needle (one-half inch) into skin-fold held between the thumb and forefinger, holding the needle during injection at a 45- to 90-degree angle.
- Do not rub injection site after administration to avoid bruising.
- Alternate administration site with each injection.

Intervention and Evaluation

- Periodically monitor the patient's CBC and stool for occult blood. There is no need for daily monitoring

in patients with normal presurgical coagulation parameters.
- Assess the patient for signs of bleeding, including bleeding at surgical or injection sites or from gums, hematuria, blood in stool, bruising, and petechiae.

Patient Teaching
- Explain to the patient that the usual length of dalteparin therapy is 5 to 10 days.
- Warn the patient to notify the physician of signs of bleeding, breathing difficulty, bruising, dizziness, fever, itching, lightheadedness, rash, and swelling.
- Advise the patient not to take other medications, including OTC drugs, without physician approval.
- Instruct the patient to rotate injection sites daily.
- Teach the patient proper injection technique.
- Instruct the patient to perform an ice massage at the injection site shortly before injection, to prevent excessive bruising.

desirudin
deh-**sear**-ew-din
(Iprivask)

CATEGORY AND SCHEDULE
Pregnancy Risk Category: C

MECHANISM OF ACTION
An anticoagulant that binds specifically and directly to thrombin, inhibiting free circulating and clot-bound thrombin. **Therapeutic Effect:** Prolongs the clotting time of human plasma.

PHARMACOKINETICS
Completely absorbed. Distributed in extracellular space. Metabolized and eliminated by the kidney. ***Half-life:*** 2–3 hr.

AVAILABILITY
Powder for Injection: 15-mg vial with diluent (diluent includes 0.6 ml mannitol (3%) in water for injection).

INDICATIONS AND DOSAGES
▸ **Prevention of deep vein thrombosis in patients undergoing hip replacement surgery**
Subcutaneous
Adults, Elderly. Initially, 15 mg q12h given 5–15 min before surgery but following induction of regional block anesthesia, if used. May administer up to 12 days postsurgery.

▸ **Moderate renal impairment (creatinine clearance 31–60 ml/min or higher)**
Subcutaneous
Adults, Elderly. 5 mg q12h.

▸ **Severe renal impairment (creatinine clearance less than 31 ml/min)**
Subcutaneous
Adults, Elderly. 1.7 mg q12h.

CONTRAINDICATIONS
Hypersensitivity to natural or recombinant hirudins (anticoagulation factors), active bleeding, irreversible coagulation disorders

INTERACTIONS
Drug
Anticoagulants, dextran 40, systemic glucocorticoids, thrombolytics: Increase the risk of bleeding and should be discontinued before start of desirudin therapy.
Herbal
None known.
Food
None known.

DIAGNOSTIC TEST EFFECTS

May increase aPTT. May decrease Hgb, and Hct concentrations.

SIDE EFFECTS

Frequent (6%)
Hematoma
Occasional (4%–2%)
Injection site mass, wound secretion, nausea, hypersensitivity reaction

SERIOUS REACTIONS

! Serious or major hemorrhage and anaphylactic reaction occur rarely.

NURSING CONSIDERATIONS

Baseline Assessment

- Before beginning desirudin therapy, discontinue any medication that may enhance the risk of hemorrhage.
- Establish the patient's aPTT and BUN and serum creatinine levels to assess hepatic and renal function.
- Avoid overinflating the cuff when monitoring the patient's BP.
- Remove adhesive tape from pressure dressings very carefully and slowly.

Lifespan Considerations

- Desirudin may be teratogenic and it is unknown if the drug is distributed in breast milk.
- Safety and efficacy of desirudin have not been established in children.
- In the elderly, age-related renal impairment may require dosage adjustment.

Precautions

- Use desirudin cautiously in patients with epidural or spinal anesthesia, renal impairment, or increased risk of hemorrhage, including bacterial endocarditis, hemophilia, history of GI or pulmonary bleeding within the past 3 months, history of hemorrhagic stroke, intracranial or intraocular bleeding, organ biopsy, puncture of a noncompressible vessel within the last month, recent major surgery, and severe uncontrolled hypertension.

Administration and Handling

Subcutaneous

- Store vials at room temperature.
- Reconstitute each vial with 0.5 ml provided diluent. Gently agitate or rotate. Use reconstituted solution immediately; however, it is stable for up to 24 hours if stored at room temperature. Discard unused portion.
- Using a 26- or 27-gauge needle about one-half inch long, withdraw reconstituted solution and administer by deep subcutaneous injection, alternating sites between left and right anterolateral and left and right posterolateral abdominal wall. Introduce entire length of needle into skin fold held between thumb and forefinger, holding skin fold during injection.

Intervention and Evaluation

- Monitor aPTT and serum creatinine level daily in patients with renal impairment or an increased risk of bleeding. Expect to reduce dosage if peak aPTT exceeds 2 times control.
- Assess the patient for abdominal or back pain, a decrease in BP and Hct, an increase in pulse rate, and severe headache because these signs may indicate hemorrhage.
- Determine the amount of female patient's menstrual discharge and monitor for an increase.
- Assess the patient's gums for erythema and gingival bleeding, skin for bruises, and urine for hematuria.
- Examine the patient for excessive bleeding from minor cuts and scratches.

Patient Teaching

- Tell the patient to use an electric razor and soft toothbrush to prevent bleeding during therapy.
- Advise the patient not to take other

medications, including OTC drugs (especially aspirin), without physician approval.

• Warn the patient to report black or red stool, coffee-ground vomitus, dark or red urine, or red-speckled mucus from cough.

• Caution female patient that her menstrual flow may be heavier than usual.

enoxaparin sodium

e-nox-ah-**pair**-in

(Clexane[AUS], Klexane[CAN], Lovenox)

Do not confuse Lovenox with Lotronex.

CATEGORY AND SCHEDULE

Pregnancy Risk Category: B

MECHANISM OF ACTION

A low-molecular-weight heparin that potentiates the action of antithrombin III and inactivates coagulation factor Xa. **Therapeutic Effect:** Produces anticoagulation. Does not significantly influence bleeding time, PT, or aPTT.

PHARMACOKINETICS

Route	Onset	Peak	Duration
Subcutaneous	N/A	3–5 hr	12 hr

Well absorbed after subcutaneous administration. Eliminated primarily in urine. Not removed by hemodialysis. ***Half-life:*** 4.5 hr.

AVAILABILITY

Injection: 30 mg/0.3 ml, 40 mg/0.4 ml, 60 mg/0.6 ml, 80 mg/0.8 ml, 100 mg/ml, 120 mg/0.8 ml, 150 mg/ml in prefilled syringes.

INDICATIONS AND DOSAGES

▸ Prevention of deep vein thrombosis (DVT) after hip and knee surgery

Subcutaneous

Adults, Elderly. 30 mg twice a day, generally for 7–10 days.

▸ Prevention of DVT after abdominal surgery

Subcutaneous

Adults, Elderly. 40 mg a day for 7–10 days.

▸ Prevention of long-term DVT in nonsurgical acute illness

Subcutaneous

Adults, Elderly. 40 mg once a day for 3 wk.

▸ Prevention of ischemic complications of unstable angina and non-Q-wave MI (with oral aspirin therapy)

Subcutaneous

Adults, Elderly. 1 mg/kg q12h.

▸ Acute DVT

Subcutaneous

Adults, Elderly. 1 mg/kg q12h or 1.5 mg/kg once daily.

▸ Usual pediatric dosage

Subcutaneous

Children. 0.5 mg/kg q12h (prophylaxis); 1 mg/kg q12h (treatment).

▸ Dosage in renal impairment

Clearance of enoxaparin is decreased when creatinine clearance is less than 30 ml/min. Monitor patient and adjust dosage as necessary. When enoxaparin is used in abdominal, hip, or knee surgery or acute illness, the dosage in renal impairment is 30 mg once a day. When enoxaparin is used to treat DVT, angina, or MI, the dosage in renal impairment is 1 mg/kg once a day.

OFF-LABEL USES

Prevention of DVT following general surgical procedures

CONTRAINDICATIONS

Active major bleeding, concurrent heparin therapy, hypersensitivity to heparin or pork products, thrombocytopenia associated with positive in vitro test for antiplatelet antibodies

INTERACTIONS

Drug

Anticoagulants, platelet inhibitors: May increase bleeding.

Herbal

None known.

Food

None known.

DIAGNOSTIC TEST EFFECTS

Increases (reversible) LDH, serum alkaline phosphatase, AST (SGOT), and ALT (SGPT) levels.

SIDE EFFECTS

Occasional (4%–1%)

Injection site hematoma, nausea, peripheral edema

SERIOUS REACTIONS

! Overdose may lead to bleeding complications ranging from local ecchymoses to major hemorrhage. Antidote: Protamine sulfate (1% solution) equal to the dose of enoxaparin injected. One mg protamine sulfate neutralizes 1 mg enoxaparin. A second dose of 0.5 mg protamine sulfate per 1 mg enoxaparin may be given if aPTT tested 2–4 hr after first injection remains prolonged.

NURSING CONSIDERATIONS

Baseline Assessment

- Assess the patient's CBC.
- Ask the patient's about allergies, especially to heparin or pork products.

Lifespan Considerations

- Enoxaparin should be used with caution in pregnant women, particularly during the last trimester and immediately postpartum because it increases the risk of maternal hemorrhage.
- It is unknown if enoxaparin is excreted in breast milk.
- Safety and efficacy of enoxaparin have not been established in children.
- The elderly may be more susceptible to bleeding.

Precautions

- Use enoxaparin cautiously in the elderly and in patients with conditions associated with increased risk of hemorrhage, history of recent GI ulceration and hemorrhage, history of heparin-induced thrombocytopenia, impaired renal function, or uncontrolled arterial hypertension.

Administration and Handling

◀ALERT▶ Do not mix with other injections or infusions. Do not give IM.

◀ALERT▶ Give initial dose as soon as possible after surgery but not more than 24 hours after surgery.

Subcutaneous

- Parenteral form normally appears clear and colorless to pale yellow.
- Store at room temperature.
- Instruct the patient to lie down before administering by deep subcutaneous injection.
- Inject between the left and right anterolateral and left and right posterolateral abdominal wall. Introduce entire length of needle (one-half inch) into skinfold held between thumb and forefinger, holding skinfold during injection.

Intervention and Evaluation

- Periodically monitor the patient's CBC and stool for occult blood; there is no need for daily monitoring in patients with normal presurgical coagulation parameters.
- Assess the patient for signs of

bleeding, including bleeding at injection or surgical sites or from gums, blood in stool, bruising, hematuria, and petechiae.

Patient Teaching

- Tell the patient that the usual length of therapy is 7 to 10 days.
- Instruct the patient to report bleeding from surgical site, chest pain, or dyspnea.
- Tell the patient to use an electric razor and soft toothbrush to prevent bleeding during therapy.
- Advise the patient not to take other medications, including OTC drugs (especially aspirin), without physician approval.
- Warn the patient to report black or red stool, coffee-ground vomitus, dark or red urine, or red-speckled mucus from cough.
- Tell female patient that her menstrual flow may be heavier than usual.

fondaparinux sodium

fawn-da-**pear**-ih-nux
(Arixtra)

CATEGORY AND SCHEDULE

Pregnancy Risk Category: B

MECHANISM OF ACTION

A factor Xa inhibitor and pentasaccharide that selectively binds to antithrombin, and increases its affinity for factor Xa, thereby inhibiting factor Xa and stopping the blood coagulation cascade. **Therapeutic Effect:** Indirectly prevents formation of thrombin and subsequently the fibrin clot.

PHARMACOKINETICS

Well absorbed after subcutaneous administration. Undergoes minimal, if any, metabolism. Highly bound to antithrombin III. Distributed mainly in blood and to a minor extent in extravascular fluid. Excreted unchanged in urine. Removed by hemodialysis. ***Half-life:*** 17–21 hr (prolonged in patients with impaired renal function).

AVAILABILITY

Injection: 2.5 mg/0.5 ml prefilled syringe.

INDICATIONS AND DOSAGES

▸ Prevention of venous thromboembolism

Subcutaneous

Adults. 2.5 mg once a day for 5–9 days after surgery. Initial dose should be given 6–8 hr after surgery. Dosage should be adjusted in the elderly and in those with renal impairment.

CONTRAINDICATIONS

Active major bleeding, bacterial endocarditis, severe renal impairment (with creatinine clearance less than 30 ml/min), thrombocytopenia associated with antiplatelet antibody formation in the presence of fondaparinux, body weight less than 50 kg

INTERACTIONS

Drug

Anticoagulants, platelet inhibitors: May increase bleeding.

Herbal

None known.

Food

None known.

DIAGNOSTIC TEST EFFECTS

Increases reversible serum creatinine, AST (SGOT), and ALT (SGPT) levels. May decrease Hgb, Hct, and platelet count.

SIDE EFFECTS

Occasional (14%)
Fever
Rare (4%–1%)
Injection site hematoma, nausea, peripheral edema

SERIOUS REACTIONS

! Accidental overdose may lead to bleeding complications ranging from local ecchymoses to major hemorrhage.
! Thrombocytopenia occurs rarely.

NURSING CONSIDERATIONS

Baseline Assessment

- Assess the patient's BUN and creatinine levels, and CBC.

Lifespan Considerations

- Fondaparinux should be used with caution in pregnant women, particularly during the last trimester and immediately postpartum because it increases the risk of maternal hemorrhage.
- It is unknown if fondaparinux is excreted in breast milk.
- Safety and efficacy of fondaparinux have not been established in children.
- In the elderly, age-related decreased renal function may increase the risk of bleeding.

Precautions

- Use fondaparinux cautiously in the elderly and patients with conditions associated with increased risk of hemorrhage, such as concurrent use of antiplatelet agents, GI ulceration, hemophilia, history of cerebrovascular accident, and severe uncontrolled hypertension; history of heparin-induced thrombocytopenia; impaired renal function; indwelling epidural catheter or neuraxial anesthesia.

Administration and Handling

Subcutaneous

- The parenteral form normally appears clear and colorless. Discard if discoloration or particulate matter is noted.
- Store at room temperature.
- Do not expel the air bubble from the prefilled syringe before injection, to avoid expelling drug.
- Pinch a fold of the patient's skin at the injection site between the thumb and forefinger. Introduce the entire length of subcutaneous needle into the skinfold. Inject into fatty tissue between the left and right anterolateral or the left and right posterolateral abdominal wall.
- Rotate injection sites.

Intervention and Evaluation

- Periodically monitor the patient's CBC and stool for occult blood, as ordered. There is no need for daily monitoring in patients with normal presurgical coagulation parameters.
- Assess the patient for signs of bleeding, including bleeding at injection or surgical sites or from gums, blood in stool, ecchymosis, hematuria, and petechiae.
- Monitor the patient's BP and pulse. Hypotension and tachycardia may indicate bleeding.

Patient Teaching

- Tell the patient that the usual length of therapy is 5 to 9 days.
- Advise the patient not to take other medications, including OTC drugs (especially aspirin and NSAIDs), without physician approval.
- Warn the patient to report severe or sudden headache, swelling in the feet or hands, unusual back pain, or unusual bleeding, bruising, or weakness.
- Instruct the patient to report bleeding from surgical site, chest pain, or dyspnea.
- Tell the patient to use an electric razor and soft toothbrush to prevent bleeding during therapy.
- Caution the patient to report black

or red stool, coffee-ground vomitus, dark or red urine, or red-speckled mucus from cough.

- Tell the female patient that her menstrual flow may be heavier than usual.

heparin sodium

hep-a-rin

(Hepalean[CAN], Heparin injection B.P.[AUS], Heparin Leo, Uniparin[AUS])

Do not confuse heparin with Hespan.

CATEGORY AND SCHEDULE

Pregnancy Risk Category: C

MECHANISM OF ACTION

A blood modifier that interferes with blood coagulation by blocking conversion of prothrombin to thrombin and fibrinogen to fibrin. **Therapeutic Effect:** Prevents further extension of existing thrombi or new clot formation. Has no effect on existing clots.

PHARMACOKINETICS

Well absorbed following subcutaneous administration. Protein binding: Very high. Metabolized in the liver. Removed from the circulation via uptake by the reticuloendothelial system. Primarily excreted in urine. Not removed by hemodialysis. ***Half-life:*** 1–6 hr.

AVAILABILITY

Injection: 10 units/ml, 100 units/ml, 1,000 units/ml, 2,500 units/ml, 5,000 units/ml, 7,500 units/ml, 10,000 units/ml, 20,000 units/ml, 25,000 units/500 ml infusion.

INDICATIONS AND DOSAGES

▸ Line flushing

IV

Adults, Elderly, Children. 100 units q6–8h.

Infants weighing less than 10 kg. 10 units q6–8h.

▸ Treatment of venous thrombosis, pulmonary embolism, peripheral arterial embolism, atrial fibrillation with embolism

Intermittent IV

Adults, Elderly. Initially, 10,000 units, then 50–70 units/kg (5,000–10,000 units) q4–6h.

Children 1 yr and older. Initially, 50–100 units/kg, then 50–100 units q4h.

IV Infusion

Adults, Elderly. Loading dose: 80 units/kg, then 18 units/kg/hr, with adjustments based on aPTT. Range: 10–30 units/kg/hr.

Children 1 yr and older. Loading dose: 75 units/kg, then 20 units/kg/hr with adjustments based on aPTT.

Children younger than 1 yr. Loading dose: 75 units/kg, then 28 units/kg/hr.

▸ Prevention of venous thrombosis, pulmonary embolism, peripheral arterial embolism, atrial fibrillation with embolism

Subcutaneous

Adult, Elderly. 5,000 units q8–12h.

CONTRAINDICATIONS

Intracranial hemorrhage, severe hypotension, severe thrombocytopenia, subacute bacterial endocarditis, uncontrolled bleeding

INTERACTIONS

Drug

Antithyroid medications, cefoperazone, cefotetan, valproic acid: May cause hypoprothrombinemia.

Other anticoagulants, platelet aggregation inhibitors, thrombolytics: May increase the risk of bleeding.
Probenecid: May increase the effects of heparin.

Herbal

Feverfew, ginkgo biloba: May have additive effect.

Food

None known.

DIAGNOSTIC TEST EFFECTS

May increase free fatty acid, AST (SGOT), and ALT (SGPT) levels. May decrease serum cholesterol and triglyceride levels.

IV INCOMPATIBILITIES

Amiodarone (Cordarone), amphotericin B complex (Abelcet, AmBisome, Amphotec), ciprofloxacin (Cipro), dacarbazine (DTIC), diazepam (Valium), dobutamine (Dobutrex), doxorubicin (Adriamycin), droperidol (Inapsine), filgrastim (Neupogen), gentamicin (Garamycin), haloperidol (Haldol), idarubicin (Idamycin), labetalol (Trandate), nicardipine (Cardene), phenytoin (Dilantin), quinidine, tobramycin (Nebcin), vancomycin (Vancocin)

IV COMPATIBILITIES

Aminophylline, ampicillin/sulbactam (Unasyn), aztreonam (Azactam), calcium gluconate, cefazolin (Ancef), ceftazidime (Fortaz), ceftriaxone (Rocephin), digoxin (Lanoxin), diltiazem (Cardizem), dopamine (Intropin), enalapril (Vasotec), famotidine (Pepcid), fentanyl (Sublimaze), furosemide (Lasix), hydromorphone (Dilaudid), insulin, lidocaine, lorazepam (Ativan), magnesium sulfate, methylprednisolone (Solu-Medrol), midazolam (Versed), milrinone (Primacor), morphine, nitroglycerin, norepinephrine (Levophed), oxytocin (Pitocin), piperacillin/tazobactam (Zosyn), procainamide (Pronestyl), propofol (Diprivan)

SIDE EFFECTS

Occasional

Itching, burning (particularly on soles of feet) caused by vasospastic reaction

Rare

Pain, cyanosis of extremity 6–10 days after initial therapy lasting 4–6 hours; hypersensitivity reaction, including chills, fever, pruritus, urticaria, asthma, rhinitis, lacrimation, and headache

SERIOUS REACTIONS

! Bleeding complications ranging from local ecchymoses to major hemorrhage occur more frequently in high-dose therapy, intermittent IV infusion, and in women 60 years of age and older.
! Antidote: Protamine sulfate 1–1.5 mg, IV, for every 100 units heparin subcutaneous within 30 minutes of overdose, 0.5–0.75 mg for every 100 units heparin subcutaneous if within 30–60 minutes of overdose, 0.25–0.375 mg for every 100 units heparin subcutaneous if 2 hours have elapsed since overdose, 25–50 mg if heparin was given by IV infusion.

NURSING CONSIDERATIONS

Baseline Assessment

• Cross-check heparin dose with another nurse before administering. Determine the patient's aPTT before administering heparin and 24 hours after administration; then every 24 to 48 hours for the first week of heparin therapy or until the maintenance dose is established.
• Monitor the patient's aPTT 1 to 2 times weekly for 3 to 4 weeks. In

long-term therapy, monitor aPTT 1 to 2 times a month.

Lifespan Considerations

- Heparin should be used with caution in pregnant women, particularly during the last trimester and immediately postpartum, because it increases the risk of maternal hemorrhage.
- Heparin does not cross the placenta and is not distributed in breast milk.
- No age-related precautions have been noted in children.
- The benzyl alcohol preservative may cause gasping syndrome in infants.
- The elderly are more susceptible to hemorrhage, and age-related decreased renal function may increase the risk of bleeding.

Precautions

- Use heparin cautiously during menstruation in patients receiving IM injections, and in those with peptic ulcer disease, recent invasive or surgical procedures, or severe hepatic or renal disease.

Administration and Handling

◀ALERT▶ Do not give by IM injection because it may cause pain, hematoma, ulceration, and erythema.

Subcutaneous

◀ALERT▶ The subcutaneous route is used for low-dose therapy.

- After withdrawing heparin from the vial, change the needle before injection to prevent leakage along the needle track.
- Inject the heparin dose above the iliac crest or in abdominal fat layer. Do not inject within 2 inches of umbilicus or scar tissue.

IV

◀ALERT▶ Continuous IV therapy is preferred because intermittent IV therapy produces a higher incidence of bleeding abnormalities.

- Store at room temperature.
- Dilute IV infusion in isotonic sterile saline, D_5W, or lactated Ringer's solution.
- Invert IV bag at least 6 times to ensure mixing, and to prevent pooling of the medication.
- Use constant-rate IV infusion pump.

Intervention and Evaluation

- Monitor the patient's aPTT diligently. Therapeutic heparin dosage produces an aPTT of 1.5–2.5 times normal.
- Assess the patient's Hct, platelet count, AST (SGOT) and ALT (SGPT) levels, and stool and urine cultures for occult blood, regardless of route of administration.
- Determine the amount of female patient's menstrual discharge and monitor for any increase.
- Assess the patient's gums for erythema and gingival bleeding, skin for ecchymosis or petechiae, and urine for hematuria.
- Examine the patient for excessive bleeding from minor cuts and scratches.
- Evaluate the patient for abdominal or back pain, a decrease in BP, an increase in pulse rate, and severe headache, which may be evidence of hemorrhage.
- Check the patient's peripheral pulses for loss of peripheral circulation.
- Avoid giving other medications by IM route because of the potential for hematomas.
- When converting to warfarin therapy, monitor the patient's PT results, as ordered. PT will be 10% to 20% higher while heparin is being given concurrently.

Patient Teaching

- Tell the patient to use an electric razor and soft toothbrush to prevent bleeding during heparin therapy.
- Advise the patient not to take other

medications, including OTC drugs, without physician approval.
• Warn the patient to report black or red stool, coffee-ground vomitus, dark or red urine, or red-speckled mucus from cough.
• Suggest that the patient carry or wear identification that notes he or she is on anticoagulant therapy.
• Advise the patient to inform his or her dentist and other physicians of heparin therapy.

lepirudin
leh-**peer**-u-din
(Refludan)

CATEGORY AND SCHEDULE
Pregnancy Risk Category: B

MECHANISM OF ACTION
An anticoagulant that inhibits thrombogenic action of thrombin (independent of antithrombin II and not inhibited by platelet factor 4). One molecule of lepirudin binds to one molecule of thrombin. **Therapeutic Effect:** Produces dose-dependent increases in aPTT.

PHARMACOKINETICS
Distributed primarily in extracellular fluid. Primarily eliminated by the kidneys. ***Half-life:*** 1.3 hr (increased in impaired renal function).

AVAILABILITY
Powder for Injection: 50 mg.

INDICATIONS AND DOSAGES
▸ **Heparin-induced thrombocytopenia and associated thromboembolic disease to prevent further thromboembolic complications**
IV, IV Infusion
Adults, Elderly. 0.2–0.4 mg/kg IV slowly over 15–20 sec, followed by IV infusion of 0.1–0.15 mg/kg/hr for 2–10 days or longer.
▸ **Dosage in renal impairment**
Initial dose is decreased to 0.2 mg/kg, with infusion rate adjusted based on creatinine clearance.

Creatinine Clearance (ml/min)	% of standard infusion rate	Infusion rate (mg/kg/hr)
45–60	50	0.075
30–44	30	0.045
15–29	15	0.0225

CONTRAINDICATIONS
None known.

INTERACTIONS
Drug
Platelet aggregation inhibitors, thrombolytics, warfarin: May increase the risk of bleeding complications.
Herbal
Ginkgo biloba: May increase the risk of bleeding.
Food
None known.

DIAGNOSTIC TEST EFFECTS
Increases aPTT and thrombin time.

IV INCOMPATIBILITIES
Do not mix with other medications.

SIDE EFFECTS
Frequent (14%–5%)
Bleeding from gums, puncture sites, or wounds, hematuria, fever, GI and rectal bleeding
Occasional (3%–1%)
Epistaxis; allergic reaction, such as rash and pruritus; vaginal bleeding

SERIOUS REACTIONS

! Overdose is characterized by excessively high aPTT.
! Intracranial bleeding occurs rarely.
! Abnormal hepatic function occurs in 6% of patients.

NURSING CONSIDERATIONS

Baseline Assessment

• Assess the patient's CBC, including platelet count, as well as aPTT and thrombin time.
• Determine the patient's initial BP.
• Obtain the patient's serum chemistry laboratory values, including BUN, serum alkaline phosphatase, creatinine, AST (SGOT), and ALT (SGPT) levels, to assess hepatic and renal function.

Lifespan Considerations

• It is unknown if lepirudin crosses the placenta or is distributed in breast milk.
• Safety and efficacy of lepirudin have not been established in children.
• In the elderly, age-related renal impairment may require dosage adjustment.

Precautions

• Use lepirudin cautiously in patients with conditions associated with increased risk of bleeding, such as bacterial endocarditis, cerebrovascular accident, hemorrhagic diathesis, intracerebral surgery, recent major bleeding, recent major surgery, and severe hypertension; severe hepatic or renal impairment, or stroke.

Administration and Handling

◀ **ALERT** ▶ Give initial dose as soon as possible after surgery but not more than 24 hours after surgery.
◀ **ALERT** ▶ Dosage adjusted according to aPTT ratio with target range of 1.5 to 2.5 normal.
◀ **ALERT** ▶ For patients weighing more than 110 kg, the maximum initial dose is 44 mg, with maximum rate of 16.5 mg/hr.

IV

• Store unreconstituted vials at room temperature.
• Reconstituted solution should be used immediately, but the IV infusion is stable for up to 24 hours at room temperature.
• To reconstitute, add 1 ml sterile water for injection or 0.9% NaCl to 50-mg vial and shake gently.
• Be aware that reconstitution normally produces a clear, colorless solution; do not use if solution is cloudy.
• For IV push, further dilute by transferring to syringe and adding sufficient sterile water for injection, 0.9% NaCl, or D_5W to produce a concentration of 5 mg/ml.
• For IV infusion, add contents of 2 vials (100 mg) to 250 or 500 ml 0.9% NaCl or D_5W, providing a concentration of 0.4 or 0.2 mg/ml, respectively.
• Give IV push over 15 to 20 seconds.
• Expect to adjust IV infusion based on aPTT or patient's body weight.

Intervention and Evaluation

• Monitor the patient's aPTT diligently.
• Assess the patient for abdominal or back pain, a decrease in BP, an increase in pulse rate, and severe headache, which may be evidence of hemorrhage.
• Determine the amount of female patient's menstrual discharge and monitor for any increase.
• Assess the patient's gums for erythema and gingival bleeding, skin for ecchymosis or petechiae, and urine for hematuria.
• Examine the patient for excessive bleeding from minor cuts and scratches.
• Assess the patient's Hct; platelet

count; renal function studies; BUN, serum creatinine, AST and ALT levels; and stool and urine specimen for occult blood.

- Check the patient's peripheral pulses for signs of diminished peripheral circulation.

Patient Teaching

- Warn the patient to report bleeding, breathing difficulty, bruising, dizziness, edema, fever, itching, lightheadedness, or rash.
- Instruct the patient to report bleeding from surgical site, chest pain, or dyspnea.
- Tell the patient to use an electric razor and soft toothbrush to prevent bleeding during lepirudin therapy.
- Advise the patient not to take other medications, including OTC drugs (especially aspirin), without physician approval.
- Warn the patient to report black or red stool, coffee-ground vomitus, dark or red urine, or red-speckled mucus from cough.
- Tell female patient that her menstrual flow may be heavier than usual.

tinzaparin sodium

tin-za-**pair**-in
(Innohep)

CATEGORY AND SCHEDULE

Pregnancy Risk Category: B

MECHANISM OF ACTION

A low-molecular-weight heparin that inhibits factor Xa. Causes less inactivation of thrombin, inhibition of platelets, and bleeding than standard heparin. Does not significantly influence bleeding time, PT, aPTT. **Therapeutic Effect:** Produces anticoagulation.

PHARMACOKINETICS

Well absorbed after subcutaneous administration. Primarily eliminated in urine. ***Half-life***: 3–4 hr.

AVAILABILITY

Injection: 20,000 anti-Xa international units/ml.

INDICATIONS AND DOSAGES

Deep vein thrombosis

Subcutaneous

Adults, Elderly. 175 anti-Xa international units/kg once a day. Continue for at least 6 days and until patient is sufficiently anticoagulated with warfarin (international normalized ratio [INR] of 2 or more for 2 consecutive days).

CONTRAINDICATIONS

Active major bleeding, concurrent heparin therapy, hypersensitivity to heparin or pork products, thrombocytopenia associated with positive in vitro test for antiplatelet antibody

INTERACTIONS

Drug

Anticoagulants, platelet inhibitors: May increase the risk of bleeding.

Herbal

Ginkgo biloba: May increase the risk of bleeding.

Food

None known.

DIAGNOSTIC TEST EFFECTS

Increases (reversible) LDH, serum alkaline phosphatase, AST (SGOT), and ALT (SGPT) levels.

SIDE EFFECTS

Frequent (16%)

Injection site reaction, such as inflammation, oozing, nodules, and skin necrosis

Rare (less than 2%)
Nausea, asthenia, constipation, epistaxis

SERIOUS REACTIONS

! Overdose may lead to bleeding complications ranging from local ecchymoses to major hemorrhage. Antidote: Dose of protamine sulfate (1% solution) should be equal to dose of tinzaparin injected. One mg protamine sulfate neutralizes 100 units of tinzaparin. A second dose of 0.5 mg tinzaparin per 1 mg protamine sulfate may be given if aPTT tested 2–4 hours after the initial infusion remains prolonged.

NURSING CONSIDERATIONS

Baseline Assessment

- Assess the patient's PT, INR and CBC, including platelet count.
- Determine the patient's initial BP.

Lifespan Considerations

- Tinzaparin should be used with caution in pregnant women, particularly during the last trimester and immediately postpartum, because it increases the risk of maternal hemorrhage.
- It is unknown if tinzaparin is excreted in breast milk.
- Safety and efficacy of tinzaparin have not been established in children.
- The elderly may be more susceptible to bleeding.

Precautions

- Use tinzaparin cautiously in the elderly and in patients with conditions associated with increased risk of hemorrhage, history of recent GI ulceration and hemorrhage, history of heparin-induced thrombocytopenia, impaired renal function, or uncontrolled arterial hypertension.

Administration and Handling

◀ **ALERT** ▶ Do not mix with other injections or infusions. Do not give IM, Subcutaneous

- The parenteral form normally appears clear and colorless to pale yellow.
- Store at room temperature.
- Instruct patient to lie down before administering by deep subcutaneous injection.

Intervention and Evaluation

- Periodically monitor the patient's CBC, including platelet count, as ordered.
- Assess the patient for signs of bleeding, including bleeding at injection or surgical sites or from gums, blood in stool, bruising, hematuria, and petechiae.

Patient Teaching

- Instruct the patient to administer tinzaparin by subcutaneous route only.
- Tell the patient that he or she may have a tendency to bleed easily. Suggest the use of an electric razor and a soft toothbrush to prevent bleeding.
- Warn the patient to report chest pain; injection site reaction, such as inflammation, nodules, or oozing; numbness, pain, swelling or tingling of joints; or unusual bleeding or bruising.

warfarin sodium

war-far-in
(Apo-Warfarin[CAN], Coumadin, Gen-Warfarin[CAN], Jantoven, Marevan[AUS], Tar-Warfarin[CAN])
Do not confuse Coumadin with Kemadrin.

CATEGORY AND SCHEDULE

Pregnancy Risk Category: D

MECHANISM OF ACTION

A coumarin derivative that interferes with hepatic synthesis of vitamin K–dependent clotting factors, resulting in depletion of coagulation factors II, VII, IX, and X. **Therapeutic Effect:** Prevents further extension of formed existing clot; prevents new clot formation or secondary thromboembolic complications.

PHARMACOKINETICS

Route	Onset	Peak	Duration
PO	1.5–3 days	5–7 days	N/A

Well absorbed from the GI tract. Metabolized in the liver. Primarily excreted in urine. Not removed by hemodialysis. ***Half-life:*** 1.5–2.5 days.

AVAILABILITY

Tablets (Coumadin, Jantoven): 1 mg, 2 mg, 2.5 mg, 3 mg, 4 mg, 5 mg, 6 mg, 7.5 mg, 10 mg.

INDICATIONS AND DOSAGES

▸ **Anticoagulant**

PO

Adults, Elderly. Initially, 5–15 mg/day for 2–5 days; then adjust based on international normalized ratio (INR). Maintenance: 2–10 mg/day.

Children. Initially, 0.1–0.2 mg/kg (maximum 10 mg). Maintenance: 0.05–0.34 mg/kg/day.

▸ **Usual elderly dosage (maintenance)**

PO, IV

Elderly. 2–5 mg/day.

OFF-LABEL USES

Prevention of recurrent cerebral embolism, myocardial reinfarction; treatment adjunct in transient ischemic attacks

CONTRAINDICATIONS

Neurosurgical procedures, open wounds, pregnancy, severe hypertension, severe hepatic or renal damage, uncontrolled bleeding, ulcers

INTERACTIONS

Drug

Acetaminophen, allopurinol, amiodarone, anabolic steroids, androgens, aspirin, cefamandole, cefoperazone, chloral hydrate, chloramphenicol, cimetidine, clofibrate, danazol, dextrothyroxine, diflunisal, disulfiram, erythromycin, fenoprofen, gemfibrozil, indomethacin, methimazole, metronidazole, oral hypoglycemics, phenytoin, plicamycin, propylthiouracil, quinidine, salicylates, sulfinpyrazone, sulfonamides, sulindac: Warfarin increases the effects of these drugs.

Alcohol: May enhance warfarin's anticoagulant effect.

Barbiturates, carbamazepine, cholestyramine, colestipol, estramustine, estrogens, griseofulvin, primidone, rifampin, vitamin K: Warfarin decreases the effects of these drugs.

Herbal

American ginseng, St. John's wort: May decrease the effectiveness of warfarin.

Feverfew, garlic, ginkgo biloba, ginseng, glucosamine-chondroitin: May increase the risk of bleeding.

Food

None known.

DIAGNOSTIC TEST EFFECTS

None known.

SIDE EFFECTS

Occasional

GI distress, such as nausea, anorexia, abdominal cramps, diarrhea

Rare

Hypersensitivity reaction, including dermatitis and urticaria, especially in those sensitive to aspirin

SERIOUS REACTIONS

! Bleeding complications ranging from local ecchymoses to major hemorrhage may occur. Drug should be discontinued immediately and vitamin K or phytonadione administered. Mild hemorrhage: 2.5–10 mg PO, IM, or IV. Severe hemorrhage: 10–15 mg IV and repeated q4h, as necessary.

! Hepatotoxicity, blood dyscrasias, necrosis, vasculitis, and local thrombosis occur rarely.

NURSING CONSIDERATIONS

Baseline Assessment

• Cross-check warfarin dosage with another nurse before administering.
• Determine the patient's INR before administration and daily after therapy begins. When INR is stabilized, follow with INR determinations every 4 to 6 weeks.

Lifespan Considerations

• Warfarin use is contraindicated in pregnancy because it causes fetal and neonatal hemorrhage and intrauterine death.
• Warfarin crosses the placenta and is distributed in breast milk.
• Children are more susceptible to the effects of warfarin.
• In the elderly, there is an increased risk of hemorrhage; a lower drug dosage is recommended.

Precautions

• Use warfarin cautiously in patients at risk for hemorrhage and in those with active tuberculosis, diabetes, gangrene, heparin-induced thrombocytopenia, and necrosis.

Administration and Handling

◀ALERT▶ Remember that warfarin dosage is highly individualized and is based on PT and INR.

PO

• Crush scored tablets as needed.
• Give warfarin without regard to food. If GI upset occurs, give with food.

IV

• Store at room temperature and protect from light. Don't refrigerate.
• To reconstitute, add 2.7 ml sterile water for injection to 5-mg vial to produce 2 mg of warfarin per ml of solution.
• Use reconstituted solution within 4 hours; discard unused portion.

Intervention and Evaluation

• Monitor the patient's INR diligently.
• Assess the patient's Hct, platelet count, AST (SGOT) and ALT (SGPT) levels, and stool and urine cultures for occult blood, regardless of administration route.
• Evaluate the patient for abdominal or back pain, a decrease in BP, an increase in pulse rate, and severe headache which can indicate hemorrhage.
• Determine the amount of female patient's menstrual discharge and monitor for any increase.
• Assess the area of thromboembolus for color and temperature.
• Check the patient's peripheral pulses.
• Assess the patient's gums for erythema and gingival bleeding, skin for ecchymosis and petechiae, and urine for hematuria.
• Examine the patient for excessive bleeding from minor cuts or scratches.

Patient Teaching

- Instruct the patient to take warfarin exactly as prescribed.
- Caution the patient against taking or discontinuing other medications without physician approval.
- Urge the patient to avoid alcohol, drastic dietary changes, and salicylates.
- Teach the patient not to change from one brand of warfarin to another.
- Instruct the patient to consult the physician before having dental work or surgery.
- Explain to the patient that his or her urine may become red-orange.
- Tell the patient to use an electric razor and soft toothbrush, to prevent bleeding during warfarin therapy.
- Advise the patient not to take take other medications, including OTC drugs, without physician approval.
- Warn the patient to report black stool, bleeding; brown, dark, or red urine; coffee-ground vomitus; or red-speckled mucus from cough.

56 Antihemophilic Agents

antihemophilic factor (factor VIII, AHF)
factor IX complex

Uses: Antihemophilic agents are used to prevent or treat bleeding episodes in patients with hemophilia A, in which factor VIII activity is deficient, or hemophilia B (also called Christmas disease), in which factor IX complex activity is deficient.

Action: Antihemophilic agents promote hemostasis by activating the intrinsic or extrinsic pathway of the coagulation cascade. Factor VIII prevents bleeding by replacing this clotting factor, which is needed to transform prothrombin into thrombin. Factor IX complex raises the plasma level of factor IX, restoring hemostasis in patients with factor IX deficiency.

antihemophilic factor (factor VIII, AHF)

an-tee-hee-moe-**fill**-ick **fak**-tor
(Alphanate, Hemofil M, Humanate P, Koate DVI, Monarc M, Monoclate-P)
Do not confuse Alphanate with Alfenta.

CATEGORY AND SCHEDULE
Pregnancy Risk Category: C

MECHANISM OF ACTION
An antihemophilic agent that assists in conversion of prothrombin to thrombin, essential for blood coagulation. Replaces missing clotting factor. **Therapeutic Effect:** Produces hemostasis; corrects or prevents bleeding episodes.

AVAILABILITY
Injection: Actual number of AHF units is listed on each vial.

INDICATIONS AND DOSAGES
▸ **Treatment and prevention of bleeding in patients with hemophilia A factor VIII deficiency, hypofibrinogenemia, von Willebrand's disease**
IV
Adults, Elderly, Children. Dosage is highly individualized and is based on patient's weight, severity of bleeding, and coagulation studies.

OFF-LABEL USES
Treatment of disseminated intravascular coagulation

CONTRAINDICATIONS
None known.

INTERACTIONS
Drug
None known.
Herbal
None known.
Food
None known.

DIAGNOSTIC TEST EFFECTS

None known.

IV INCOMPATIBILITIES

Do not mix with other IV solutions or medications.

SIDE EFFECTS

Occasional

Allergic reaction, including fever, chills, urticaria, wheezing, hypotension, nausea, feeling of chest tightness; stinging at injection site; dizziness; dry mouth; headache; altered taste

SERIOUS REACTIONS

! There is a risk of transmitting viral hepatitis.
! Intravascular hemolysis may occur if large or frequent doses are used with blood group A, B, or AB.

NURSING CONSIDERATIONS

Baseline Assessment

• Avoid overinflating cuff when monitoring the patient's BP. Take BP manually, avoiding automatic BP cuffs.
• Remove adhesive tape from pressure dressings very carefully and slowly.

Precautions

• Use AHF cautiously in patients with hepatic disease and in those with blood type A, B, or AB. If large doses are given to patients with these blood types, expect to monitor Hct and direct Coombs test to check for hemolytic anemia. If hemolytic anemia occurs, expect to give transfusions with type O blood.

Administration and Handling

IV

• Refer to individual vials for specific storage requirements.
• Warm concentrate and diluent to room temperature.
• Gently agitate or rotate to dissolve. Do not shake vigorously. Complete dissolution may take 5 to 10 minutes.
• Filter before administering.
• Administer IV at a rate of approximately 2 ml/minute. Can give up to 10 ml/minute.

Intervention and Evaluation

• Monitor the IV site for oozing.
• Assess the patient for allergic reactions.
• Monitor the patient's vital signs, and urine for hematuria.
• Assess the patient for abdominal or back pain, severe headache, a decrease in BP, and an increase in pulse rate, which can indicate hemorrhage.
• Determine the amount of female patient's menstrual discharge and monitor for any increase.
• Assess the patient's gums for erythema and gingival bleeding and skin for bruises and petechiae.
• Examine the patient for excessive bleeding from minor cuts or scratches.
• Evaluate the patient for therapeutic response (reduction of swelling, easier joint movement, relief of pain).

Patient Teaching

• Tell the patient to use an electric razor and soft toothbrush to prevent bleeding.
• Warn the patient to report black or red stool, coffee-ground emesis, dark or red urine, or red-speckled mucus from cough.

factor IX complex

fak-tor nine **calm**-plex
(Benefix, Propex T, Konyne)

CATEGORY AND SCHEDULE

Pregnancy Risk Category: C

MECHANISM OF ACTION

A blood modifier that raises plasma levels of factor IX, restoring hemostasis in patients with factor IX deficiency. **Therapeutic Effect:** Increases blood clotting factors II, VII, IX, and X.

AVAILABILITY

Injection: Number of units is indicated on each vial.

INDICATIONS AND DOSAGES

▸ **Reversal of anticoagulant effect of coumarin anticoagulants; bleeding caused by hemophilia B; bleeding in patients with hemophilia A who have factor VIII inhibitors**

IV

Adults, Elderly, Children. Amount of factor IX required is individualized. Dosage depends on degree of deficiency, level of each factor desired, patient's weight, and severity of bleeding.

CONTRAINDICATIONS

Sensitivity to mouse protein

INTERACTIONS

Drug

Aminocaproic acid: May increase the risk of thrombosis.

Herbal

None known.

Food

None known.

DIAGNOSTIC TEST EFFECTS

None known.

IV INCOMPATIBILITIES

Do not mix with other medications.

SIDE EFFECTS

Rare

Mild hypersensitivity reaction, marked by, fever, chills, change in BP and pulse rate, rash, and urticaria

SERIOUS REACTIONS

! There is a high risk of venous thrombosis during the postoperative period.

! Acute hypersensitivity reaction or anaphylactic reaction may occur.

! There is a risk of transmitting viral hepatitis and other viral diseases.

NURSING CONSIDERATIONS

Baseline Assessment

- Assess the patient's coagulation studies and the extent of existing bleeding, joint pain, overt bleeding or bruising, and swelling.

Precautions

- Use factor IX complex cautiously in patients with hepatic impairment, recent surgery, or sensitivity to factor IX.

Administration and Handling

IV

- Store in refrigerator.
- Reconstituted solution is stable for 12 hours at room temperature; do not refrigerate.
- Before reconstitution, warm diluent to room temperature.
- Gently agitate vial until powder is completely dissolved, so that the active components won't be removed when the solution is filtered during administration.
- Filter before administration.
- Begin administration within 3 hours of reconstitution.
- Administer by slow IV push or IV infusion.
- Infuse slowly, no faster than 3

ml/minute. Too rapid an IV infusion may produce a change in BP and pulse rate, headache, flushing, and a tingling sensation.

Intervention and Evaluation

- Monitor the patient's intake and output and vital signs.
- Assess the patient for hypersensitivity reaction.
- Monitor the patient's coagulation studies closely.
- Avoid administering other medications by the IM or subcutaneous route.
- Monitor the patient's IV site for oozing every 5 to 15 minutes for 1 to 2 hours after administration.
- Report hematuria or change in vital signs immediately.

Patient Teaching

- Tell the patient to use an electric razor and soft toothbrush to prevent bleeding.
- Warn the patient to report black or red stool, coffee-ground emesis, dark or red urine, or red-speckled mucus from cough.
- Caution the patient against using OTC medications without physician approval.
- Instruct the patient to carry identification that indicates his or her condition or disease.

57 Antiplatelet Agents

abciximab
anagrelide
aspirin
cilostazol
clopidogrel
dipyridamole
eptifibatide
ticlopidine hydrochloride
tirofiban
treprostinil sodium

Uses: Most antiplatelet agents are used to prevent myocardial infarction (MI) or stroke, repeat MI, and stroke in patients with transient ischemic attacks (TIAs). *Cilostazol* is prescribed to reduce symptoms of intermittent claudication. The *glycoprotein (GP) IIb/IIIa receptor inhibitors* are used to prevent ischemic events in patients with acute coronary syndrome and those undergoing percutaneous coronary intervention.

Action: The three major groups of antiplatelet drugs inhibit platelet aggregation by different mechanisms. *Aspirin* irreversibly inhibits cyclooxygenase, thereby blocking the synthesis of thromboxane A_2. *Adenosine diphosphate (ADP) receptor antagonists,* such as clopidogrel, irreversibly block ADP receptors. *GP IIb/IIIa receptor inhibitors,* such as abciximab and tirofiban, reversibly block GP IIb/IIIa receptors. (See the illustration *Mechanisms and Sites of Action: Hematologic Agents,* page 1036.)

COMBINATION PRODUCTS

AGGRENOX: dipyridamole/aspirin (an antiplatelet agent) 200 mg/25 mg.

abciximab

ab-**six**-ih-mab
(c7E3 Fab, ReoPro)

CATEGORY AND SCHEDULE

Pregnancy Risk Category: C

MECHANISM OF ACTION

A glycoprotein IIb/IIIa receptor inhibitor that rapidly inhibs platelet aggregation by preventing the binding of fibrinogen to GP IIb/IIIa receptor sites on platelets. **Therapeutic Effect:** Prevents closure of treated coronary arteries. Prevents acute cardiac ischemic complications.

PHARMACOKINETICS

Rapidly cleared from plasma. Initial-phase half-life is less than 10 min; second-phase half-life is 30 min. Platelet function generally returns within 48 hr.

AVAILABILITY

Injection: 2 mg/ml (5-ml vial).

INDICATIONS AND DOSAGES

▸ **Percutaneous coronary intervention (PCI)**

IV Bolus

Adults. 0.25 mg/kg 10–60 min before angioplasty or atherectomy, then 12-hr IV infusion of 0.125

mcg/kg/min. Maximum: 10 mcg/min.

▸ **PCI (unstable angina)**

IV Bolus

Adults. 0.25 mg/kg, followed by 18- to 24-hr infusion of 10 mcg/min, ending 1 hr after procedure.

CONTRAINDICATIONS

Active internal bleeding, arteriovenous malformation or aneurysm, cerebrovascular accident (CVA) with residual neurologic defect, history of CVA (within the past 2 years) or oral anticoagulant use within the past 7 days unless PT is less than 1.2 × control, history of vasculitis, intracranial neoplasm, prior IV dextran use before or during PTCA, recent surgery or trauma (within the past 6 weeks), recent (within the past 6 weeks or less) GI or GU bleeding, thrombocytopenia (less than 100,000 cells/mcl), and severe uncontrolled hypertension

INTERACTIONS

Drug

Anticoagulants, including heparin: May increase risk of hemorrhage.

Platelet aggregation inhibitors (such as aspirin, dextran, thrombolytic agents): May increase risk of bleeding.

Herbal

None known.

Food

None known.

DIAGNOSTIC TEST EFFECTS

Increases activated clotting time (ACT), aPTT, and PT. Decreases platelet count.

IV INCOMPATIBILITIES

Administer in separate line; no other medication should be added to infusion solution.

SIDE EFFECTS

Frequent

Nausea (16%), hypotension (12%)

Occasional (9%)

Vomiting

Rare (3%)

Bradycardia, confusion, dizziness, pain, peripheral edema, urinary tract infection

SERIOUS REACTIONS

! Major bleeding complications may occur. If complications occur, stop the infusion immediately.

! Hypersensitivity reaction may occur.

! Atrial fibrillation or flutter, pulmonary edema, and complete atrioventricular block occur occasionally.

NURSING CONSIDERATIONS

Baseline Assessment

- Expect to discontinue heparin 4 hours before the arterial sheath is removed.
- Maintain patient on bed rest for 6 to 8 hours after the sheath is removed or the drug is discontinued, whichever is later.
- To assess for preexisting blood abnormalities, check aPTT, platelet count, and PT before abciximab infusion, 2 to 4 hours after treatment, and 24 hours after treatment or before discharge, whichever is first.
- Check the insertion site and the distal pulse of the affected limb while the femoral artery sheath is in place. Check site and distal pulse routinely for 6 hours after the femoral artery sheath has been removed.
- Minimize the need for invasive procedures, such as blood draws, catheter placements, intubations, and numerous injections.

Lifespan Considerations

- It is unknown if abciximab is distributed in breast milk.

• Safety and efficacy have not been established in children.
• There is an increased risk of bleeding in the elderly.

Precautions

• Use abciximab cautiously in patients who weigh less than 75 kg and in those who are over age 65, have a history of GI disease, or are receiving aspirin, heparin, or thrombolytics. Also use abciximab cautiously in patients who've had a PTCA within 12 hours of the onset of signs and symptoms of acute MI, who've had a prolonged PTCA (greater than 70 minutes), or who've had a failed PTCA, because they are at increased risk for bleeding.

Administration and Handling

IV

• Store vials in refrigerator.
• Solution normally appears clear and colorless. Do not shake.
• Discard any unused portion or any preparation that contains opaque particles.
• For bolus injection and continuous infusion, use a sterile, nonpyrogenic, low protein-binding 0.2- or 0.22-micron filter. The continuous infusion may be filtered either during drug preparation or at the time of administration.
• Withdraw the desired dose and dilute in 250 ml of 0.9% NaCl or D_5W (for example, 10 mg in 250 ml equals a concentration of 40 mcg/ml).
• The bolus dose may be given undiluted.
• Give in separate IV line; do not add other medications to infusion.
• While femoral artery sheath is in position, maintain patient on complete bed rest with head of bed elevated at 30 degrees.
• Maintain affected limb in straight position.
• After the sheath has been removed, apply femoral pressure for 30 minutes, either manually or mechanically; then apply a pressure dressing.

Intervention and Evaluation

• Stop abciximab and heparin infusion if serious bleeding uncontrolled by pressure occurs.
• Assess skin for ecchymosis and petechiae. Also, assess for GI, GU, and retroperitoneal bleeding and for bleeding at all puncture sites.
• Avoid IM injections and venipunctures; also avoid using indwelling urinary catheters and nasogastric tubes.
• Handle the patient carefully and as infrequently as possible, to prevent bleeding.
• Do not obtain BP in the lower extremities because the patient may have deep vein thrombi.
• Assess for signs and symptoms of hemorrhage, including a decrease in BP, increase in pulse rate, abdominal or back pain, and severe headache. Also, monitor laboratory test results, including ACT, aPTT, platelet count, and PT.
• Determine the amount of female patient's menstrual discharge and monitor for any increase.
• Assess urine for hematuria.
• Monitor for any new or expanding hematomas.
• Gently remove dressings and tape.

Patient Teaching

• Instruct the patient to use electric razor and soft toothbrush to prevent bleeding.
• Warn the patient to report signs of bleeding, including black or red stool, coffee-ground emesis, red or dark urine, or red-speckled mucus from cough.

anagrelide

ah-**na**- greh-lide
(Agrylin)

CATEGORY AND SCHEDULE

Pregnancy Risk Category: C

MECHANISM OF ACTION

A hematologic agent that reduces platelet production and prevents platelet shape changes caused by platelet aggregating agents. **Therapeutic Effect:** Inhibits platelet aggregation.

PHARMACOKINETICS

After oral administration, plasma concentration peak within 1 hr. Extensively metabolized. Primarily excreted in urine. ***Half-life:*** About 3 days.

AVAILABILITY

Capsules: 0.5 mg, 1 mg.

INDICATIONS AND DOSAGES

▸ Thrombocythemia

PO

Adults, Elderly. Initially, 0.5 mg 4 times a day or 1 mg twice a day. Adjust to lowest effective dosage, increasing by up to 0.5 mg/day or less in any 1 wk. Maximum: 10 mg/day or 2.5 mg/dose.

CONTRAINDICATIONS

None known.

INTERACTIONS

Drug

None known.

Herbal

None known.

Food

None known.

DIAGNOSTIC TEST EFFECTS

May increase hepatic enzymes levels (rare).

SIDE EFFECTS

Frequent (5% or more)

Headache, palpitations, diarrhea, abdominal pain, nausea, flatulence, bloating, asthenia, pain, dizziness

Occasional (less than 5%)

Tachycardia, chest pain, vomiting, paresthesia, peripheral edema, anorexia, dyspepsia, rash

Rare

Confusion, insomnia

SERIOUS REACTIONS

! Angina, heart failure, and arrhythmias occur rarely.

NURSING CONSIDERATIONS

Baseline Assessment

- Expect to obtain Hgb, Hct, and platelet and WBC counts before treatment, every 2 days during the first week of treatment, and weekly thereafter until therapeutic range is achieved.
- Determine if the patient is or plans to become pregnant or is breast-feeding because anagrelide may cause fetal harm.

Lifespan Considerations

- It is unknown if anagrelide crosses the placenta or is distributed in breast milk. Anagrelide may cause fetal harm.
- Safety and efficacy of anagrelide have not been established in children younger than 16 years.
- Use anagrelide cautiously in the elderly, who may have age-related cardiac disease and decreased renal and hepatic function.

Precautions

- Use anagrelide cautiously in patients with cardiac disease or hepatic or renal impairment.

Administration and Handling

PO

- May give without regard to food.

Intervention and Evaluation

- Expect to monitor BUN and serum creatinine levels and hepatic enzyme test results.
- Assess the patient with suspected heart disease for tachycardia, palpitations, and signs and symptoms of CHF, such as dypsnea.
- Assess the patient's skin for bruises or petechiae, and inspect catheter and needle insertion sites for bleeding. Also assess the patient for signs and symptoms of GI bleeding.

Patient Teaching

- Inform the patient that his or her platelet count should respond within 7 to 14 days of beginning therapy.

◀ **ALERT** ▶ Warn the female patient that anagrelide is not recommended in pregnant women. Strongly urge her to use contraceptives while taking anagrelide.

aspirin

See Non-Narcotic Analgesics

cilostazol

sil-**os**-tah-zol

(Pletal)

Do not confuse Pletal with Plendil.

CATEGORY AND SCHEDULE

Pregnancy Risk Category: C

MECHANISM OF ACTION

A phosphodiesterase III inhibitor that inhibits platelet aggregation. Dilates vascular beds with greatest dilation in femoral beds. **Therapeutic Effect:** Improves walking distance in patients with intermittent claudication.

PHARMACOKINETICS

Moderately absorbed from the GI tract. Protein binding: 95%–98%. Extensively metabolized in the liver. Excreted primarily in the urine and, to a lesser extent, in the feces. Not removed by hemodialysis. ***Half-life:*** 11–13 hr. Therapeutic effect is usually noted in 2–4 wk but may take as long as 12 wk.

AVAILABILITY

Tablets: 50 mg, 100 mg.

INDICATIONS AND DOSAGES

▸ **Intermittent claudication**

PO

Adults, Elderly. 100 mg twice a day at least 30 min before or 2 hr after meals.

CONTRAINDICATIONS

CHF of any severity

INTERACTIONS

Drug

Clarithromycin, diltiazem, erythromycin, fluconazole, fluoxetine, omeprazole, sertraline: May incease concentration of cilostazol.

Aspirin: May potentiate inhibition of platelet aggregation.

Herbal

None known.

Food

Grapefruit, grapefruit juice: May increase blood concentration and risk of toxicity of cilostazol.

DIAGNOSTIC TEST EFFECTS

May increase BUN and serum creatinine levels. May decrease Hgb and Hct.

SIDE EFFECTS

Frequent (34%–10%)

Headache, diarrhea, palpitations, dizziness, pharyngitis

Occasional (7%–3%)

Nausea, rhinitis, back pain, peripheral edema, dyspepsia, abdominal pain, tachycardia, cough, flatulence, myalgia

Rare (2%–1%)

Leg cramps, paresthesia, rash, vomiting

SERIOUS REACTIONS

! Signs and symptoms of overdose are noted by severe headache, diarrhea, hypotension, and cardiac arrhythmias.

NURSING CONSIDERATIONS

Baseline Assessment

- Assess the patient's Hgb, Hct, and platelet count before and periodically during cilostazol treatment.

Lifespan Considerations

- It is unknown if cilostazol crosses the placenta or is distributed in breast milk.
- Safety and efficacy of cilostazol have not been established in children.
- No age-related precautions have been noted in the elderly.

Administration and Handling

PO

- Give cilostazol at least 30 minutes before or 2 hours after meals.
- Do not give with grapefruit juice.

Intervention and Evaluation

- Assess the patient for relief of cramping in the feet, calf muscles, thighs, and buttocks during exercise. Also assess for improved walking endurance.

Patient Teaching

- Instruct the patient to take cilostazol on an empty stomach at least 30 minutes before or 2 hours after meals.
- Advise the patient to avoid taking cilostazol with grapefruit juice because it may increase the drug's blood concentration and risk of toxicity.

clopidogrel

clo-**pid**-o-grill

(Iscover[AUS], Plavix)

Do not confuse Plavix with Paxil.

CATEGORY AND SCHEDULE

Pregnancy Risk Category: B

MECHANISM OF ACTION

A thienopyridine derivative that inhibits binding of the enzyme adenosine phosphate (ADP) to its platelet receptor and subsequent ADP-mediated activation of a glycoprotein complex. **Therapeutic Effect:** Inhibits platelet aggregation.

PHARMACOKINETICS

Route	Onset	Peak	Duration
PO	1 hr	2 hr	N/A

Rapidly absorbed. Protein binding: 98%. Extensively metabolized by the liver. Eliminated equally in the urine and feces. ***Half-life:*** 8 hr.

AVAILABILITY

Tablets: 75 mg.

INDICATIONS AND DOSAGES

Myocardial infarction (MI), stroke reduction

PO

Adults, Elderly. 75 mg once a day.

▸ **Acute coronary syndrome**
PO
Adults, Elderly. Initially, 300 mg loading dose, then 75 mg once a day (in combination with aspirin).

CONTRAINDICATIONS

Active bleeding, coagulation disorders, severe hepatic disease

INTERACTIONS

Drug

Fluvastatin, other NSAIDs, phenytoin, tamoxifen, tolbutamide, torsemide, warfarin: May interfere with metabolism of these drugs.

Herbal

Ginger, ginkgo biloba: May increase the risk of bleeding.

Food

None known.

DIAGNOSTIC TEST EFFECTS

Prolongs bleeding time.

SIDE EFFECTS

Frequent (15%)

Skin disorders

Occasional (8%–6%)

Upper respiratory tract infection, chest pain, flulike symptoms, headache, dizziness, arthralgia

Rare (5%–3%)

Fatigue, edema, hypertension, abdominal pain, dyspepsia, diarrhea, nausea, epistaxis, dyspnea, rhinitis

SERIOUS REACTIONS

! None known.

NURSING CONSIDERATIONS

Baseline Assessment

- Obtain a platelet count before clopidogrel therapy, every 2 days during the first week of treatment and weekly thereafter until therapeutic maintenance dose is reached.
- Abrupt discontinuation of clopidrogel produces an elevated platelet count within 5 days.

Lifespan Considerations

- It is unknown if clopidogrel crosses the placenta or is distributed in breast milk.
- Safety and efficacy of clopidogrel have not been established in children.
- No age-related precautions have been noted in the elderly.

Precautions

- Use clopidrogel cautiously in preoperative patients and in those with hematologic disorders, history of bleeding, hypertension, or hepatic or renal impairment.

Administration and Handling

PO

- Give clopidogrel without regard to food.
- Do not crush coated tablets.

Intervention and Evaluation

- Monitor the patient's platelet count for thrombocytopenia.
- Assess the patient's Hgb, WBC count, and BUN, serum bilirubin, creatinine, AST (SGOT) and ALT (SGPT) levels.
- Evaluate the patient for signs and symptoms of hepatic insufficiency during clopidogrel therapy.

Patient Teaching

- Inform the patient that it may take longer to stop bleeding during drug therapy.
- Warn the patient to report unusual bleeding.
- Tell the patient to notify his or her dentist and other physicians of clopidogrel therapy before surgery is scheduled or new drugs are prescribed.

dipyridamole

dye-peer-**id**-a-mole
(Apo-Dipyridamole[CAN], Novodipiradol[CAN], Persantin[AUS], Persantin 100[AUS], Persantin SR[AUS], Persantine)
Do not confuse Aggrenox with Aggrastat, dipyridamole with disopyramide, or Persantin with Periactin.

CATEGORY AND SCHEDULE

Pregnancy Risk Category: C

MECHANISM OF ACTION

A blood modifier and platelet aggregation inhibitor that inhibits the activity of adenosine deaminase and phosphodiesterase, enzymes causing accumulation of adenosine and cyclic adenosine monophosphate. **Therapeutic Effect:** Inhibits platelet aggregation; may cause coronary vasodilation.

PHARMACOKINETICS

Slowly, variably absorbed from the GI tract. Widely distributed. Protein binding: 91%–99%. Metabolized in the liver. Primarily eliminated via biliary excretion. ***Half-life:*** 10–15 hr.

AVAILABILITY

Tablets: 25 mg, 50 mg, 75 mg.
Injection: 5 mg/ml.

INDICATIONS AND DOSAGES

▸ Prevention of thromboembolic disorders

PO

Adults, Elderly. 75–400 mg/day in combination with other medications.
Children. 3–6 mg/kg/day in 3 divided doses.

▸ Diagnostic aid

IV

Adults, Elderly (based on weight). 0.142 mg/kg/min infused over 4 min; although a maximum hasn't been determined, doses greater than 60 mg have been determined to be unnecessary for any patient.

OFF-LABEL USES

Prevention of myocardial reinfarction, treatment of transient ischemic attacks

CONTRAINDICATIONS

None known.

INTERACTIONS

Drug

Anticoagulants, aspirin, heparin, salicylates, thrombolytics: May increase the risk of bleeding with these drugs.

Herbal

None known.

Food

None known.

DIAGNOSTIC TEST EFFECTS

None known.

IV INCOMPATIBILITIES

No information available via Y-site administration.

SIDE EFFECTS

Frequent (14%)
Dizziness
Occasional (6%–2%)
Abdominal distress, headache, rash
Rare (less than 2%)
Diarrhea, vomiting, flushing, pruritus

SERIOUS REACTIONS

! Overdose produces peripheral vasodilation, resulting in hypotension.

NURSING CONSIDERATIONS

Baseline Assessment

- Assess the patient for chest pain.
- Obtain the patient's BP and pulse.
- When dipyridamole is used as an antiplatelet, check the patient's hematologic laboratory values.

Lifespan Considerations

- Dipyridamole is distributed in breast milk.
- Safety and efficacy of dipyridamole have not been established in children.
- No age-related precautions have been noted in the elderly.

Precautions

- Use dipyridamole cautiously in patients with hypotension.

Administration and Handling

PO

- Give on an empty stomach with full glass of water.

IV

- Dilute to at least 1:2 ratio with 0.9% NaCl or D_5W for total volume of 20 to 50 ml because undiluted solution may cause irritation.
- Infuse over 4 minutes.
- Inject thallium within 5 minutes after dipyridamole infusion has ended, as prescribed.

Intervention and Evaluation

- Assist the patient with ambulation if he or she experiences dizziness.
- Assess the patient's BP for hypotension.
- Examine the patient's skin for erythema and rash.

Patient Teaching

- Urge the patient to avoid alcohol during dipyridamole therapy. Explain that drinking three or more alcoholic beverages a day increases the risk of stomach bleeding and dizziness, possibly resulting in a fall.
- Suggest dry toast and unsalted crackers to relieve nausea.
- Tell the patient that therapeutic response may not be achieved before 2 to 3 months of continuous therapy.
- Warn the patient to use caution when rising suddenly from a lying or sitting position.

eptifibatide

ep-tih-**fib**-ah-tide
(Integrilin)

CATEGORY AND SCHEDULE

Pregnancy Risk Category: B

MECHANISM OF ACTION

A glycoprotein IIb/IIIa inhibitor that rapidly inhibits platelet aggregation by preventing binding of fibrinogen to receptor sites on platelets. **Therapeutic Effect:** Prevents closure of treated coronary arteries. Also prevents acute cardiac ischemic complications.

AVAILABILITY

Injection solution: 0.75 mg/ml, 2 mg/ml.

INDICATIONS AND DOSAGES

▸ Adjunct to percutaneous coronary intervention

IV Bolus, IV Infusion

Adults, Elderly. 180 mcg/kg before PCI initiation; then continuous drip of 2 mcg/kg/min and a second 180 mcg/kg bolus 10 min after the first. Maximum: 15 mg/hr. Continue until hospital discharge or for up to 18–24 hours. Minimum 12 hours is recommended. Concurrent aspirin and heparin therapy is recommended.

▸ Acute coronary syndrome

IV Bolus, IV Infusion

Adults, Elderly. 180 mcg/kg bolus then 2 mcg/kg/min until discharge or coronary artery bypass graft, up to 72 hr. Maximum: 15 mg/hr. Concurrent aspirin and heparin therapy is recommended.

▸ **Dosage in renal impairment**

Creatinine clearance less than 50 ml/min. Use 180 mcg/kg bolus (maximum 22.6 mg) and 1 mcg/kg/min infusion (maximum: 7.5 mg/hr).

CONTRAINDICATIONS

Active internal bleeding, AV malformation or aneurysm, history of cerebrovascular accident (CVA) within 2 years or CVA with residual neurologic defect, history of vasculitis, intracranial neoplasm, oral anticoagulant use within last 7 days unless PT is less than 1.22 times the control, recent (6 wk or less) GI or GU bleeding, recent (6 wk or less) surgery or trauma, prior IV dextran use before or during PTCA, severe uncontrolled hypertension, thrombocytopenia (less than 100,000 cells/mcl)

INTERACTIONS

Drug

Anticoagulants, heparin: May increase the risk of hemorrhage.

Dextran, other platelet aggregation inhibitors (such as aspirin), thrombolytic agents: May increase the risk of bleeding.

Herbal

None known.

Food

None known.

DIAGNOSTIC TEST EFFECTS

Increases aPTT, PT, and clotting time. Decreases platelet count.

IV INCOMPATIBILITIES

Administer in separate line; do not add other medications to infusion solution.

SIDE EFFECTS

Occasional (7%)

Hypotension

SERIOUS REACTIONS

! Minor to major bleeding complications may occur, most commonly at arterial access site for cardiac catheterization.

NURSING CONSIDERATIONS

Baseline Assessment

• Obtain the patient's Hgb, Hct, and platelet count before treatment. If platelet count is less than 90,000/mm^3, obtain additional platelet counts routinely to avoid development of thrombocytopenia.

Lifespan Considerations

• It is unknown if eptifibatide causes fetal harm or can affect reproduction capacity.

• It is unknown if eptifibatide is distributed in breast milk.

• Safety and efficacy of eptifibatide have not been established in children.

• In the elderly, the risk of major bleeding is increased.

Precautions

• Use eptifibatide cautiously in patients who weigh less than 75 kg, are older than 65 years, have a history of GI disease, or are receiving aspirin, heparin, or thrombolytics.

• Use cautiously in patients with PTCA less than 12 hours from the onset of symptoms of acute MI, prolonged PTCA that's greater than 70 minutes, and failed PTCA.

Administration and Handling

IV

• Store vials in refrigerator. Solution normally appears clear and is colorless. Do not shake. Discard unused portions. Also discard if preparation contains any opaque particles.

• Withdraw bolus dose from 10-ml

vial (2 mg/ml); for IV infusion withdraw from 100-ml vial (0.75 mg/ml). May give IV push and infusion undiluted.
- Give bolus dose IV push over 1 to 2 minutes.

Intervention and Evaluation
- Diligently monitor the patient for bleeding, particularly at other arterial and venous puncture sites.
- Avoid NG tube and urinary catheter use, if possible.

Patient Teaching
- Instruct the patient to report bleeding from surgical site, chest pain, or dyspnea.
- Tell the patient to use an electric razor and soft toothbrush, to prevent bleeding during eptifibatide therapy.
- Advise the patient not to take other medications, including OTC drugs (especially aspirin), without physician approval.
- Warn the patient to report black or red stool, coffee-ground emesis, dark or red urine, or red-speckled mucus from cough.
- Tell the female patient that her menstrual flow may be heavier than usual.

ticlopidine hydrochloride

tye-**klo**-pa-deen
(Apo-Ticlopidine[CAN], Ticlid, Tilodene[AUS])

CATEGORY AND SCHEDULE
Pregnancy Risk Category: B

MECHANISM OF ACTION
An aggregation inhibitor that inhibits the release of adenosine diphosphate from activated platelets, which prevents fibrinogen from binding to glycoprotein IIb/IIIa receptors on the surface of activated platelets. **Therapeutic Effect:** Inhibits platelet aggregation and thrombus formation.

AVAILABILITY
Tablets: 250 mg.

INDICATIONS AND DOSAGES
▸ **Prevention of stroke**
PO
Adults, Elderly. 250 mg twice a day.

OFF-LABEL USES
Treatment of intermittent claudication, sickle cell disease, subarachnoid hemorrhage

CONTRAINDICATIONS
Active pathologic bleeding, such as bleeding peptic ulcer and intracranial bleeding, hematopoietic disorders, including neutropenia and thrombocytopenia; presence of hemostatic disorder; severe hepatic impairment

INTERACTIONS
Drug
Aspirin, heparin, oral anticoagulants, thrombolytics: May increase the risk of bleeding with these drugs.
Herbal
None known.
Food
None known.

DIAGNOSTIC TEST EFFECTS
May increase serum cholesterol, serum alkaline phosphatase, bilirubin, triglyceride, AST (SGOT), and ALT (SGPT) levels. May prolong bleeding time. May decrease neutrophil and platelet counts.

SIDE EFFECTS
Frequent (13%–5%)
Diarrhea, nausea, dyspepsia, including heartburn, indigestion, GI discomfort, and bloating

Rare (2%–1%)
Vomiting, flatulence, pruritus, dizziness

SERIOUS REACTIONS

! Neutropenia occurs in approximately 2% of patients.
! Thrombotic thrombocytopenia purpura, agranulocytosis, hepatitis, cholestatic jaundice, and tinnitus occur rarely.

NURSING CONSIDERATIONS

Baseline Assessment

- Discontinue ticlopidine 10–14 days before surgery if antiplatelet effect is not desired.
- Plan to obtain laboratory studies, particularly hepatic enzyme tests and CBC.

Lifespan Considerations

- The safety and efficacy of ticlopidine in children has not been established.
- No age-related precautions have been noted in the elderly.

Precautions

- Use ticlopidine cautiously in patients with an increased risk of bleeding or severe hepatic or renal disease.

Administration and Handling

PO

- Give ticlopidine with food or just after meals to increase bioavailability and decrease GI discomfort.

Intervention and Evaluation

- Assess the patient's pattern of daily bowel activity and stool consistency.
- Assist the patient with ambulation if he or she experiences dizziness.
- Monitor the patient's heart sounds.
- Assess the patient's BP for hypotension and skin for erythema and rash.
- Monitor the patient's CBC and hepatic enzyme levels.
- Observe the patient for signs of bleeding.

Patient Teaching

- Instruct the patient to take ticlopidine with food to decrease GI symptoms.
- Stress to the patient that periodic blood tests are essential to treatment.
- Warn the patient to report chills, fever, sore throat, or unusual bleeding.

tirofiban

tye-roe-**fye**-ban
(Aggrastat)
Do not confuse Aggrastat with Aggrenox.

CATEGORY AND SCHEDULE

Pregnancy Risk Category: B

MECHANISM OF ACTION

An antiplatelet and antithrombotic agent that binds to platelet receptor glycoprotein IIb/IIIa, preventing binding of fibrinogen. **Therapeutic Effect:** Inhibits platelet aggregation and thrombus formation.

PHARMACOKINETICS

Poorly bound to plasma proteins; unbound fraction in plasma: 35%. Limited metabolism. Primarily eliminated in the urine (65%) and, to a lesser amount, in the feces. Removed by hemodialysis. ***Half-life:*** 2 hr. Clearance is significantly decreased in severe renal impairment (creatinine clearance less than 30 ml/min).

AVAILABILITY

Injection Premix: 12.5 mg/250 ml, 25 mg/500 ml (50 mcg/ml).
Vial: 250 mcg/ml.

INDICATIONS AND DOSAGES

▸ Inhibition of platelet aggregation

IV

Adults, Elderly. Initially, 0.4 mcg/kg/min for 30 min; then continue at 0.1 mcg/kg/min through procedure and for 12–24 hr after procedure.

▸ Severe renal insufficiency (creatinine clearance less than 30 ml/min)

Adults, Elderly. Half the usual rate of infusion.

CONTRAINDICATIONS

Active internal bleeding or a history of bleeding diathesis within previous 30 days, arteriovenous malformation or aneurysm, history of intracranial hemorrhage, history of thrombocytopenia after prior exposure to tirofiban, intracranial neoplasm, major surgical procedure within previous 30 days, severe hypertension, stroke

INTERACTIONS

Drug

Drugs that affect hemostasis (such as aspirin, heparin, NSAIDs, and warfarin): May increase the risk of bleeding.

Herbal

None known.

Food

None known.

DIAGNOSTIC TEST EFFECTS

Decreases Hct, Hgb and platelet count.

IV INCOMPATIBILITIES

Do not mix with other medications.

SIDE EFFECTS

Occasional (6%–3%)

Pelvis pain, bradycardia, dizziness, leg pain

Rare (2%–1%)

Edema and swelling, vasovagal reaction, diaphoresis, nausea, fever, headache

SERIOUS REACTIONS

! Signs and symptoms of overdose include generally minor mucocutaneous bleeding and bleeding at the femoral artery access site.

! Thrombocytopenia occurs rarely.

NURSING CONSIDERATIONS

Baseline Assessment

- Assess the patient's aPTT, Hct, Hgb, platelet count, and serum creatinine level before tirofiban administration, within 6 hours after the loading dose, and then at least daily during therapy. If the patient's platelet count is less than 90,000/mm^3, obtain additional platelet counts routinely to avoid thrombocytopenia. If the patient develops thrombocytopenia, discontinue tirofiban and heparin, as prescribed.

Lifespan Considerations

- It is unknown if tirofiban is distributed in breast milk.
- Safety and efficacy of tirofiban have not been established in children.
- There is an increased risk of bleeding in the elderly. Use tirofiban with caution in this patient population.

Precautions

- Use tirofiban cautiously in patients with hemorrhagic retinopathy, platelet counts less than 150,000/mm^3, or renal impairment.
- Use cautiously in patients who are also receiving drugs affecting hemostasis, such as warfarin.

Administration and Handling

◂ALERT▸ Heparin and tirofiban can be administered through the same IV line.

IV

- Store at room temperature and

protect from light. Use only clear solution.
• Discard unused solution 24 hours after start of infusion.
• For injection for solution (250 mcg/ml), withdraw and discard 100 ml from a 500-ml bag of 0.9% NaCl or D_5W and replace this volume with 100 ml of tirofiban drawn from two 50-ml vials, or withdraw and discard 50 ml from a 250-ml bag and replace with 50 ml of tirofiban drawn from one 50-ml vial to achieve a final concentration of 50 mcg/ml.
• Mix injection for solution (250 mcg/ml) well before administration.
• For injection (50 mcg/ml) premix in 500-ml IntraVia container, tear off the dust cover to open the IntraVia container.
• Check the IntraVia container for leaks by squeezing the inner bag firmly; if a leak is found or if the solution is not clear, discard the solution.
• Do not add other drugs or remove injection (50 mcg/ml) premix solution directly from the bag with a syringe. Do not use plastic containers in series connections because doing so may result in air embolism caused by drawing air from the first container that holds no solution.
• For loading dose, give 0.4 mcg/kg/min for 30 minutes. For maintenance infusion, give 0.1 mcg/kg/min.

Intervention and Evaluation
• Monitor the patient's aPTT 6 hours after the beginning of the heparin infusion. Adjust heparin dosage to maintain aPTT at approximately 2 times control.
• Closely monitor the patient for bleeding, particularly at other arterial and venous puncture sites and IM injection sites.
• Avoid NG tube and urinary catheter use, if possible.
• Maintain the patient on complete bed rest, with the head of the bed elevated at 30 degrees.

Patient Teaching
• Inform the patient that it may take longer to stop bleeding during tirofiban therapy.
• Warn the patient to report unusual bleeding.
• Tell the patient to notify his or her dentist and other physicians of tirofiban therapy before surgery is scheduled or new drugs are prescribed.

treprostinil sodium

treh-**prost**-in-ill
(Remodulin)

CATEGORY AND SCHEDULE
Pregnancy Risk Category: B

MECHANISM OF ACTION
An antiplatelet that directly dilates pulmonary and systemic arterial vascular beds, inhibiting platelet aggregation. **Therapeutic Effect:** Reduces symptoms of pulmonary arterial hypertension associated with exercise.

PHARMACOKINETICS
Rapidly, completely absorbed after subcutaneous infusion; 91% bound to plasma protein. Metabolized by the liver. Excreted mainly in the urine with a lesser amount eliminated in the feces. ***Half-life:*** 2–4 hr.

AVAILABILITY
Injection: 1 mg/ml, 2.5 mg/ml, 5 mg/ml, 10 mg/ml.

INDICATIONS AND DOSAGES
▸ **Pulmonary arterial hypertension**
Continuous subcutaneous infusion
Adults, Elderly. Initially, 1.25 ng/kg/

min. Reduce infusion rate to 0.625 ng/kg/min if initial dose cannot be tolerated. Increase infusion rate in increments of no more than 1.25 ng/kg/min per week for the first 4 wk and then no more than 2.5 ng/kg/min per week for the duration of infusion.

▸ Hepatic impairment (mild to moderate)

Adults, Elderly. Decrease the initial dose to 0.625 ng/kg/min based on ideal body weight and increase cautiously.

CONTRAINDICATIONS

None known.

INTERACTIONS

Drug

Anticoagulants, aspirin, heparin, thrombolytics: May increase the risk of bleeding.

Drugs that alter BP, including antihypertensive agents, diuretics, vasodilators: Reduced BP caused by treprostinil may be exacerbated by these drugs.

Herbal

None known.

Food

None known.

DIAGNOSTIC TEST EFFECTS

None known.

SIDE EFFECTS

Frequent

Infusion site pain, erythema, induration, rash

Occasional

Headache, diarrhea, jaw pain, vasodilation, nausea

Rare

Dizziness, hypotension, pruritus, edema

SERIOUS REACTIONS

! Abrupt withdrawal or sudden large reductions in dosage may result in worsening of pulmonary arterial hypertension symptoms.

NURSING CONSIDERATIONS

Baseline Assessment

• Expect to obtain laboratory test results, including BUN, hepatic enzyme, and serum creatinine levels.

Lifespan Considerations

• It is unknown if treprostinil is distributed in breast milk.
• Safety and efficacy of treprostinil have not been established in children.
• In the elderly, age-related decreased cardiac, hepatic, and renal function as well as concurrent disease or other drug therapy may require dosage adjustment.
• Consider dosage selection carefully in the elderly, because of the increased incidence of diminished organ function.

Precautions

• Use treprostinil cautiously in elderly patients older than 65 years of age with liver or renal impairment.

Administration and Handling

Subcutaneous

• Store at room temperature and administer without further dilution.
• Do not use a single vial for longer than 14 days after initial use.
• Give as a continuous subcutaneous infusion via a subcutaneous catheter, using an infusion pump designed for subcutaneous drug delivery.
• Calculate the infusion rate using following formula: Infusion rate (ml/hr) = Dose (ng/kg/min) multiplied by Weight (kg) multiplied by (0.00006/treprostinil dosage strength concentration [mg/ml]).
• To avoid potential interruptions in drug delivery, provide the patient with immediate access to a backup

infusion pump and spare subcutaneous infusion sets.

Patient Teaching

- Show the patient how to administer tresprostinil via a self-inserted subcutaneous catheter using an ambulatory pump.
- Teach the patient how to care for the subcutaneous catheter and troubleshoot infusion pump problems.
- Tell the patient to report signs of increased pulmonary artery pressure, such as dyspnea, cough, or chest pain.

58 Hematinics

ferrous fumarate,
ferrous gluconate,
ferrous sulfate
iron dextran
iron sucrose
sodium ferric gluconate complex

Uses: Hematinics (iron supplements) are used to prevent and treat iron deficiency, which may result from improper diet, pregnancy, impaired absorption, or prolonged blood loss.

Action: Hematinics provide supplementary iron to ensure adequate supplies for the formation of hemoglobin, which is needed for erythropoiesis and oxygen transport.

COMBINATION PRODUCTS

FERRO-SEQUELS: ferrous fumarate/docusate (a stool softener) 150 mg/100 mg.

ferrous fumarate

fer-rous **fume**-ah-rate
(Feostat, Femiron, Ferro-Sequels, Nephro-Fer, Palafer[CAN])

ferrous gluconate

fer-rous **glue**-kuh-nate
(Apo-Ferrous Gluconate[CAN], Fergon)

ferrous sulfate

fer-rous **sul**-fate
(Apo-Ferrous Sulfate[CAN], Fer-In-Sol, Fer-Iron, Ferro-Gradumet[AUS], Slow-Fe)

CATEGORY AND SCHEDULE

Pregnancy Risk Category: A
OTC

MECHANISM OF ACTION

An enzymatic mineral that is as an essential component in the formation of Hgb, myoglobin, and enzymes. Promotes effective erythropoiesis and transport and utilization of oxygen (O_2). **Therapeutic Effect:** Prevents iron deficiency.

PHARMACOKINETICS

Absorbed in the duodenum and upper jejunum. Ten percent absorbed in patients with normal iron stores; increased to 20%–30% in those with inadequate iron stores. Primarily bound to serum transferrin. Excreted in urine, sweat, and sloughing of intestinal mucosa and by menses. ***Half-life:*** 6 hr.

AVAILABILITY

Ferrous fumarate
Tablets (Femiron): 63 mg (20 mg elemental iron).
Tablets (Nephro-Fer): 350 mg (115 mg elemental iron).
Tablets (Chewable [Feostat]): 100 mg (33 mg elemental iron).
Tablet (Time-Release [Ferro-Sequels]): 150 mg (50 mg elemental iron).
Ferrous gluconate
Tablets: 325 mg (36 mg elemental iron).
Tablets (Fergon): 240 mg (27 mg elemental iron).
Ferrous sulfate
Tablets: 325 mg (65 mg elemental iron).
Tablets (Timed-Release [Slow FE]): 160 mg (50 mg elemental iron).
Elixir: 220 mg/5 ml (44 mg elemental iron per 5 ml).
*Oral Drops (Ferr-In-Sol, Fer-Iron):*75 mg/0.6 ml.

INDICATIONS AND DOSAGES

▸ Iron deficiency anemia

Dosage is expressed in terms of milligrams of elemental iron, degree of anemia, patient weight, and presence of any bleeding. Expect to use periodic hematologic determinations as guide to therapy.

PO (ferrous fumarate)
Adults, Elderly. 60–100 mg twice a day.
Children. 3–6 mg/kg/day in 2–3 divided doses.
PO (ferrous gluconate)
Adults, Elderly. 60 mg 2–4 times a day.
Children. 3–6 mg/kg/day in 2–3 divided doses.
PO (ferrous sulfate)
Adults, Elderly. 325 mg 2–4 times a day.
Children. 3–6 mg/kg/day in 2–3 divided doses.

▸ Prevention of iron deficiency

PO (ferrous fumarate)
Adults, Elderly. 60–100 mg/day.
Children. 1–2 mg/kg/day.
PO (ferrous gluconate)
Adults, Elderly. 60 mg/day.
Children. 1–2 mg/kg/day.
PO (ferrous sulfate)
Adults, Elderly. 325 mg/day.
Children. 1–2 mg/kg/day.

CONTRAINDICATIONS

Hemochromatosis, hemosiderosis, hemolytic anemias, peptic ulcer disease, regional enteritis, ulcerative colitis

INTERACTIONS

Drug

Antacids, calcium supplements, pancreatin, pancrelipase: May decrease the absorption of ferrous fumarate, ferrous gluconate, and ferrous sulfate.

Etidronate, quinolones, tetracyclines: May decrease the absorption of etidronate, quinolones, and tetracyclines.

Herbal

None known.

Food

Eggs, milk: Inhibit ferrous fumarate absorption.

DIAGNOSTIC TEST EFFECTS

May increase serum bilirubin and iron levels. May decrease serum calcium level. May obscure occult blood in stools.

SIDE EFFECTS

Occasional

Mild, transient nausea

Rare

Heartburn, anorexia, constipation, diarrhea

SERIOUS REACTIONS

! Large doses may aggravate existing GI tract disease, such as peptic ulcer disease, regional enteritis, and ulcerative colitis.

! Severe iron poisoning occurs most often in children and is manifested as vomiting, severe abdominal pain, diarrhea, and dehydration, followed by hyperventilation, pallor or cyanosis, and cardiovascular collapse.

NURSING CONSIDERATIONS

Baseline Assessment

- Monitor blood test results, including Hgb and Hct, before and during therapy.
- Assess the patient's nutritional status and dietary intake.

Lifespan Considerations

- Ferrous fumarate, ferrous sulfate, and ferrous gluconate cross the placenta and are distributed in breast milk.
- No age-related precautions have been noted in children or the elderly.

Precautions
- Use these drugs cautiously in patients with bronchial asthma or iron hypersensitivity.

Administration and Handling
PO
- Store all forms, including tablets, capsules, suspension, and drops, at room temperature.
- Give between meals with water unless GI discomfort occurs; if so, give with meals.
- Use dropper or straw to administer the liquid preparation and allow the drug solution to drop on the back of the patient's tongue, to prevent mucous membrane and teeth staining.
- To avoid transient staining of mucous membranes and teeth, place liquid on back of tongue with dropper or straw.
- Avoid simultaneous administration of antacids or tetracycline.
- Do not crush sustained-release form.

Intervention and Evaluation
- Monitor the patient's Hgb, reticulocyte count, ferritin and serum iron levels, and total iron-binding capacity.
- Assess the patient's pattern of daily bowel activity and stool consistency.
- Know that eggs and milk inhibit drug absorption.
- Evaluate the patient for clinical improvement and record relief of iron deficiency symptoms (fatigue, headache, irritability, pallor, and paresthesia of extremities).

Patient Teaching
- Tell the patient that his or her stools will darken in color.
- Teach the patient to take the drug after meals, or with food if GI discomfort occurs.
- Instruct the patient not to take the drug within 2 hours of antacids because antacids prevent drug absorption of ferrous.
- Teach the patient not to take the drug with milk or eggs.

iron dextran
iron **dex**-tran
(Dexiron[CAN], Infed, Infufer[CAN])

CATEGORY AND SCHEDULE
Pregnancy Risk Category: C

MECHANISM OF ACTION
A trace element and essential component in the formation of Hgb. Necessary for effective erythropoiesis and transport and utilization of oxygen. Serves as cofactor of several essential enzymes. **Therapeutic Effect:** Replenishes Hgb and depleted iron stores.

PHARMACOKINETICS
Readily absorbed after IM administration. Most absorption occurs within 72 hr; remainder within 3–4 wk. Bound to protein to form hemosiderin, ferritin, or transferrin. No physiologic system of elimination. Small amounts lost daily in shedding of skin, hair, and nails and in feces, urine, and perspiration. ***Half-life:*** 5–20 hr.

AVAILABILITY
Injection: 50 mg/ml.

INDICATIONS AND DOSAGES
▸ **Iron deficiency anemia (no blood loss)**

Dosage is expressed in terms of milligrams of elemental iron, degree of anemia, patient weight, and presence of any bleeding. Expect to use periodic hematologic determinations as guide to therapy.

IV, IM
Adults, Elderly. Mg iron = 0.66 × weight (kg) × (100 – Hgb [g/dl]/ 14.8)

▸ **Iron replacement secondary to blood loss**
IV, IM
Adults, Elderly. Replacement iron (mg) = blood loss (ml) times Hct.

Maximum daily dosages
Adults weighing more than 50 kg. 100 mg.
Children weighing 10-50 kg. 100 mg.
Children weighing 5-less than 10 kg. 50 mg.
Infants weighing less than 5 kg. 25 mg.

CONTRAINDICATIONS

All anemias except iron deficiency anemia, including pernicious, aplastic, normocytic, and refractory

INTERACTIONS

Drug
None known.

Herbal
None known.

Food
None known.

DIAGNOSTIC TEST EFFECTS

None known.

IV INCOMPATIBILITIES

No information available via Y-site administration.

SIDE EFFECTS

Frequent
Allergic reaction (such as rash and itching), backache, myalgia, chills, dizziness, headache, fever, nausea, vomiting, flushed skin, pain or redness at injection site, brown discoloration of skin, metallic taste

SERIOUS REACTIONS

! Anaphylaxis has occurred during the first few minutes after injection, causing death rarely.
! Leukocytosis and lymphadenopathy occur rarely.

NURSING CONSIDERATIONS

Baseline Assessment
- Do not give concurrently with oral iron form because excessive iron may produce excessive iron storage, called hemosiderosis.
- Assess the patient for adequate muscle mass before injecting medication.

Lifespan Considerations
- Iron dextran may cross the placenta in some form and trace amounts of the drug are distributed in breast milk.
- No age-related precautions have been noted in children and the elderly.

Precautions
- Use iron dextran extremely cautiously in patients with serious hepatic impairment.
- Use cautiously in patients with bronchial asthma, a history of allergies, or rheumatoid arthritis.

Administration and Handling
◂ **ALERT** ▸ Plan to discontinue oral iron before administering iron dextran because excessive iron intake may produce excessive iron storage (hemosiderosis).
◂ **ALERT** ▸ Know that a test dose is generally given before the full dose; stay with the patient for several minutes after injection of the test dose because of the potential for anaphylactic reaction.

IV
- Store at room temperature.
- May give undiluted or dilute in 0.9% NaCl for infusion.

• Do not exceed an administration rate of 50 mg/min (1 ml/min). A too-rapid IV rate may produce flushing, chest pain, shock, hypotension, and tachycardia.
• Keep patient recumbent for 30 to 45 minutes after IV administration to minimize orthostatic hypotension.
IM
• Draw up medication with one needle; use new needle for injection, to minimize skin staining.
• Use Z-tract technique by displacing subcutaneous tissue lateral to injection site before inserting needle, to minimize skin staining.
• Administer deep into upper outer quadrant of buttock only.

Intervention and Evaluation
• Be alert for acute exacerbation of joint pain and swelling in patients with rheumatoid arthritis and iron deficiency anemia.
• Inguinal lymphadenopathy may occur with IM injection.
• Monitor the patient's IM site for abscess formation, atrophy, brownish skin color, necrosis, and swelling.
• Evaluate the patient for inflammation, pain, and soreness at or near IM injection site.
• Examine the patient's IV site for phlebitis.
• Monitor the patient's serum ferritin level.

Patient Teaching
• Tell the patient that pain and brown staining of the skin may occur at the injection site.
• Caution the patient not to take oral iron while receiving iron injections.
• Instruct the patient that stools may become black during iron therapy. Explain that this side effect is harmless unless accompanied by abdominal cramping or pain and red streaking or sticky consistency of stool.
• Warn the patient to report abdominal cramping or pain, back pain, fever, headache, or red streaking and a sticky consistency of stool.
• Suggest chewing gum, sucking on hard candy, and maintaining good oral hygiene to prevent or reduce the metallic taste.

iron sucrose
iron **sue**-crose
(Venofer)

CATEGORY AND SCHEDULE
Pregnancy Risk Category: B

MECHANISM OF ACTION
A trace element that is an essential component in the formation of Hgb. It's necessary for effective erythropoiesis and oxygen transport capacity of blood, and transport and utilization of oxygen, and serves as cofactor of several essential enzymes. **Therapeutic Effect:** Replenishes body iron stores in patients on long-term hemodialysis who have iron deficiency anemia and are receiving erythropoietin.

AVAILABILITY
Injection: 20 mg/ml or 100 mg elemental iron in 5-ml single-dose vial.

INDICATIONS AND DOSAGES
▸ **Iron deficiency anemia**
Dosage is expressed in terms of milligrams of elemental iron.
IV
Adults, Elderly. 5 ml iron sucrose, or 100 mg elemental iron, delivered during dialysis; administer 1–3 times a wk to total dose of 1,000 mg in 10 doses. Give no more than 3 times a wk.

OFF-LABEL USES

Treatment of dystrophic epidermolysis bullosa

CONTRAINDICATIONS

All anemias except iron deficiency anemia, including pernicious, aplastic, normocytic, and refractory anemia; evidence of iron overload

INTERACTIONS

Drug

None known.

Herbal

None known.

Food

None known.

DIAGNOSTIC TEST EFFECTS

Increases Hgb and Hct, serum ferritin level, and serum transferrin saturation.

IV INCOMPATIBILITIES

Do not mix with other medications or add to parenteral nutrition solution for IV infusion.

SIDE EFFECTS

Frequent (36%–23%)

Hypotension, leg cramps, diarrhea

SERIOUS REACTIONS

! Too rapid IV administration may produce severe hypotension, headache, vomiting, nausea, dizziness, paresthesia, abdominal and muscle pain, edema, and cardiovascular collapse.

! Hypersensitivity reaction occurs rarely.

NURSING CONSIDERATIONS

Baseline Assessment

- Plan to obtain laboratory test results, including Hgb and Hct, serum ferritin level, and serum transferrin saturation.
- Make sure the patient has patent dialysis access before preparing drug.

Precautions

- Use iron sucrose cautiously in patients with cardiac dysfunction, bronchial asthma, history of allergies, or hepatic or renal impairment.

Administration and Handling

◀ALERT▶ Administer directly into dialysis line during hemodialysis, as prescribed.

IV

- Store at room temperature.
- May be given as undiluted, slow IV injection. For IV infusion, dilute each vial in maximum of 100 ml 0.9% NaCl immediately before infusion.
- For IV injection, administer into the dialysis line at a rate of 1 ml, or 20 mg iron, undiluted solution per minute. Allow 5 minutes per vial; do not exceed 1 vial per injection.
- For IV infusion, administer into dialysis line at a rate of 100 mg iron over at least 15 minutes, to reduce the risk of hypotensive episodes.

Intervention and Evaluation

- Initially, monitor the patient's Hct, Hgb, serum ferritin, and serum transferrin levels monthly, then every 2 to 3 months as determined by the physician.
- Obtain reliable patient serum iron levels 48 hours after iron sucrose administration.

Patient Teaching

- Tell the patient to expect follow-up blood tests to monitor the results of treatment.
- Explain that iron sucrose is administered during dialysis.
- Ask the patient to report leg cramps or diarrhea.

sodium ferric gluconate complex

sew-**dee**-um **fair**-ick **glue**-koe-nate **calm**-plex
(Ferrlecit)

CATEGORY AND SCHEDULE

Pregnancy Risk Category: B

MECHANISM OF ACTION

A trace element that repletes total iron content in body. Replaces iron found in Hgb, myoglobin, and specific enzymes; allows oxygen transport via Hgb. **Therapeutic Effect:** Prevents and corrects iron deficiency.

AVAILABILITY

Ampules: 12.5 mg/ml elemental iron.

INDICATIONS AND DOSAGES

▸ Iron deficiency anemia

IV Infusion

Adults, Elderly. 125 mg in 100 ml 0.9% NaCl infused over 1 hr. Minimum cumulative dose 1 g elemental iron given over 8 sessions at sequential dialysis treatments. May be given during dialysis session.

CONTRAINDICATIONS

All anemias not associated with iron deficiency

INTERACTIONS

Drug

None known.

Herbal

None known.

Food

None known.

DIAGNOSTIC TEST EFFECTS

None known.

IV INCOMPATIBILITIES

Do not mix with other medications.

SIDE EFFECTS

Frequent (greater than 3%)

Flushing, hypotension, hypersensitivity reaction

Occasional (3%–1%)

Injection site reaction, headache, abdominal pain, chills, flulike syndrome, dizziness, leg cramps, dyspnea, nausea, vomiting, diarrhea, myalgia, pruritus, edema

SERIOUS REACTIONS

! A potentially fatal hypersensitivity reaction occurs rarely, characterized by cardiovascular collapse, cardiac arrest, dyspnea, bronchospasm, angioedema, and urticaria.

! Rapid administration may cause hypotension associated with flushing, lightheadedness, fatigue, weakness, or severe pain in the chest, back, or groin.

NURSING CONSIDERATIONS

Baseline Assessment

- Assess patient's nutritional status and dietary intake.

Lifespan Considerations

- It is unknown if sodium ferric gluconate complex is distributed in breast milk.
- Safety and efficacy of sodium ferric gluconate complex have not been established in children.
- No age-related precautions have been noted in the elderly. However, lower initial dosages of sodium ferric gluconate complex are recommended in the elderly.

Precautions

- Use sodium ferric gluconate complex cautiously in patients with asthma, iron overload, hepatic impairment, rheumatoid arthritis, or significant allergies.

Administration and Handling

◀ALERT▶ Plan to initially administer a 25-mg test dose that's diluted in 50 ml 0.9% NaCl and given over 60 minutes.

• May give undiluted as slow IV injection without test dose.

IV

• Store at room temperature.
• Use immediately after dilution.
• Remember that the standard recommended dose is 125 mg (10 ml) diluted with 100 ml 0.9% NaCl.
• Infuse both test dose and standard dose over 1 hour.
• Do not give concurrently with oral iron because excessive iron intake may produce excessive iron storage (hemosiderosis).

Intervention and Evaluation

• Monitor the patient's laboratory test results, especially CBC, serum iron concentrations, and vital signs. Test results may not be meaningful for 3 weeks after beginning sodium ferric gluconate complex therapy.
• Assess patients with rheumatoid arthritis or iron deficiency anemia for acute exacerbation of joint pain and swelling.

Patient Teaching

• Tell the patient that his or her stools may become black during iron therapy. Explain that this effect is harmless unless accompanied by abdominal cramping or pain and red streaking and sticky consistency of stool.
• Warn the patient to report abdominal cramping or pain and red streaking and sticky consistency of stool.
• Tell the patient that the drug may be administered during dialysis treatments.

59 Hematopoietic Agents

darbepoetin alfa
epoetin alfa
filgrastim
oprelvekin (interleukin-2, IL-2)
pegfilgrastim
sargramostim (granulocyte macrophage colony-stimulating factor, GM-CSF)

Uses: Hematopoietic agents are used to accelerate neutrophil repopulation after chemotherapy, to accelerate bone marrow recovery after autologous bone marrow transplant, and to stimulate erythrocyte production in patients with chronic renal failure.

Action: Hematopoietic agents act by stimulating the proliferation and differentiation of hematopoietic growth factors (naturally occurring hormones) and by enhancing the function of mature forms of neutrophils, monocytes, macrophages, and erythrocytes.

darbepoetin alfa

dar-beh-**poe**-ee-tin
(Aranesp)
Do not confuse Aranesp with Aricept.

CATEGORY AND SCHEDULE
Pregnancy Risk Category: C

MECHANISM OF ACTION
A glycoprotein that stimulates formation of RBCs in bone marrow; increases serum half-life of epoetin. **Therapeutic Effect:** Induces erythropoiesis and release of reticulocytes from bone marrow.

PHARMACOKINETICS
Well absorbed after subcutaneous administration. ***Half-life:*** 48.5 hr.

AVAILABILITY
Injection: 25 mcg/ml, 40 mcg/ml, 60 mcg/ml, 100 mcg/ml, 150 mcg/ml, 200 mcg/ml, 300 mcg/ml.

INDICATIONS AND DOSAGES
▸ **Anemia in chronic renal failure**
IV Bolus, Subcutaneous
Adults, Elderly. Initially, 0.45 mcg/kg once weekly. Adjust dosage to achieve and maintain a target Hgb not to exceed 12 g/dl. Do not increase dosage more frequently than once monthly. Limit increases in Hgb by less than 1 g/dl over any 2-week period.

▸ **Anemia associated with chemotherapy**
IV, Subcutaneous
Adults, Elderly. 2.25 mcg/kg/dose once a week.

CONTRAINDICATIONS
History of sensitivity to mammalian cell-derived products or human albumin, uncontrolled hypertension

INTERACTIONS
Drug

None known.

Herbal

None known.

Food

None known.

DIAGNOSTIC TEST EFFECTS
May increase BUN, serum phosphorus, potassium, serum creatinine, serum uric acid, and sodium levels. May decrease bleeding time, serum

iron concentration, and serum ferritin.

IV INCOMPATIBILITIES

Do not mix with other medications.

SIDE EFFECTS

Frequent

Myalgia, hypertension or hypotension, headache, diarrhea

Occasional

Fatigue, edema, vomiting, reaction at administration site, asthenia, dizziness

SERIOUS REACTIONS

! Vascular access thrombosis, CHF, sepsis, arrhythmias, and anaphylactic reaction occur rarely.

NURSING CONSIDERATIONS

Baseline Assessment

- Assess the patient's BP before administering darbepoetin. Because 80% of patients with chronic renal failure have a history of hypertension, expect that BP will rise during early therapy.
- Assess the patient's serum iron level. Keep in mind that transferrin saturation should be greater than 20%, and serum ferritin level should be greater than 100 ng/ml before and during therapy.
- Consider that all patients will eventually need supplemental iron therapy.
- Establish the patient's baseline CBC; especially note the patient's Hct.

Lifespan Considerations

- It is unknown if darbepoetin alfa crosses the placenta or is distributed in breast milk.
- Safety and efficacy of darbepoetin alfa have not been established in children.
- In the elderly, age-related renal impairment may require dosage adjustment.

Precautions

- Use darbepoetin alfa cautiously in patients with hemolytic anemia, history of seizures, known porphyria (impairment of erythrocyte formation in bone marrow), sickle cell anemia, or thalassemia.

Administration and Handling

◀ALERT▶ Avoid excessive agitation of vial; do not shake because it will cause foaming.

IV

- Refrigerate vials. Do not shake vials vigorously because doing so may denature medication, rendering it inactive.
- Reconstitution is not necessary.
- May be given as an IV bolus.

Subcutaneous

- Use one dose per vial; do not reenter vial. Discard unused portion. May be mixed in a syringe with bacteriostatic 0.9% NaCl with benzyl alcohol 0.9% or bacteriostatic saline at a 1:1 ratio. Benzyl alcohol acts as a local anesthetic and may reduce injection site discomfort.

Intervention and Evaluation

- Monitor the patient's Hct level diligently. Reduce the dosage if Hct level increases more than 4 points in 2 weeks.
- Monitor the patient's CBC with differential, Hgb, reticulocyte count, and BUN, phosphorus, potassium, serum creatinine, and serum ferritin levels.
- Monitor the patient's BP aggressively for an increase because 25% of patients taking darbepoietin alfa require antihypertensive therapy and dietary restrictions.

Patient Teaching

- Stress to the patient that frequent blood tests will be needed to determine correct dosage.

- Warn the patient to report severe headache.
- Warn the patient to avoid tasks that require mental alertness or motor skills until his or her response to the drug is established.

epoetin alfa

eh-**poh**-ee-tin **al**-fa
(Epogen, Eprex[CAN], Procrit)
Do not confuse Epogen with Neupogen.

CATEGORY AND SCHEDULE

Pregnancy Risk Category: C

MECHANISM OF ACTION

A glycoprotein that stimulates division and differentiation of erythroid progenitor cells in bone marrow. **Therapeutic Effect:** Induces erythropoiesis and releases reticulocytes from bone marrow.

PHARMACOKINETICS

Well absorbed after subcutaneous administration. Following administration, an increase in reticulocyte count occurs within 10 days, and increases in Hgb, Hct, and RBC count are seen within 2–6 wk. ***Half-life:*** 4–13 hr.

AVAILABILITY

Injection: 2,000 units/ml, 3,000 units/ml, 4,000 units/ml, 10,000 units/ml, 20,000 units/ml, 40,000 units/ml.

INDICATIONS AND DOSAGES

▸ Treatment of anemia in chemotherapy patients

IV, Subcutaneous
Adults, Elderly, Children. 150 units/kg/dose 3 times a wk. Maximum: 1,200 units/kg/wk.

▸ Reduction of allogenic blood transfusions in elective surgery

Subcutaneous
Adults, Elderly. 300 units/kg/day 10 days before day of, and 4 days after surgery.

▸ Chronic renal failure

IV Bolus, Subcutaneous
Adults, Elderly. Initially, 50–100 units/kg 3 times a wk. Target Hct range: 30%–36%. Adjust dosage no earlier than 1-mo intervals unless prescribed. Decrease dosage if Hct is increasing and approaching 36%. Plan to temporarily withhold doses if Hct continues to rise and to reinstate lower dosage when Hct begins to decrease. If Hct increases by more than 4 points in 2 wk, monitor Hct twice a wk for 2–6 wk. Increase dose if Hct does not increase 5–6 points after 8 wk (with adequate iron stores) and if Hct is below target range. Maintenance: *For patients on dialysis:* 75 units/kg 3 times a wk. Range: 12.5–525 units/kg. *For patients not on dialysis:* 75–150 units/kg/wk.

▸ HIV infection in patients treated with AZT

IV, Subcutaneous
Adults. Initially, 100 units/kg 3 times a wk for 8 wk; may increase by 50–100 units/kg 3 times a wk. Evaluate response q4–8wk thereafter. Adjust dosage by 50–100 units/kg 3 times a wk. If dosages larger than 300 units/kg 3 times a wk are not eliciting response, it is unlikely patient will respond. Maintenance: Titrate to maintain desired Hct.

OFF-LABEL USES

Prevention of anemia in patients donating blood before elective surgery or autologous transfusion, treatment of anemia associated with neoplastic diseases

CONTRAINDICATIONS

History of sensitivity to mammalian cell-derived products or human albumin, uncontrolled hypertension

INTERACTIONS

Drug

Heparin: An increase in RBC volume may enhance blood clotting. Heparin dosage may need to be increased.

Herbal

None known.

Food

None known.

DIAGNOSTIC TEST EFFECTS

May increase BUN, serum phosphorus, serum potassium, serum creatinine, serum uric acid, and sodium levels. May decrease bleeding time, iron concentration, and serum ferritin levels.

IV INCOMPATIBILITIES

Do not mix with other medications.

SIDE EFFECTS

▸ Patients receiving chemotherapy

Frequent (20%–17%)

Fever, diarrhea, nausea, vomiting, edema

Occasional (13%–11%)

Asthenia, shortness of breath, paresthesia

Rare (5%–3%)

Dizziness, trunk pain

▸ Patients with chronic renal failure

Frequent (24%–11%)

Hypertension, headache, nausea, arthralgia

Occasional (9%–7%)

Fatigue, edema, diarrhea, vomiting, chest pain, skin reactions at administration site, asthenia, dizziness

▸ Patients with HIV infection treated with AZT

Frequent (38%–15%)

Fever, fatigue, headache, cough, diarrhea, rash, nausea

Occasional (14%–9%)

Shortness of breath, asthenia, skin reaction at injection site, dizziness

SERIOUS REACTIONS

! Hypertensive encephalopathy, thrombosis, cerebrovascular accident, MI, and seizures have occurred rarely.

! Hyperkalemia occurs occasionally in patients with chronic renal failure, usually in those who do not conform to medication regimen, dietary guidelines, and frequency of dialysis regimen.

NURSING CONSIDERATIONS

Baseline Assessment

- Assess the patient's BP before administering epoetin. Because 80% of patients with chronic renal failure have a history of hypertension, expect that BP will rise during early therapy.
- Assess the patient's serum iron level. Keep in mind that transferrin saturation should be greater than 20%, and serum ferritin level should be greater than 100 ng/ml before and during therapy.
- Consider that all patients will eventually need supplemental iron therapy.
- Establish the patient's CBC; especially note the patient's Hct.
- Monitor the patient aggressively for increased BP. Know that 25% of patients receiving epoetin alfa also require antihypertensive therapy and dietary restrictions.

Lifespan Considerations

- It is unknown if epoetin alfa

crosses the placenta or is distributed in breast milk.

• Safety and efficacy of epoetin alfa have not been established in children 12 years of age and younger.

• No age-related precautions have been noted in the elderly.

Precautions

• Use epoetin alfa cautiously in patients with a history of seizures and known porphyria (an impairment of erythrocyte formation in bone marrow).

Administration and Handling

◀ALERT▶ Avoid excessive agitation of vial; do not shake because it can cause foaming. Also, vigorous shaking may denature medication, rendering it inactive.

◀ALERT▶ Patients receiving AZT who have serum erythropoietin levels greater than 500 milliunits are not likely to respond to therapy.

IV

• Refrigerate vials. Do not shake vials.

• Reconstitution is not necessary.

• May be given as an IV bolus.

Subcutaneous

• Use one dose per vial; do not reenter vial. Discard unused portion. May be mixed in a syringe with bacteriostatic 0.9% NaCl with benzyl alcohol 0.9% or bacteriostatic saline at a 1:1 ratio. Benzyl alcohol acts as a local anesthetic and may reduce injection site discomfort.

Intervention and Evaluation

• Monitor the patient's Hct level diligently. Reduce the dosage if the patient's Hct level increases more than 4 points in 2 weeks.

• Assess the patient's CBC routinely.

• Monitor the patient's body temperature, especially in patients receiving chemotherapy and in patients with HIV infection treated with zidovudine, and serum BUN, serum phosphorus, serum potassium, serum creatinine, and serum uric acid levels, especially in patients with chronic renal failure.

Patient Teaching

• Stress to the patient that frequent blood tests will be needed to determine correct dosage.

• Warn the patient to report severe headache.

• Caution the patient to avoid potentially hazardous activities during the first 90 days of therapy. There is an increased risk of seizure development in patients with chronic renal failure during the first 90 days of therapy.

filgrastim

fill-**grass**-tim

(Neupogen)

Do not confuse Neupogen with Epogen or Nutramigen.

CATEGORY AND SCHEDULE

Pregnancy Risk Category: C

MECHANISM OF ACTION

A biologic modifier that stimulates production, maturation, and activation of neutrophils to increase their migration and cytotoxicity. **Therapeutic Effect:** Decreases incidence of infection.

PHARMACOKINETICS

Readily absorbed after subcutaneous administration. Not removed by hemodialysis. ***Half-life:*** 3.5 hr.

AVAILABILITY

Injection: 300 mcg/ml, 480 mcg/0.8 ml.

INDICATIONS AND DOSAGES

▸ **Myelosuppression**

IV or Subcutaneous Infusion, Subcutaneous Injection

Adults, Elderly. Initially, 5 mcg/kg/day. May increase by 5 mcg/ kg for each chemotherapy cycle based on duration or severity of absolute neutrophil count nadir.

▸ **Bone marrow transplant**

IV or Subcutaneous Infusion

Adults, Elderly. 5–10 mcg/kg/day. Adjust dosage daily during period of neutrophil recovery based on neutrophil response.

▸ **Mobilization progenitor cells**

IV or Subcutaneous Infusion

Adults. 10 mcg/kg/day beginning at least 4 days before first leukapheresis and continuing until last leukapheresis.

▸ **Chronic neutropenia, congenital neutropenia**

Subcutaneous

Adults, Children. 6 mcg/kg/dose twice a day.

▸ **Idiopathic or cyclic neutropenia**

Subcutaneous

Adults, Children. 5 mcg/kg/dose once a day.

OFF-LABEL USES

Treatment of AIDS-related neutropenia; drug-induced neutropenia; myelodysplastic syndrome

CONTRAINDICATIONS

Hypersensitivity to *Escherichia coli*–derived proteins, 24 hours before or after cytotoxic chemotherapy, concurrent use of other drugs that may result in lowered platelet count

INTERACTIONS

Drug

None known.

Herbal

None known.

Food

None known.

DIAGNOSTIC TEST EFFECTS

May increase LDH concentrations, leukocyte alkaline phosphatase (LAP) scores, and serum alkaline phosphatase and uric acid levels.

IV INCOMPATIBILITIES

Amphotericin (Fungizone), cefepime (Maxipime), cefotaxime (Claforan), cefoxitin (Mefoxin), ceftizoxime (Cefizox), ceftriaxone (Rocephin), cefuroxime (Zinacef), clindamycin (Cleocin), dactinomycin (Cosmegen), etoposide (VePesid), fluorouracil, furosemide (Lasix), heparin, mannitol, methylprednisolone (Solu-Medrol), mitomycin (Mutamycin), prochlorperazine (Compazine)

IV COMPATIBILITIES

Bumetanide (Bumex), calcium gluconate, hydromorphone (Dilaudid), lorazepam (Ativan), morphine, potassium chloride

SIDE EFFECTS

Frequent

Nausea or vomiting (57%), mild to severe bone pain (22%) that occurs more frequently with high-dose IV form less frequently with low-dose subcutaneous form; alopecia (18%), diarrhea (14%), fever (12%), fatigue (11%)

Occasional (9%–5%)

Anorexia, dyspnea, headache, cough, rash

Rare (less than 5%)

Psoriasis, hematuria or proteinuria, osteoporosis

SERIOUS REACTIONS

! Long-term administration

occasionally produces chronic neutropenia and splenomegaly.
! Thrombocytopenia, MI, and arrhythmias occur rarely.
! Adult respiratory distress syndrome may occur in patients with sepsis.

NURSING CONSIDERATIONS

Baseline Assessment

• Obtain a CBC before the start of filgrastim therapy, and twice weekly thereafter.

Lifespan Considerations

• It is unknown if filgrastim crosses the placenta or is distributed in breast milk.
• No age-related precautions have been noted in children or the elderly.

Precautions

• Use filgrastim cautiously in patients with gout, malignancy with myeloid characteristics (because of the potential for granulocyte-colony-stimulating factor potential to act as a growth factor), preexisting cardiac conditions, and psoriasis.

Administration and Handling

◀ **ALERT** ▶ May be given by subcutaneous injection or short IV infusion (15–30 minutes) or by continuous IV infusion.
◀ **ALERT** ▶ Begin filgrastim therapy at least 24 hours after last dose of chemotherapy; discontinue at least 24 hours before next dose of chemotherapy.
◀ **ALERT** ▶ Begin therapy at least 24 hours after bone marrow infusion.

IV

• Refrigerate vials.
• Filgrastim is stable for up to 24 hours at room temperature, provided vial contents are clear and contain no particulate matter. The drug remains stable if accidentally exposed to freezing temperature.
• Use single-dose vial. Do not reenter vial. Do not shake.
• Dilute with 10 to 50 ml D_5W to a concentration of 15 mcg/ml or higher. For a concentration from 5 to 14 mcg/ml, add 2 ml of 5% albumin to each 50 ml D_5W to provide a final concentration of 2 mg/ml. Do not dilute to a final concentration of less than 5 mcg/ml.
• For intermittent infusion (piggyback), infuse over 15 to 30 minutes. For continuous infusion, give single dose over 4 to 24 hours.
• In all situations, flush IV line with D_5W before and after administration.

Subcutaneous

• Store in refrigerator, but remove before use and allow to warm to room temperature.
• Aspirate syringe before injecting drug to avoid intra-arterial administration.

Intervention and Evaluation

• In patients with sepsis, be alert for adult respiratory distress syndrome.
• Closely monitor patients with preexisting cardiac conditions.
• Monitor the patient's BP for a transient decrease. Also assess body temperature, Hct, CBC, and hepatic enzyme and serum uric acid levels.

Patient Teaching

• Warn the patient to report chest pain, chills, fever, palpitations, or severe bone pain.
• Instruct the patient to avoid situations that might place him or her at risk for contracting an infectious disease, such as influenza.

oprelvekin (interleukin-2, IL-2)

oh-**prel**-vee-kinn
(Neumega)
Do not confuse Neumega with Neupogen.

CATEGORY AND SCHEDULE
Pregnancy Risk Category: C

MECHANISM OF ACTION
A hematopoietic that stimulates production of blood platelets, essential to the blood-clotting process. **Therapeutic Effect:** Increases platelet production.

AVAILABILITY
Injection: 5 mg.

INDICATIONS AND DOSAGES
▸ **Prevention of thrombocytopenia**
Subcutaneous
Adults. 50 mcg/kg once a day.
Children. 75–100 mcg/kg once a day. Continue for 14–28 days or until platelet count reaches 50,000 cells/mcl after its nadir.

CONTRAINDICATIONS
None known.

INTERACTIONS
Drug
None known.
Herbal
None known.
Food
None known.

DIAGNOSTIC TEST EFFECTS
May decrease Hgb and Hct, usually within 3–5 days of initiation of therapy; reverses about 1 week after discontinuance of therapy.

SIDE EFFECTS
Frequent
Nausea or vomiting (77%); fluid retention (59%); neutropenic fever (48%); diarrhea (43%); rhinitis (42%); headache (41%); dizziness (38%); fever (36%); insomnia (33%); cough (29%); rash, pharyngitis (25%); tachycardia (20%); vasodilation (19%)

SERIOUS REACTIONS
! Transient atrial fibrillation or flutter occurs in 10% of patients and may be caused by increased plasma volume; oprelvekin is not directly arrhythmogenic. Arrhythmias usually are brief in duration and spontaneously convert to normal sinus rhythm.
! Papilledema may occur in children.

NURSING CONSIDERATIONS

Baseline Assessment
- Plan to obtain the patient's CBC before chemotherapy and at regular intervals thereafter.
- Expect to obtain an EKG to assess for an underlying arrhythmia.

Precautions
- Use oprelvekin cautiously in patients with or susceptible to developing CHF and in those with a history of atrial arrhythmia or heart failure.

Administration and Handling
◂ **ALERT** ▸ Begin oprelvekin administration 6 to 24 hours following completion of chemotherapy dose.
Subcutaneous
- Store in refrigerator. Once reconstituted, use within 3 hours.
- Add 1 ml sterile water for injection to provide concentration of 5 mg/ml oprelvekin. Inject along inside surface of vial, and swirl contents gently to avoid excessive agitation.
- Discard unused portion.

• Give single injection in the abdomen, thigh, hip, or upper arm.

Intervention and Evaluation

• Closely monitor the patient's fluid and electrolyte status, particularly if he or she is receiving diuretic therapy.
• Assess the patient for fluid retention evidenced by dyspnea on exertion and peripheral edema. Fluid retention generally occurs during the first week of therapy and continues for the duration of treatment.
• Monitor the patient's platelet count periodically to assess therapeutic response. Continue drug dosing until postnadir platelet count is greater than 50,000 cells/mcl.
• Discontinue oprelvekin more than 2 days before starting next round of chemotherapy.

Patient Teaching

• Tell the patient that follow-up blood tests will be performed to assess the results of therapy.
• Instruct the patient to use an electric razor and soft toothbrush to prevent bleeding until platelet count is within normal range.
• Tell the patient to report palpitations or dyspnea.

pegfilgrastim

pehg-phil-**gras**-tim
(Neulasta)
Do not confuse Neulasta with Neumega.

CATEGORY AND SCHEDULE

Pregnancy Risk Category: C

MECHANISM OF ACTION

A colony-stimulating factor that regulates production of neutrophils within bone marrow. Also a glycoprotein that primarily affects neutrophil progenitor proliferation, differentiation, and selected end-cell functional activation. **Therapeutic Effect:** Increases phagocytic ability and antibody-dependent destruction; decreases incidence of infection.

PHARMACOKINETICS

Readily absorbed after subcutaneous administration. ***Half-life:*** 15–80 hr.

AVAILABILITY

Solution for Injection: 10 mg/ml.

INDICATIONS AND DOSAGES

▸ Myelosuppression

Subcutaneous

Adults, Elderly. Give as a single 6-mg injection once per chemotherapy cycle.

CONTRAINDICATIONS

Hypersensitivity to *Escherichia coli*–derived proteins, within 14 days before and 24 hours after cytotoxic chemotherapy

INTERACTIONS

Drug

Lithium: May potentiate the release of neutrophils.

Herbal

None known.

Food

None known.

DIAGNOSTIC TEST EFFECTS

May increase LDH concentrations, leukocyte alkaline phosphatase scores, and serum alkaline phosphatase and uric acid levels.

SIDE EFFECTS

Frequent (72%–15%)

Bone pain, nausea, fatigue, alopecia, diarrhea, vomiting, constipation, anorexia, abdominal pain, arthralgia, generalized weakness, peripheral edema, dizziness, stomatitis, mucositis, neutropenic fever

SERIOUS REACTIONS

! Allergic reactions, such as anaphylaxis, rash, and urticaria, occur rarely.
! Cytopenia resulting from an antibody response to growth factors occurs rarely.
! Splenomegaly occurs rarely; assess for left upper abdominal or shoulder pain.
! Adult respiratory distress syndrome (ARDS) may occur in patients with sepsis.

NURSING CONSIDERATIONS

Baseline Assessment

- Obtain a CBC and platelet count before initiation of pegfilgrastim therapy and routinely thereafter.

Lifespan Considerations

- It is unknown if pegfilgrastim crosses the placenta or is distributed in breast milk.
- Safety and efficacy of pegfilgrastim have not been established in children. Its use should be avoided in infants, children, and adolescents weighing less than 45 kg
- No age-related precautions have been noted in the elderly.

Precautions

- Use pegfilgrastim cautiously in patients who concurrently use medications with mycelioid properties and in those with sickle cell disease.

Administration and Handling

◀ **ALERT** ▶ Do not administer from 14 days before to 24 hours after cytotoxic chemotherapy, as prescribed.
◀ **ALERT** ▶ Do not use pegfilgrastim in infants, children, and adolescents weighing less than 45 kg.

Subcutaneous

- Store in refrigerator, but may warm to room temperature up to 48 hours before use. Discard if left at room temperature for longer than 48 hours.
- Protect from light.
- Avoid freezing, but if accidentally frozen, may allow to thaw in refrigerator before administration. Discard if freezing takes place a second time.
- Discard if discoloration or precipitate is present.

Intervention and Evaluation

- Monitor the patient for allergic reactions.
- Examine the patient for peripheral edema, particularly behind the medial malleolus, which is usually the first area to show peripheral edema.
- Assess the patient's mucous membranes for evidence of mucositis (such as red mucous membranes, white patches, and extreme mouth soreness) and stomatitis.
- Evaluate the patient's muscle strength.
- Assess the patient's pattern of daily bowel activity and stool consistency.
- Evaluate patients with sepsis for signs and symptoms of ARDS, such as dyspnea.

Patient Teaching

- Tell the patient of pegfilgrastim's possible side effects, as well as the signs and symptoms of allergic reactions.
- Stress to the patient the importance of compliance with pegfilgrastim regimen, including regular monitoring of blood counts.

sargramostim (granulocyte macrophage colony-stimulating factor, GM-CSF)

sar-gra-**moh**-stim
(Leukine)
Do not confuse Leukine with Leukeran.

CATEGORY AND SCHEDULE
Pregnancy Risk Category: C

MECHANISM OF ACTION
A colony-stimulating factor that stimulates proliferation and differentiation of hematopoietic cells to activate mature granulocytes and macrophages. **Therapeutic Effect:** Assists bone marrow in making new WBCs and increases their chemotactic, antifungal, and antiparasitic activity. Increases cytoneoplastic cells and activates neutrophils to inhibit tumor cell growth.

PHARMACOKINETICS

Effect	Onset	Peak	Duration
Increase WBCs	7–14 days	N/A	1 wk

Detected in serum within 5 min after subcutaneous administration. ***Half-life:*** IV, 1 hr; subcutaneous, 3 hr.

AVAILABILITY
Injection Solution: 500 mcg/ml.
Injection Powder for Reconstitution: 250 mcg.

INDICATIONS AND DOSAGES
▸ **Myeloid recovery following bone marrow transplant (BMT)**
IV Infusion
Adults, Elderly. Usual parenteral dosage: 250 mcg/m^2/day for 21 days (as 2-hr infusion). Begin 2–4 hr after autologous bone marrow infusion and not less than 24 hr after last dose of chemotherapy or not less than 12 hr after last radiation treatment. Discontinue if blast cells appear or underlying disease progresses.

▸ **Bone marrow transplant failure, engraftment delay**
IV Infusion
Adults, Elderly. 250 mcg/m^2/day for 14 days. Infuse over 2 hr. May repeat after 7 days off therapy if engraftment has not occurred with 500 mcg/m^2/day for 14 days.

▸ **Stem cell transplant**
IV, Subcutaneous
Adults. 250 mcg/m^2/day.

OFF-LABEL USES
Treatment of AIDS-related neutropenia; chronic, severe neutropenia; drug-induced neutropenia; myelodysplastic syndrome

CONTRAINDICATIONS
Twelve hours before or after radiation therapy; 24 hours before or after chemotherapy; excessive leukemic myeloid blasts in bone marrow or peripheral blood (greater than 10%); known hypersensitivity to GM-CSF, yeast-derived products, or components of drug

INTERACTIONS
Drug
Lithium, steroids: May increase the effects of sargramostim.
Herbal
None known.
Food
None known.

DIAGNOSTIC TEST EFFECTS
May increase serum bilirubin, creatinine, and hepatic enzyme levels. May decrease serum albumin level.

IV INCOMPATIBILITIES

Amphotericin B complex (Abelcet, AmBisome, Amphotec), hydromorphone (Dilaudid), lorazepam (Ativan), morphine

IV COMPATIBILITIES

Calcium gluconate, dopamine (Intropin), heparin, magnesium, potassium chloride

SIDE EFFECTS

Frequent

GI disturbances, including nausea, diarrhea, vomiting, stomatitis, anorexia, and abdominal pain; arthralgia or myalgia; headache; malaise; rash; pruritus

Occasional

Peripheral edema, weight gain, dyspnea, asthenia, fever, leukocytosis, capillary leak syndrome (such as fluid retention, irritation at local injection site, and peripheral edema)

Rare

Rapid or irregular heartbeat, thrombophlebitis

SERIOUS REACTIONS

! Pleural or pericardial effusion occurs rarely after infusion.

NURSING CONSIDERATIONS

Baseline Assessment

- Monitor the patient for supraventricular arrhythmias during administration, especially if the patient has a history of cardiac arrhythmias.
- Assess the patient closely for dyspnea during and immediately after infusion, particularly if the patient has a history of lung disease. Expect to slow the infusion rate by half if dyspnea occurs during infusion. Stop the infusion immediately if dyspnea continues, and notify the physician.
- If the patient's neutrophil count exceeds 20,000 cells/mm^3 or platelet count exceeds 500,000/mm^3, stop the infusion or reduce the rate by half, as prescribed, based on the patient's clinical condition.
- The patient's blood counts will return to normal or to baseline 3 to 7 days after discontinuation of therapy.

Lifespan Considerations

- It is unknown if sargramostim crosses the placenta or is distributed in breast milk.
- Safety and efficacy of this drug have not been established in children.
- No age-related precautions have been noted in the elderly.

Precautions

- Use sargramostim cautiously in patients with CHF, hypoxia, impaired hepatic or renal function, preexisting cardiac disease, preexisting fluid retention, or pulmonary infiltrates.

Administration and Handling

IV

- Refrigerate powder, reconstituted solution, and diluted solution for injection. Do not shake. Do not use past expiration date.
- Reconstituted solution is normally clear and colorless.
- Use reconstituted solution within 6 hours; discard unused portion. Use one dose/vial; do not reenter vial.
- To reconstitute, add 1 ml preservative-free sterile water for injection to 250-mcg or 500-mcg vial.
- Direct sterile water for injection to side of vial, and gently swirl contents to avoid foaming. Do not shake or vigorously agitate.
- After reconstitution, further dilute with 0.9% NaCl. If final concentration is less than 10 mcg/ml, add 1 mg albumin per ml 0.9% NaCl to provide a final albumin concentration of 0.1%.

◀ **ALERT** ▶ Albumin is added before sargramostim to prevent drug adsorption to components of drug delivery system.

- Give each single dose over 2, 4, or 24 hours, as directed by physician.

Intervention and Evaluation

- Monitor the patient's CBC, pulmonary, liver, and kidney function test results, platelet count, vital signs, and weight.

Patient Teaching

- Tell the patient to expect frequent follow-up blood tests to evaluate the effectiveness of drug therapy.
- Warn the patient to report chest pain, chills, fever, palpitations, or dyspnea.
- Instruct the patient to avoid situations that might place him or her at risk for contracting an infectious disease such as influenza.

60 Plasma Expanders

albumin, human
dextran, low molecular weight (dextran 40); high molecular weight (dextran 75)
hetastarch

Uses: Plasma expanders are used to treat hypovolemia, to expand plasma volume and maintain cardiac output in shock or impending shock, and to treat hypoproteinemia-induced edema or decreased intravascular volume.

Action: Plasma expanders stay in the vascular space and restore plasma volume by maintaining the colloidal osmotic pressure.

albumin, human

al-**byew**-min
(Albumex[AUS], Albuminar, Albutein, Buminate, Plasbumin)
Do not confuse albumin or Albuminar with albuterol.

CATEGORY AND SCHEDULE

Pregnancy Risk Category: C

MECHANISM OF ACTION

A plasma protein fraction that acts as a blood volume expander. **Therapeutic Effect:** Provides temporary increase in blood volume; reduces hemoconcentration and blood viscosity.

PHARMACOKINETICS

Route	Onset	Peak	Duration
IV	15 min (in well-hydrated patient)	N/A	N/A

Distributed throughout extracellular fluid. ***Half-life:*** 15–20 days.

AVAILABILITY

Injection: 5%, 25%.

INDICATIONS AND DOSAGES

▸ **Hypovolemia**
IV
Adults, Elderly. Initially, 25 g; may repeat in 15–30 min. Maximum: 250 g within 48 hr.
Children. 0.5–1 g/kg/dose (10–20 ml/kg/dose of 5% albumin) Maximum: 6 g/kg/day.

▸ **Hypoproteinemia**
IV
Adults, Elderly, Children. 0.5–1 g/kg/dose (10–20 ml/kg/dose of 5% albumin). Repeat in 1–2 days.

▸ **Burns**
IV
Adults, Elderly, Children. Initially, give large volumes of crystalloid infusion to maintain plasma volume. After 24 hr, give 25 g, then adjust dosage to maintain plasma albumin concentration of 2–2.5 g/100 ml.

▸ **Cardiopulmonary bypass**
IV
Adults, Elderly. 5% or 25% albumine with crystalloid to maintain plasma albumin concentration of 2.5 g/100 ml.

▸ **Acute nephrosis, Nephrotic syndrome**
IV
Adults, Elderly. 25 g of 25% injection, with diuretic once a day for 7–10 days.

▸ **Hemodialysis**
IV
Adults, Elderly. 100 ml (25 g) of 25% albumin.

▸ **Hyperbilirubinemia, Erythroblastosis fetalis**
IV
Infants. 1 g/kg 1–2 hr before transfusion.

CONTRAINDICATIONS

Heart failure, history of allergic reaction to albumin level, hypervolemia, normal serum albumin, pulmonary edema, severe anemia

INTERACTIONS

Drug
None known.
Herbal
None known.
Food
None known.

DIAGNOSTIC TEST EFFECTS

May increase serum alkaline phosphatase concentration.

IV INCOMPATIBILITIES

Midazolam (Versed), vancomycin (Vancocin), verapamil (Isoptin)

IV COMPATIBILITIES

Diltiazem (Cardizem), lorazepam (Ativan)

SIDE EFFECTS

Occasional
Hypotension
Rare
High dose in repeated therapy: altered vital signs, chills, fever, increased salivation, nausea, vomiting, urticaria, tachycardia

SERIOUS REACTIONS

! Fluid overload may occur, marked by increased BP, and distended neck veins. Neurological changes that may occur include headache, weakness, blurred vision, behavioral changes, incoordination, and isolated muscle twitching. Pulmonary edema may also occur, evidenced by rapid breathing, rales, wheezing, and coughing.

NURSING CONSIDERATIONS

Baseline Assessment
- Expect to obtain BP and pulse and respiration rates immediately before administration.
- Ensure adequate hydration before albumin is administered.

Lifespan Considerations
- It is unknown if albumin crosses the placenta or is distributed in breast milk.
- No age-related precautions have been noted in children or the elderly.

Precautions
- Use human albumin cautiously in patients with hepatic or renal impairment, hypertension, normal serum albumin level, poor heart function, or pulmonary disease.

Administration and Handling
IV
◂ **ALERT** ▸ Dosage is based on the patient's condition; duration of administration is based on the patient's response.
- Store at room temperature. Albumin normally appears as a clear, brownish, odorless, and moderately viscous fluid.
- Do not use if the solution has been frozen, appears turbid, or contains sediment, or if the vial has been open 4 hours or more.
- Make a 5% solution from 25% solution by adding 1 volume 25% solution to 4 volumes 0.9% NaCl (preferred) or D_5W. Do not use sterile water for injection because life-threatening acute renal failure and hemolysis can occur.
- Give by IV infusion. Rate varies depending on therapeutic use, patient's blood volume, and concentration of the solute.

- Give 5% solution at 5 to 10 ml/minute. Give 25% at a usual rate of 2 to 3 ml/minute.
- Administer 5% solution undiluted; administer 25% solution undiluted or diluted with 0.9% NaCl (preferred) or D_5W.
- May give without regard to patient's blood group or Rh factor.

Intervention and Evaluation

- Monitor BP for hypertension or hypotension.
- Assess the patient frequently for signs and symptoms of fluid overload and pulmonary edema.
- Check the patient's skin for flushing and urticaria.
- Monitor the patient's intake and output; especially watch for decreased urine output.
- Assess for therapeutic response as evidenced by increased BP and decreased edema.

Patient Teaching

- Advise the patient to immediately report difficulty breathing, itching, or rash.

dextran, low molecular weight (dextran 40)

dex-tran

(Gentran, Rheomacrodex[CAN])

dextran, high molecular weight (dextran 75)

(Macrodex)

Do not confuse Gentran with Genprine.

CATEGORY AND SCHEDULE

Pregnancy Risk Category: C

MECHANISM OF ACTION

A branched polysaccharide that produces plasma volume expansion due to high colloidal osmotic effect. Draws interstitial fluid into the intravascular space. May also increase blood flow in microcirculation. **Therapeutic Effect:** Increases central venous pressure, cardiac output, stroke volume, BP, urine output, capillary perfusion, and pulse pressure. Decreases heart rate, peripheral resistance, and blood viscosity. Corrects hypovolemia.

AVAILABILITY

Injection (High Molecular Weight [Gentran]): 6% dextran 70 in 500 ml 0.9% NaCl.

Injection (Low Molecular Weight [Gentran LMD]): 10% dextran 40 in 500 ml D_5W, 10% dextran 40 in 500 ml 0.9% NaCl.

INDICATIONS AND DOSAGES

▸ **Volume expansion, shock**

IV

Adults, Elderly. 500–1,000 ml at a rate of 20–40 ml/min. Maximum: 20 ml/kg for first 24 hr, and 10 ml/kg thereafter.

Children. Total dose not to exceed 20 ml/kg on day 1 and 10 ml/kg/day thereafter.

CONTRAINDICATIONS

Hypervolemia, renal failure, severe bleeding disorders, severe CHF, severe thrombocytopenia

INTERACTIONS

Drug

None known.

Herbal

None known.

Food

None known.

DIAGNOSTIC TEST EFFECTS

Prolongs bleeding time and depresses platelet count. Decreases clotting factors V, VIII, and IX.

IV INCOMPATIBILITIES

Do not add medications to dextran solution.

SIDE EFFECTS

Occasional

Mild hypersensitivity reaction, including urticaria, nasal congestion, wheezing

SERIOUS REACTIONS

! Severe or fatal anaphylaxis, manifested by marked hypotension and cardiac or respiratory arrest, may occur early during IV infusion, generally in those not previously exposed to IV dextran.

NURSING CONSIDERATIONS

Baseline Assessment

- Expect to obtain laboratory values, such as bleeding time, platelet count, and clotting factors.

Precautions

- Use dextran cautiously in patients with chronic hepatic disease or extreme dehydration.

Administration and Handling

◀ ALERT ▶ Therapy should not continue longer than 5 days.

IV

- Store at room temperature. Use only clear solutions, and discard partially used containers.
- Give by IV infusion only.
- Monitor the patient closely during first 15 minutes of infusion for anaphylactic reaction.
- Monitor the patient's vital signs every 5 minutes.
- Monitor the patient's urine flow rate during administration. Discontinue dextran 40 and give an osmotic diuretic, as prescribed, if oliguria or anuria occur to minimize vascular overloading.
- If dextran is given by rapid injection, monitor the patient's central venous pressure (CVP). Immediately discontinue the drug and notify the physician if CVP rises precipitously.
- Monitor the patient's BP diligently during infusion. Stop the infusion immediately if marked hypotension occurs, a sign of imminent anaphylactic reaction.
- If evidence of blood volume overexpansion occurs, discontinue the drug until blood volume is adjusted by diuresis.

Intervention and Evaluation

- Monitor the patient's urine output closely. An increase in output generally occurs in patients with oliguria after dextran administration. If urine output does not increase after 500 ml dextran has been infused, discontinue the drug until diuresis occurs.
- Monitor the patient for signs and symptoms of fluid overload, such as peripheral or pulmonary edema, and impending CHF.
- Assess the patient's lung sounds for crackles.
- Monitor the patient's CVP to detect blood volume overexpansion.
- Monitor the patient's vital signs and observe closely for signs and symptoms of allergic reaction.
- Assess the patient for overt bleeding, especially at the surgical site, as well as bruising and petechiae development, especially following surgery and in patients on anticoagulant therapy.

Patient Teaching

- Instruct the patient to report bleeding from the surgical site, chest pain, or dyspnea.
- Tell the patient to use an electric razor and soft toothbrush, to prevent bleeding during dextran therapy.
- Advise the patient not to take any medications, including OTC drugs (especially aspirin), without physician approval.
- Warn the patient to report black or

red stool, coffee-ground emesis, dark or red urine, or red-speckled mucus from cough.

• Tell the female patient that her menstrual flow may be heavier than usual.

hetastarch

het-ah-starch
(Hespan, Hextend)

CATEGORY AND SCHEDULE

Pregnancy Risk Category: C

MECHANISM OF ACTION

A plasma volume expander that exerts osmotic pull on tissue fluids. **Therapeutic Effect:** Reduces hemoconcentration and blood viscosity; increases circulating blood volume.

PHARMACOKINETICS

Smaller molecules, less than 50,000 molecular weight, rapidly excreted by kidneys; larger molecules, 50,000 molecular weight and greater, slowly degraded to smaller-sized molecules, then excreted. ***Half-life:*** 17 days.

AVAILABILITY

Injection: 6 g/100 ml 0.9% NaCl (500 ml infusion container)

INDICATIONS AND DOSAGES

▸ Plasma volume expansion

IV

Adults, Elderly. 500–1000 ml/day up to 1,500 ml/day (20 mg/kg) at a rate up to 20 ml/kg/hr in hemorrhagic shock and at a slower rate in burns and septic shock.

▸ Leukapheresis

IV

Adults, Elderly. 250–700 ml infused at a constant rate, usually 1:8 to venous whole blood.

CONTRAINDICATIONS

Anuria, oliguria, severe bleeding disorders, severe CHF

INTERACTIONS

Drug

None significant.

Herbal

None known.

Food

None known.

DIAGNOSTIC TEST EFFECTS

May prolong bleeding, and clotting times, aPTT, and PT. May decrease Hct concentration.

IV INCOMPATIBILITIES

Amikacin (Amikin), ampicillin (Polycillin), cefazolin (Ancef, Kefzol), cefotaxime (Claforan), cefoxitin (Mefoxin), gentamicin (Garamycin), ranitidine (Zantac), tobramycin (Nebcin)

SIDE EFFECTS

Rare

Allergic reaction resulting in vomiting, mild temperature elevation, chills, itching, submaxillary and parotid gland enlargement, peripheral edema of lower extremities, mild flulike symptoms, headache, muscle aches

SERIOUS REACTIONS

! Fluid overload, marked by increased BP and distended neck veins, may occur. Neurologic changes that may occur include headache, weakness, blurred vision, behavioral changes, incoordination, and isolated muscle twitching. Pulmonary edema may also occur, manifested by rapid breathing, crackles, wheezing, and coughing.

! Anaphylactic reaction, including periorbital edema, urticaria, and wheezing, may occur.

NURSING CONSIDERATIONS

Baseline Assessment

• Expect to obtain laboratory tests, including coagulation studies and CBC.

• Assess the patient's vitals signs, including BP, as well as central venous pressure (CVP).

Precautions

• Use hetastarch cautiously in patients with CHF, hepatic disease, pulmonary edema, sodium-restricted diets, or thrombocytopenia.

• Use cautiously in the elderly or children.

Administration and Handling

IV

• Store solution at room temperature.

• Solution normally appears clear, pale yellow to amber. Do not use if discolored a deep turbid brown, or if precipitate forms.

• Administer only by IV infusion.

• Do not add drugs to IV line or mix with other IV fluids.

• In acute hemorrhagic shock, administer at a rate approaching 1.2 g/kg/hr (20 ml/kg/hr), as prescribed. Expect to use slower rates in burns and septic shock.

• Monitor the patient's CVP when giving by rapid infusion. If CVP rises precipitously, immediately discontinue the drug, as prescribed, to prevent blood volume overexpansion.

Intervention and Evaluation

• Monitor the patient for signs and symptoms of fluid overload, such as peripheral and pulmonary edema, and impending CHF.

• Assess the patient's lung sounds for crackles and wheezing.

• During leukapheresis, monitor the patient's aPTT; Hct and Hgb; fluid intake and output; leukocyte and platelet counts; and PT.

• Monitor the patient's CVP to detect blood volume overexpansion.

• Monitor the patient's urine output closely. An increase in output generally occurs in patients with oliguria after hetastarch administration.

• Assess the patient for itching, periorbital edema, wheezing, and urticaria, signs of an allergic reaction.

• Monitor the patient for anuria, changes in output ratio, and oliguria and for bleeding from surgical or trauma sites.

Patient Teaching

• Tell the patient to use an electric razor and soft toothbrush to prevent bleeding.

• Warn the patient to report black or red stool, coffee-ground vomitus, dark or red urine, or red-speckled mucus from cough.

61 Thrombolytic Agents

alteplase, recombinant
reteplase, recombinant
streptokinase
tenecteplase

Uses: Thrombolytic agents are used to treat acute and severe thrombotic diseases, including acute coronary thrombosis, acute MI, massive pulmonary emboli, and ischemic stroke.

Action: Thrombolytics act directly or indirectly on the fibrinolytic system to convert plasminogen to plasmin, an enzyme that degrades the fibrin matrix of thrombi, or clots. (See the illustration *Mechanisms and Sites of Action: Hematologic Agents,* page 1036.) This action dissolves thrombi that have already formed.

alteplase, recombinant

al-teep-lase
(Activase, Actilyse[AUS], Cathflo Activase)
Do not confuse alteplase or Activase with Altace.

CATEGORY AND SCHEDULE

Pregnancy Risk Category: C

MECHANISM OF ACTION

A tissue plasminogen activator that acts as a thrombolytic by binding to the fibrin in a thrombus and converting entrapped plasminogen to plasmin. This process initiates fibrinolysis. **Therapeutic Effect:** Degrades fibrin clots, fibrinogen, and other plasma proteins.

PHARMACOKINETICS

Rapidly metabolized in the liver. Primarily excreted in urine. ***Half-life:*** 35 min.

AVAILABILITY

Powder for Injection (Cathflo Activase): 2 mg.
Powder for Injection (Activase): 50 mg, 100 mg.

INDICATIONS AND DOSAGES

▸ **Acute MI**

IV Infusion

Adults weighing greater than 67 kg. 100 mg over 90 min, starting with 15-mg bolus over 1–2 min, then 50 mg over 30 min, then 35 mg over 60 min. Or a 3-hour infusion, giving 60 mg over first hr (6–10 mg as bolus over 1–2 min), 20 mg over second hr, and 20 mg over third hr.

Adults weighing 67 kg or less: 100 mg over 90 min, starting with 15-mg bolus, then 0.75 mg/kg over 30 min (maximum: 50 mg), then 0.5 mg/kg over 60 min (maximum: 35 mg). Or 3-hour infusion of 1.25 mg/kg giving 60% of dose over first hr (6%–10% as 1- to 2-min bolus), 20% over second hr, and 20% over third hr.

▸ **Acute pulmonary emboli**

IV Infusion

Adults. 100 mg over 2 hr. Institute or reinstitute heparin near end or immediately after infusion when aPTT or thrombin time (TT) returns to twice normal or less.

Acute ischemic stroke
IV Infusion
Adults. 0.9 mg/kg over 60 min (10% total dose as initial IV bolus over 1 min).
Central venous catheter clearance
IV
Adults, Elderly. 2 mg; may repeat after 2 hr.

OFF-LABEL USES

Coronary thrombolysis, to decrease ischemic events in unstable angina

CONTRAINDICATIONS

Active internal bleeding, AV malformation or aneurysm, bleeding diathesis, intracranial neoplasm, intracranial or intraspinal surgery or trauma, recent (within past 2 months) cerebrovascular accident, severe uncontrolled hypertension

INTERACTIONS

Drug

Anticoagulants, including cefotetan, heparin, plicamycin, valproic acid: May increase risk of hemorrhage.
Platelet aggregation inhibitors, including aspirin, NSAIDs, ticlopidine: May increase risk of bleeding.

Herbal

None known.

Food

None known.

DIAGNOSTIC TEST EFFECTS

Decreases plasminogen and fibrinogen levels during infusion, which decreases clotting time (and confirms the presence of lysis). Decreases Hgb and Hct.

IV INCOMPATIBILITIES

Dobutamine (Dobutrex), dopamine (Intropin), heparin, nitroglycerin

IV COMPATIBILITIES

Lidocaine, metoprolol (Lopressor), morphine, nitroglycerin, propranolol (Inderal)

SIDE EFFECTS

Frequent

Superficial bleeding at puncture sites, decreased BP

Occasional

Allergic reaction, such as rash or wheezing; bruising

SERIOUS REACTIONS

! Severe internal hemorrhage may occur.
! Lysis of coronary thrombi may produce atrial or ventricular arrhythmias or stroke.

NURSING CONSIDERATIONS

Baseline Assessment

- Obtain baseline apical pulse rate and BP and record patient's weight.
- Expect to evaluate the patient's 12-lead EKG, serum creatine kinase (CK), and CK-MB concentrations, and electrolyte levels.
- Assess Hct, platelet count, TT, aPTT, PT, and fibrinogen level before therapy starts.
- Expect to obtain a blood sample for blood type, crossmatch, and hold.

Lifespan Considerations

- Alteplase is used only when the benefit to the mother outweighs the risk to a fetus. Also, it is unknown if alteplase crosses the placenta or is distributed in breast milk.
- Safety and efficacy have not been established in children.
- In the elderly, there is an increased risk of bleeding. Patients must be carefully selected and monitored.

Precautions

- Use alteplase cautiously in patients who are pregnant or within the first 10 postpartum days. Also use cautiously in patients with recent (within past 10 days) major surgery or GI bleeding, organ biopsy, trauma, cerebrovascular disease, or cardiopulmonary resuscitation; in patients with diabetic retinopathy, endocarditis, left heart thrombus, occluded AV cannula at infected site, severe hepatic or renal disease, or thrombophlebitis; and in the elderly.

Administration and Handling

IV

- Store vials at room temperature. Reconstitute immediately before use with sterile water for injection.
- Reconstitute 100-mg vial with 100 ml sterile water for injection (50-mg vial with 50 ml sterile water for injection) without preservative to provide a concentration of 1 mg/ml. May dilute further with equal volume D_5W or 0.9% NaCl to provide a concentration of 0.5 mg/ml.
- Gently swirl or slowly invert vial; avoid excessive agitation.
- After reconstitution, solution normally appears colorless to pale yellow.
- Solution is stable for 8 hours after reconstitution. Discard unused portion.
- Give by IV infusion via infusion pump. (See individual dosages above.)
- If minor bleeding occurs at puncture site, apply pressure for 30 seconds; if unrelieved, apply a pressure dressing.
- If uncontrolled hemorrhage occurs, discontinue the infusion immediately. Slowing the rate of infusion may worsen the hemorrhage.
- Avoid undue pressure when injecting the drug into the catheter because the catheter can rupture or expel a clot into circulation.

Intervention and Evaluation

- Perform continuous cardiac monitoring and assess for arrhythmias. Check the patient's BP and pulse and respiration rates every 15 minutes until stable; then check hourly.
- Assess the patient's peripheral pulses and heart and breath sounds.
- Monitor the patient for relief of chest pain and notify the physician if it continues or recurs. Note the pain's location, type, and intensity.
- Assess for bleeding, including overt blood and blood in body substances.
- Monitor aPTT per facility protocol.
- Monitor the patient's BP for signs of hypotension.
- Avoid procedures that may increase risk of bleeding, such as IM injections or invasive procedures.
- Assess the patient's neurologic status frequently.

Patient Teaching

- Encourage the patient to strictly follow measures to reduce the risk of bleeding, such as using an electric razor and a soft toothbrush.
- Advise the patient to immediately report signs of bleeding, such as oozing from cuts or gums.

reteplase, recombinant

reh-te-place

(Rapilysin[AUS], Retavase)

Do not confuse reteplase or Retavase with Restasis.

CATEGORY AND SCHEDULE

Pregnancy Risk Category: C

MECHANISM OF ACTION

A tissue plasminogen activator that activates the fibrinolytic system by directly cleaving plasminogen to generate plasmin, an enzyme that degrades the fibrin of the thrombus.

Therapeutic Effect: Exerts thrombolytic action.

PHARMACOKINETICS

Rapidly cleared from plasma. Eliminated primarily by the liver and kidney. ***Half-life:*** 13–16 min.

AVAILABILITY

Powder for Injection: 10.4 units (18.1 mg).

INDICATIONS AND DOSAGES

▸ Acute MI, CHF

IV Bolus

Adults, Elderly. 10 units over 2 min; repeat in 30 min.

CONTRAINDICATIONS

Active internal bleeding, AV malformation or aneurysm, bleeding diathesis, history of cerebrovascular accident, intracranial neoplasm, recent intracranial or intraspinal surgery or trauma, severe uncontrolled hypertension

INTERACTIONS

Drug

Heparin, platelet aggregation antagonists (such as abciximab, aspirin, dipyridamole), warfarin: Increase the risk of bleeding.

Herbal

Ginkgo biloba: May increase the risk of bleeding.

Food

None known.

DIAGNOSTIC TEST EFFECTS

May decrease fibrinogen and serum plasminogen levels.

IV INCOMPATIBILITIES

Do not mix with other medications.

SIDE EFFECTS

Frequent

Bleeding at superficial sites, such as venous injection sites, catheter insertion sites, venous cutdowns, arterial punctures, and sites of recent surgical procedures, gingival bleeding

SERIOUS REACTIONS

! Bleeding at internal sites may occur, including intracranial, retroperitoneal, GI, GU, and respiratory sites.

! Lysis or coronary thrombi may produce atrial or ventricular arrhythmias and stroke.

NURSING CONSIDERATIONS

Baseline Assessment

- Obtain the patient's apical pulse and BP.
- Evaluate the patient's 12-lead EKG, creatine kinase (CK), and CK-MB concentrations, and electrolyte levels.
- Assess the patient's aPTT, Hct, plasminogen and fibrinogen levels, platelet count, PT, and thrombin time before therapy starts.
- Type and hold patient's blood sample.

Lifespan Considerations

- It is unknown if reteplase is distributed in breast milk.
- Safety and efficacy of reteplase have not been established in children.
- The elderly are more susceptible to bleeding. Use reteplase cautiously in this patient population.

Precautions

- Use reteplase cautiously in patients with acute pericarditis; bacterial endocarditis; cerebrovascular disease; diabetic retinopathy; hepatic or renal impairment; hypertension; major surgery, including coronary artery bypass graft, obstetric delivery, and organ biopsy; mitral stenosis with atrial fibrillation, occluded AV

cannula at an infected site, ophthalmic hemorrhage, recent GI or GU bleeding, or septic thrombophlebitis.
• Use cautiously in patients of advanced age and in patients receiving oral anticoagulants.

Administration and Handling

◀ALERT▶ Withhold the second dose if the patient experiences anaphylaxis or bleeding.

IV

• Use within 4 hours of reconstitution. Discard any unused portion.
• Reconstitute only with sterile water for injection immediately before use.
• Reconstituted solution contains 1 unit/ml.
• Do not shake the vial.
• Slight foaming may occur; let stand for a few minutes to allow bubbles to dissipate.
• Give through a dedicated IV line.
• Give as a 10-unit plus 10-unit double bolus, with each IV bolus administered over 2 minutes.
• Give the second bolus 30 minutes after the first bolus injection.
• Do not add other medications to the bolus injection solution.
• Do not give second IV bolus if serious bleeding occurs after first bolus.

Intervention and Evaluation

• Carefully monitor all needle puncture sites and catheter insertion sites for bleeding.
• Perform continuous cardiac monitoring for arrhythmias, BP, and pulse and respiration rates until the patient is stable.
• Evaluate the patient's breath sounds and peripheral pulses.
• Monitor the patient for relief of chest pain. Notify the physician if chest pain continues or recurs. Note pain's intensity, location, and quality.
• Avoid procedures that may increase risk of bleeding, such as injections and shaving.

Patient Teaching

• Tell the patient to use an electric razor and soft toothbrush to prevent bleeding during drug therapy.
• Warn the patient to report black or red stool, coffee-ground vomitus, dark or red urine, red-speckled mucus from cough, or other signs of bleeding.
• Tell the patient to immediately report chest pain, headache, palpitations, or shortness of breath.

streptokinase

strep-toe-**kye**-nase
(Streptase)

CATEGORY AND SCHEDULE

Pregnancy Risk Category: C

MECHANISM OF ACTION

An enzyme that activates the fibrinolytic system by converting plasminogen to plasmin, an enzyme that degrades fibrin clots. Acts indirectly by forming a complex with plasminogen, which converts plasminogen to plasmin. Action occurs within the thrombus, on its surface, and in circulating blood. **Therapeutic Effect:** Destroys thrombi.

PHARMACOKINETICS

Rapidly cleared from plasma by antibodies and the reticuloendothelial system. Route of elimination unknown. Duration of action continues for several hours after drug has been discontinued. ***Half-life:*** 23 min.

AVAILABILITY

Powder for Injection: 250,000 units, 750,000 units, 1.5 million units.

INDICATIONS AND DOSAGES

▸ **Acute evolving transmural MI (given as soon as possible after symptoms occur)**

IV Infusion

Adults, Elderly (1.5 million units diluted to 45 ml). 1.5 million units infused over 60 min.

Intracoronary Infusion

Adults, Elderly (250,000 units diluted to 125 ml). Initially, 20,000-units (10-ml) bolus; then, 2,000 unit/min for 60 min. Total dose: 140,000 units.

▸ **Pulmonary embolism, deep vein thrombosis (DVT), arterial thrombosis and embolism (given within 7 days of onset)**

IV Infusion

Adults, Elderly (1.5 million units diluted to 90 ml). Initially, 250,000 units infused over 30 min; then, 100,000 unit/hr for 24–72 hr for arterial thrombosis or embolism, and pulmonary embolism, 72 hr for DVT.

Intra-Arterial Infusion

Adults, Elderly (1.5 million units diluted to 45 ml). Initially, 250,000 units infused over 30 min; then 100,000 unit/hr for maintenance.

CONTRAINDICATIONS

Carcinoma of the brain, cerebrovascular accident, internal bleeding, intracranial surgery, recent streptococcal infection, severe hypertension

INTERACTIONS

Drug

Anticoagulants, heparin: May increase the risk of hemorrhage.

Platelet aggregation inhibitors such as aspirin: May increase the risk of bleeding.

Herbal

None known.

Food

None known.

DIAGNOSTIC TEST EFFECTS

Decreases serum plasminogen and fibrinogen level during infusion, decreasing clotting time and confirming presence of lysis

IV INCOMPATIBILITIES

Do not mix with medications other than dobutamine, dopamine, heparin, lidocaine, and nitroglycerin.

IV COMPATIBILITIES

Dobutamine (Dobutrex), dopamine (Intropin), heparin, lidocaine, nitroglycerin

SIDE EFFECTS

Frequent

Fever, superficial bleeding at puncture sites, decreased BP

Occasional

Allergic reaction, including rash and wheezing; ecchymosis

SERIOUS REACTIONS

! Severe internal hemorrhage may occur.

! Lysis of coronary thrombi may produce life-threatening arrhythmias.

NURSING CONSIDERATIONS

Baseline Assessment

- Assess the patient's aPTT, Hct, fibrinogen level, platelet count, and PT before therapy starts.
- Discontinue heparin (if heparin is a component of treatment) before giving streptokinase. PT or aPTT should be less than twice normal value before therapy starts.
- Determine the female patient's usual discharge amount during menses.

Lifespan Considerations

- Streptokinase should be used during pregnancy only when the benefit to the mother outweighs the risk to the fetus.

• It is unknown if streptokinase crosses the placenta or is distributed in breast milk.
• Safety and efficacy of streptokinase have not been established in children.
• The elderly may have an increased risk of intracranial hemorrhage. Streptokinase should be used cautiously in this patient population.

Precautions

• Use streptokinase cautiously in patients with GI bleeding or recent trauma and in those who have had major surgery within past 10 days.

Administration and Handling

◀ALERT▶ Streptokinase must be administered within 12 to 14 hours of clot formation. It has little effect on older, organized clots.

◀ALERT▶ Do not use within 5 days to 6 months of previous streptokinase treatment if administered for streptococcal infection, such as acute glomerulonephritis secondary to streptococcal infection, pharyngitis, and rheumatic fever.

IV

• Store unopened vials at room temperature. Refrigerate reconstituted solution and use within 24 hours.
• Reconstitute vial with 5 ml D_5W or 0.9% NaCl (preferred). Add diluent slowly to side of vial; roll and tilt to avoid foaming. Do not shake vial. May dilute further with 50 to 500 ml of D_5W or 0.9% NaCl in 45-ml increments.
• For peripheral IV administration for coronary artery thrombi, give 1.5 million units over 60 minutes.
• For direct intracoronary administration of coronary artery thrombi, give bolus dose over 25 to 30 seconds using coronary catheter. Follow with 2,000 unit/minute for 60 minutes.
• For treatment of DVT, pulmonary arterial embolism, or arterial thrombi, give single dose over 25 to 30 minutes. Follow with maintenance dose of 100,000 or more units every hour for 24 to 72 hours (72 hours for DVT).
• Monitor the patient's BP during infusion. Hypotension, which may be severe, occurs in 1% to 10% of patients. If necessary, decrease the infusion rate, as prescribed.
• Discontinue the infusion immediately and notify the physician if uncontrolled hemorrhage occurs. Be aware that slowing the rate of infusion instead of discontinuing it may produce worsening hemorrhage. Do not use dextran to control hemorrhage.

Intervention and Evaluation

• Evaluate the patient for clinical response and monitor vital signs per protocol.
• Handle the patient carefully and as infrequently as possible, to prevent bleeding and ecchymosis.
• Monitor the patient's Hgb and Hct, BP, and platelet count. Do not obtain BP in lower extremities because a deep vein thrombus may be present.
• Monitor the patient's aPTT, fibrinogen level, PT, and thrombin every 4 hours after therapy begins.
• Examine the patient's stool for occult blood.
• Assess the patient for abdominal or back pain, a decrease in BP, an increase in pulse rate, and severe headache, which may indicate hemorrhage.
• Monitor the female patient for an increase in menstrual flow.
• Assess the patient's area of peripheral thromboembolus for color and temperature.
• Assess the patient's peripheral pulses, skin for bruises and petechiae, and urine for hematuria.
• Examine the patient for exces-

sive bleeding from minor cuts and scratches and other signs of bleeding.

Patient Teaching

- Tell the patient to use an electric razor and soft toothbrush to prevent bleeding during drug therapy.
- Warn the patient to report black or red stool, coffee-ground vomitus, dark or red urine, red-speckled mucus from cough, or other signs of bleeding.
- Tell the patient to immediately report chest pain, headache, palpitations or shortness of breath.

tenecteplase

ten-**eck**-teh-place
(Metalyse[AUS], TNKase)

CATEGORY AND SCHEDULE

Pregnancy Risk Category: C

MECHANISM OF ACTION

A tissue plasminogen activator produced by recombinant DNA that binds to fibrin and converts plasminogen to plasmin. Initiates fibrinolysis by degrading fibrin clots, fibrinogen, other plasma proteins. **Therapeutic Effect:** Exerts thrombolytic action.

PHARMACOKINETICS

Extensively distributed to tissues. Completely eliminated by hepatic metabolism. ***Half-life:*** 11–20 min.

AVAILABILITY

Powder for Injection: 50 mg.

INDICATIONS AND DOSAGES

▸ Acute MI

IV

Adults. Dosage is based on patient's weight. Treatment should be initiated as soon as possible after onset of symptoms.

Weight (kg)	(mg)	(ml)
90 or more	50	10
80 to less than 90	45	9
70 to less than 80	40	8
60 to less than 70	35	7
less than 60	30	6

CONTRAINDICATIONS

Active internal bleeding, aneurysm, AV malformation, bleeding diathesis, history of cerebrovascular accident, intracranial or intraspinal surgery or trauma within past 2 months, intracranial neoplasm, severe uncontrolled hypertension

INTERACTIONS

Drug

Anticoagulants (such as heparin, warfarin), aspirin, dipyridamole, glycoprotein IIb/IIIa inhibitors: Increase the risk of bleeding.

Herbal

Ginkgo biloba: May increase the risk of bleeding.

Food

None known.

DIAGNOSTIC TEST EFFECTS

Decreases plasminogen and fibrinogen levels during infusion, decreasing clotting time and confirming presence of lysis. Decreases Hct and Hgb.

IV INCOMPATIBILITIES

Do not mix with other medications.

SIDE EFFECTS

Frequent

Bleeding (major, 4.7%; minor, 21.8%)

SERIOUS REACTIONS

! Bleeding at internal sites may occur, including intracranial, retroperitoneal, GI, GU, and respiratory sites.

! Lysis or coronary thrombi may produce atrial or ventricular arrhythmias and stroke.

NURSING CONSIDERATIONS

Baseline Assessment

- Obtain the patient's apical pulse and BP and record the patient's weight.
- Evaluate the patient's 12-lead EKG, cardiac enzyme concentrations, and electrolyte levels.
- Assess the patient's aPTT, Hct, fibrinogen level, Hgb, platelet count, and thrombin time before therapy starts.
- Type and hold patient's blood sample.

Lifespan Considerations

- It is unknown if tenecteplase is distributed in breast milk.
- Safety and efficacy of tenecteplase have not been established in children.
- The elderly may have an increased risk of intracranial hemorrhage, major bleeding, and stroke. Tenecteplase should be used cautiously in this patient population.

Precautions

- Use tenecteplase cautiously in patients who previously received tenecteplase and in patients with severe hepatic impairment.

Administration and Handling

◀ALERT▶ Give as a single IV bolus over 5 seconds. Precipitate may occur when given in an IV line containing dextrose. Flush line with saline before and after administration.

IV

- Store at room temperature.
- If possible, use immediately after reconstitution but may refrigerate for up to 8 hours. Discard after 8 hours.
- Tenecteplase is normally a colorless to pale yellow solution. Do not use if solution is discolored or contains particulates.
- Add 10 ml sterile water for injection without preservative to vial to provide concentration of 5 mg/ml. Gently swirl until dissolved. Do not shake. If foaming occurs, allow vial to sit undisturbed for several minutes.
- Administer as IV push over 5 seconds.

Intervention and Evaluation

- Perform continuous cardiac monitoring for arrhythmias, BP, and pulse and respiration rates every 15 minutes until the patient is stable, then hourly.
- Evaluate the patient's heart and breath sounds and peripheral pulses.
- Monitor the patient for relief of chest pain, and notify the physician if it continues or recurs. Note the pain's intensity, location, and quality.
- Assess the patient for bleeding, including blood in body substances and overt blood.
- Monitor the patient's aPTT per protocol.
- Monitor the patient's BP for signs of hypotension.
- Avoid procedures that might increase the risk of bleeding, such as injections and shaving.
- Assess the patient's neurologic status.

Patient Teaching

- Tell the patient to use an electric razor and soft toothbrush, to prevent bleeding during drug therapy.
- Warn the patient to report black or red stool, coffee-ground vomitus, dark or red urine, red-speckled mucus from cough, or other signs of bleeding.
- Tell the patient to immediately report chest pain, headache, palpitations, or shortness of breath.

62 Miscellaneous Hematologic Agents

aminocaproic acid
pentoxifylline
protamine sulfate

Uses: Miscellaneous hematologic agents serve different purposes. *Aminocaproic acid* is used to treat excessive bleeding from hyperfibrinolysis or urinary fibrinolysis. The hemorheologic drug *pentoxifylline* is used to treat the symptoms of intermittent claudication. *Protamine* is used to treat severe heparin overdose and neutralize the effects of heparin given during extracorporeal circulation.

Action: Each miscellaneous agent acts in a different way on the hematologic system. *Aminocaproic acid* inhibits the activation of plasminogen activator substances and blocks antiplasmin activity by inhibiting fibrinolysis. *Pentoxifylline* alters erythrocyte flexibility and inhibits tumor necrosis factor production, neutrophil activation, and platelet aggregation; these actions reduce blood viscosity. *Protamine* complexes with heparin to form a stable salt, which reduces heparin's anticoagulant activity.

aminocaproic acid

a-mee-noe-ka-**proe**-ik
(Amicar)
Do not confuse Amicar with amikacin or Amikin.

CATEGORY AND SCHEDULE

Pregnancy Risk Category: C

MECHANISM OF ACTION

A systemic hemostatic that acts as an antifibrinolytic and antihemorrhagic by inhibiting the activation of plasminogen activator substances. **Therapeutic Effect:** Prevents formation of fibrin clots.

AVAILABILITY

Syrup: 250 mg/ml.
Tablets: 500 mg.
Injection: 250 mg/ml.

INDICATIONS AND DOSAGES

▸ **Acute bleeding**

PO, IV Infusion

Adults, Elderly. 4–5 g over first hr; then 1–1.25 g/hr. Continue for 8 hr or until bleeding is controlled. Maximum: 30 g/24 hr.

Children. 3 g/m^2 over first hr; then 1 $g/m^2/hr$. Maximum: 18 $g/m^2/24$ hr.

▸ **Dosage in renal impairment**

Decrease dose to 25% of normal.

OFF-LABEL USES

Prevention of recurrence of subarachnoid hemorrhage, prevention of hemorrhage in hemophiliacs following dental surgery

CONTRAINDICATIONS

Evidence of active intravascular clotting process, disseminated intravascular coagulation without concurrent heparin therapy, hematuria of upper urinary tract origin (unless benefit outweighs risk); newborns (parenteral form)

INTERACTIONS

Drug

None known.

Herbal

None known.

Food

None known.

DIAGNOSTIC TEST EFFECTS

May elevate serum potassium level.

IV INCOMPATIBILITIES

Sodium lactate

SIDE EFFECTS

Occasional

Nausea, diarrhea, cramps, decreased urination, decreased BP, dizziness, headache, muscle fatigue and weakness, myopathy, bloodshot eyes

SERIOUS REACTIONS

! Too-rapid IV administration produces tinnitus, rash, arrhythmias, unusual fatigue, and weakness.

! Rarely, a grand mal seizure occurs, generally preceded by weakness, dizziness, and headache.

NURSING CONSIDERATIONS

Baseline Assessment

- Obtain vital signs and assess the patient's neurologic status before and regularly during therapy.

Lifespan Considerations

- No information is available concerning the distribution of aminocaproic acid in breast milk.
- There is no documented evidence of adverse effects in children.
- Although no elderly-related problems have been noted, cautious use is advised because of the risk of age-related renal impairment, which may require dosage reduction.

Precautions

- Use aminocaproic acid cautiously in patients with hyperfibrinolysis or impaired cardiac, hepatic, or renal function.

Administration and Handling

◀ALERT▶ Expect to administer a reduced dose if the patient has cardiac, renal, or hepatic impairment.

PO (Tablets)

- Store in a tight container.

PO (Syrup)

- The syrup may be given as an oral rinse for the control of bleeding during dental and oral surgery in hemophilic patients.
- Protect from freezing.

IV

- Dilute each 1 g in up to 50 ml 0.9% NaCl, D_5W, Ringer's solution, or sterile water for injection. Do not use sterile water for injection in patients with subarachnoid hemorrhage.
- Do not give by direct injection. Give only by IV infusion.
- Infuse 5 g or less over the first hour in 250 ml of solution. Give each succeeding 1 g over 1 hour in 50 to 100 ml of solution.
- Monitor the patient for hypotension during the infusion.
- Be aware that rapid infusion may produce arrhythmias, including bradycardia.

Intervention and Evaluation

- Assess the patient for severe and continuous muscular pain or weakness, which may indicate myopathy.
- Monitor serum creatine kinase and AST (SGOT) levels frequently to determine the presence of skeletal myopathy which is characterized by an increase in these levels.
- Monitor the patient's BP, heart rate and rhythm, and pulse rate. Abdomi-

nal or back pain, decrease in BP, increase in pulse rate, and severe headache may indicate hemorrhage.
• Assess the patient's peripheral pulses.
• Check for skin ecchymoses, excessive bleeding from minor cuts or scratches, and petechiae.
• Monitor the female patient for an increase in menstrual flow.
• Evaluate the patient's gums for erythema and gingival bleeding.
• Examine the patient's urine for hematuria.

Patient Teaching
• Instruct the patient to report red or dark urine, black or red stool, coffee-ground vomitus, or blood-tinged mucus from cough.

pentoxifylline

pen-tox-**if**-ih-lin
(Albert[CAN], Apo-Pentoxifylline SR[CAN], Pentoxifylline[CAN], Pentoxyl, Trental)
Do not confuse Trental with Tegretol or Trandate.

CATEGORY AND SCHEDULE
Pregnancy Risk Category: C

MECHANISM OF ACTION
A blood viscosity-reducing agent that alters the flexibility of RBCs; inhibits production of tumor necrosis factor, neutrophil activation, and platelet aggregation. **Therapeutic Effect:** Reduces blood viscosity and improves blood flow.

PHARMACOKINETICS
Well absorbed after oral administration. Undergoes first-pass metabolism in the liver. Primarily excreted in urine. Unknown if removed by hemodialysis. ***Half-life:*** 24–48 min; metabolite, 60–90 min.

AVAILABILITY
Tablets (Controlled-Release [Pentoxil, Trental]): 400 mg.

INDICATIONS AND DOSAGES
▸ **Intermittent claudication**
PO
Adults, Elderly. 400 mg 3 times a day. Decrease to 400 mg twice a day if GI or CNS adverse effects occur. Continue for at least 8 wk.

CONTRAINDICATIONS
History of intolerance to xanthine derivatives, such as caffeine, theophylline, or theobromine; recent cerebral or retinal hemorrhage

INTERACTIONS
Drug
Antihypertensives: May increase the effects of antihypertensives.
Herbal
None known.
Food
None known.

DIAGNOSTIC TEST EFFECTS
None known.

SIDE EFFECTS
Occasional (5%–2%)
Dizziness, nausea, altered taste, dyspepsia, marked by heartburn, epigastric pain, and indigestion
Rare (less than 2%)
Rash, pruritus, anorexia, constipation, dry mouth, blurred vision, edema, nasal congestion, anxiety

SERIOUS REACTIONS
! Angina and chest pain occur rarely and may be accompanied by palpitations, tachycardia, and arrhythmias.
! Signs and symptoms of overdose,

such as flushing, hypotension, nervousness, agitation, hand tremor, fever, and somnolence, appear 4–5 hours after ingestion and last for 12 hours.

NURSING CONSIDERATIONS

Baseline Assessment

- Determine if the patient has a sensitivity or is allergic to xanthine derivatives, such as caffeine, theophylline, or theobromine.
- Ask the patient about his or her signs and symptoms of intermittent claudication, such as aching, cramping, and pain in calf muscles, buttocks, thighs, and feet.

Lifespan Considerations

- It is unknown if pentoxifylline crosses the placenta and is distributed in breast milk.
- Safety and efficacy of pentoxifylline have not been established in children.
- In the elderly, age-related renal impairment may require cautious use.

Precautions

- Use pentoxifylline cautiously in patients with chronic occlusive arterial disease, insulin-treated diabetes, hepatic or renal impairment, peptic ulcer disease, or recent surgery.

Administration and Handling

PO

- Do not crush or break film-coated tablets.
- Give with meals to avoid GI upset.

Intervention and Evaluation

- Assist the patient with ambulation if dizziness occurs.
- Assess the patient for hand tremor.
- Monitor the patient for relief of signs and symptoms of intermittent claudication. Symptoms generally occur while walking or exercising or with weight bearing in the absence of walking or exercising.

Patient Teaching

- Tell the patient that pentoxifylline's therapeutic effect is generally noted in 2 to 4 weeks.
- Warn the patient to avoid tasks requiring mental alertness or motor skills until his or her response has been established.
- Urge the patient not to smoke and to limit caffeine intake. Explain that smoking causes constriction and occlusion of peripheral blood vessels.

protamine sulfate

proe-ta-meen

(Protamine[CAN], Protamine sulfate)

Do not confuse protamine with ProAmatine, Protopam, or Protropin.

CATEGORY AND SCHEDULE

Pregnancy Risk Category: C

MECHANISM OF ACTION

A protein that complexes with heparin to form a stable salt. **Therapeutic Effect:** Reduces anticoagulant activity of heparin.

AVAILABILITY

Injection: 10 mg/ml.

INDICATIONS AND DOSAGES

▸ Heparin oversode (antidote and treatment)

IV

Adults, Elderly. 1 mg protamine sulfate neutralizes 90–115 units of heparin. Heparin disappears rapidly from circulation, reducing the dosage demand for protamine as time elapses.

OFF-LABEL USES
Treatment of enoxaparin toxicity

CONTRAINDICATIONS
None known.

INTERACTIONS
Drug
None known.
Herbal
None known.
Food
None known.

DIAGNOSTIC TEST EFFECTS
None known.

SIDE EFFECTS
Frequent
Decreased BP, dyspnea
Occasional
Hypersensitivity reaction (urticaria, angioedema); nausea and vomiting, which generally occur in those sensitive to fish and seafood, vasectomized men, infertile men, those on isophane (NPH) insulin, or those previously on protamine therapy
Rare
Back pain

SERIOUS REACTIONS
! Too-rapid IV administration may produce acute hypotension, bradycardia, pulmonary hypertension, dyspnea, transient flushing, and feeling of warmth.

! Heparin rebound may occur several hours after heparin has been neutralized (usually 8–9 hours after protamine administration). Heparin rebound occurs most often after arterial or cardiac surgery.

NURSING CONSIDERATIONS
Baseline Assessment
- Evaluate the patient's aPTT, Hct, and PT.
- Assess the patient for bleeding.

Precautions
- Use protamine cautiously in patients with a history of allergy to fish and seafood and in those previously on protamine therapy because of a propensity to hypersensitivity reaction.
- Use cautiously in infertile or vasectomized men and patients on isophane (NPH) or insulin therapy.

Administration and Handling
IV
- Store vials at room temperature.
- May give undiluted over 10 minutes. Do not exceed 5 mg/min or 50 mg in any 10-minute period.
- Make sure the patient is supine while protamine is being administered, to prevent injury from a hypotensive episode or other complication.

Intervention and Evaluation
- Monitor the patient's activated clotting time, aPTT, BP, cardiac function, and other coagulation tests.

Patient Teaching
- Tell the patient to use an electric razor and soft toothbrush to prevent bleeding until coagulation studies normalize.
- Warn the patient to report black or red stool, coffee-ground vomitus, dark or red urine, or red-speckled mucus from cough.

63 Adrenocortical Steroids

betamethasone
cortisone acetate
dexamethasone
fludrocortisone
hydrocortisone
methylprednisolone, methylprednisolone acetate, methylprednisolone sodium succinate
prednisolone
prednisone
triamcinolone, triamcinolone acetonide, triamcinolone diacetate, triamcinolone hexacetonide

Uses: Adrenocortical steroids are used as replacement therapy in adrenal insufficiency, including Addison's disease. Because these agents have anti-inflammatory and immunosuppressant properties, they're also used to treat the symptoms of multiorgan diseases and conditions, such as rheumatoid arthritis, osteoarthritis, severe psoriasis, ulcerative colitis, lupus erythematosus, anaphylactic shock, and status asthmaticus, and to prevent the rejection of transplanted organs.

Action: Adrenocortical steroids suppress the migration of polymorphonuclear leukocytes and reverse increased capillary permeability by their anti-inflammatory effects. They suppress the immune system by decreasing lymphatic system activity. (See the illustration *Mechanisms of Action: Adrenocortical Steroids,* page 1121.)

COMBINATION PRODUCTS

BLEPHAMIDE: prednisolone/sulfacetamide (an anti-infective) 0.2%/10%.
CIPRO HC OTIC: hydrocortisone/ciprofloxacin (an anti-infective) 1%/0.2%.
CIPRODEX OTIC: dexamethasone/ciprofloxacin (an anti-infective) 0.1%/0.3%.
CORTISPORIN: hydrocortisone/neomycin (an anti-infective)/polymyxin (an anti-infective) 5 mg/10,000 units/5 mg; 10 mg/10,000 units/5 mg.
DEXACIDIN: dexamethasone/neomycin (an anti-infective)/polymyxin (an anti-infective): 0.1%/3.5 mg/10,000 units per g or ml.
LOTRISONE: betamethasone/clotrimazole (an antifungal) 0.05%/1%.
MAXITROL: dexamethasone/neomycin (an anti-infective)/polymyxin (an anti-infective) 0.1%/3.5 mg/10,000 units per g or ml.
MYCO-II: triamcinolone/nystatin (an antifungal) 0.1%/100,000 units/g.
MYCOLOG II: triamcinolone/nystatin (an antifungal) 0.1%/100,000 units/g.
MYCO-TRIACET: triamcinolone/nystatin (an antifungal) 0.1%/100,000 units/g.
TOBRADEX: dexamethasone/tobramycin (an aminoglycoside) 1%/3%.
VASOCIDIN: prednisolone/sulfacetamide (an anti-infective) 0.25%/10%.

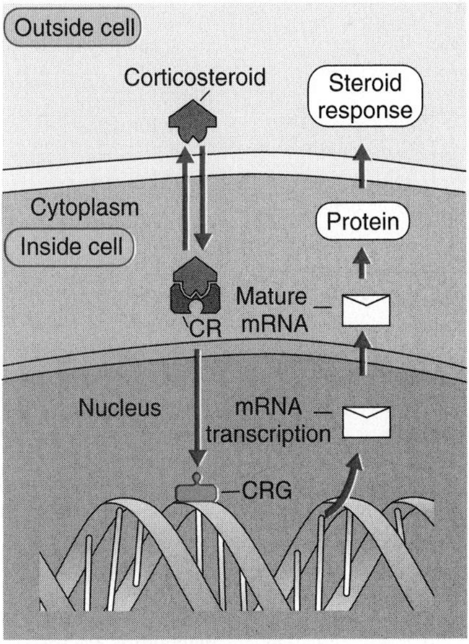

Mechanisms of Action: Adrenocortical Steroids

Adrenocortical steroids (also called corticosteroids) are available in many forms, such as prednisone, and produce a wide range of effects, such as immunosuppression and anti-inflammation. Here's how these drugs work at the cellular level.

Corticosteroids are hormones that are naturally produced by the body (endogenous hormones). Synthetic corticosteroids work much the same as the endogenous hormones. When a corticosteroid enters a cell, it binds to corticosteroid receptors (CRs) in the cell's cytoplasm, forming a complex. The complex moves to the nucleus where it causes the transcription of corticosteroid responsive genes (CRGs) to messenger ribonucleic acid (mRNA), eventually translating to a protein that produces a steroid response in target tissues.

betamethasone

bay-ta-**meth**-a-sone
(Alphatrex, Betaderm[CAN], Betatrex, Beta-Val, Betnesol[CAN], Celestone, Diprolene, Luxiq, Maxivate)

CATEGORY AND SCHEDULE

Pregnancy Risk Category: C (D if used in first trimester)

MECHANISM OF ACTION

An adrenocortical steroid that controls the rate of protein synthesis, depresses the migration of polymorphonuclear leukocytes and fibroblasts, reduces capillary permeability and prevents or controls inflammation. **Therapeutic Effect:** Decreases tissue response to inflammatory process.

AVAILABILITY

Tablet (Celestone): 0.6 mg.
Cream: (Alphatrex, Diprolene, Maxivate) 0.05%.
Cream (Betatrex, Beta-Val): 0.1%.
Foam (Luxiq): 0.12%.
Gel (Diprolene): 0.05%.
Lotion: (Alphatrex, Diprolene, Maxivate): 0.05%.
Lotion (Betatrex, Beta-Val): 0.1%.
Ointment: (Alphatrex, Diprolene, Maxivate): 0.05%.
Ointment (Betatrex): 0.1%.
Syrup (Celestone): 0.6 mg/5 ml.
Injection (Celestone, Soluspan): 6 mg/ml.

INDICATIONS AND DOSAGES

▸ **Anti-inflammation, immunosuppression, corticosteroid replacement therapy**

PO

Adults, Elderly. 0.6–7.2 mg/day.
Children. 0.063–0.25 mg/kg/day in 3–4 divided doses.

▸ **Relief of inflammed and pruritic dermatoses**

Topical

Adults, Elderly. 1–3 times a day.
Foam: Apply twice a day.

CONTRAINDICATIONS

Hypersensitivity to betamethasone, systemic fungal infections

INTERACTIONS

Drug

Amphotericin: May increase hypokalemia.
Digoxin: May increase digoxin toxicity secondary to hypokalemia.
Diuretics, insulin, oral hypoglycemics, potassium supplements: May decrease the effects of these drugs.
Hepatic enzyme inducers: May decrease the effect of betamethasone.
Live-virus vaccines: May decrease the patient's antibody response to vaccine, increase vaccine side effects, and potentiate virus replication.

Herbal

None known.

Food

None known.

DIAGNOSTIC TEST EFFECTS

May increase blood glucose levels and serum lipids, amylase, and sodium levels. May decrease serum calcium, potassium, and thyroxine levels.

SIDE EFFECTS

Frequent

Systemic: Increased appetite, abdominal distention, nervousness, insomnia, false sense of well-being
Topical: Burning, stinging, pruritus

Occasional

Systemic: Dizziness, facial flushing, diaphoresis, decreased or blurred vision, mood swings
Topical: Allergic contact dermatitis, purpura or blood-containing blisters, thinning of skin with easy bruising, telangiectasis or raised, dark-red spots on skin

SERIOUS REACTIONS

! Overdose may cause systemic hypercorticism and adrenal suppression.

NURSING CONSIDERATIONS

Baseline Assessment

- Determine if the patient has a hypersensitivity to corticosteroids and sulfite.
- Obtain the patient's blood glucose level, BP, serum electrolyte levels, height, and weight.
- Evaluate the results of initial tests, such as tuberculosis skin test, x-rays, and EKG.
- Determine if the patient has diabe-

tes mellitus, and anticipate an increase in his or her antidiabetic drug regimen due to raised blood glucose level.
- If the patient is taking digoxin, plan to draw blood to determine serum digoxin level.

Lifespan Considerations
- Monitor growth and development of children receiving long-term steroid therapy.

Precautions
- Use betamethasone cautiously in patients at increased risk for peptic ulcer disease and in those with cirrhosis, hypothyroidism, or nonspecific ulcerative colitis.

Administration and Handling

PO
- Give betamethasone with milk or food to decrease GI upset.
- Give single doses before 9 a.m.; give multiple doses at evenly spaced intervals.

Topical
- Gently cleanse area before applying drug. Apply sparingly and rub into area thoroughly.
- Use occlusive dressings only as ordered.
- When using aerosol, spray area for 3 seconds from a 15-cm distance; avoid inhalation.

Intervention and Evaluation
- Monitor the patient's BP and blood glucose and electrolyte levels. If the patient is taking digoxin, closely monitor his or her digoxin level.
- Apply topical preparation sparingly. Do not use topical form on broken skin or in areas of infection and do not apply to the face or inguinal areas, or to wet skin.

Patient Teaching
- Instruct the patient to take betamethasone with food or milk.
- Teach the patient to take a single daily dose in the morning.
- Instruct the patient to apply topical form in a thin layer.
- Caution the patient against abruptly discontinuing the drug.
- Explain that steroids often cause mood swings, ranging from euphoria to depression.

cortisone acetate

kor-ti-sone

(Cortate[AUS], Cortone[CAN])

Do not confuse cortisone with Cort-Dome.

CATEGORY AND SCHEDULE

Pregnancy Risk Category: C (D if used in the first trimester)

MECHANISM OF ACTION

An adrenocortical steroid that inhibits the accumulation of inflammatory cells at inflammation sites, phagocytosis, lysosomal enzyme release and synthesis, and release of mediators of inflammation. **Therapeutic Effect:** Prevents or suppresses cell-mediated immune reactions. Decreases or prevents tissue response to inflammatory process.

AVAILABILITY

Tablets: 25 mg.

INDICATIONS AND DOSAGES

Dosage is dependent on the condition being treated and patient response.

▸ **Anti-inflammation, immunosuppression**

PO

Adults, Elderly. 25–300 mg/day in divided doses q12-24h.

Children. 2.5–10 mg/kg/day in divided doses q6-8h.

▸ **Physiologic replacement**
PO
Adults, Elderly. 25–35 mg/day.
Children. 0.5–0.75 mg/kg/day in divided doses q8h.

CONTRAINDICATIONS

Hypersensitivity to corticosteroids, administration of live-virus vaccine, peptic ulcers (except in life-threatening situations), systemic fungal infection

INTERACTIONS

Drug

Amphotericin: May increase hypokalemia.
Digoxin: May increase digoxin toxicity caused by hypokalemia.
Diuretics, insulin, oral hypoglycemics, potassium supplements: May decrease the effects of these drugs.
Hepatic enzyme inducers: May decrease the effects of cortisone.
Live-virus vaccines: May decrease the patient's antibody response to vaccine, increase vaccine side effects, and potentiate virus replication.

Herbal

None known.

Food

None known.

DIAGNOSTIC TEST EFFECTS

May increase blood glucose and serum lipid, amylase, and sodium levels. May decrease serum calcium, potassium, and thyroxine levels.

SIDE EFFECTS

Frequent

Insomnia, heartburn, anxiety, abdominal distention, increased diaphoresis, acne, mood swings, increased appetite, facial flushing, delayed wound healing, increased susceptibility to infection, diarrhea or constipation

Occasional

Headache, edema, change in skin color, frequent urination

Rare

Tachycardia, allergic reaction (such as rash and hives), psychological changes, hallucinations, depression

SERIOUS REACTIONS

! Long-term therapy may cause hypocalcemia, hypokalemia, muscle wasting in arms and legs, osteoporosis, spontaneous fractures, amenorrhea, cataracts, glaucoma, peptic ulcer disease, and CHF.
! Abrupt withdrawal following long-term therapy may cause anorexia, nausea, fever, headache, joint pain, rebound inflammation, fatigue, weakness, lethargy, dizziness, and orthostatic hypotension.

NURSING CONSIDERATIONS

Baseline Assessment

- Determine if the patient is hypersensitive to corticosteroids.
- Obtain the patient's BP, blood glucose and serum electrolyte levels, height, and weight.
- Determine if the patient has diabetes mellitus, and anticipate an increase in his or her antidiabetic drug regimen because of raised blood glucose levels.
- If the patient is taking digoxin, plan to draw blood for determining serum digoxin level.

Lifespan Considerations

- Monitor growth and development of children receiving long-term steroid therapy.

Precautions

- Use cortisone cautiously in patients with cirrhosis, CHF, history of tuberculosis (it may reactivate disease), hypertension, hypothyroidism, nonspecific ulcerative colitis, psychosis, seizure disorders, or thromboembolic disorders.

Intervention and Evaluation

- Be alert to signs and symptoms of infection caused by reduced immune response, including fever, sore throat, and vague symptoms.
- Monitor patients on long-term therapy, for signs and symptoms of hypocalcemia (such as muscle twitching, cramps, and positive Chvostek's or Trousseau's signs), or hypokalemia (such as EKG changes, nausea and vomiting, irritability, weakness and muscle cramps, and numbness or tingling, especially in the lower extremities).
- Expect to continue prolonged therapy slowly.
- Assess the patient's ability to sleep and emotional status.

Patient Teaching

- Instruct the patient not to change the dosage of or schedule for cortisone.
- Caution the patient against abruptly discontinuing the drug. Explain to the patient that the drug must be withdrawn gradually under medical supervision.
- Warn the patient to report fever, muscle aches, sore throat, and sudden weight gain or swelling.
- Tell the patient to inform his or her dentist and other physicians that he or she is taking cortisone or has taken it within the past 12 months.
- Explain that steroids often cause mood swings, ranging from euphoria to depression.

dexamethasone

dex-a-**meth**-a-sone

(Decadron, Desamethsone Intensol, Dexasone, Dexasone LA, Dexmethsone[AUS], Diodex[CAN], Hexadrol[CAN], Maxidex, Solurex, Solurex LA)

Do not confuse dexamethasone with desoximetasone or dextramethophan, or Maxidex with Maxzide.

CATEGORY AND SCHEDULE

Pregnancy Risk Category: C (D if used in the first trimester)

MECHANISM OF ACTION

A long-acting glucocorticoid that inhibits accumulation of inflammatory cells at inflammation sites, phagocytosis, lysosomal enzyme release and synthesis, and release of mediators of inflammation. **Therapeutic Effect:** Prevents and suppresses cell and tissue immune reactions and inflammatory process.

PHARMACOKINETICS

Rapidly, completely absorbed from the GI tract after oral administration. Widely distributed. Protein binding: High. Metabolized in the liver. Primarily excreted in urine. Minimally removed by hemodialysis. ***Half-life:*** 3–4.5 hr.

AVAILABILITY

Elixir: 0.5 mg/5 ml, 1 mg/ml.
Inhalant, Intranasal: Solution, suspension, ointment.
Ophthalmic Ointment.
Ophthalmic Suspension.
Oral Solution: 0.5 mg/5 ml, 0.5 mg/0.5 ml.
Tablets: 0.25 mg, 0.5 mg, 0.75 mg, 1 mg, 1.5 mg, 2 mg, 4 mg, 6 mg.

Topical Aerosol.
Topical Cream.
Injection: 4 mg/ml.

INDICATIONS AND DOSAGES

▸ Anti-inflammatory

PO, IV, IM

Adults, Elderly. 0.75–9 mg/day in divided doses q6–12h.

Children. 0.08–0.3 mg/kg/day in divided doses q6–12h.

▸ Cerebral edema

IV

Adults, Elderly. Initially, 10 mg, then 4 mg (IV or IM) q6h.

PO, IV, IM

Children. Loading dose of 1–2 mg/kg, then 1–1.5 mg/kg/day in divided doses q4–6h.

▸ Nausea and vomiting in chemotherapy patients

IV

Adults, Elderly. 8–20 mg once, then 4 mg (PO) q4–6h or 8 mg q8h.

Children. 10 mg/m^2/dose (Maximum: 20 mg), then 5 mg/m^2/dose q6h.

▸ Physiologic replacement

PO, IV, IM

Children. 0.03–0.15 mg/kg/day in divided doses q6–12h.

▸ Usual ophthalmic dosage, ocular inflammatory conditions

Ointment

Adults, Elderly, Children. Thin coating 3–4 times/day.

Suspension

Adults, Elderly, Children. Initially, 2 drops q1h while awake and q2h at night for 1 day, then reduce to 3–4 times/day.

CONTRAINDICATIONS

Active untreated infections, fungal, tuberculosis, or viral diseases of the eye

INTERACTIONS

Drug

Amphotericin: May increase hypokalemia.

Digoxin: May increase digoxin toxicity caused by hypokalemia.

Diuretics, insulin, oral hypoglycemics, potassium supplements: May decrease the effects of these drugs.

Hepatic enzyme inducers: May decrease the effects of dexamethasone.

Live-virus vaccines: May decrease the patient's antibody response to vaccine, increase vaccine side effects, and potentiate virus replication.

Herbal

None known.

Food

None known.

DIAGNOSTIC TEST EFFECTS

May increase blood glucose and serum lipid, amylase, and sodium levels. May decrease serum calcium, potassium, and thyroxine levels.

IV INCOMPATIBILITIES

Ciprofloxacin (Cipro), daunorubicin (Cerubidine), idarubicin (Idamycin), midazolam (Versed)

IV COMPATIBILITIES

Aminophylline, cimetidine (Tagamet), cisplatin (Platinol), cyclophosphamide (Cytoxan), cytarabine (Cytosar), docetaxel (Taxotere), doxorubicin (Adriamycin), etoposide (VePesid), granisetron (Kytril), heparin, hydromorphone (Dilaudid), lorazepam (Ativan), morphine, ondansetron (Zofran), paclitaxel (Taxol), potassium chloride, propofol (Diprivan)

SIDE EFFECTS

Frequent

Inhalation: Cough, dry mouth, hoarseness, throat irritation
Intranasal: Burning, mucosal dryness
Ophthalmic: Blurred vision
Systemic: Insomnia, facial swelling or cushingoid appearance, moderate abdominal distention, indigestion, increased appetite, nervousness, facial flushing, diaphoresis

Occasional

Inhalation: Localized fungal infection, such as thrush
Intranasal: Crusting inside nose, nosebleed, sore throat, ulceration of nasal mucosa.
Ophthalmic: Decreased vision, watering of eyes, eye pain, burning, stinging, redness of eyes, nausea, vomiting
Systemic: Dizziness, decreased or blurred vision
Topical: Allergic contact dermatitis, purpura or blood-containing blisters, thinning of skin with easy bruising, telangiectasis or raised, dark-red spots on skin

Rare

Inhalation: Increased bronchospasm, esophageal candidiasis
Intranasal: Nasal and pharyngeal candidiasis, eye pain
Systemic: General allergic reaction (such as rash and hives); pain, redness, or swelling at injection site; psychological changes; false sense of well-being; hallucinations; depression

SERIOUS REACTIONS

! Long-term therapy may cause muscle wasting (especially in the arms and legs), osteoporosis, spontaneous fractures, amenorrhea, cataracts, glaucoma, peptic ulcer disease, and CHF.

! The ophthalmic form may cause glaucoma, ocular hypertension, and cataracts.

! Abrupt withdrawal following long-term therapy may cause severe joint pain, severe headache, anorexia, nausea, fever, rebound inflammation, fatigue, weakness, lethargy, dizziness, and orthostatic hypotension.

NURSING CONSIDERATIONS

Baseline Assessment

- Determine if the patient is hypersensitive to any corticosteroids.
- Obtain the patient's baselines for blood glucose levels, BP, serum electrolyte levels, height, and weight.
- Evaluate the results of initial tests, such as tuberculosis skin test, x-rays, and EKG.
- Determine if the patient has diabetes mellitus, and anticipate an increase in his or her antidiabetic drug regimen because of raised blood glucose levels.
- If the patient is taking digoxin, plan to draw blood to determine serum digoxin level.

Lifespan Considerations

- Dexamethasone crosses the placenta and is distributed in breast milk.
- Prolonged treatment with high dosages may decrease the short-term growth rate and cortisol secretion in children.
- The elderly are at higher risk for developing hypertension or osteoporosis.

Precautions

- Use dexamethasone cautiously in patients with cirrhosis, CHF, diabetes mellitus, high thromboembolic risk, hypertension, hyperthyroidism, ocular herpes simplex, osteoporosis, peptic ulcer disease, respiratory tuberculosis, seizure disorders, ulcerative colitis, or untreated systemic infections.

- Use the ophthalmic form cautiously in patients on long-term therapy because prolonged use may result in cataracts or glaucoma.

Administration and Handling

PO

- Give dexamethasone with milk or food.

IV

◀ALERT▶ Dexamethasone sodium phosphate may be given by IV push or IV infusion.

- For IV push, give over 1 to 4 minutes.
- For IV infusion, mix with 0.9% NaCl or D_5W and infuse over 15 to 30 minutes.
- If administering to a neonate, solution must be preservative free.
- IV solution must be used within 24 hours.

IM

- Give deep IM, preferably in the gluteus maximus.

Ophthalmic

- To administer the solution or ointment, place a gloved finger on the patient's lower eyelid and pull it out until a pocket is formed between the patient's eye and lower lid. Hold the dropper above the pocket and place the correct number of drops (or one quarter to one half inch ointment) into the pocket. Close the patient's eye gently.
- For the ophthalmic solution, apply digital pressure to the lacrimal sac for 1 to 2 minutes to minimize the drainage to the nose and throat, thereby reducing the risk of systemic effects.
- For the ophthalmic ointment, close the patient's eye for 1 to 2 minutes. Instruct the patient to roll his or her eyeball to increase the contact area of drug to eye.
- Remove excess solution or ointment around the patient's eye with a tissue.
- Use ointment at night to reduce the frequency of solution administration.
- Expect to taper the dosage slowly when discontinuing the drug.

Topical

- Gently cleanse the area before applying drug. Apply sparingly and rub into area thoroughly.
- Use occlusive dressings only as ordered.

Intervention and Evaluation

- Monitor the patient's intake and output and record weight daily.
- Evaluate the patient's food tolerance. Assess the patient's pattern of daily bowel activity.
- If the patient experiences hyperacidity, report it promptly.
- Check the patient's vital signs at least 2 times a day.
- Be alert to signs and symptoms of infection such as fever, sore throat, and vague symptoms.
- Monitor the patient's electrolyte levels.
- Monitor the patient for signs and symptoms of hypercalcemia (such as cramps and muscle twitching) or hypokalemia (such as irritability, nausea and vomiting, muscle cramps and weakness, and numbness or tingling, especially of the lower extremities).
- Assess the patient's ability to sleep and emotional status.

Patient Teaching

- Caution the patient against abruptly discontinuing the drug or changing the dosage or schedule. Explain to the patient that the drug must be withdrawn gradually under medical supervision.
- Warn the patient to report fever, muscle aches, sore throat, and sudden weight gain or swelling.
- Explain to the patient that severe stress, including serious infection, surgery, or trauma, may require an increase in dexamethasone dosage.

- Tell the patient to inform his or her dentist and other physicians that he or she is taking dexamethasone or has taken it within the past 12 months.
- Instruct the patient using the topical form to apply the drug after a bath or shower for best absorption.
- Explain that steroids often cause mood swings, ranging from euphoria to depression.

fludrocortisone

floo-droe-**kor**-ti-sone
(Florinef)
Do not confuse Florinef with Fioricet or Florinal.

CATEGORY AND SCHEDULE

Pregnancy Risk Category: C

MECHANISM OF ACTION

A mineralocorticoid that acts at distal tubules. **Therapeutic Effect:** Increases potassium and hydrogen ion excretion. Replaces sodium loss and raises blood pressure (with low dosages). Inhibits endogenous adrenal cortical secretion, thymic activity, and secretion of corticotropin by pituitary gland (with higher dosages).

PHARMACOKINETICS

Well absorbed from the GI tract. Protein binding: 42%. Widely distributed. Metabolized in the liver and kidney. Primarily excreted in urine. ***Half-life:*** 3.5 hr.

AVAILABILITY

Tablets: 0.1 mg.

INDICATIONS AND DOSAGES

▸Addison's disease

PO

Adults, Elderly. 0.05–0.1 mg/day. Range: 0.1 mg 3 times a wk to 0.2 mg/day. Administration with cortisone or hydrocortisone preferred.

▸Salt-losing adrenogenital syndrome

PO

Adults, Elderly. 0.1–0.2 mg/day.

▸Usual pediatric dosage

Children. 0.05–0.1 mg/day.

OFF-LABEL USES

Treatment of acidosis in renal tubular disorders, idiopathic orthostatic hypotension

CONTRAINDICATIONS

CHF, systemic fungal infection

INTERACTIONS

Drug

Digoxin: May increase the risk of digoxin toxicity caused by hypokalemia.
Hepatic enzyme inducers (such as phenytoin): May increase the metabolism of fludrocortisone.
Hypokalemia-causing medications: May increase the effects of fludrocortisone.
Sodium-containing medications: May increase BP, incidence of edema, and serum sodium level.

Herbal

None known.

Food

None known.

DIAGNOSTIC TEST EFFECTS

May increase serum sodium level. May decrease Hct and serum potassium level.

SIDE EFFECTS

Frequent

Increased appetite, exaggerated sense of well-being, abdominal distention, weight gain, insomnia, mood swings
High dosages, prolonged therapy, too-rapid withdrawal: Increased

susceptibility to infection with masked signs and symptoms, delayed wound healing, hypokalemia, hypocalcemia, GI distress, diarrhea or constipation, hypertension

Occasional

Headache, dizziness, menstrual difficulty or amenorrhea, gastric ulcer development

Rare

Hypersensitivity reaction

SERIOUS REACTIONS

! Long-term therapy may cause muscle wasting (especially in the arms and legs), osteoporosis, spontaneous fractures, amenorrhea, cataracts, glaucoma, peptic ulcer disease, and CHF.

! Abruptly withdrawing the drug after long-term therapy may cause anorexia, nausea, fever, headache, joint pain, rebound inflammation, fatigue, weakness, lethargy, dizziness, and orthostatic hypotension.

NURSING CONSIDERATIONS

Baseline Assessment

- Obtain the patient's BP, blood glucose and serum electrolyte levels, chest x-ray, EKG, height, and weight.

Lifespan Considerations

- It is unknown if fludrocortisone crosses the placenta or is distributed in breast milk.
- Fludrocortisone use in children may suppress growth and inhibit endogenous steroid production.
- Effects of fludrocortisone use in the elderly are unknown.

Precautions

- Use fludrocortisone cautiously in patients with edema, hypertension, or impaired renal function.

Administration and Handling

PO

- Give fludrocortisone with food or milk.

Intervention and Evaluation

- Monitor the patient's BP and blood glucose, serum renin, and electrolyte levels.
- Expect to taper the dosage slowly if fludrocortisone is to be discontinued.

Patient Teaching

- Warn the patient against abruptly discontinuing the drug or altering the dosage or schedule. Explain to the patient that the drug must be withdrawn gradually under medical supervision.
- Tell the patient to report continuing headaches, fever, muscle aches, sore throat, or sudden weight gain or swelling.
- Instruct the patient to maintain careful personal hygiene and to avoid exposure to disease or trauma.
- Explain that severe stress, such as serious infection, surgery, or trauma may require an increase in the fludrocortisone dosage.
- Explain that steroids often cause mood swings, ranging from euphoria to depression.

hydrocortisone

hye-dro-**kor**-ti-sone
(A-HydroCort, Anusol-HC, Colifoam[AUS], Cortaid, Cortef cream[AUS], Cortic cream[AUS], Cortic DS[AUS], Cortifoam, Cortizone-5, Cortizone-10, Derm-Aid cream[AUS], Dermaid[AUS], Dermaid soft cream[AUS], Egocort cream[AUS], Emcort, Hycor[AUS], Hycor eye ointment[AUS], Hysone[AUS], Hytone, Locoid, Nupercainal Hydrocortisone Cream, Preparation H Hydrocortisone, Protocort, Siquent Hycor[AUS], Solu-Cortef, Squibb HC[AUS], WestCort)

CATEGORY AND SCHEDULE

Pregnancy Risk Category: C (D if used in first trimester)
OTC (Hydrocortisone 0.5% and 1% Cream, Gel, and Ointment)

MECHANISM OF ACTION

An adrenocortical steroid that inhibits accumulation of inflammatory cells at inflammation sites, phagocytosis, lysosomal enzyme release and synthesis and release of mediators of inflammation. **Therapeutic Effect:** Prevents or suppresses cell-mediated immune reactions. Decreases or prevents tissue response to inflammatory process.

PHARMACOKINETICS

Route	Onset	Peak	Duration
IV	N/A	4–6 hr	8–12 hr

Well absorbed after IM administration. Widely distributed. Metabolized in the liver. ***Half-life:*** Plasma, 1.5–2 hr; biologic, 8–12 hr.

AVAILABILITY

Tablet (Cortef): 5 mg, 10 mg, 20 mg.
Cream (Rectal [Nupercainal Hydrocortisone Cream, Cortizone-10, Preparation H Hydrocortisone]): 1%.
Cream (Topical [Cortizone-5]): 0.5%.
Cream (Topical [Caldecort, Cortizone-10]): 1%.
Cream (Topical [Hytone]): 2.5%.
Ointment (Topical [Locoid]): 0.1%.
Ointment (Topical [Westcort]): 0.2%.
Ointment (Topical [Cortizone-5]): 0.5%.
Ointment (Topical [Anusol-HC, Cortaid, Cortizone-10]): 1%.
Ointment (Topical [Hytone]): 2.5%.
Suppositories (Anusol-HC): 25 mg.
Suppositories (Emcort, Protocort): 30 mg.
Injection (A-hydro-Cort, Solu-Cortef): 100 mg, 250 mg, 500 mg, 1 g.

INDICATIONS AND DOSAGES

▸ Acute adrenal insufficiency
IV
Adults, Elderly. 100 mg IV bolus; then 300 mg/day in divided doses q8h.
Children. 1–2 mg/kg IV bolus; then 150–250 mg/day in divided doses q6–8h.
Infants. 1–2 mg/kg/dose IV bolus; then 25–150 mg/day in divided doses q6–8h.

▸ Anti-inflammation, immunosuppression
IV, IM
Adults, Elderly. 15–240 mg q12h.
Children. 1–5 mg/kg/day in divided doses q12h.

▸ Physiologic replacement
PO
Children. 0.5–0.75 mg/kg/day in divided doses q8h.

IM
Children. 0.25–0.35 mg/kg/day as a single dose.

▸ **Status asthmaticus**
IV
Adults, Elderly. 100–500 mg q6h.
Children. 2 mg/kg/dose q6h.

▸ **Shock**
IV
Adults, Elderly, Children 12 yr and older. 100–500 mg q6h.
Children younger than 12 yr. 50 mg/kg. May repeat in 4 hr, then q24h as needed.

▸ **Adjunctive treatment of ulcerative colitis**
Rectal
Adults, Elderly. 100 mg at bedtime for 21 nights or until clinical and proctologic remission occurs (may require 2–3 mo of therapy).
Rectal (Cortifoam)
Adults, Elderly. 1 applicator 1–2 times a day for 2–3 wk, then every second day until therapy ends.
Topical
Adults, Elderly. Apply sparingly 2–4 times a day.

CONTRAINDICATIONS

Fungal, tuberculosis, or viral skin lesions; serious infections

INTERACTIONS

Drug

Amphotericin: May increase hypokalemia.
Digoxin: May increase the risk of digoxin toxicity caused by hypokalemia.
Diuretics, insulin, oral hypoglycemics, potassium supplements: May decrease the effects of these drugs.
Hepatic enzyme inducers: May decrease the effects of hydrocortisone.
Live-virus vaccines: May decrease the patient's antibody response to vaccine, increase vaccine side effects, and potentiate virus replication.

Herbal

None known.

Food

None known.

DIAGNOSTIC TEST EFFECTS

May increase blood glucose and serum lipid, amylase, and sodium levels. May decrease serum calcium, potassium, and thyroxine levels.

IV INCOMPATIBILITIES

Ciprofloxacin (Cipro), diazepam (Valium), idarubicin (Idamycin), midazolam (Versed), phenytoin (Dilantin)

IV COMPATIBILITIES

Aminophylline, amphotericin, calcium gluconate, cefepime (Maxipime), digoxin (Lanoxin), diltiazem (Cardizem), diphenhydramine (Benadryl), dopamine (Intropin), insulin, lidocaine, lorazepam (Ativan), magnesium sulfate, morphine, norepinephrine (Levophed), procainamide (Pronestyl), potassium chloride, propofol (Diprivan)

SIDE EFFECTS

Frequent

Insomnia, heartburn, nervousness, abdominal distention, diaphoresis, acne, mood swings, increased appetite, facial flushing, delayed wound healing, increased susceptibility to infection, diarrhea or constipation

Occasional

Headache, edema, change in skin color, frequent urination
Topical: Itching, redness, irritation

Rare

Tachycardia, allergic reaction (such as rash and hives), psychological changes, hallucinations, depression

Topical: Allergic contact dermatitis, purpura
Systemic: Absorption more likely with use of occlusive dressings or extensive application in young children

SERIOUS REACTIONS

! Long-term therapy may cause hypocalcemia, hypokalemia, muscle wasting (especially in arms and legs), osteoporosis, spontaneous fractures, amenorrhea, cataracts, glaucoma, peptic ulcer disease, and CHF.
! Abruptly withdrawing the drug after long-term therapy may cause anorexia, nausea, fever, headache, sudden severe joint pain, rebound inflammation, fatigue, weakness, lethargy, dizziness, and orthostatic hypotension.

NURSING CONSIDERATIONS

Baseline Assessment

- Determine if the patient has a hypersensitivity to corticosteroids.
- Obtain the patient's BP, blood glucose and serum electrolyte levels, height, and weight.
- Evaluate the results of initial tests, such as tuberculosis skin test, x-rays, and EKG.
- Determine if the patient has diabetes mellitus, and anticipate an increase in his or her antidiabetic drug regimen because of raised blood glucose level.
- If the patient is taking digoxin, plan to draw blood to determine serum digoxin level.

Lifespan Considerations

- Hydrocortisone crosses the placenta and is distributed in breast milk. Patients taking hydrocortisone should not breast-feed.
- Prolonged hydrocortisone use during the first trimester of pregnancy may produce cleft palate in the neonate.
- Prolonged treatment or high dosages may decrease the cortisol secretion and short-term growth rate in children.
- The elderly may be more susceptible to developing hypertension or osteoporosis.

Precautions

- Use hydrocortisone cautiously in patients with cirrhosis, CHF, diabetes mellitus, hypertension, hyperthyroidism, osteoporosis, peptic ulcer disease, seizure disorders, thromboembolic tendencies, thrombophlebitis, or ulcerative colitis.

Administration and Handling

IV
- Store at room temperature.
- After reconstitution, store hydrocortisone sodium succinate solution at room temperature and use within 72 hours. Use immediately if further diluted with D_5W, 0.9% NaCl, or other compatible diluent. For hydrocortisone sodium succinate IV push, dilute to 50 mg/ml; for intermittent infusion dilute to 1 mg/ml.
- Administer hydrocortisone sodium succinate solution IV push over 3 to 5 minutes. Give intermittent infusion over 20 to 30 minutes.

Topical
- Gently cleanse area before applying drug. Apply sparingly and rub into area thoroughly.
- Use occlusive dressings only as ordered.

Rectal
- Shake homogeneous suspension well.
- Instruct patient to lie on his or her left side with left leg extended and right leg flexed.
- Gently insert applicator tip into rectum, pointed slightly toward umbilicus, and slowly instill medication.

Intervention and Evaluation

- Examine the patient for edema.
- Be alert to signs and symptoms of infection, such as fever and sore throat, that indicate reduced immune response.
- Assess the patient's pattern of daily bowel activity and stool consistency.
- Monitor the patient's electrolyte levels.
- Monitor the patient for signs and symptoms of hypocalcemia (such as cramps and muscle twitching), or hypokalemia (such as EKG changes, irritability, nausea and vomiting, numbness or tingling of lower extremities, and weakness).
- Evaluate the patient's ability to sleep and emotional status.

Patient Teaching

- Warn the patient to report fever, muscle aches, sore throat, or sudden weight gain or swelling.
- Instruct the patient to consult the physician before taking aspirin or other medications during hydrocortisone therapy.
- Urge the patient to avoid alcohol and limit caffeine intake during hydrocortisone therapy.
- Tell the patient to notify his or her dentist and other physicians that he or she is taking cortisone or has taken it within the past 12 months.
- Caution the patient against overuse of joints injected with hydrocortisone for symptomatic relief.
- Instruct the patient to apply topical hydrocortisone valerate after a bath or shower for best absorption. Teach the patient not to cover the affected area with plastic pants, tight diapers, or other types of coverings unless the physician instructs otherwise.
- Warn the patient to avoid contacting his or her eyes with the medication.
- Explain that steroids often cause mood swings, ranging from euphoria to depression.

methylprednisolone

meth-il-pred-**niss**-oh-lone
(Medrol)

methylprednisolone acetate

(Depo-Medrol, Depo-Nisolone [AUS])

methylprednisolone sodium succinate

(A-Methapred, Solu-Medrol)

Do not confuse methylprednisolone with medroxyprogesterone, or Medrol with Mebaral.

CATEGORY AND SCHEDULE

Pregnancy Risk Category: C

MECHANISM OF ACTION

An adrenocortical steroid that suppresses migration of polymorphonuclear leukocytes and reverses increased capillary permeability. **Therapeutic Effect:** Decreases inflammation.

PHARMACOKINETICS

Route	Onset	Peak	Duration
PO	N/A	1–2 hr	30–36 hr
IM	N/A	4–8 days	1–4 wk

Well absorbed from the GI tract after IM administration. Widely distributed. Metabolized in the liver. Excreted in urine. Removed by hemodialysis. ***Half-life:*** 3.5 hr.

AVAILABILITY

Tablets (Medrol): 2 mg, 4 mg, 8 mg, 16 mg, 32 mg.

Injection Powder for Reconstitution (A-Methapred, Solu-Medrol): 40 mg, 125 mg, 500 mg, 1 g.
Injection Suspension (Depo-Medrol): 20 mg/ml, 40 mg/ml, 80 mg/ml.

INDICATIONS AND DOSAGES

▸ Substitution therapy for deficiency states: acute or chronic adrenal insufficiency, adrenal insufficiency secondary to pituitary insufficiency, and congenital adrenal hyperplasia; nonendocrine disorders: allergic, collagen, hepatic, intestinal tract, ocular, renal, and skin diseases; arthritis; bronchial asthma; cerebral edema; malignancies; and rheumatic carditis
PO
Adults, Elderly. Initially, 4–48 mg/day.
IV (Methylprednisolone sodium succinate)
Adults, Elderly. 40–250 mg q4–6h. High dosage: 30 mg/kg over at least 30 min. Repeat q4–6h for 48–72 hr.

▸ Spinal cord injury
IV Bolus
Adults, Elderly. 30 mg/kg over 15 min. Maintenance dose: 5.4 mg/kg/hr over 23 hr, to be given within 45 min of bolus dose.
IM (Methylprednisolone acetate)
Adults, Elderly. 10–80 mg/day.
Intra-Articular, Intralesional
Adults, Elderly. 4–40 mg, up to 80 mg q1–5wk.

CONTRAINDICATIONS

Administration of live virus vaccines, systemic fungal infection

INTERACTIONS

Drug

Amphotericin: May increase hypokalemia.
Digoxin: May increase the risk of digoxin toxicity caused by hypokalemia
Diuretics, insulin, oral hypoglycemics, potassium supplements: May decrease the effects of these drugs.
Hepatic enzyme inducers: May decrease the effects of methylprednisolone.
Live-virus vaccines: May decrease the patient's antibody response to vaccine, increase vaccine side effects, and potentiate virus replication.

Herbal

None known.

Food

None known.

DIAGNOSTIC TEST EFFECTS

May increase blood cholesterol, glucose and serum lipid, amylase, and sodium levels. May decrease serum calcium, potassium, and thyroxine levels.

IV INCOMPATIBILITIES

Ciprofloxacin (Cipro), diltiazem (Cardizem), docetaxel (Taxotere), etoposide (VePesid), filgrastim (Neupogen), gemcitabine (Gemzar), paclitaxel (Taxol), potassium chloride, propofol (Diprivan), vinorelbine (Navelbine)

IV COMPATIBILITIES

Dopamine (Intropin), heparin, midazolam (Versed), theophylline

SIDE EFFECTS

Frequent

Insomnia, heartburn, anxiety, abdominal distention, diaphoresis, acne, mood swings, increased appetite, facial flushing, GI distress, delayed wound healing, increased susceptibility to infection, diarrhea or constipation

Occasional

Headache, edema, tachycardia,

change in skin color, frequent urination, depression

Rare

Psychosis, increased blood coagulability, hallucinations

SERIOUS REACTIONS

! Long-term therapy may cause hypocalcemia, hypokalemia, muscle wasting (especially in arms and legs), osteoporosis, spontaneous fractures, amenorrhea, cataracts, glaucoma, peptic ulcer disease, and CHF.

! Abruptly withdrawing the drug after long-term therapy may cause anorexia, nausea, fever, headache, sudden severe myalgia, rebound inflammation, fatigue, weakness, lethargy, dizziness, and orthostatic hypotension.

NURSING CONSIDERATIONS

Baseline Assessment

- Determine if the patient has a hypersensitivity to corticosteroids.
- Obtain the patient's BP, blood glucose and serum electrolyte levels, height, and weight.
- Evaluate the results of initial tests, such as tuberculosis skin test, x-rays, and EKG.
- Determine if the patient has diabetes mellitus, and anticipate an increase in his or her antidiabetic drug regimen because of raised blood glucose levels.
- If the patient is taking digoxin, plan to draw blood to determine serum digoxin level.

Lifespan Considerations

- Methylprednisolone crosses the placenta and is distributed in breast milk. Patients taking methylprednisolone should not breast-feed.
- Prolonged methylprednisolone use in the first trimester of pregnancy may cause cleft palate in the neonate.
- Prolonged treatment or high dosages may decrease cortisol secretion and short-term growth rate in children.
- No age-related precautions have been noted in the elderly.

Precautions

- Use methylprednisolone cautiously in patients with cirrhosis, CHF, diabetes mellitus, hypertension, hypothyroidism, thromboembolic disorders, or ulcerative colitis.

Administration and Handling

◀ALERT▶ Individualize dosage based on the disease, patient, and response.

PO

- Give methylprednisolone with food or milk.
- Give single doses before 9 a.m.; give multiple doses at evenly spaced intervals.

IV

- Store vials at room temperature.
- Follow directions with Mix-o-vial.
- For infusion, add to D_5W or 0.9% NaCl. Give IV push over 2 to 3 minutes. Give IV piggyback over 10 to 20 minutes.
- Do not give methylprednisolone acetate via IV line.

IM

- Methylprednisolone acetate should not be further diluted.
- Reconstitute methylprednisolone sodium succinate with bacteriostatic water for injection.
- Give deep IM injection into gluteus maximus.

Intervention and Evaluation

- Monitor the patient's intake and output and record daily weight.
- Assess the patient for edema.
- Evaluate the patient's pattern of daily bowel activity.
- Check the patient's vital signs at least 2 times a day.
- Be alert to signs and symptoms of infection, such as fever, sore throat, and vague symptoms.

- Monitor the patient's electrolyte levels.
- Monitor the patient for signs and symptoms of hypocalcemia (such as cramps and muscle twitching), or hypokalemia (such as EKG changes, irritability, nausea and vomiting, numbness or tingling of lower extremities, and weakness).
- Assess the patient's ability to sleep and emotional status.
- Check the patient's laboratory results for blood coagulability and evidence of thromboembolism.

Patient Teaching

- Instruct the patient to take oral methylprednisolone with food or milk.
- Caution the patient against abruptly discontinuing the drug or changing the dosage or schedule. Explain to the patient that the drug must be withdrawn gradually under medical supervision.
- Warn the patient to report fever, muscle aches, sore throat, or sudden weight gain or edema.
- Tell the patient to maintain good personal hygiene and to avoid exposure to disease or trauma. Explain to the patient that severe stress, such as serious infection, surgery, or trauma may require an increase in methylprednisolone dosage.
- Stress to the patient that follow-up visits and laboratory tests are a necessary part of treatment and that children must be assessed for growth retardation.
- Tell the patient to inform his or her dentist or other physicians that he or she is taking methylprednisolone or has taken it within the past 12 months.
- Explain that steroids often cause mood swings, ranging from euphoria to depression.

prednisolone

pred-**niss**-oh-lone
(AK-Pred, AK-Tate[CAN], Inflamase Forte, Inflamase Mild, Minims-Prednisolone[CAN], Novo-Prednisolone[CAN], Orapred, Pediapred, Pred Forte, Pred Mild, Prelone, Solone[AUS])
Do not confuse prednisolone with prednisone or primidone.

CATEGORY AND SCHEDULE

Pregnancy Risk Category: C (D if used in first trimester)

MECHANISM OF ACTION

An adrenocortical steroid that inhibits accumulation of inflammatory cells at inflammation sites, phagocytosis, lysosomal enzyme release and synthesis, and release of mediators of inflammation. **Therapeutic Effect:** Prevents or suppresses cell-mediated immune reactions. Decreases or prevents tissue response to inflammatory process.

AVAILABILITY

Oral Solution (Pediapred): 6.7 mg/5 ml.
Oral Solution (Orapred): 20 mg/5 ml.
Tablets: 5 mg.
Syrup (Prelone): 5 mg/5 ml.
Ophthalmic Solution (Inflamase Mild): 0.125%.
Ophthalmic Solution (AK-Pred, Inflamase Forte): 1%.
Ophthalmic Suspension (Pred Mild): 0.12%.
Ophthalmic Suspension (Pred Forte): 1%.

INDICATIONS AND DOSAGES

▸ Substitution therapy for deficiency states: acute or chronic adrenal insufficiency, congenital adrenal hyperplasia, and adrenal insufficiency secondary to pituitary insufficiency; nonendocrine disorders: arthritis; rheumatic carditis; allergic, collagen, intestinal tract, liver, ocular, renal, skin diseases; bronchial asthma; cerebral edema; malignancies

PO

Adults, Elderly. 5–60 mg/day in divided doses.

Children. 0.1–2 mg/kg/day in 1–4 divided doses.

▸ Treatment of conjuctivitis and corneal injury

Ophthalmic

Adults, Elderly. 1–2 drops every hr during day and q2h during night. After response, decrease dosage to 1 drop q4h, then 1 drop 3–4 times a day.

CONTRAINDICATIONS

Acute superficial herpes simplex keratitis, systemic fungal infections, varicella

INTERACTIONS

Drug

Amphotericin: May increase hypokalemia.

Digoxin: May increase the risk of digoxin toxicity caused by hypokalemia

Diuretics, insulin, oral hypoglycemics, potassium supplements: May decrease the effects of these drugs.

Hepatic enzyme inducers: May decrease the effects of prednisolone.

Live-virus vaccines: May decrease the patient's antibody response to vaccine, increase vaccine side effects, and potentiate virus replication.

Herbal

None known.

Food

None known.

DIAGNOSTIC TEST EFFECTS

May increase blood glucose and serum lipid, amylase, and sodium levels. May decrease serum calcium, potassium, and thyroxine levels.

SIDE EFFECTS

Frequent

Insomnia, heartburn, nervousness, abdominal distention, increased sweating, acne, mood swings, increased appetite, facial flushing, delayed wound healing, increased susceptibility to infection, diarrhea or constipation

Occasional

Headache, edema, change in skin color, frequent urination

Rare

Tachycardia, allergic reaction (such as rash and hives), psychological changes, hallucinations, depression

Ophthalmic: stinging or burning, posterior subcapsular cataracts

SERIOUS REACTIONS

! Long-term therapy may cause hypocalcemia, hypokalemia, muscle wasting (especially in the arms and legs), osteoporosis, spontaneous fractures, amenorrhea, cataracts, glaucoma, peptic ulcer disease, and CHF.

! Abruptly withdrawing the drug after long-term therapy may cause anorexia, nausea, fever, headache, severe or sudden joint pain, rebound inflammation, fatigue, weakness, lethargy, dizziness, and orthostatic hypotension.

! Suddenly discontinuing prednisolone may be fatal.

NURSING CONSIDERATIONS

Baseline Assessment

- Determine if the patient has a hypersensitivity to corticosteroids.
- Obtain the patient's BP, blood glucose and serum electrolyte levels, height, and weight.
- Evaluate the results of initial tests, such as tuberculosis skin test, x-rays, and EKG.
- Determine if the patient has diabetes mellitus, and anticipate an increase in his or her antidiabetic drug regimen because of raised blood glucose level.
- If the patient is taking digoxin, plan to draw blood to determine serum digoxin levels.
- Keep in mind that patients taking prednisolone should never be given live-virus vaccines, such as smallpox vaccine.

Lifespan Considerations

- Monitor growth and development of children receiving long-term steriod therapy.

Precautions

- Use prednisolone cautiously in patients with cirrhosis, CHF, diabetes mellitus, hypertension, hypothyroidism, myasthenia gravis, ocular herpes simplex, osteoporosis, peptic ulcer disease, thromboembolic disorders, or ulcerative colitis.

Administration and Handling

Ophthalmic

- For ophthalmic solution, shake well before using.
- Instill drops into conjunctival sac, as prescribed. Avoid touching the applicator tip to the conjunctiva to avoid contamination.

Intervention and Evaluation

- Be alert to signs and symptoms of infection, such as fever, sore throat, and vague symptoms.
- Assess the patient's mouth daily for signs and symptoms of candidal infection, such as white patches and painful mucous membranes and tongue.

Patient Teaching

- Warn the patient to report fever, muscle aches, sore throat, and sudden weight gain, or swelling.
- Urge the patient to avoid alcohol and to limit caffeine intake during prednisolone therapy.
- Caution the patient against abruptly discontinuing the drug without physician approval.
- Tell the patient to avoid exposure to chickenpox or measles.
- Explain that steroids often cause mood swings, ranging from euphoria to depression.

prednisone

pred-ni-sone
(Apo-Prednisone[CAN], Deltasone, Panafcort[AUS], Prednisone Intensol, Sone[AUS], Sterapred, Sterapred DS, Winpred[CAN])
Do not confuse prednisone with prednisolone or primidone.

CATEGORY AND SCHEDULE

Pregnancy Risk Category: C (D if used in first trimester)

MECHANISM OF ACTION

An adrenocortical steroid that inhibits accumulation of inflammatory cells at inflammation sites, phagocytosis, lysosomal enzyme release and synthesis, and release of mediators of inflammation. **Therapeutic Effect:** Prevents or suppresses cell-mediated immune reactions. Decreases or prevents tissue response to inflammatory process.

PHARMACOKINETICS

Well absorbed from the GI tract.

Protein binding: 70%–90%. Widely distributed. Metabolized in the liver and converted to prednisolone. Primarily excreted in urine. Not removed by hemodialysis. ***Half-life:*** 3.4–3.8 hr.

AVAILABILITY

Oral Concentrate (Prednisone Intensol): 5 mg/ml.
Oral Solution: 5 mg/5 ml.
Tablets (Deltasone): 2.5 mg, 5 mg, 10 mg, 20 mg, 50 mg.
Tablets (Sterapred): 5 mg, 10 mg.

INDICATIONS AND DOSAGES

▸ **Substitution therapy in deficiency states: acute or chronic adrenal insufficiency, congenital adrenal hyperplasia, and adrenal insufficiency secondary to pituitary insufficiency; nonendocrine disorders: arthritis; rheumatic carditis; allergic, collagen, intestinal tract, liver, ocular, renal, skin diseases; bronchial asthma; cerebral edema; malignancies**
PO
Adults, Elderly. 5–60 mg/day in divided doses.
Children. 0.05–2 mg/kg/day in 1–4 divided doses.

CONTRAINDICATIONS

Acute superficial herpes simplex keratitis, systemic fungal infections, varicella

INTERACTIONS

Drug

Amphotericin: May increase hypokalemia.
Digoxin: May increase the risk of digoxin toxicity caused by hypokalemia
Diuretics, insulin, oral hypoglycemics, potassium supplements: May decrease the effects of these drugs.
Hepatic enzyme inducers: May decrease the effects of prednisone.
Live-virus vaccines: May decrease the patient's antibody response to vaccine, increase vaccine side effects, and potentiate virus replication.

Herbal

None known.

Food

None known.

DIAGNOSTIC TEST EFFECTS

May increase blood glucose and serum lipid, amylase, and sodium levels. May decrease serum calcium, potassium, and thyroxine levels.

SIDE EFFECTS

Frequent

Insomnia, heartburn, nervousness, abdominal distention, increased sweating, acne, mood swings, increased appetite, facial flushing, delayed wound healing, increased susceptibility to infection, diarrhea or constipation

Occasional

Headache, edema, change in skin color, frequent urination

Rare

Tachycardia, allergic reaction (including rash and hives), psychological changes, hallucinations, depression

SERIOUS REACTIONS

! Long-term therapy may cause muscle wasting in the arms and legs, osteoporosis, spontaneous fractures, amenorrhea, cataracts, glaucoma, peptic ulcer disease, and CHF.
! Abruptly withdrawing the drug following long-term therapy may cause anorexia, nausea, fever, headache, sudden or severe joint pain, rebound inflammation, fatigue, weakness, lethargy, dizziness, and orthostatic hypotension.

! Suddenly discontinuing prednisone may be fatal.

NURSING CONSIDERATIONS

Baseline Assessment

- Determine if the patient has a hypersensitivity to corticosteroids.
- Obtain the patient's BP, blood glucose and serum electrolyte levels, height, and weight.
- Determine if the patient has diabetes mellitus, and anticipate an increase in his or her antidiabetic drug regimen because of raised blood glucose level.
- If the patient is taking digoxin, plan to draw blood to determine serum digoxin levels.
- Check the results of initial tests, such as tuberculosis skin test, x-rays, and EKG.
- Keep in mind that patients taking prednisone should never be given live-virus vaccines, such as smallpox vaccine.

Lifespan Considerations

- Prednisone crosses the placenta and is distributed in breast milk.
- Prolonged prednisone use in the first trimester of pregnancy causes cleft palate in the neonate.
- Prolonged treatment or high dosages may decrease the cortisol secretion and short-term growth rate in children.
- The elderly may be more susceptible to developing hypertension or osteoporosis.

Precautions

- Use prednisone cautiously in patients with CHF, cirrhosis, hypertension, hyperthyroidism, myasthenia gravis, ocular herpes simplex, osteoporosis, peptic ulcer disease, thromboembolic disorders, or ulcerative colitis.

Administration and Handling

PO

- Give prednisone without regard to meals; give with food if GI upset occurs.
- Give single doses before 9 a.m.; give multiple doses at evenly spaced intervals.

Intervention and Evaluation

- Monitor the patient's BP, blood glucose, and serum electrolyte levels, height, and weight.
- Be alert to signs and symptoms of infection such as fever, sore throat, and vague symptoms.
- Assess the patient's mouth daily for signs and symptoms of candidal infection, such as white patches and painful mucous membranes and tongue.

Patient Teaching

- Warn the patient to report fever, muscle aches, sore throat, or sudden weight gain or swelling.
- Urge the patient to avoid alcohol and limit caffeine intake during prednisone therapy.
- Caution the patient against abruptly discontinuing prednisone without physician approval.
- Warn the patient to avoid exposure to chickenpox or measles.
- Explain that steroids often cause mood swings, ranging from euphoria to depression.

triamcinolone

trye-am-**sin**-oh-lone
(Aristocort)

triamcinolone acetonide

(Aristocort, Azmacort, Kenacort A[AUS], Kenalog, Kenalog in Orabase[AUS], Nasacort AQ, Triaderm[CAN])

triamcinolone diacetate

(Amcort, Aristocort Intralesional)

triamcinolone hexacetonide

(Aristospan)

Do not confuse triamcinolone with Triaminicin or Triaminicol.

CATEGORY AND SCHEDULE

Pregnancy Risk Category: C (D if used in first trimester)

MECHANISM OF ACTION

An adrenocortical steroid that inhibits accumulation of inflammatory cells at inflammation sites, phagocytosis, lysosomal enzyme release and synthesis, and release of mediators of inflammation. **Therapeutic Effect:** Prevents or suppresses cell-mediated immune reactions. Decreases or prevents tissue response to inflammatory process.

AVAILABILITY

Oral (Topical Paste [Kenalog in Orabase]): 0.1% or 5 g.
Tablets (Aristocort): 4 mg.
Inhalation (Oral [Azmacort]): 100 mcg/actuation.
Nasal Spray (Tri-Nasal): 50 mcg/inhalation.
Nasal Spray (Vasacort AQ): 55 mcg/inhalation.
Cream (Aristocort A): 0.025%, 0.05%, 0.1%.
Cream (Kenalog, Triderm): 0.1%.
Ointment (Aristocort A, Kenalog): 0.025%, 0.1%.
Injection (acetonide, Kenalog): 10 mg/ml, 40 mg/ml.
Injection (diacetate, Aristocort): 25 mg/ml), 40 mg/ml.
Injection (hexacetonide, Aristospan): 5 mg/ml, 20 mg/ml.

INDICATIONS AND DOSAGES

▸ **Immunosuppression, relief of acute inflammation**

PO
Adults, Elderly. 4–60 mg/day.
IM
Adults, Elderly. 40 mg/wk (triamcinolone diacetate). Initially, 2.5–60 mg/day (triamcinolone acetonide). Initially, 2.5–40 mg up to 100 mg; 2–20 mg (triamcinolone hexacetonide).
Intra-Articular, Intralesional
Adults, Elderly. 5–40 mg.

▸ **Control of bronchial asthma**

Inhalation
Adults, Elderly. 2 inhalations 3–4 times a day.
Children 6–12 yr. 1–2 inhalations 3–4 times a day. Maximum: 12 inhalations/day.

▸ **Rhinitis**

Intranasal
Adults, Children 6 yr and older. 2 sprays each nostril each day.

▸ **Relief of inflammation or pruritus associated with corticoid-responsive dermatoses**

Topical
Adults, Elderly. 2–4 times a day. May give 1–2 times a day or as intermittent therapy.

CONTRAINDICATIONS

Administration of live-virus vaccines, especially smallpox vaccine; hypersensitivity to corticosteroids or

tartrazine; IM injection or oral inhalation in children younger than 6 years; peptic ulcer disease (except life-threatening situations); systemic fungal infection
Topical: Marked circulation impairment

INTERACTIONS
Drug
Amphotericin: May increase hypokalemia.
Digoxin: May increase the risk of digoxin toxicity caused by hypokalemia.
Diuretics, insulin, oral hypoglycemics, potassium supplements: May decrease the effects of these drugs.
Hepatic enzyme inducers: May decrease the effects of triamcinolone.
Live-virus vaccines: May decrease the patient's antibody response to vaccine, increase vaccine side effects, and potentiate virus replication.
Herbal
None known.
Food
None known.

DIAGNOSTIC TEST EFFECTS
May increase blood glucose and serum lipid, amylase, and sodium levels. May decrease serum calcium, potassium, and thyroxine levels.

SIDE EFFECTS
Frequent
Insomnia, dry mouth, heartburn, nervousness, abdominal distention, diaphoresis, acne, mood swings, increased appetite, facial flushing, delayed wound healing, increased susceptibility to infection, diarrhea or constipation
Occasional
Headache, edema, change in skin color, frequent urination
Rare
Tachycardia, allergic reaction (including rash and hives), mental changes, hallucinations, depression
Topical: Allergic contact dermatitis

SERIOUS REACTIONS
! Long-term therapy may cause muscle wasting in the arms or legs, osteoporosis, spontaneous fractures, amenorrhea, cataracts, glaucoma, peptic ulcer disease, and CHF.
! Abruptly withdrawing the drug following long-term therapy may cause anorexia, nausea, fever, headache, arthralgia, rebound inflammation, fatigue, weakness, lethargy, dizziness, and orthostatic hypotension.
! Anaphylaxis occurs rarely with parenteral administration.
! Suddenly discontinuing triamcinolone may be fatal.
! Blindness has occurred rarely after intralesional injection around face and head.

NURSING CONSIDERATIONS
Baseline Assessment
- Determine if the patient is hypersensitive to corticosteroids or tartrazine (Kenacort).
- Obtain the patient's baselines for BP, blood glucose and serum electrolyte levels, height, and weight.
- Determine if the patient has diabetes mellitus, and anticipate an increase in his or her antidiabetic drug regimen because of raised blood glucose level.
- If the patient is taking digoxin, plan to draw blood to determine serum digoxin level.
- Check the results of initial tests, such as tuberculosis skin test, x-rays, and EKG.
- Keep in mind that patients taking triamcinolone should never be given

live-virus vaccines, such as smallpox vaccine.

Lifespan Considerations

- Monitor growth and development in children receiving long-term steroid therapy.

Precautions

- Use triamcinolone cautiously in patients with CHF, cirrhosis, history of tuberculosis (it may reactivate disease), hypertension, hypothyroidism, nonspecific ulcerative colitis, psychosis, or renal insufficiency.
- Discontinue prolonged therapy slowly.

Administration and Handling

PO

- Give triamcinolone with food or milk.
- Give single doses before 9 a.m.; give multiple doses at evenly spaced intervals.

IM

- Do not give IV.
- Give deep IM injection into gluteus maximus.

Inhalation

- Shake container well. Instruct the patient to exhale as completely as possible.
- Place mouthpiece fully into the patient's mouth and, while holding the inhaler upright, have the patient inhale deeply and slowly while pressing the top of the canister. Instruct the patient to hold his or her breath as long as possible before slowly exhaling.
- Wait 1 minute between inhalations when multiple inhalations have been ordered to allow for deeper bronchial penetration.
- Rinse the patient's mouth with water immediately after inhalation to prevent thrush.

Topical

- Gently cleanse area before applying drug. Apply sparingly and rub into area thoroughly.
- Use occlusive dressings only as ordered.

Intervention and Evaluation

- Monitor the patient's blood glucose level, BP, and intake and output. Record the patient's weight daily.
- Assess the patient for edema.
- Check the patient's vital signs at least 2 times a day.
- Be alert to signs and symptoms of infection such as fever, pharyngitis, and vague symptoms.
- Evaluate the patient for signs and symptoms of hypocalcemia (such as cramps, muscle twitching, and positive Chvostek's or Trousseau's signs), or hypokalemia (such as EKG changes, irritability, muscle cramps and weakness, nausea and vomiting, and numbness and tingling in the lower extremities).
- Assess the patient's ability to sleep and emotional status.
- Check the mucous membranes for signs and symptoms of fungal infection in patients using inhaled triamcinolone.
- Monitor the growth rate in children.
- Check the patient's laboratory results for blood coagulability and evidence of thromboembolism.
- Assist the patient with ambulation.

Patient Teaching

- Tell the patient taking oral triamcinolone to report difficulty breathing, muscle weakness, sudden weight gain, or facial edema.
- Instruct the patient taking oral triamcinolone to take the drug with food or after meals.
- Warn the patient to notify the physician if his or her condition worsens.
- Caution the patient against abruptly discontinuing oral triamcinolone without physician approval.

- Explain to the patient that oral triamcinolone may cause dry mouth.
- Urge the patient to avoid alcohol during oral triamcinolone therapy.
- Instruct patients taking inhaled triamcinolone not to use the drug for acute asthma attacks.
- Tell the patient taking inhaled triamcinolone to rinse his or her mouth after drug administration to decrease the risk of mouth soreness.
- Warn the patient taking inhaled triamcinolone to notify the physician stomatitis occurs.
- Warn the patient taking nasal triamcinolone to notify the physician if unusual cough or spasm or persistent nasal bleeding, burning, or infection occurs.
- Explain that steroids often cause mood swings, ranging from euphoria to depression.

64 Antidiabetic Agents

acarbose
glimepiride
glipizide
glyburide
insulin
metformin hydrochloride
miglitol
nateglinide
pioglitazone
repaglinide
rosiglitazone maleate

Uses: All antidiabetic agents are used to treat diabetes. *Insulin* is used to manage insulin-dependent (type 1) diabetes mellitus and non-insulin-dependent (type 2) diabetes mellitus. It's also used in acute situations, such as ketoacidosis, severe infections, and major surgery in otherwise non-insulin-dependent diabetes mellitus. It's administered to patients receiving parenteral nutrition and is the drug of choice during pregnancy.

Sulfonylureas, such as glimepiride and glyburide, are used to control hyperglycemia in type 2 diabetes mellitus that's not controlled by weight management and diet alone.

Alpha-glucosidase inhibitors, such as acarbose and miglitol, and *biguanides,* such as metformin, are used along with diet to lower the blood glucose level in patients with type 2 diabetes mellitus whose hyperglycemia can't be managed by diet alone.

Meglitinides, such as nateglinide and repaglinide, are used alone or with other antidiabetic agents to control the blood glucose level in patients with type 2 diabetes mellitus whose hyperglycemia can't be managed by diet and exercise.

Thiazolidinediones, such as pioglitazone and rosiglitazone, are used as adjunct therapy in patients with type 2 diabetes mellitus who are currently receiving insulin.

Action: Antidiabetic agents act in different ways to control diabetes. (See the illustration *Mechanisms of Action: Antidiabetic Agents,* page 1148.) *Insulin* is a hormone synthesized and secreted by beta cells in the islets of Langerhans in the pancreas. It controls the storage and use of glucose, amino acids, and fatty acids by activated transport systems and enzymes. It also inhibits the breakdown of glycogen, fat, and protein. Insulin lowers the blood glucose level by inhibiting glycogenolysis and gluconeogenesis in the liver and by stimulating glucose uptake by muscle and adipose tissue. Insulin activity is initiated by binding to cell surface receptors.

Sulfonylureas stimulate insulin release from beta cells and increase insulin sensitivity in peripheral tissues. Endogenous insulin must be present for these oral drugs to be effective.

Alpha-glucosidase inhibitors work locally in the small intestine, slowing carbohydrate breakdown and glucose absorption.

Biguanides decrease hepatic glucose output and enhance peripheral glucose uptake.

Meglitinides stimulate the release of insulin by depolarizing beta cells in the pancreas, which prompts their calcium channels to open. This action causes an influx of intracellular calcium and stimulates insulin secretion.

Thiazolidinediones decrease insulin resistance.

COMBINATION PRODUCTS

AVANDAMET: metformin/rosiglitazone (an antidiabetic) 500 mg/1 mg; 500 mg/2 mg; 500 mg/4 mg; 1 g/2 mg; 1 g/4 mg.
GLUCOVANCE: glyburide/metformin (an antidiabetic) 1.25 mg/250 mg; 2.5 mg/500 mg; 5 mg/500 mg.
HUMALOG MIX 75/25: lispro suspension 75% and lispro solution 25%.
HUMULIN 50/50: NPH 50% and regular 50%.
HUMULIN 70/30: NPH 70% and rapid-acting regular 30%.
METAGLIP: glipizide/metformin (an antidiabetic) 2.5 mg/250 mg; 2.5 mg/500 mg; 5 mg/500 mg.
NOVOLIN 70/30: NPH 70% and rapid-acting regular 30%.
NOVOLOG 70/30: aspart suspension 70% and aspart solution 30%.

acarbose

a-**car**-bose
(Glucobay[AUS], Prandase[CAN], Precose)
Do not confuse Precose with PreCare.

CATEGORY AND SCHEDULE

Pregnancy Risk Category: B

MECHANISM OF ACTION

An alpha glucosidase inhibitor that delays glucose absorption and digestion of carbohydrates, resulting in a smaller rise in blood glucose concentration after meals. **Therapeutic Effect:** Lowers postprandial hyperglycemia.

AVAILABILITY

Tablets: 25 mg, 50 mg, 100 mg.

INDICATIONS AND DOSAGES

Diabetes mellitus

PO

Adults, Elderly. Initially, 25 mg 3 times a day with first bite of each main meal. Increase at 4- to 8-wk intervals. Maximum: For patients weighing more than 60 kg, 100 mg 3

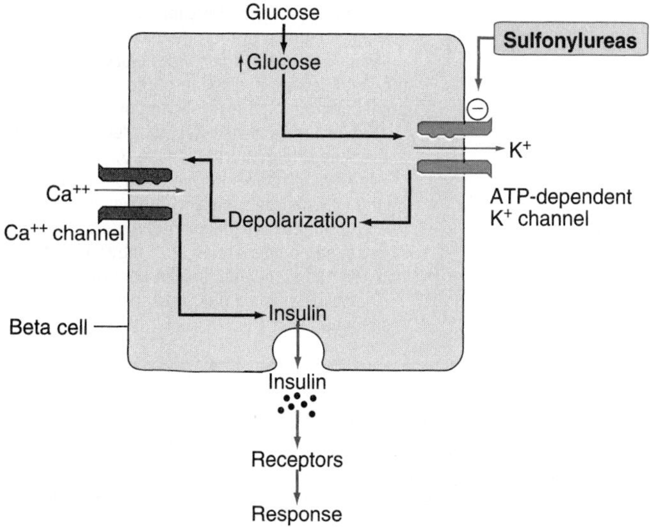

Mechanisms of Action: Antidiabetic Agents

Diabetes mellitus takes two forms: type 1 diabetes characterized by a complete lack of insulin and type 2 diabetes marked by insufficient insulin secretion, insulin resistance in peripheral tissues, or both. Normally, the beta cells in the pancreatic islets of Langerhans are responsible for secreting insulin. When glucose levels rise in the beta cell, it triggers adenosine triphosphate (ATP)-dependent potassium (K^+) channels in the membranes of beta cells to close. Then the beta cells depolarize and calcium (Ca^{++}) enters the cell through the Ca^{++} channel, and insulin is released from the cell. When circulating insulin engages with insulin receptors on cell membranes, it facilitates the movement of glucose into the cell, among other actions.

Type 1 diabetes is treated with the use of exogenous insulin, which mimics natural insulin in the body. Insulin takes many forms with varying degrees of onset, peak, and duration, including rapid, regular, intermediate, and long-acting.

Type 2 diabetes is usually treated with oral agents. Sulfonylureas, such as glyburide, block ATP-dependent K^+ channels in the cell membranes of beta cells, ultimately resulting in the release of insulin.

times a day; for patients weighing 60 kg or less, 50 mg 3 times a day.

CONTRAINDICATIONS

Chronic intestinal diseases associated with marked disorders of digestion or absorption, cirrhosis, colonic ulceration, conditions that may deteriorate as a result of increased gas formation in the intestine, diabetic ketoacidosis, hypersensitivity to acarbose, inflammatory bowel disease, partial intestinal obstruction or predisposition to intestinal obstruction, significant renal dysfunction (serum creatinine level greater than 2 mg/dl)

INTERACTIONS

Drug

Digestive enzymes, intestinal absorbents (such as charcoal): Reduces effects of acarbose.

Herbal

None known.

Food

None known.

DIAGNOSTIC TEST EFFECTS

May increase AST (SGOT) levels.

SIDE EFFECTS

Side effects diminish in frequency and intensity over time.

Frequent

Transient GI disturbances: flatulence (77%), diarrhea (33%), abdominal pain (21%)

SERIOUS REACTIONS

! None known.

NURSING CONSIDERATIONS

Baseline Assessment

- Expect to check blood glucose level.
- Discuss lifestyle to determine the extent of the patient's learning and emotional needs.

Lifespan Considerations

- Acarbose use is not recommended during pregnancy. It is unknown if acarbose is distributed in breast milk.
- Safety and efficacy have not been established in children.
- Hypoglycemia may be difficult to recognize in the elderly. Also, age-related renal impairment may increase sensitivity to the glucose-lowering effect of acarbose.

Precautions

- Use acarbose cautiously in patients with fever or infection or in those who've had surgery or trauma because these states may cause loss of glycemic control.

Administration and Handling

PO

- Give with the first bite of each main meal.

Intervention and Evaluation

- Monitor food intake and blood glucose, glycosylated hemoglobin, and AST (SGOT) levels.
- Assess for signs and symptoms of hypoglycemia (anxiety, cool wet skin, diplopia, dizziness, headache, hunger, numbness in mouth, tachycardia, tremors) or hyperglycemia (deep rapid breathing, dim vision, fatigue, nausea, polydipsia, polyphagia, polyuria, vomiting).
- Be alert to conditions that alter glucose requirements, including fever, increased activity or stress, or a surgical procedure.

Patient Teaching

- Advise the patient not to skip or delay meals.
- Stress that the patient consult the physician when glucose demands are altered (such as with fever, heavy physical activity, infection, stress, trauma).
- Warn the patient to avoid alcoholic beverages.
- Explain to the patient that exercise, good personal hygiene (including foot care), not smoking, and weight control are essential parts of therapy.

glimepiride

gly-**mep**-er-ide

(Amaryl)

Do not confuse glimepiride with glipizide or glyburide.

CATEGORY AND SCHEDULE

Pregnancy Risk Category: C

MECHANISM OF ACTION

A second-generation sulfonylurea that promotes release of insulin from beta cells of the pancreas and increases insulin sensitivity at peripheral sites. **Therapeutic Effect:** Lowers blood glucose concentration.

PHARMACOKINETICS

Route	Onset	Peak	Duration
PO	N/A	2–3 hr	24 hr

Completely absorbed from the GI tract. Protein binding: greater than 99%. Metabolized in the liver. Excreted in urine and eliminated in feces. ***Half-life:*** 5–9.2 hr.

AVAILABILITY

Tablets: 1 mg, 2 mg, 4 mg.

INDICATIONS AND DOSAGES

▸ **Diabetes mellitus**

PO

Adults, Elderly. Initially, 1–2 mg once a day, with breakfast or first main meal. Maintenance: 1–4 mg once a day. After dose of 2 mg is reached, dosage should be increased in increments of up to 2 mg q1–2wk, based on blood glucose response. Maximum: 8 mg/day.

▸ **Dosage in renal impairment**

PO

Adults. 1 mg once/day.

CONTRAINDICATIONS

Diabetic complications, such as ketosis, acidosis, and diabetic coma; severe hepatic or renal impairment; monotherapy for type 1 diabetes mellitus; stress situations, including severe infection, trauma, and surgery

INTERACTIONS

Drug

Beta blockers: May increase the hypoglycemic effect of glimepiride and mask signs of hypoglycemia.
Cimetidine, ciprofloxacin, fluconazole, MAOIs, quinidine, ranitidine, large doses of salicylates: May increase the effects of glimepiride.
Corticosteroids, lithium, thiazide diuretics: May decrease the effects of glimepiride.
Oral anticoagulants: May increase the effects of oral anticoagulants.

Herbal

None known.

Food

None known.

DIAGNOSTIC TEST EFFECTS

May increase BUN and LDH concentrations and serum alkaline phosphatase, creatinine, and AST (SGOT) levels.

SIDE EFFECTS

Frequent

Altered taste sensation, dizziness, somnolence, weight gain, constipation, diarrhea, heartburn, nausea, vomiting, stomach fullness, headache

Occasional

Increased sensitivity of skin to sunlight, peeling of skin, itching, rash

SERIOUS REACTIONS

! Overdose or insufficient food intake may produce hypoglycemia, especially with increased glucose demands.

! GI hemorrhage, cholestatic hepatic jaundice, leukopenia, thrombocytopenia, pancytopenia, agranulocytosis, and aplastic or hemolytic anemia occur rarely.

NURSING CONSIDERATIONS

Baseline Assessment

- Check the patient's blood glucose levels, as ordered.
- Discuss lifestyle to determine the extent of the patient's emotional and learning needs regarding diabetes mellitus.

Lifespan Considerations

- Glimepiride use is not recommended during pregnancy. It is unknown if glimepiride is distributed in breast milk.
- Safety and efficacy of glimepiride have not been established in children.
- Hypoglycemia may be difficult to recognize in the elderly. Also, age-related renal impairment may increase sensitivity to glucose-lowering effect.

Precautions

- Use glimepiride cautiously in patients with adrenal insufficiency, debilitation, hepatic disease, impaired renal function, intestinal obstruction, malnutrition, pituitary insufficiency, prolonged vomiting, severe diarrhea, or uncontrolled hyperthyroidism.

Administration and Handling

PO

- Give glimepiride with breakfast or first main meal.

Intervention and Evaluation

- Monitor the patient's blood glucose level and food intake.
- Assess the patient for signs and symptoms of hypoglycemia (anxiety, cool wet skin, diplopia, dizziness, headache, hunger, numbness in mouth, tachycardia, tremors), or hyperglycemia (deep rapid breathing, dim vision, fatigue, nausea, polydipsia, polyphagia, polyuria, vomiting).
- Be alert to conditions that alter blood glucose requirements, such as fever, increased activity, stress, or a surgical procedure.

Patient Teaching

- Stress to the patient that the prescribed diet is a principal part of treatment. Warn the patient not to skip or delay meals.
- Make sure the patient is aware of the typical signs and symptoms of hypoglycemia and hyperglycemia.
- Instruct the patient to carry candy, sugar packets, or other sugar supplements for immediate response to hypoglycemia and urge the patient to wear medical alert identification stating he or she has diabetes.
- Stress that the patient consult the physician when glucose demands are altered, such as with fever, heavy physical activity, infection, stress, or trauma.
- Ensure follow-up instruction if the patient or family does not thoroughly understand diabetes management or blood glucose–testing technique.
- Teach the patient to wear sunscreen and protective eyewear to prevent the effects of light sensitivity.

glipizide

glip-i-zide

(Glucotrol, Glucotrol XL, Melizide[AUS], Minidiab[AUS])

Do not confuse glipizide with glimepiride or glyburide.

CATEGORY AND SCHEDULE

Pregnancy Risk Category: C

MECHANISM OF ACTION

A second-generation sulfonylurea that promotes the release of insulin from beta cells of the pancreas and increases insulin sensitivity at peripheral sites. **Therapeutic Effect:** Lowers blood glucose concentration.

PHARMACOKINETICS

Route	Onset	Peak	Duration
PO	15–30 min	2–3 hr	12–24 hr
Extended-release	2–3 hr	6–12 hr	24 hr

Well absorbed from the GI tract. Protein binding: 99%. Metabolized in the liver. Excreted in urine. ***Half-life:*** 2–4 hr.

AVAILABILITY

Tablets (Glucotrol): 5 mg, 10 mg.
Tablets (Extended-Release [Glucotrol XL]): 2.5 mg, 5 mg, 10 mg.

INDICATIONS AND DOSAGES

▸Diabetes mellitus

PO

Adults. Initially, 5 mg/day or 2.5 mg in the elderly or those with hepatic disease. Adjust dosage in 2.5- to 5-mg increments at intervals of several days. Maximum single dose: 15 mg. Maximum dose/day: 40 mg. Maintenance (extended-release tablet): 20 mg/day.
Elderly. Initially, 2.5–5 mg/day. May increase by 2.5–5 mg/day q1–2wk.

CONTRAINDICATIONS

Diabetic ketoacidosis with or without coma, type 1 diabetes mellitus

INTERACTIONS

Drug

Beta blockers: May increase the hypoglycemic effect of glipizide and mask signs of hypoglycemia.
Cimetidine, ciprofloxacin, fluconazole, MAOIs, quinidine, ranitidine, large doses of salicylates: May increase the effects of glipizide.
Corticosteroids, lithium, thiazide diuretics: May decrease the effects of glipizide.
Oral anticoagulants: May increase the effects of oral anticoagulants.

Herbal

None known.

Food

None known.

DIAGNOSTIC TEST EFFECTS

May increase BUN and LDH concentrations and serum alkaline phosphatase, creatinine, and AST (SGOT) levels.

SIDE EFFECTS

Frequent

Altered taste sensation, dizziness, somnolence, weight gain, constipation, diarrhea, heartburn, nausea, vomiting, stomach fullness, headache

Occasional

Increased sensitivity of skin to sunlight, peeling of skin, itching, rash

SERIOUS REACTIONS

! Overdose or insufficiet food intake may produce hypoglycemia, especially with increased glucose demands.

! GI hemorrhage, cholestatic hepatic jaundice, leukopenia, thrombocytopenia, pancytopenia, agranulocytosis, and aplastic or hemolytic anemia occurs rarely.

NURSING CONSIDERATIONS

Baseline Assessment

- Check the patient's blood glucose level, as ordered.
- Discuss lifestyle to determine the extent of the patient's emotional and learning needs.

Lifespan Considerations

- Insulin is the drug of choice during pregnancy.

- Glipizide given within 1 month of delivery may produce neonatal hypoglycemia.
- Glipizide crosses the placenta and is distributed in breast milk.
- Safety and efficacy of glipizide have not been established in children.
- Hypoglycemia may be difficult to recognize in the elderly. Also, age-related renal impairment may increase sensitivity to the glucose-lowering effect.

Precautions

- Use glipizide cautiously in patients with adrenal or pituitary insufficiency, hypoglycemic reactions, or impaired hepatic or renal function.

Administration and Handling

PO

- May give glipizide with food; however, the response is better if given 15 to 30 minutes before meals.
- Do not crush extended-release tablets.

Intervention and Evaluation

- Monitor the patient's blood glucose level and food intake.
- Assess the patient for signs and symptoms of hypoglycemia (anxiety, cool wet skin, diplopia, dizziness, headache, hunger, numbness in mouth, tachycardia, tremors), or hyperglycemia (deep rapid breathing, dim vision, fatigue, nausea, polydipsia, polyphagia, polyuria, vomiting).
- Be alert to conditions that alter blood glucose requirements, such as fever, increased activity, stress, or a surgical procedure.

Patient Teaching

- Stress to the patient that the prescribed diet is a principal part of treatment. Warn the patient not to skip or delay meals.
- Make sure the patient is aware of the typical signs and symptoms of hypoglycemia and hyperglycemia.
- Instruct the patient to carry candy, sugar packets, or other sugar supplements for immediate response to hypoglycemia and urge the patient to wear medical alert identification stating that he or she has diabetes.
- Stress that the patient consult the physician when glucose demands are altered, such as with fever, heavy physical activity, infection, stress, or trauma.
- Ensure follow-up instruction if the patient or family does not thoroughly understand diabetes management or blood glucose-testing technique.
- Teach the patient to wear sunscreen and protective eyewear to prevent the effects of light sensitivity.

glyburide

glye-byoor-ide
(Daonil[CAN], DiaBeta, Euglucon[CAN], Glimel[AUS], Glynase, Micronase, Semi-Daonil[AUS], Semi-Euglucon[AUS])
Do not confuse glyburide with glimepiride or glipizide, or Micronase with Micro-K or Micronor.

CATEGORY AND SCHEDULE

Pregnancy Risk Category: C

MECHANISM OF ACTION

A second-generation sulfonylurea that promotes release of insulin from beta cells of the pancreas and increases insulin sensitivity at peripheral sites. **Therapeutic Effect:** Lowers blood glucose concentration.

PHARMACOKINETICS

Route	Onset	Peak	Duration
PO	0.25–1 hr	1–2 hr	12–24 hr

Well absorbed from the GI tract. Protein binding: 99%. Metabolized in the liver to weakly active metabolite. Primarily excreted in urine. Not removed by hemodialysis. ***Half-life:*** 1.4–1.8 hr.

AVAILABILITY

Tablets (DiaBeta, Micronase): 1.25 mg, 2.5 mg, 5 mg.
Tablets (Glynase): 1.5 mg, 3 mg, 6 mg.

INDICATIONS AND DOSAGES

▸ Diabetes mellitus

PO

Adults. Initially 2.5–5 mg. May increase by 2.5 mg/day at weekly intervals. Maintenance: 1.25–20 mg/day. Maximum: 20 mg/day.
Elderly. Initially, 1.25–2.5 mg/day. May increase by 1.25–2.5 mg/day at 1- to 3-wk intervals.

PO (micronized tablets [Glynase])

Adults, Elderly. Initially 0.75–3 mg/day. May increase by 1.5 mg/day at weekly intervals. Maintenance: 0.75–12 mg/day as a single dose or in divided doses.

▸ Dosage in renal impairment

Glyburide is not recommended in patients with creatinine clearance less than 50 ml/min.

CONTRAINDICATIONS

Diabetic ketoacidosis with or without coma, monotherapy for type 1 diabetes mellitus

INTERACTIONS

Drug

Beta blockers: May increase the hypoglycemic effect of glyburide and mask signs of hypoglycemia.
Cimetidine, ciprofloxacin, fluconazole, MAOIs, quinidine, ranitidine, large doses of salicylates: May increase the effects of glyburide.
Corticosteroids, lithium, thiazide diuretics: May decrease the effects of glyburide.
Oral anticoagulants: May increase the effects of oral anticoagulants.

Herbal

None known.

Food

None known.

DIAGNOSTIC TEST EFFECTS

May increase BUN and LDH concentrations and serum alkaline phosphatase, creatinine, and AST (SGOT) levels.

SIDE EFFECTS

Frequent

Altered taste sensation, dizziness, somnolence, weight gain, constipation, diarrhea, heartburn, nausea, vomiting, stomach fullness, headache

Occasional

Increased sensitivity of skin to sunlight, peeling of skin, itching, rash

SERIOUS REACTIONS

! Overdose or insufficient food intake may produce hypoglycemia, especially in patients with increased glucose demands.
! Cholestatic jaundice, leukopenia, thrombocytopenia, pancytopenia, agranulocytosis, and aplastic or hemolytic anemia occur rarely.

NURSING CONSIDERATIONS

Baseline Assessment

- Check the patient's blood glucose level, as ordered.
- Discuss lifestyle to determine the extent of the patient's emotional and learning needs.

Lifespan Considerations

- Glyburide crosses the placenta and is distributed in breast milk.

- Glyburide use within 2 weeks of delivery may produce neonatal hypoglycemia.
- Safety and efficacy of glyburide have not been established in children.
- Hypoglycemia may be difficult to recognize in the elderly. Also, age-related renal impairment may increase sensitivity to the glucose-lowering effect.

Precautions

- Use glyburide cautiously in patients with adrenal or pituitary insufficiency, hypoglycemic reactions, or impaired hepatic or renal function.

Administration and Handling

PO

- May give glyburide with food to reduce GI symptoms.
- Store at room temperature in a tightly closed container.

Intervention and Evaluation

- Monitor the patient's blood glucose and food intake.
- Assess the patient for signs and symptoms of hypoglycemia (anxiety, cool wet skin, diplopia, dizziness, headache, hunger, perioral numbness, tachycardia, tremors), or hyperglycemia (deep rapid breathing, dim vision, fatigue, nausea, polydipsia, polyphagia, polyuria, vomiting).
- Be alert to conditions that alter blood glucose requirements, such as fever, increased activity, stress, or a surgical procedure.

Patient Teaching

- Stress to the patient that the prescribed diet is a principal part of treatment. Warn the patient not to skip or delay meals.
- Make sure the patient is aware of the typical signs and symptoms of hypoglycemia and hyperglycemia.
- Instruct the patient to carry candy, sugar packets, or other sugar supplements for immediate response to hypoglycemia and urge the patient to wear medical alert identification stating that he or she has diabetes.
- Stress that the patient consult the physician when glucose demands are altered, such as with fever, heavy physical activity, infection, stress, or trauma.
- Ensure follow-up instruction if the patient or family does not thoroughly understand diabetes management or blood glucose–testing technique.
- Teach the patient to wear sunscreen and protective eyewear to prevent the effects of light sensitivity.

insulin

in-sull-in

Rapid acting: Insulin Lispro (Humalog), Insulin Aspart (Novolog, NovoMix 30[AUS], Novorapid[AUS]), Regular Insulin (Actrapid[AUS], Humulin R, Novolin R, Regular Iletin II)
Intermediate acting: NPH (Humulin N, Novolin N, NPH Iletin II), Lente: (Humulin L, Lente Iletin II, Monotard[AUS], Novolin L)
Long acting: Insulin Glargine (Lantus)

CATEGORY AND SCHEDULE

Pregnancy Risk Category: B
OTC

MECHANISM OF ACTION

An exogenous insulin that facilitates passage of glucose, potassium, and magnesium across the cellular membranes of skeletal and cardiac muscle and adipose tissue. Controls storage and metabolism of carbohydrates, protein, and fats. Promotes conversion of glucose to glycogen in the liver. **Therapeutic Effect:** Controls glucose levels in diabetic patients.

PHARMACOKINETICS

Drug Form	Onset (hr)	Peak (hr)	Duration (hr)
Lispro	0.25	0.5–1.5	4–5
Insulin aspart	1/6	1–3	3–5
Regular	0.5–1	2–4	5–7
NPH	1–2	6–14	24+
Lente	1–3	6–14	24+
Insulin glargine	N/A	N/A	24

AVAILABILITY

All insulins are available as 100 units/ml concentrations.
Rapid Acting: Humulin R, Novolin R, Novolog, Humalog, Regular Iletin II.
Intermediate Acting: Humulin L, Novolin L, Lente Iletin II, Humulin N, Novolin N, NPH Illetin II.
Long Acting: Lantus.

INDICATIONS AND DOSAGES

▸ **Treatment of insulin-dependent type 1 diabetes mellitus and non–insulin-dependent type 2 diabetes mellitus when diet or weight control has failed to maintain satisfactory blood glucose levels or in event of fever, infection, pregnancy, surgery, or trauma, or severe endocrine, hepatic or renal dysfunction; emergency treatment of ketoacidosis (regular insulin); to promote passage of glucose across cell membrane in hyperalimentation (regular insulin): to facilitate intracellular shift of potassium in hyperkalemia (regular insulin)**
Subcutaneous
Adults, Elderly, Children. 0.5–1 unit/kg/day.
Adolescents (during growth spurt). 0.8–1.2 unit/kg/day.

CONTRAINDICATIONS

Hypersensitivity or insulin resistance may require change of type or species source of insulin

INTERACTIONS

Drug

Alcohol: May increase the effects of insulin.
Beta-adrenergic blockers: May increase the risk of hyperglycemia or hypoglycemia; may mask signs and prolong periods of hypoglycemia.
Glucocorticoids, thiazide diuretics: May increase blood glucose level.

Herbal

None known.

Food

None known.

DIAGNOSTIC TEST EFFECTS

May decrease serum magnesium, phosphate, and potassium concentrations.

IV INCOMPATIBILITIES

Diltiazem (Cardizem), dopamine (Intropin), nafcillin (Nafcil)

IV COMPATIBILITIES

Amiodarone (Cordarone), ampicillin/sulbactam (Unasyn), cefazolin (Ancef), cimetidine (Tagamet), digoxin (Lanoxin), dobutamine (Dobutrex), famotidine (Pepcid), gentamicin, heparin, magnesium sulfate, metoclopramide (Reglan), midazolam (Versed), milrinone (Primacor), morphine, nitroglycerin, potassium chloride, propofol (Diprivan), vancomycin (Vancocin)

SIDE EFFECTS

Occasional

Localized redness, swelling, and itching caused by improper injection technique or allergy to cleansing solution or insulin

Infrequent

Somogyi effect, including rebound hyperglycemia with chronically excessive insulin dosages: systemic allergic reaction, marked by rash, angioedema, and anaphylaxis; lipodystrophy or depression at injection site due to breakdown of adipose tissue; lipohypertrophy or accumulation of subcutaneous tissue at injection site due to inadequate site rotation

Rare

Insulin resistance

SERIOUS REACTIONS

! Severe hypoglycemia caused by hyperinsulinism may occur with insulin overdose, decrease or delay of food intake, or excessive exercise and in those with brittle diabetes.

! Diabetic ketoacidosis may result from stress, illness, omission of insulin dose, or long-term poor insulin control.

NURSING CONSIDERATIONS

Baseline Assessment

- Check the patient's blood glucose level, as ordered.
- Discuss lifestyle to determine the extent the patient's emotional and learning needs.

Lifespan Considerations

- Insulin is the drug of choice for treating diabetes mellitus during pregnancy but close medical supervision is needed. The patient's insulin needs may drop for 24 to 72 hours postpartum, then rise to pre-pregnancy levels.
- Insulin is not secreted in breast milk. Lactation may decrease insulin requirements.
- No age-related precautions have been noted in children.
- Decreased vision and shakiness in the elderly may lead to inaccurate insulin self-dosing.

Administration and Handling

◀ALERT▶ Insulin dosages are individualized and monitored. Adjust dosage, as prescribed, to achieve premeal and bedtime glucose levels of 80 to140 mg/dl (100 to 200 mg/dl in children younger than 5 years).

Subcutaneous

- Store currently used insulin at room temperature; avoid extreme temperatures and direct sunlight. Store extra vials in refrigerator. Discard unused vials if not used for several weeks.
- Give subcutaneous only. Regular insulin is the only insulin that may be given IV or IM for ketoacidosis or other specific situations.
- Warm the drug to room temperature; do not give cold insulin.
- Roll the drug vial gently between hands; do not shake. Regular insulin normally appears clear.
- Administer insulin approximately 30 minutes before a meal. Insulin Lispro may be given up to 15 minutes before meals. Check the patient's blood glucose concentration before administration. Insulin dosages are highly individualized.
- Always draw regular insulin first when insulin is mixed. Mixtures must be administered at once because binding can occur within 5 minutes. Humalog may be mixed with Humulin N and Humulin L.
- Give subcutaneous injections in the abdomen, buttocks, thigh, upper arm, or upper back if there is adequate adipose tissue.
- Maintain a careful record of rotated injection sites.
- For home situations, prefilled syringes are stable for 1 week when refrigerated, including mixtures once they have stabilized; for example, NPH/Regular stabilizes after 15 minutes and Lente/Regular stabilizes after 24 hours. Prefilled syringes should be stored in the vertical or oblique position to avoid plugging.

The plunger should be pulled back slightly and the syringe rocked to remix the solution before injection.

IV (Regular)

- Use only if solution is clear.
- May give undiluted.

Intervention and Evaluation

- Monitor the sleeping patient for diaphoresis and restlessness.
- Assess the patient for signs and symptoms of hypoglycemia (anxiety, cool wet skin, diplopia, dizziness, headache, hunger, numbness in mouth, tachycardia, tremors), or hyperglycemia, (deep rapid breathing [Kussmaul's respirations], dim vision, fatigue, nausea, polydipsia, polyphagia, polyuria, vomiting).
- Be alert to conditions that alter blood glucose requirements, such as fever, increased activity, stress, or a surgical procedure.

Patient Teaching

- Make sure that the patient is adept at drawing up the prescribed dosage of insulin, as well as the proper injection technique. Also ensure that he or she can perform self-testing for blood glucose at the prescribed intervals.
- Stress to the patient that the regimen of exercise, good hygiene (including foot care), prescribed diet, and weight control is an integral part of treatment. Warn the patient to avoid smoking and not to skip or delay meals.
- Ensure that the patient knows the signs and symptoms of hypoglycemia and hyperglycemia.
- Tell the patient to carry candy, sugar packets, or other sugar supplements for immediate response to hypoglycemia and urge the patient to wear medical alert identification stating that he or she has diabetes.
- Stress that the patient consult the physician when glucose demands are altered, such as with fever, heavy physical activity, infection, stress, and trauma.
- Tell the patient to inform his or her dentist, other physicians, or surgeons of insulin therapy before any treatment is given.

metformin hydrochloride

met-**for**-min

(Diabex[AUS], Diaformin[AUS], Fortamet, Glucohexal[AUS], Glucomet[AUS], Glucophage, Glucophage XL, Glycon[CAN], Novo-Metformin[CAN], Riomet)

CATEGORY AND SCHEDULE

Pregnancy Risk Category: B

MECHANISM OF ACTION

An antihyperglycemic that decreases hepatic production of glucose. Decreases absorption of glucose and improves insulin sensitivity. **Therapeutic Effect:** Improves glycemic control, stabilizes or decreases body weight, and improves lipid profile.

PHARMACOKINETICS

Slowly, incompletely absorbed after oral administration. Food delays or decreases the extent of absorption. Protein binding: Negligible. Primarily distributed to intestinal mucosa and salivary glands. Primarily excreted unchanged in urine. Removed by hemodialysis. ***Half-life:*** 3–6 hr.

AVAILABILITY

Oral Solution (Riomet): 100 mg/ml.
Tablets (Glucophage): 500 mg, 850 mg, 1,000 mg.
Tablets (Extended-Release [Glucophage XL]): 500 mg, 750 mg.

Tablets (Extended-Release [Fortamet]): 500 mg, 1000 mg.

INDICATIONS AND DOSAGES

▸ **Diabetes mellitus**

PO (500-mg, 1,000-mg tablet)

Adults, Elderly. Initially, 500 mg twice a day, with morning and evening meals. May increase in 500-mg increments every week, in divided doses. May give twice a day up to 2,000 mg/day (for example, 1,000 mg twice a day [with morning and evening meals]). If 2,500 mg/day is required, give 3 times a day with meals. Maximum: 2,500 mg/day.

Children 10–16 yr. Initially, 500 mg twice a day. May increase by 500 mg/day at weekly intervals. Maximum: 2,000 mg/day.

PO (850-mg tablet)

Adults, Elderly. Initially, 850 mg/day, with morning meal. May increase dosage in 850-mg increments every other week, in divided doses. Maintenance: 850 mg twice a day, with morning and evening meals. Maximum: 2,550 mg/day (850 mg 3 times a day).

PO (Extended-Release tablets)

Adults, Elderly. Initially, 500 mg once a day. May increase by 500 mg/day at weekly intervals. Maximum: 2,000 mg once a day.

▸ **Adjunct to insulin therapy**

PO

Adults, Elderly. Initially, 500 mg/day. May increase by 500 mg at 7-day intervals. Maximum: 2,500 mg/day (2,000 mg/day for extended-release form).

OFF-LABEL USES

Treatment of metabolic complications of AIDS, prediabetes, weight reduction

CONTRAINDICATIONS

Acute CHF, MI, cardiovascular collapse, renal disease or dysfunction, respiratory failure, septicemia

INTERACTIONS

Drug

Alcohol, amiloride, cimetidine, digoxin, furosemide, morphine, nifedipine, procainamide, quinidine, quinine, ranitidine, triamterene, trimethoprim, vancomycin: Increase metformin blood concentration.

Furosemide, hypoglycemia-causing medications: May require a decrease in metformin dosage.

Iodinated contrast studies: May cause acute renal failure and increased risk of lactic acidosis.

Herbal

None known.

Food

None known.

DIAGNOSTIC TEST EFFECTS

None known.

SIDE EFFECTS

Occasional (greater than 3%)

GI disturbances (including diarrhea, nausea, vomiting, abdominal bloating, flatulence, and anorexia) that are transient and resolve spontaneously during therapy.

Rare (3%–1%)

Unpleasant or metallic taste that resolves spontaneously during therapy

SERIOUS REACTIONS

! Lactic acidosis occurs rarely but is a fatal complication in 50% of cases. Lactic acidosis is characterized by an increase in blood lactate levels (greater than 5 mmol/L), a decrease in blood pH, and electrolyte disturbances. Signs and symptoms of lactic acidosis include unexplained hyperventilation, myalgia, malaise, and somnolence, which may advance to cardiovascular collapse (shock), acute CHF, acute MI, and prerenal azotemia.

NURSING CONSIDERATIONS

Baseline Assessment

- Inform the patient of the potential advantages and risks of metformin therapy and of alternative modes of treatment.
- Assess the patient's Hgb and Hct, RBC count, and serum creatinine level before beginning metformin therapy and annually thereafter.

Lifespan Considerations

- Insulin is the drug of choice during pregnancy.
- Metformin is distributed in breast milk in animals.
- Safety and efficacy of metformin have not been established in children.
- In the elderly, age-related renal impairment or peripheral vascular disease may require dosage adjustment or discontinuation of drug.

Precautions

- Use metformin cautiously in patients with conditions that cause hyperglycemia or hypoglycemia or delay food absorption, such as diarrhea, high fever, malnutrition, gastroparesis, and vomiting.
- Use cautiously in cardiovascular patients; in debilitated, elderly, or malnourished patients with renal impairment; in patients with hepatic impairment; and in patients concurrently taking drugs that affect renal function.
- Use cautiously in patients with CHF, chronic respiratory difficulty, or uncontrolled hyperthyroidism or hypothyroidism.
- Use cautiously in patients who consume excessive amounts of alcohol.

Administration and Handling

◀ **ALERT** ▶ Plan to decrease the insulin dosage if blood glucose level falls below 120 mg/dl.

◀ **ALERT** ▶ Lactic acidosis is a rare but potentially severe consequence of metformin therapy. Expect to withhold metformin in patients with conditions that may predispose to lactic acidosis, such as dehydration, hypoperfusion, hypoxemia, and sepsis.

PO

- Give metformin with meals.
- Do not crush film-coated tablets.

Intervention and Evaluation

- Monitor the patient's fasting blood glucose level, glycosylated Hgb, folic acid level, and renal function.
- Assess the patient concurrently taking oral sulfonylureas for signs and symptoms of hypoglycemia, including anxiety, cool wet skin, diplopia, dizziness, headache, hunger, numbness in mouth, tachycardia, and tremors.
- Be alert to conditions that alter blood glucose requirements, such as fever, increased activity, stress, or a surgical procedure.

Patient Teaching

- Warn the patient to notify the physician and discontinue metformin therapy, as prescribed, if he or she experiences signs or symptoms of lactic acidosis, such as drowsiness, extreme fatigue, muscle aches, and unexplained hyperventilation.
- Stress to the patient that the prescribed diet is a principal part of treatment. Warn the patient not to skip or delay meals.
- Tell the patient that diabetes mellitus requires lifelong control.
- Urge the patient to avoid consuming alcohol.
- Instruct the patient to report diarrhea, easy bleeding or bruising, change in color of stool or urine,

headache, nausea, persistent rash, and vomiting.

miglitol
mig-lee-tall
(Glyset)

CATEGORY AND SCHEDULE
Pregnancy Risk Category: B

MECHANISM OF ACTION
An alpha-glucosidase inhibitor that delays the digestion of ingested carbohydrates into simple sugars such as glucose. **Therapeutic Effect:** Produces smaller rise in blood glucose concentration after meals.

AVAILABILITY
Tablets: 25 mg, 50 mg, 100 mg.

INDICATIONS AND DOSAGES
Diabetes mellitus
PO
Adults, Elderly. Initially, 25 mg 3 times a day with first bite of each main meal. Maintenance: 50 mg 3 times a day. Maximum: 100 mg 3 times a day.

CONTRAINDICATIONS
Colonic ulceration, diabetic ketoacidosis, hypersensitivity to miglitol, inflammatory bowel disease, partial intestinal obstruction

INTERACTIONS
Drug
Digoxin, propranolol, ranitidine: May decrease the blood concentrations and effects of these drugs.
Herbal
None known.
Food
None known.

DIAGNOSTIC TEST EFFECTS
None known.

SIDE EFFECTS
Frequent (40%–10%)
Flatulence, loose stools, diarrhea, abdominal pain
Occasional (5%)
Rash

NURSING CONSIDERATIONS
Baseline Assessment
- Check the patient's blood glucose level, as ordered.
- Discuss lifestyle to determine the extent of the patient's emotional and learning needs.
- Establish the patient's use of medications, especially digoxin, propranolol, and ranitidine.

Lifespan Considerations
- Adequate studies have not been done in pregnant patients.
- Miglitol is distributed in breast milk; breast-feeding is not recommended during miglitol therapy.
- Safety and efficacy have not been established in children.

Precautions
- Use miglitol cautiously in patients with renal impairment.

Administration and Handling
PO
- Give with the first bite of each main meal.

Intervention and Evaluation
- Monitor the patient's blood glucose level and food intake.
- Assess the patient for signs and symptoms of hypoglycemia (anxiety, cool wet skin, diplopia, dizziness, headache, hunger, numbness in mouth, tachycardia, tremors), or hyperglycemia, (deep rapid breathing, dim vision, fatigue, nausea, polydipsia, polyphagia, polyuria, vomiting).
- Be alert to conditions that alter

blood glucose requirements, such as fever, increased activity, stress, or a surgical procedure.

Patient Teaching

- Instruct the patient to take miglitol with the first bite of food at each meal because taking the drug later will greatly alter its effectiveness.
- Stress to the patient that the prescribed diet is a principal part of treatment. Warn the patient not to skip or delay meals.
- Urge the patient to wear medical alert identification stating that he or she has diabetes.
- Stress that the patient consult the physician when glucose demands are altered, such as with fever, heavy physical activity, infection, stress, or trauma.

nateglinide

na-**teg**-lin-ide
(Starlix)

CATEGORY AND SCHEDULE

Pregnancy Risk Category: C

MECHANISM OF ACTION

An antihyperglycemic that stimulates release of insulin from beta cells of the pancreas by depolarizing beta cells, leading to an opening of calcium channels. Resulting calcium influx induces insulin secretion. **Therapeutic Effect:** Lowers blood glucose concentration.

AVAILABILITY

Tablets: 60 mg, 120 mg.

INDICATIONS AND DOSAGES

▸ Diabetes mellitus

PO

Adult, Elderly. 120 mg 3 times a day before meals. Initially, 60 mg may be given.

CONTRAINDICATIONS

Diabetic ketoacidosis, type 1 diabetes mellitus

INTERACTIONS

Drug

Beta blockers, MAOIs, NSAIDs, salicylates: May increase hypoglycemic effect of nateglinide.

Corticosteroids, thiazide diuretics, thyroid medication, sympathomimetics: May decrease hypoglycemic effect of nateglinide.

Herbal

None known.

Food

Liquid meal: Peak plasma levels may be significantly reduced if administered 10 minutes before a liquid meal.

DIAGNOSTIC TEST EFFECTS

None known.

SIDE EFFECTS

Frequent (10%)

Upper respiratory tract infection

Occasional (4%–3%)

Back pain, flu symptoms, dizziness, arthropathy, diarrhea

Rare (3% or less)

Bronchitis, cough

SERIOUS REACTIONS

! Hypoglycemia occurs in less than 2% of patients.

NURSING CONSIDERATIONS

Baseline Assessment

- Expect to check the patient's fasting blood glucose level and glycosylated Hgb periodically to determine minimum effective dosage.
- Discuss lifestyle to determine the

extent of the patient's emotional and learning needs.
• Expect to allow at least 1 week to elapse to assess the patient's response to drug before new dose adjustment is made.

Precautions

• Use nateglinide cautiously in patients with hepatic or renal impairment.

Administration and Handling

PO

• Ideally, give within 15 minutes of a meal; however, may give immediately to as long as 30 minutes before a meal.

Intervention and Evaluation

• Monitor the patient's blood glucose level and food intake.
• Assess the patient for signs and symptoms of hypoglycemia (anxiety, cool wet skin, diplopia, dizziness, headache, hunger, numbness in mouth, tachycardia, tremors), or hyperglycemia (deep rapid breathing, dim vision, fatigue, nausea, polydipsia, polyphagia, polyuria, vomiting).
• Be alert to conditions that alter blood glucose requirements, such as fever, increased activity, stress, or a surgical procedure.

Patient Teaching

• Stress to the patient that the prescribed diet is a principal part of treatment. Warn the patient not to skip or delay meals.
• Make sure the patient is aware of the typical signs and symptoms of hypoglycemia and hyperglycemia.
• Instruct the patient to carry candy, sugar packets, or other sugar supplements for immediate response to hypoglycemia and urge the patient to wear medical alert identification stating that he or she has diabetes.
• Stress that the patient consult the physician when glucose demands are altered, such as with fever, heavy physical activity, infection, stress, or trauma.
• Ensure follow-up instruction if the patient or family does not thoroughly understand diabetes management or blood glucose–testing technique.

pioglitazone

pye-oh-**gli**-ta-zone
(Actos)

CATEGORY AND SCHEDULE

Pregnancy Risk Category: C

MECHANISM OF ACTION

An antidiabetic that improves target-cell response to insulin without increasing pancreatic insulin secretion. Decreases hepatic glucose output and increases insulin-dependent glucose utilization in skeletal muscle. **Therapeutic Effect:** Lowers blood glucose concentration.

PHARMACOKINETICS

Rapidly absorbed. Highly protein bound (99%), primarily to albumin. Metabolized in the liver. Excreted in urine. Unknown if removed by hemodialysis. ***Half-life:*** 16–24 hr.

AVAILABILITY

Tablets: 15 mg, 30 mg, 45 mg.

INDICATIONS AND DOSAGES

▸ **Diabetes mellitus, combination therapy**

PO

Adult, Elderly. With insulin: Initially, 15–30 mg once a day. Initially continue current insulin dosage; then decrease insulin dosage by 10% to 25% if hypoglycemia occurs or plasma glucose level decreases to less than 100 mg/dl. Maximum: 45 mg/day. With sulfonylureas: Initially, 15–30 mg/day. Decrease sulfonylurea dosage if hypoglycemia occurs. Wtih metformin: Initially, 15–30 mg/day. As monotherapy: Monotherapy is not to be used if patient is well controlled with diet and exercise alone. Initially, 15–30 mg/day. May increase dosage in increments until 45 mg/day is reached.

CONTRAINDICATIONS

Active hepatic disease; diabetic ketoacidosis; increased serum transaminase levels, including ALT (SGPT) greater than 2.5 times normal serum level; type 1 diabetes mellitus

INTERACTIONS

Drug

Gemfibrizol: May increase the effect and toxicity of pioglitazone.
Ketoconazole: May significantly inhibit metabolism of pioglitazone.
Oral Contraceptives: May alter the effects of oral contraceptives.

Food

None known.

Herbal

None known.

DIAGNOSTIC TEST EFFECTS

May increase creatine kinase (CK) level. May decrease Hgb levels by 2% to 4% and serum alkaline phosphatase, bilirubin, and ALT (SGOT) levels. Less than 1% of patients experience ALT values 3 times the normal level.

SIDE EFFECTS

Frequent (13%–9%)

Headache, upper respiratory tract infection

Occasional (6%–5%)

Sinusitis, myalgia, pharyngitis, aggravated diabetes mellitus

SERIOUS REACTIONS

! None known.

NURSING CONSIDERATIONS

Baseline Assessment

• Check the patient's hepatic enzyme levels, as ordered, before beginning pioglitazone therapy and periodically thereafter.

Lifespan Considerations

• It is unknown if pioglitazone crosses the placenta or is distributed in breast milk. Pioglitazone use is not recommended in pregnant or breast-feeding women.
• Safety and efficacy of pioglitazone have not been established in children.
• No age-related precautions have been noted in the elderly.

Precautions

• Use pioglitazone cautiously in patients with CHF, edema, and hepatic impairment.

Administration and Handling

PO
• Give pioglitazone without regard to meals.

Intervention and Evaluation

• Monitor the patient's blood glucose level, Hgb, and hepatic function test results, especially AST and ALT levels.
• Assess the patient for signs and symptoms of hypoglycemia (anxiety, cool wet skin, diplopia, dizziness, headache, hunger, numbness in mouth, tachycardia, tremors), or hyperglycemia (deep rapid breathing, dim vision, fatigue, nausea, polydipsia, polyphagia, polyuria, vomiting).
• Be alert to conditions that alter blood glucose requirements, such as fever, increased activity, stress, or a surgical procedure.

Patient Teaching

• Ensure follow-up instruction if the patient or family does not thoroughly

understand diabetes management or blood glucose-testing technique.
- Stress to the patient that the prescribed diet is a principal part of treatment. Warn the patient not to skip or delay meals.
- Make sure the patient is aware of the typical signs and symptoms of hypoglycemia and hyperglycemia.
- Instruct the patient to carry candy, sugar packets, or other sugar supplements for immediate response to hypoglycemia.
- Urge the patient to avoid alcohol.
- Warn the patient to report abdominal or chest pain, dark urine or light stool, hypoglycemic reactions, fever, nausea, palpitations, rash, vomiting, or yellowing of the eyes or skin.

repaglinide

re-**pag**-lih-nide
(GlucoNorm[CAN], NovoNorm[AUS], Prandin)

CATEGORY AND SCHEDULE

Pregnancy Risk Category: C

MECHANISM OF ACTION

An antihyperglycemic that stimulates release of insulin from beta cells of the pancreas by depolarizing beta cells, leading to an opening of calcium channels. Resulting calcium influx induces insulin secretion. **Therapeutic Effect:** Lowers blood glucose concentration.

PHARMACOKINETICS

Rapidly, completely absorbed from the GI tract. Protein binding: 98%. Metabolized in the liver to inactive metabolites. Excreted primarily in feces with a lesser amount in urine. Unknown if removed by hemodialysis. ***Half-life:*** 1 hr.

AVAILABILITY

Tablets: 0.5 mg, 1 mg, 2 mg.

INDICATIONS AND DOSAGES

▸ **Diabetes mellitus**

PO

Adults, Elderly. 0.5–4 mg 2–4 times a day. Maximum: 16 mg/day.

CONTRAINDICATIONS

Diabetic ketoacidosis, type 1 diabetes mellitus

INTERACTIONS

Drug

Beta blockers, chloramphenicol, gemfibrozil, MAOIs, NSAIDs, probenecid, salicylates, sulfonamides, warfarin: May increase the effects of repaglinide.

Herbal

None known.

Food

Food: Decreases repaglinide plasma concentration.

DIAGNOSTIC TEST EFFECTS

None known.

SIDE EFFECTS

Frequent (10%–6%)

Upper respiratory tract infection, headache, rhinitis, bronchitis, back pain

Occasional (5%–3%)

Diarrhea, dyspepsia, sinusitis, nausea, arthralgia, urinary tract infection

Rare (2%)

Constipation, vomiting, paresthesia, allergy

SERIOUS REACTIONS

! Hypoglycemia occurs in 16% of patients.

! Chest pain occurs rarely.

NURSING CONSIDERATIONS

Baseline Assessment

- Expect to check the patient's fasting blood glucose level and glycosylated Hgb periodically to determine the minimum effective dosage of repaglinide.
- Expect to allow at least 1 week to elapse to assess the patient's response to drug before new dosage adjustment is made.

Lifespan Considerations

- It is unknown if repaglinide is distributed in breast milk.
- Safety and efficacy of repaglinide have not been established in children.
- No age-related precautions have been noted in the elderly, but hypoglycemia may be more difficult to recognize in this patient population.

Precautions

- Use repaglinide cautiously in patients with hepatic or renal impairment.

Administration and Handling

PO

- Ideally, give repaglinide within 15 minutes of a meal; however, it may be given immediately to as long as 30 minutes before a meal.

Intervention and Evaluation

- Monitor the patient's blood glucose level and food intake.
- Assess the patient for signs and symptoms of hypoglycemia (anxiety, cool wet skin, diplopia, dizziness, headache, hunger, numbness in mouth, tachycardia, tremors), or hyperglycemia (deep rapid breathing, dim vision, fatigue, nausea, polydipsia, polyphagia, polyuria, vomiting).
- Be alert to conditions that alter blood glucose requirements, such as fever, increased activity, stress, or a surgical procedure.

Patient Teaching

- Stress to the patient that the prescribed diet is a principal part of treatment. Warn the patient not to skip or delay meals.
- Make sure the patient is aware of the typical signs and symptoms of hypoglycemia and hyperglycemia.
- Urge the patient to wear medical alert identification stating that he or she has diabetes.
- Stress that the patient consult the physician when glucose demands are altered, such as with fever, heavy physical activity, infection, stress, or trauma.
- Explain to the patient that diabetes mellitus requires lifelong control. Urge the patient to continue to adhere to dietary instructions, a regular exercise program, and regular testing of urine or blood glucose.
- Tell the patient taking repaglinide with insulin or a sulfonylurea to always have a source of glucose available to treat symptoms of low blood sugar.

rosiglitazone maleate

roz-ih-**gli**-ta-zone
(Avandia)

Do not confuse Avandia with Avalide, Avinza, or Prandin.

CATEGORY AND SCHEDULE

Pregnancy Risk Category: C

MECHANISM OF ACTION

An antidiabetic that improves target-cell response to insulin without increasing pancreatic insulin secretion. Decreases hepatic glucose output and increases insulin-dependent glucose utilization in skeletal muscle. **Therapeutic Effect:** Lowers blood glucose concentration.

PHARMACOKINETICS

Rapidly absorbed. Protein binding: 99%. Metabolized in the liver. Excreted primarily in urine, with a lesser amount in feces. Not removed by hemodialysis. ***Half-life:*** 3–4 hr.

AVAILABILITY

Tablets: 2 mg, 4 mg, 8 mg.

INDICATIONS AND DOSAGES

▸ Diabetes mellitus, combination therapy

PO

Adults, Elderly. Initially, 4 mg as a single daily dose or in divided doses twice a day. May increase to 8 mg/day after 12 wk of therapy if fasting glucose level is not adequately controlled.

▸ Diabetes mellitus, monotherapy

Adults, Elderly. Initially, 4 mg as single daily dose or in divided doses twice a day. May increase to 8 mg/day after 12 wk of therapy.

CONTRAINDICATIONS

Active hepatic disease, diabetic ketoacidosis, increased serum transaminase levels, including ALT (SGPT) greater than 2.5 times the normal serum level, type 1 diabetes mellitus

INTERACTIONS

Drug

None known.

Herbal

None known.

Food

None known.

DIAGNOSTIC TEST EFFECTS

May decrease Hct and Hgb and serum alkaline phosphatase, bilirubin, and AST (SGOT) levels. Less than 1% of patients experience ALT values that are 3 times the normal level.

SIDE EFFECTS

Frequent (9%)

Upper respiratory tract infection

Occasional (4%–2%)

Headache, edema, back pain, fatigue, sinusitis, diarrhea

SERIOUS REACTIONS

! None known.

NURSING CONSIDERATIONS

Baseline Assessment

- Expect to obtain the patient's hepatic enzyme levels before beginning rosiglitazone therapy and periodically thereafter.

Lifespan Considerations

- It is unknown if rosiglitazone crosses the placenta or is distributed in breast milk. Rosiglitazone use is not recommended in pregnant or breast-feeding women.
- Safety and efficacy of rosiglitazone have not been established in children.
- No age-related precautions have been noted in the elderly.

Precautions

- Use rosiglitazone cautiously in patients with CHF, edema, or hepatic impairment.

Administration and Handling

PO

- Give rosiglitazone without regard to meals.

Intervention and Evaluation

- Monitor the patient's blood glucose levels, Hgb, and hepatic enzyme test results, especially ALT and AST levels.
- Assess the patient for signs and symptoms of hypoglycemia (anxiety, cool wet skin, diplopia, dizziness, headache, hunger, numbness in mouth, tachycardia, tremors), or hyperglycemia (deep rapid breathing, dim vision, fatigue, nausea, polydipsia, polyphagia, polyuria, vomiting).

• Be alert to conditions that alter blood glucose requirements, such as fever, increased activity, stress, or a surgical procedure.

Patient Teaching

• Stress to the patient that the prescribed diet is a principal part of treatment. Warn the patient not to skip or delay meals.
• Make sure the patient is aware of the typical signs and symptoms of hypoglycemia and hyperglycemia.
• Instruct the patient to carry candy, sugar packets, or other sugar supplements for immediate response to hypoglycemia and urge the patient to wear medical alert identification stating he or she has diabetes.
• Urge the patient to avoid alcohol.
• Warn the patient to report abdominal or chest pain, dark urine or light stool, hypoglycemic reactions, fever, nausea, palpitations, rash, vomiting, and yellowing of the eyes or skin.
• Ensure follow-up instruction if the patient or family does not thoroughly understand diabetes management or blood glucose–testing technique.
• Instruct the patient taking rosiglitazone with insulin or a sulfonylurea to always have a source of glucose available to treat symptoms of low blood sugar.

65 Antigout Agents

allopurinol
colchicine
probenecid

Uses: Antigout agents play different roles in the treatment of gout. *Allopurinol* and *probenecid* are used to reduce hyperuricemia, which helps prevent acute gout attacks. *Colchicine* is used to treat acute gout attacks, reduce the incidence of attacks in chronic gout, and abort an impending gout attack. In addition, probenecid may be given with penicillins or cephalosporins to increase and prolong the plasma antibiotic levels.

Action: Antigout agents act in slightly different ways. *Allopurinol* reduces hyperuricemia by inhibiting uric acid formation. *Colchicine* provides an anti-inflammatory action specific to gout. *Probenecid* reduces hyperuricemia by promoting uric acid excretion. (See the illustration *Mechanism of Action: Antigout Agents,* page 1170.)

allopurinol

al-oh-**pure**-i-nole
(Aloprim, Allohexal[AUS], Allosig [AUS], Apo-Allopurinol[CAN], Capurate[AUS], Progout[AUS] Purinol[CAN], Zyloprim)
Do not confuse Zyloprim with ZORprin.

CATEGORY AND SCHEDULE

Pregnancy Risk Category: C

MECHANISM OF ACTION

A xanthine oxidase inhibitor that decreases uric acid production by inhibiting xanthine oxidase, an enzyme. **Therapeutic Effect:** Reduces uric acid concentrations in both serum and urine.

PHARMACOKINETICS

Route	Onset	Peak	Duration
PO, IV	2–3 days	1–3 wk	1–2 wk

Well absorbed from the GI tract. Widely distributed. Metabolized in the liver to active metabolite. Excreted primarily in urine. Removed by hemodialysis. ***Half-life:*** 1–3 hr; metabolite, 12–30 hr.

AVAILABILITY

Tablets (Zyloprim): 100 mg, 300 mg.
Powder for Injection (Aloprim): 500 mg.

INDICATIONS AND DOSAGES

▸ **Chronic gouty arthritis**

PO

Adults, Children older than 10 yr. Initially, 100 mg/day; may increase by 100 mg/day at weekly intervals. Maximum: 800 mg/day. Maintenance: 100–200 mg 2–3 times a day or 300 mg/day.

▸ **To prevent uric acid nephropathy during chemotherapy**

PO

Adults: Initially, 600–800 mg/day

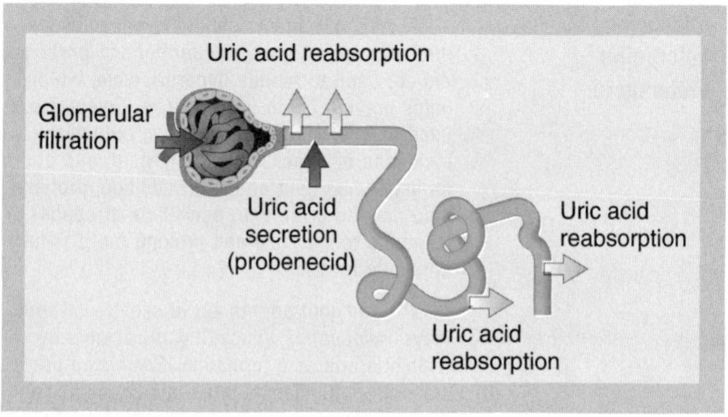

Mechanism of Action: Antigout Agents

Several drugs are used to manage gout, a disorder of purine metabolism that increases uric acid production or decreases its renal excretion. The result is hyperuricemia (an increased serum uric acid level). When the balance between uric acid formation and excretion is disturbed, uric acid precipitates and forms urate crystals. Then leukocytes and other inflammatory cells move to the area, producing inflammation that can cause gout attacks.

Three drugs are commonly used to manage gout: allopurinol, probenecid, and colchicine. Allopurinol and probenecid help prevent gout attacks by decreasing the uric acid level. Allopurinol interferes with uric acid production by binding to and inhibiting xanthine oxidase, an enzyme that converts adenine and guanine to uric acid. This action leads to decreased uric acid levels in blood and urine. Probenecid competitively inhibits uric acid reabsorption in the proximal tubules of the nephrons, as illustrated here. This action increases uric acid excretion.

Unlike the other antigout agents, colchicine doesn't influence uric acid synthesis or reabsorption. Instead, it acts as an anti-inflammatory agent to treat a gout attack. It does this by inhibiting the action of leukocytes on urate crystals and diminishing inflammation.

---

starting 2–3 days before initiation of chemotherapy or radiation therapy.
Children 6–10 yr. 100 mg 3 times a day or 300 mg once a day.
Children less than 6 yr. 50 mg 3 times a day.
IV
Adults. 200–400 mg/m^2/day beginning 24–48 hr before initiation of chemotherapy.
Children. 200 mg/m^2/day. Maximum: 600 mg/day.

▸ **Prevention of uric acid calculi**
PO
Adults. 100–200 mg 1–4 times a day or 300 mg once a day.

▸ **Recurrent calcium oxalate calculi**
PO
Adults. 200–300 mg/day.
Elderly. Initially, 100 mg/day, gradually increased until optimal uric acid level is reached.

▸ **Dosage in renal impairment**
Dosage is modified based on creatinine clearance.

Creatinine Clearance	Dosage Adjustment
10–20 ml/min	200 mg/day
3–9 ml/min	100 mg/day
Less than 3 ml/min	100 mg at extended intervals

OFF-LABEL USES
In mouthwash following fluorouracil therapy to prevent stomatitis

CONTRAINDICATIONS
Asymptomatic hyperuricemia

INTERACTIONS
Drug
Amoxicillin, ampicillin: May increase incidence of rash.
Azathioprine, mercaptopurine: May increase therapeutic effect and toxicity of azathioprine and mercaptopurine.
Oral anticoagulants: May increase anticoagulant effect.
Thiazide diuretics: May decrease the effect of allopurinol.
Herbal
None known.
Food
None known.

DIAGNOSTIC TEST EFFECTS
May increase BUN, serum creatinine, serum alkaline phosphatase, AST (SGOT), and ALT (SGPT) levels.

IV INCOMPATIBILITIES
Amikacin (Amikin), carmustine (BiCNU), cefotaxime (Claforan), chlorpromazine (Thorazine), cimetidine (Tagamet), clindamycin (Cleocin), cytarabine (Ara-C), dacarbazine (DTIC), diphenhydramine (Benadryl), doxorubicin (Adriamycin), doxycycline (Vibramycin), droperidol (Inapsine), fludarabine (Fludara), gentamicin (Garamycin), haloperidol (Haldol), hydroxyzine (Vistaril), idarubicin (Idamycin), imipenem-cilastatin (Primaxin), meperidine (Demerol), methylprednisolone (Solu-Medrol), metoclopramide (Reglan), ondansetron (Zofran), prochlorperazine (Compazine), promethazine (Phenergan), streptozocin (Zanosar), tobramycin (Nebcin), vinorelbine (Navelbine)

IV COMPATIBILITIES
Bumetanide (Bumex), calcium gluconate, furosemide (Lasix), heparin, hydromorphone (Dilaudid), lorazepam (Ativan), morphine, potassium chloride

SIDE EFFECTS
Occasional
Oral: Somnolence, unusual hair loss
IV: Rash, nausea, vomiting
Rare
Diarrhea, headache

SERIOUS REACTIONS
! Pruritic maculopapular rash possibly accompanied by malaise, fever, chills, joint pain, nausea, and vomiting should be considered a toxic reaction.
! Severe hypersensitivity may follow appearance of rash.
! Bone marrow depression, hepatic toxicity, peripheral neuritis, and acute renal failure occur rarely.

NURSING CONSIDERATIONS
Baseline Assessment
- Ensure that the patient drinks 10 to 12 eight-ounce glasses of fluid daily while taking allopurinol.
Lifespan Considerations
- It is unknown if allopurinol crosses placenta or is distributed in breast milk.
- No age-related precautions have been noted in children or the elderly.

Precautions

• Use allopurinol cautiously in patients with CHF, diabetes mellitus, hypertension, or impaired renal or hepatic function.

Administration and Handling

PO

• May give with or immediately after meals or milk.
• Ensure that the patient drinks at least 10 to 12 eight-ounce glasses of fluid each day.
• Administer dosages greater than 300 mg/day in divided doses.

IV

• Store unreconstituted vials at room temperature.
• May store reconstituted solution at room temperature; give within 10 hours. Do not use if precipitate forms or solution is discolored.
• Reconstitute 500-mg vial with 25 ml sterile water for injection, which produces a clear, almost colorless solution (concentration of 20 mg/ml).
• Further dilute with 0.9% NaCl or D_5W (19 ml of added diluent yields 1 mg/ml, 9 ml yields 2 mg/ml, and 2.3 ml yields maximum concentration of 6 mg/ml).
• Infuse over 30 to 60 minutes.

Intervention and Evaluation

• Discontinue drug immediately if rash or other evidence of allergic reaction appears.
• Encourage high fluid intake (3,000 ml/day). Monitor the patient's intake and output. The patient's output should be at least 2,000 ml/day.
• Assess the patient's CBC, hepatic enzyme test results, and serum uric acid level.
• Examine the patient's urine for cloudiness and unusual color and odor.
• Assess the patient for signs and symptoms of a therapeutic response, including improved joint range of motion and reduced redness, swelling, and tenderness.

Patient Teaching

• Explain to the patient that it may take 1 week or more or the full therapeutic effect of the drug to be evident.
• Encourage the patient to drink 10 to 12 eight-ounce glasses of fluid daily while allopurinol.
• Warn the patient to avoid tasks that require mental alertness or motor skills until his or her response to the drug has been established.

colchicine

kol-chi-seen
(Colchicine, Colgout[AUS])

CATEGORY AND SCHEDULE

Pregnancy Risk Category: D

MECHANISM OF ACTION

An alkaloid that decreases leukocyte motility, phagocytosis, and lactic acid production. **Therapeutic Effect:** Decreases urate crystal deposits and reduces inflammatory process.

PHARMACOKINETICS

Rapidly absorbed from the GI tract. Highest concentration is in the liver, spleen, and kidney. Protein binding: 30%–50%. Reenters the intestinal tract by biliary secretion and is reabsorbed from the intestines. Partially metabolized in the liver. Eliminated primarily in feces.

AVAILABILITY

Tablets: 0.6 mg.
Injection: 1 mg.

INDICATIONS AND DOSAGES

Acute gouty arthritis

PO

Adults, Elderly. 0.6–1.2 mg; then 0.6 mg q1–2h or 1–1.2 mg q2h, until pain is relieved or nausea, vomiting, or diarrhea occurs. Total dose: 4–8 mg.

IV

Adults, Elderly. Initially, 2 mg; then 0.5 mg q6h until satisfactory response. Maximum: 4 mg/wk or 4 mg/one course of treatment. If pain recurs, may give 1–2 mg/day for several days but no sooner than 7 days after a full course of IV therapy (total of 4 mg).

Chronic gouty arthritis

PO

Adults, Elderly. 0.5–0.6 mg once weekly up to once a day, depending on number of attacks per year.

OFF-LABEL USES

To reduce frequency of recurrence of familial Mediterranean fever; treatment of acute calcium pyrophosphate deposition, amyloidosis, biliary cirrhosis, recurrent pericarditis, sarcoid arthritis

CONTRAINDICATIONS

Blood dyscrasias; severe cardiac, GI, hepatic, or renal disorders

INTERACTIONS

Drug

Bone marrow depressants: May increase the risk of blood dyscrasias.
NSAIDs: May increase the risk of bone marrow depression, neutropenia, and thrombocytopenia.

Herbal

None known.

Food

None known.

DIAGNOSTIC TEST EFFECTS

May increase serum alkaline phosphatase and AST (SGOT) levels. May decrease platelet count.

IV INCOMPATIBILITIES

No information available via Y-site administration.

SIDE EFFECTS

Frequent

PO: Nausea, vomiting, abdominal discomfort

Occasional

PO: Anorexia

Rare

Hypersensitivity reaction, including angioedema
Parenteral: Nausea, vomiting, diarrhea, abdominal discomfort, pain or redness at injection site, neuritis in injected arm

SERIOUS REACTIONS

! Bone marrow depression, including aplastic anemia, agranulocytosis, and thrombocytopenia, may occur with long-term therapy.

! Overdose initially causes a burning feeling in the skin or throat, severe diarrhea, and abdominal pain. The patient then experiences fever, seizures, delirium, and renal impairment, marked by hematuria and oliguria. The third stage of overdose causes hair loss, leukocytosis, and stomatitis.

NURSING CONSIDERATIONS

Baseline Assessment

- Instruct the patient to drink 8 to 10 eight-ounce glasses of fluid each day while taking colchicine to aid renal excretion of uric acid.

Lifespan Considerations

- It is unknown if colchicine crosses the placenta or is distributed in breast milk.
- Safety and efficacy of colchicine

have not been established in children.

- The elderly may be more susceptible to cumulative toxicity and age-related renal impairment may increase risk of myopathy.

Precautions

- Use colchicine cautiously in debilitated or elderly patients and in patients with impaired hepatic function.

Administration and Handling

◀ALERT▶ Patients with impaired renal function may experience myopathy and neuropathy manifested as generalized weakness.

◀ALERT▶ Subcutaneous or IM administration produces severe local reaction. Administer via IV route only.

PO

- Give colchicine without regard to meals.

IV

- Store at room temperature.
- May dilute with 0.9% NaCl or sterile water for injection; do not dilute with D_5W.
- Administer over 2 to 5 minutes.

Intervention and Evaluation

- Discontinue colchicine immediately if GI symptoms occur.
- Encourage the patient to maintain a high fluid intake (3,000 ml/day). Monitor the patient's fluid intake and output; output should be at least 2,000 ml/day.
- Monitor the patient's serum uric acid level.
- Assess the patient for evidence of therapeutic response, including improved joint range of motion and reduced joint tenderness, redness, and swelling.

Patient Teaching

- Encourage the patient to limit his intake of high purine foods, such as fish and organ meats, and to drink 8 to 10 eight-ounce glasses of fluid daily while taking colchicine.
- Warn the patient to notify the physician if fever, numbness, skin rash, sore throat, fatigue, unusual bleeding or bruising, or weakness occurs.
- Instruct the patient to discontinue colchicine as soon as gout pain is relieved, or at the first appearance of diarrhea, nausea, or vomiting.

probenecid

proe-**ben**-e-sid

(Benuryl[CAN], Pro-Cid[AUS])

Do not confuse probenecid with procainamide.

CATEGORY AND SCHEDULE

Pregnancy Risk Category: C

MECHANISM OF ACTION

An uricosuric that competitively inhibits reabsorption of uric acid at the proximal convoluted tubule. Also, inhibits renal tubular secretion of weak organic acids, such as penicillins. **Therapeutic Effect:** Promotes uric acid excretion, reduces serum uric acid level, and increases plasma levels of penicillins and cephalosporins.

AVAILABILITY

Tablets: 500 mg.

INDICATIONS AND DOSAGES

▸ **Gout**

PO

Adults, Elderly. Initially, 250 mg twice a day for 1 wk; then 500 mg twice a day. May increase by 500 mg q4wk. Maximum: 2–3 g/day. Maintenance: Dosage that maintains normal uric acid level.

▸ As adjunct to penicillin or cephalosporin therapy to prolong antibiotic plasma levels

PO

Adults, Elderly. 2 g/day in divided doses.

Children weighing more than 50 kg. Receive adult dosage.

Children 2–14 yr. Initially, 25 mg/kg. Maintenance: 40 mg/kg/day in 4 divided doses.

▸ Gonorrhea

PO

Adults, Elderly. 1 g 30 min before penicillin, ampicillin, or amoxicillin.

CONTRAINDICATIONS

Blood dyscrasias, children younger than 2 years, concurrent high-dose aspirin therapy, severe renal impairment, uric acid calculi

INTERACTIONS

Drug

Alcohol: May increase serum urate level.

Antineoplastics: May increase the risk of uric acid nephropathy.

Cephalosporins, methotrexate, nitrofurantoin, NSAIDs, penicillins, zidovudine: May increase blood concentrations of these drugs.

Heparin: May increase and prolong the effects of heparin.

Salicylates: May decrease uricosuric effect.

Herbal

None known.

Food

None known.

DIAGNOSTIC TEST EFFECTS

May inhibit renal excretion of serum PSP (phenolsulfonphthalein), 17-ketosteroids, and BSP (sulfobromophthalein).

SIDE EFFECTS

Frequent (10%–6%)

Headache, anorexia, nausea, vomiting

Occasional (5%–1%)

Lower back or side pain, rash, hives, itching, dizziness, flushed face, frequent urge to urinate, gingivitis

SERIOUS REACTIONS

! Severe hypersensitivity reactions, including anaphylaxis, occur rarely and usually within a few hours after administration following previous use. If severe hypersensitivity reactions develop, discontinue the drug immediately and contact the physician.

! Pruritic maculopapular rash, possibly accompanied by malaise, fever, chills, arthralgia, nausea, vomiting, leukopenia, and aplastic anemias should be considered a toxic reaction.

NURSING CONSIDERATIONS

Baseline Assessment

- Expect not to start therapy until acute gouty attack has subsided.
- Determine if the patient is hypersensitive to probenecid or is taking cephalosporins or penicillins.

Precautions

- Use probenecid cautiously in patients with hematuria, peptic ulcer disease, or renal colic.

Administration and Handling

◀ALERT▶ Do not start giving probenecid until acute gouty attack has subsided; continue drug if acute attack occurs during therapy.

◀ALERT▶ Probenecid should not be used in patients with renal impairment.

PO

- Give probenecid with or immediately after meals or milk.
- Instruct the patient to drink at least

6 to 8 eight-ounce glasses of fluid each day to prevent renal calculi.

Intervention and Evaluation

- Use other agents for gout, as prescribed, if the patient experiences an exacerbation of gout after therapy.
- Discontinue probenecid immediately if rash or other evidence of an allergic reaction occurs.
- Encourage the patient to maintain a high fluid intake (3,000 ml/day). Monitor the patient's intake and urine output. Output should be at least 2,000 ml/day.
- Assess the patient's CBC and serum uric acid level.
- Evaluate the patient's urine for cloudiness, odor, and unusual color.
- Assess the patient for therapeutic response, including improved joint range of motion and reduced joint tenderness, redness, and swelling.

Patient Teaching

- Tell the patient to drink plenty of fluids to decrease risk of uric acid calculi.
- Urge the patient to avoid alcohol and large doses of aspirin or other salicylates.
- Tell the patient to avoid eating high-purine foods, such as anchovies, kidneys, liver, meat extracts, sardines, and sweetbreads.
- Explain to the patient that it may take more than 1 week for the full therapeutic effect of the drug to be evident.
- Instruct the patient to drink 6 to 8 eight-ounce glasses of fluid each day during probenecid therapy.

66 Bisphosphonates

alendronate sodium
etidronate disodium
ibandronate sodium
pamidronate disodium
risedronate sodium
tiludronate
zoledronic acid

Uses: Bisphosphonates are used to treat Paget's disease and hypercalcemia. Some of these agents can be used to prevent and treat postmenopausal and other forms of osteoporosis. Pamidronate can also be used to treat breast cancer and osteolytic bone lesions of multiple myeloma.

Action: Bisphosphonates primarily act on bone. Their major effect is inhibition of normal and abnormal bone resorption, which leads to increased bone mineral density and a decreased serum calcium level.

alendronate sodium

a-**len**-dro-nate
(Fosamax)
Do not confuse Fosamax with Flomax.

CATEGORY AND SCHEDULE

Pregnancy Risk Category: C

MECHANISM OF ACTION

A bisphosphonate that inhibits normal and abnormal bone resorption, without retarding mineralization. **Therapeutic Effect:** Leads to significantly increased bone mineral density; reverses the progression of osteoporosis.

PHARMACOKINETICS

Poorly absorbed after oral administration. Protein binding: 78%. After oral administration, rapidly taken into bone, with uptake greatest at sites of active bone turnover. Excreted in urine. ***Terminal half-life:*** Greater than 10 yr (reflects release from skeleton as bone is resorbed).

AVAILABILITY

Tablets: 5 mg, 10 mg, 35 mg, 40 mg, 70 mg.
Oral Solution: 70 mg/75 ml.

INDICATIONS AND DOSAGES

‣ **Osteoporosis (in men)**
PO
Adults, Elderly. 10 mg once a day in the morning.

‣ **Glucocorticoid-induced osteoporosis**
PO
Adults, Elderly. 5 mg once a day in the morning.
Postmenopausal women not receiving estrogen. 10 mg once a day in the morning.

‣ **Postmenopausal osteoporosis**
PO (treatment)
Adults, Elderly. 10 mg once a day in the morning or 70 mg weekly.
PO (prevention)
Adults, Elderly. 5 mg once a day in the morning or 35 mg weekly.

‣ **Paget's disease**
PO
Adults, Elderly. 40 mg once a day in the morning.

OFF-LABEL USES

Treatment of breast cancer

CONTRAINDICATIONS

GI disease, including dysphagia, frequent heartburn, gastrointestinal reflux disease, hiatal hernia, and ulcers, inability to stand or sit upright for at least 30 minutes; renal impairment; sensitivity to alendronate

INTERACTIONS

Drug

Aspirin: May increase GI disturbances.

IV ranitidine: May double the bioavailability of alendronate.

Herbal

None known.

Food

Beverages other than plain water, dietary supplements, food: May interfere with absorption of alendronate.

DIAGNOSTIC TEST EFFECTS

Reduces serum calcium and serum phosphate concentrations. Significantly decreases serum alkaline phosphatase level in patients with Paget's disease.

SIDE EFFECTS

Frequent (8%–7%)

Back pain, abdominal pain

Occasional (3%–2%)

Nausea, abdominal distention, constipation, diarrhea, flatulence

Rare (Less than 2%)

Rash

SERIOUS REACTIONS

! Overdose causes hypocalcemia, hypophosphatemia, and significant GI disturbances.

! Esophageal irritation occurs if alendronate is not given with 6–8 ounces of plain water or if the patient lies down within 30 minutes of drug administration.

NURSING CONSIDERATIONS

Baseline Assessment

- Plan to correct hypocalcemia and vitamin D deficiency, if present, before starting alendronate therapy.

Lifespan Considerations

- Alendronate may cause decreased maternal weight gain and incomplete fetal ossification and delay delivery.
- It is unknown if alendronate is excreted in breast milk. Do not give to women who are breast-feeding.
- Safety and efficacy of alendronate have not been established in children.
- No age-related precautions have been noted in the elderly.

Precautions

- Use alendronate cautiously in patients with hypocalcemia or vitamin D deficiency.

Administration and Handling

PO

◀ALERT▶ Give at least 30 minutes before the first food, beverage, or medication of the day.

- Give with 6 to 8 ounces of plain water because mineral water, coffee, tea, and juice will decrease the drug's absorption.
- Make sure that the patient does not lie down or eat for at least 30 minutes after receiving the medication. By drinking plain water and remaining upright, the medication will reach the stomach quickly, which minimizes the risk of esophageal irritation.

Intervention and Evaluation

- Monitor the patient's serum electrolytes, including serum alkaline phosphatase and serum calcium levels.

Patient Teaching

- Instruct the patient that expected benefits occur only when alendronate is taken with a full glass (6–8 ounces) of plain water first thing in the morning and at least 30 minutes before the first food, beverage, or medication of the day. Explain that taking alendronate with beverages other than plain water, including mineral water, orange juice, and coffee, significantly reduces absorption of the medication.

- Advise the patient not to lie down for at least 30 minutes after taking the medication. Explain that remaining upright helps the drug move quickly to the stomach and reduces the risk of esophageal irritation.
- Encourage the patient to consider beginning weight-bearing exercises and modifying behavioral factors, such as reducing alcohol consumption and stopping cigarette smoking.

etidronate disodium

ee-**tid**-roe-nate

(Didronel)

Do not confuse etidronate with etidocaine or etomidate.

CATEGORY AND SCHEDULE

Pregnancy Risk Category: C (parenteral), B (oral)

MECHANISM OF ACTION

A bisphosphonate that decreases mineral release and matrix in bone and inhibits osteocytic osteolysis. **Therapeutic Effect:** Decreases bone resorption.

AVAILABILITY

Tablets: 200 mg, 400 mg.
Injection: 300-mg ampule (50 mg/ml).

INDICATIONS AND DOSAGES

▸ **Paget's disease**

PO

Adults, Elderly. Initially, 5–10 mg/kg/day not to exceed 6 mo, or 11–20 mg/kg/day not to exceed 3 mo. Repeat only after drug-free period of at least 90 days.

▸ **Heterotopic ossification caused by spinal cord injury**

PO

Adult, Elderly. 20 mg/kg/day for 2 wk; then 10 mg/kg/day for 10 wk.

▸ **Heterotopic ossification complicating total hip replacement**

PO

Adults, Elderly. 20 mg/kg/day for 1 mo before surgery; then 20 mg/kg/day for 3 mo after surgery.

▸ **Hypercalcemia associated with malignancy**

IV

Adults, Elderly. 7.5 mg/kg/day for 3 days. For retreatment, allow 7 days between treatment courses. Follow with oral therapy on day after last infusion. Begin with 20 mg/kg/day for 30 days; may extend up to 90 days.

CONTRAINDICATIONS

Clinically overt osteomalacia

INTERACTIONS

Drug

Antacids containing aluminum, calcium, magnesium mineral supplements: May decrease the absorption of etidronate.

Herbal

None known.

Food

Foods with calcium: May decrease the absorption of etidronate.

DIAGNOSTIC TEST EFFECTS

None known.

IV INCOMPATIBILITIES

Do not mix with other medications.

SIDE EFFECTS

Frequent

Nausea; diarrhea; continuing or more frequent bone pain in patients with Paget's disease

Occasional

Bone fractures, especially of the femur

Parenteral: Metallic, altered taste

Rare

Hypersensitivity reaction

SERIOUS REACTIONS

! Nephrotoxicity, including hematuria, dysuria, and proteinuria, has occurred with parenteral route.

NURSING CONSIDERATIONS

Baseline Assessment

- Expect to obtain the patient's laboratory values, especially serum electrolyte levels and kidney function test results.

Lifespan Considerations

- Adequate studies have not been done regarding the effect of oral etidronate use during pregnancy. Parenteral etidronate may cause skeletal malformations in the fetus.
- It is unknown if etidronate is excreted in breast milk. Do not give to women who are breast-feeding.
- Safety and efficacy of etidronate have not been established in children.
- Elderly patients may be prone to overhydration when treated with parenteral etidronate in conjunction with hydration therapy.

Precautions

- Use etidronate cautiously in patients with hyperphosphatemia, impaired renal function, or restricted calcium and vitamin D intake.

Administration and Handling

PO

- Administer on an empty stomach.
- Give etidronate 2 hours before antacids, food, or vitamins.

IV

- Store at room temperature.
- Must dilute with at least 250 ml 0.9% NaCl or D_5W.
- Infuse over at least 2 hours.

Intervention and Evaluation

- Assess the patient for diarrhea.
- Monitor the patient's electrolyte levels.
- Monitor BUN, and fluid intake and output in the patient with impaired renal function.
- Evaluate pain in the patient with Paget's disease.

Patient Teaching

- Tell the patient that it may take up to 3 months for a noticeable therapeutic response.
- Instruct the patient to consume calcium-rich foods, such as dairy products and milk.
- Teach the patient to take oral etidronate on an empty stomach, 2 hours before ingesting antacids, food, or vitamins.

ibandronate sodium

eye-**band**-droh-nate

(Boniva)

CATEGORY AND SCHEDULE

Pregnancy Risk Category: C

MECHANISM OF ACTION

A bisphosphonate that binds to bone hydroxyapatite (part of the mineral matrix of bone) and inhibits osteoclast activity. **Therapeutic Effect:** Reduces rate of bone turnover and bone resorption, resulting in a net gain in bone mass.

PHARMACOKINETICS

Absorbed in the upper GI tract. Extent of absorption impaired by food or beverages (other than plain water). Rapidly binds to bone. Unabsorbed portion is eliminated in urine. Protein binding: 90%. ***Half-life:*** 10–60 hr.

AVAILABILITY

Tablets: 2.5 mg

INDICATIONS AND DOSAGES

▸ **Osteoporosis**

PO

Adults, Elderly. 2.5 mg daily.

CONTRAINDICATIONS

Hypersensitivity to other bisphosphonates, including alendronate, etidronate, pamidronate, risedronate, and tiludronate; inability to stand or sit upright for at least 60 minutes; severe renal impairment with creatinine clearance less than 30 ml/min; uncorrected hypocalcemia

INTERACTIONS

Drug

Antacids containing aluminum, calcium, magnesium; vitamin D: Decrease the absorption of ibandronate.

Herbal

None known.

Food

Beverages other than plain water, dietary supplements, food: Interfere with the absorption of ibandronate.

DIAGNOSTIC TEST EFFECTS

May decrease serum alkaline phosphatase level. May increase blood cholesterol level.

SIDE EFFECTS

Frequent (13%–6%)

Back pain; dyspepsia, including epigastric distress and heartburn; peripheral discomfort; diarrhea; headache; myalgia

Occasional (4%–3%)

Dizziness, arthralgia, asthenia

Rare (2% or less)

Vomiting, hypersensitivity reaction

SERIOUS REACTIONS

! Upper respiratory tract infection occurs occasionally.

! Overdose causes hypocalcemia, hypophosphatemia, and significant GI disturbances

NURSING CONSIDERATIONS

Baseline Assessment

- Plan to correct hypocalcemia and vitamin D deficiencies, if present, before beginning ibandronate therapy.
- Expect to obtain the patient's laboratory studies, especially BUN and serum electrolyte and creatinine levels.
- Prepare the patient for a bone density study.

Lifespan Considerations

- Ibandronate may have teratogenic effects.
- It is unknown if ibandronate is excreted in breast milk. Breastfeeding is not recommended for female patients taking ibandronate.
- Safety and efficacy of ibandronate have not been established in children.
- No age-related precautions have been noted in the elderly.

Precautions

- Use ibandronate cautiously in patients with GI diseases, including duodenitis, dysphagia, esophagitis, gastritis, and ulcers, and mild to moderate renal impairment.

Administration and Handling

PO

- Give ibandronate on an empty

stomach with 6–8 ounces of plain—not mineral—water 60 minutes before the patient receives his or her first food or beverage of the day. Make sure the patient is standing or sitting in an upright position and that he or she does not lie down for 60 minutes after drug administration.

• The patient should not chew or suck the tablet because of the potential for oropharyngeal ulceration.

Intervention and Evaluation

• Monitor the patient's serum electrolytes, especially calcium and serum alkaline phosphatase levels.

Patient Teaching

• Tell the patient that the drug's expected benefits occur only when the medication is taken with a full glass (6–8 ounces) of plain water first thing in the morning and at least 60 minutes before the first beverage, food, or medications of the day. Explain to the patient that taking ibandronate with beverages other than plain water, including coffee, mineral water, and orange juice, significantly reduces the absorption of the drug.

• Instruct the patient not to lie down for at least 60 minutes after taking ibandronate to potentiate delivery to the stomach and reduce the risk of esophageal irritation.

• Encourage the patient to consider beginning weight-bearing exercises and modifying behavioral factors, such as reducing alcohol consumption and stopping cigarette smoking.

pamidronate disodium

pam-**id**-drow-nate

(Aredia, Pamisol[AUS])

Do not confuse Aredia with Adriamcyin.

CATEGORY AND SCHEDULE

Pregnancy Risk Category: D

MECHANISM OF ACTION

A bisphosphate that binds to bone and inhibits osteoclast-mediated calcium resorption. **Therapeutic Effect:** Lowers serum calcium concentrations.

PHARMACOKINETICS

Route	Onset	Peak	Duration
IV	24–48 hr	5–7 days	N/A

After IV administration, rapidly absorbed by bone. Slowly excreted unchanged in urine. Unknown if removed by hemodialysis. ***Half-life:*** bone, 300 days; unmetabolized, 2.5 hr.

AVAILABILITY

Powder for Injection: 30 mg, 90 mg. *Injection Solution:* 3 mg/ml, 6 mg/ml, 9 mg/ml.

INDICATIONS AND DOSAGES

▸ Hypercalcemia

IV Infusion

Adults, Elderly. Moderate hypercalcemia (corrected serum calcium level 12–13.5 mg/dl): 60–90 mg. Severe hypercalcemia (corrected serum calcium level greater than 13.5 mg/dl): 90 mg.

▸ Paget's disease

IV Infusion

Adults, Elderly. 30 mg/day for 3 days.

▸ **Osteolytic bone lesion**
IV Infusion
Adults, Elderly. 90 mg over 2–4 hr once a month.

CONTRAINDICATIONS
Hypersensitivity to other bisphosphonates, such as etidronate, tiludronate, risedronate, and alendronate

INTERACTIONS
Drug
Calcium-containing medications, vitamin D: May antagonize effects of pamidronate in treatment of hypercalcemia.
Herbal
None known.
Food
None known.

DIAGNOSTIC TEST EFFECTS
May decrease serum phosphate, magnesium, calcium, and potassium levels.

IV INCOMPATIBILITIES
Calcium-containing IV fluids

SIDE EFFECTS
Frequent (greater than 10%)
Temperature elevation (at least 1°C) 24–48 hr after administration (27%); redness, swelling, induration, pain at catheter site in patients receiving 90 mg (18%); anorexia, nausea, fatigue
Occasional (10%–1%)
Constipation, rhinitis

SERIOUS REACTIONS
! Hypophosphatemia, hypokalemia, hypomagnesemia, and hypocalcemia occur more frequently with higher dosages.
! Anemia, hypertension, tachycardia, atrial fibrillation, and somnolence occur more frequently with 90-mg doses.
! GI hemorrhage occurs rarely.

NURSING CONSIDERATIONS
Baseline Assessment
• Establish the patient's serum electrolyte levels, including BUN and serum calcium and creatinine levels.
Lifespan Considerations
• Because there are no adequate and well-controlled studies in pregnant women, it is unknown if pamidronate causes fetal harm or is excreted in breast milk. Do not give to women who are breast-feeding.
• Safety and efficacy of pamidronate have not been established in children.
• The elderly may become overhydrated and require careful monitoring of fluid and electrolytes. Dilute the drug in a smaller volume for elderly patients.
Precautions
• Use pamidronate cautiously in patients with cardiac failure or renal impairment.
Administration and Handling
IV
• Store parenteral form at room temperature.
• The reconstituted vial is stable for 24 hours when refrigerated; the IV solution is stable for 24 hours after dilution.
• Reconstitute each 30-mg vial with 10 ml sterile water for injection to provide concentration of 3 mg/ml. Allow the drug to dissolve before withdrawing. Further dilute with 1,000 ml sterile 0.45% or 0.9% NaCl or D_5W.
• Administer as IV infusion over 2 to 24 hours for treatment of hypercalcemia and over 2 to 4 hours for other indications.

- Adequate hydration is essential during pamidronate administration. Avoid overhydration in patients with the potential for heart failure.

Intervention and Evaluation

- Monitor the patient's Hct, Hgb, and serum magnesium and creatinine levels.
- Provide the patient with adequate hydration, and take precautions to avoid overhydrating the patient.
- Monitor the patient's fluid intake and output carefully.
- Examine the patient's lungs for crackles and dependent body parts for edema.
- Monitor the patient's BP, pulse, and temperature.
- Assess the patient's catheter site for pain, redness, and swelling.
- Assess the patient's pattern of daily bowel activity and stool consistency.
- Be alert for potential GI hemorrhage in patients receiving 90-mg dose.

Patient Teaching

- Explain to the patient the need for follow-up testing.
- Tell the patient to avoid drugs containing calcium and vitamin D, such as antacids, because they might antagonize the effects of pamidronate.

risedronate sodium

rye-se-**droe**-nate
(Actonel)

CATEGORY AND SCHEDULE

Pregnancy Risk Category: C

MECHANISM OF ACTION

A bisphosphonate that binds to bone hydroxyapatite and inhibits osteoclasts. **Therapeutic Effect:** Reduces bone turnover (the number of sites at which bone is remodeled) and bone resorption.

AVAILABILITY

Tablets: 5 mg, 30 mg, 35 mg.

INDICATIONS AND DOSAGES

▸ **Paget's disease**

PO

Adults, Elderly. 30 mg/day for 2 mo. Retreatment may occur after 2-mo post-treatment observation period.

▸ **Prevention and treatment of postmenopausal osteoporosis**

PO

Adults, Elderly. 5 mg/day or 35 mg once weekly.

▸ **Glucocorticoid-induced osteoporosis**

PO

Adults, Elderly. 5 mg/day.

CONTRAINDICATIONS

Hypersensitivity to other bisphosphonates, including etidronate, tiludronate, risedronate, and alendronate; hypocalcemia; inability to stand or sit upright for at least 20 minutes; renal impairment when serum creatinine clearance is greater than 5 mg/dl

INTERACTIONS

Drug

Antacids containing aluminum, calcium, magnesium; vitamin D: May decrease the absorption of risedronate.

Herbal

None known.

Food

None known.

DIAGNOSTIC TEST EFFECTS

None known.

SIDE EFFECTS

Frequent (30%)
Arthralgia

Occasional (12%–8%)
Rash, flulike symptoms, peripheral edema

Rare (5%–3%)
Bone pain, sinusitis, asthenia, dry eye, tinnitus

SERIOUS REACTIONS

! Overdose causes hypocalcemia, hypophosphatemia, and significant GI disturbances.

NURSING CONSIDERATIONS

Baseline Assessment

- Expect to correct hypocalcemia and vitamin D deficiency, if present, before beginning risedronate therapy.
- Plan to obtain the patient's laboratory studies, especially serum electrolyte levels and kidney function test results.

Lifespan Considerations

- Because there are no adequate and well-controlled studies in pregnant women, it is unknown if risedronate causes fetal harm or is excreted in breast milk.
- Safety and efficacy of risedronate have not been established in children. Do not give to women who are breast-feeding.
- No age-related precautions have been noted in the elderly.

Precautions

- Use risedronate cautiously in patients with GI disease, including duodenitis, dysphagia, esophagitis, gastritis, and ulcers, or severe renal impairment.

Administration and Handling

PO

- Administer 30 to 60 minutes before patient consumes drink, food, or other oral medications, to avoid interference with absorption.
- Give on an empty stomach with a full glass of plain water; do not give with mineral water.
- Make sure the patient does not lie down for 30 minutes after swallowing tablet to help drug delivery to the stomach and reduce the risk of esophageal irritation.

Intervention and Evaluation

- Expect to check the patient's serum electrolytes, especially alkaline phosphatase and calcium levels.
- Monitor BUN, intake and output, and serum creatinine levels in patients with renal impairment, as ordered.

Patient Teaching

- Instruct the patient to take the drug with a full glass (6–8 ounces) of plain water first thing in the morning and at least 30 minutes before first beverage, food, or medication of the day. Explain to the patient that taking risedronate with other beverages, including coffee, mineral water, and orange juice, significantly reduces the absorption of the drug.
- Teach the patient not to lie down for at least 30 minutes after taking risedronate to potentiate delivery to the stomach and reduce the risk of esophageal irritation.
- Explain to the patient that the drug's therapeutic effect depends on his or her adherence to administration instructions.
- Urge the patient to consider beginning weight-bearing exercises and modifying his or her behavioral factors, such as avoiding alcohol consumption and cigarette smoking.

tiludronate

ti-**loo**-dro-nate
(Skelid)

CATEGORY AND SCHEDULE

Pregnancy Risk Category: C

MECHANISM OF ACTION

A calcium regulator that inhibits functioning osteoclasts through disruption of cytoskeletal ring structure and inhibition of osteoclastic proton pump. **Therapeutic Effect:** Inhibits bone resorption.

AVAILABILITY

Tablets: 200 mg.

INDICATIONS AND DOSAGES

▸ Paget's disease

PO

Adults, Elderly. 400 mg once a day for 3 mo. Must take with 6–8 ounces plain water. Do not give within 2 hr of food intake. Avoid giving aspirin, calcium supplements, mineral supplements, or antacids within 2 hr of tiludronate administration.

CONTRAINDICATIONS

GI disease, such as dysphagia and gastric ulcer, impaired renal function

INTERACTIONS

Drug

Antacids containing aluminum or magnesium, calcium, salicylates: May interfere with the absorption of tiludronate.

Herbal

None known.

Food

None known.

DIAGNOSTIC TEST EFFECTS

None known.

SIDE EFFECTS

Frequent (9%–6%)

Nausea, diarrhea, generalized body pain, back pain, headache

Occasional

Rash, dyspepsia, vomiting, rhinitis, sinusitis, dizziness

NURSING CONSIDERATIONS

Baseline Assessment

- Determine if the patient is pregnant or using other medications, especially aluminum, magnesium, calcium, and salicylates.
- Obtain the patient's BUN and serum creatinine level to assess renal function.
- Assess the patient for evidence of GI abnormalities.

Lifespan Considerations

- Because there are no adequate and well-controlled studies in pregnant women, it is unknown if tiludronate causes fetal harm or is excreted in breast milk. Do not give to women who are breast-feeding.
- Safety and efficacy of tiludronate have not been established in children.
- No age-related precautions have been noted in the elderly.

Precautions

- Use tiludronate cautiously in patients with hyperparathyroidism, hypocalcemia, and vitamin D deficiency.

Administration and Handling

- Give tiludronate at least 2 hours before or after beverages, food, other medications, calcium or other mineral supplements, and vitamin D.
- Administer with 6 to 8 ounces of plain water (not mineral water).

Intervention and Evaluation

- Monitor the patient's adjusted serum calcium, serum alkaline phosphatase, osteocalcin, and urinary hydroxyproline levels to assess the effectiveness of tiludronate.

Patient Teaching

- Instruct the patient take the drug with 6 to 8 ounces of plain water.
- Warn the patient to avoid taking other medications or food for 2 hours before or after taking tiludronate.
- Instruct the patient to consult the physician to determine if he or she

needs calcium and vitamin D supplements.

zoledronic acid

zole-eh-**drone**-ick
(Zometa)

CATEGORY AND SCHEDULE

Pregnancy Risk Category: C

MECHANISM OF ACTION

A bisphosphonate that inhibits the resorption of mineralized bone and cartilage; inhibits increased osteoclastic activity and skeletal calcium release induced by stimulatory factors produced by tumors. **Therapeutic Effect:** Increases urinary calcium and phosphorus excretion; decreases serum calcium and phosphorus levels.

AVAILABILITY

Injection Powder for Reconstitution: 4 mg.
Injection Solution: 4 mg/5 ml.

INDICATIONS AND DOSAGES

▸ **Hypercalcemia**

IV Infusion

Adults, Elderly. 4 mg IV infusion given over no less than 15 min. Re-treatment may be considered, but at least 7 days should elapse to allow for full response to initial dose.

▸ **Multiple Myeloma**

IV

Adults, Elderly. 4 mg q3–4wk.

CONTRAINDICATIONS

Hypersensitivity to other bisphosphonates, including alendronate, etidronate, pamidronate, risedronate, and tiludronate

INTERACTIONS

Drug

Calcium-containing medications, vitamin D: May antagonize the effects of zoledronic acid in treatment of hypercalcemia.

Herbal

None known.

Food

None known.

DIAGNOSTIC TEST EFFECTS

May decrease serum magnesium, calcium, and phosphate levels.

IV INCOMPATIBILITIES

Do not mix with other medications.

SIDE EFFECTS

Frequent (44%–26%)

Fever, nausea, vomiting, constipation

Occasional (15%–10%)

Hypotension, anxiety, insomnia, flulike symptoms (fever, chills, bone pain, myalgia, and arthralgia)

Rare

Conjunctivitis

SERIOUS REACTIONS

! Renal toxicity may occur if IV infusion is administered in less than 15 minutes.

NURSING CONSIDERATIONS

Baseline Assessment

• Establish the patient's serum electrolyte levels, including serum calcium, as well as renal function test results.

◂ **ALERT** ▸ Make sure the patient is adequately hydrated before administering zoledronic acid.

Lifespan Considerations

• Because there are no adequate and well-controlled studies in pregnant women, it is unknown if zoledronic acid causes fetal harm or is excreted in breast milk. Do not give to women who are breast-feeding.

- Safety and efficacy of zoledronic acid have not been established in children.
- Age-related renal impairment may require cautious use or dosage adjustment in the elderly.

Precautions

- Use zoledronic acid cautiously in patients with history of aspirin-sensitive asthma or hypoparathyroidism, renal impairment, or risk of hypocalcemia.

Administration and Handling

IV

- Store at room temperature.
- If not used immediately, reconstituted solution should be refrigerated; time from reconstitution to end of administration should not exceed 24 hours.
- Reconstitute 4-mg vial with 5 ml sterile water for injection. Allow drug to dissolve before withdrawing. Further dilute with 100 ml 0.9% NaCl or D_5W.
- Adequate hydration is essential during zoledronic acid administration.
- Administer as an IV infusion over not less than 15 minutes. Infusing over less than 15 minutes increases the risk of renal function deterioration.

Intervention and Evaluation

- Monitor the patient's CBC, Hgb, Hct, renal function test results, and serum electrolytes, including, serum calcium, magnesium, and phosphate levels.
- Assess the patient's vertebral bone mass and document its improvement or stabilization.
- Assess the patient for fever.
- Monitor fluid intake and output, especially in patients with impaired renal function.

Patient Teaching

- Explain to the patient the need for follow-up testing.
- Tell the patient to avoid drugs containing calcium and vitamin D, such as antacids, because they might antagonize the effects of zoledronic acid.

67 Estrogens and Progestins

conjugated estrogens
estradiol
estropipate
medroxyprogesterone acetate
megestrol acetate
progesterone

Uses: Estrogens and progestins are commonly used for contraception and hormone replacement therapy after menopause. They're also used to treat dysfunctional uterine bleeding, female hypogonadism, and prostate and other forms of cancer.

Actions: As ovarian sex hormones, estrogens and progestins provide different actions. *Estrogens,* such as estradiol, mainly promote proliferation and growth of specific cells in the body and are responsible for the development of most secondary sex characteristics, such as the breasts and milk-producing apparatus. These agents primarily cause the cellular proliferation and growth of female reproductive organs, including the ovaries, fallopian tubes, uterus, and vagina. *Progestins,* such as progesterone, stimulate secretion by the uterine endometrium during the latter half of the female sexual cycle, preparing the uterus for implantation of the fertilized ovum. These hormones decrease the frequency of uterine contractions, which helps prevent expulsion of the implanted ovum. Progesterone also promotes breast development. Both types of hormones protect women against coronary heart disease and osteoporosis.

COMBINATION PRODUCTS

ACTIVELLA: estradiol/norethindrone (a hormone) 1 mg/0.5 mg.
COMBIPATCH: estradiol/norethindrone (a hormone) 0.05 mg/0.14 mg; 0.05 mg/0.25 mg.
FEMHRT: estradiol/norethindrone (a hormone) 5 mcg/1 mg.
LUNELLE: estradiol/ medroxyprogesterone (a progestin) 5 mg/25 mg per 0.5 ml.
PREMPHASE: conjugated estrogens/ medroxyprogesterone (an androgen): 0.625 mg/5 mg.
PREMPRO: conjugated estrogens/ medroxyprogesterone (an androgen): 0.3 mg/1.5 mg; 0.45 mg/1.5 mg; 0.625 mg/2.5 mg; 0.625 mg/5 mg.
MEGESTROL ACETATE: See hormones

conjugated estrogens

ess-troe-jenz
(Cenestin, C.E.S.[CAN], Congest[CAN], Enjuvia, Premarin, Premarin Crème[AUS])
Do not confuse Premarin with Primaxin or Remeron.

CATEGORY AND SCHEDULE

Pregnancy Risk Category: X

MECHANISM OF ACTION

An estrogen that increases synthesis of DNA, RNA, and various proteins in target tissues; reduces release of gonadotropin-releasing hormone from the hypothalamus; and reduces follicle-stimulating hormone (FSH) and leuteinizing hormone (LH) release from the pituitary gland. **Therapeutic Effect:** Promotes normal growth, promotes development of femal sex organs, and maintains GU function and vasomotor stability. Prevents accelerated bone loss by inhibiting bone resorption, restoring balance of bone resorption and formation. Inhibits LH and decreases serum concentration of testosterone.

PHARMACOKINETICS

Well absorbed from the GI tract. Widely distributed. Protein binding: 50%–80%. Metabolized in the liver. Primarily excreted in urine.

AVAILABILITY

Tablets (Cenestin, Premarin): 0.3 mg, 0.45 mg, 0.625 mg, 0.9 mg, 1.25 mg.
Tablets (Enjuvia): 0.625 mg, 1.25 mg.
Injection: 25 mg.
Vaginal Cream: 0.625 mg/g.

INDICATIONS AND DOSAGES

▸ Vasomotor symptoms associated with menopause, atrophic vaginitis, kraurosis vulvae
PO
Adults, Elderly. 0.3–0.625 mg/day cyclically (21 days on, 7 days off) or continuously.
Intravaginal
Adults, Elderly. 0.5–2 g/day cyclically, such as 21 days on and 7 days off.

▸ Female hypogonadism
PO
Adults. 0.3–0.625 mg/day in divided doses for 20 days; then a rest period of 10 days.

▸ Female castration, primary ovarian failure
PO
Adults. Initially, 1.25 mg/day cyclically. Adjust dosage, upward or downward, according to severity of symptoms and patient response. For maintenance, adjust dosage to lowest level that will provide effective control.

▸ Osteoporosis
PO
Adults, Elderly. 0.3–0.625 mg/day, cyclically, such as 25 days on and 5 days off.

▸ Breast cancer
PO
Adults, Elderly. 10 mg 3 times a day for at least 3 mo.

▸ Prostate cancer
PO
Adults, Elderly. 1.25–2.5 mg 3 times a day.

▸ Abnormal uterine bleeding
PO
Adults. 1.25 mg q4h for 24 hr, then 1.25 mg/day for 7–10 days.
IV, IM
Adults. 25 mg; may repeat once in 6–12 hr.

OFF-LABEL USES

Prevention of estrogen deficiency–induced premenopausal osteoporosis
Cream: Prevention of nosebleeds

CONTRAINDICATIONS

Breast cancer with some exceptions, hepatic disease, thrombophlebitis, undiagnosed vaginal bleeding

INTERACTIONS

Drug

Bromocriptine: May interfere with the effects of bromocriptine.
Cyclosporine: May increase blood cyclosporine concentration and the risk of hepatotoxicity and nephrotoxicity.
Hepatotoxic medications: May increase the risk of hepatotoxicity.

Herbal

None known.

Food

None known.

DIAGNOSTIC TEST EFFECTS

May increase blood glucose, HDL, serum calcium, and triglyceride levels. May decrease serum cholesterol levels and LDH concentrations. May affect serum metapyrone testing and thyroid function tests.

IV INCOMPATIBILITIES

No information available via Y-site administration.

SIDE EFFECTS

Frequent

Vaginal bleeding, such as spotting or breakthrough bleeding; breast pain or tenderness; gynecomastia

Occasional

Headache, hypertension, intolerance to contact lenses
High-doses: Anorexia, nausea

Rare

Loss of scalp hair, depression

SERIOUS REACTIONS

! Prolonged administration may increase the risk of gallbladder disease, thromboembolic disease, and breast, cervical, vaginal, endometrial, and hepatic carcinoma.

NURSING CONSIDERATIONS

Baseline Assessment

- Determine if the patient is hypersensitive to estrogen and whether he or she has had previous jaundice or thromboembolic disorders associated with pregnancy or estrogen therapy.

Lifespan Considerations

- Conjugated estrogens are distributed in breast milk and may be harmful to the fetus. They should not be used during breast-feeding.
- Safety and efficacy of conjugated estrogens have not been established in children.
- No age-related precautions have been noted in the elderly.

Precautions

- Use conjugated estrogens cautiously in patients with asthma, cardiac dysfunction, diabetes mellitus, epilepsy, migraine headaches, or renal impairment.

Administration and Handling

PO

- Administer at the same time each day.
- Give conjugated estrogens with food or milk if nausea occurs.

IV, IM

- Refrigerate vials.
- Reconstitute with 5 ml sterile water for injection containing benzyl alcohol (provided).
- Slowly add diluent, shaking gently. Avoid vigorous shaking.
- The reconstituted solution is stable for 60 days refrigerated. Do not use if solution darkens or precipitate forms.
- For the IV form, give slowly to prevent flushing.

Intervention and Evaluation

- Assess the patient's BP periodically.

• Examine the patient for edema and record his or her weight.
• Promptly report signs and symptoms of thromboembolic or thrombotic disorders, including loss of coordination, numbness or weakness of an extremity, shortness of breath, speech or vision disturbance, sudden severe headache, and pain in the chest, leg, or groin.

Patient Teaching

• Urge the patient to avoid smoking because of the increased risk of blood clot formation and MI.
• Explain to the patient the importance of diet and exercise when conjugated estrogens are taken to retard osteoporosis.
• Teach the patient how to recognize the signs and symptoms of blood clots, such as tenderness and swelling.
• Warn the patient to report abnormal vaginal bleeding, depression, or signs and symptoms of blood clots.
• Teach the female patient to perform a breast self-examination monthly.
• Instruct the patient to report weekly weight gain of more than 5 pounds.
• Instruct the female patient to notify the physician and to discontinue the drug, as prescribed if she suspects she is pregnant.

estradiol

ess-tra-**dye**-ole
(Aerodil[AUS], Alora, Climara, Delestrogen, Depo-Estradiol, Esclim, Estrace, Estraderm, Estraderm MX[AUS], Estradot[CAN], Estrasorb, Estrogel, Estring, Femring, Kliovance[AUS], Menostar, Oesclim[CAN], Primogyn Depot[AUS], Progynova[AUS], Sandrena Gel[AUS], Vagifem, Vivelle, Vivelle Dot, Zumenon[AUS])
Do not confuse Estraderm with Testoderm.

CATEGORY AND SCHEDULE

Pregnancy Risk Category: X

MECHANISM OF ACTION

An estrogen that increases synthesis of DNA, RNA, and proteins in target tissues; reduces release of gonadotropin-releasing hormone from the hypothalamus; and reduces follicle-stimulating hormone and luteinizing hormone (LH) release from the pituitary. **Therapeutic Effect:** Promotes normal growth, promotes development of female sex organs, and maintains GU function and vasomotor stability. Prevents accelerated bone loss by inhibiting bone resorption, restoring balance of bone resorption and formation. Inhibits LH and decreases serum testosterone concentration.

PHARMACOKINETICS

Well absorbed from the GI tract. Widely distributed. Protein binding: 50%–80%. Metabolized in the liver. Primarily excreted in urine. ***Half-life:*** Unknown.

AVAILABILITY

Tablets (Estrace): 0.5 mg, 1 mg, 2 mg.

Emulsion (Topical [Estrasorb]): 2.5 mg/g.
Injection (Cypionate [Depo-Estradiol]): 5 mg/ml.
Injection (Valerate [Delestrogen]): 10 mg/ml.
Topical Gel (EstroGel): 1.25 g.
Transdermal System (Alora): twice weekly: 0.025 mg, 0.05 mg, 0.075 mg, 0.1 mg.
Transdermal System (Climara): once weekly: 0.025 mg, 0.0375 mg, 0.05 mg, 0.06 mg, 0.075 mg, 0.1 mg.
Transdermal System (Esclim): twice weekly: 0.025 mg, 0.0375 mg, 0.05 mg, 0.075 mg, 0.1 mg.
Transdermal System (Estraderm): twice weekly: 0.05 mg, 0.1 mg.
Transdermal System (Menostar): once a week: 1 mg.
Transdermal System (Vivelle): twice weekly: 0.025 mg, 0.0375 mg, 0.05 mg, 0.075 mg, 0.1 mg.
Transderamal System (Vivelle Dot): twice weekly: 0.0375 mg, 0.05 mg, 0.075 mg, 0.1 mg.
Vaginal Cream (Estrace): 0.1 mg/g.
Vaginal Ring (Estring): 2 mg.
Vaginal Ring (Femring): 0.05 mg.
Vaginal Tablet (Vagifem): 25 mcg.

INDICATIONS AND DOSAGES

▸ Prostate cancer
IM (estradiol valerate)
Adults, Elderly. 30 mg or more q1–2 wk.
PO
Adults, Elderly. 10 mg 3 times a day for at least 3 mo.

▸ Breast cancer
PO
Adults, Elderly. 10 mg 3 times a day for at least 3 mo.

▸ Osteoporosis prophylaxis in postmenopausal females
PO
Adults, Elderly. 0.5 mg/day cyclically (3 weeks on, 1 week off).
Transdermal (Climara)
Adults, Elderly. Initially, 0.025 mg weekly, adjust dose as needed.
Transdermal (Alora, Vivelle, Vivelle-Dot):
Adults, Elderly. Initially, 0.025 mg patch twice weekly, adjust dose as needed.
Transdermal (Estraderm)
Adults, Elderly. 0.05 mg twice weekly.
Transdermal (Menostar)
Adults, Elderly. 1 mg weekly.

▸ Female hypoestrogenism
PO
Adults, Elderly. 1–2 mg/day, adjust dose as needed.
IM (cypionate)
Adults, Elderly. 1.5–2 mg monthly.
IM (estradiol valerate)
Adults, Elderly. 10–20 mg q4wk.

▸ Vasomotor symptoms associated with menopause
PO
Adults, Elderly. 1–2 mg/day cyclically (3 weeks on, 1 week off), adjust dose as needed.
IM (estradiol cypionate)
Adults, Elderly. 1–5 mg q3–4wk.
IM (estradiol valerate)
Adults, Elderly. 10–20 mg q4wk.
Topical Emulsion (Estrasorb)
Adults, Elderly. 3.84 g once a day in the morning.
Topical Gel (Estrogel)
Adults, Elderly. 1.25 g/day.
Transdermal (Climara)
Adults, Elderly. 0.025 mg weekly. Adjust dose as needed.
Transdermal (Alora, Esclim, Estrader, Vivelle-Dot)
Adults, Elderly. 0.05 mg twice a week.
Transdermal (Vivelle)
Adults, Elderly. 0.0375 mg twice a week.
Vaginal Ring (Femring)
Adults, Elderly. 0.05 mg. May increase to 0.1 mg if needed.

▸ **Vaginal atrophy**
Vaginal Ring (Estring)
Adults, Elderly. 2 mg.
▸ **Atrophic vaginitis**
Vaginal Tablet (Vagifem)
Adults, Elderly. Initially, 1 tablet/day for 2 weeks. Maintenance: 1 tablet twice a week.

OFF-LABEL USES

Treatment of Turner's syndrome

CONTRAINDICATIONS

Abnormal vaginal bleeding, active arterial thrombosis, blood dyscrasias, estrogen-dependent cancer, known or suspected breast cancer, pregnancy, thrombophlebitis or thromboembolic disorders, thyroid dysfunction

INTERACTIONS

Drug

Bromocriptine: May interfere with the effects of bromocriptine.
Cyclosporine: May increase blood cyclosporine concentration and the risk of hepatotoxicity and nephrotoxicity.
Hepatotoxic medications: May increase the risk of hepatotoxicity.

Herbal

Saw palmetto: Increases the effects of saw palmetto.

Food

None known.

DIAGNOSTIC TEST EFFECTS

May increase blood glucose, HDL, serum calcium, and triglyceride levels. May decrease serum cholesterol levels and LDH concentrations. May affect metapyrone testing and thyroid function tests.

SIDE EFFECTS

Frequent

Anorexia, nausea, swelling of breasts, peripheral edema marked by swollen ankles and feet
Transdermal: Skin irritation, redness

Occasional

Vomiting, especially with high doses; headache that may be severe; intolerance to contact lenses; hypertension; glucose intolerance; brown spots on exposed skin
Vaginal: Local irritation, vaginal discharge, changes in vaginal bleeding, including spotting, and breakthrough or prolonged bleeding

Rare

Chorea or involuntary movements, hirsutism or abnormal hairiness, loss of scalp hair, depression

SERIOUS REACTIONS

! Prolonged administration increases the risk of gallbladder disease, thromboembolic disease, and breast, cervical, vaginal, endometrial, and hepatic carcinoma.
! Cholestatic jaundice occurs rarely.

NURSING CONSIDERATIONS

Baseline Assessment

• Determine if the patient is hypersensitive to estrogen and whether she has had previous jaundice or thromboembolic disorders associated with pregnancy or estrogen therapy.
• Determine if the patient is pregnant.

Lifespan Considerations

• Estradiol is distributed in breast milk and may be harmful to the infant. Estradiol should not be used during breast-feeding.
• Estradiol should be used cautiously in children whose bone growth is not complete because the drug may accelerate epiphyseal closure.
• No age-related precautions have been noted in the elderly.

Precautions

• Use estradiol cautiously in children whose bone growth is incomplete.
• Use cautiously in patients with

diseases exacerbated by fluid retention and in those with hepatic or renal insufficiency.

Administration and Handling

PO

- Administer estradiol at the same time each day.

IM

- Rotate the vial to disperse drug in solution.
- Give deep IM injection into the gluteus maximus.

Vaginal

- Apply estradiol cream at bedtime for best absorption.
- To administer, insert the end of the filled applicator into the patient's vagina, directing the applicator slightly toward the sacrum; push the plunger down completely.
- Do not let the cream contact the skin to prevent topical absorption of the drug.

Transdermal

◀ **ALERT** ▶ Transdermal Climara is administered once weekly; other transdermal forms of estradiol are applied twice weekly.

- To apply, remove the old patch and select a new site. Consider using the buttocks as an alternative application site. Peel off the protective strip on the patch to expose the adhesive surface. Apply to clean, dry, intact skin on the trunk of the patient's body in an area with as little hair as possible. Press in place for at least 10 seconds.
- Do not apply the patch to the patient's breasts or waistline.

Intervention and Evaluation

- Monitor the patient's BP, weight, and blood glucose, hepatic enzyme, and serum calcium levels.

Patient Teaching

- Urge the patient to limit alcohol and caffeine intake.
- Encourage the patient to stop smoking tobacco if he or she is a smoker.
- Warn the patient to report calf or chest pain, depression, numbness or weakness of an extremity, severe abdominal pain, shortness of breath, speech or vision disturbance, sudden headache, unusual bleeding, or vomiting.

estropipate

es-tro-**pip**-ate

(Genoral[AUS], Ogen, Ortho-Est)

CATEGORY AND SCHEDULE

Pregnancy Risk Category: X

MECHANISM OF ACTION

An estrogen that increases synthesis of DNA, RNA, abd proteins in target tissues; reduces release of gonadotropin-releasing hormone from the hypothalamus; and reduces follicle-stimulating hormone (FSH) and luteinizing hormone (LH) from the pituitary. **Therapeutic Effect:** Promotes normal growth, promotes development of female sex organs, and maintains GU function and vasomotor stability. Prevents accelerated bone loss by inhibiting bone resorption, restoring balance of bone resorption and formation. Inhibits LH and decreases serum testosterone concentration.

AVAILABILITY

Tablets (Ogen, Ortho-Est): 0.625 mg (0.75 mg estropipate), 1.25 mg (1.5 mg estropipate), 2.5 mg (3 mg estropipate).

Vaginal Cream (Ogen): 1.5 mg/g.

INDICATIONS AND DOSAGES

▸ **Vasomotor symptoms, atrophic vaginitis, kraurosis vulvae**
PO
Adults, Elderly. 0.625–5 mg/day cyclically.

▸ **Atrophic vaginitis, kraurosis vulvae**
Intravaginal
Adults, Elderly. 2–4 g/day cyclically.

▸ **Female hypogonadism, castration, primary ovarian failure**
PO
Adults, Elderly. 1.25–7.5 mg/day for 21 days; then off for 8–10 days. Repeat if bleeding does not occur by end of off cycle.

▸ **Prevention of osteoporosis**
PO
Adults, Elderly. 0.625 mg/day (25 days of 31-day cycle/mo).

CONTRAINDICATIONS

Abnormal vaginal bleeding, active arterial thrombosis, blood dyscrasias, estrogen-dependent cancer, known or suspected breast cancer, pregnancy, thrombophlebitis or thromboembolic disorders, thyroid dysfunction

INTERACTIONS

Drug

Bromocriptine: May interfere with the effects of bromocriptine.
Cyclosporine: May increase blood cyclosporine concentration and the risk of hepatotoxicity and nephrotoxicity.
Hepatotoxic medications: May increase the risk of hepatotoxicity.

Herbal

Saw palmetto: Increases the effects of saw palmetto.

Food

None known.

DIAGNOSTIC TEST EFFECTS

May increase blood glucose, HDL, serum calcium, and triglyceride levels. May decrease serum cholesterol and LDH concentrations. May affect metapyrone testing and thyroid function tests.

SIDE EFFECTS

Frequent

Anorexia, nausea, swelling of breasts, peripheral edema marked by swollen ankles and feet

Occasional

Vomiting, especially with high doses; headache that may be severe; intolerance to contact lenses; hypertension; glucose intolerance; brown spots on exposed skin
Vaginal: Local irritation, vaginal discharge, changes in vaginal bleeding, including spotting, and breakthrough or prolonged bleeding

Rare

Chorea or involuntary movements, hirsutism or abnormal hairiness, loss of scalp hair, depression

SERIOUS REACTIONS

! Prolonged administration increases the risk of gallbladder disease, thromboembolic disease and breast, cervical, vaginal, endometrial, and hepatic carcinoma.
! Cholestatic jaundice occurs rarely.

NURSING CONSIDERATIONS

Baseline Assessment

• Determine if the patient is hypersensitive to estrogen and whether she has had jaundice or thromboembolic disorders associated with pregnancy or estrogen therapy.
• Determine if the patient is pregnant.

Lifespan Considerations

• Estropipate is distributed in breast milk and may be harmful to the

infant. Estropipate should not be used during breast-feeding.
- Estropipate should be used cautiously in children whose bone growth is not complete because the drug may accelerate epiphyseal closure.
- No age-related precautions have been noted in the elderly.

Precautions
- Use estropipate cautiously in patients with diseases exacerbated by fluid retention and in those with hepatic or renal insufficiency.

Administration and Handling
- Store in a tightly-closed container.
- Administer estropipate at the same time each day.

Intervention and Evaluation
- Promptly report signs and symptoms of thromboembolic or thrombotic disorders, including peripheral paresthesia, shortness of breath, speech or vision disturbance, and sudden headache.

Patient Teaching
- Urge the patient to avoid smoking because of the increased risk of blood clot formation and MI.
- Warn the patient to report depression or abnormal vaginal bleeding.
- Teach the patient to remain recumbent for at least 30 minutes after vaginal application and not to use tampons during estropipate therapy.
- Instruct the female patient to notify the physician and discontinue the drug, as prescribed, if she suspects she is pregnant.

medroxyprogesterone acetate

me-**drox**-ee-proe-**jess**-te-rone (Depo-Provera, Depo-Provera Contraceptive, Novo-Medrone[CAN], Provera, Ralovera[AUS])

Do not confuse medroxyprogesterone with hydroxyprogesterone, methylprednisolone, or methyltestosterone.

CATEGORY AND SCHEDULE

Pregnancy Risk Category: X

MECHANISM OF ACTION

A hormone that transforms endometrium from proliferative to secretory in an estrogen-primed endometrium. Inhibits secretion of pituitary gonadotropins. **Therapeutic Effect:** Prevents follicular maturation and ovulation. Stimulates growth of mammary alveolar tissue and relaxes uterine smooth muscle. Corrects hormonal imbalance.

PHARMACOKINETICS

Slowly absorbed after IM administration. Protein binding: 90%. Metabolized in the liver. Primarily excreted in urine. ***Half-life:*** 30 days.

AVAILABILITY

Tablets (Provera): 2.5 mg, 5 mg, 10 mg.
Injection (Depo-Provera Contraceptive): 150 mg/ml.
Injection (Depo-Provera): 400 mg/ml.

INDICATIONS AND DOSAGES

▸ **Endometrial hyperplasia**

PO

Adults. 2.5–10 mg/day for 14 days.

▸ **Secondary amenorrhea**
PO
Adults. 5–10 mg/day for 5–10 days, beginning at any time during menstrual cycle or 2.5 mg/day.
▸ **Abnormal uterine bleeding**
PO
Adults. 5–10 mg/day for 5–10 days, beginning on calculated day 16 or day 21 of menstrual cycle.
▸ **Endometrial, renal carcinoma**
IM
Adults, Elderly. Initially, 400–1,000 mg; repeat at 1-wk intervals. If improvement occurs and disease is stabilized, begin maintenance with as little as 400 mg/mo.
▸ **Prevention of pregnancy**
IM
Adults. 150 mg q3mo.

OFF-LABEL USES
Hormone replacement therapy in estrogen-treated menopausal women, treatment of endometriosis

CONTRAINDICATIONS
Carcinoma of breast; estrogen-dependent neoplasm; history of or active thrombotic disorders, such as cerebral apoplexy, thrombophlebitis, or thromboembolic disorders; hypersensitivity to progestins; known or suspected pregnancy; missed abortion; severe hepatic dysfunction; undiagnosed abnormal genital bleeding; use as pregnancy test

INTERACTIONS
Drug
Bromocriptine: May interfere with the effects of bromocriptine.
Herbal
None known.
Food
None known.

DIAGNOSTIC TEST EFFECTS
May alter results for serum thyroid and liver function tests, prothrombin time, and metapyrone test

SIDE EFFECTS
Frequent
Transient menstrual abnormalities (including spotting, change in menstrual flow or cervical secretions, and amenorrhea) at initiation of therapy
Occasional
Edema, weight change, breast tenderness, nervousness, insomnia, fatigue, dizziness
Rare
Alopecia, depression, dermatologic changes, headache, fever, nausea

SERIOUS REACTIONS
! Thrombophlebitis, pulmonary or cerebral embolism, and retinal thrombosis occur rarely.

NURSING CONSIDERATIONS
Baseline Assessment
- Determine if the patient is hypersensitive to progestins or pregnant before beginning medroxyprogesterone therapy.
- Plan to obtain the patient's blood glucose level, BP, and weight.

Lifespan Considerations
- Medroxyprogesterone use should be avoided during pregnancy, especially in the first 4 months because the drug may cause congenital heart and limb reduction defects in the neonate.
- Medroxyprogesterone is distributed in breast milk.
- Safety and efficacy of medroxyprogesterone have not been established in children.
- No age-related precautions have been noted in the elderly.

Precautions
- Use medroxyprogesterone cautiously in patients with conditions aggravated by fluid retention, includ-

ing asthma, seizures, migraine, and cardiac or renal dysfunction, and in those with diabetes mellitus or history of depression.

Administration and Handling

PO

- Give medroxyprogesterone without regard to meals.

IM

- Shake vial immediately before administering to ensure complete suspension.
- Inject IM only in upper arm or upper outer aspect of buttock. Rarely, a residual lump, change in skin color, or sterile abscess occurs at injection site.

Intervention and Evaluation

- Monitor the patient's weight daily and report weekly gain of 5 pounds or more.
- Monitor the patient's BP periodically.
- Assess the patient for rash and urticaria.
- Immediately report chest pain, migraine headache, numbness of an arm or leg, sudden decrease in vision, sudden shortness of breath, and pain, redness, swelling, or warmth in the calf.

Patient Teaching

- Warn the patient to report chest pain, blood-tinged expectorants, hemoptysis, numbness in the arm or leg, severe headache, severe pain or swelling in the calf, severe abdominal pain or tenderness, sudden loss of vision, or unusually heavy vaginal bleeding.
- Encourage the patient to stop smoking tobacco if he or she is a smoker.

megestrol acetate

See Hormones

progesterone

proe-**jess**-ter-one

(Crinone, Prochieve, Prometrium)

CATEGORY AND SCHEDULE

Pregnancy Risk Category: D

MECHANISM OF ACTION

A natural steroid hormone that promotes mammary gland development and relaxes uterine smooth muscle. **Therapeutic Effect:** Decreases abnormal uterine bleeding; transforms endometrium from proliferative to secretory in an estrogen-primed endometrium.

AVAILABILITY

Capsules (Prometrium): 100 mg, 200 mg.
Injection: 50 mg/ml.
Vaginal Gel (Crinone, Prochieve): 4% (45 mg), 8% (90 mg).

INDICATIONS AND DOSAGES

▸ **Amenorrhea**

PO

Adults. 400 mg daily in evening for 10 days.

IM

Adults. 5–10 mg for 6–8 days. Withdrawal bleeding expected in 48–72 hr if ovarian activity produced proliferative endometrium.

Vaginal

Adults. Apply 45 mg (4% gel) every other day for 6 or fewer doses.

▸ **Abnormal uterine bleeding**

IM

Adults. 5–10 mg for 6 days. When estrogen given concomitantly, begin progesterone after 2 wk of estrogen therapy; discontinue when menstrual flow begins.

▸ Prevention of endometrial hyperplasia

PO

Adults. 200 mg in evening for 12 days per 28-day cycle in combination with daily conjugated estrogen.

▸ Infertility

Vaginal

Adults. 90 mg (8% gel) once a day (twice a day in women with partial or complete ovarian failure).

OFF-LABEL USES

Treatment of corpus luteum dysfunction

CONTRAINDICATIONS

Breast cancer; history of active cerebral apoplexy; thromboembolic disorders or thrombophlebitis; missed abortion; severe hepatic dysfunction; undiagnosed vaginal bleeding; use as a pregnancy test

INTERACTIONS

Drug

Bromocriptine: May interfere with the effects of bromocriptine.

Herbal

None known.

Food

None known.

DIAGNOSTIC TEST EFFECTS

May increase serum LDL and serum alkaline phosphatase levels. May decrease glucose tolerance and HDL concentrations. May cause abnormal serum thyroid, metapyrone, hepatic, and endocrine function test results.

SIDE EFFECTS

Frequent

Breakthrough bleeding or spotting at beginning of therapy, amenorrhea, change in menstrual flow, breast tenderness

Gel: drowsiness

Occasional

Edema, weight gain or loss, rash, pruritus, photosensitivity, skin pigmentation

Rare

Pain or swelling at injection site, acne, depression, alopecia, hirsutism

SERIOUS REACTIONS

! Thrombophlebitis, cerebrovascular disorders, retinal thrombosis, and pulmonary embolism occur rarely.

NURSING CONSIDERATIONS

Baseline Assessment

- Determine if the patient is hypersensitive to progestins or pregnant before beginning progesterone therapy.
- Plan to obtain the patient's blood glucose level, BP, and weight.

Lifespan Considerations

- Progesterone use should be avoided during pregnancy.
- Progesterone is distributed in breast milk.
- Safety and efficacy of progesterone have not been established in children.
- No age-related precautions have been noted in the elderly.

Precautions

- Use progesterone cautiously in patients with conditions aggravated by fluid retention, diabetes mellitus, or a history of depression.

Administration and Handling

PO

- Administer the daily dose in the evening to minimize the effects of dizziness and drowsiness.
- If the dose is taken in the morning, administer it 2 hours after breakfast.

IM

- Store progesterone at room temperature. Shake vial well before withdrawing dose.

• Administer deep IM injection in a large muscle mass. Rarely, a residual lump, change in skin color, or sterile abscess occurs at the injection site.
• Rotate injection sites.

Intervention and Evaluation

• Monitor the patient's weight daily and report weekly gain of more than 5 pounds.
• Monitor the patient's BP periodically.
• Assess the patient for rash and urticaria.
• Immediately report chest pain, migraine headache, peripheral paresthesia, sudden decrease in vision, and sudden shortness of breath, and pain, redness, swelling, or warmth in the calf.
• Note that the patient is receiving progesterone on pathology specimens.

Patient Teaching

• Tell the patient to use sunscreen and to wear protective clothing until her tolerance to sunlight and ultraviolet light has been determined.
• Warn the patient to report abnormal vaginal bleeding or other symptoms.
• Instruct the patient to contact the physician, and stop taking the drug, as prescribed, if she suspects she is pregnant.
• Encourage the patient to stop smoking tobacco if she is a smoker.
• Warn the patient using progesterone vaginal gel form to avoid performing tasks that require mental alertness or motor skills until her response to the drug has been established.

68 Oxytocics

dinoprostone
methylergonovine
mifepristone
oxytocin

Uses: Oxytocic agents are used to induce or augment labor when maternal or fetal need exists. They're also used to control postpartum hemorrhage, cause uterine contractions after cesarean delivery or during other uterine surgery, and to induce therapeutic abortion. In addition, oxytocin is used to promote release of breast milk.

Action: Oxytocics stimulate the frequency and force of contractions of uterine smooth muscle and increase the responsiveness of the uterus closer to term. Some agents, such as oxytocin, stimulate the breasts to release milk by causing myoepithelial cells around the mammary glands to contract.

dinoprostone

dye-noe-**prost**-one
(Cervidil, Prepidil Gel, Prostin E_2)
Do not confuse Cervidil or Prepidil with bepridil, or Prostin with Prostigmin.

CATEGORY AND SCHEDULE

Pregnancy Risk Category: C

MECHANISM OF ACTION

A prostaglandin that directly acts on the myometrium, causing softening and dilation effect of the cervix. **Therapeutic Effect:** Stimulates myometrial contractions in gravid uterus.

PHARMACOKINETICS

Undergoes rapid enzymatic deactivation primarily in maternal lungs. Protein binding: 73%. Primarily excreted in urine. ***Half-life:*** Less than 5 min.

AVAILABILITY

Vaginal Gel (Prepidil): 0.5 mg.
Vaginal Inserts (Cervidil): 10 mg.
Vaginal Suppositories: 20 mg.

INDICATIONS AND DOSAGES

▸ **Abortifacient**

Intravaginal

Adults. 20 mg or one suppository high into vagina. May repeat at 3- to 5-hr intervals until abortion occurs. Do not administer for longer than 2 days.

▸ **Ripening of unfavorable cervix**

Intracervical

Adults. Initially, 0.5 mg (2.5 ml) (Prepidil); if no cervical or uterine response, may repeat 0.5-mg dose in 6 hr. Maximum: 1.5 mg (7.5 ml) for a 24-hr period. Or 10 mg (Cervidil) over 12-hr period; remove upon onset of active labor or 12 hr after insertion.

CONTRAINDICATIONS

Active cardiac, hepatic, pulmonary or renal disease; acute pelvic inflammatory disease; fetal malpresentation; hypersensitivity to dinoprostone or other prostaglandins; significant cephalopelvic disproportion

INTERACTIONS

Drug

Oxytocics: May cause uterine hypertonus, possibly resulting in uterine rupture or cervical laceration.

Herbal

None known.

Food

None known.

DIAGNOSTIC TEST EFFECTS

None known.

SIDE EFFECTS

Frequent

Vomiting (66%), diarrhea (40%), nausea (33%)

Occasional

Headache (10%), chills or shivering (10%), hives, bradycardia, increased uterine pain accompanying abortion, peripheral vasoconstriction

Rare

Flushing, vulvae edema

SERIOUS REACTIONS

! Overdose may cause uterine hypertonicity with spasm and tetanic contraction, leading to cervical laceration or perforation, and uterine rupture or hemorrhage.

NURSING CONSIDERATIONS

Baseline Assessment

- Offer the patient emotional support.
- Obtain orders for antidiarrheals, antiemetics, meperidine, and other pain medication for abdominal cramps when giving the suppository form.
- Assess the patient for uterine activity or vaginal bleeding.
- Assess the patient's Bishop score when giving the vaginal gel. Also, assess the patient's degree of effacement to determine the size of shielded endocervical catheter.

Lifespan Considerations

- The suppository form of dinoprostone is teratogenic; therefore, the abortion must be complete.
- Sustained uterine hyperstimulation due to dinoprostone gel administration may cause adverse effects in the fetus, such as an abnormal heart rate.
- Dinoprostone is not used in children or the elderly.

Precautions

- Use dinoprostone cautiously in patients with anemia, cardiovascular disease, cervicitis, compromised or scarred uterus, diabetes mellitus, epilepsy, hepatic disease, history of asthma, hypertension or hypotension, infected endocervical lesions or acute vaginitis, jaundice, renal disease, or uterine fibroids.

Administration and Handling

Gel

- Refrigerate. Bring to room temperature just before use to avoid forcing warming process.
- Use caution when handling to prevent skin contact. Wash hands thoroughly with soap and water following administration.
- Assemble dosing apparatus as described in manufacturer's insert.
- Place the patient in the dorsal position and use a speculum to visualize the cervix.
- Introduce gel into cervical canal just below level of internal os.
- After administration, have the patient remain in the supine position for at least 15 to 30 minutes to minimize leakage of the drug from the cervical canal.

Suppository

- Keep frozen (less than 4°F [15.6°C]); bring to room temperature just before use. Remove foil wrapper after suppository reaches room temperature.
- Administer only in a hospital

setting, with emergency equipment available.
- Avoid skin contact because of risk of absorption.
- Insert high in the patient's vagina.
- Keep patient supine for 10 minutes after administration.

Intervention and Evaluation

- Check the duration, frequency, and strength of contractions in the patient receiving the suppository form.
- Monitor vital signs of the patient receiving the suppository form every 15 minutes until stable, then hourly until abortion is complete.
- Check the resting uterine tone of the patient receiving the suppository form.
- Expect to give medications to relieve GI adverse effects, if indicated, or abdominal cramps in the patient receiving the suppository form.
- Monitor character of the cervix, including dilation and effacement; fetal status, including heart rate; and uterine activity, including the onset of uterine contractions, of the patient receiving the vaginal gel.
- Have the patient receiving the vaginal gel remain recumbent for 12 hours after application with continuous electronic monitoring of fetal heart rate and uterine activity.
- Record vital signs of the patient receiving he vaginal gel at least hourly in the presence of uterine activity.
- Reassess the Bishop score of the patient receiving the vaginal gel.

Patient Teaching

- Warn the patient receiving the suppository form to notify the physician if chills, fever, foul-smelling or increased vaginal discharge, or uterine cramps or pain occurs.

methylergonovine

meth-ill-er-goe-**noe**-veen
(Methergine)

CATEGORY AND SCHEDULE

Pregnancy Risk Category: C

MECHANISM OF ACTION

An ergot alkaloid that stimulates alpha-adrenergic and serotonin receptors, producing arterial vasoconstriction. Causes vasospasm of coronary arteries and directly stimulates uterine muscle. **Therapeutic Effect:** Increases strength and frequency of uterine contractions. Decreases uterine bleeding.

PHARMACOKINETICS

Route	Onset	Peak	Duration
PO	5–10 min	N/A	N/A
IV	Immediate	N/A	3 hr
IM	2–5 min	N/A	N/A

Rapidly absorbed from the GI tract after IM administration. Distributed rapidly to plasma, extracellular fluid, and tissues. Metabolized in the liver and undergoes first-pass effect. Primarily excreted in urine. ***Half-life:*** IV (alpha phase), 2–3 min or less; IV (beta phase), 20–30 min or longer.

AVAILABILITY

Tablets: 0.2 mg.
Injection: 0.2 mg/ml.

INDICATIONS AND DOSAGES

▸ **Prevention and treatment of postpartum and postabortion hemorrhage due to atony or involution**

PO

Adults. 0.2 mg 3–4 times a day. Continue for up to 7 days.

IV, IM
Adults. Initially, 0.2 mg. May repeat q2–4h for no more than a total of 5 doses.

OFF-LABEL USES
Treatment of incomplete abortion

CONTRAINDICATIONS
Hypertension, pregnancy, toxemia, untreated hypocalcemia

INTERACTIONS
Drug
Vasoconstrictors, vasopressors: May increase the effects of methylergonovine.
Herbal
None known.
Food
None known.

DIAGNOSTIC TEST EFFECTS
May decrease serum prolactin concentration.

IV INCOMPATIBILITIES
No information available for Y-site administration.

IV COMPATIBILITIES
Heparin, potassium

SIDE EFFECTS
Frequent
Nausea, uterine cramping, vomiting
Occasional
Abdominal pain, diarrhea, dizziness, diaphoresis, tinnitus, bradycardia, chest pain
Rare
Allergic reaction, such as rash and itching; dyspnea; severe or sudden hypertension

SERIOUS REACTIONS
! Severe hypertensive episodes may result in CVA, serious arrhythmias, and seizures. Hypertensive effects are more frequent with patient susceptibility, rapid IV administration, and concurrent use of regional anesthesia or vasoconstrictors.
! Peripheral ischemia may lead to gangrene.

NURSING CONSIDERATIONS
Baseline Assessment
- Determine the patient's BP, pulse rate, and serum calcium level.
- Assess the patient's bleeding before methylergonovine administration.

Lifespan Considerations
- Methylergonovine use is contraindicated during pregnancy. Small amounts of the drug are distributed in breast milk.
- Safety and efficacy of methylergonovine use in children or the elderly are unknown.

Precautions
- Use methylergonovine cautiously in patients with coronary artery disease, hepatic or renal impairment, occlusive peripheral vascular disease, or sepsis.

Administration and Handling
◀ALERT▶ Methylergonovine should never be used for induction or augmentation of labor.
- May give PO, IV, or IM.
- Refrigerate ampules.
- Initial dose may be given parenterally, followed by an oral regimen.

IV
- Use IV route in life-threatening situations only, as prescribed.
- Dilute drug with 0.9% NaCl to a volume of 5 ml.
- Give over at least 1 minute, carefully monitoring the patient's BP.

Intervention and Evaluation
- Monitor the patient's bleeding, BP, pulse rate, and uterine tone every 15 minutes until she has been stable for 1 to 2 hours.

• Assess the patient's extremities for color, movement, pain, and warmth.
• Report chest pain promptly.
• Assist the patient with ambulation if dizziness occurs.

Patient Teaching

• Urge the patient to avoid smoking because of added effects of vasoconstriction.
• Warn the patient to report increased bleeding, cold or pale feet or hands, cramping, or foul-smelling lochia.
• Instruct the patient to report if pale cold extremeties occur. Explain to the patient that this drug may diminish circulation.

mifepristone

miff-eh-**pris**-tone
(Mifeprex)
Do not confuse Mifeprex with Mirapex, or mifepristone with misoprostol.

CATEGORY AND SCHEDULE

Pregnancy Risk Category: X

MECHANISM OF ACTION

An abortifacient that has antiprogestational activity resulting from competitive interaction with progesterone. Inhibits the activity of endogenous or exogenous progesterone. Also has antiglucocorticoid and weak antiandrogenic activity. **Therapeutic Effect:** Terminates pregnancy.

AVAILABILITY

Tablets: 200 mg.

INDICATIONS AND DOSAGES

▸ **Termination of pregnancy**

PO

Adults. Day 1: 600 mg as single dose. Day 3: 400 mcg misoprostol. Day 14: Post-treatment examination.

OFF-LABEL USES

Cushing's syndrome, endometriosis, intrauterine fetal death or nonviable early pregnancy, postcoital contraception or contragestation, unresectable meningioma

CONTRAINDICATIONS

Chronic adrenal failure, concurrent long-term steroid or anticoagulant therapy, confirmed or suspected ectopic pregnancy, intrauterine device (IUD) in place, hemorrhagic disorders, inherited porphyria

INTERACTIONS

Drug

Carbamazepine, phenobarbital, phenytoin, rifampin: May increase the metabolism of mifepristone.
Erythromycin, itraconazole, ketoconazole: May inhibit the metabolism of mifepristone.

Herbal

St. John's wort: May increase the metabolism of mifepristone.

Food

Grapefruit, grapefruit juice: May inhibit the metabolism of mifepristone.

DIAGNOSTIC TEST EFFECTS

May decrease Hgb level and Hct and RBC count.

SIDE EFFECTS

Frequent (greater than 10%)

Headache, dizziness, abdominal pain, nausea, vomiting, diarrhea, fatigue

Occasional (10%–3%)

Uterine hemorrhage, insomnia, vaginitis, dyspepsia, back pain, fever, viral infections, rigors

Rare (2%–1%)
Anxiety, syncope, anemia, asthenia, leg pain, sinusitis, leukorrhea

SERIOUS REACTIONS

! None known.

NURSING CONSIDERATIONS

Baseline Assessment

- Determine if the patient is taking anticonvulsants, erythromycin, itraconazole, ketoconazole, or rifampin because these drugs may inhibit the metabolism of mifepristone.
- Ask the patient if she has an IUD in place. Mifepristone should not be given until an in-place IUD has been removed.
- Make sure that an ectopic pregnancy has been ruled out.

Precautions

- Use mifepristone cautiously in patients older than 35 years of age or who smoke more than 10 cigarettes a day.
- Use cautiously in patients with cardiovascular disease, diabetes, hepatic or renal impairment, hypertension, or severe anemia.

Administration and Handling

◀ALERT▶ Treatment with mifepristone and misoprostol requires three office visits.

Intervention and Evaluation

- Monitor the patient's Hgb level and Hct.

Patient Teaching

- Explain the treatment procedure, its effects, and the need for a follow-up visit.
- Tell the patient that she may experience uterine cramping and vaginal bleeding.

oxytocin

ox-ee-**toe**-sin
(Pitocin, Syntocinon INJ[AUS])
Do not confuse Pitocin with Pitressin.

CATEGORY AND SCHEDULE

Pregnancy Risk Category: X

MECHANISM OF ACTION

An oxytocic that affects uterine myofibril activity and stimulates mammary smooth muscle.
Therapeutic Effect: Contracts uterine smooth muscle. Enhances lactation.

PHARMACOKINETICS

Route	Onset	Peak	Duration
IV	Immediate	N/A	1 hr
IM	3–5 min	N/A	2–3 hr

Rapidly absorbed through nasal mucous membranes. Protein binding: 30%. Distributed in extracellular fluid. Metabolized in the liver and kidney. Primarily excreted in urine. ***Half-life:*** 1–6 min.

AVAILABILITY

Injection: 10 units/ml.
Nasal Spray: 40 units/ml

INDICATIONS AND DOSAGES

▸ **Induction or stimulation of labor**
IV
Adults. 0.5–1 milliunits/min. May gradually increase in increments of 1–2 milliunits/min. Rates of 9–10 milliunits/min are rarely required.

▸ **Abortion**
IV
Adults. 10–20 milliunits/min. Maximum: 30 units/12 hr dose.

▸ **Control of postpartum bleeding**
IV Infusion
Adults. 10–40 units in 1,000 ml IV fluid at a rate sufficient to control uterine atony.
IM
Adults. 10 units (total dose) after delivery.

CONTRAINDICATIONS

Adequate uterine activity that fails to progress, cephalopelvic disproportion, fetal distress without imminent delivery, grand multiparity, hyperactive or hypertonic uterus, obstetric emergencies that favor surgical intervention, prematurity, unengaged fetal head, unfavorable fetal position or presentation, when vaginal delivery is contraindicated, such as active genital herpes infection, placenta previa, or cord presentation

INTERACTIONS

Drug

Caudal block anesthetics, vasopressors: May increase pressor effects.
Other oxytocics: May cause cervical lacerations, uterine hypertonus, or uterine rupture.

Herbal

None known.

Food

None known.

DIAGNOSTIC TEST EFFECTS

None known.

IV INCOMPATIBILITIES

No known incompatibilities via Y-site administration.

IV COMPATIBILITIES

Heparin, insulin, multivitamins, potassium chloride

SIDE EFFECTS

Occasional

Tachycardia, premature ventricular contractions, hypotension, nausea, vomiting

Rare

Nasal: Lacrimation or tearing, nasal irritation, rhinorrhea, unexpected uterine bleeding or contractions

SERIOUS REACTIONS

! Hypertonicity may occur with tearing of the uterus, increased bleeding, abruptio placentae, and cervical and vaginal lacerations.
! In the fetus, bradycardia, CNS or brain damage, trauma due to rapid propulsion, low Apgar score at 5 minutes, and retinal hemorrhage occur rarely.
! Prolonged IV infusion of oxytocin with excessive fluid volume has caused severe water intoxication with seizures, coma, and death.

NURSING CONSIDERATIONS

Baseline Assessment

- Assess the patient's BP and pulse rate, and fetal heart rate.
- Determine the duration, frequency, and strength of uterine contractions.

Lifespan Considerations

- Oxytocin should be used as indicated, and is not known to cause fetal abnormalities.
- Oxytocin is present in small amounts in breast milk. Nasal oxytocin is used only for initial breast milk propulsion and ejection during the first postpartal week, and is not meant for continued use. Oxytocin is not recommended for use in pregnant patients because it may precipitate contractions and abortions.
- Oxytocin is not used in children or the elderly.

Precautions

- Induction of labor should be for medical, not elective, reasons.

Administration and Handling

IV

- Store at room temperature.
- Dilute 10 to 40 units (1 to 4 ml) in 1,000 ml of 0.9% NaCl, lactated Ringer's solution, or D_5W to provide a concentration of 10 to 40 milliunits/ml solution.
- Give by IV infusion and use an infusion device to carefully control prescribed rate of flow.

Intervention and Evaluation

- Monitor the patient's BP and pulse and respiration rates; uterine contractions, including duration, frequency, and strength; and fetal heart rate every 15 minutes.
- Notify the physician of uterine contractions that last longer than 1 minute, occur more frequently than every 2 minutes, or stop.
- Carefully monitor and record the patient's intake and output.
- Be alert to potential water intoxication.
- Carefully monitor the patient for unexpected or increased blood loss.

Patient Teaching

- Inform the patient and family about the progress of labor.
- Teach the patient the proper use of oxytocin nasal spray.
- Explain that the drug will be present in breast milk, so breast-feeding isn't recommended.
- Tell the patient that oxytocin can be used during the first postpartal week to promote milk ejection but that its use beyond the first postpartal week isn't recommended.

69 Pituitary Hormones

desmopressin
somatrem, somatropin
vasopressin

Uses: Pituitary hormones have various uses. *Antidiuretic hormones,* such as desmopressin and vasopressin, are used to treat diabetes insipidus, postoperative abdominal distention, nocturnal enuresis, hemophilia A, and von Willebrand's disease. *Growth hormones,* such as somatrem and somatropin, are used to treat pediatric growth hormone (GH) deficiency, chronic renal insufficiency, Turner's syndrome, and cachexia or wasting in patients with acquired immunodeficiency syndrome.

Action: The actions of pituitary hormones also vary greatly. *Antidiuretic hormones* act on the collecting ducts of the kidneys to increase their permeability to water, resulting in increased water reabsorption. In higher concentrations, these agents constrict arterioles throughout the body, which increases blood pressure. *Growth hormones* cause growth in almost all body tissues: a childhood deficiency of GH results in dwarfism; an excess results in acromegaly. Metabolic effects of these agents include an increased rate of protein synthesis, mobilization of fatty acids from adipose tissue, and a decreased rate of glucose use.

desmopressin

des-moe-**press**-in
(DDAVP, Minirin[AUS], Octostim [CAN], Stimate)

CATEGORY AND SCHEDULE

Pregnancy Risk Category: B

MECHANISM OF ACTION

A synthetic pituitary hormone that increases reabsorption of water by increasing permeability of collecting ducts of the kidneys. Also serves as a plasminogen activator. **Therapeutic Effect:** Increases plasma factor VIII (antihemophilic factor). Decreases urinary output.

PHARMACOKINETICS

Route	Onset	Peak	Duration
PO	1 hr	2–7 hr	6–8 hr
IV	15–30 min	1.5–3 hr	N/A
Intranasal	15 min–1 hr	1–5 hr	5–21 hr

Poorly absorbed after oral or nasal administration. Metabolism: Unknown. ***Half-life:*** Oral: 1.5–2.5 hr. Intranasal: 3.3–3.5 hr. IV: 0.4–4 hr.

AVAILABILITY

Tablets (DDAVP): 0.1 mg, 0.2 mg.
Injection (DDAVP): 4 mcg/ml.
Nasal Solution (DDAVP): 100 mcg/ml.

Nasal Spray (Stimate): 1.5 mg/ml (150 mcg/spray).
Nasal Spray (DDAVP): 100 mcg/ml (10 mcg/spray).

INDICATIONS AND DOSAGES

▸ **Primary nocturnal enuresis**

PO

Children 12 yr and older. 0.2–0.6 mg once before bedtime.

Intranasal

Children 6 yr and older. Initially, 20 mcg (0.2 ml) at bedtime; use one-half dose in each nostril. Adjust to maximum of 40 mcg/day.

▸ **Central cranial diabetes insipidus**

PO

Adults, Elderly, Children 12 yr and older. Initially, 0.05 mg twice a day. Range: 0.1–1.2 mg/day in 2–3 divided doses.

Children younger than 12 yr. Initially, 0.05 mg; then twice a day. Range: 0.1–0.8 mg daily.

Intranasal

Adults, Elderly, Children older than 12 yr. 5–40 mcg (0.05–0.4 ml) in 1–3 doses/day.

Children 3 mo–12 yr. Initially, 5 mcg (0.05 ml)/day. Range: 5–30 mcg (0.05–0.3 ml)/day.

IV, Subcutaneous

Adults, Elderly, Children 12 yr and older. 2–4 mcg/day in 2 divided doses or 1/10 of maintenance intranasal dose.

▸ **Hemophilia A, Von Willebrand's Disease (Type I)**

IV Infusion

Adults, Elderly, Children weighing more than 10 kg. 0.3 mcg/kg diluted in 50 ml 0.9% NaCl.

Children weighing 10 kg and less. 0.3 mcg/kg diluted in 10 ml 0.9% NaCl.

Intranasal

Adults, Elderly, Children 12 yr and older weighing more than 50 kg. 300 mcg; use 1 spray in each nostril.

Adults, Elderly, Children 12 yr and older weighing 50 kg and less. 150 mcg as a single spray.

CONTRAINDICATIONS

Hemophilia A with factor VIII levels less than 5%; hemophilia B; severe type I, type IIB, or platelet-type von Willebrand's disease

INTERACTIONS

Drug

Carbamazepine, chlorpropamide, clofibrate: May increase the effects of desmopressin.

Demeclocycline, lithium, norepinephrine: May decrease effects of desmopressin.

Herbal

None known.

Food

None known.

DIAGNOSTIC TEST EFFECTS

None known.

SIDE EFFECTS

Occasional

IV: Pain, redness, or swelling at injection site; headache; abdominal cramps; vulval pain; flushed skin; mild BP elevation; nausea with high dosages

Nasal: Rhinorrhea, nasal congestion, slight BP elevation

SERIOUS REACTIONS

! Water intoxication or hyponatremia, marked by headache, somnolence, confusion, decreased urination, rapid weight gain, seizures, and coma, may occur in overhydration. Children, elderly patients, and infants are especially at risk.

NURSING CONSIDERATIONS

Baseline Assessment

• Establish the patient's BP, serum electrolyte levels, pulse rate, urine specific gravity, and weight.
• Plan to check the patient's laboratory values for factor VIII coagulant concentration (in hemophilia A and von Willebrand's disease), and bleeding times.

Lifespan Considerations

• Use cautiously in neonates younger than 3 months old because this age-group is at increased risk for fluid balance problems.
• Careful fluid restrictions are recommended in infants.
• The elderly are at increased risk for hyponatremia and water intoxication.

Precautions

• Use desmopressin cautiously in patients with fluid or electrolyte imbalances, coronary artery disease, hypertensive cardiovascular disease, or predisposition to thrombus formation.

Administration and Handling

PO
• Store away from light and excessive heat.

IV
• Refrigerate. Desmopressin is stable for 2 weeks at room temperature.
• For IV infusion, dilute in 10 to 50 ml 0.9% NaCl and prepare to infuse over 15 to 30 minutes.
• For preoperative use, administer 30 minutes before procedure, as prescribed.
• Monitor the patient's BP and pulse during infusion.
• Remember that the IV dose is one tenth the intranasal dose.

Intranasal
• Refrigerate DDAVP nasal solution and Stimate nasal spray. Nasal solution and Stimate nasal spray are stable for 3 weeks at room temperature if unopened.
• DDAVP nasal spray is stable at room temperature.
• To administer, draw up a measured quantity of desmopressin with a calibrated catheter (rhinyle). Insert one end in the patient's nose and have the patient blow on the other end to deposit the solution deep in the nasal cavity. For infants, young children, and obtunded patients, an air-filled syringe may be attached to the catheter to deposit the solution.

Subcutaneous
• Estimate therapeutic response by adequacy of sleep duration.
• Expect to adjust morning and evening dosages separately.

Intervention and Evaluation

• Check the patient's BP and pulse rate during IV infusion.
• Monitor the patient for signs and symptoms of diabetes insipidus. Also assess serum electrolyte levels, fluid intake, serum osmolality, urine volume, urine specific gravity, and weight.
• Assess the patient's factor VIII antigen level, APTT, and factor VIII activity level for hemophilia.

Patient Teaching

• Caution the patient to avoid overhydration.
• Teach the patient the proper technique for intranasal administration.
• Warn the patient to report abdominal cramps, headache, heartburn, nausea, or shortness of breath.
• Tell the parent of a child treated for nocturnal enuresis to carefully monitor the child's sleep pattern.

somatrem

soe-ma-trem
(Protropin)
Do not confuse Protropin with Proloprim, Protamine, or Protopam.

somatropin

soe-mah-**troe**-pin
(Genotropin, Humatrope, Norditropin, Nutropin, Nutropin AQ, Nutropin Depot, Saizen, Serostim, Zorbtive)
Do not confuse somatropin with sumatriptan.

CATEGORY AND SCHEDULE

Pregnancy Risk Category: B (for Genotropin, Saizen, Serostim, Zorbtive); C (for Humatrope, Norditropin, Nutropin, Nutropin AQ, Nutropin Depot, Protopin)

MECHANISM OF ACTION

A polypeptide hormone that stimulates cartilagenous growth areas of long bones, increases the number and size of skeletal muscle cells, influences the size of organs, and increases RBC mass by stimulating erythropoietin. Influences the metabolism of carbohydrates (decreases insulin sensitivity), fats (mobilizes fatty acids), minerals (retains phosphorus, sodium, potassium by promotion of cell growth), and proteins (increases protein synthesis). **Therapeutic Effect:** Stimulates growth.

PHARMACOKINETICS

Well absorbed after subcutaneous or IM administration. Localized primarily in the kidneys and liver. ***Half-life:*** IV, 20–30 min; subcutaneous, IM, 3–5 hr.

AVAILABILITY

Injection, Powder for Reconstitution (somatrem [Protropin]): 5 mg.
Injection, Powder for Reconstitution (somatropin [Genotropin]): 1.5 mg, 5.8 mg.
Injection, Powder for Reconstitution (somatropin [Humatrope]): 5 mg, 6 mg, 12 mg, 24 mg.
Injection, Powder for Reconstitution (somatropin [Norditropin]): 4 mg, 8 mg.
Injection, Powder for Reconstitution (somatropin [Nutropin]): 5 mg, 10 mg.
Injection, Powder for Reconstitution (somatropin [Nutropin Depot]): 13.5 mg, 18 mg, 22.5 mg.
Injection, Powder for Reconstitution (somatropin [Saizen]): 5 mg, 8.8 mg.
Injection, Powder for Reconstitution (somatropin [Serostim]): 4 mg, 5 mg, 6 mg.
Injection, Powder for Reconstitution (somatropin [Zorbtive]): 4 mg, 5 mg, 6 mg, 8.8 mg.
Injection Solution: (somatropin [Nutropin AQ]): 5 mg/ml.

INDICATIONS AND DOSAGES

▸ **Growth hormone deficiency**

Subcutaneous

Adults. 0.006 mg/kg Humatrope, Nutropin, or Nutropin AQ once daily; or 0.04–0.08 mg/kg Genotropin weekly divided into 6–7 equal doses/wk.

Children. 0.3 mg/kg Protopin weekly divided into daily doses; 0.16–0.24 mg/kg Genotropin weekly divided into daily doses; 0.18–0.3 mg/kg Humatrope weekly divided into alternate-day doses or 6 doses/wk; 0.024–0.036 mg/kg/dose Norditropin 6–7 times/wk; 0.3–0.7 mg/kg Nutropin weekly divided into daily doses; 0.06 mg/kg Saizen 3 times/wk; or 0.75 mg/kg Nutropin

Depot twice monthly or 1.5 mg/kg once monthly.

▸ **Chronic renal insufficiency**
Subcutaneous
Children. 0.35 mg/kg Nutropin or Nutropin AQ weekly divided into daily doses.

▸ **Turner syndrome**
Subcutaneous
Children. 0.375 mg/kg Humatrope, Nutropin, or Nutropin AQ weekly divided into equal doses 3–7 times/wk.

▸ **AIDS-related wasting**
Subcutaneous
Adults weighing more than 55 kg. 6 mg once a day at bedtime.
Adults weighing 45–55 kg. 5 mg once a day at bedtime.
Adults weighing 35–44 kg. 4 mg once a day at bedtime.
Adults weighing less than 35 kg. 0.1 mg/kg once a day at bedtime.

▸ **Short bowel syndrome**
Subcutaneous
Adults. 0.1 mg/kg/day (Zorbtive). Maximum: 8 mg/day.

CONTRAINDICATIONS

None known.

INTERACTIONS

Drug

Corticosteroids: May inhibit growth response.

Herbal

None known.

Food

None known.

DIAGNOSTIC TEST EFFECTS

May increase serum alkaline phosphatase, inorganic phosphorus, and parathyroid hormone levels. May decrease glucose tolerance. May slightly decrease thyroid function.

SIDE EFFECTS

Frequent
Otitis media, other ear disorders (with Turner's syndrome)

Occasional
Carpal tunnel syndrome; gynecomastia; myalgia; swelling of hands, feet, or legs; fatigue; asthenia

Rare
Rash, pruritus, altered vision, headache, nausea, vomiting, injection site pain and swelling, abdominal pain, hip or knee pain

SERIOUS REACTIONS

! None known.

NURSING CONSIDERATIONS

Baseline Assessment

• Obtain the patient's baseline thyroid function results and blood glucose level.

Lifespan Considerations

• It is unknown if somatrem and somatropin are distributed in breast milk.
• No age-related considerations have been noted in children or the elderly.

Precautions

• Use somatrem and somatropin cautiously in patients with diabetes mellitus, malignancy, or untreated hypothyroidism.

Administration and Handling

◂ **ALERT** ▸ If somatrem will be administered to a neonate, reconstitute it only with sterile water for injection because the preservative benzyl alcohol has been associated with fatal toxicity (such as gasping syndrome) in premature infants. Use only 1 dose per vial and discard any unused portion.

Subcutaneous (somatrem [Protopin])
• Store somatrem in the refrigerator. Do not freeze. Use reconstituted vials within 14 days. Don't use the solution if it becomes cloudy.

• Reconstitute each 5-mg vial of somatrem with 1 to 5 ml bacteriostatic water for injection (containing benzyl alcohol) or each 10-mg vial with 1 to 10 ml bacteriostatic water for injection (containing benzyl alcohol). Aim the stream of diluent against the glass wall of the vial. Swirl the vial gently until the contents have completely dissolved. Don't shake the vial (results in a cloudy solution). The solution should be clear immediately after reconstitution. If the solution is cloudy immediately after reconstitution or refrigeration, do not use it.

Subcutaneous (somatropin [Humatrope])

• Refrigerate—don't freeze—vials of Humatrope. The reconstituted solution is stable for 14 days if reconstituted with bacteriostatic water for injection and refrigerated, or for 24 hours if reconstituted with sterile water for injection and refrigerated. Discard the reconstituted solution if it becomes cloudy or contains precipitate.

• Reconstitute Humatrope vials with 1.5 to 5 ml of the diluent provided. Aim the stream of diluent against the glass wall of the vial. Swirl the vial gently until the contents have completely dissolved. Don't shake the vial.

• To reconstitute Humatrope cartridges, use only the diluent syringe and diluent connector. Don't reconstitute with the diluent provided with Humatrope vials.

Subcutaneous (somatropin [Nutropin])

• Refrigerate—don't freeze—vials of Nutropin. The reconstituted solution is stable for 14 days if reconstituted with bacteriostatic water for injection and stored in the refrigerator. Discard the reconstituted solution if it becomes cloudy or contains precipitate.

• Reconstitute each 5-mg vial of Nutropin with 1 to 5 ml bacteriostatic water for injection (containing benzyl alcohol) or each 10-mg vial with 1 to 10 ml bacteriostatic water for injection (containing benzyl alcohol). Aim the stream of diluent against the glass wall of the vial. Swirl the vial gently until the contents have completely dissolved. Don't shake the vial (results in a cloudy solution). The solution should be clear immediately after reconstitution. Discard the solution if it's cloudy immediately after reconstitution or refrigeration.

Intervention and Evaluation

• Monitor the patient's bone density, growth rate, parathyroid and thyroid function, renal function, blood glucose level, and serum calcium and phosphorus levels.

• Observe the AIDS patient for decreased wasting.

Patient Teaching

• Teach the patient how to reconstitute the drug for administration and how to handle and dispose of needles.

• Advise the patient to report a limp, pain in the hip or knee, severe headache, or visual disturbances.

• Explain the need for regular follow-up visits with the physician.

vasopressin

vay-soe-**press**-in
(Pitressin, Pressyn[CAN])
Do not confuse Pitressin with Pitocin.

CATEGORY AND SCHEDULE

Pregnancy Risk Category: B

MECHANISM OF ACTION

A posterior pituitary hormone that increases reabsorption of water by the renal tubules. Increases water permeability at the distal tubule and collecting duct. Directly stimulates smooth muscle in the GI tract.
Therapeutic Effect: Causes peristalsis and vasoconstriction.

PHARMACOKINETICS

Route	Onset	Peak	Duration
IV	N/A	N/A	0.5–1 hr
IM, Subcutaneous	1–2 hr	N/A	2–8 hr

Distributed throughout extracellular fluid. Metabolized in the liver and kidney. Primarily excreted in urine. ***Half-life:*** 10–20 min.

AVAILABILITY

Injection: 20 units/ml.

INDICATIONS AND DOSAGES

▸ **Cardiac arrest**
IV
Adults, Elderly. 40 units as a one-time bolus.
▸ **Diabetes insipidus**
IV Infusion
Adults, Children. 0.5 mUnits/kg/hr. May double dose q30min. Maximum: 10 mUnits/kg/hr.
IM, Subcutaneous
Adults, Elderly. 5–10 units 2–4 times a day. Range: 5–60 unit/day.
Children. 2.5–10 units, 2–4 times a day.
▸ **Abdominal distention, intestinal paresis**
IM
Adults, Elderly. Initially, 5 units. Subsequent doses, 10 units q3–4h.
▸ **GI hemorrhage**
IV Infusion
Adults, Elderly. Initially, 0.2–0.4 unit/min progressively increased to 0.9 unit/min.
Children. 0.002–0.005 unit/kg/min. Titrate as needed. Maximum: 0.01 unit/kg/min.
▸ **Vasodilatory shock**
IV
Adults, Elderly. Initially, 0.04 - 0.1 unit/min. Titrate to desired effect.

OFF-LABEL USES

Adjunct in treatment of acute, massive hemorrhage

CONTRAINDICATIONS

None known.

INTERACTIONS

Drug
Alcohol, demeclocycline, lithium, norepinephrine: May decrease the effects of vasopressin.
Carbamazepine, chlorpropamide, clofibrate: May increase the effects of vasopressin.
Herbal
None known.
Food
None known.

DIAGNOSTIC TEST EFFECTS

None known.

IV INCOMPATIBILITIES

Amphotericin B complex (Abelcet, AmBisome, Amphotec), diazepam

(Valium), etomidate (Amidate), furosemide (Lasix), thiopentothal

IV COMPATIBILITIES

Dobutamine (Dobutrex), dopamine (Intropin), heparin, lorazepam (Ativan), midazolam (Versed), milrinone (Primacor), verapamil (Calan, Isoptin)

SIDE EFFECTS

Frequent

Pain at injection site (with vasopressin tannate)

Occasional

Abdominal cramps, nausea, vomiting, diarrhea, dizziness, diaphoresis, pale skin, circumoral pallor, tremors, headache, eructation, flatulence

Rare

Chest pain; confusion; allergic reaction, including rash or hives, pruritus, wheezing or difficulty breathing, facial and peripheral edema; sterile abscess (with vasopressin tannate)

SERIOUS REACTIONS

! Anaphylaxis, MI, and water intoxication have occurred.

! The elderly and very young are at higher risk for water intoxication.

NURSING CONSIDERATIONS

Baseline Assessment

• Establish the patient's BP, serum electrolyte levels, pulse rate, urine specific gravity, and weight.

Lifespan Considerations

• Vasopressin should be used cautiously in breast-feeding women.

• Vasopressin should be used cautiously in children and the elderly because of the risk of water intoxication and hyponatremia in these age-groups.

Precautions

• Use vasopressin cautiously in patients with arteriosclerosis, asthma, cardiac disease, goiter with cardiac complications, migraine, nephritis, renal disease, seizures, or vascular disease.

Administration and Handling

◀ALERT▶ May administer intranasally on cotton pledgets, or by nasal spray; individualize dosage.

IV

• Store at room temperature.

• Dilute with D_5W or 0.9% NaCl to concentration of 0.1 to 1 unit/ml.

• Give as IV infusion.

IM, Subcutaneous

• Give with 1 to 2 glasses of water to reduce side effects.

Intervention and Evaluation

• Monitor the patient's fluid intake and output closely, and restrict the patient's intake, as ordered, to prevent water intoxication.

• Weigh the patient daily, if indicated.

• Check the patient's BP and pulse rate 2 times a day.

• Monitor the patient's serum electrolyte levels and urine specific gravity.

• Evaluate the patient's injection site for abscess, erythema, and pain.

• Report side effects experienced by the patient; a reduced dosage may be required.

• Be alert for early signs of water intoxication, such as somnolence, headache, and listlessness.

• If allergic symptoms or chest pain occurs, withhold the medication, as prescribed, and notify the physician immediately.

Patient Teaching

• Warn the patient to report chest pain, headache, shortness of breath, or other symptoms.

• Stress to the patient the importance of monitoring his or her fluid intake and output.

• Urge the patient to avoid alcohol during vasopressin therapy.

70 Thyroid Agents

levothyroxine
liothyronine (T3)
methimazole
propylthiouracil

Uses: Two *thyroid hormones*—levothyroxine and liothyronine—are used to treat primary or secondary hypothyroidism, myxedema, cretinism, or simple goiter. Levothyroxine is also used in thyroid cancer management. Levothyroxine and liothyronine are used in thyroid suppression tests. *Propylthiouracil* and *methimazole* are used to treat hyperthyroidism, especially before thyroid surgery or radioactive iodine therapy.

Action: *Thyroid hormones* are essential for normal growth, development, and energy metabolism. They promote growth and development by controlling DNA transcription and protein synthesis, which are required for nervous system development. These agents stimulate energy use by increasing the basal metabolic rate, which increases oxygen consumption and heat production. They also act as cardiac stimulants by increasing the heart rate, force of cardiac contractions, and cardiac output. *Propylthiouracil* blocks the oxidation of iodine in the thyroid gland, thereby preventing the synthesis of thyroid hormones.

COMBINATION PRODUCTS

THYROLAR: levothyroxine/liothyronine 12.5 mcg/3.1 mcg; 25 mcg/6.25 mcg; 50 mcg/12.5 mcg; 100 mcg/25 mcg; 150 mcg/37.5 mcg.

levothyroxine

lee-voe-thye-**rox**-een
(Droxine[AUS], Eltroxin[CAN], Eutroxsig [AUS], Levothroid, Levoxyl, Novothyrox[CAN], Oroxine[AUS], Synthroid, Unithroid)
Do not confuse levothyroxine with liothyronine.

CATEGORY AND SCHEDULE

Pregnancy Risk Category: A

MECHANISM OF ACTION

A synthetic isomer of thyroxine involved in normal metabolism, growth, and development, especially of the CNS in infants. Possesses catabolic and anabolic effects. **Therapeutic Effect:** Increases basal metabolic rate, enhances gluconeogenesis and stimulates protein synthesis.

PHARMACOKINETICS

Variable, incomplete absorption from the GI tract. Protein binding: greater than 99%. Widely distributed. Deiodinated in peripheral tissues, minimal metabolism in the liver. Eliminated by biliary excretion. ***Half-life:*** 6–7 days.

AVAILABILITY

Tablets (Levo-T, Levothroid, Levoxyl, Synthroid, Unithroid): 0.025 mg, 0.05 mg, 0.075 mg, 0.088 mg, 0.1 mg, 0.112 mg, 0.125 mg, 0.137 mg, 0.15 mg, 0.175 mg, 0.2 mg, 0.3 mg.
Injection (Synthroid): 200 mcg, 500 mcg.

INDICATIONS AND DOSAGES

▸ **Hypothyroidism**
PO
Adults, Elderly. Initially, 12.5–50 mcg. May increase by 25–50 mcg/day q2–4wk. Maintenance: 100–200 mcg/day.
Children 13 yr and older. 150 mcg/day.
Children 6–12 yr. 100–125 mcg/day.
Children 1–5 yr. 75–100 mcg/day.
Children 7-11 mo. 50–75 mcg/day.
Children older than 3–6 mo. 25–50 mcg/day.
Children 3 mo and younger. 10–15 mcg/day.

▸ **Thyroid suppression therapy**
PO
Adults, Elderly. 2–6 mcg/kg/day for 7–10 days.

▸ **Thyroid stimulating hormone suppression in thyroid cancer, nodules, euthyroid goiters**
PO
Adults, Elderly. 2–6 mcg/kg/day for 7–10 days.
IV
Adults, Elderly, Children. Initial dosage approximately half the previously established oral dosage.

CONTRAINDICATIONS

Hypersensitivity to tablet components, such as tartrazine; allergy to aspirin; lactose intolerance; MI and thyrotoxicosis uncomplicated by hypothyroidism; treatment of obesity

INTERACTIONS

Drug

Cholestyramine, colestipol: May decrease the absorption of levothyroxine.
Oral anticoagulants: May alter the effects of oral anticoagulants
Sympathomimetics: May increase the risk of coronary insufficiency and the effects of levothyroxine.

Herbal

None known.

Food

None known.

DIAGNOSTIC TEST EFFECTS

None known.

IV INCOMPATIBILITIES

Do not use or mix with other IV solutions.

SIDE EFFECTS

Occasional

Reversible hair loss at the start of therapy (in children)

Rare

Dry skin, GI intolerance, rash, hives, pseudotumor cerebri or severe headache in children

SERIOUS REACTIONS

! Excessive dosage produces signs and symptoms of hyperthyroidism, including weight loss, palpitations, increased appetite, tremors, nervousness, tachycardia, hypertension, headache, insomnia, and menstrual irregularities.
! Cardiac arrhythmias occur rarely.

NURSING CONSIDERATIONS

Baseline Assessment

- Determine if the patient is hypersensitive to aspirin, lactose, or tartrazine.
- Obtain the patient's weight and vital signs.

• Levothyroxine therapy may intensify the signs and symptoms of adrenal insufficiency, diabetes insipidus, diabetes mellitus, and hypopituitarism.
• Administer adrenocortical steroids, as prescribed, before thyroid therapy in patients with coexisting hypoadrenalism and hypothyroidism.

Lifespan Considerations

• Levothyroxine does not cross the placenta and is minimally excreted in breast milk.
• No age-related precautions have been noted in children.
• Use caution in interpreting thyroid function tests in neonates.
• The elderly may be more sensitive to thyroid effects. Individualized dosages are recommended for this patient population.

Precautions

• Use levothyroxine cautiously in elderly patients and patients with angina pectoris, hypertension, or other cardiovascular disease.

Administration and Handling

◀ **ALERT** ▶ Do not use different brands of levothyroxine interchangeably because of problems with bioequivalence among manufacturers.

◀ **ALERT** ▶ Begin therapy with small doses and increase the dosage gradually, as prescribed.

PO

• Give at same time each day to maintain hormone levels.
• Administer before breakfast to prevent insomnia.
• Crush tablets, as needed.

IV

• Store vials at room temperature.
• Reconstitute 200 or 500-mcg vial with 5 ml 0.9% NaCl to provide a concentration of 40 or 100 mcg/ml, respectively; shake until clear.
• Use immediately, and discard unused portion.
• Give each 100 mcg or less over 1 minute.

Intervention and Evaluation

• Monitor the patient's pulse for rate and rhythm. Report a marked increase in pulse rate or one that exceeds 100 beats/minute.
• Assess the patient for nervousness and tremors.
• Evaluate the patient's appetite and sleep pattern.

Patient Teaching

• Caution the patient against discontinuing the drug. Explain to the patient that replacement therapy for hypothyroidism is life-long.
• Stress to the patient that follow-up office visits and thyroid function tests are essential.
• Instruct the patient to take the drug at the same time each day, preferably in the morning.
• Teach the patient to monitor his or her pulse for rate and rhythm. Advise the patient to report a change in rhythm or a pulse rate of 100 beats/minute or more.
• Instruct the patient not to change brands of the drug.
• Warn the patient to promptly report chest pain, insomnia, nervousness, tremors, or weight loss.
• Tell the pediatric patient and his or her caregiver that children may experience reversible hair loss or increased aggressiveness during the first few months of therapy.
• Warn the patient that the full therapeutic effect of the drug may take 1 to 3 weeks to appear.

liothyronine (T3)

lye-oh-**thye**-roe-neen
(Cytomel, Tertroxin[AUS], Triostat)
Do not confuse liothyronine with levothyroxine.

CATEGORY AND SCHEDULE
Pregnancy Risk Category: A

MECHANISM OF ACTION
A synthetic form of triiodothyronine (T_3), a thyroid hormone involved in normal metabolism, growth, and development, especially of the CNS in infants. Possesses catabolic and anabolic effects. **Therapeutic Effect:** Increases basal metabolic rate, enhances gluconeogenesis, and stimulates protein synthesis.

AVAILABILITY
Tablets (Cytomel): 5 mcg, 25 mcg, 50 mcg.
Injection (Triostat): 10 mcg/ml.

INDICATIONS AND DOSAGES
▸ Hypothyroidism
PO
Adults, Elderly. Initially, 25 mcg/day. May increase in increments of 12.5–25 mcg/day q1–2wk. Maximum 100 mcg/day.
Children. Initially, 5 mcg/day. May increase by 5 mcg/day q3–4wk. Maintenance: 100 mcg/day (children older than 3 yr); 50 mcg/day (children 1–3 yr); 20 mcg/day (infants).
▸ Myxedema
PO
Adults, Elderly. Initially, 5 mcg/day. Increase by 5–10 mcg q1–2wk (after 25 mcg/day has been reached, may increase in 12.5-mcg increments). Maintenance: 50–100 mcg/day.
▸ Nontoxic goiter
PO
Adults, Elderly. Initially, 5 mcg/day. Increase by 5–10 mcg/day q1–2wk. When 25 mcg/day has been reached, may increase by 12.5–25 mcg/day q1–2wk. Maintenance: 75 mcg/day.
Children. 5 mcg/day. May increase by 5 mcg q1–2wk. Maintenance: 15–20 mcg/day.
▸ Congenital hypothyroidism
PO
Children. Initially, 5 mcg/day. Increase by 5 mcg/day q3–4 days. Maintenance: Full adult dosage (children older than 3 yr); 50 mcg/day (children 1–3 yr); 20 mcg/day (infants).
▸ T_3 suppression test
PO
Adults, Elderly. 75–100 mcg/day for 7 days; then repeat ^{131}I thyroid uptake test.
▸ Myxedema coma, precoma
IV
Adults, Elderly. Initially, 25–50 mcg (10–20 mcg in patients with cardiovascular disease). Total dose at least 65 mcg/day.

CONTRAINDICATIONS
MI and thyrotoxicosis uncomplicated by hypothyroidism; obesity

INTERACTIONS
Drug
Cholestyramine, colestipol: May decrease the absorption of liothyronine.
Oral anticoagulants: May alter the effects of these drugs.
Sympathomimetics: May increase the risk of coronary insufficiency and the effects of liothyronine.
Herbal
None known.
Food
None known.

DIAGNOSTIC TEST EFFECTS
None known.

SIDE EFFECTS
Occasional
Reversible hair loss at start of therapy (in children)
Rare
Dry skin, GI intolerance, rash, hives, pseudotumor cerebri or severe headache in children

SERIOUS REACTIONS
! Excessive dosage produces signs and symptoms of hyperthyroidism, including weight loss, palpitations, increased appetite, tremors, nervousness, tachycardia, hypertension, headache, insomnia, and menstrual irregularities.
! Cardiac arrhythmias occur rarely.

NURSING CONSIDERATIONS
Baseline Assessment
- Determine if the patient is hypersensitive to aspirin or tartrazine.
- Obtain the patient's weight and vital signs.
- Liothyronine therapy may intensify the signs and symptoms of adrenal insufficiency, diabetes insipidus, diabetes mellitus, and hypopituitarism.
- Administer adrenocortical steroids, as prescribed, before thyroid therapy in patients with coexisting hypoadrenalism and hypothyroidism.

Lifespan Considerations
- Liothyronine does not cross the placenta and is minimally excreted in breast milk.
- No age-related precautions have been noted in children.
- Use caution in interpreting thyroid function test results in neonates.
- The elderly may be more sensitive to thyroid effects. Individualized dosages are recommended for this patient population.

Precautions
- Use liothyronine cautiously in patients with adrenal insufficiency, cardiovascular disease, coronary artery disease, diabetes insipidus, or diabetes mellitus.

Administration and Handling
◀ALERT▶ Initial and subsequent dosages are based on the patient's clinical status and response.
◀ALERT▶ Do not use different brands of liothyronine interchangeably because of problems with bioequivalence among manufacturers.

IV
- Administer IV dose over 4 hours but no longer than 12 hours apart.

Intervention and Evaluation
- Monitor the patient's pulse for rate and rhythm. Report a marked increase in pulse rate or one that exceeds 100 beats/minute.
- Assess the patient for nervousness and tremors.
- Evaluate the patient's appetite and sleep pattern.

Patient Teaching
- Caution the patient against discontinuing the drug. Explain to the patient that replacement therapy for hypothyroidism is life-long.
- Stress to the patient that follow-up office visits and thyroid function tests are essential.
- Instruct the patient to take the drug at the same time each day, preferably in the morning.
- Teach the patient to monitor his or her pulse. Advise the patient to report a change in rhythm, a marked increase in rate, or a pulse of 100 beats/minute or more.
- Tell the patient not to change brands of the drug.
- Warn the patient to promptly report chest pain, insomnia, nervousness, tremors, or weight loss.

• Explain to the pediatric patient and his or her caregiver that children may experience reversible hair loss or increased aggressiveness during the first few months of therapy.

methimazole

meth-**im**-a-zole
(Tapazole)

CATEGORY AND SCHEDULE

Pregnancy Risk Category: D

MECHANISM OF ACTION

A thiomidazole derivative that inhibits synthesis of thyroid hormone by interfering with the incorporation of iodine into tyrosyl residues. **Therapeutic Effect:** Effectively treats hyperthyroidism by decreasing thyroid hormone levels.

AVAILABILITY

Tablets: 5 mg, 10 mg.

INDICATIONS AND DOSAGES

▸ **Hyperthyroidism**

PO

Adults, Elderly. Initially, 15–60 mg/day in 3 divided doses. Maintenance: 5–15 mg/day.

Children. Initially, 0.4 mg/kg/day in 3 divided doses. Maintenance: One-half the initial dose.

CONTRAINDICATIONS

None known.

INTERACTIONS

Drug

Amiodarone, iodinated glycerol, iodine, potassium iodide: May decrease response to methimazole.

Digoxin: May increase the blood concentration of digoxin as patient becomes euthyroid.

^{131}I: May decrease thyroid uptake of ^{131}I.

Oral anticoagulants: May decrease the effects of oral anticoagulants.

Herbal

None known.

Food

None known.

DIAGNOSTIC TEST EFFECTS

May increase LDH, serum alkaline phosphatase, bilirubin, AST (SGOT), and ALT (SGPT) levels and prothrombin time. May decrease prothrombin level and WBC count.

SIDE EFFECTS

Frequent (5%–4%)

Fever, rash, pruritus

Occasional (3%–1%)

Dizziness, loss of taste, nausea, vomiting, stomach pain, peripheral neuropathy or numbness in fingers, toes, face

Rare (less than 1%)

Swollen lymph nodes or salivary glands

SERIOUS REACTIONS

! Agranulocytosis as long as 4 months after therapy, pancytopenia, and hepatitis have occurred.

NURSING CONSIDERATIONS

Baseline Assessment

• Obtain the patient's pulse and weight.
• Expect to perform thyroid function studies.

Lifespan Considerations

• Methimazole crosses the placenta and should be avoided during pregnancy.
• Methimazole should be avoided in patients who are breast-feeding.

Precautions

• Use methimazole cautiously in patients older than 40 years of age, in patients taking methimazole with other agranulocytosis-inducing drugs, and in patients with impaired hepatic function.

Administration and Handling

• Store at room temperature in a light-resistant container.
• Administer with food if GI symptoms occur.

Intervention and Evaluation

• Monitor the patient's pulse and weigh daily.
• Assess the patient's skin for rash, pruritus, and lymphadenopathy.
• Monitor the patient's CBC, prothrombin time, and serum hepatic enzymes.
• Evaluate the patient for signs and symptoms of bleeding and infection.

Patient Teaching

• Caution the patient against exceeding the prescribed dosage.
• Instruct the patient to space doses evenly around the clock.
• Teach the patient to take his or her resting pulse daily to monitor therapeutic results.
• Urge the patient to restrict consumption of iodine products and seafood.
• Warn the patient to immediately report illness or unusual bleeding or bruising.

propylthiouracil

proe-pill-thye-oh-**yoor**-a-sill
(Propylthiouracil, Propyl-Thyracil[CAN])

CATEGORY AND SCHEDULE

Pregnancy Risk Category: D

MECHANISM OF ACTION

A thiourea derivative that blocks oxidation of iodine in the thyroid gland and blocks synthesis of thyroxine and triiodothyronine. **Therapeutic Effect:** Inhibits synthesis of thyroid hormone.

AVAILABILITY

Tablets: 50 mg.

INDICATIONS AND DOSAGES

▸ Hyperthyroidism

PO

Adults, Elderly. Initially: 300–450 mg/day in divided doses q8h. Maintenance: 100–150 mg/day in divided doses q8–12h.
Children. Initially: 5–7 mg/kg/day in divided doses q8h. Maintenance: 33%–66% of initial dose in divided doses q8–12h.
Neonates. 5–10 mg/kg/day in divided doses q8h.

CONTRAINDICATIONS

None known.

INTERACTIONS

Drug

Amiodarone, iodinated glycerol, iodine, potassium iodide: May decrease response of propylthiouracil.
Digoxin: May increase digoxin blood concentration as patient becomes euthyroid.
^{131}I: May decrease thyroid uptake of ^{131}I.
Oral anticoagulants: May decrease the effects of oral anticoagulants.

Herbal

None known.

Food

None known.

DIAGNOSTIC TEST EFFECTS

May increase LDH, serum alkaline phosphatase, bilirubin, AST (SGOT), and ALT (SGPT) levels and prothrombin time.

SIDE EFFECTS

Frequent

Urticaria, rash, pruritus, nausea, skin pigmentation, hair loss, headache, paraesthesia

Occasional

Somnolence, lymphadenopathy, vertigo

Rare

Drug fever, lupus-like syndrome

SERIOUS REACTIONS

! Agranulocytosis as long as 4 months after therapy, pancytopenia, and fatal hepatitis have occurred.

NURSING CONSIDERATIONS

Baseline Assessment

- Obtain the patient's pulse and weight.
- Expect to obtain laboratory test results, including LDH, serum alkaline phosphatase, bilirubin, AST, and ALT levels and prothrombin time.

Lifespan Considerations

- Propylthiouracil crosses the placenta and should be avoided during pregnancy.
- Propylthiouracil should be avoided in patients who are breast-feeding.
- Use cautiously in children because of the risk of hepatic dysfunction.

Precautions

- Use propylthiouracil cautiously in patients older than 40 years of age and in patients taking propylthiouracil with other agranulocytosis-inducing drugs.

Intervention and Evaluation

- Monitor the patient's pulse and weight daily.
- Assess the patient's skin for eruptions, itching, and swollen lymph glands.
- Monitor the patient's blood study results for bone marrow suppression.
- Be alert to signs and symptoms of hepatitis, including somnolence, jaundice, nausea, and vomiting.
- Evaluate the patient for signs and symptoms of bleeding and infection.

Patient Teaching

- Instruct the patient to space doses evenly around the clock.
- Teach the patient to take his or her resting pulse daily to monitor therapeutic results. Tell the patient to report a pulse rate of less than 60 beats per minute.
- Urge the patient to restrict consumption of iodine products and seafood.
- Warn the patient to immediately report cold intolerance, depression, and weight gain.

71 Miscellaneous Hormonal Agents

agalsidase beta
calcitonin
cinacalcet
dutasteride
finasteride
glucagon hydrochloride
imiglucerase
laronidase
miglustat
octreotide acetate
pegvisomant
raloxifene
teriparatide acetate
testosterone

Uses: Miscellaneous hormonal agents have a wide variety of indications. *Agalsidase beta* is an enzyme used to treat Fabry disease, an X-linked genetic disorder. *Calcitonin* is used to treat Paget's disease, osteoporosis in postmenopausal women, and (as an adjunct) hypercalcemia. *Cinacalcet* is used to treat hypercalcemia in patients with parathyroid cancer. *Dutasteride* and *finasteride* are prescribed to treat benign prostatic hyperplasia (BPH). *Glucagon* is used to treat severe hypoglycemia in diabetic patients and as a diagnostic aid in GI tract radiography. *Imiglucerase* and *miglustat* are helpful in managing Gaucher's disease. *Laronidase* is used to improve pulmonary function and walking capacity in patients with Hurler and Hurler-Scheie forms of mucopolysaccharidosis I and for patients with moderate to severe symptoms of the Scheie form. *Octreotide* is prescribed to control the symptoms of metastatic carcinoid tumors, vasoactive intestinal peptic-secreting tumors, secretory diarrhea, and acromegaly. *Pegvisomant* is used to normalize the serum level of insulin-like growth factor-I (IGF-I) in patients with acromegaly who've had an inadequate response to surgery, radiation therapy, or other medical treatments. *Raloxifene* is used to prevent and treat osteoporosis in postmenopausal women: *Teriparatide* is indicated to treat osteoporosis in patients at high risk for fractures. *Testosterone* is used to treat male hypogonadism, delayed male puberty, and inoperable breast cancer.

Action: Because miscellaneous hormonal agents belong to different subclasses, their actions vary widely. *Agalsidase beta* provides an exogenous source of alpha-galactosidase A, an enzyme missing in patients with Fabry disease. This drug catalyzes the hydrolysis of glycosphingolipids, reducing their accumulation in the capillary endothelium of the kidneys and in other cells. *Calcitonin* decreases osteoclast activity, decreases sodium and calcium reabsorption in the kidneys, and increases calcium absorption in the GI tract. *Cinacalcet,* a calcium-receptor agonist, increases the calcium sensing of the receptor on the parathyroid gland, thus lowering the serum calcium and parathyroid hormone levels. *Dutasteride* and *finasteride* inhibit the enzyme that converts testosterone to dihydrotestosterone (DHT) in the prostate gland, thus reducing the serum DHT level. *Glucagon* promotes hepatic glycogenolysis and gluconeogenesis. *Imiglucerase* catalyzes the hydrolysis of the glycolipid glucocerebrosidase to glucose and ceramide. *Miglustat* reduces the formation of glucosylceramide, which isn't broken down effectively in patients with Gaucher's disease. *Laronidase* provides exogenous lysosomal enzymes, which are needed for the catabolism of glycosaminoglycans. *Octreotide* suppresses the secretion of serotonin and gastroenteropancreatic peptides, which enhances fluid and electrolyte absorption from the GI tract. *Pegvisomant* selectively binds to growth hormone (GH) receptors on cell surfaces, where it blocks the binding and action of endogenous GH and decreases the serum level of IGF-I and other GH-responsive serum proteins. *Raloxifene* affects some receptors as estrogen, thereby preventing bone loss. *Teriparatide* acts on bone to mobilize calcium and on the kidneys to decrease calcium clearance and increase phosphate excretion. *Testosterone* mimics endogenous androgen, promoting the development of male sex organs and maintaining secondary sex characteristics in androgen-deficient men.

---

agalsidase beta

ah-**gull**-sigh-dase
(Fabrazyme)

CATEGORY AND SCHEDULE

Pregnancy Risk Category: B

MECHANISM OF ACTION

An enzyme that treats Fabry disease, an X-linked genetic disorder, by catalyzing the hydrolysis of glycosphingolipids, reducing their accumulation in the kidneys' capillary endothelium and other body tissues. **Therapeutic Effect:** Provides an exogenous source of alpha-galactosidase A, an enzyme missing in those with Fabry disease.

AVAILABILITY

Powder for Injection: 37 mg (5 mg/ml when reconstituted).

INDICATIONS AND DOSAGES

▸ **Fabry disease**

IV

Adults, Elderly. 1 mg/kg q2wk. Give no more than 0.25 mg/min (15 mg/hr). May slow infusion rate if infusion-related reaction occurs. If no reaction occurs, infusion rate may be increased in increments of 0.05 to 0.08 mg/min (3 to 5 mg/hr).

CONTRAINDICATIONS

None known.

INTERACTIONS

Drug

None known.

Herbal

None known.

Food

None known.

DIAGNOSTIC TEST EFFECTS

None known.

IV INCOMPATIBILITIES

Don't mix any other medications with agalsidase beta.

SIDE EFFECTS

Expected (52%–45%)

Infusion reactions (rigors, fever, headache)

Frequent (38%–21%)

Rhinitis, nausea, anxiety, pharyngitis, edema, skeletal pain

Occasional (17%–14%)

Temperature change sensation, hypotension, pallor, paresthesia, pruritus, urticaria, bronchitis

Rare (10%–7%)

Depression, arthralgia, dyspepsia, laryngitis, sinusitis

SERIOUS REACTIONS

! Serious infusion reactions, such as tachycardia, hypertension, throat tightness, chest pain, dyspnea, vomiting, lip edema, and rash occur frequently.

! Other serious reactions include bradycardia, arrhythmias, vertigo, nephrotic syndrome, CVA, and cardiac arrest.

NURSING CONSIDERATIONS

Baseline Assessment

• Pretreat the patient with antipyretics before administering agalsidase, as prescribed.

Precautions

• Use agalsidase beta cautiously in febrile patients and patients with compromised cardiac function, moderate to severe hypertension, or renal impairment.

Administration and Handling

◂ **ALERT** ▸ Give the patient an antipyretic before the infusion, as prescribed.

IV

• Store vials in the refrigerator. Allow them to reach room temperature before reconstitution, which takes about 30 minutes.

• Reconstitute each vial by slowly injecting 7.2 ml sterile water for injection. Roll and tilt gently.

• Before adding the reconstituted solution to 500 ml 0.9% NaCl, remove an equal volume from the 500-ml infusion bag, and then add it to the 500-ml 0.9% NaCl infusion bag.

• The reconstituted and diluted solution should be used immediately; if this is not possible, the solution may be stored in the refrigerator for 24 hours.

• Administer at a rate of no more than 0.25 mg/minute (15 mg/hour). Expect to decrease the infusion rate if the patient has an infusion reaction. If no reaction occurs, the infusion rate may be increased in increments of 0.05 to 0.08 mg/minute (3 to 5 mg/hour).

Intervention and Evaluation

- Monitor the patient for an infusion reaction. Plan to decrease the infusion rate or temporarily stop the infusion if the patient experiences a reaction. As prescribed, give additional antipyretics, antihistamines, or steroids to alleviate these symptoms.
- Closely monitor patients with compromised cardiac function because they're at increased risk for severe complications from infusion reactions.

Patient Teaching

- Tell the patient to let you know as soon as adverse reactions occur.
- Inform the patients that a registry has been established to better understand Fabry disease and to evaluate the long-term effects of agalsidase.

calcitonin

kal-si-**toe**-nin
(Calcimar, Caltine[CAN], Cibacalcin, Miacalcin)
Do not confuse calcitonin with calcitriol.

CATEGORY AND SCHEDULE

Pregnancy Risk Category: C

MECHANISM OF ACTION

A synthetic hormone that decreases osteoclast activity in bones, decreases tubular reabsorption of sodium and calcium in the kidneys, and increases absorption of calcium in the GI tract. **Therapeutic Effect:** Regulates serum calcium concentrations.

PHARMACOKINETICS

Injection form rapidly metabolized (primarily in kidneys); primarily excreted in urine. Nasal form rapidly absorbed. ***Half-life:*** 70–90 min (injection); 43 min (nasal).

AVAILABILITY

Injection: 200 international units/ml (calcitonin-salmon), 500 mg (calcitonin-human).
Nasal Spray: 200 international units/activation (calcitonin-salmon).

INDICATIONS AND DOSAGES

▸ **Skin testing before treatment in patients with suspected sensitivity to calcitonin-salmon**

Intracutaneous

Adults, Elderly. Prepare a 10-international units/ml dilution; withdraw 0.05 ml from a 200-international units/ml vial in a tuberculin syringe; fill up to 1 ml with 0.9% NaCl. Take 0.1 ml and inject intracutaneously on inner aspect of forearm. Observe after 15 min; a positive response is the appearance of more than mild erythema or wheal.

▸ **Paget's disease**

IM, Subcutaneous

Adults, Elderly. Initially, 100 international units/day. Maintenance: 50 international units/day or 50–100 international units every 1–3 days.

Intranasal

Adults, Elderly. 200–400 international units/day.

▸ **Osteoporosis imperfecta**

IM, Subcutaneous

Adults. 2 international units/kg 3 times a week.

▸ **Postmenopausal osteoporosis**

IM, Subcutaneous

Adults, Elderly. 100 international units/day with adequate calcium and vitamin D intake.

Intranasal

Adults, Elderly. 200 international units/day as a single spray, alternating nostrils daily.

▸ **Hypercalcemia**
IM, Subcutaneous
Adults, Elderly. Initially, 4 international units/kg q12h; may increase to 8 international units/kg q12h if no response in 2 days; may further increase to 8 international units/kg q6h if no response in another 2 days.

OFF-LABEL USES

Treatment of secondary osteoporosis due to drug therapy or hormone disturbance

CONTRAINDICATIONS

Hypersensitivity to gelatin desserts or salmon protein

INTERACTIONS

Drug
None known.

Herbal
None known.

Food
None known.

DIAGNOSTIC TEST EFFECTS

None known.

SIDE EFFECTS

Frequent
IM, Subcutaneous (10%): Nausea (may occur 30 min after injection, usually diminishes with continued therapy), inflammation at injection site
Nasal (12%–10%): Rhinitis, nasal irritation, redness, sores

Occasional
IM, Subcutaneous (5%–2%): Flushing of face or hands
Nasal (5%–3%): Back pain, arthralgia, epistaxis, headache

Rare
IM, Subcutaneous: Epigastric discomfort, dry mouth, diarrhea, flatulence
Nasal: Itching of earlobes, edema of feet, rash, diaphoresis

SERIOUS REACTIONS

! Patients with a protein allergy may develop a hypersensitivity reaction.

NURSING CONSIDERATIONS

Baseline Assessment
- Check the patient's electrolyte levels.
- If the patient is suspected of having a sensitivity to calcitonin, perform a skin test before beginning calcitonin therapy.

Lifespan Considerations
- Calcitonin does not cross the placenta.
- It is unknown if calcitonin is distributed in breast milk; its safety in breast-feeding women has not been established.
- The safety and efficacy of this drug have not been established in children.
- No age-related precautions have been noted in the elderly.

Precautions
- Use calcitonin cautiously in patients with a history of allergy or renal dysfunction.

Administration and Handling
IM, Subcutaneous
- Calcitonin may be administered subcutaneously or IM. No more than 2 ml should be given IM at any one site.
- Bedtime administration may reduce flushing and nausea.

Intranasal
- Refrigerate the nasal spray. It may be stored at room temperature once the pump has been activated.
- Have the patient clear his or her nasal passages as much as possible.
- Tilt the patient's head slightly forward and insert the spray tip into the nostril, pointing toward the nasal passages and away from the septum.
- Spray into the nostril while holding the other nostril closed, and at the

same time have the patient inhale through the nose to deliver the drug as high into the nasal passage as possible.

Intervention and Evaluation

- Rotate injection sites and check them for inflammation.
- Assess the patient's vertebral bone mass, and document its improvement or stabilization.
- Assess the patient for an allergic reaction, such as rash, urticaria, dyspnea, swelling, hypotension, and tachycardia.
- Improvement in biochemical abnormalities and bone pain usually occurs in the first few months of treatment; in patients with neurologic lesions, improvement may take more than a year.

Patient Teaching

- Teach the patient and family how to administer the drug. Stress the need to use aseptic technique and rotate injection sites.
- Tell the patient that nausea usually decreases with continued therapy.
- Warn the patient to notify the physician immediately of itching, rash, shortness of breath, or significant nasal irritation.

cinacalcet

sin-ah-**kal**-set
(Sensipar)

CATEGORY AND SCHEDULE

Pregnancy Risk Category: C

MECHANISM OF ACTION

A calcium receptor agonist that increases the sensitivity of the calcium-sensing receptor on the parathyroid gland to extracellular calcium, thus lowering the parathyroid hormone (PTH) levels.
Therapeutic Effect: Decreases serum calcium and PTH levels.

PHARMACOKINETICS

Extensively distributed after PO administration. Protein binding: 93%–97%. Rapidly and extensively metabolized by multiple enzymes. Primarily eliminated in urine with a lesser amount excreted in feces.
Half-life: 30–40 hr.

AVAILABILITY

Tablets: 30 mg, 60 mg, 90 mg.

INDICATIONS AND DOSAGES

▸ Hypercalcemia in parathyroid carcinoma

PO

Adults, Elderly. Initially, 30 mg twice a day. Titrate dosage sequentially (60 mg twice a day, 90 mg twice a day, and 90 mg 3–4 times a day) every 2–4 wk as needed to normalize serum calcium levels.

▸ Secondary hyperparathyroidism in patients on dialysis

PO

Adults, Elderly. Initially, 30 mg once a day. Titrate dosage sequentially (60, 90, 120, and 180 mg once a day) every 2–4 wk.

CONTRAINDICATIONS

None known.

INTERACTIONS

Drug

Amitriptyline: Increases amitriptyline plasma concentration.
Flecainide, thioridazine, tricyclic antidepressants, vinblastine: May require dosage adjustment of these drugs.
Erythromycin, itraconazole, ketoconazole: Increase cinacalcet plasma concentration.

Herbal

None known.

Food

High-fat meals: Increase cinacalcet plasma concentration.

DIAGNOSTIC TEST EFFECTS

Reduces serum calcium level.

SIDE EFFECTS

Frequent (31%–21%)
Nausea, vomiting, diarrhea
Occasional (15%–10%)
Myalgia, dizziness
Rare (7%–5%)
Asthenia, hypertension, anorexia, noncardiac chest pain

SERIOUS REACTIONS

! Overdose may lead to hypocalcemia.

NURSING CONSIDERATIONS

Baseline Assessment

- Obtain the patient's baseline serum electrolyte levels.

Lifespan Considerations

- Cinacalcet may cross the placental barrier.
- Cincalcet's safe use during breast-feeding has not been established; the drug may cause adverse reactions in breast-fed infants.
- The safety and efficacy of cinacalcet have not been established in children.
- No age-related precautions have been noted in the elderly.

Precautions

- Use cinacalcet cautiously in patients with hepatic function impairment.

Administration and Handling

PO

- Store tablets at room temperature.
- Don't break or crush film-coated tablets.
- Give the drug with food or shortly after a meal.

Intervention and Evaluation

- Monitor the patient's serum calcium level.
- Assess the patient's pattern of daily bowel activity and stool consistency.
- Administer an antidiarrheal or antiemetic, as prescribed, to prevent an electrolyte imbalance.
- Assess the patient for dizziness and institute safety precautions.

Patient Teaching

- Instruct the patient to take cinacalcet with food or shortly after a meal.
- Advise the patient to notify the health care provider immediately if he or she experiences diarrhea or vomiting.

dutasteride

do-tah-**stir**-eyed
(Avodart)

CATEGORY AND SCHEDULE

Pregnancy Risk Category: X

MECHANISM OF ACTION

An androgen hormone inhibitor that inhibits 5-alpha reductase, an intracellular enzyme that converts testosterone into dihydrotestosterone (DHT) in the prostate gland, reducing the serum DHT level. **Therapeutic Effect:** Reduces size of the prostate gland.

PHARMACOKINETICS

Route	Onset	Peak	Duration
PO	24 hr	N/A	3–8 wk

Moderately absorbed after PO administration. Widely distributed. Protein binding: 99%. Metabolized in the liver. Primarily excreted in feces. ***Half-life:*** Up to 5 wk.

AVAILABILITY

Capsule: 0.5 mg.

INDICATIONS AND DOSAGES

▸ Benign prostatic hyperplasia (BPH)

PO

Adults, Elderly. 0.5 mg once a day.

OFF-LABEL USES

Treatment of hair loss

CONTRAINDICATIONS

Females, physical handling of tablets by those who are or may be pregnant

INTERACTIONS

Drug

None known.

Herbal

None known.

Food

None known.

DIAGNOSTIC TEST EFFECTS

Decreases the serum prostate-specific antigen (PSA) level

SIDE EFFECTS

Occasional

Gynecomastia, sexual dysfunction (decreased libido, impotence, and decreased volume of ejaculate)

SERIOUS REACTIONS

! Toxicity may be manifested as rash, diarrhea, and abdominal pain.

NURSING CONSIDERATIONS

Baseline Assessment

- Assess the patient for signs and symptoms of BPH, including urinary hesitancy, post-void dribbling, reduced force of urinary stream, and sensation of incomplete bladder emptying.
- Expect to obtain serum PSA determinations before and periodically during therapy.

Precautions

- Use dutasteride cautiously in patients with hepatic disease or impairment, pre-existing sexual dysfunction (such as impotence and decreased libido), or obstructive uropathy.

Administration and Handling

PO

- Don't break, crush, or open capsules.
- Give dutasteride without regard to food.

Intervention and Evaluation

- Diligently monitor the patient's fluid intake and output.
- Assess the patient for improvement of BPH signs and symptoms.

Patient Teaching

- Inform the patient that dutasteride may cause impotence and decrease ejaculate volume.
- Tell the patient that urinary flow may not improve for up to 6 months after beginning treatment.
- Caution the patient not to let women who are or may be pregnant handle dutasteride capsules. Explain that the drug has a pregnancy risk category of X and carries the risk of causing anomalies in the male fetus.

finasteride

feen-**as**-ter-ide

(Propecia, Proscar)

Do not confuse Proscar with Posicor, ProSom, Prozac, or Psorcon.

CATEGORY AND SCHEDULE

Pregnancy Risk Category: X

MECHANISM OF ACTION

An androgen hormone inhibitor that inhibits 5-alpha reductase, an intracellular enzyme that converts testosterone into dihydrotestosterone (DHT) in the prostate gland, resulting in a decreased serum DHT level. **Therapeutic Effect:** Reduces size of the prostate gland.

PHARMACOKINETICS

Route	Onset	Peak	Duration
PO	24 hr	1–2 days	5–7 days

Rapidly absorbed from the GI tract. Protein binding: 90%. Widely distributed. Metabolized in the liver. ***Half-life:*** 6–8 hr. Onset of clinical effect: 3–6 mo of continued therapy.

AVAILABILITY

Tablets (Propecia): 1 mg.
Tablets (Proscar): 5 mg.

INDICATIONS AND DOSAGES

▸ **Benign prostatic hyperplasia (BPH)**
PO
Adults, Elderly. 5 mg once a day (for a minimum of 6 mo).
▸ **Hair loss**
PO
Adults. 1 mg/day.

OFF-LABEL USES

Adjuvant monotherapy after radical prostatectomy in treatment of prostate cancer

CONTRAINDICATIONS

Exposure to the patient's semen or handling of finasteride tablets by those who are or may be pregnant

INTERACTIONS

Drug
None known.
Herbal
None known.
Food
None known.

DIAGNOSTIC TEST EFFECTS

Decreases the serum prostate-specific antigen (PSA) level, even in patients with prostate cancer

SIDE EFFECTS

Rare (4%–2%)
Gynecomastia, sexual dysfunction (impotence, decreased libido, decreased volume of ejaculate)

SERIOUS REACTIONS

! None known.

NURSING CONSIDERATIONS

Baseline Assessment
- Expect to perform a digital rectal exam and obtain serum PSA determinations in patients with BPH before and periodically during finasteride therapy.
- Obtain liver function test results before starting therapy.

Lifespan Considerations
- Women who are or may be pregnant should not handle finasteride tablets because the drug may produce abnormal external genitalia in the male fetus.
- Finasteride is not indicated for use in children.
- The efficacy of this drug has not been established in the elderly.

Precautions
- Use finasteride cautiously in patients with hepatic impairment.

Administration and Handling
PO
- Don't break or crush film-coated tablets.
- Give finasteride without regard to food.

Intervention and Evaluation
- Diligently monitor the patient's fluid intake and output, especially in

patients with signs of obstructed uropathy, such as large residual urinary volume or severely diminished urinary flow.

Patient Teaching

- Inform the patient that finasteride may cause impotence and decrease ejaculate volume.
- Stress the need to take the drug for at least 6 months.
- Inform the patient that he may not notice improved urinary flow even if the prostate gland shrinks.
- Explain to the patient that it is unknown if taking this drug decreases the need for surgery.
- Warn the patient not to let women who are or may be pregnant handle finasteride tablets or be exposed to his semen because of the potential risk to a male fetus.

glucagon hydrochloride

glue-ka-gon

(GlucaGen, GlucaGen Diagnostic Kit, Glucagen[AUS], Glucagon, Glucagon Diagnostic Kit, Glucagon Emergency Kit)

Do not confuse glucagon with Glaucon.

CATEGORY AND SCHEDULE

Pregnancy Risk Category: B

MECHANISM OF ACTION

A glucose elevating agent that promotes hepatic glycogenolysis, gluconeogenesis. Stimulates production of cyclic adenosine monophosphate (cAMP), which results in increased plasma glucose concentration, smooth muscle relaxation, and an inotropic myocardial effect. **Therapeutic Effect:** Increases plasma glucose level.

AVAILABILITY

Powder for Injection: 1 mg.

INDICATIONS AND DOSAGES

▸ Hypoglycemia

IV, IM, Subcutaneous

Adults, Elderly, Children weighing more than 20 kg. 0.5–1 mg. May give 1 or 2 additional doses if response is delayed.

Children weighing 20 kg or less. 0.5 mg.

▸ Diagnostic aid

IV, IM

Adults, Elderly. 0.25–2 mg 10 min prior to procedure.

OFF-LABEL USES

Treatment of esophageal obstruction due to foreign bodies, toxicity associated with beta blockers or calcium channel blockers

CONTRAINDICATIONS

Hypersensitivity to glucagon or beef or pork proteins, known pheochromocytoma

INTERACTIONS

Drug

Anticoagulants: May increase the effects of these drugs.

Herbal

None known.

Food

None known.

DIAGNOSTIC TEST EFFECTS

May decrease serum potassium level.

IV INCOMPATIBILITIES

Don't mix glucagon with any other medications.

SIDE EFFECTS

Occasional

Nausea, vomiting

Rare
Allergic reaction, such as urticaria, respiratory distress, and hypotension

SERIOUS REACTIONS

! Overdose may produce persistent nausea and vomiting and hypokalemia, marked by severe weakness, decreased appetite, irregular heartbeat, and muscle cramps.

NURSING CONSIDERATIONS

Baseline Assessment

• Obtain an immediate assessment of the patient, including clinical signs and symptoms and history.
• Give glucagon immediately, as prescribed, if hypoglycemic coma is established.

Precautions

• Use glucagon cautiously in patients with a history suggestive of insulinoma or pheochromocytoma.

Administration and Handling

◀ALERT▶ Place the patient on his or her side to avoid aspiration because glucagon (as well as hypoglycemia) may produce nausea and vomiting.
◀ALERT▶ Administer IV dextrose if the patient fails to respond to glucagon.

IV, IM, Subcutaneous

• Store vials at room temperature.
• After reconstitution, the solution is stable for 48 hours if refrigerated. If reconstituted with sterile water for injection, use it immediately. Do not use glucagon solution unless it's clear.
• Reconstitute the powder with the diluent supplied by the manufacturer when preparing doses of 2 mg or less. For doses greater than 2 mg, dilute with sterile water for injection.
• To provide 1 mg glucagon/ml, reconstitute the 1-mg vial with 1 ml diluent.
• The patient will usually awaken in 5 to 20 minutes. If the patient fails to respond after 1 or 2 additional doses, give IV glucose as prescribed.
• When the patient awakens, give oral carbohydrates to restore hepatic glycogen stores and prevent secondary hypoglycemia.

Intervention and Evaluation

• Monitor the patient's response time carefully.
• Have IV dextrose readily available in case the patient does not awaken within 20 minutes.
• Assess the patient for evidence of an allergic reaction, including hypotension, respiratory difficulty, and urticaria.

Patient Teaching

• Teach the patient to recognize symptoms of hypoglycemia, including anxiety, increased sweating, difficulty concentrating, headache, hunger, nausea, nervousness, pale and cool skin, shakiness, unusual fatigue, unusual weakness, and unconsciousness.
• Instruct the patient and caregivers to treat early signs of hypoglycemia with a simple sugar first, such as hard candy, honey, orange juice, sugar cubes, or table sugar dissolved in water or juice, followed by a protein source, such as cheese and crackers, half a sandwich, or a glass of milk.
• Urge the patient to wear a medical identification bracelet.

imiglucerase

im-ih-**gloo**-sir-ace
(Cerezyme)
Do not confuse Cerezyme with Cerebyx or Ceredase.

CATEGORY AND SCHEDULE

Pregnancy Risk Category: C

MECHANISM OF ACTION
An enzyme analogue of the enzyme beta-glucocerebrosidase, which catalyzes hydrolysis of the glycolipid glucocerebroside to glucose and ceramide. **Therapeutic Effect:** Minimizes conditions associated with Gaucher's disease, such as anemia and bone disease.

AVAILABILITY
Powder for Injection: 212 units (equivalent to a withdrawal dose of 200 units), 424 units (equivalent to a withdrawal dose of 400 units).

INDICATIONS AND DOSAGES
▸ Gaucher's disease

IV

Adults, Elderly, Children. Initially, 2.5 units/kg infused over 1–2 hr 3 times a week up to 60 units/kg/wk. Maintenance: Progressive reduction in dosage while monitoring patient response.

CONTRAINDICATIONS
None known.

INTERACTIONS
Drug

None known.

Herbal

None known.

Food

None known.

DIAGNOSTIC TEST EFFECTS
None known.

IV INCOMPATIBILITIES
Don't mix imiglucerase with any solution other than 0.9% NaCl.

SIDE EFFECTS
Frequent (3%)

Headache

Occasional (less than 3%–1%)

Nausea, abdominal discomfort, dizziness, pruritus, rash, small decrease in BP, urinary frequency

NURSING CONSIDERATIONS
Baseline Assessment

- Expect to obtain CBC, platelet count, and liver function test results.

Administration and Handling

IV

- Refrigerate vials.
- The reconstituted solution is stable for 24 hours if refrigerated.
- Reconstitute the 200-unit vial with 5.1 ml sterile water (or the 400-unit vial with 10.2 ml) to provide a concentration of 40 units/ml. Further dilute with 100 to 200 ml 0.9% NaCl.
- Infuse the solution over 1 to 2 hours.

Intervention and Evaluation

- Monitor the patient's CBC, platelet count, and liver function test results.

Patient Teaching

- Instruct the patient to tell you about any side effects, such as headache.
- Let the patient know about any required follow-up tests.

laronidase
lar-**on**-ih-dase

(Aldurazyme)

CATEGORY AND SCHEDULE
Pregnancy Risk Category: B

MECHANISM OF ACTION
An enzyme that increases the catabolism of glycosaminoglycans in those with a deficiency of the lysosomal enzymes required for glycosaminoglycan catabolism. **Therapeutic Effect:** Prevents glycosaminogly-

cans from causing widespread cellular, tissue, and organ dysfunction.

AVAILABILITY

Injection: 2.9 mg/5 ml.

INDICATIONS AND DOSAGES

▸ Mucopolysaccharidosis

IV

Adults, Elderly. 0.58 mg/kg infused once weekly.

CONTRAINDICATIONS

None known.

INTERACTIONS

Drug

None known.

Herbal

None known.

Food

None known.

DIAGNOSTIC TEST EFFECTS

None known.

SIDE EFFECTS

Frequent (36%–18%)

Infusion-related reactions, such as facial flushing, rash, fever, and headache

Occasional (9%)

Cough, bronchospasm, urticaria, pruritus, angioedema, dependent edema, hypotension, hyperreflexia

SERIOUS REACTIONS

! Upper respiratory tract infection occurs commonly.

! Anaphylactic reactions, such as angioedema, severe bronchospasm, and dyspnea, occurs rarely.

NURSING CONSIDERATIONS

Baseline Assessment

• Pre-treat the patient with antipyretics and antihistamines 60 minutes before starting the IV infusion.

Administration and Handling

• Refrigerate vials.
• Once reconstituted, the solution should be used immediately. If this isn't possible, refrigerate the solution for no longer than 36 hours from the time of preparation to completion of administration.
• Pre-treat the patient with antipyretics and antihistamines, as prescribed, 60 minutes before starting the IV infusion.
• The total volume of the infusion is determined by the patient's weight. Patients who weigh 20 kg or less should receive a total volume of 100 ml. Patients who weigh more than 20 kg should receive a total volume of 250 ml.
• Dilute with 0.1% albumin (human) in 0.9% NaCl. Take care not to shake the solution. Administer using a 0.2-micrometer filter.
• Begin the infusion at a rate of 10 mcg/kg/hour, and increase it in 15-minute increments to 20 mcg/kg/hour, then 50 mcg/kg/hour, and then 100 mcg/kg/hour during the first hour, as prescribed.
• Give the remainder of the infusion at 200 mcg/kg/hour over 2 to 3 hours for a total infusion time of 3 to 4 hours.

Intervention and Evaluation

• Assess the patient's skin for facial flushing and rash.
• Closely monitor the patient for infusion-related reactions. Slowing the infusion rate, temporarily stopping the infusion, or administering additional antipyretics and antihistamines may ameliorate such reactions.

Patient Teaching

• Instruct the patient or the patient's parent to report side effects immediately.
• Urge the patient to ask his orher physician about the registry program

that has been established for patients with mucopolysaccharidosis to monitor and evaluate treatments.

miglustat

mig-**lew**-stat
(Zavesca)

CATEGORY AND SCHEDULE

Pregnancy Risk Category: X

MECHANISM OF ACTION

A Gaucher disease agent that inhibits the enzyme, glucosylceramide synthase, reducing the rate of synthesis of most glycosphingolipids. Allows the residual activity of the deficient enzyme, glucocerebrosidase, to be more effective in degrading lysosomal storage within tissues.
Therapeutic Effect: Minimizes conditions associated with Gaucher's disease, such as anemia and bone disease.

AVAILABILITY

Capsules: 100 mg.

INDICATIONS AND DOSAGES

▸ Gaucher's disease

PO

Adults, Elderly. One 100-mg capsule 3 times a day at regular intervals.

▸ Dosage in renal impairment

For patients with creatinine clearance of 50–70 ml/min, dosage is reduced to 100 mg twice a day.
For patients with creatinine clearance of 30–49 ml/min dosage is 100 mg once a day.

CONTRAINDICATIONS

Women who are or may become pregnant

INTERACTIONS

Drug

Imiglucerase: May decrease the effects of imiglucerase.

Herbal

None known.

Food

None known.

DIAGNOSTIC TEST EFFECTS

None known.

SIDE EFFECTS

Expected (89%–65%)
Diarrhea, weight loss

Frequent (39%–11%)
Hand tremor, flatulence, headache, abdominal pain, nausea

Occasional (7%–4%)
Paresthesia, anorexia, dyspepsia, leg cramps, vomiting

SERIOUS REACTIONS

! Thrombocytopenia occurs in 7% of patients.
! Overdose produces dizziness and neutropenia.

NURSING CONSIDERATIONS

Baseline Assessment

- Plan to perform a baseline neurologic evaluation, with follow-up evaluations every 6 months throughout treatment.

Precautions

- Use miglustat cautiously in patients with impaired fertility or renal function.

Administration and Handling

- Give miglustat without regard to food.
- Don't open, crush, or break capsules.

Intervention and Evaluation

- Encourage the patient to maintain adequate fluid intake.
- Assess the patient's bowel sounds for peristalsis.

• Assess the patient's pattern of daily bowel activity and stool consistency.
• Weigh the patient weekly.
• Observe the patient for a hand tremor.

Patient Teaching

• Instruct the patient to avoid high-carbohydrate foods during miglustat treatment if he or she experiences diarrhea.
• Stress the need to use reliable contraceptive methods during miglustat treatment and for 3 months afterward. Warn the patient to notify the physician and plan to stop miglustat therapy before trying to conceive.

octreotide acetate

ok-**tree**-oh-tide
(Sandostatin, Sandostatin LAR)
Do not confuse octreotide with OctreoScan, or Sandostatin with Sandimmune or Sandoglobulin.

CATEGORY AND SCHEDULE

Pregnancy Risk Category: B

MECHANISM OF ACTION

An antidiarrheal and growth hormone suppressant that suppresses the secretion of serotonin and gastroenteropancreatic peptides and enhances fluid and electrolyte absorption from the GI tract. **Therapeutic Effect:** Prolongs intestinal transit time.

PHARMACOKINETICS

Route	Onset	Peak	Duration
Subcutaneous	N/A	N/A	Up to 12 hr

Rapidly and completely absorbed from injection site. Excreted in urine. Removed by hemodialysis. ***Half-life:*** 1.5 hr.

AVAILABILITY

Injection (Sandostatin): 0.05 mg/ml, 0.1 mg/ml, 0.2 mg/ml, 0.5 mg/ml, 1 mg/ml.
Suspension for Injection (Sandostatin LAR): 10-mg, 20-mg, 30-mg vials.

INDICATIONS AND DOSAGES

▸ **Diarrhea**

IV (Sandostatin)
Adults, Elderly. Initially, 50–100 mcg q8h. May increase by 100 mcg/dose q48h. Maximum: 500 mcg q8h.
Subcutaneous (Sandostatin)
Adults, Elderly. 50 mcg 1–2 times a day.
IV, Subcutaneous (Sandostatin)
Children. 1–10 mcg/kg q12h.

▸ **Carcinoid tumors**

IV, Subcutaneous (Sandostatin)
Adults, Elderly. 100–600 mcg/day in 2–4 divided doses.
IM (Sandostatin LAR)
Adults, Elderly. 20 mg q4wk.

▸ **Vipomas**

IV, Subcutaneous (Sandostatin)
Adults, Elderly. 200–300 mcg/day in 2–4 divided doses.
IM (Sandostatin LAR)
Adults, Elderly. 20 mg q4wk.

▸ **Esophageal varices**

IV (Sandostatin)
Adults, Elderly. Bolus of 25–50 mcg followed by IV infusion of 25–50 mcg/hr.

▸ **Acromegaly**

IV, Subcutaneous (Sandostatin)
Adults, Elderly. 50 mcg 3 times a day. Increase as needed. Maximum: 500 mcg 3 times a day.

▸ **Acromegaly**

IM (Sandostatin LAR)
Adults, Elderly. 20 mg q4wk for 3 mo. Maximum: 40 mg q4wk.

OFF-LABEL USES
Treatment of AIDS-associated secretory diarrhea, chemotherapy-induced diarrhea, insulinomas, small-bowel fistulas, control of bleeding esophageal varices

CONTRAINDICATIONS
None known.

INTERACTIONS
Drug
Glucagon, growth hormone, insulin, oral antidiabetics: May alter glucose concentrations.
Herbal
None known.
Food
None known.

DIAGNOSTIC TEST EFFECTS
May decrease serum thyroxine (T_4) concentration.

SIDE EFFECTS
Frequent (10%–6%, 58%–30% in acromegaly patients)
Diarrhea, nausea, abdominal discomfort, headache, injection site pain
Occasional (5%–1%)
Vomiting, flatulence, constipation, alopecia, facial flushing, pruritus, dizziness, fatigue, arrhythmias, ecchymosis, blurred vision
Rare (less than 1%)
Depression, diminished libido, vertigo, palpitations, dyspnea

SERIOUS REACTIONS
! Patients using octreotide may develop cholelithiasis or, with prolonged high dosages, hypothyroidism.
! GI bleeding, hepatitis, and seizures occur rarely.

NURSING CONSIDERATIONS
Baseline Assessment
- Establish the patient's BP, weight, blood glucose level, and serum electrolyte levels.

Lifespan Considerations
- It is unknown if octreotide is excreted in breast milk.
- The children's dosage has not been established.
- No age-related precautions have been noted in the elderly.

Precautions
- Use octreotide cautiously in patients with insulin-dependent diabetes or renal failure.

Administration and Handling
◀ **ALERT** ▶ Sandostatin may be given IV, IM, or subcutaneously. Sandostatin LAR may be given only IM.

IM
- Give the drug immediately after mixing.
- Inject octreotide deep IM in a large muscle mass at 4-week intervals. Avoid deltoid injections.

Subcutaneous
- Don't use solution if it becomes discolored or contains particulates.
- Avoid multiple injections at the same site within short period.

Intervention and Evaluation
- Monitor the patient's blood glucose levels, fecal fat, fluid and electrolyte balance, and thyroid function test results.
- Monitor growth hormone levels in acromegaly patients.
- Weigh the patient every 2 to 3 days; report weight gain of more than 5 lb a week.
- Monitor the patient's BP, pulse rate, and respiratory rate periodically during treatment.
- Be alert for decreased urine output and peripheral edema, especially of the ankles.

• Assess the patient's pattern of daily bowel activity and stool consistency.

Patient Teaching

• Advise the patient to notify the physician about any unusual signs or symptoms, such as palpitations or unusual bleeding.
• Tell the patient to weigh himself or herself daily; and to report a weight gain of more than 5 lb per week.

pegvisomant

peg-**vis**-oh-mant
(Somavert)
Do not confuse Somavert with somatrem or somatropin.

CATEGORY AND SCHEDULE

Pregnancy Risk Category: B

MECHANISM OF ACTION

A protein that selectively binds to growth hormone (GH) receptors on cell surfaces, blocking the binding of endogenous growth hormones and interfering with growth hormone signal transduction. **Therapeutic Effect:** Decreases serum concentrations of insulin-like growth factor 1 (IGF-1) and other GH-responsive serum proteins.

PHARMACOKINETICS

Not distributed extensively into tissues after subcutaneous administration. Less than 1% excreted in urine. ***Half-life:*** 6 days.

AVAILABILITY

Powder for Injection: 10-mg, 15-mg, 20-mg vials.

INDICATIONS AND DOSAGES

▸ Acromegaly

Subcutaneous

Adults, Elderly. Initially, 40 mg, as a loading dose, then 10 mg daily. After 4–6 wk, adjust dosage in 5-mg increments if serum IGF-1 level is still elevated, or in 5-mg decrements if IGF-1 level has decreased below the normal range. Maximum: 30 mg daily.

CONTRAINDICATIONS

Latex allergy (stopper on vial contains latex)

INTERACTIONS

Drug

Insulin, oral antidiabetics: May enhance effects of these drugs, possibly resulting in hypoglycemia. Dosage should be decreased when initiating pegvisomant therapy.
Opioids: Decrease serum pegvisomant level.

Herbal

None known.

Food

None known.

DIAGNOSTIC TEST EFFECTS

Interferes with measurement of serum growth hormone concentration. May increase AST (SGOT), ALT (SGPT), and transaminase levels. Decreases effect of insulin on carbohydrate metabolism.

SIDE EFFECTS

Frequent (23%)

Infection (cold symptoms, upper respiratory tract infection, blister, ear infection)

Occasional (8%–5%)

Back pain, dizziness, injection site reaction, peripheral edema, sinusitis, nausea

Rare (less than 4%)

Diarrhea, paresthesia

SERIOUS REACTIONS

! Pegvisomant use may markedly

elevate liver function test results, including serum transaminase levels.
! Substantial weight gain occurs rarely.

NURSING CONSIDERATIONS

Baseline Assessment
- Expect to obtain the patient's serum alkaline phosphatase, bilirubin, AST (SGOT), and ALT (SGPT) levels.

Lifespan Considerations
- It is unknown if pegvisomant is excreted in breast milk.
- The safety and efficacy of pegvisomant have not been established in children.
- In the elderly, treatment should begin at the low end of the dosage range.

Precautions
- Use pegvisomant cautiously in elderly patients and patients with diabetes mellitus.

Administration and Handling
Subcutaneous
- Store unreconstituted vials in the refrigerator.
- Administer the drug within 6 hours of reconstitution.
- The solution normally appears clear after reconstitution. Discard the solution if it appears cloudy or contains particles.
- Withdraw 1 ml sterile water for injection and inject it into the vial of pegvisomant, aiming the stream against the glass wall.
- Hold the vial between the palms of both hands and roll it gently to dissolve the powder; do not shake.
- Administer only one dose from each vial.

Intervention and Evaluation
- Plan to obtain the patient's serum IGF-1 concentrations 4 to 6 weeks after therapy begins and periodically thereafter. Adjust the drug dosage based on these results, not on growth hormone assays, as prescribed.
- For patients with tumors that secrete growth hormone, expect to monitor for progressive tumor growth with periodic imaging scans of the sella turcica, as ordered.
- Monitor diabetic patients for hypoglycemia.

Patient Teaching
- Inform the patient that routine monitoring of liver function test results is essential during pegvisomant treatment.
- Urge the patient to notify the physician if he or she experiences yellowing of the skin or sclera of eyes or any other adverse effects.
- Make sure that patients with diabetes mellitus know the signs and symptoms of hypoglycemia and how to treat it.

raloxifene

ra-**lox**-i-feen
(Evista)
Do not confuse raloxifene with propoxyphene.

CATEGORY AND SCHEDULE
Pregnancy Risk Category: X

MECHANISM OF ACTION
A selective estrogen receptor modulator that affects some receptors like estrogen. **Therapeutic Effect:** Like estrogen, prevents bone loss and improves lipid profiles.

PHARMACOKINETICS
Rapidly absorbed after PO administration. Highly bound to plasma proteins (greater than 95%) and albumin. Undergoes extensive first-pass metabolism in liver. Excreted mainly in feces and, to a lesser

extent, in urine. Unknown if removed by hemodialysis. ***Half-life:*** 27.7 hr.

AVAILABILITY

Tablets: 60 mg.

INDICATIONS AND DOSAGES

▸ Prevention or treatment of osteoporosis

PO

Adults, Elderly. 60 mg a day.

OFF-LABEL USES

Treatment of breast cancer in postmenopausal women, prevention of fractures

CONTRAINDICATIONS

Active or history of venous thromboembolic events, such as deep vein thrombosis, pulmonary embolism, and retinal vein thrombosis; women who are or may become pregnant

INTERACTIONS

Drug

Ampicillin, cholestyramine: Reduce raloxifene absorption.

Hormone replacement therapy, systemic estrogen: Don't use raloxifene concurrently with these drugs.

Warfarin: May decrease PT and the effects of warfarin.

Herbal

None known.

Food

None known.

DIAGNOSTIC TEST EFFECTS

Lowers serum total cholesterol and LDL levels, but does not affect HDL or triglyceride levels. Slightly decreases platelet count and serum inorganic phosphate, albumin, calcium, and protein levels.

SIDE EFFECTS

Frequent (25%–10%)

Hot flashes, flulike symptoms, arthralgia, sinusitis

Occasional (9%–5%)

Weight gain, nausea, myalgia, pharyngitis, cough, dyspepsia, leg cramps, rash, depression

Rare (4%–3%)

Vaginitis, UTI, peripheral edema, flatulence, vomiting, fever, migraine, diaphoresis

SERIOUS REACTIONS

! Pneumonia, gastroenteritis, chest pain, vaginal bleeding, and breast pain occur rarely.

NURSING CONSIDERATIONS

Baseline Assessment

- Determine if the patient is pregnant before starting raloxifene therapy.
- Establish the patient's total and LDL cholesterol serum levels before beginning raloxifene therapy and routinely thereafter.

Lifespan Considerations

- It is unknown if raloxifene is distributed in breast milk. However, this drug is not recommended for breast-feeding women.
- Raloxifene is not used in children.
- No age-related precautions have been noted in the elderly.

Precautions

- Use raloxifene cautiously in patients with cardiovascular disease, hepatic or renal impairment, or a history of cervical or uterine cancer.

Administration and Handling

PO

- Give raloxifene without regard to food at any time of day.
- Discontinue the drug 72 hours before and during prolonged immobilization, such as postoperative recovery and prolonged bed rest.

Resume therapy, as prescribed, only after the patient is fully ambulatory.

Intervention and Evaluation

• Monitor the patient's bone mineral density, platelet count, and serum levels of inorganic phosphate, calcium, total and LDL cholesterol, and protein.

Patient Teaching

• Warn the patient to avoid prolonged immobility during travel because limited movement increases the risk of venous thromboembolic events.
• Instruct the patient to take supplemental calcium and vitamin D if his or her daily dietary intake is inadequate.
• Encourage the patient to avoid alcohol consumption and cigarette smoking during raloxifene therapy.
• Instruct the patient to engage in regular exercise.

teriparatide acetate

tear-ee-**pear**-ah-tide
(Forteo)

CATEGORY AND SCHEDULE

Pregnancy Risk Category: C

MECHANISM OF ACTION

A synthetic hormone that acts on bone to mobilize calcium; also acts on kidney to reduce calcium clearance and increase phosphate excretion. **Therapeutic Effect:** Increases the rate at which calcium is released from bone into blood; stimulates new bone formation.

AVAILABILITY

Injection: 750 mg in 3-ml prefilled pen delivers 20 mcg/dose.

INDICATIONS AND DOSAGES

▸ **Osteoporosis**

Subcutaneous

Adults, Elderly. 20 mcg once a day into thigh or abdominal wall.

CONTRAINDICATIONS

Conditions that increase the risk of osteosarcoma (including Paget's disease, unexplained elevations of alkaline phosphatase level, open epiphyses, and prior skeletal radiation therapy), hypercalcemia, hypercalcemic disorders (such as hyperparathyroidism)

INTERACTIONS

Drug

Digoxin: May increase serum digoxin concentration.

Herbal

None known.

Food

None known.

DIAGNOSTIC TEST EFFECTS

May increase the serum calcium level.

SIDE EFFECTS

Occasional

Leg cramps, nausea, dizziness, headache, orthostatic hypotension, tachycardia

SERIOUS REACTIONS

! None known.

NURSING CONSIDERATIONS

Baseline Assessment

• Expect to check the patient's urinary and serum calcium levels and blood parathyroid hormone level.

Precautions

• Use teriparatide cautiously in patients with bone metastases, a history of skeletal malignancies, or metabolic bone diseases other than osteoporosis and in patients receiving concurrent digoxin therapy.

Administration and Handling

Subcutaneous

- Keep teriparatide refrigerated, minimizing the time out of the refrigerator. Don't freeze the drug; discard if if it becomes frozen.
- Inject teriparatide into the thigh or abdominal wall.

Intervention and Evaluation

- Plan to monitor the patient's bone mineral density, parathyroid hormone level, and urinary and serum calcium levels.
- Monitor the patient's BP for hypotension and pulse rate for tachycardia.
- Observe the patient for signs and symptoms of hypercalcemia.

Patient Teaching

- Instruct the patient to immediately sit or lie down if he or she experiences symptoms of orthostatic hypotension, such as dizziness or lightheadedness.
- Warn the patient to notify the physician if he or she experiences persistent symptoms of hypercalcemia, including loss of energy or strength, lethargy, constipation, nausea, and vomiting.

testosterone

tess-**toss**-ter-one

(Andriol[CAN], Androderm, AndroGel, Andropository[CAN], Delatestryl, Depotest[CAN], Depo-Testosterone, Everone[CAN], Striant, Testim, Testoderm, Testoprel, Virilon IM[CAN])

Do not confuse testosterone with testolactone.

CATEGORY AND SCHEDULE

Pregnancy Risk Category: X

MECHANISM OF ACTION

A primary endogenous androgen that promotes growth and development of male sex organs and maintains secondary sex characteristics in androgen-deficient males. **Therapeutic Effect:** Helps relieve androgen deficiency.

PHARMACOKINETICS

Well absorbed after IM administration. Protein binding: 98%. Undergoes first-pass metabolism in the liver. Primarily excreted in urine. Unknown if removed by hemodialysis. ***Half-life:*** 10–20 min.

AVAILABILITY

Cypionate Injection (Depo-Testosterone): 100 mg/ml, 200 mg/ml.
Ethanate Injection (Delatestryl): 200 mg/ml.
Subcutaneous Pellets (Testopel): 75 mg.
Topical Gel (AndroGel): 25 mg/2.5 g, 50 mg/5 g.
Topical Gel (Testim): 50 mg/5 g.
Transdermal Patch (Androderm): 2.5 mg/day, 5 mg/day.
Transdermal Patch (Testoderm): 4 mg/day, 6 mg/day.
Buccal (Striant): 30 mg.

INDICATIONS AND DOSAGES

▸ Male hypogonadism

IM

Adults. 50–400 mg q2–4wk.
Adolescents. Initially 40–50 mg/m^2/dose monthly until growth rate falls to prepubertal levels. 100 mg/m^2/dose until growth ceases. Maintenance virilizing dose: 100 mg/m^2/dose twice a month.

Subcutaneous (Pellets)

Adults, adolescents. 150–450 mg q3–6mo.

Transdermal (Patch [Testoderm])
Adults, Elderly. Start therapy with 6 mg/day patch. Apply patch to scrotal skin.
Transdermal (Patch [Testoderm TTS])
Adults, Elderly. Apply TTS patch to arm, back, or upper buttocks.
Transdermal (Patch [Androderm])
Adults, Elderly. Start therapy with 5 mg/day patch applied at night. Apply patch to abdomen, back, thighs, or upper arms.
Transdermal (Gel [AndroGel])
Adults, Elderly. Initial dose of 5 mg delivers 50 mg testosterone and is applied once daily to the abdomen, shoulders, or upper arms. May increase to 7.5 g, then to 10 g, if necessary.
Transdermal (Gel [Testim])
Adults, Elderly. Initial dose of 5 g delivers 50 mg testosterone and is applied once a day to the shoulders or upper arms. May increase to 10 g.
Buccal System (Striant)
Adults, Elderly: 30 mg q12h.

▸ **Delayed puberty**
IM
Adults. 50–200 mg q2–4wk.
Adolescents. 40–50 mg/m^2/dose every month for 6 mo.
Subcutaneous (Pellets)
Adults, Adolescents. 150–450 mg q3–6mo.

▸ **Breast carcinoma**
IM (testosterone aqueous)
Adults. 50–100 mg 3 times a week.
IM (testosterone cypionate or ethanate)
Adults. 200–400 mg q2–4wk.
IM (testosterone propionate)
Adults. 50–100 mg 3 times a week.

CONTRAINDICATIONS
Cardiac impairment, hypercalcemia, pregnancy, prostate or breast cancer in males, severe hepatic or renal disease

INTERACTIONS
Drug
Hepatotoxic medications: May increase the risk of hepatotoxicity.
Oral anticoagulants: May increase the effects of oral anticoagulants.
Herbal
None known.
Food
None known.

DIAGNOSTIC TEST EFFECTS
May increase blood Hgb level and Hct, as well as serum LDL, alkaline phosphatase, bilirubin, calcium, potassium, sodium, and AST (SGOT) levels. May decrease serum HDL level.

SIDE EFFECTS
Frequent
Gynecomastia, acne
Females: Hirsutism, amenorrhea or other menstrual irregularities, deepening of voice, clitoral enlargement that may not be reversible when drug is discontinued
Occasional
Edema, nausea, insomnia, oligospermia, priapism, male-pattern baldness, bladder irritability, hypercalcemia (in immobilized patients or those with breast cancer), hypercholesterolemia, inflammation and pain at IM injection site
Transdermal: Pruritus, erythema, skin irritation
Rare
Polycythemia (with high dosage), hypersensitivity

SERIOUS REACTIONS
! Peliosis hepatitis (presence of blood-filled cysts in parenchyma of liver), hepatic neoplasms, and hepatocellular carcinoma have been associated with prolonged high-dose therapy.

! Anaphylactic reactions occur rarely.

NURSING CONSIDERATIONS

Baseline Assessment

- Establish the patient's blood Hgb and Hct, BP, and weight.
- If ordered, check the patient's serum cholesterol and electrolyte and liver function test results.
- Wrist x-rays may be ordered to determine bone maturation in children.

Precautions

- Use testosterone cautiously in patients with diabetes and hepatic or renal impairment.

Lifespan Considerations

- Testosterone use is contraindicated during breast-feeding.
- Use testosterone with caution in children because its safety and efficacy have not been established.
- Testosterone use in the elderly may increase the risk of hyperplasia or stimulate growth of occult prostate carcinoma.

Administration and Handling

IM

- Inject testosterone deep into the gluteal muscle.
- Do not give testosterone IV.
- Warming and shaking redissolves crystals that may form in long-acting preparations.
- A wet needle may cause the solution to become cloudy; this does not affect potency.

Transdermal Patches (Testoderm, Testoderm TTS, Androderm)

- Apply Testoderm to clean, dry scrotal skin that has been dry-shaved for optimal skin contact. Apply Testoderm TTS to the arm, back, or upper buttocks.
- Apply Androderm to clean, dry skin on the back, abdomen, upper arms, or thighs. Don't apply it to the scrotum; bony prominences, such as the shoulder; or oily, damaged, or irritated skin. Don't apply Androderm to the same site for 7 days.

Transdermal Gel (AndroGel, Testim)

- Apply the gel to clean, dry, intact skin of shoulder or upper arm, preferably in the morning. Androgel may also be applied to the abdomen.
- Open the packet, squeeze the entire contents into the palm of the hand, and apply at once to the affected site.
- Allow the gel to dry.
- Don't apply the gel to the genital areas.

Buccal (Striant)

- Apply Striant to the gum area above the incisor tooth, alternating sides of the mouth with each application.
- Striant is not affected by consumption of alcohol or food, gum chewing, or tooth brushing.
- Remove Striant product before placing the new one.

Intervention and Evaluation

- Examine the patient's injection site for pain, redness, or swelling.
- Check the patient's BP at least twice a day.
- Weigh the patient daily and report weekly gains of more than 5 lb.
- Evaluate the patient for edema.
- Monitor the patient's intake and output and sleep patterns.
- Assess the patient's blood Hgb and Hct periodically when giving high doses, as ordered. Also plan to check serum cholesterol and electrolyte levels, as well as liver function test results.
- Expect to obtain hand or wrist x-rays when using the drug in prepubertal children.
- Monitor patients with breast cancer or immobility for hypercalcemia, confusion, irritability, lethargy, and muscle weakness.

- Ensure that the patient consumes adequate calories and protein.
- Assess the patient for signs of virilization, such as deepening of the voice.

Patient Teaching

- Instruct the patient to apply the patch to a clean, dry, hairless area of the skin, avoiding bony prominences.
- Caution the patient not to take any other medications, including OTC drugs, without first consulting the physician.
- Advise the patient to consume a diet high in calories and protein. Tell the patient that food may be better tolerated if he or she eats small, frequent meals.
- Instruct the patient to weigh himself or herself every day and to report to the physician weight gain of 5 lb or more per week.
- Warn the patient to notify the physician if he or she experiences acne, nausea, vomiting, or foot swelling. Tell female patients to also promptly report deepening of the voice, hoarseness, and menstrual irregularities. Tell male patients to report difficulty urinating, frequent erections, and gynecomastia.
- Stress to the patient the importance of regular monitoring tests and visits to the physician.

72 Antirheumatic Agents

auranofin
aurothioglucose
gold sodium thiomalate
hydroxychloroquine sulfate
leflunomide
methotrexate sodium
sulfasalazine

Uses: Antirheumatic agents are used to relieve symptoms of rheumatoid arthritis, especially in patients who have had an insufficient therapeutic response to NSAIDs. Specific antirheumatic agents may be used to treat malaria (hydroxychloroquine), trophoblastic neoplasms and other cancers (methotrexate), and ulcerative colitis and inflammatory bowel disease (sulfasalazine).

Action: Disease-modifying antirheumatic drugs include gold compounds and immunosuppressive and antimalarial agents. *Gold compounds,* such as auranofin, aurothioglucose, and gold sodium thiomalate, depress leukocyte migration and suppress prostaglandin activity. They may also inhibit the destructive lysosomal enzymes in leukocytes, which are released at joints. Some *immunosuppressive agents,* such as methotrexate, suppress the inflammatory process of rheumatoid arthritis; others, such as leflunomide, inhibit enzymes in the pathway of pyrimidine synthesis. *Antimalarial agents,* such as hydroxychloroquine, act by an unknown mechanism in rheumatoid arthritis.

auranofin

ah-**ran**-oh-fin
(Ridaura)
Do not confuse Ridaura with Cardura.

aurothioglucose

ah-row-thigh-oh-**glue**-cose
(Gold-50[AUS], Solganal)

CATEGORY AND SCHEDULE

Pregnancy Risk Category: C

MECHANISM OF ACTION

Gold compounds that alter cellular mechanisms, collagen biosynthesis, enzyme systems, and immune responses. **Therapeutic Effect:** Suppresses synovitis in the active stage of rheumatoid arthritis.

PHARMACOKINETICS

Auranofin (29% gold): Moderately absorbed from the GI tract. Protein binding: 60%. Rapidly metabolized. Primarily excreted in urine. ***Half-life:*** 21–31 days. Aurothioglucose (50% gold): Slowly and erraticly absorbed after IM administration. Protein binding: 95%–99%. Primarily excreted in urine. ***Half-life:*** 3–27 days (increased with increased number of doses).

AVAILABILITY

Capsules (Ridaura): 3 mg.
Injection (Solganal): 50-mg/ml suspension.

INDICATIONS AND DOSAGES

▸ Rheumatoid arthritis

PO

Adults, Elderly. 6 mg/day as a single or 2 divided doses. If there is no response in 6 mo, may increase to 9 mg/day in 3 divided doses. If response is still inadequate, discontinue.

Children. 0.1 mg/kg/day as a single or 2 divided doses. Maintenance: 0.15 mg/kg/day. Maximum: 0.2 mg/kg/day.

IM

Adults, Elderly. Initially, 10 mg, followed by 25 mg for 2 doses, then 50 mg weekly until total dose of 0.8–1 g has been given. If patient has improved and shows no signs of toxicity, may give 50 mg q3–4wk for many months.

Children. 0.25 mg/kg; may increase by 0.25 mg/kg each week. Maintenance: 0.75–1 mg/kg/dose. Maximum: 25 mg/dose for 20 doses, then repeated q2–4wk.

OFF-LABEL USES

Treatment of pemphigus, psoriatic arthritis

CONTRAINDICATIONS

Bone marrow aplasia, history of gold-induced pathologies (including blood dyscrasias, exfoliative dermatitis, necrotizing enterocolitis, and pulmonary fibrosis), severe blood dyscrasias

INTERACTIONS

Drug

Bone marrow depressants; hepatotoxic and nephrotoxic medications: May increase the risk of aurothioglucose toxicity.

Penicillamine: May increase the risk of hematologic or renal adverse effects.

Herbal

None known.

Food

None known.

DIAGNOSTIC TEST EFFECTS

May decrease Hgb level, Hct, and WBC and platelet counts. May increase urine protein level. May alter hepatic function test results.

SIDE EFFECTS

Frequent

Auranofin: Diarrhea (50%), pruritic rash (26%), abdominal pain (14%), stomatitis (13%), nausea (10%)

Aurothioglucose: Rash (39%), stomatitis (19%), diarrhea (13%).

Occasional

Aurothioglucose: Nausea, vomiting, anorexia, abdominal cramps

SERIOUS REACTIONS

! Signs and symptoms of gold toxicity, the primary serious reaction, include decreased Hgb level, decreased granulocyte count (less than 150,000/mm^3), proteinuria, hematuria, stomatitis, blood dyscrasias (anemia, leukopenia [WBC count less than 4,000/mm^3], thrombocytopenia, and eosinophilia), glomerulonephritis, nephrotic syndrome, and cholestatic jaundice.

NURSING CONSIDERATIONS

Baseline Assessment

- Determine if the patient is pregnant before beginning treatment.
- Check the results of the patient's urinalysis, CBC (particularly Hgb level, Hct, and WBC and platelet counts), and renal and liver function tests (especially BUN level and serum alkaline phosphatase, creatinine, AST [SGOT], and ALT [SGPT] levels) before beginning therapy.

Lifespan Considerations

• Auranofin and aurothioglucose cross the placenta and are distributed in breast milk. These drugs should be used only when their benefits outweigh the possible risks to the fetus.
• No age-related precautions have been noted in children.
• Use these drugs cautiously in the elderly, who may have age-related renal impairment.

Precautions

• Use gold compounds cautiously in patients with blood dyscrasias, compromised cerebral or cardiovascular circulation, eczema, a history of sensitivity to gold compounds, marked hypertension, renal or liver impairment, severe debilitation, Sjögren's syndrome in rheumatoid arthritis, or systemic lupus erythematosus.

Administration and Handling

PO
• Give these drugs without regard to food.
IM
◀ **ALERT** ▶ Give auranofin or aurothioglucose as weekly injections.
• Inject the drug in the upper outer quadrant of the gluteus maximus.

Intervention and Evaluation

• Assess the patient's pattern of daily bowel activity and stool consistency.
• Test the patient's urine for hematuria and proteinuria.
• Monitor the patient's CBC and renal and liver function tests.
• Assess the patient for pruritus, which may be the first sign of an impending rash, and examine the patient's skin daily for ecchymoses, purpura, and rash.
• Examine the patient's oral mucous membranes, palate, pharynx, and tongue borders for ulceration and investigate any complaints of a metallic taste. These may be signs of stomatitis.
• Evaluate the patient for the expected therapeutic response, including improved grip strength, increased joint mobility, reduced joint tenderness, and relief of pain, stiffness, and swelling.

Patient Teaching

• Inform the patient that he or she should experience a therapeutic response to the drug in 3 to 6 months.
• Advise the patient to avoid exposure to sunlight, which may turn skin gray or blue.
• Urge the patient to notify the physician if he or she develops GI symptoms (nausea, vomiting, or abdominal cramps), metallic taste, sore mouth, pruritus, or rash.
• Stress the importance of maintaining diligent oral hygiene to help prevent stomatitis.

aurothioglucose

(Gold-50[AUS], Solganal)
See auranofin

gold sodium thiomalate

gold sodium thigh-oh-**mal**-ate
(Myochrysine, Myocrisin[AUS])

CATEGORY AND SCHEDULE

Pregnancy Risk Category: C

MECHANISM OF ACTION

A gold compound whose mechanism of action is unknown. May decrease prostaglandin synthesis or alter cellular mechanisms by inhibiting sulfhydryl systems. **Therapeutic Effect:** Decreases synovial inflammation, retards cartilage and bone destruction, suppresses or prevents—

but does not cure—arthritis and synovitis.

AVAILABILITY

Injection: 50 mg/ml.

INDICATIONS AND DOSAGES

▸ Rheumatoid arthritis

IM

Adults, Elderly. Initially, 10 mg, followed by 25 mg for second dose, then 25–50 mg/wk until improvement noted or total of 1 g has been administered. Maintenance: 25–50 mg q2wk for 2–20 wk; if stable, may increase intervals to q3–4wk.
Children. Initially, 10 mg, then 1 mg/kg/wk up to a maximum single dose of 50 mg. Maintenance: 1 mg/kg/dose q2–4wk.

▸ Dosage in renal impairment

Dosage is modified based on creatinine clearance.

Creatinine Clearance	Dosage
50–80 ml/min	50% of usual dose
less than 50 ml/min	not recommended

OFF-LABEL USES

Treatment of psoriatic arthritis

CONTRAINDICATIONS

Colitis; concurrent use of antimalarials, immunosuppressive agents, penicillamine, or phenylbutazone; CHF; exfoliative dermatitis; history of blood dyscrasias; severe hepatic or renal impairment; systemic lupus erythematosus

INTERACTIONS

Drug

Bone marrow depressants, hepatotoxic and nephrotoxic medications: May increase the risk of toxicity.
Penicillamine: May increase the risk of adverse hematologic or renal effects.

Herbal

None known.

Food

None known.

DIAGNOSTIC TEST EFFECTS

May decrease Hgb level, Hct, and WBC and platelet counts. May increase urine protein level. May alter liver function test results.

SIDE EFFECTS

Frequent

Pruritic dermatitis, stomatitis, diarrhea, abdominal pain, nausea

Occasional

Vomiting, anorexia, flatulence, dyspepsia, conjunctivitis, photosensitivity

Rare

Constipation, urticaria, rash

SERIOUS REACTIONS

! Signs and symptoms of gold toxicity include decreased Hgb level, decreased granulocyte count (less than 150,000/mm^3), proteinuria, hematuria, blood dyscrasias (anemia, leukopenia [WBC less than 4,000 mm^3], thrombocytopenia, and eosinophilia), glomerulonephritis, nephrotic syndrome, and cholestatic jaundice.

NURSING CONSIDERATIONS

Baseline Assessment

- Determine if the patient is pregnant before beginning treatment.
- Check the results of the patient's urinalysis, CBC (particularly Hgb level, Hct, and WBC and platelet counts), and renal and liver function tests (especially BUN level and serum alkaline phosphatase, creatinine, AST [SGOT], and ALT [SGPT] levels) before beginning therapy.

Administration and Handling

◀ **ALERT** ▶ Give gold sodium thiomalate as weekly injections, as prescribed.

Intervention and Evaluation

- Assess the patient's pattern of daily bowel activity and stool consistency.
- Test the patient's urine for hematuria or proteinuria.
- Monitor the patient's CBC and liver and renal function test results.
- Examine the patient's skin frequently for ecchymoses, purpura, and rash.
- Assess the patient's oral mucous membranes, palate, pharynx, and tongue borders for ulceration, and investigate any complaints of a metallic taste. These may be signs of stomatitis.
- Evaluate the patient for the expected therapeutic response, including improved grip strength, increased joint mobility, reduced joint tenderness, and relief of joint pain, stiffness, and swelling.

Patient Teaching

- Inform the patient that the drug's therapeutic effect may take 6 months or longer to appear.
- Warn the patient to avoid exposure to sunlight, which may turn skin gray or blue.
- Stress the importance of maintaining diligent oral hygiene during gold sodium thiomalate therapy.

hydroxychloroquine sulfate

See Miscellaneous Anti-infective Agents

leflunomide

le-**flu**-na-mide
(Arava)

CATEGORY AND SCHEDULE

Pregnancy Risk Category: X

MECHANISM OF ACTION

An immunomodulatory agent that inhibits dihydroorotate dehydrogenase, the enzyme involved in autoimmune process that leads to rheumatoid arthritis. **Therapeutic Effect:** Reduces signs and symptoms of rheumatoid arthritis and slows structural damage.

PHARMACOKINETICS

Well absorbed after PO administration. Protein binding: greater than 99%. Metabolized to active metabolite in the GI wall and liver. Excreted through both renal and biliary systems. Not removed by hemodialysis. ***Half-life:*** 16 days.

AVAILABILITY

Tablets: 10 mg, 20 mg.

INDICATIONS AND DOSAGES

▸ **Rheumatoid arthritis**

PO

Adults, Elderly. Initially, 100 mg/day for 3 days, then 10–20 mg/day.

CONTRAINDICATIONS

Pregnancy or plans to become pregnant

INTERACTIONS

Drug

Rifampin: Increases the blood concentration of leflunomide.
Warfarin: May increase the effects of warfarin.

Herbal

None known.

Food

None known.

DIAGNOSTIC TEST EFFECTS

May increase hepatic enzyme levels, especially AST (SGOT), and ALT (SGPT).

SIDE EFFECTS

Frequent (20%–10%)

Diarrhea, respiratory tract infection, alopecia, rash, nausea

SERIOUS REACTIONS

! Transient thrombocytopenia and leukopenia occur rarely.

NURSING CONSIDERATIONS

Baseline Assessment

- Determine if the patient is pregnant before beginning treatment.
- Assess the patient's limitations in activities of daily living due to rheumatoid arthritis.

Lifespan Considerations

- Leflunomide may cause fetal harm. Although it is not known whether leflunomide is excreted in breast milk, the drug is not recommended for breast-feeding women.
- The safety and efficacy of leflunomide have not been established in children younger than 18 years.
- No age-related precautions have been noted in the elderly.

Precautions

- Use leflunomide cautiously in patients with immunodeficiency, bone marrow dysplasia, impaired hepatic or renal function, or positive serology for hepatitis B or C.

Administration and Handling

PO

- Give leflunomide without regard to food.

Intervention and Evaluation

- Monitor the patient's tolerance of the drug.
- Assess the patient for symptomatic relief of rheumatoid arthritis including relief of pain and improved range of motion, grip strength, and mobility.
- Monitor the patient's liver function test results.

Patient Teaching

- Teach the patient that leflunomide may be taken with or without food.
- Inform the patient that the drug's therapeutic effect may take longer than 8 weeks to appear.
- Warn the patient to avoid becoming pregnant during leflunomide therapy. Explain that this drug has a pregnancy risk category of X.

methotrexate sodium

See Antimetabolites

sulfasalazine

See Miscellaneous Anti-infective Agents

73 Immune Globulins

hepatitis B immune globulin (human)
immune globulin IV (IGIV)
lymphocyte immune globulin N
respiratory syncytial immune globulin
Rh_o(D) immune globulin

Uses: Immune globulins are used primarily to immunize patients against infectious diseases, such as hepatitis B virus and respiratory syncytial virus infections. In addition, *immune globulin IV* is used to treat primary immunodeficiency syndromes, Kawasaki disease, and idiopathic thrombocytopenic purpura; to prevent bacterial infections in patients with hypogammaglobulinemia; and as an adjunct in bone marrow transplantation. *Lymphocyte immune globulin N* is used to prevent and treat allograft rejection, to treat aplastic anemia, and to prevent graft vs. host disease after bone marrow transplantation. *Rh_o(D) immune globulin* is used to prevent isoimmunization in Rh-negative patients exposed to Rh-positive blood.

Action: These immune globulins provide passive immunity, which involves administration of preformed antibodies. Passive immunity isn't permanent and doesn't last as long as active immunity, which results from immunization with an antigen to develop defenses against a future exposure.

hepatitis B immune globulin (human)

hep-ah-**tie**-tis **B** ih-**mewn glah**-byew-lin
(Bayhep B, H-B-Vax II [AUS], Nabi-HB)

CATEGORY AND SCHEDULE

Pregnancy Risk Category: C

MECHANISM OF ACTION

An immune globulin of inactivated hepatitis B virus that provides passive immunity against hepatitis B virus.

AVAILABILITY

Injection: 5-ml vial.

INDICATIONS AND DOSAGES

▸ Prevention of hepatitis B infection

IM

Adults, Elderly. Usual 0.06 ml/kg; for acute exposure 3–5 ml. Repeat 28–30 days after exposure.

CONTRAINDICATIONS

Allergies to gamma globulin or thimerosal, IgA deficiency, IM injection in patients with coagulation disorders or thrombocytopenia

INTERACTIONS

Drug

None known.

Herbal

None known.

Food

None known.

DIAGNOSTIC TEST EFFECTS

None known.

SIDE EFFECTS

Frequent

Headache (26%), injection site pain (12%)

Occasional (5%)

Malaise, nausea, myalgia

SERIOUS REACTIONS

! None known.

NURSING CONSIDERATIONS

Baseline Assessment

- Ask the patient if he or she is allergic to gamma globulin, thimerosal, eggs, or chicken products before administering this drug.
- Expect to obtain baseline liver function studies and hepatitis B antibody levels.

Lifespan Considerations

- None known.

Precautions

- Use hepatitis B immune globulin cautiously in patients with coagulation disorders or thrombocytopenia.
- This drug is contraindicated in patients with IgA deficiency or allergies to gamma globulin or thimerosal.

Administration and Handling

IM

◀ALERT▶ Avoid giving IM injections to patients with coagulation disorders or thrombocytopenia

- Refrigerate this drug; do not freeze it.
- Administer by IM injection only in the gluteal or deltoid area.

Intervention and Evaluation

◀ALERT▶ This drug is for IM injection only.

- Use care when administering this drug to patients with bleeding disorders or thrombocytopenia.
- Obtain periodic liver function studies and hepatitis B antibody levels.

Patient Teaching

- Advise the patient to complete the full course of immunization.
- Instruct the patient to promptly report any side effects, including headache or injection site pain.
- Teach the patient how hepatitis B is transmitted, for example, by blood and body fluids.

immune globulin IV (IGIV)

ih-**mewn glah**-byew-lin (Baygam[CAN], Carimune, Gamimune N, Gammagard S/D, Gammar-P-IV, Gamunex, Iveegam EN, Octagam, Panglobulin, Polygam S/D, Sandoglobulin[AUS], Venoglobulin-S)

Do not confuse Sandoglobulin with Sandimmune or Sandostatin.

CATEGORY AND SCHEDULE

Pregnancy Risk Category: C

MECHANISM OF ACTION

An immune serum that increases antibody titer and antigen-antibody reaction. **Therapeutic Effect:** Provides passive immunity against infection; induces rapid increase in platelet count; produces anti-inflammatory effect.

PHARMACOKINETICS

Evenly distributed between intravascular and extravascular space. ***Half-life:*** 21–23 days.

AVAILABILITY

Injection Solution (Gamimune N, Gamunex): 10%.
Injection Solution (Octagam): 5%.
Injection Solution (Venoglobulin-S): 5%, 10%.
Injection Powder for Reconstitution (Carimune, Panglobulin): 1 g, 3 g, 6 g, 12 g.
Injection Powder for Reconstitution (Gammagard S/D, Polygam S/D): 2.5 g, 5 g, 10 g.
Injection Powder for Reconstitution (Gammar-P-IV): 1 g, 2.5 g, 5 g, 10 g.
Injection Powder for Reconstitution (Iveegam EN): 0.5 g, 1g, 2.5 g, 5g.

INDICATIONS AND DOSAGES

▸ **Primary immunodeficiency syndrome**
IV
Adults, Elderly, Children. 200–400 mg/kg once monthly.

▸ **Idiopathic thrombocytopenic purpura (ITP)**
IV
Adults, Elderly, Children. 400–1,000 mg/kg/day for 2–5 days.

▸ **Kawasaki disease**
IV
Adults, Elderly, Children. 2 g/kg as a single dose.

▸ **Chronic lymphocytic leukemia**
IV
Adults, Elderly, Children. 400 mg/kg q3–4wk.

▸ **Bone marrow transplant**
IV
Adults, Elderly, Children. 400–500 mg/kg/dose every week for 12 wk, then every month.

OFF-LABEL USES

Control and prevention of infections in infants and children with immunosuppression due to AIDS or AIDS-related complex; prevention of acute infections in immunosuppressed patients; prevention and treatment of infections in high-risk, preterm, low-birth-weight neonates; treatment of chronic inflammatory demyelinating polyneuropathies and multiple sclerosis

CONTRAINDICATIONS

Allergies to gamma globulin, thimerosal, or anti-IgA antibodies; isolated IgA deficiency

INTERACTIONS

Drug

Live-virus vaccines: May increase vaccine side effects, potentiate virus replication, and decrease the patient's antibody response to the vaccine.

Herbal

None known.

Food

None known.

DIAGNOSTIC TEST EFFECTS

None known.

IV INCOMPATIBILITIES

Do not mix IGIV with any other medications.

SIDE EFFECTS

Frequent

Tachycardia, backache, headache, arthralgia, myalgia

Occasional

Fatigue, wheezing, injection site rash or pain, leg cramps, urticaria, bluish lips and nailbeds, light-headedness

SERIOUS REACTIONS

! Anaphylactic reactions are rare, but the incidence increases with repeated injections of IGIV. Keep epinephrine readily available.
! Overdose may produce chest tightness, chills, diaphoresis, dizziness, facial flushing, nausea, vomiting, fever, and hypotension.

! Hypersensitivity reaction, characterized by anxiety, arthralgia, dizziness, flushing, myalgia, palpitations, and pruritus, occurs rarely.

NURSING CONSIDERATIONS

Baseline Assessment

• Make sure the patient is well hydrated before giving IGIV.

Lifespan Considerations

• It is unknown if IGIV crosses the placenta or is distributed in breast milk.
• No age-related precautions have been noted in children or the elderly.

Precautions

• Use IGIV cautiously in patients with cardiovascular disease, diabetes mellitus, history of thrombosis, impaired renal function, sepsis, or volume depletion and in those who use nephrotoxic drugs concurrently.

Administration and Handling

IV

• Refer to individual IV preparations for storage requirements and information about stability after reconstitution.
• Reconstitute IGIV only with the diluent provided by the manufacturer.
• Discard partially used or turbid preparations.
• Administer IGIV by infusion only through separate tubing. Avoid mixing IGIV with other medications or IV infusion fluids.
• The infusion rate varies among products.
• Monitor the patient's BP and vital signs diligently during and immediately after IV administration. A precipitous fall in BP may indicate an anaphylactic reaction.
• Stop the infusion immediately if you suspect an anaphylactic reaction. Keep epinephrine readily available.

Intervention and Evaluation

• Control the infusion rate carefully. A too-rapid infusion increases the risk of a precipitous drop in BP, and an anaphylactic reaction, marked by chest tightness, chills, diaphoresis, facial flushing, fever, nausea, and vomiting. Stop the infusion temporarily if such signs occur.
• Assess the patient closely during the infusion, especially in the first hour.
• Monitor the patient's vital signs continuously.
• Monitor the platelet count of patient's being treated for ITP.

Patient Teaching

• Explain the rationale for IGIV therapy to the patient.
• Inform the patient that he or she should have a rapid response to therapy, which will last 1 to 3 months.
• Advise the patient to notify the physician if he or she experiences dyspnea, decreased urine output, fluid retention, edema, or sudden weight gain.

lymphocyte immune globulin N

lym-phow-site
(Atgam)
Do not confuse Atgam with Ativan.

CATEGORY AND SCHEDULE

Pregnancy Risk Category: C

MECHANISM OF ACTION

A biological response modifier that acts as a lymphocyte selective immunosuppressant, reducing the number and altering the function of T lymphocytes, which are responsible for cell-mediated and humoral immunity. Lymphocyte immune globulin N also stimulates the release of hematopoietic growth factors. **Therapeutic Effect:** Prevents allograft rejection; treats aplastic anemia.

AVAILABILITY

Injection: 250 mg/5 ml.

INDICATIONS AND DOSAGES

▸ **To delay onset of renal allograft rejection**

IV

Adults, Elderly, Children. 15 mg/kg/day for 14 days, then every other day for 14 days. First dose within 24 hr before or after transplantation.

▸ **Treatment of renal allograft rejection**

IV

Adults, Elderly, Children. 10–15 mg/kg/day for 14 days, then every other day for 14 more days. Maximum: 21 doses.

▸ **Aplastic anemia**

IV

Adults, Elderly, Children. 10–20 mg/kg once a day for 8–14 days, then every other day. Maximum: 21 doses.

OFF-LABEL USES

Immunosuppressant in bone marrow, heart, and liver transplants, treatment of pure red cell aplasia, multiple sclerosis, myasthenia gravis, and scleroderma

CONTRAINDICATIONS

Systemic hypersensitivity reaction to previous injection of lymphocyte immune globulin N

INTERACTIONS

Drug

None known.

Herbal

None known.

Food

None known.

DIAGNOSTIC TEST EFFECTS

May alter renal function test results.

IV INCOMPATIBILITIES

No information is available for Y-site administration.

SIDE EFFECTS

Frequent

Fever (51%), thrombocytopenia (30%), rash (2%), chills (16%), leukopenia (14%), systemic infection (13%)

Occasional (10%–5%)

Serum sickness–like reaction, dyspnea, apnea, arthralgia, chest pain, back pain, flank pain, nausea, vomiting, diarrhea, phlebitis.

SERIOUS REACTIONS

! Thrombocytopenia may occur but is generally transient.

! A severe hypersensitivity reaction, including anaphylaxis, occurs rarely.

NURSING CONSIDERATIONS

Baseline Assessment

• To prevent chemical phlebitis, avoid using a peripheral vein for IV infusion. Instead, expect to use a central venous catheter, a Groshong catheter, or a peripherally inserted central catheter.

Precautions

• Use lymphocyte immune globulin N cautiously in patients receiving concurrent immunosuppressive therapy.

Administration and Handling

IV

• Keep the drug refrigerated before and after dilution.

• Discard the diluted solution after 24 hours.

- Dilute the total daily dose with 0.9% NaCl, as prescribed, to a final concentration of no more than 4 mg/ml.
- Gently rotate the diluted solution; avoid shaking it.
- Use a 0.2- to 1-micron filter, and infuse the total daily dose over at least 4 hours.

Intervention and Evaluation

- Expect to monitor the patient frequently for chills, fever, erythema, and pruritus. Obtain an order for prophylactic antihistamines or corticosteroids to treat these potential side effects.

Patient Teaching

- Instruct the patient to immediately report chest pain, rapid or irregular heartbeat, shortness of breath, wheezing, or swelling of the face or throat, which may occur during the IV infusion.
- Stress the importance of avoiding exposure to people with colds or infections and of notifying the physician as soon as signs or symptoms of infection develop.

respiratory syncytial immune globulin

res-purr-ah-tore-ee sin-**sish**-ee-al ih-**mewn glah**-byew-lin
(RespiGam)

CATEGORY AND SCHEDULE

Pregnancy Risk Category: C

MECHANISM OF ACTION

An immune serum with a high concentration of neutralizing and protective antibodies specific for respiratory syncytial virus (RSV). **Therapeutic Effect:** Provides protection against RSV infection and decreases the severity of existing infection.

AVAILABILITY

Injection: 2,500 mcg RSV immune globulin.

INDICATIONS AND DOSAGES

▸ **Prevention of RSV in children with bronchopulmonary dysplasia and history of premature birth**

IV

Children younger than 24 mo. 750 mg/kg (15 ml/kg) administered at a rate of 1.5 ml/kg/hr for the first 15 min, then 3.6 ml/kg/hr for remainder of infusion. Given once monthly for 5 doses beginning in September or October.

CONTRAINDICATIONS

IgA deficiency

INTERACTIONS

Drug

Live-virus vaccines: May decrease the patient's antibody response to the vaccine.

Herbal

None known.

Food

None known.

DIAGNOSTIC TEST EFFECTS

None known.

SIDE EFFECTS

Occasional (6%–2%)
Fever, vomiting, wheezing

Rare (less than 1%)
Diarrhea, rash, tachycardia, hypertension, hypoxia, injection site inflammation

SERIOUS REACTIONS

! Hypersensitivity reactions, characterized by dizziness, flushing, anxiety, palpitations, pruritus, myalgia, and arthralgia, occur rarely.

NURSING CONSIDERATIONS

Baseline Assessment

- Assess the patient's ABG, blood chemistry, electrolyte and total protein levels as well as serum osmolality.
- Determine the patient's cardiopulmonary status and vital signs before giving the drug, before each dosage or rate increase, every 30 minutes during the infusion, and 30 minutes after the infusion is completed.
- Record the child's body weight in kilograms.
- Perform a baseline pulmonary assessment, including breath sounds, presence of intercostal retractions, and respiratory rate.

Precautions

- Use RSV immune globulin cautiously in patients with pulmonary disease.

Administration and Handling

IV

- Refrigerate vials. Do not freeze.
- Do not shake the vials.
- Start the infusion within 6 hours and complete it within 12 hours of opening the vial.
- Administer the infusion at a rate of 1.5 ml/kg/hr for the first 15 minutes, then 3.6 ml/kg/hr until the end of the infusion.

Intervention and Evaluation

- Monitor the patient's ABG levels, BP, heart and respiratory rates, RSV antibody titers, and temperature.
- Observe the patient for crackles, intercostal or supraventricular retractions, and wheezing.

Patient Teaching

- Advise the parents to notify the physician if the child has any heart or lung impairment.
- Warn the parents to notify the physician if the child experiences any allergic reaction (such as chest tightness, facial swelling, itching, or tingling in the mouth or throat), drowsiness, fever, muscle stiffness, nausea, or vomiting.
- Teach the parents how to minimize the child's exposure to infected individuals.
- Encourage the parents to have the child immunized, as recommended.
- Advise the parents to monitor the child for signs of infection, including fever.

Rh_o(D) immune globulin

row D ih-**mewn glah**-byew-lin
(BayRho-D Full Dose, BayRho Minidose, MICRhogam, RhoGAM, Rhophylac,WinRho SDF)

CATEGORY AND SCHEDULE

Pregnancy Risk Category: C

MECHANISM OF ACTION

Rh_o(D) immune globulin contains anti-Rh_o(D) antibody to the RBC antigen Rh_o(D). Rh_o(D) immune globulin suppresses the active antibody response and formation of anti-Rh_o(D) in Rh_o(D)-negative women exposed to Rh_o-positive blood from a pregnancy with an Rh_o(D)-positive fetus or transfusion with Rh_o(D)-positive blood. The anti-Rh_o(D) antibody in Rh_o(D) immune globulin may bind to Rh_o(D) antigen in maternal circulation, preventing stimulation of the primary immune response to Rh_o(D) and subsequent active production of anti-Rh_o(D). Injection of Rh_o(D) immune globulin into an Rh-positive patient with idiopathic thrombocytopenic purpura (ITP) may result in the formation of anti-Rh_o(D)-coated RBC complexes; as the RBCs are cleared by the spleen, they saturate the capacity of the spleen to clear antibody-coated cells, sparing antibody-coated platelets. **Therapeutic Effect:** Prevents antibody response and hemolytic disease of the newborn in women who have previously conceived an Rh_o(D)-positive fetus. Prevents Rh_o(D) sensitization in patients who have received Rh_o(D)-positive blood. Decreases bleeding in patients with ITP.

AVAILABILITY

Injection, Powder for Reconstitution (WinRho SDF): 120 mcg, 300 mcg.
Injection Solution (BayRho D Full Dose, RhoGAM): 300 mcg.
Injection Solution (BayRho D Mini-Dose, MICRORhoGAM): 50 mcg.
Injection Solution (Rhophylac): 300 mcg/2 ml.

INDICATIONS AND DOSAGES

▸ ITP
IV (WinRho SDF)
Adults, Elderly, Children. Initially, 50 mcg/kg as single dose (reduce to 25–40 mcg/kg if Hgb is less than 10 g/dl) Maintenance: 25–60 mcg/kg based on platelet count and Hgb level.

▸ Suppression of the active antibody response and formation of anti-Rh_o(D) in Rh_o(D)-negative women exposed to Rh_o-positive blood from a pregnancy with an Rh_o(D)-positive fetus
IM (BayRho-D Full Dose, RhoGAM)
Adults. 300 mcg preferably within 72 hr of delivery.
IV, IM (WinRho SDF)
Adults. 300 mcg at 28 wk gestation. After delivery: 120 mcg preferably within 72 hr.

▸ Suppression of active antibody response and formation of anti-Rh_o(D) in Rh_o(D)-negative women exposed to Rh_o-positive blood from a miscarriage with an Rh_o(D)-positive fetus
IM (BayRho-D Full Dose, RhoGAM)
Adults. 300 mcg as soon as possible.

▸ Suppresson of the active antibody response and formation of anti-Rh_o(D) in Rh_o(D)-negative women exposed to Rh_o-positive blood from an abortion, miscarriage, or termination of an ectopic pregnancy with an Rh_o(D)-positive fetus
IM (BayRho-D, RhoGAM)
Adults. 300 mcg if more than 13 wk gestation, 50 mcg if less than 13 wk gestation.
IV, IM (WinRho SDF)
Adults. 120 mcg after 34 wk gestation.

▸ Transfusion incompatibility
IV
Adults. 3,000 units (600 mcg) q8h until total dose given.
IM
Adults. 6,000 units (1,200 mcg) q12h until total dose given.

CONTRAINDICATIONS

Hypersensitivity to any component, IgA deficiency, mothers whose Rh group or immune status is uncertain, prior sensitization to Rh_o(D), Rh_o(D)-positive mother or pregnant woman, transfusion of Rh_o(D)-positive blood in previous 3 months

INTERACTIONS

Drug
Live-virus vaccines: May interfere with the patient's immune response to the vaccine.

Herbal
None known.

Food
None known.

DIAGNOSTIC TEST EFFECTS

None known.

SIDE EFFECTS

Hypotension, pallor, vasodilation (IV formulation), fever, headache, chills, dizziness, somnolence, lethargy, rash, pruritus, abdominal pain, diarrhea, discomfort and swelling at injection site, back pain, myalgia, arthralgia, asthenia

SERIOUS REACTIONS

! None known.

NURSING CONSIDERATIONS

Baseline Assessment

- Assess the patient for bleeding disorders.
- Assess the patient's Hgb level. Administer this drug cautiously to patients with an Hgb level less than 8 g/dl.

Precautions

- Use Rh_o(D) immune globulin cautiously in patients with bleeding disorders, particularly thrombocytopenia, and blood Hgb less than 8 g/dl.

Administration and Handling

◀ALERT▶ Give this drug within 72 hours after exposure to an incompatible blood transfusion or massive fetal hemorrhage.

IV

- Refrigerate vials; do not freeze.
- Reconstitute the 120-mcg and 300-mcg vials with 2.5 ml 0.9% NaCl (the 1,000-mcg vials with 8.5 ml 0.9% NaCl).
- Gently swirl—do not shake—the vial.
- Once reconstituted, the solution is stable for 12 hours at room temperature.
- Infuse the solution over 3 to 5 minutes.

IM

- Reconstitute the 120-mcg and 300-mcg vials with 2.5 ml 0.9% NaCl (the 1,000-mg vials with 8.5 ml 0.9% NaCl).
- Inject the IM solution into the deltoid muscle of the upper arm or the anterolateral aspect of the upper thigh.

Intervention and Evaluation

- Monitor the patient's CBC (especially Hgb and platelet count), BUN and serum creatinine levels, reticulocyte count, and urinalysis results.
- Assess the patient for signs and symptoms of hemolysis.

Patient Teaching

- Teach the patient that this drug is given only by injection, which may be painful.
- Advise the patient to notify the physician if he or she experiences chills, dizziness, fever, headache, or rash.

74 Immunologic Agents

- adalimumab
- alefacept
- anakinra
- azathioprine
- basiliximab
- cyclosporine
- daclizumab
- etanercept
- glatiramer
- interferon alfa-2a
- interferon alfa-2b
- interferon alfa-n3
- interferon alfacon-1
- interferon beta-1a
- interferon beta-1b
- interferon gamma-1b
- muromonab-CD3
- mycophenolate mofetil
- natalizumab
- peginterferon alfa-2a
- peginterferon alfa-2b
- sirolimus
- tacrolimus
- thalidomide

Uses: Immunologic agents can stimulate or suppress immune function. *Immunostimulants,* such as inteferons and peginterferons, are used to treat infection, immunodeficiency disorders, and cancer. *Immunosuppressants,* such as basiliximab and tacrolimus, are used to inhibit the immune response in autoimmune diseases and to improve short-term and long-term allograft survival. For additional uses, see the specific entries in this chapter.

Action: *Immunostimulants* enhance immune activity, including increased phagocytosis by macrophages and augmentation of specific cytotoxicity by T-lymphocytes. *Immunosuppressants* dampen the immune response; most of them do this by affecting interleukin-2, others by affecting inosine monophosphate dehydrogenase. For additional actions, see the specific entries in this chapter.

COMBINATION PRODUCTS

REBETRON: interferon alfa-2b/ribavirin (an antiviral) 3 million units/200 mg.

adalimumab

ah-dah-**lim**-you-mab
(Humira)

CATEGORY AND SCHEDULE

Pregnancy Risk Category: B

MECHANISM OF ACTION

A monoclonal antibody that binds specifically to tumor necrosis factor (TNF) alpha, blocking its interaction with cell surface TNF receptors. **Therapeutic Effect:** Reduces inflammation, tenderness, and swelling of joints; slows or prevents progressive destruction of joints in rheumatoid arthritis.

PHARMACOKINETICS

Half-life: 10–20 days.

AVAILABILITY

Injection: 40 mg/0.8 ml in prefilled syringes.

INDICATIONS AND DOSAGES

▸ **Rheumatoid arthritis**

Subcutaneous

Adults, Elderly. 40 mg every other week. Dose may be increased to 40 mg/wk in those not taking methotrexate.

CONTRAINDICATIONS

Active infections

INTERACTIONS

Drug

Methotrexate: Reduces the absorption of adalimumab by 29%–40%, but dosage adjustment is unnecessary if given concurrently.

Herbal

None known.

Food

None known.

DIAGNOSTIC TEST EFFECTS

May increase levels of blood cholesterol, other lipids, and serum alkaline phosphatase

SIDE EFFECTS

Frequent (20%)

Injection site, erythema, pruritus, pain, and swelling

Occasional (12%–9%)

Headache, rash, sinusitis, nausea

Rare (7%–5%)

Abdominal or back pain, hypertension

SERIOUS REACTIONS

! Rare reactions include hypersensitivity reactions, malignancies, respiratory tract infections, bronchitis, UTIs, and more serious infections (such as pneumonia, tuberculosis, cellulitus, pyelonephritis, and septic arthritis).

NURSING CONSIDERATIONS

Baseline Assessment

- Assess the duration, location, onset, and type of inflammation or pain.
- Inspect the patient's affected joints for deformities, immobility, and skin condition.
- Expect to obtain baseline laboratory values, including liver function test results and a lipid profile.

Lifespan Considerations

- It is unknown if adalimumab is excreted in breast milk.
- The safety and efficacy of adalimumab have not been established in children.
- Cautious use in the elderly is necessary because they're at increased risk for serious infection and malignancy.

Precautions

- Use adalimumab cautiously in elderly patients, pregnant women, and patients with cardiovascular disease, demyelinating disorders, history of sensitivity to monoclonal antibodies, and pre-existing or recent onset of CNS disturbances.

Administration and Handling

Subcutaneous

- Refrigerate adalimumab. Do not freeze it.
- Discard any unused portion.
- Rotate injection sites. Administer each injection at least 1 inch from previous site. Never inject drug into bruised, hard, red, or tender areas.

Intervention and Evaluation

- Monitor the patient's laboratory values, particularly serum alkaline phosphatase levels.
- Assess the patient for evidence of a therapeutic response, such as improved grip strength, increased joint mobility, reduced joint tenderness, and relief of pain, stiffness, and swelling.

Patient Teaching

- Teach the patient how to administer subcutaneous injections and to rotate injection sites.
- Inform the patient that injection site reactions generally occur in the first month of treatment and decrease with continued therapy.
- Instruct the patient to avoid receiving live-vaccines during adalimumab treatment.

alefacept

ale-fah-cept
(Amevive)

CATEGORY AND SCHEDULE

Pregnancy Risk Category: B

MECHANISM OF ACTION

An immunologic agent that interferes with the activation of T lymphocytes by binding to the lymphocyte antigen, thus reducing the number of circulating T lymphocytes. **Therapeutic Effect:** Prevents T cells from becoming overactive, which may help reduce symptoms of chronic plaque psoriasis.

PHARMACOKINETICS

Half-life: 270 hr.

AVAILABILITY

Powder for Injection: 7.5 mg, 15 mg.

INDICATIONS AND DOSAGES

▸ **Plaque psoriasis**

IV

Adults, Elderly. 7.5 mg once weekly for 12 wk.

IM

Adults, Elderly. 15 mg once weekly for 12 wk.

CONTRAINDICATIONS

History of systemic malignancy, concurrent use of immunosuppressive agents or phototherapy

INTERACTIONS

Drug

None known.

Herbal

None known.

Food

None known.

DIAGNOSTIC TEST EFFECTS

Decreases serum T-lymphocyte levels. May increase serum AST (SGOT) and ALT (SGPT) levels.

IV INCOMPATIBILITIES

Don't mix alefacept with any other medications. Don't reconstitute it with any diluent other than that supplied by the manufacturer.

SIDE EFFECTS

Frequent (16%)

Injection site pain and inflammation (with IM administration)

Occasional (5%)

Chills

Rare (2% or less)

Pharyngitis, dizziness, cough, nausea, myalgia

SERIOUS REACTIONS

! Rare reactions include hypersensitivity reactions, lymphopenia, malignancies, and serious infections requiring hospitalization (such as abscess, pneumonia, and postoperative wound infection).

! Coronary artery disease and MI occur in fewer than 1% of patients.

NURSING CONSIDERATIONS

Baseline Assessment

- Obtain the patient's $CD4^+$ T-lymphocyte count before and weekly during the 12-week treatment period.

Lifespan Considerations

- It is unknown if alefacept crosses the placenta or is distributed in breast milk.
- The safety and efficacy of this drug have not been established in children.
- Cautious use is necessary in the elderly because they're at increased risk for infections and certain malignancies.

Precautions

- Use alefacept cautiously in elderly patients, patients at high risk for malignancy, and patients with chronic infections or a history of recurrent infections.

Administration and Handling

◀ALERT▶ The patient may be retreated for an additional 12 weeks, as prescribed, if at least 12 weeks have elapsed since the previous course of therapy and the patient's $CD4^+$ T-lymphocyte count is within normal limits.

IV, IM

- Store unopened vials at room temperature.

◀ALERT▶ For both IV and IM administration, withdraw 0.6 ml of the supplied diluent and, with the needle pointed at the sidewall of the vial, slowly inject the diluent into the vial of alefacept. Swirl the vial gently to dissolve the contents; don't shake or vigorously agitate the vial, to avoid excessive foaming.

- The reconstituted solution should be clear and colorless to slightly yellow. Don't use if it becomes discolored or cloudy or contains undissolved material.
- Use the drug immediately after reconstitution or within 4 hours if refrigerated. Discard unused portion within 4 hours of reconstitution.

IV

- Reconstitute the 7.5-mg vial with 0.6 ml of the supplied diluent (sterile water for injection); 0.5 ml of the reconstituted solution contains 7.5 mg alefacept.
- Prepare two syringes with 3 ml 0.9% NaCl for a pre- and post-administration flush.
- Prime the winged infusion set with 3 ml 0.9% NaCl and insert the set into the vein.
- Attach the drug-filled syringe to the infusion set, and administer the solution over no more than 5 seconds.
- Flush the infusion set with 3 ml 0.9% NaCl.

IM

- Reconstitute 15-mg vial with 0.6 ml of the supplied diluent (sterile water for injection); 0.5 ml of reconstituted solution contains 15 mg alefacept.
- Inject the full 0.5 ml of solution.
- Use a different IM site for each new IM injection. Administer each injection at least 1 inch from an old site, avoiding tender, bruised, red, or hard areas.

Intervention and Evaluation

- Closely monitor $CD4^+$ T-lymphocyte counts.
- Withhold the dose if the $CD4^+$ count is less than 250 cells/microliter. Discontinue treatment if the count remains below 250 cells/microliter.

Patient Teaching

- Inform the patient that regular monitoring of WBC count is necessary during alefacept therapy.
- Advise the patient to notify the physician if he or she experiences any signs of infection or malignancy.
- Urge the patient to avoid contact with infected individuals and situations that might place him or her at risk for infection.

anakinra

an-a-**kin**-ra

(Kineret)

CATEGORY AND SCHEDULE

Pregnancy Risk Category: B

MECHANISM OF ACTION

An interleukin-1 (IL-1) receptor antagonist that blocks the binding of IL-1, a protein that is a major mediator of joint disease and is present in excess amounts in patients with rheumatoid arthritis. **Therapeutic Effect:** Inhibits the inflammatory response.

PHARMACOKINETICS

No accumulation of anakinra in tissues or organs was observed after daily subcutaneous doses. Excreted in urine. ***Half-life:*** 4–6 hr.

AVAILABILITY

Solution: 100-mg syringe.

INDICATIONS AND DOSAGES

▸ **Rheumatoid arthritis**

Subcutaneous

Adults, Children older than 18 yr, Elderly. 100 mg/day, given at same time each day.

CONTRAINDICATIONS

Known hypersensitivity to *Escherichia coli*–derived proteins, serious infection

INTERACTIONS

Drug

Live-virus vaccines: May cause the vaccines to be ineffective.

Herbal

None known.

Food

None known.

DIAGNOSTIC TEST EFFECTS

May increase the eosinophil count. May decrease WBC, platelet, and absolute neutrophil counts.

SIDE EFFECTS

Occasional

Injection site ecchymosis, erythema, and inflammation

Rare

Headache, nausea, diarrhea, abdominal pain

SERIOUS REACTIONS

! Infections, including upper respiratory tract infection, sinusitis, flulike symptoms, and cellulitis, have been noted.

! Neutropenia may occur, particularly when anakinra is used in combination with tumor necrosis factor-blocking agents.

NURSING CONSIDERATIONS

Baseline Assessment

- Assess the patient's level of pain and inflammation, stiffness, and range of motion before and regularly during treatment to determine the patient's response to anakinra therapy.

Lifespan Considerations

- It is unknown if anakinra is distributed in breast milk.
- The safety and efficacy of anakinra have not been established in children.
- Use anakinra cautiously in the elderly, who may experience age-related renal impairment.

Precautions

- Use anakinra cautiously in patients with asthma or renal impairment. Asthmatic patients are at increased risk for serious infection, and patients with renal impairment are at increased risk for a toxic reaction.

Administration and Handling
Subcutaneous
- Keep the drug refrigerated. Don't freeze or shake it.
- Don't use the drug if it becomes discolored or contains particles.
- Give the drug by subcutaneous injection.
- Don't administer live-virus vaccines concurrently with anakinra because the vaccines may not be effective.

Intervention and Evaluation
- Expect to monitor the patient's neutrophil count before therapy begins, monthly for 3 months during therapy, and then quarterly for up to 1 year.
- Evaluate the patient for inflammatory reactions, especially during the first 4 weeks of therapy. Inflammation is uncommon after the first month of therapy.

Patient Teaching
- Teach the patient the proper drug dosage and the correct procedure for a subcutaneous injection.
- Explain the importance of proper disposal of syringes and needles.

azathioprine

ay-za-**thye**-oh-preen
(Alti-Azathioprine[CAN], Azasan, Imuran, Thioprine[AUS])
Do not confuse azathioprine with Azulfidine or azatadine, or Imuran with Elmiron or Imferon.

CATEGORY AND SCHEDULE
Pregnancy Risk Category: D

MECHANISM OF ACTION
An immunologic agent that antagonizes purine metabolism and inhibits DNA, protein, and RNA synthesis. **Therapeutic Effect:** Suppresses cell-mediated hypersensitivities; alters antibody production and immune response in transplant recipients; reduces the severity of arthritis symptoms.

AVAILABILITY
Tablets (Azasan): 25 mg, 50 mg, 75 mg, 100 mg.
Tablets (Imuran): 50 mg.
Injection: 100-mg vial.

INDICATIONS AND DOSAGES
▸ **Adjunct in prevention of renal allograft rejection**
PO, IV
Adults, Elderly, Children. 2–5 mg/kg/day on day of transplant, then 1–3 mg/kg/day as maintenance dose.

▸ **Rheumatoid arthritis**
PO
Adults. Initially, 1 mg/kg/day as a single dose or in 2 divided doses. May increase by 0.5 mg/kg/day after 6–8 wk at 4-wk intervals up to maximum of 2.5 mg/kg/day. Maintenance: Lowest effective dosage. May decrease dose by 0.5 mg/kg or 25 mg/day q4wk (while other therapies, such as rest, physiotherapy, and salicylates, are maintained).
Elderly. Initially, 1 mg/kg/day (50–100 mg); may increase by 25 mg/day until response or toxicity.

▸ **Dosage in renal impairment**
Dosage is modified based on creatinine clearance.

Creatinine Clearance	Dose
10–50 ml/min	75% of usual dose
less than 10 ml/min	50% of usual dose

OFF-LABEL USES
Treatment of biliary cirrhosis, chronic active hepatitis, glomerulo-

nephritis, inflammatory bowel disease, inflammatory myopathy, multiple sclerosis, myasthenia gravis, nephrotic syndrome, pemphigoid, pemphigus, polymyositis, systemic lupus erythematosus

CONTRAINDICATIONS

Pregnant patients with rheumatoid arthritis

INTERACTIONS

Drug

Allopurinol: May increase activity and risk of toxicity of azathioprine.
Bone marrow depressants: May increase myelosuppression.
Live-virus vaccines: May potentiate virus replication, increase the vaccine's side effects, and decrease the patient's antibody response to the vaccine.
Other immunosuppressants: May increase the risk of infection or neoplasms.

Herbal

None known.

Food

None known.

DIAGNOSTIC TEST EFFECTS

May decrease serum albumin, Hgb, and serum uric acid levels. May increase serum alkaline phosphatase, amylase, bilirubin, AST (SGOT), and ALT (SGPT) levels.

IV INCOMPATIBILITIES

Methyl and propyl parabens, phenol

SIDE EFFECTS

Frequent

Nausea, vomiting, anorexia (particularly during early treatment and with large doses)

Occasional

Rash

Rare

Severe nausea and vomiting with diarrhea, abdominal pain, hypersensitivity reaction

SERIOUS REACTIONS

! Azathioprine use increases the risk of developing neoplasia (new abnormal-growth tumors).
! Significant leukopenia and thrombocytopenia may occur, particularly in those undergoing kidney transplant rejection.
! Hepatotoxicity occurs rarely.

NURSING CONSIDERATIONS

Baseline Assessment

- If azathioprine is being given for arthritis, assess the duration, location, onset, and type of fever, inflammation, and pain. Inspect affected joints for deformities, immobility, and skin condition.

Precautions

- Use azathioprine cautiously in immunosuppressed patients; patients previously treated for rheumatoid arthritis with alkylating agents (such as chlorambucil, cyclophosphamide, and melphalan); and patients with current or recent chickenpox.

Administration and Handling

PO

- Give azathioprine during or after meals to reduce the risk of GI disturbances.
- Store the tablets at room temperature.

IV

- Store the parenteral form at room temperature.
- After reconstitution, the IV solution is stable for 24 hours at room temperature.
- Reconstitute the 100-mg vial with 10 ml sterile water for injection to provide a concentration of 10 mg/ml.
- Swirl the vial gently to dissolve the solution.

- The solution may be further diluted in 50 ml D_5W or 0.9% NaCl.
- Infuse the solution over 30 to 60 minutes (range is 5 minutes to 8 hours).

Intervention and Evaluation

- Monitor the patient's CBC (especially platelet count) and serum hepatic enzyme levels weekly during the first month of therapy, twice monthly during the second and third months of treatment, and monthly thereafter.
- Expect to reduce the dosage or discontinue the drug if the WBC count falls rapidly.
- Assess the patient's laboratory test results, as well as signs and symptoms, for delayed myelosuppression.
- In patients receiving azathioprine for arthritis, evaluate for signs of a therapeutic response, including improved grip strength, increased joint mobility, reduced joint tenderness, and relief of pain, stiffness, and swelling.

Patient Teaching

- Explain to the patient with rheumatoid arthritis that the drug's therapeutic response may take up to 12 weeks to appear.
- Instruct the patient to notify the physician if abdominal pain, fever, mouth sores, sore throat, or unusual bleeding occurs.
- Caution women of childbearing age to avoid pregnancy during treatment.

basiliximab

bay-zul-**ix**-ah-mab
(Simulect)
Do not confuse basiliximab with daclizumab.

CATEGORY AND SCHEDULE

Pregnancy Risk Category: B

MECHANISM OF ACTION

A monoclonal antibody that binds to and blocks the receptor of interleukin-2, a protein that stimulates the proliferation of T lymphocytes, which play a major role in organ transplant rejection. **Therapeutic Effect:** Prevents lymphocytic activity and impairs response of the immune system to antigens, which prevents acute renal transplant rejection.

PHARMACOKINETICS

Half-life: Adults, 4–10 days; children, 5–17 days.

AVAILABILITY

Powder for Injection: 10 mg, 20 mg.

INDICATIONS AND DOSAGES

▸ Prevention of acute organ rejection in patients receiving a kidney transplant

IV

Adults, Elderly, Children weighing 35 kg or more. 20 mg within 2 hr before transplant surgery and 20 mg 4 days after transplant.

Children weighing less than 35 kg. 10 mg within 2 hr before transplant surgery and 10 mg 4 days after transplant.

CONTRAINDICATIONS

None known.

INTERACTIONS

Drug

None known.

Herbal

None known.

Food

None known.

DIAGNOSTIC TEST EFFECTS

May increase BUN and serum cholesterol, creatinine, and uric acid levels. May decrease platelet count and serum magnesium and phosphate levels. May increase or decrease blood glucose, Hct, Hbg level, and serum calcium and potassium levels.

IV INCOMPATIBILITIES

Specific information is not available. Don't infuse other drugs through the same IV line.

SIDE EFFECTS

Frequent (greater than 10%)

GI disturbances (constipation, diarrhea, dyspepsia), CNS effects (dizziness, headache, insomnia, tremor), respiratory tract infection, dysuria, acne, leg or back pain, peripheral edema, hypertension

Occasional (10%–3%)

Angina, neuropathy, abdominal distention, tachycardia, rash, hypotension, urinary disturbances (urinary frequency, genital edema, hematuria), arthralgia, hirsutism, myalgia

SERIOUS REACTIONS

! None known.

NURSING CONSIDERATIONS

Baseline Assessment

- Expect to obtain the patient's baseline BUN, blood glucose, and serum calcium, creatinine, alkaline phosphatase, potassium, and uric acid levels.
- Obtain the patient's vital signs, particularly BP and pulse rate, before beginning therapy.

Lifespan Considerations

- It is unknown if basiliximab crosses the placenta or is distributed in breast milk. Basiliximab is not recommended for breast-feeding or pregnant patients.
- No age-related precautions have been noted in children or the elderly.

Precautions

- Use basiliximab cautiously in patients with an infection or a history of malignancy.

Administration and Handling

IV

- Refrigerate unopened vials.
- Discard the solution if a precipitate forms.
- Reconstitute with 5 ml sterile water for injection. Shake gently to dissolve.
- Further dilute with 50 ml 0.9% NaCl or D_5W. Gently invert to avoid foaming.
- Use drug within 4 hours after reconstitution (within 24 hours if refrigerated).
- Infuse over 20 to 30 minutes.

Intervention and Evaluation

- Diligently monitor all of the patient's laboratory test results, especially CBC.
- Assess the patient's BP for hypertension or hypotension, and pulse rate for evidence of tachycardia.
- Determine if the patient is experiencing adverse CNS, GI, or urinary reactions.
- Monitor the patient for signs or symptoms of a wound or systemic infection, including fever, sore throat, and unusual bleeding or bruising.

Patient Teaching

- Warn the patient to notify the physician if he or she experiences difficulty breathing or swallowing, itching, rapid heartbeat, rash, swelling of lower extremities, or weakness.

- Caution women of childbearing age to avoid pregnancy while taking basiliximab.

cyclosporine

sye-kloe-**spor**-in

(Cysporin[AUS], Gengraf, Neoral, Restasis, Sandimmune, Sandimmune Neoral[AUS])

Do not confuse cyclosporine with cycloserine, cyclophosphamide, or Cyklokapron.

CATEGORY AND SCHEDULE

Pregnancy Risk Category: C

MECHANISM OF ACTION

A cyclic polypeptide that inhibits both cellular and humoral immune responses by inhibiting interleukin-2, a proliferative factor needed for T-cell activity. **Therapeutic Effect:** Prevents organ rejection and relieves symptoms of psoriasis and arthritis.

PHARMACOKINETICS

Variably absorbed from the GI tract. Protein binding: 90%. Widely distributed. Metabolized in the liver. Eliminated primarily by biliary or fecal excretion. Not removed by hemodialysis. ***Half-life:*** Adults, 10–27 hr; children, 7–19 hr.

AVAILABILITY

Capsules (Softgel [Gengraf, Neoral, Sandimmune]): 25 mg, 100 mg.
Oral Solution (Sandimmune): 50-ml bottle with calibrated liquid measuring device.
Injection (Sandimmune): 50 mg/ml.
Ophthalmic Emulsion (Restasis): 0.05%.

INDICATIONS AND DOSAGES

▸ Transplantation, prevention of organ rejection

PO

Adults, Elderly, Children. 10–18 mg/kg/dose given 4–12 hr prior to organ transplantation. Maintenance: 5–15 mg/kg/day in divided doses, then tapered to 3–10 mg/kg/day.

IV

Adults, Elderly, Children. Initially, 5–6 mg/kg/dose given 4–12 hr prior to organ transplantation. Maintenance: 2–10 mg/kg/day in divided doses.

▸ Rheumatoid arthritis

PO

Adults, Elderly. Initially, 2.5 mg/kg a day in 2 divided doses. May increase by 0.5–0.75 mg/kg/day. Maximum: 4 mg/kg/day.

▸ Psoriasis

PO

Adults, Elderly. Initially, 2.5 mg/kg/day in 2 divided doses. May increase by 0.5 mg/kg/day. Maximum: 4 mg/kg/day.

▸ Dry eye

Ophthalmic

Adults, Elderly. Instill 1 drip in each affected eye q12h.

OFF-LABEL USES

Treatment of alopecia areata, aplastic anemia, atopic dermatitis, Behçet's disease, biliary cirrhosis, prevention of corneal transplant rejection

CONTRAINDICATIONS

History of hypersensitivity to cyclosporine or polyoxyethylated castor oil

INTERACTIONS

Drug

ACE inhibitors, potassium-sparing diuretics, potassium supplements: May cause hyperkalemia.

Cimetidine, danazol, diltiazem, erythromycin, ketoconazole: May increase cyclosporine concentration and risk of hepatotoxicity and nephrotoxicity.
Immunosuppressants: May increase risk of infection and lymphoproliferative disorders.
Live-virus vaccines: May increase vaccine side effects, potentiate virus replication, and decrease the patient's antibody response to the vaccine.
Lovastatin: May increase the risk of acute renal failure and rhabdomyolysis.

Herbal

St. John's wort: May alter cyclosporine absorption.

Food

Grapefruit, grapefruit juice: May increase the absorption and risk of toxicity of cyclosporine.

DIAGNOSTIC TEST EFFECTS

May increase BUN and serum alkaline phosphatase, amylase, bilirubin, creatinine, potassium, uric acid, AST (SGOT), and ALT (SGPT) levels. May decrease serum magnesium level. Therapeutic peak serum level is 50–300 ng/ml; toxic serum level is greater than 400 ng/ml.

IV INCOMPATIBILITIES

Amphotericin B complex (Abelcet, AmBisome, Amphotec), magnesium

IV COMPATIBILITIES

Propofol (Diprivan)

SIDE EFFECTS

Frequent

Mild to moderate hypertension (26%), hirsutism (21%), tremor (12%)

Occasional (4%–2%)

Acne, leg cramps, gingival hyperplasia (marked by red, bleeding, and tender gums), paresthesia, diarrhea, nausea, vomiting, headache

Rare (less than 1%)

Hypersensitivity reaction, abdominal discomfort, gynecomastia, sinusitis

SERIOUS REACTIONS

! Mild nephrotoxicity occurs in 25% of renal transplant patients, 38% of cardiac transplant patients, and 37% of liver transplant patients, generally 2 to 3 months after transplantation (more severe toxicity is generally occurs soon after transplantation). Hepatotoxicity occurs in 4% of renal transplant patients, 7% of cardiac transplant patients, and 4% of liver transplant patients, generally within the first month after transplantation. Both toxicities usually respond to dosage reduction.

! Severe hyperkalemia and hyperuricemia occur occasionally.

NURSING CONSIDERATIONS

Baseline Assessment

- Monitor blood test results, including renal function studies, liver function tests, and drug blood levels, before beginning cyclosporine therapy and regularly during treatment.

Lifespan Considerations

- Cyclosporine readily crosses the placenta and is distributed in breast milk. Women taking this drug should not breast-feed.
- No age-related precautions have been noted in pediatric transplant patients.
- Elderly patients are at increased risk for hypertension and an increased serum creatinine level.

Precautions

- Use cyclosporine cautiously in pregnant patients and patients with cardiac impairment, chickenpox, herpes zoster infection, hypokalemia,

malabsorption syndrome, or renal or hepatic impairment.
• Use ophthalmic form cautiously in patients with an active eye infection.

Administration and Handling

◀ **ALERT** ▶ The oral solution is available in 50-ml bottles and comes with a calibrated liquid measuring device. Expect to begin therapy with the oral form as soon as possible.

◀ **ALERT** ▶ Expect to give cyclosporine with adrenal corticosteroids. Know that administering other immunosuppressive agents with cyclosporine increases the patient's susceptibility to infection and lymphoma.

PO
• In a glass container, mix oral solution with room-temperature milk, chocolate milk, or orange juice. Stir the mixture well and have the patient drink it immediately. Avoid using Styrofoam containers because the liquid form of the drug may adhere to the wall of the container.
• Add more diluent to the glass container and mix it with the remaining solution to ensure that the patient swallows the total amount of cyclosporine.
• Dry the outside of the measuring device before replacing it in its cover. Don't rinse it with water.
• Don't refrigerate the oral solution because it may separate. Discard the oral solution 2 months after the bottle has been opened.

IV
• Store the parenteral form at room temperature and protect it from light.
• Dilute each milliliter of concentrate with 20 to 100 ml 0.9% NaCl or D_5W.
• After diluted, solution is stable for 24 hours.
• Infuse the solution over 2 to 6 hours.
• Monitor the patient continuously for the first 30 minutes of the infusion, and frequently thereafter for a hypersensitivity reaction, marked by facial flushing and dyspnea.

Ophthalmic
• Invert vial several times to obtain a uniform suspension.
• Instruct the patient to remove any contact lenses prior to administration. May re-insert lenses 15 min after drug administration.
• May use with artificial tears.

Intervention and Evaluation

• Diligently monitor the patient's BUN and serum LDH, bilirubin, creatinine, AST (SGOT), and ALT (SGPT) levels for hepatotoxicity or nephrotoxicity. Mild toxicity is characterized by a slow rise in serum levels; more overt toxicity, by a rapid rise in serum levels. Hematuria is also noted in nephrotoxicity.
• Monitor the patient's serum potassium level for hyperkalemia.
• Monitor the patient's BP for hypertension.
• Know that the therapeutic peak serum level of cyclosporine is 50 to 300 ng/ml and the toxic serum level is over 400 ng/ml.

Patient Teaching

• Instruct the patient to take the drug at the same times each day and to consult the physician for further instructions if he or she forgets to take a dose.
• Tell the patient to take the dose after a trough serum level has been drawn.
• Inform the patient that routine blood testing is essential during cyclosporine therapy.
• Advise the patient that the drug's side effects may include headache, excessive hair growth, gum disease, and tremor. Urge the patient to maintain good oral hygiene to prevent gingivitis.
• Caution the patient to avoid con-

suming grapefruit and grapefruit juice because they increase the drug's blood concentration and risk of side effects.
• Tell the patient to keep the capsules in their original foil wrapping and to store them in a dry, cool environment, away from direct light. Tell the patient to keep the liquid form in the amber-colored glass container.

daclizumab

day-**cly**-zu-mab
(Zenapax)

CATEGORY AND SCHEDULE

Pregnancy Risk Category: C

MECHANISM OF ACTION

A monoclonal antibody that binds to the interleukin-2 (IL-2) receptor complex, inhibiting the IL-2–mediated activation of T lymphocytes, a critical pathway in the cellular immune response involved in allograft rejection. **Therapeutic Effect:** Prevents organ rejection.

PHARMACOKINETICS

Half-life: Adults, 20 days.

AVAILABILITY

Injection: 25 mg/5 ml.

INDICATIONS AND DOSAGES

▸ **Prevention of acute renal transplant rejection (in combination with an immunosuppressive)**

IV

Adults, Children. 1 mg/kg over 15 min q14 days for 5 doses, beginning no more than 24 hr before transplantation. Maximum: 100 mg.

OFF-LABEL USES

Treatment of graft vs. host disease

CONTRAINDICATIONS

None known.

INTERACTIONS

Drug

None known.

Herbal

None known.

Food

None known.

DIAGNOSTIC TEST EFFECTS

None known.

IV INCOMPATIBILITIES

Don't mix daclizumab with any other drugs.

SIDE EFFECTS

Occasional (greater than 2%)

Constipation, nausea, diarrhea, vomiting, abdominal pain, edema, headache, dizziness, fever, pain, fatigue, insomnia, weakness, arthralgia, myalgia, diaphoresis

SERIOUS REACTIONS

! Hypersensitivity reaction, which occurs rarely, is characterized by dyspnea, tachycardia, dysphagia, peripheral edema, rash, and pruritus.

NURSING CONSIDERATIONS

Baseline Assessment

• Expect to obtain the patient's baseline laboratory values, including a CBC, and vital signs, particularly BP and pulse rate.

Lifespan Considerations

• It is unknown if daclizumab crosses the placenta or is distributed in breast milk.
• No age-related precautions have been noted in children or the elderly.

Precautions

• Use daclizumab cautiously in patients with an infection or a history of malignancy.

Administration and Handling

◀ **ALERT** ▶ Daclizumab is given in combination with an immunosuppressive regimen (cyclosporine, corticosteroids) for prevention of organ rejection.

IV

• Refrigerate vials and protect them from light.
• Dilute the drug in 50 ml 0.9% NaCl. Invert the vial gently. Avoid shaking it.
• Infuse the drug over 15 minutes.
• Once reconstituted, the solution is stable for 4 hours at room temperature, 24 hours if refrigerated.

Intervention and Evaluation

• Diligently monitor all blood test results, including CBC.
• Assess the patient's BP for hypertension and hypotension and pulse-rate for tachycardia.
• Determine if the patient is experiencing GI disturbances or urinary changes.
• Monitor the patient for signs and symptoms of systemic infection, such as fever or sore throat, unusual bleeding or bruising, and wound infection.

Patient Teaching

• Warn the patient to notify the physician if he or she experiences difficulty breathing or swallowing, itching or swelling of the lower extremities, rash, rapid heartbeat, or weakness.
• Caution the patient to avoid pregnancy during daclizumab therapy.
• Urge the patient to avoid crowded areas and other circumstances that place him or her at risk for infection.

etanercept

e-**tan**-er-cept
(Enbrel)

CATEGORY AND SCHEDULE

Pregnancy Risk Category: B

MECHANISM OF ACTION

A protein that binds to tumor necrosis factor (TNF), blocking its interaction with cell surface receptors. Elevated levels of TNF, which is involved in inflammatory and immune responses, are found in the synovial fluid of rheumatoid arthritis patients. **Therapeutic Effect:** Relieves symptoms of rheumatoid arthritis.

PHARMACOKINETICS

Well absorbed after subcutaneous administration. ***Half-life:*** 115 hr.

AVAILABILITY

Powder for Injection: 25 mg.
Prefilled Syringe: 50 mg.

INDICATIONS AND DOSAGES

▸ **Rheumatoid arthritis, psoriatic arthritis, ankylosing spondylitis**

Subcutaneous

Adults, Elderly. 25 mg twice weekly given 72–96 hr apart. Alternative weekly dosing: 0.8 mg/kg/dose once a week. Maximum: 50 mg/week. Maximum: 25 mg/dose.

▸ **Juvenile rheumatoid arthritis**

Children 4–17 yr. 0.4 mg/kg (Maximum: 25 mg dose) twice weekly given 72–96 hr apart. Alternative weekly dosing: 50 mg once weekly. Maximum: 25 mg/dose.

▸ **Plaque psoriasis**

Subcutaneous

Adults, Elderly. 50 mg twice a week (give 3–4 days apart) for 3 mo. Maintenance: 50 mg once a week.

OFF-LABEL USES

Treatment of Crohn's disease

CONTRAINDICATIONS

Serious active infection or sepsis

INTERACTIONS

Drug

None known.

Herbal

None known.

Food

None known.

DIAGNOSTIC TEST EFFECTS

None known.

SIDE EFFECTS

Frequent (37%)

Injection site erythema, pruritus, pain, and swelling; abdominal pain, vomiting (more common in children than adults)

Occasional (16%–4%)

Headache, rhinitis, dizziness, pharyngitis, cough, asthenia, abdominal pain, dyspepsia

Rare (less than 3%)

Sinusitis, allergic reaction

SERIOUS REACTIONS

! Infections (such as pyelonephritis, cellulitis, osteomyelitis, wound infection, leg ulcer, septic arthritis, diarrhea, bronchitis, and pneumonia), occur in 38%–29% of patients.

! Rare adverse effects include heart failure, hypertension, hypotension, pancreatitis, GI hemorrhage, and dyspnea. The patient also may develop autoimmune antibodies.

NURSING CONSIDERATIONS

Baseline Assessment

- Assess the duration, location, onset, and type of inflammation or pain the patient is experiencing.

Lifespan Considerations

- It is unknown if etanercept is excreted in breast milk.
- No age-related precautions have been noted in the elderly or in children 4 years and older.

Precautions

- Use etanercept cautiously in patients with a history of recurrent infections or illnesses that predispose to infection, such as diabetes mellitus.

Administration and Handling

◀ALERT▶ Don't add other medications to the solution. Don't use a filter during reconstitution or administration.

Subcutaneous

- Refrigerate unopened vials.
- Once reconstituted, the drug may be stored for up to 6 hours in the refrigerator.
- Reconstitute only with 1 ml sterile bacteriostatic water for injection (containing 0.9% benzyl alcohol). Don't use other diluents.
- Slowly inject the diluent into the vial. Some foaming will occur. To avoid excessive foaming, slowly swirl the contents until the powder is dissolved (less than 5 minutes).
- The reconstituted solution normally appears clear and colorless. Discard the solution if it contains particles or becomes cloudy or discolored.
- Withdraw all the solution into the syringe. The final volume should be approximately 1 ml.
- Inject the drug into the patient's abdomen, thigh, or upper arm.
- Rotate injection sites. Administer each new injection at least 1 inch from an old site, avoiding tender, bruised, hard, or red areas.

Intervention and Evaluation

- Evaluate the patient for signs of a therapeutic response, including improved grip strength, increased joint mobility, reduced joint tenderness, and relief of pain, stiffness, and swelling.

- Obtain the patient's CBC and erythrocyte sedimentation rate or C-reactive protein level.
- Temporarily discontinue therapy and expect to treat the patient with varicella-zoster immune globulin, as prescribed, if the patient experiences significant exposure to varicella virus during treatment.

Patient Teaching

- Teach the patient and caregiver how to prepare and inject the drug as well as preferred injection sites if the patient will be taking etanercept at home.
- Reassure the patient that injection site reactions generally occur in the first month of treatment and decrease in frequency with continued etanercept therapy.
- Caution the patient against receiving live-virus vaccines during treatment.
- Advise the patient to notify the physician if he or she experiences bleeding, bruising, pallor, or persistent fever.

glatiramer

gla-**teer**-a-mer
(Copaxone)
Do not confuse Copaxone with Compazine.

CATEGORY AND SCHEDULE

Pregnancy Risk Category: B

MECHANISM OF ACTION

An immunosuppressive whose exact mechanism is unknown. May act by modifying immune processes thought to be responsible for the pathogenesis of multiple sclerosis (MS). **Therapeutic Effect:** Slows progression of MS.

PHARMACOKINETICS

Substantial fraction of glatiramer is hydrolyzed locally. Some fraction of injected material enters lymphatic circulation, reaching regional lymph nodes; some may enter systemic circulation intact.

AVAILABILITY

Injection: 20 mg/ml in prefilled syringes.

INDICATIONS AND DOSAGES

▸ MS

Subcutaneous
Adults, Elderly. 20 mg once a day.

CONTRAINDICATIONS

Hypersensitivity to glatiramer or mannitol

INTERACTIONS

Drug

None known.

Herbal

None known.

Food

None known.

DIAGNOSTIC TEST EFFECTS

None known.

SIDE EFFECTS

Expected (73%–40%)

Pain, erythema, inflammation, or pruritus at injection site; asthenia

Frequent (27%–18%)

Arthralgia, vasodilation, anxiety, hypertonia, nausea, transient chest pain, dyspnea, flulike symptoms, rash, pruritus

Occasional (17%–10%)

Palpitations, back pain, diaphoresis, rhinitis, diarrhea, urinary urgency

Rare (8%–6%)

Anorexia, fever, neck pain, peripheral edema, ear pain, facial edema, vertigo, vomiting

SERIOUS REACTIONS

! Infection is a common effect.
! Lymphadenopathy occurs occasionally.

NURSING CONSIDERATIONS

Baseline Assessment

- Obtain baseline vital signs, including temperature.
- Assess the patient's baseline knowledge about administering subcutaneous injections, and develop an appropriate teaching plan.

Lifespan Considerations

- It is unknown if glatiramer is distributed in breast milk.
- The safety and efficacy of glatiramer have not been established in children.
- No information is available on glatiramer use in the elderly.

Precautions

- Use glatiramer cautiously in patients with an immediate post-injection reaction, including anxiety, chest pain, dyspnea, flushing, palpitations, and urticaria. This reaction is usually transient and self-limiting.

Administration and Handling

Subcutaneous

- Refrigerate syringes.

Intervention and Evaluation

- Assess the patient for injection site reactions.
- Monitor the patient for fever, chills, and other evidence of infection.

Patient Teaching

- Teach the patient and caregiver how to administer subcutaneous injections and properly dispose of needles.
- Warn the patient to notify the physician if he or she experiences a rash, weakness, difficulty breathing or swallowing, or itching or swelling of the legs.
- Caution the patient to avoid pregnancy during glatiramer therapy.

interferon alfa-2a

inn-ter-**fear**-on
(Roferon-A)
Do not confuse interferon alfa-2a with interferon alfa-2b.

CATEGORY AND SCHEDULE

Pregnancy Risk Category: C

MECHANISM OF ACTION

A biological response modifier that inhibits viral replication in virus-infected cells, suppresses cell proliferation, increases phagocytic action of macrophage, and augments specific lymphocytic cell toxicity. **Therapeutic Effect:** Prevents rapid growth of malignant cells; inhibits hepatitis virus.

PHARMACOKINETICS

Well absorbed after IM and subcutaneous administration. Undergoes proteolytic degradation during reabsorption in kidneys. ***Half-life:*** 2 hr (IM); 3 hr (subcutaneous).

AVAILABILITY

Injection, vial: 6 million units/ml.
Injection (Pre-filled Syringe): 3 million units/0.5 ml, 6 million units/0.5 ml, 9 million units/0.5 ml.
Injection (Single Dose Vial): 36 million units/ml.

INDICATIONS AND DOSAGES

▸ Hairy cell leukemia

IM, Subcutaneous

Adults. Initially, 3 million units/day for 16–24 wk. Maintenance: 3 million units 3 times a wk. Do not use 36-million-unit vial.

Chronic myelocytic leukemia

IM, Subcutaneous

Adults. 9 million units/day.

Melanoma

IM, Subcutaneous

Adults, Elderly. 12 million units/m^2 3 times a week for 3 mo.

AIDS-related Kaposi's sarcoma

IM, Subcutaneous

Adults. Initially, 36 million units/day for 10–12 wk, may give 3 million units on day 1, 9 million units on day 2, 18 million units on day 3, then 36 million units/day for remaining of 10–12 wk. Maintenance: 36 million units/day 3 times a wk.

Chronic hepatitis C

IM, Subcutaneous

Adults, Elderly. 6 million units 3 times a week for 3 mo, then 3 million units 3 times a week for 9 mo.

OFF-LABEL USES

Treatment of active, chronic hepatitis; bladder or renal carcinoma; malignant melanoma; multiple myeloma; mycosis fungoides; non-Hodgkin's lymphoma

CONTRAINDICATIONS

Autoimmune hepatitis

INTERACTIONS

Drug

Bone marrow depressants: May increase myelosuppression.

Herbal

None known.

Food

None known.

DIAGNOSTIC TEST EFFECTS

May increase serum LDH, alkaline phosphatase, AST (SGOT), and ALT (SGPT) levels. May decrease Hct, blood Hgb level, and leukocyte and platelet counts.

SIDE EFFECTS

Frequent (greater than 20%)

Flulike symptoms, nausea, vomiting, cough, dyspnea, hypotension, edema, chest pain, dizziness, diarrhea, weight loss, altered taste, abdominal discomfort, confusion, paresthesia, depression, visual and sleep disturbances, diaphoresis, lethargy

Occasional (20%–5%)

Alopecia (partial), rash, dry throat or skin, pruritus, flatulence, constipation, hypertension, palpitations, sinusitis

Rare (less than 5%)

Hot flashes, hypermotility, Raynaud's syndrome, bronchospasm, earache, ecchymosis

SERIOUS REACTIONS

! Arrhythmias, CVA, transient ischemic attacks, CHF, pulmonary edema, and MI occur rarely.

NURSING CONSIDERATIONS

Baseline Assessment

• Plan to obtain urinalysis, CBC, platelet count, BUN level, and serum alkaline phosphatase, creatinine, AST (SGOT), and ALT (SGPT) levels before and routinely during therapy.

Lifespan Considerations

• Interferon alfa-2a should not be used by pregnant or breast-feeding women.

• The safety and efficacy of interferon alfa-2a have not been established in children.

• Elderly patients are more prone to cardiotoxicity and neurotoxicity.

• Age-related renal impairment may require cautious use of interferon alfa-2a in the elderly.

Precautions

• Use interferon alfa-2a cautiously in patients with cardiac diseases or abnormalities, compromised CNS function, hepatic or renal impairment, myelosuppression, or seizure disorders.

Administration and Handling

◀ALERT▶ Subcutaneous administration is preferred for thrombocytopenic patients and other patients at risk for bleeding.

◀ALERT▶ Dosage is individualized based on the patient's clinical response and tolerance of the drug's adverse effects. When used in combination therapy, expect to consult specific protocols for optimum dosage and sequence of drug administration. If severe adverse reactions occur, modify the dosage or temporarily discontinue the drug, as prescribed.

IM, Subcutaneous

- Refrigerate the drug.

◀ALERT▶ Don't shake the vial.

- The solution normally appears colorless; don't use it if it contains precipitate or becomes discolored.

Intervention and Evaluation

- Monitor all levels of the patient's clinical function, and assess for the numerous side effects.
- Encourage the patient to drink ample fluids, particularly during early therapy.
- Offer the patient emotional support.

Patient Teaching

- Inform the patient that the drug's therapeutic effects may take 1 to 3 months to appear.
- Advise the patient that flulike symptoms tend to diminish with continued therapy.
- Caution the patient to avoid tasks that require mental alertness or motor skills until his or her response to the drug has been established.
- Advise the patient to notify the physician if nausea or vomiting continues at home.
- Urge the patient not to consume alcohol during drug therapy.
- Instruct the female patient to use an effective contraceptive method during therapy, and to notify the physician if she becomes or may be pregnant.

interferon alfa-2b

inn-ter-**fear**-on

(Intron-A)

Do not confuse interferon alfa-2b with interferon alfa-2a.

CATEGORY AND SCHEDULE

Pregnancy Risk Category: C

MECHANISM OF ACTION

A biological response modifier that inhibits viral replication in virus-infected cells, suppresses cell proliferation, increases phagocytic action of macrophages, and augments specific cytotoxicity of lymphocytes for target cells. **Therapeutic Effect:** Prevents rapid growth of malignant cells; inhibits hepatitis virus.

PHARMACOKINETICS

Well absorbed after IM and subcutaneous administration. Undergoes proteolytic degradation during reabsorption in kidneys. ***Half-life:*** 2–3 hr.

AVAILABILITY

Injection (Multidose Vial): 6 million units/ml, 10 million units/ml.
Injection (Single Dose Vial): 3 million units/0.5 ml, 5 million units/0.5 ml, 10 million units/ml.
Injection (Pre-filled Solution): 3 million units/0.2 ml, 5 million units/0.2 ml, 10 million units/0.2 ml.

INDICATIONS AND DOSAGES

▸ Hairy cell leukemia

IM, Subcutaneous

Adults. 2 million units/m^2 3 times a week. If severe adverse reactions occur, modify dose or temporarily discontinue drug.

▸ Condyloma acuminatum

Intralesional

Adults. 1 million units/lesion 3 times a week for 3 wk. Use only 10-million-unit vial, and reconstitute with no more than 1 ml diluent.

▸ AIDS-related Kaposi's sarcoma

IM, Subcutaneous

Adults. 30 million units/m^2 3 times a week. Use only 50-million-unit vials. If severe adverse reactions occur, modify dose or temporarily discontinue drug.

▸ Chronic hepatitis C

IM, Subcutaneous

Adults. 3 million units 3 times a week for up to 6 mo. For patients who tolerate therapy and whose ALT (SGPT) level normalizes within 16 weeks, therapy may be extended for up to 18–24 mo.

▸ Chronic hepatitis B

IM, Subcutaneous

Adults. 30–35 million units weekly, either as 5 million units/day or 10 million units 3 times a week.

▸ Malignant melanoma

IV

Adults. Initially, 20 million units/m^2 5 times a week for 4 wk. Maintenance: 10 million units IM or subcutaneously 3 times a week for 48 wk.

▸ Follicular lymphoma

Subcutaneous

Adults. 5 million units 3 times a week for up to 18 mo.

OFF-LABEL USES

Treatment of bladder, cervical, or renal carcinoma; chronic myelocytic leukemia; laryngeal papillomatosis; multiple myeloma; mycosis fungoides

CONTRAINDICATIONS

None known.

INTERACTIONS

Drug

Bone marrow depressants: May increase myelosuppression.

Herbal

None known.

Food

None known.

DIAGNOSTIC TEST EFFECTS

May increase PT, aPTT, and serum LDH, alkaline phosphatase, AST (SGOT), and ALT (SGPT) levels. May decrease blood Hgb level, Hct, and leukocyte and platelet counts.

IV INCOMPATIBILITIES

No information available. Do not mix with other medications for Y-site administration.

SIDE EFFECTS

Frequent

Flulike symptoms, rash (only in patients with hairy cell leukemia, Kaposi's sarcoma)

Patients with Kaposi's sarcoma: All previously mentioned side effects plus depression, dyspepsia, dry mouth or thirst, alopecia, rigors

Occasional

Dizziness, pruritus, dry skin, dermatitis, altered taste

Rare

Confusion, leg cramps, back pain, gingivitis, flushing, tremor, nervousness, eye pain

SERIOUS REACTIONS

! Hypersensitivity reactions occur rarely.

! Severe flulike symptoms may occur at higher doses.

NURSING CONSIDERATIONS

Baseline Assessment

• Plan to obtain urinalysis, CBC, platelet count, BUN level, and serum alkaline phosphatase, creatinine, AST (SGOT), and ALT (SGPT) levels before and routinely during therapy.

Lifespan Considerations

• Interferon alfa-2b should not be used by pregnant or breast-feeding women.
• The safety and efficacy of interferon alfa-2b have not been established in children.
• Elderly patients are more prone to cardiotoxicity and neurotoxicity.
• Age-related renal impairment may require cautious use of interferon alfa-2b in the elderly.

Precautions

• Use interferon alfa-2b cautiously in patients with cardiac disease or abnormalities, compromised CNS function, hepatic or renal impairment, myelosuppression, or seizure disorders.

Administration and Handling

◀ALERT▶ Dosage is individualized based on the patient's clinical response and tolerance of the drug's adverse effects. When used in combination therapy, consult specific protocols for optimum dosage and sequence of drug administration, as prescribed.

◀ALERT▶ Remember that side effects are dose-related.

IV

• Refrigerate unopened vials; however, the drug remains stable for 7 days at room temperature.
• Prepare the solution immediately before use.
• Reconstitute with the diluent provided by the manufacturer.
• Withdraw the desired dose and further dilute with 100 ml 0.9% NaCl to provide final concentration of at least 10 million units/100 ml.
• Administer the drug over 20 minutes.

IM, Subcutaneous

• Don't administer interferon alfa-2b by IM injection if the patient's platelet count is less than 50,000/m^3; instead give it subcutaneously.
• For patients with hairy cell leukemia, reconstitute as follows: add 1 ml bacteriostatic water for injection to each 3-million-unit vial to provide a concentration of 3 million units/ml, or add 1 ml to each 5-million-unit vial, 2 ml to each 10-million-unit vial, or 5 ml to each 25-million-unit vial to provide a concentration of 5 million units/ml.
• For patients with condylomata acuminata, reconstitute each 10 million unit vial with 1 ml bacteriostatic water for injection to provide a concentration of 10 million units/ml. Use a tuberculin syringe with a 25- or 26-gauge needle. Give the drug in the evening with acetaminophen, which alleviates side effects.
• For patients with AIDS-related Kaposi's sarcoma, reconstitute each 50-million-unit vial with 1 ml bacteriostatic water for injection to provide a concentration of 50 million units/ml.
• Agitate the vial gently and withdraw the solution with a sterile syringe.

Intervention and Evaluation

• Monitor all levels of the patient's clinical function, and assess for the numerous side effects.
• Encourage the patient to drink ample fluids, particularly during early therapy.
• Offer the patient emotional support.

Patient Teaching

• Inform the patient that the drug's

therapeutic effect may take 1 to 3 months to appear.

- Tell the patient that flulike symptoms may be minimized by taking the drug at bedtime and tend to diminish with continued therapy.
- Caution the patient to avoid receiving immunizations without the physician's approval and coming in contact with people who have recently received a live-virus vaccine because interferon alfa-2b lowers the body's resistance.
- Advise the patient to avoid tasks that require mental alertness or motor skills until his or her response to the drug has been established.
- Suggest that the patient take sips of tepid water to relieve dry mouth.
- Instruct the female patient to use effective contraceptive measures during therapy and to notify the physician if she is or may be pregnant.

interferon alfa-n3

in-ter-**fear**-on
(Alferon N)

CATEGORY AND SCHEDULE

Pregnancy Risk Category: C

MECHANISM OF ACTION

A biological response modifier that inhibits viral replication in virus-infected cells, suppresses cell proliferation, increases phagocytic action of macrophages, and augments specific cytotoxicity of lymphocytes for target cells. **Therapeutic Effect:** Inhibits viral growth in condylomata acuminatum.

AVAILABILITY

Injection: 5 million international units/ml.

INDICATIONS AND DOSAGES

▸ Condyloma acuminatum

Intralesional

Adults, Children 18 yr and older. 0.05 ml (250,000 international units) per wart twice a week up to 8 wk. Maximum dose/treatment session: 0.5 ml (2.5 million international units). Do not repeat for 3 mo after initial 8 wk course unless warts enlarge or new warts appear.

OFF-LABEL USES

Treatment of active chronic hepatitis, bladder carcinoma, chronic myelocytic leukemia, laryngeal papillomatosis, malignant melanoma, multiple myeloma, mycosis fungoides, non-Hodgkin's lymphoma

CONTRAINDICATIONS

Previous history of anaphylactic reaction to egg protein, mouse immunoglobulin, or neomycin

INTERACTIONS

Drug

Bone marrow depressants: May increase myelosuppression.

Herbal

None known.

Food

None known.

DIAGNOSTIC TEST EFFECTS

May increase serum LDH, alkaline phosphatase, AST (SGOT), and ALT (SGPT) levels. May decrease blood Hgb level, Hct, and leukocyte and platelet counts.

SIDE EFFECTS

Frequent

Flu-like symptoms

Occasional

Dizziness, pruritus, dry skin, dermatitis, altered taste

Rare

Confusion, leg cramps, back pain,

gingivitis, flushing, tremor, nervousness, eye pain

SERIOUS REACTIONS

! Hypersensitivity reaction occurs rarely.

! Severe flulike symptoms may occur at higher doses.

NURSING CONSIDERATIONS

Baseline Assessment

• Obtain and monitor the results of diagnostic tests, such as a CBC, before and regularly during therapy.

Precautions

• Use interferon alfa-n3 cautiously in patients with diabetes mellitus and ketoacidosis, hemophilia, pulmonary embolism, seizure disorders, severe myelosuppression, severe pulmonary disease, thrombophlebitis, uncontrolled CHF, or unstable angina.

Administration and Handling

Intralesional

• Refrigerate vials. Do not freeze or shake them.

• Using a 30-gauge needle, inject the drug into the base of each wart.

Intervention and Evaluation

• Monitor all levels of the patient's clinical function, and assess for side effects.

• Encourage the patient to drink ample fluids, particularly during early therapy.

Patient Teaching

• Inform the patient that flulike symptoms may be alleviated or minimized by taking doses at bedtime and that they tend to diminish with continued therapy.

• Inform the patient about any follow-up testing.

interferon alfacon-1

in-ter-**fear**-on

(Infergen)

CATEGORY AND SCHEDULE

Pregnancy Risk Category: C

MECHANISM OF ACTION

A biological response modifier that stimulates the immune system. **Therapeutic Effect:** Inhibits hepatitis C virus.

AVAILABILITY

Injection: 9 mcg/0.3 ml, 15 mcg/0.5 ml.

INDICATIONS AND DOSAGES

▸ **Chronic hepatitis C**

Subcutaneous

Adults. 9 mcg 3 times a week for 24 wk. May increase to 15 mcg 3 times a week in patients who tolerate but fail to respond to 9-mcg dose.

CONTRAINDICATIONS

History of autoimmune hepatitis or severe psychiatric disorders

SIDE EFFECTS

Frequent (greater than 50%)

Headache, fatigue, fever, depression

NURSING CONSIDERATIONS

Baseline Assessment

• Expect to obtain serum alkaline phosphatase, AST (SGOT), and ALT (SGPT), hepatitis C virus (HCV) antibody, and HCV-RNA levels.

Precautions

• Use interferon alfacon-1 cautiously in patients with a history of autoimmune disease, cardiac disease, depression, endocrine disorders, hepatic disorders, or myelosuppression.

Administration and Handling
Subcutaneous
◀ALERT▶ Make sure at least 48 hours elapse between doses of interferon alfacon-1.
Intervention and Evaluation
- Plan to obtain liver function test results and HCV antibody levels periodically.

Patient Teaching
- Instruct the patient to report any side effects, including headache or injection site pain as soon as possible.
- Teach the patient how hepatitis C is thought to be transmitted, such as by blood and body fluid.

interferon beta-1a
inn-ter-**fear**-on
(Avonex, Rebif)
Do not confuse interferon beta-1a with interferon beta-1b, or Avonex with Avelox.

CATEGORY AND SCHEDULE
Pregnancy Risk Category: C

MECHANISM OF ACTION
A biological response modifier that interacts with specific cell receptors found on the surface of human cells. **Therapeutic Effect:** Produces antiviral and immunoregulatory effects.

PHARMACOKINETICS
Peak serum levels attained 3–15 hr after IM administration. Biological markers increase within 12 hr and remain elevated for 4 days. ***Half-life:*** 10 hr (Avonex); 69 hr (Rebif).

AVAILABILITY
Injection, Powder for Reconstitution (Avonex): 30 mcg.
Injection Solution (Pre-filled Syringe [Avonex]): 30 mcg/0.5 ml.
Injection Solution (Pre-filled Syringe [Rebif]): 22 mcg/ml, 44 mcg/ml.
Titration Pack (Pre-filled Syringes [Rebif]): 8.8 mcg and 22 mcg.

INDICATIONS AND DOSAGES
▸ **Relapsing-remitting multiple sclerosis**
IM (Avonex)
Adults. 30 mcg once weekly.
Subcutaneous (Rebif)
Adults. Initially 8.8 mcg 3 times a week, may increase to 44 mcg 3 times a week over 4–6 wk.

OFF-LABEL USES
Treatment of AIDS, AIDS-related Kaposi's sarcoma, malignant melanoma, renal cell carcinoma

CONTRAINDICATIONS
Hypersensitivity to albumin or interferon

INTERACTIONS
Drug
None known.
Herbal
None known.
Food
None known.

DIAGNOSTIC TEST EFFECTS
May increase blood glucose and BUN levels, and serum alkaline phosphatase, bilirubin, calcium, AST (SGOT), and ALT (SGPT) levels. May decrease blood Hgb level and neutrophil, platelet, and WBC counts.

SIDE EFFECTS
Frequent
Headache (67%), flulike symptoms (61%), myalgia (34%), upper respiratory tract infection (31%), generalized pain (24%), asthenia, chills

(21%), sinusitis (18%), infection (11%)

Occasional

Abdominal pain, arthralgia (9%), chest pain, dyspnea (6%), malaise, syncope (4%)

Rare

Injection site reaction, hypersensitivity reaction (3%)

SERIOUS REACTIONS

! Anemia occurs in 8% of patients.

NURSING CONSIDERATIONS

Baseline Assessment

- Obtain CBC and serum alkaline phosphatase, AST (SGOT), and ALT (SGPT) levels.
- Assess the patient's home situation for support of therapy.

Lifespan Considerations

- Interferon beta-1a may cause spontaneous abortion.
- It is unknown if interferon beta-1a is distributed in breast milk.
- Interferon beta-1a should be used cautiously in children because its safety and efficacy have not been established in this age-group.
- No information is available on the use of interferon beta-1a in the elderly.

Precautions

- Use interferon beta-1a cautiously in children younger than 18 years and patients with chronic, progressive multiple sclerosis.

Administration and Handling

IM (Avonex powder for injection)

- Refrigerate unopened vials.
- Warm vials to room temperature before use.
- Reconstitute 30 mcg *MicroPin* (6.6 million unit) vial with 1.1 ml of the diluent provided by the manufacturer.

◀ **ALERT** ▶ Gently swirl—do not shake—the vial to dissolve the drug.

- If the drug is not used immediately after reconstitution, refrigerate it and use it within 6 hours. Discard it if it becomes discolored or contains a precipitate.
- After 6 hours, discard any unused portion because the drug contains no preservative.

IM (Avonex prefilled syringes)

- Allow the drug to warm to room temperature prior to use.
- Use syringe within 12 hr after removal from refrigerator.

Subcutaneous (Rebif prefilled syringes)

- Refigerate vials. If refrigeration is unavailable, the drug may be stored at room temperature, away from heat and light, up to 30 days.
- Administer the drug at the same time of day 3 days each week. Separate doses by at least 48 hours.

Intervention and Evaluation

- Assess the patient for flulike symptoms, headache, and myalgia.
- Periodically monitor the patient's laboratory results and reevaluate injection technique.
- Evaluate the patient for depression and suicidal ideation.

Patient Teaching

- Caution the patient against changing the drug dosage or administration schedule without consulting the physician.
- Teach the patient how to reconstitute and administer the drug, including aseptic technique and proper disposal of needles and syringes.
- Instruct the patient to document the type and severity of injection site reactions. Explain that these reactions will not require discontinuation of therapy, but should be reported immediately.

interferon beta-1b

inn-ter-**fear**-on

(Betaferon[AUS], Betaseron)

Do not confuse interferon beta-1b with interferon beta-1a.

CATEGORY AND SCHEDULE

Pregnancy Risk Category: C

MECHANISM OF ACTION

A biological response modifier that interacts with specific cell receptors found on the surface of human cells. **Therapeutic Effect:** Produces antiviral and immunoregulatory effects.

PHARMACOKINETICS

Half-life: 8 min–4.3 hr.

AVAILABILITY

Powder for Injection: 0.3 mg (9.6 million units).

INDICATIONS AND DOSAGES

▸ Relapsing-remitting multiple sclerosis

Subcutaneous

Adults. 0.25 mg (8 million units) every other day.

OFF-LABEL USES

Treatment of acute non-A and non-B hepatitis, AIDS, AIDS-related Kaposi's sarcoma, malignant melanoma, renal cell carcinoma

CONTRAINDICATIONS

Hypersensitivity to albumin or interferon

INTERACTIONS

Drug

None known.

Herbal

None known.

Food

None known.

DIAGNOSTIC TEST EFFECTS

May increase blood glucose and BUN levels, and serum alkaline phosphatase, bilirubin, calcium, AST (SGOT), and ALT (SGPT) levels. May decrease blood Hgb level and neutrophil, platelet, and WBC counts.

SIDE EFFECTS

Frequent

Injection site reaction (85%), headache (84%), flulike symptoms (76%), fever (59%), asthenia (49%), myalgia (44%), sinusitis (36%), diarrhea, dizziness (35%), mental status changes (29%), constipation (24%), diaphoresis (23%), vomiting (21%)

Occasional

Malaise (15%), somnolence (6%), alopecia (4%)

SERIOUS REACTIONS

! Seizures occur rarely.

NURSING CONSIDERATIONS

Baseline Assessment

- Obtain CBC and serum alkaline phosphatase, AST (SGOT), and ALT (SGPT) levels.
- Assess the patient's home situation for support of therapy.

Lifespan Considerations

- It is unknown if interferon beta-1b is distributed in breast milk.
- The safety and efficacy of interferon beta-1b have not been established in children.
- No information is available on the use of interferon beta-1b in the elderly.

Precautions

- Use interferon beta-1b cautiously in children younger than 18 years and patients with chronic, progressive multiple sclerosis.

Administration and Handling

Subcutaneous

- Store vials at room temperature.
- After reconstitution, the solution is stable for 3 hours if refrigerated.
- Reconstitute the 0.3-mg (9.6-million-unit) vial with 1.2 ml of the diluent supplied by the manufacturer to provide a concentration of 0.25 mg/ml (8 million units/ml).

◀ALERT▶ Gently swirl—do not shake—the vial to dissolve the drug.

- Use the solution within 3 hours of reconstitution.
- Discard the solution if it becomes discolored or contains a precipitate.
- Using a 27-gauge needle, inject 1 ml of the solution subcutaneously into the patient's abdomen, arms, hips, or thighs.
- Discard any unused portion because the solution contains no preservative.

Intervention and Evaluation

- Periodically monitor laboratory results and reevaluate injection technique.
- Assess the patient for flulike symptoms, most commonly nausea.
- Monitor the patient's sleep pattern.
- Assess the patient's pattern of daily bowel activity and stool consistency.
- Assist the patient with ambulation if he or she experiences dizziness.
- Determine if the patient experiences GI discomfort.
- Monitor the patient's food intake.
- Evaluate the patient for depression and suicidal ideation.

Patient Teaching

- Teach the patient how to reconstitute and administer the drug, including aseptic technique and proper disposal of needles and syringes.
- Tell the patient to notify the physician if he or she experiences flulike symptoms. Explain that these symptoms are a common side effect but decrease as therapy continues.
- Warn the patient to wear sunscreen and protective clothing when exposed to sunlight or ultraviolet light until the extent of his or her photosensitivity has been determined.
- Instruct the patient to avoid becoming pregnant during therapy.

interferon gamma-1b

in-ter-**fear**-on
(Actimmune, Imukin[AUS])

CATEGORY AND SCHEDULE

Pregnancy Risk Category: C

MECHANISM OF ACTION

A biological response modifier that induces activation of macrophages in blood monocytes to phagocytes, which is necessary in the body's cellular immune response to intracellular and extracellular pathogens. Enhances phagocytic function and antimicrobial activity of monocytes. **Therapeutic Effect:** Decreases signs and symptoms of serious infections in chronic granulomatous disease.

PHARMACOKINETICS

Slowly absorbed after subcutaneous administration.

AVAILABILITY

Injection: 100 mcg (2 million units).

INDICATIONS AND DOSAGES

▸ **Chronic granulomatous disease; severe, malignant osteopetrosis**

Subcutaneous

Adults, Children older than 1 yr. 50 mcg/m^2 (1.5 million units/m^2) in patients with body surface area

(BSA) greater than 0.5 m^2; 1.5 mcg/kg/dose in patients with BSA 0.5 m^2 or less. Give 3 times a week.

CONTRAINDICATIONS

Hypersensitivity to *Escherichia coli*–derived products

INTERACTIONS

Drug

Bone marrow depressants: May increase myelosuppression.

Herbal

None known.

Food

None known.

DIAGNOSTIC TEST EFFECTS

None known.

SIDE EFFECTS

Frequent

Fever (52%); headache (33%); rash (17%); chills, fatigue, diarrhea (14%)

Occasional (13%–10%)

Vomiting, nausea

Rare (6%–3%)

Weight loss, myalgia, anorexia

SERIOUS REACTIONS

! Interferon gamma-1b may exacerbate pre-existing CNS disturbances, including decreased mental status, gait disturbance, and dizziness, as well as cardiac disorders.

NURSING CONSIDERATIONS

Baseline Assessment

- Plan to obtain CBC, urinalysis, BUN level and serum alkaline phosphatase, creatinine, AST (SGOT), and ALT (SGPT) levels, before and every 3 months during therapy.

Lifespan Considerations

- It is unknown if interferon gamma-1b crosses the placenta or is distributed in breast milk.
- The safety and efficacy of interferon gamma-1b have not been established in children younger than 1 year.
- Children are more likely to experience flulike symptoms.
- No information is available on the use of interferon gamma-1b in the elderly.

Precautions

- Use interferon gamma-1b cautiously in patients with compromised CNS function, myelosuppression, pre-existing cardiac disorders (including arrhythmias, CHF, and myocardial ischemia), or seizure disorders.

Administration and Handling

◀ ALERT ▶ Avoid excessive agitation of the vial; don't shake it.

Subcutaneous

- Refrigerate unopened vials; don't freeze them.
- Discard vials kept at room temperature for longer than 12 hours.
- Vials come in single doses; discard any unused portion.
- The solution normally appears clear and colorless. Do not use it if it becomes discolored or contains a precipitate.
- Administer the drug 3 times a week. Rotate injection sites.

Intervention and Evaluation

- Monitor the patient for flulike symptoms, including chills, fatigue, fever, and myalgia.
- Examine the patient's skin for rash.

Patient Teaching

- Instruct the patient to store vials in the refrigerator.
- Teach the patient how to properly administer the drug and dispose of needles and syringes.
- Reassure the patient that flulike symptoms are generally mild and tend to disappear as treatment continues. Explain that these symptoms

may be minimized by giving the drug at bedtime.

- Advise the patient to avoid performing tasks that require mental alertness or motor skills until his or her response to the drug has been established.

muromonab-CD3

mur-oo-**mon**-ab
(Orthoclone, OKT3)

CATEGORY AND SCHEDULE

Pregnancy Risk Category: C

MECHANISM OF ACTION

A monoclonal antibody derived from purified IgG_2 that reacts with a T-3 (CD3) antigen of human T-cell membranes, blocking the production and function of T cells, which play a major role in acute organ rejection.
Therapeutic Effect: Reverses organ rejection.

AVAILABILITY

Injection: 1 mg/ml.

INDICATIONS AND DOSAGES

▸ Treatment of acute renal allograft rejection

IV

Adults, Elderly, Children 12 yr and older. 5 mg/day for 10–14 days, beginning as soon as acute renal rejection is diagnosed.
Children younger than 12 yr. 0.1 mg/kg/day for 10–14 days, beginning as soon as acute renal rejection is diagnosed.

CONTRAINDICATIONS

History of hypersensitivity to muromonab-CD3 or any murine-derived product, fluid overload (as evidenced by chest X-ray or weight gain of more than 3%) in the week before initial treatment

INTERACTIONS

Drug

Live-virus vaccines: May potentiate virus replication, increase the vaccine's side effects, and decrease the patient's response to the vaccine.
Other immunosuppressants: May increase the risk of infection or lymphoproliferative disorders.

Herbal

Echinacea: May decrease the effects of muromonab-CD3.

Food

None known.

DIAGNOSTIC TEST EFFECTS

None known.

IV INCOMPATIBILITIES

Do not mix muromonab with any other medications.

SIDE EFFECTS

Frequent

Fever, chills, dyspnea, malaise frequently occurs 30 min–6 hr after first dose. This reaction markedly diminishes after the 2nd day of treatment.

Occasional

Chest pain, nausea, vomiting, diarrhea, tremor

SERIOUS REACTIONS

! Symptoms of cytokine release syndrome, a common reaction, may range from mild flulike symptoms to a life-threatening, shocklike reaction.

! Infection due to immunosuppression generally occurs within 45 days after initial treatment. Cytomegalovirus occurs in 19% of patients, and herpes simplex occurs in 27% of patients. A severe, life-threatening

infection occurs in fewer than 5% of patients.
! Severe pulmonary edema occurs in fewer than 2% of patients.
! Fatal hypersensitivity reactions occur occasionally.

NURSING CONSIDERATIONS

Baseline Assessment

• Plan to obtain a chest X-ray within 24 hours of beginning muromonab-CD3 therapy to ensure that the patient's lungs are free of fluid.
• Monitor the patient's immunologic test results (including plasma drug levels and quantitative T-lymphocyte surface phenotyping), liver and renal function test results, and WBC count before and during therapy.
• Check for fluid overload before beginning muromonab-CD3 treatment to decrease the risk of pulmonary edema.

Precautions

• Use muromonab-CD3 cautiously in patients with impaired cardiac, hepatic, or renal function.

Administration and Handling

IV
• Have resuscitative drugs and equipment immediately available.
• Refrigerate ampules. Don't use the drug if it has been left out of the refrigerator for longer than 4 hours.
• Don't shake the ampule before using.
• The solution may develop fine translucent particles, which won't affect potency.
• Draw the solution into the syringe through a 0.22-micron filter. Discard the filter; use a needle for IV administration.
• Administer by IV push over less than 1 minute.
• Give 1 mg/kg methylprednisolone 1-4 hours before and 100 mg hydrocortisone 30 minutes after the first dose of muromonab-CD3, as prescribed, to decrease the risk and severity of cytokine release syndrome.

Intervention and Evaluation

• Give antipyretics to patients with a fever above 100°F.
• Obtain chest X-rays and auscultate the patient's breath sounds to detect fluid overload. Also, be alert for weight gain of more than 3% over pre-therapy weight.
• Monitor the patient's intake and output.
• Assess the patient's pattern of daily bowel activity and stool consistency.

Patient Teaching

• Tell the patient to expect a first-dose reaction, including chest tightness, chills, fever, diarrhea, nausea, vomiting, and wheezing.
• Urge the patient to avoid receiving immunizations and coming in contact with crowds and people with known infections during muromonab-CD3 therapy.

mycophenolate mofetil

my-co-**fen**-o-late
(CellCept)

CATEGORY AND SCHEDULE

Pregnancy Risk Category: C

MECHANISM OF ACTION

An immunologic agent that suppresses the immunologically mediated inflammatory response by inhibiting inosine monophosphate dehydrogenase, an enzyme that deprives lymphocytes of nucleotides necessary for DNA and RNA synthesis, thus inhibiting the proliferation of T and B lymphocytes. **Therapeutic Effect:** Prevents transplant rejection.

PHARMACOKINETICS

Rapidly and extensively absorbed after PO administration (food decreases drug plasma concentration but doesn't affect absorption). Protein binding: 97%. Completely hydrolyzed to active metabolite mycophenolic acid. Primarily excreted in urine. Not removed by hemodialysis. ***Half-life:*** 17.9 hr.

AVAILABILITY

Capsules: 250 mg.
Oral Suspension: 200 mg/ml.
Tablets: 500 mg.
Injection: 500 mg.

INDICATIONS AND DOSAGES

▸ Prevention of renal transplant rejection
PO, IV
Adults, Elderly. 1 g twice a day.

▸ Prevention of heart transplant rejection
PO, IV
Adults, Elderly. 1.5 g twice a day.

▸ Prevention of liver transplant rejection
PO
Adults, Elderly. 1.5 g twice a day.
IV
Adults, Elderly. 1 g twice a day.

▸ Usual pediatric dosage
PO
Children. 600 mg/m^2/dose twice a day. Maximum: 2 g/day.

OFF-LABEL USES

Treatment of liver transplantation rejection, mild heart transplant rejection, moderate to severe psoriasis

CONTRAINDICATIONS

Hypersensitivity to mycophenolic acid

INTERACTIONS

Drug

Acyclovir, ganciclovir: May increase plasma concentrations of both drugs in patients with renal impairment.
Antacids (aluminum- and magnesium-containing), cholestyramine: May decrease the absorption of mycophenolate.
Live-virus vaccines: May potentiate virus replication, increase vaccine side effects, and decrease the patient's antibody response to the vaccine.
Other immunosuppressants: May increase the risk of infection or lymphomas.
Probenecid: May increase mycophenolate plasma concentration.

Herbal

Echinacea: May decrease the effects of mycophenolate.

Food

All foods: May decrease mycophenolate plasma concentration.

DIAGNOSTIC TEST EFFECTS

May increase serum cholesterol, alkaline phosphatase, creatinine, AST (SGOT), and ALT (SGPT) levels. May increase or decrease blood glucose as well as serum lipid, calcium, potassium, phosphate, and uric acid levels.

IV INCOMPATIBILITIES

Mycophenolate is compatible only with D_5W. Do not infuse it concurrently with other drugs or IV solutions.

SIDE EFFECTS

Frequent (37%–20%)
UTI, hypertension, peripheral edema, diarrhea, constipation, fever, headache, nausea
Occasional (18%–10%)
Dyspepsia; dyspnea; cough;

hematuria; asthenia; vomiting; edema; tremors; abdominal, chest, or back pain; oral candidiasis; acne

Rare (9%–6%)

Insomnia, respiratory tract infection, rash, dizziness

SERIOUS REACTIONS

! Significant anemia, leukopenia, thrombocytopenia, neutropenia, and leukocytosis may occur, particularly in those undergoing renal transplant rejection.

! Sepsis and infection occur occasionally.

! GI tract hemorrhage occurs rarely.

! Patients receiving mycophenolate have an increased risk of developing neoplasms.

NURSING CONSIDERATIONS

Baseline Assessment

• Plan to perform a pregnancy test in female patients of childbearing potential within 1 week before beginning mycophenolate therapy.

• Assess the patient's medical history, especially for renal function and active digestive disease, and drug history, including the use of other immunosuppressants.

Lifespan Considerations

• It is unknown if mycophenolate crosses the placenta or is distributed in breast milk. Patients taking this drug should avoid breast-feeding.

• The safety and efficacy of mycophenolate have not been established in children.

• Age-related renal impairment may require a dosage adjustment in the elderly.

Precautions

• Use mycophenolate cautiously in female patients of childbearing potential and in patients with active serious digestive disease, neutropenia, or renal impairment.

Administration and Handling

PO

• Give mycophenolate on an empty stomach.

• Do not open or crush capsules.

• Avoid inhaling the powder in capsules and keep the powder away from skin and mucous membranes. If contact occurs, wash thoroughly with soap and water, and rinse the eyes profusely with plain water.

• Store the reconstituted suspension in the refrigerator or at room temperature. It remains stable for 60 days after reconstitution.

• The suspension can be administered orally or by nasogastric tube (minimum size: 8 French).

IV

• Store vials at room temperature.

• Reconstitute each 500-mg vial with 14 ml D_5W. Gently agitate the vial.

• For a 1-g dose, further dilute with 140 ml D_5W; for a 1.5-g dose, further dilute with 210 ml D_5W to provide a concentration of 6 mg/ml.

• Infuse the drug over at least 2 hours.

Intervention and Evaluation

• Plan to obtain the patient's CBC weekly during the first month of therapy, twice monthly during the second and third months, then monthly for the rest of the first year.

• Reduce the dosage or discontinue the drug if the patient experiences a rapid fall in WBC count.

• Assess the patient for delayed myelosuppression.

Patient Teaching

• Instruct the female patient (unless she has had a hysterectomy) to use effective contraception before, during, and for 6 weeks after discontinuing mycophenolate therapy, even if she has had a history of infertility. Advise her to use two forms of contraception concurrently unless she will remain abstinent.

• Advise the patient to notify the physician if he or she experiences abdominal pain, fever, sore throat, or unusual bleeding or bruising.
• Stress the need for regular laboratory tests during mycophenolate therapy.
• Inform the patient that malignancies may occur. Be prepared to answer questions and provide additional information.

natalizumab

nat-ah-**lih**-zoo-mab
(Tysabri)

CATEGORY AND SCHEDULE

Pregnancy Risk Category: C

◀ALERT▶ Marketing of this drug has been suspended to evaluate the adverse effects that have been reported related to its use (as of this writing).

MECHANISM OF ACTION

A monoclonal antibody that binds to the surface of leukocytes, inhibiting their adhesion to the vascular endothelial cells of the GI tract and preventing them from migrating across the endothelium into inflamed parenchymal tissue. **Therapeutic Effect:** Decreases clinical exacerbations of multiple sclerosis.

PHARMACOKINETICS

Half-life: 11 days.

AVAILABILITY

Injection Solution: 300 mg/15 ml concentrate.

INDICATIONS AND DOSAGES

▸ **Relapses of multiple sclerosis**

IV

Adults 18 yr and older, Elderly. 300 mg every 4 wk.

CONTRAINDICATIONS

None known.

INTERACTIONS

Drug

None known.

Herbal

None known.

Food

None known.

DIAGNOSTIC TEST EFFECTS

Increases basophil, eosinophil, lymphocyte, monocyte, and RBC counts (increases are reversible, usually within 16 wk after last natalizumab dose). May alter liver function test results.

IV INCOMPATIBILITIES

Don't mix natalizumab with any other medications or dilute it with anything other than 0.9% NaCl.

SIDE EFFECTS

Frequent (35%–15%)

Headache, fatigue, depression, arthralgia

Occasional (10%–5%)

Abdominal discomfort, rash, urinary frequency or urgency, menstrual irregularities, dysmenorrhea, dermatitis

Rare (4%–2%)

Pruritus, chest discomfort, local bleeding, rigors, tremor, syncope

SERIOUS REACTIONS

! UTI, lower respiratory tract infection, gastroenteritis, vaginitis, allergic reaction, and tonsillitis occur occasionally.

NURSING CONSIDERATIONS

Baseline Assessment

- Obtain the patient's blood chemistry studies, including CBC and liver function test results.
- Assess the patient's home situation for support of therapy.

Lifespan Considerations

- It is unknown if natalizumab crosses the placenta or is distributed in breast milk.
- The safety and efficacy of natalizumab have not been established in children younger than 18 years.
- No age-related precautions have been noted for elderly patients.

Precautions

- Use natalizumab cautiously in children younger than 18 years and in patients with chronic progressive multiple sclerosis.

Administration and Handling

IV

- Protect natalizumab vials from light. Don't freeze them.
- To reconstitute, withdraw 15 ml natalizumab from the vial and inject it into 100 ml 0.9% NaCl.
- Invert the vial to mix the solution completely. Do not shake it.
- Inspect the solution for particles. Discard it if it contains particles or becomes discolored.
- After reconstitution, the solution is stable for 8 hours if refrigerated.
- Infuse natalizumab over 1 hour.
- Following the infusion, flush the IV line with 0.9% NaCl.

Intervention and Evaluation

- Periodically monitor the patient's laboratory test results and reevaluate the infusion technique.
- Assess the patient for arthralgia, depression, menstrual irregularities, and urinary changes.
- Examine the patient's skin for dermatitis and rash, and ask about pruritus.
- Monitor the patient for signs and symptoms of a respiratory or urinary tract infection.

Patient Teaching

- If the patient will receive the drug at home, make sure he or she knows how to handle and prepare it properly. Review infusion techniques before discharge.
- Instruct the patient to report side effects to the physician.
- Inform the patient when to obtain follow-up blood work.

peginterferon alfa-2a

peg-inn-ter-**fear**-on
(Pegasys)

CATEGORY AND SCHEDULE

Pregnancy Risk Category: C

MECHANISM OF ACTION

An immunomodulator that binds to specific membrane receptors on the cell surface, inhibiting viral replication in virus-infected cells, suppressing cell proliferation, and producing reversible decreases in leukocyte and platelet counts. **Therapeutic Effect:** Inhibits hepatitis C virus.

PHARMACOKINETICS

Readily absorbed after subcutaneous administration. Excreted by the kidneys. ***Half-life:*** 80 hr.

AVAILABILITY

Injection: 180 mcg/ml.

INDICATIONS AND DOSAGES

▸ **Hepatitis C**

Subcutaneous

Adults 18 yr and older, Elderly. 180 mcg (1 ml) injected in abdomen or thigh once weekly for 48 wk.

▸ **Dosage in renal impairment**
For patients who require hemodialysis, dosage is 135 mg injected in abdomen or thigh once weekly for 48 wk.

▸ **Dosage in hepatic impairment**
For patients with progressive ALT (SGPT) increases above baseline values, dosage is 90 mcg injected in abdomen or thigh once weekly for 48 wk.

CONTRAINDICATIONS

Autoimmune hepatitis, decompensated hepatic disease, infants, neonates

INTERACTIONS

Drug

Bone marrow depressants: May increase myelosuppression.
Theophylline: May increase the serum level of theophylline.

Herbal

None known.

Food

None known.

DIAGNOSTIC TEST EFFECTS

May increase ALT (SGPT) level. May decrease the absolute neutrophil, platelet, and WBC counts. May cause a slight decrease in blood Hgb level and Hct.

SIDE EFFECTS

Frequent (54%)

Headache

Occasional (23%–13%)

Alopecia, nausea, insomnia, anorexia, dizziness, diarrhea, abdominal pain, flulike symptoms, psychiatric reactions (depression, irritability, anxiety), injection site reaction

Rare (8%–5%)

Impaired concentration, diaphoresis, dry mouth, nausea, vomiting

SERIOUS REACTIONS

! Serious, acute hypersensitivity reactions, such as urticaria, angioedema, bronchoconstriction, and anaphylaxis, may occur. Other rare reactions include pancreatitis, colitis, endocrine disorders (e.g., diabetes mellitus), hyperthyroidism or hypothyroidism, ophthalmologic disorders, and pulmonary disorders.

NURSING CONSIDERATIONS

Baseline Assessment

- Plan to obtain CBC, EKG, urinalysis, BUN level, and serum alkaline phosphatase, creatinine, AST (SGOT), and ALT (SGPT) levels before and routinely during therapy.
- Ensure that patients with diabetes mellitus or hypertension have an ophthalmologic exam before beginning therapy.

Lifespan Considerations

- Peginterferon alfa-2a may cause spontaneous abortion.
- It is unknown if peginterferon alfa-2a is distributed in breast milk.
- The safety and efficacy of peginterferon alfa-2a have not been established in children younger than 18 years.
- Cardiac, CNS, and systemic effects may be more severe in the elderly, particularly in those with renal impairment.

Precautions

- Use peginterferon alfa-2a extremely cautiously in patients with a history of neuropsychiatric disorders.
- Use the drug cautiously in elderly patients and in patients with autoimmune, cardiac, endocrine (diabetes mellitus, hyperthyroidism, hypothyroidism), pulmonary, or ophthalmic disorders; colitis; compromised CNS function; myelosuppression; or renal impairment (creatinine clearance less than 50 ml/minute).

Administration and Handling

◀ **ALERT** ▶ For patients with moderate to severe adverse reactions, expect to decrease the dose to 135 mcg (0.75 ml) or 90 mcg (0.5 ml), as prescribed. For patients with an absolute neutrophil count less than 750 cells/mm^3, reduce dose to 135 mcg (0.75 ml). For those with an absolute neutrophil count less than 500 cells/mm^3, discontinue treatment until the count returns to 1,000 cells/mm^3. For those with a platelet count less than 50,000 cells/mm^3, reduce dose to 90 mcg.

Subcutaneous

- Refrigerate vials.
- Vials are for single use only; discard unused portions.
- Inject the drug subcutaneously in the abdomen or thigh.

Intervention and Evaluation

- Monitor the patient for abdominal pain and bloody diarrhea, evidence of colitis.
- Monitor the patient's chest X-ray for pulmonary infiltrates.
- Assess the patient for pulmonary function impairment.
- Encourage the patient to drink ample fluids, particularly during early therapy.
- Assess the patient's serum hepatitis C virus RNA levels after 24 weeks of treatment.
- Monitor the patient for depression.
- Offer the patient emotional support.

Patient Teaching

- Inform the patient that the drug's therapeutic effect should appear in 1 to 3 months.
- Explain that flulike symptoms tend to diminish with continued therapy.
- Urge the patient to immediately notify the physician if he or she experiences depression or suicidal thoughts.
- Caution the patient to avoid performing tasks requiring mental alertness or motor skills until his or her response to the drug has been established.

peginterferon alfa-2b

peg-inn-ter-**fear**-on

(PEG-Intron)

CATEGORY AND SCHEDULE

Pregnancy Risk Category: C

MECHANISM OF ACTION

An immunomodulator that inhibits viral replication in virus-infected cells, suppresses cell proliferation, increases phagocytic action of macrophages, and augments specific cytotoxicity of lymphocytes for target cells. **Therapeutic Effect:** Inhibits hepatitis C virus.

AVAILABILITY

Injection Powder for Reconstitution: 50 mcg, 80 mcg, 120 mcg, 150 mcg.

INDICATIONS AND DOSAGES

▸ **Chronic hepatitis C, monotherapy**

Subcutaneous

Adults 18 yr and older, Elderly. Administer appropriate dosage (see chart below) once weekly for 1 yr on the same day each wk.

Vial Strength	Weight (kg)	mcg*	ml*
100 mcg/ml	37–45	40	0.4
	46–56	50	0.5
160 mcg/ml	57–72	64	0.4
	73–88	80	0.5
240 mcg/ml	89–106	96	0.4
	107–136	120	0.5
300 mcg/ml	137–160	150	0.5

*of peginterferon alpha-2b to administer

▸ Chronic hepatitis C
Subcutaneous
Combination therapy with ribavirin (400 mg twice a day). Initially, 1.5 mcg/kg/wk.

CONTRAINDICATIONS

Autoimmune hepatitis, decompensated hepatic disease, history of psychiatric disorders

INTERACTIONS

Drug

Bone marrow depressants: May increase myelosuppression.

Herbal

None known.

Food

None known.

DIAGNOSTIC TEST EFFECTS

May increase blood glucose and ALT (SGPT) levels. May decrease blood neutrophil and platelet counts.

SIDE EFFECTS

Frequent (50%–47%)
Flu-like symptoms; inflammation, bruising, pruritus, and irritation at injection site
Occasional (29%–18%)
Psychiatric reactions (depression, anxiety, emotional lability, irritability), insomnia, alopecia, diarrhea
Rare
Rash, diaphoresis, dry skin, dizziness, flushing, vomiting, dyspepsia

SERIOUS REACTIONS

! Serious, acute hypersensitivity reactions (such as urticaria, angioedema, bronchoconstriction, and anaphylaxis), pulmonary disorders, endocrine disorders (e.g., diabetes mellitus), hypothyroidism, hyperthyroidism, and pancreatitis occur rarely.

! Ulcerative colitis may occur within 12 weeks of starting treatment.

NURSING CONSIDERATIONS

Baseline Assessment

- Plan to obtain CBC, EKG, urinalysis, BUN level, and serum alkaline phosphatase, creatinine, AST (SGOT), and ALT (SGPT) levels before and routinely during therapy.
- Ensure that patients with diabetes mellitus or hypertension have an ophthalmologic exam before beginning therapy.

Lifespan Considerations

- Peginterferon alfa-2b may cause spontaneous abortion.
- It is unknown if peginterferon alfa-2b is distributed in breast milk.
- The safety and efficacy of peginterferon alfa-2b have not been established in children younger than 18 years.
- Cardiac, CNS, and systemic effects may be more severe in the elderly, particularly in patients with renal impairment.

Precautions

- Use peginterferon alfa-2b cautiously in elderly patients and patients with autoimmune, cardiac, endocrine (diabetes mellitus, hyperthyroidism, hyperthyroidism), pulmonary, or ophthalmic disorders; colitis; compromised CNS function; myelosuppression; or renal impairment (creatinine clearance less than 50 ml/minute).

Administration and Handling

◂ALERT▸ If severe adverse reactions occur, modify the dosage dose or temporarily discontinue the drug, as prescribed. Know that the dosage is based on weight.

◂ALERT▸ Remember that the drug's side effects are dose-related.

Subcutaneous
- Store vials at room temperature.
- Reconstitute the drug by adding 0.7 ml sterile water for injection (the supplied diluent) to the vial. Use it

immediately or after reconstitution or, if necessary, refrigerate it for up to 24 hours.

Intervention and Evaluation

- Monitor the patient for abdominal pain and bloody diarrhea, evidence of colitis.
- Monitor the patient's chest x-ray for pulmonary infiltrates.
- Assess the patient for pulmonary function impairment.
- Encourage the patient to drink adequate fluids, particularly during early therapy.
- Assess the patient's serum hepatitis C virus RNA levels after 24 weeks of treatment.
- Monitor the patient for depression.
- Offer the patient emotional support.

Patient Teaching

- Instruct the patient to consume adequate fluids and to avoid alcohol.
- Inform the patient that flulike symptoms, such as body aches, headache, and nausea, tend to diminish with continued therapy.
- Advise the patient to notify the physician if he or she experiences bloody diarrhea, fever, persistent abdominal pain, depression, signs of infection, or unusual bruising or bleeding.

sirolimus

sir-oh-**leem**-us
(Rapamune)

CATEGORY AND SCHEDULE

Pregnancy Risk Category: C

MECHANISM OF ACTION

An immunosuppressant that inhibits T-lymphocyte proliferation induced by stimulation of cell surface receptors, mitogens, alloantigens, and lymphokines. Prevents activation of the enzyme target of rapamycin, a key regulatory kinase in cell cycle progression. **Therapeutic Effect:** Inhibits proliferation of T and B cells, essential components of the immune response; prevents organ transplant rejection.

AVAILABILITY

Oral Solution: 1 mg/ml.
Tablets: 1 mg, 2 mg.

INDICATIONS AND DOSAGES

▸ **Prevention of organ transplant rejection**

PO

Adults. Loading dose: 6 mg. Maintenance: 2 mg/day.

Children 13 yr and older weighing less than 40 kg. Loading dose: 3 mg/m^2. Maintenance: 1 mg/m^2/day.

CONTRAINDICATIONS

Hypersensitivity to sirolimus, malignancy

INTERACTIONS

Drug

Cyclosporine, diltiazem, ketoconazole: May increase the blood concentration and risk of toxicity of sirolimus.

Rifampin: May decrease the blood concentration and effects of sirolimus.

Herbal

None known.

Food

Grapefruit, grapefruit juice: May decrease the metabolism of sirolimus.

DIAGNOSTIC TEST EFFECTS

May decrease blood Hgb level, Hct, and platelet count. May increase serum cholesterol, creatinine, and triglyceride levels.

SIDE EFFECTS

Occasional

Hypercholesterolemia, hyperlipidemia, hypertension, rash; with high doses (5 mg/day): anemia, arthralgia, diarrhea, hypokalemia, and thrombocytopenia

SERIOUS REACTIONS

! None known.

NURSING CONSIDERATIONS

Baseline Assessment

- Determine if the female patient is pregnant or breast-feeding.
- Determine if the patient is taking other medications, especially cyclosporine, diltiazem, ketoconazole, and rifampin.
- Determine if the patient has chickenpox, herpes zoster, an infection, or a malignancy.
- Expect to perform baseline laboratory tests, including a CBC and serum lipid profile.

Precautions

- Use sirolimus cautiously in patients with chickenpox, herpes zoster, hepatic impairment, or an infection.

Intervention and Evaluation

- Monitor the patient's liver function test results periodically.

Patient Teaching

- Instruct the patient to take the drug at the same time each day, and to notify the physician if he or she misses a dose.
- Tell the patient to avoid consuming grapefruit or grapefruit juice during therapy.
- Urge the patient to avoid coming in contact with people with colds or other infections.
- Inform the patient that strict monitoring is an essential part of sirolimus therapy identifying and preventing symptoms of organ rejection.

tacrolimus

tak-roe-**leem**-us

(Prograf, Protopic)

Do not confuse Protopic with Protonix, Protopam, Protopin.

CATEGORY AND SCHEDULE

Pregnancy Risk Category: C

MECHANISM OF ACTION

An immunologic agent that inhibits T-lymphocyte activation by binding to intracellular proteins, forming a complex, and inhibiting phosphatase activity. **Therapeutic Effect:** Suppresses the immunologically mediated inflammatory response; prevents organ transplant rejection.

PHARMACOKINETICS

Variably absorbed after PO administration (food reduces absorption). Protein binding: 75%–97%. Extensively metabolized in the liver. Excreted in urine. Not removed by hemodialysis. ***Half-life:*** 11.7 hr.

AVAILABILITY

Capsules (Prograf): 0.5 mg, 1 mg, 5 mg.
Injection (Prograf): 5 mg/ml.
Ointment (Protopic): 0.03%, 0.1%.

INDICATIONS AND DOSAGES

▸Prevention of liver transplant rejection

PO

Adults, Elderly. 0.1–0.15 mg/kg/day in 2 divided doses 12 hr apart.
Children. 0.15–0.2 mg/kg/day in 2 divided doses 12 hr apart.

IV

Adults, Elderly, Children. 0.03–0.15 mg/kg/day as a continuous infusion.

▸ **Prevention of kidney transplant rejection**
PO
Adults, Elderly. 0.2 mg/kg/day in 2 divided doses 12 hr apart
IV
Adults, Elderly. 0.03–0.15 mg/kg/day as continuous infusion.

▸ **Atopic dermatitis**
Topical
Adults, Elderly, Children 2 yr and older. Apply 0.03% ointment to affected area twice a day. 0.1% ointment may be used in adults and the elderly. Continue until 1 wk after symptoms have cleared.

OFF-LABEL USES

Prevention of organ rejection in patients receiving allogeneic bone marrow, heart, pancreas, pancreatic island cell, or small-bowel transplant, treatment of autoimmune disease, severe recalcitrant psoriasis

CONTRAINDICATIONS

Concurrent use with cyclosporine (increases the risk of nephrotoxicity), hypersensitivity to HCO-60 polyoxyl 60 hydrogenated castor oil (used in solution for injection), hypersensitivity to tacrolimus

INTERACTIONS

Drug

Aminoglycosides, amphotericin B, cisplatin: Increase the risk of renal dysfunction.
Antacids: Decrease the absorption of tacrolimus.
Antifungals, bromocriptine, calcium channel blockers, cimetidine, clarithromycin, cyclosporine, danazol, diltiazem, erythromycin, methylprednisolone, metoclopramide: Increase tacrolimus blood concentration.
Carbamazepine, phenobarbital, phenytoin, rifamycin: Decrease tacrolimus blood concentration.
Cyclosporine: Increases the risk of nephrotoxicity.
Live-virus vaccines: May potentiate virus replication, increase vaccine side effects, and decrease the patient's antibody response to the vaccine.
Other immunosuppressants: May increase the risk of infection or lymphomas.

Herbal

Echinacea: May decrease the effects of tacrolimus.

Food

Grapefruit, grapefruit juice: May alter the effects of the drug.

DIAGNOSTIC TEST EFFECTS

May increase blood glucose, BUN, and serum creatinine levels, as well as WBC count. May decrease serum magnesium level and RBC and thrombocyte counts. May alter serum potassium level.

IV INCOMPATIBILITIES

No known drug incompatibilities. Do not mix tacrolimus with other medications if possible.

IV COMPATIBILITIES

Calcium gluconate, dexamethasone (Decadron), diphenhydramine (Benadryl), dobutamine (Dobutrex), dopamine (Intropin), furosemide (Lasix), heparin, hydromorphone (Dilaudid), insulin, leucovorin, lorazepam (Ativan), morphine, nitroglycerin, potassium chloride

SIDE EFFECTS

Frequent (greater than 30%)
Headache, tremor, insomnia, paresthesia, diarrhea, nausea, constipation, vomiting, abdominal pain, hypertension

Occasional (29%–10%)
Rash, pruritus, anorexia, asthenia, peripheral edema, photosensitivity

SERIOUS REACTIONS

! Nephrotoxicity (characterized by increased serum creatinine level and decreased urine output), neurotoxicity (including tremor, headache, and mental status changes), and pleural effusion are common adverse reactions.
! Thrombocytopenia, leukocytosis, anemia, atelectasis, sepsis, and infection occur occasionally.

NURSING CONSIDERATIONS

Baseline Assessment

• Assess the patient's drug history, especially for other immunosuppressants, and medical history, especially renal function.
• Obtain baseline laboratory tests, including BUN, CBC, and hepatic enzyme, serum creatinine, and serum electrolyte levels.

Lifespan Considerations

• Tacrolimus crosses the placenta and is distributed in breast milk. Patients taking this drug should not breast-feed.
• Hyperkalemia and renal dysfunction have been noted in neonates.
• Children may require a higher dosage because of decreased bioavailability and increased clearance of the drug.
• Post-transplant lymphoproliferative disorder is more common in children, especially children younger than 3 years.
• Age-related renal impairment may require a dosage adjustment in the elderly.

Precautions

• Use tacrolimus cautiously in patients with immunosuppression or hepatic or renal impairment.

Administration and Handling

◀ALERT▶ For patients unable to take capsules, initiate therapy with IV infusion. Give oral dose 8 to 12 hours after discontinuing IV infusion. Titrate dosage based on clinical assessments of rejection and patient tolerance. For patients with hepatic or renal impairment, give the lowest IV and oral doses, as prescribed. Plan to delay administration for 48 hours or longer in patients with postoperative oliguria.

PO
• Administer tacrolimus on an empty stomach.
• Don't give this drug with grapefruit or grapefruit juice or within 2 hours of antacids.

IV
• Store the diluted solution in a glass or polyethylene containers and discard it after 24 hours. Don't store it in a polyvinyl chloride container because the container may absorb the drug or affect its stability.
• Keep oxygen and an aqueous solution of epinephrine 1:1,000 available at the bedside before beginning the IV infustion.
• Dilute the drug with 250 to 1,000 ml 0.9% NaCl or D_5W, depending on the desired dose, to provide a concentration of 0.004 to 0.02 mg/ml.
• Administer tacrolimus as a continuous IV infusion.
• Monitor the patient continuously for the first 30 minutes of the infusion and at frequent intervals thereafter.
• Stop the infusion immediately at the first sign of a hypersensitivity reaction.

Topical
• Tacrolimus ointment is for external use only.
• Rub the ointment gently and completely into clean, dry skin.

- Don't cover the treated area with an occlusive dressing.

Intervention and Evaluation

- Closely monitor patients with impaired renal function.
- Obtain a CBC weekly during the first month of therapy, twice monthly during the second and third months of treatment, then monthly for the rest of the first year. Also monitor the patient's liver function test results and serum creatinine and potassium levels.
- Closely monitor the patient's intake and output.
- Assess the patient for signs and symptoms of serious adverse effects, such as a change in mental status or a decrease in urine output. Immediately report your findings to the physician.

Patient Teaching

- Teach the patient to take the capsules on an empty stomach and not to mix them with grapefruit juice.
- Instruct the patient to take the drug at the same time each day and to notify the physician if he or she misses a dose.
- Caution the patient to avoid crowds and people with infections.
- Advise the patient to notify the physician if he or she experiences chest pain, dizziness, headache, decreased urination, rash, respiratory infection, or unusual bleeding or bruising.
- Urge the patient to avoid exposure to sunlight and artificial light because this may cause a photosensitivity reaction.

thalidomide

thah-**lid**-owe-mide
(Thalomid)

CATEGORY AND SCHEDULE

Pregnancy Risk Category: X

MECHANISM OF ACTION

An immunomodulator whose exact mechanism is unknown. Has sedative, anti-inflammatory, and immunosuppressive activity, which may be due to selective inhibition of the production of tumor necrosis factor-alpha. **Therapeutic Effect:** Improves muscle wasting in HIV patients; reduces local and systemic effects of leprosy.

AVAILABILITY

Capsules: 50 mg.

INDICATIONS AND DOSAGES

▸ **AIDS-related muscle wasting**

PO

Adults. 100–300 mg a day.

▸ **Leprosy**

PO

Adults, Elderly. Initially, 100–300 mg/day as single bedtime dose, at least 1 hr after the evening meal. Continue until active reaction subsides, then reduce dose q2–4 wk in 50-mg increments.

OFF-LABEL USES

Treatment of Crohn's disease, recurrent aphthous ulcers in HIV patients, wasting syndrome associated with HIV or cancer

CONTRAINDICATIONS

Neutropenia, peripheral neuropathy; pregnancy, sensitivity to thalidomide

INTERACTIONS

Drug

Alcohol, other CNS depressants: May increase sedative effects.
Medications associated with peripheral neuropathy (such as isoniazid, lithium, metronidazole, phenytoin): May increase peripheral neuropathy.
Medications that decrease effectiveness of hormonal contraceptives (such as carbamazepine, protease inhibitors, rifampin): May decrease the effectiveness of the contraceptive; patient must use two other methods of contraception.

Herbal

None known.

Food

None known.

DIAGNOSTIC TEST EFFECTS

None known.

SIDE EFFECTS

Frequent

Somnolence, dizziness, mood changes, constipation, dry mouth, peripheral neuropathy

Occasional

Increased appetite, weight gain, headache, loss of libido, edema of face and limbs, nausea, alopecia, dry skin, rash, hypothyroidism

SERIOUS REACTIONS

! Neutropenia, peripheral neuropathy, and thromboembolism occur rarely.

NURSING CONSIDERATIONS

Baseline Assessment

- Determine if the female patient is pregnant. Thalidomide use is contraindicated in pregnant women.
- Determine if the patient is using other medications.
- Assess the patient for hypersensitivity to thalidomide.

Precautions

- Use thalidomide cautiously in patients with a history of seizures.

Administration and Handling

- Administer thalidomide with water at least 1 hour after the evening meal and, if possible, at bedtime because of the risk of developing somnolence.

Intervention and Evaluation

- Monitor the patient's HIV viral load, nerve conduction studies, and WBC count.
- Observe the patient for signs and symptoms of peripheral neuropathy.

Patient Teaching

- Urge the patient to avoid consuming alcohol or using other drugs that cause drowsiness during thalidomide therapy.
- Instruct female patients of childbearing age to perform a pregnancy test within 24 hours before beginning thalidomide therapy, and then every 2 to 4 weeks.
- Advise the patient to discontinue the drug and notify the physician if he or she experiences symptoms of peripheral neuropathy.
- Caution the patient to avoid performing tasks that require mental alertness or motor skills until his or her response to the drug has been established.

75 Herbals

black cohosh
chamomile
DHEA
dong quai
echinacea
feverfew
garlic
ginger
ginkgo biloba
ginseng
glucosamine and chondroitin
kava kava
melatonin
saw palmetto
St. John's wort
valerian
yohimbe

Uses: Many patients take herbal supplements because they believe these natural medicines are safer and healthier than conventional drugs, because cultural influences and recommendations from family members and friends make these remedies attractive, or because herbal preparations offer convenience and relatively low cost. Herbals are used for various purposes, ranging from menopausal symptom relief and immune system stimulation to memory enhancement and sleep promotion. For specific uses, see the entries in this chapter.

Action: Herbal supplements are plant-derived products that promote health and relieve disease symptoms. Although some are effective, many aren't and a few can be harmful. Their actions vary greatly. For example, *black cohosh* is a phytoestrogen that may have estrogen-like effects. However, its exact mechanism of action is unknown. *Echinacea* may increase phagocytosis and lymphocyte activity, possibly by releasing tumor necrosis factor, interleukin-1, and interferon. *Ginkgo biloba* possesses antioxidant and free radical-scavenging properties, which protect tissues from oxidative damage. *Melatonin* is a pineal hormone that interacts with melatonin receptors in the brain to regulate the body's circadian rhythm and sleep patterns. For additional mechanisms of action, see the entries in this chapter.

black cohosh

blak coe-hosh
(Black Cohosh Softgel, Remifemin)
Also known as baneberry, bugbane, bugwort, fairy candles

CATEGORY AND SCHEDULE

Pregnancy Risk Category: N/A
OTC

MECHANISM OF ACTION

An herb that may have estrogen-like effects. **Effect:** Reduces symptoms of menopause, such as hot flashes.

AVAILABILITY

Softgel Capsules: 40 mg.
Tablets: 20 mg.

INDICATIONS AND DOSAGES

▸ To treat symptoms of menopause, to induce labor, to reduce lipid levels and BP, to provide sedation

PO

Adults, Elderly. 20–80 mg twice a day.

CONTRAINDICATIONS

Breast-feeding, preterm pregnancy (may increase risk of miscarriage); use for longer than 6 months

INTERACTIONS

Drug

Antihypertensives: May increase the action of these drugs.

Tamoxifen: May have additive antiproliferative effect.

Herbal

None known.

Food

None known.

DIAGNOSTIC TEST EFFECTS

May decrease serum luteinizing hormone concentration.

SIDE EFFECTS

Nausea, headache, dizziness, weight gain, visual changes, migraines

SERIOUS REACTIONS

! Overdose may cause nausea or vomiting, bradycardia, and diaphoresis.

! May produce hepatotoxicity.

NURSING CONSIDERATIONS

Baseline Assessment

• Determine if the patient is pregnant or breast-feeding.

Lifespan Considerations

• The use of black cohosh is contraindicated in pregnant and breast-feeding women.

• The safety and efficacy of this herb have not been established in children.

• No age-related precautions have been noted in the elderly.

Precautions

• Use black cohosh cautiously in patients with breast, ovarian, or uterine cancer; endometriosis; or uterine fibroids.

Intervention and Evaluation

• Monitor the patient's BP and serum lipid levels.

Patient Teaching

• Urge the patient to notify the physician immediately if she is or plans to become pregnant, or is breast-feeding.

• Advise the patient not to take black cohosh for longer than 6 months.

chamomile

ka-mow-meal

Also known as German chamomile, pinheads

CATEGORY AND SCHEDULE

Pregnancy Risk Category: N/A

OTC

MECHANISM OF ACTION

An herb that inhibits the release of histamine. **Effect:** Produces antihistaminic, antiflatulent, antispasmodic, mild sedative, and anti-inflammatory effects.

AVAILABILITY

Whole Flowers: 30 g/jar, 45 g/jar, 120 g/jar.

INDICATIONS AND DOSAGES

▸ To treat symptoms of flatulence, travel sickness, diarrhea, insomnia, GI spasms

PO

Adults, Elderly. 2–8 g of dried

flower heads 3 times a day or 1 cup of tea 3–4 times a day.

CONTRAINDICATIONS
Pregnancy

INTERACTIONS
Drug
Aspirin, clopidogrel, dalteparin, enoxaparin, heparin, warfarin: May increase anticoagulation and risk of bleeding.
Benzodiazepines: May increase sedation.
Herbal
Feverfew, garlic, ginger, ginkgo, licorice: May increase the risk of bleeding.
Ginseng, kava kava, St. John's wort, valerian: May increase the sedative effects of these herbs.
Food
None known.

DIAGNOSTIC TEST EFFECTS
None known.

SIDE EFFECTS
Allergic reaction (contact dermatitis, severe hypersensitivity reaction, anaphylactic reaction), eye irritation

SERIOUS REACTIONS
! An anaphylactic reaction (bronchospasm, severe pruritus, angioedema) may occur.

NURSING CONSIDERATIONS
Baseline Assessment
- Determine if the patient is asthmatic, breast-feeding, or pregnant.
- Determine if the patient is taking other medications, such as those that increase the risk of bleeding or have sedative effects.
- Assess the patient for allergies to asters, daisies, chrysanthemums, or ragweed.

Lifespan Considerations
- Because chamomile has teratogenic, menstrual, and uterine stimulant effects, its use is contraindicated in pregnant or breast-feeding women.
- The safety and efficacy of chamomile have not been established in children.
- No age-related precautions have been noted in the elderly.

Precautions
- Use chamomile cautiously in patients with asthma (because this herb may exacerbate the condition), and in patients allergic to asters, daisies, chrysanthemums, or ragweed.

Intervention and Evaluation
- Monitor the patient for signs and symptoms of an allergic reaction.

Patient Teaching
- Urge the patient to notify the physician immediately if she is or plans to become pregnant or is breast-feeding.
- Inform the patient that chamomile may cause mild sedation. Advise the patient not to perform activities requiring mental alertness or motor skills until his or her response to the herb has been established.
- Urge the patient to avoid alcohol, anticoagulants, and other sedatives during chamomile therapy.

DHEA
dee-ach-ee-aye
Also known as prasterone

CATEGORY AND SCHEDULE
Pregnancy Risk Category: N/A
OTC

MECHANISM OF ACTION
An herb that is produced in the

adrenal glands and liver and is metabolized to androstenedione, a major precursor to androgens and estrogens. Also produced in the CNS and concentrated in the limbic regions; may function as an excitatory neuroregulator. **Effect:** Androgen or estrogen-like hormonal effects may be responsible for DHEA benefits.

AVAILABILITY

Capsules: 25 mg.
Tablets: 25 mg.

INDICATIONS AND DOSAGES

▸ **To improve depressed mood and fatigue in HIV patients**
PO
Adults, Elderly. 30–90 mg/day.

▸ **Improvement of cognitive function and memory, increase bone mineral density, energy, muscle mass, strength, stimulate immune system, prevention of osteoporosis, treatment of atherosclerosis, cancer, hyperglycemia, prevention of osteoporosis**
PO
Adults, Elderly. 25–50 mg/day.

CONTRAINDICATIONS

None known.

INTERACTIONS

Drug

Androgen and estrogen therapy: May interfere with these therapies.
Triazolam: May increase blood concentration of triazolam.

Herbal

None known.

Food

None known.

DIAGNOSTIC TEST EFFECTS

None known.

SIDE EFFECTS

Acne, hair loss, hirsutism, voice deepening, insulin resistance, altered menstrual cycle, hypertension, abdominal pain, fatigue, headache, nasal congestion.

SERIOUS REACTIONS

! None known.

NURSING CONSIDERATIONS

Baseline Assessment

- Assess the patient for hormone-sensitive tumors because DHEA may stimulate their growth.
- Avoid use of hormone replacement therapy.

Lifespan Considerations

- Be aware that DHEA may adversely effect pregnancy by increasing androgen levels and that its use should be avoided during pregnancy.
- Be aware that the safety and efficacy of DHEA have not been established in children.
- In the elderly, age-related liver impairment may require caution.

Precautions

- DHEA use may increase the risk of breast, hormone-sensitive, and prostate cancers.
- Avoid DHEA use in patients with breast, ovarian, or uterine cancer, diabetes mellitus (can increase insulin resistance or sensitivity), depression (may increase risk of adverse psychiatric effects), endometriosis, and uterine fibroids.

Intervention and Evaluation

- Assess the patient for changes in mood and sleep pattern.
- Monitor the patient for aggressiveness, irritability, and restlessness.

Patient Teaching

- Warn patients to avoid DHEA use during breast-feeding, concurrent hormone replacement therapy, and pregnancy.

• Advise the patient that if he or she experiences acne, a lower DHEA dosage may provide relief from the condition.

dong quai

dong quay

Also known as Chinese angelica, dang gui, tang kuei, toki

CATEGORY AND SCHEDULE

Pregnancy Risk Category: N/A

OTC

MECHANISM OF ACTION

An herb that competitively inhibits estradiol binding to estrogen receptors. Has vasodilation, antispasmodic, and central nervous system (CNS) stimulant activity. **Effect:** Reduces symptoms of menopause.

AVAILABILITY

Softgel: 200 mg, 530 mg, 565 mg.

INDICATIONS AND DOSAGES

▸ **Gynecologic ailments, including menstrual cramps and menopause symptoms; uterine stimulant; control hypertension; as an antiinflammatory, vasodilator, immunosuppressant, analgesic, and antipyretic**

PO

Adults, Elderly. 3–4 g/day in divided doses with meals.

CONTRAINDICATIONS

Bleeding disorders, excessive menstrual flow, pregnancy due to uterine stimulant effect

INTERACTIONS

Drug

Warfarin: Increases anticoagulant effect and risk of bleeding with this drug.

Herbal

Feverfew, garlic, ginger, ginkgo, ginseng: May increase the risk of bleeding.

Food

None known.

DIAGNOSTIC TEST EFFECTS

May increase prothrombin time and international normalized ratio (INR).

SIDE EFFECTS

Diarrhea, photosensitivity, nausea, vomiting, anorexia, increased menstrual flow

SERIOUS REACTIONS

! None known.

NURSING CONSIDERATIONS

Baseline Assessment

• Determine if the patient is breast-feeding, pregnant, or plans to become pregnant.

• Determine if the patient is taking other medications, especially those that increase risk of bleeding.

Lifespan Considerations

• Be aware that dong quai use is contraindicated in pregnancy and breast-feeding.

• Be aware that the safety and efficacy of dong quai have not been established in children.

• There are no age-related precautions noted in the elderly.

Precautions

• Use cautiously in patients who are breast-feeding and patients with breast, ovarian, and uterine cancer.

Intervention and Evaluation

• Assess the patient for hypersensitivity reaction.

Patient Teaching

• Warn the patient to notify the physician immediately if she becomes or plans to become pregnant.

• Caution the patient not to breast-feed during dong quai therapy.
• Advise the patient that dong quai use may cause a photosensitivity reaction. Instruct the patient to wear protective clothing and sunscreen to protect against a photosensitivity reaction.

echinacea

eck-in-**ay**-see-ah
Also known as black susans, comb flower, red sunflower, scurvy root

CATEGORY AND SCHEDULE

Pregnancy Risk Category: N/A
OTC

MECHANISM OF ACTION

An herb that stimulates the immune system and has antiviral effects. Increases phagocytosis and lymphocyte activity, possibly by releasing tumor necrosis factor, interleukin-1, and interferon. **Effect:** Prevents or reduces symptoms associated with upper respiratory tract infections.

AVAILABILITY

Capsules: 200 mg, 380 mg, 400 mg, 500 mg.
Powder: 25 g, 100 g, 500 g.
Tincture: 475 mg/ml.
Juice.

INDICATIONS AND DOSAGES

▸ **Prevention and treatment of the common cold, other upper respiratory tract infections, UTIs, and vaginal candidiasis**

PO

Adults, Elderly. 6–9 ml herbal juice for up to 8 wk.

CONTRAINDICATIONS

Autoimmune disease, breast-feeding, children 2 years and younger, history of allergic conditions, pregnancy, tuberculosis

INTERACTIONS

Drug

Immunosuppressant (such as corticosteroids, cyclosporine, mycophenolate): May interfere with the effects of these drugs.
Econazole vaginal cream: May reduce the action of this drug.

Herbal

None known.

Food

None known.

DIAGNOSTIC TEST EFFECTS

None known.

SIDE EFFECTS

Allergic reaction (urticaria, acute asthma or dyspnea, angioedema), fever, nausea, vomiting, diarrhea, unpleasant taste, abdominal pain, dizziness.

SERIOUS REACTIONS

! None known.

NURSING CONSIDERATIONS

Baseline Assessment

• Determine if the patient is pregnant or breast-feeding, has a history of autoimmune disease, or is receiving concurrent immunosuppressant therapy.

Lifespan Considerations

• Echinacea use is contraindicated during pregnancy and breast-feeding.
• The safety and efficacy of echinacea have not been established in children younger than 2 years.
• No age-related precautions have been noted in the elderly.

Precautions

• Use echinacea cautiously in patients with diabetes mellitus because this herb may alter blood glucose control.
• Don't administer echinacea for more than 8 weeks because doing so may decrease the herb's effectiveness.

Administration and Handling

◂ALERT▸ A variety of doses have been used depending on the preparation.

Intervention and Evaluation

• Assess the patient for a hypersensitivity reaction.
• Assess the patient for improvement in symptoms of infection.

Patient Teaching

• Warn the patient not to use echinacea while pregnant or breast-feeding.
• Caution the patient against administering echinacea to children younger than 2 years.
• Advise the patient not to use echinacea for longer than 8 weeks without at least a 1-week rest period.

feverfew

fee-vir-fyoo

Also known as bachelor's button, featherfew, midsummer daisy, Santa Maria

CATEGORY AND SCHEDULE

Pregnancy Risk Category: N/A
OTC

MECHANISM OF ACTION

An herb whose exact mechanism is unknown. May inhibit platelet aggregation and serotonin release from platelets and leukocytes. May also inhibit or block prostaglandin synthesis. **Effect:** Reduces pain intensity, vomiting, and noise sensitivity in severe migraine headaches.

AVAILABILITY

Capsules: 100 mg.
Chewing Leaf: 380 mg.
Extract.

INDICATIONS AND DOSAGES

▸ **Migraine headache**

PO

Adults, Elderly. 50–100 mg extract/day or 50–125 mg leaf/day.

CONTRAINDICATIONS

Allergies to chrysanthemums, daisies, marigolds, or ragweed; breast-feeding; pregnancy (may cause uterine contraction or miscarriage)

INTERACTIONS

Drug

Anticoagulants, antiplatelet agents: May increase the risk of bleeding.
NSAIDs: May decrease the effectiveness of feverfew.

Herbal

Garlic, ginger, ginkgo biloba: May increase the risk of bleeding.

Food

None known.

DIAGNOSTIC TEST EFFECTS

None known.

SIDE EFFECTS

Capsules: Abdominal pain, muscle stiffness, arthralgia, indigestion, diarrhea, flatulence, nausea, vomiting
Chewing leaf: Mouth ulceration, inflammation of oral mucosa and tongue, swelling of lips, loss of taste

SERIOUS REACTIONS

! A hypersensitivity reaction may occur.

NURSING CONSIDERATIONS

Baseline Assessment

- Determine if the patient is breast-feeding or pregnant before administering feverfew.

Lifespan Considerations

- Feverfew use is contraindicated during pregnancy and breast-feeding.
- The safety and efficacy of feverfew have not been established in children. Children should not use feverfew.
- No age-related precautions have been noted in the elderly.

Precautions

- Use chewing leaf cautiously in patients with a history of oral inflammation or ulceration.
- Use feverfew cautiously in patients taking anticoagulants or antiplatelet inhibitors because concurrent use may increase the risk of bleeding.

Intervention and Evaluation

- Assess the patient for a hypersensitivity reaction.
- Evaluate the patient for joint or muscle pain and mouth ulcers.

Patient Teaching

- Warn the patient not to use feverfew while breast-feeding or pregnant.
- Caution the patient to avoid giving feverfew to children.

garlic

gar-lick

Also known as ail, allium, nectar of the gods, poor man's treacle, stinking rose

CATEGORY AND SCHEDULE

Pregnancy Risk Category: N/A
OTC

MECHANISM OF ACTION

An herb that possesses antithrombotic properties, increases fibrinolytic activity, decreases platelet aggregation, and increases PT. Also acts as an HMG-CoA reductase inhibitor. **Effect:** Lowers cholesterol levels, reduces BP, prevents age-related vascular changes and atherosclerosis, produces antioxidant effect.

AVAILABILITY

Capsules: 100 mg, 300 mg, 500 mg, 1,000 mg, 1.5 g.
Tablets: 400 mg, 1,250 mg.
Extract.
Oil.
Powder.
Tea.

INDICATIONS AND DOSAGES

▸ **Hyperlipidemia, hypertension**

PO (capsules, powder, tea)
Adults, Elderly. 600–1,200 mg/ day in divided doses 3 times a day.

CONTRAINDICATIONS

Bleeding disorders

INTERACTIONS

Drug

Anticoagulants, antiplatelet agents (such as aspirin, clopidogrel, enoxaparin, warfarin): May increase the risk of bleeding.
Cyclosporine, oral contraceptives: May decrease the effects of these drugs.
Insulin, oral antidiabetic agents: May increase the hypoglycemic effect of these drugs.
Saquinavir, other HIV antiretrovirals: May decrease the blood concentration and effects of these drugs.

Herbal
Feverfew, ginger, ginkgo biloba, ginseng: May increase the risk of bleeding.
Food
None known.

DIAGNOSTIC TEST EFFECTS
May decrease blood glucose and serum cholesterol levels and increase international normalized ratio.

SIDE EFFECTS
Breath or body odor, oropharyngeal or esophageal burning, heartburn, nausea, vomiting, diarrhea, allergic reactions (rhinitis, urticaria, angioedema).

SERIOUS REACTIONS
! None known.

NURSING CONSIDERATIONS
Baseline Assessment
- Assess the patient's serum lipid levels and determine whether the patient is taking anticoagulants or antiplatelet agents before beginning therapy.
- Determine if the patient is a diabetic or taking insulin or oral antidiabetic agents.

Lifespan Considerations
- Garlic use may stimulate labor and cause colic in infants.
- The safety and efficacy of garlic have not been established in children; however, garlic may be beneficial for children with hypercholesterolemia.
- No age-related precautions have been noted in the elderly.

Precautions
- Use garlic cautiously in patients with diabetes mellitus because it may decrease blood glucose levels; in hypothyroidism because it may reduce iodine uptake; and in inflammatory GI conditions, because it may irritate the GI tract.
- Use garlic with caution because it may prolong bleeding time. Have the patient discontinue its use 1 to 2 weeks before surgery.

Administration and Handling
◀ALERT▶ Appropriate dosages for conditions other than hyperlipidemia and hypertension vary, depending on the preparation used.

Intervention and Evaluation
- Monitor the patient's blood glucose levels, coagulation studies, CBC, and serum lipid levels.
- Assess the patient for allergic reactions.

Patient Teaching
- Warn the patient to avoid garlic use during breast-feeding and pregnancy.
- Advise the patient to inform all of health care providers about garlic use.
- Instruct the patient to discontinue garlic use 1 to 2 weeks before any procedure in which excessive bleeding may occur.

ginger
jin-jer
Also known as black ginger, race ginger, zingiber

CATEGORY AND SCHEDULE
Pregnancy Risk Category: N/A
OTC

MECHANISM OF ACTION
An herb that possesses antipyretic, analgesic, antitussive, and sedative properties. Increases GI motility; may act on serotonin receptors, primarily 5-HT_3. **Effect:** Reduces nausea and vomiting.

AVAILABILITY

Capsules: 470 mg, 550 mg.
Root: 470 mg, 550 mg.
Extract.
Powder.
Tablets.
Tea.
Tincture.

INDICATIONS AND DOSAGES

▸ **Prevention of nausea and vomiting in early pregnancy**
PO
Adults. 250 mg 4 times a day. Maximum: 4 g/day.

▸ **Prevention of nausea and vomiting from motion sickness**
PO
Adults. 1 g (dried powder root) 30 min before travel.

▸ **Nausea**
PO
Adults. 550–1,100 mg 3 times a day.

▸ **Arthritis**
PO
Adults. 170 mg 3 times a day or 255 mg twice a day.

CONTRAINDICATIONS

None known.

INTERACTIONS

Drug

Anticoagulants, antiplatelet agents: May increase the risk of bleeding (with large amounts of ginger).

Herbal

Feverfew, garlic, ginkgo biloba, ginseng: May increase the risk of bleeding.

Food

None known.

DIAGNOSTIC TEST EFFECTS

None known.

SIDE EFFECTS

Abdominal discomfort, heartburn, diarrhea, hypersensitivity reaction, nausea

SERIOUS REACTIONS

! CNS depression and arrhythmias may occur.

NURSING CONSIDERATIONS

Baseline Assessment

• Determine if the patient is taking anticoagulants and antiplatelet agents before beginning therapy because these drugs may increase the risk of bleeding.

Lifespan Considerations

• Ginger use during pregnancy is controversial; large amounts of ginger may cause miscarriage.
• The safety and efficacy of ginger have not been established in children.
• No age-related precautions have been noted in the elderly.

Precautions

• Use ginger cautiously in pregnant patients and patients with bleeding conditions or diabetes mellitus (may cause hypoglycemia).

Intervention and Evaluation

• Monitor the patient for a hypersensitivity reaction.

Patient Teaching

• Advise patients to use ginger cautiously during breast-feeding and pregnancy.

ginkgo biloba

gink-go bye-**loe**-buh
Also known as fossil tree, maidenhair tree, tanakan

CATEGORY AND SCHEDULE

Pregnancy Risk Category: N/A
OTC

MECHANISM OF ACTION

An herb that possesses antioxidant and free radical scavenging properties. Protects tissues from oxidative damage and may prevent progression of tissue degeneration in patients with dementia. May increase the release of neurotransmitters, including catecholamines, and inhibition of monoamine oxidase (MAO). **Effect:** Enhances cognitive ability in dementia syndromes.

AVAILABILITY

Capsules: 40 mg, 60 mg.
Tablets: 40 mg, 60 mg.
Fluid Extract.
Tincture.

INDICATIONS AND DOSAGES

▸ **Dementia syndromes, including Alzheimer's disease**
PO (extract)
Adults, Elderly. 120–240 mg/day in 2–3 doses.
▸ **Vertigo, tinnitus**
PO
Adults, Elderly. 120–160 mg/day.
▸ **Cognitive function**
PO
Adults, Elderly. 120–600 mg a day.

CONTRAINDICATIONS

Breast-feeding, pregnancy

INTERACTIONS

Drug

Anticoagulants, antiplatelet agents (such as aspirin, heparin, clopidogrel, warfarin): May increase the risk of bleeding.
MAOIs: May increase the effects of these drugs.

Herbal

Feverfew, garlic, ginger, ginseng: May increase the risk of bleeding.

Food

None known.

DIAGNOSTIC TEST EFFECTS

May alter blood glucose levels.

SIDE EFFECTS

Headache, dizziness, palpitations, constipation, allergic skin reactions; with large doses, nausea, vomiting, diarrhea, weakness, lack of muscle tone.

SERIOUS REACTIONS

! A hypersensitivity reaction may occur.

NURSING CONSIDERATIONS

Baseline Assessment

- Determine if the patient is taking anticoagulants, antiplatelet agents, or MAOIs before beginning therapy.
- Assess the patient for a history of bleeding disorders, diabetes mellitus, and seizures.

Lifespan Considerations

- Ginkgo biloba use is contraindicated in breast-feeding and pregnancy.
- The safety and efficacy of ginkgo biloba have not been established in children. Children should not use ginkgo biloba.
- No age-related precautions have been noted in the elderly.

Precautions

- Use ginkgo biloba cautiously in patients with bleeding disorders, diabetes mellitus, or epilepsy and in patients who are prone to seizures.
- Couples having difficulty conceiving should avoid ginkgo biloba.

Administration and Handling

◀ **ALERT** ▶ Appropriate dosing for various indications vary. The patient should be started at low doses of ginkgo biloba, with the dose titrated higher as needed.

Intervention and Evaluation

- Monitor the patient's blood glucose level.

• Assess the patient for signs and symptoms of a hypersensitivity reaction.

Patient Teaching

• Warn the patient not to use ginkgo biloba during breast-feeding and pregnancy or while taking anticoagulants or antiplatelet agents.
• Inform the patient that it may take up to 6 months for the herb to become effective.
• Caution the patient not to give ginkgo biloba to children.

ginseng

jin-sing
Also known as Asian ginseng, Chinese ginseng, red ginseng

CATEGORY AND SCHEDULE

Pregnancy Risk Category: N/A
OTC

MECHANISM OF ACTION

An herb that affects the hypothalamic-pituitary-adrenal axis and appears to stimulate natural killer cells. **Effect:** Reduces stress; affects immune function.

AVAILABILITY

Capsules: 100 mg, 250 mg, 410 mg, 500 mg.
Tablets: 250 mg, 1,000 mg.
Dried Root.
Extract.
Powder.
Tea: 1,500 mg/bag (usually).
Tincture.

INDICATIONS AND DOSAGES

▸ **To assist in blood glucose control; to boost energy level; to enhance brain activity, cognitive function, concentration, memory, and work efficiency; to increase physical endurance and resistance to stress**

PO (tablets or capsules)
Adults, Elderly. 200–600 mg/day.
PO (powder root)
Adults, Elderly. 0.6–3 g 1–3 times a day.
PO (tea)
Adults, Elderly. 1,500 mg 1–3 times a day.

CONTRAINDICATIONS

Bleeding tendencies or thrombosis, breast-feeding, pregnancy

INTERACTIONS

Drug

Anticoagulants, antiplatelet agents (such as aspirin, clopidogrel, enoxaparin, heparin, warfarin): May increase the risk of bleeding.
Furosemide: May decrease the effects of furosemide.
Immunosuppressants (such as cyclosporine, prednisone): May interfere with these drugs.
Insulin, oral antidiabetic agents: May increase the effects of these drugs.

Herbal

Chamomile, feverfew, garlic, ginger, ginkgo biloba: May increase the risk of bleeding.

Food

Coffee, tea: May increase the effects of ginseng.

DIAGNOSTIC TEST EFFECTS

May decrease blood glucose level. May prolong aPTT.

SIDE EFFECTS

Frequent
Insomnia
Occasional
Vaginal bleeding, amenorrhea, palpitations, hypertension, diarrhea, headache, allergic reactions

SERIOUS REACTIONS

! None known.

NURSING CONSIDERATIONS

Baseline Assessment

- Determine if the patient is breast-feeding, pregnant, or taking anticoagulants or immunosuppressants before starting therapy.
- Determine if the patient has diabetes mellitus or is taking insulin or other oral antidiabetics.
- Obtain the patient's baseline blood glucose level.

Lifespan Considerations

- Breast-feeding or pregnant women should not use ginseng because the herb's safety for these patients has not been determined.
- The safety and efficacy of this herb have not been established in children.
- No age-related precautions have been noted in the elderly.

Precautions

- Use ginseng cautiously in patients with cardiac disorders, diabetes mellitus, endometriosis, hormone-sensitive cancers (including breast, ovarian, and uterine cancer), or uterine fibroids.

Intervention and Evaluation

- Monitor the patient's blood glucose level and coagulation studies.
- Assess the patient for signs and symptoms of a hypersensitivity reaction, including a rash.

Patient Teaching

- Warn the patient to avoid ginseng use during breast-feeding and pregnancy.
- Advise the patient not to give ginseng to children.
- Caution the patient to avoid using ginseng continuously for longer than 3 months.

glucosamine and chondroitin

glue-**koe**-sah-meen and **con**-droy-tin

CATEGORY AND SCHEDULE

Pregnancy Risk Category: N/A
OTC

MECHANISM OF ACTION

Glucosamine is necessary for synthesis of mucopolysaccharides, which make up the body's tendons, ligaments, cartilage, and synovial fluid. It may also decrease glucose-induced insulin secretion. Chondroitin, which is found endogenously in cartilage tissue, is a substrate that is necessary to maintain and repair bone and cartilage. It may also have some anticoagulant properties. **Effect:** Relieves symptoms of osteoarthritis.

AVAILABILITY

Glucosamine
Capsules: 500 mg.
Tablets: 500 mg.
Chondroitin
Capsules: 250 mg.

INDICATIONS AND DOSAGES

▸ **Osteoarthritis**

PO (Glucosamine)
Adults, Elderly. 500 mg 3 times a day or 1–2 g/day.
PO (Chondroitin)
Adults, Elderly. 200–400 mg 2–3 times a day.

CONTRAINDICATIONS
None known.

INTERACTIONS
Drug
Chondroitin
Anticoagulants: Monitor anticoagulant therapy in patients taking chrondroitin.
Glucosamine
Warfarin: Glucosamine use may increase the effects of warfarin.
Herbal
None known.
Food
None known.

DIAGNOSTIC TEST EFFECTS
Glucosamine may increase the blood glucose level. Chondroitin may increase the antifactor Xa level.

SIDE EFFECTS
Glucosamine: Mild GI symptoms, such as flatulence, bloating, and cramps
Chondroitin: Nausea, diarrhea, constipation, edema, alopecia, allergic reactions

SERIOUS REACTIONS
! None known.

NURSING CONSIDERATIONS
Baseline Assessment
- Determine if the patient is taking anticoagulants, antidiabetics, or antiplatelet agents before starting therapy.
- Determine if the patient is breast-feeding or pregnant.
Lifespan Considerations
- Breast-feeding or pregnant women should avoid using glucosamine and chondroitin.
- The safety and efficacy of glucosamine and chondroitin have not been established in children.
- No age-related precautions have been noted in the elderly.
Precautions
- Use glucosamine cautiously in patients with diabetes mellitus because it may increase insulin resistance.
Administration and Handling
◀ ALERT ▶ Many combination products containing both glucosamine and chrondroitin are available.
Intervention and Evaluation
- Monitor the patient to determine the effectiveness of glucosamine and chrondroitin therapy in relieving osteoarthritis symptoms.
Patient Teaching
- Warn the patient not to use glucosamine or chondroitin during breast-feeding and pregnancy.
- Caution the patient not to give glucosamine or chondroitin to children.
- Inform the patient that it may take several months of therapy for these herbs to be effective.
- Advise the patient that glucosamine may alter blood glucose levels.

kava kava
ka-vah **ka**-vah
Also known as ava, kew, sakau, tonga, yagona

CATEGORY AND SCHEDULE
Pregnancy Risk Category: N/A
OTC

MECHANISM OF ACTION
An herb whose exact mechanism of action is unknown, but which is known to possess CNS effects.
Effect: Produces anxiolytic, sedative, and analgesic effects.

AVAILABILITY

Capsules: 140 mg, 150 mg, 250 mg, 300 mg, 425 mg, 500 mg.
Extract.
Liquid.
Tea.
Tincture.

INDICATIONS AND DOSAGES

▸ Anxiety disorders, stress, restlessness, sedation, sleep enhancement

PO

Adults, Elderly. 100 mg 3 times a day or 1 cup of the tea 3 times a day.

CONTRAINDICATIONS

Breast-feeding, pregnancy (may cause loss of uterine tone)

INTERACTIONS

Drug

Alcohol, benzodiazepines: May increase the risk of drowsiness.

Herbal

Chamomile, ginseng, goldenseal, melatonin, St. John's wort, valerian: May increase the risk of drowsiness.

Food

None known.

DIAGNOSTIC TEST EFFECTS

May increase liver function test results.

SIDE EFFECTS

GI upset; headache; dizziness; vision changes (blurred vision, red eyes); allergic skin reactions; dry, flaky skin; yellowing of eyes, skin, hair, and nails; nausea; vomiting; weight loss; shortness of breath

SERIOUS REACTIONS

! None known.

NURSING CONSIDERATIONS

Baseline Assessment

- Determine if the patient is breast-feeding, pregnant, or using CNS depressants before starting therapy.
- Obtain liver function test results.

Lifespan Considerations

- Kava kava use is contraindicated in breast-feeding and pregnant women.
- The safety and efficacy of kava kava have not been established in children.
- No age-related precautions have been noted in the elderly.

Precautions

- Use kava kava cautiously in patients with depression or a history of recurrent hepatitis.

Administration and Handling

◂ALERT▸ Be aware that kava kava may be removed from the market.

Intervention and Evaluation

- Monitor the patient's liver function test results.
- Examine the patient for allergic skin reactions.

Patient Teaching

- Warn the patient not to use kava kava if she is breast-feeding, pregnant, or planning to become pregnant.
- Advise the patient not to give kava kava to children 12 years and younger.
- Inform the patient not to use kava kava for longer than 3 months because it may be habit-forming.
- Caution the patient to avoid tasks that require mental alertness or motor skills until his or her response to the herb has been established.

melatonin

mel-ah-**tone**-in
Also known as pineal hormone

CATEGORY AND SCHEDULE

Pregnancy Risk Category: N/A
OTC

MECHANISM OF ACTION

A hormone synthesized endogenously by the pineal gland that interacts with melatonin receptors in the brain. **Effect:** Regulates the body's circadian rhythm and sleep patterns. Acts as an antioxidant, protecting cells from oxidative damage by free radicals.

AVAILABILITY

Lozenges: 3 mg.
Powder.
Tablets: 0.5 mg, 3 mg.

INDICATIONS AND DOSAGES

▸ **Insomnia**

PO

Adults, Elderly. 0.5–5 mg at bedtime.

▸ **Jet lag**

PO

Adults, Elderly. 5 mg/day beginning 3 days before flight and continuing until 3 days after flight.

CONTRAINDICATIONS

Breast-feeding, pregnancy

INTERACTIONS

Drug

Alcohol, benzodiazepines: May increase CNS depressant effects.
Immunosuppressants: May interfere with the effects of these drugs.
Isoniazid: May enhance the effects of isoniazid.

Herbal

Chamomile, ginseng, goldenseal, kava kava, valerian: May increase sedative effects.

Food

None known.

DIAGNOSTIC TEST EFFECTS

May increase human growth hormone levels. May decrease luteinizing hormone levels.

SIDE EFFECTS

Headache, transient depression, fatigue, somnolence, dizziness, abdominal cramps, decreased alertness, hypersensitivity reaction, tachycardia, nausea, vomiting, anorexia, changes in sleep patterns, confusion

SERIOUS REACTIONS

! None known.

NURSING CONSIDERATIONS

Baseline Assessment

• Determine if the patient is breastfeeding, pregnant, or using other medications, especially CNS depressants, before starting therapy.
• Determine if the patient has a history of depression or seizures.
• Assess the patient's sleep pattern if melatonin is used for insomnia.

Lifespan Considerations

• Melatonin use is contraindicated in breast-feeding and pregnant women.
• The safety and efficacy of melatonin have not been established in children.
• No age-related precautions have been noted in the elderly.

Precautions

• Use melatonin cautiously in patients with cardiovascular disease, depression (may worsen dysphoria), hepatic disease, or seizures (may increase incidence).

Administration and Handling
- Store melatonin in a sealed container away from heat and moisture.

Intervention and Evaluation
- Monitor the herb's effectiveness in improving the patient's insomnia.
- Assess the patient for CNS effects and hypersensitivity reactions.

Patient Teaching
- Warn the female patient not to take melatonin if she is breast-feeding, pregnant, or planning to become pregnant.
- Encourage an environment conducive to sleep (low lighting, quiet).
- Caution the patient to avoid performing tasks that require mental alertness or motor skills until his or her response to the herb has been established.

saw palmetto

saw pall-**meh**-toe
Also known as American dwarf palm tree, cabbage palm, sabal, zu-zhong

CATEGORY AND SCHEDULE

Pregnancy Risk Category: N/A
OTC

MECHANISM OF ACTION

An herb that appears to inhibit 5-alpha-reductase and prevent conversion of testosterone to dihydrotestosterone (DHT). Has antiandrogenic, antiproliferative, and anti-inflammatory properties. **Effect:** Reduces prostate growth.

AVAILABILITY

Capsules: 80 mg, 160 mg, 500 mg.
Berries.
Fluid Extract.
Tea.

INDICATIONS AND DOSAGES

▸ Benign prostatic hyperplasia (BPH)
PO
Adults, Elderly. 160 mg twice a day or 320 mg once a day using a liquid extract or 1-2 g of whole berries.

▸ Diuretic, sedative, anti-inflammatory, antiseptic
PO
Adults, Elderly. 0.6-1.5 ml liquid extract or 0.5-1 g dried berries 3 times a day.

CONTRAINDICATIONS

Because saw palmetto is used in men, it should not be used by women who are breast-feeding (due to anti-androgenic and estrogenic activity) or pregnant

INTERACTIONS

Drug
Hormone replacement therapy, oral contraceptives: May interfere with the effects of these drugs.
Herbal
None known.
Food
None known.

DIAGNOSTIC TEST EFFECTS

None known.

SIDE EFFECTS

Mild anorexia, dizziness, nausea, vomiting, constipation, diarrhea, headache, impotence, hypersensitivity reactions, back pain

SERIOUS REACTIONS

! None known.

NURSING CONSIDERATIONS

Baseline Assessment
- Determine if the patient is using oral contraceptives or receiving hormone replacement therapy be-

cause saw palmetto may interfere with these therapies.
- Assess the patient's symptoms, including frequent or painful urination and urinary hesitancy or urgency.
- Test the male patient and obtain a prostate-specific antigen (PSA) test before administering saw palmetto.

Lifespan Considerations
- Saw palmetto use is contraindicated for breast-feeding and pregnant women.
- The safety and efficacy of saw palmetto have not been established in children.
- No age-related precautions have been noted in the elderly.

Precautions
- Use saw palmetto cautiously in patients with hepatic or renal disorders because the herb's safety has not been established in these patients.

Administration and Handling
PO
- Store saw palmetto in a cool, dry place away from heat and moisture.
- Administer this herb with meals to minimize GI symptoms.

Intervention and Evaluation
- Assess the patient for signs and symptoms of hypersensitivity reactions.
- Assess the patient for decreased nocturia, decreased residual urine volume, and improved urinary flow.

Patient Teaching
- Instruct the patient to take saw palmetto with food.

St. John's wort

say-nt **jonz wurd**
Also known as amber, demon chaser, goatweed, hardhay, rosin rose, tipton weed

CATEGORY AND SCHEDULE

Pregnancy Risk Category: N/A
OTC

MECHANISM OF ACTION

An herb that inhibits catechol-*O*-methyl transferase (COMT) and monoamine oxidase (MAO) and modulates the effects of serotonin by inhibiting serotonin reuptake and 5-HT_3 and 5-HT_4 antagonism.
Effect: Relieves depression.

AVAILABILITY

Capsules: 150 mg, 300 mg,
Liquid Extract.
Tincture.

INDICATIONS AND DOSAGES

▸ **Depression**
PO
Adults, Elderly. 300 mg 3 times a day (usually).

CONTRAINDICATIONS

Breast-feeding (may increase uterine muscle tone in mother and cause colic, drowsiness, and lethargy in infants), pregnancy

INTERACTIONS

Drug
ACE inhibitors: May cause hypertension.
Antidepressants: May increase the therapeutic effect of St. John's wort.
Cyclosporine: May decrease the effectiveness of this drug, resulting in organ rejection.
Digoxin: May exacerbate CHF.
Indinavir: May decrease the blood

concentration and effects of indinavir.

Herbal

Chamomile, ginseng, goldenseal, kava kava, valerian: May increase the therapeutic and adverse effects of St. John's wort.

Food

Tyramine-containing foods: May cause a hypertensive crisis (with large doses of herb).

DIAGNOSTIC TEST EFFECTS

May increase international normalized ratio and PT in patients treated with warfarin.

SIDE EFFECTS

Abdominal cramps, insomnia, vivid dreams, restlessness, anxiety, agitation, irritability, fatigue, dry mouth, headache, dizziness, photosensitivity, confusion

SERIOUS REACTIONS

! None known.

NURSING CONSIDERATIONS

Baseline Assessment

- Determine if the patient is breast-feeding, pregnant, or taking other medications before starting therapy.
- Determine the patient's history of psychiatric disorders.
- Assess the patient's anxiety level, memory, mental status, and mood.

Lifespan Considerations

- St. John's wort use is contraindicated in breast-feeding and pregnant women.
- The safety and efficacy of St. John's wort have not been established in children.
- No age-related precautions have been noted in the elderly.

Precautions

- Use St. John's wort cautiously in patients with bipolar disorder or schizophrenia.

Intervention and Evaluation

- Monitor for improvement in the patient's behavior and depressive state.
- Monitor the patient for side effects.

Patient Teaching

- Inform the patient that the herb's therapeutic effect may take 4 to 6 weeks to appear.
- Caution the patient against abruptly discontinuing St. John's wort.
- Warn the patient not to take any medications, including OTC drugs, without first consulting the physician.
- Advise the patient to avoid foods high in tyramine, such as aged cheese, pickled products, beer, and wine, while taking St. John's wort.
- Urge the patient to wear protective clothing and sunscreen when outdoors and to avoid overexposure to sunlight.

valerian

vah-**leh**-ree-un

Also known as all-heal, amantilla, garden heliotrope, valeriana.

CATEGORY AND SCHEDULE

Pregnancy Risk Category: N/A

OTC

MECHANISM OF ACTION

An herb that appears to inhibit the enzyme system responsible for catabolism of gamma-aminobutyric acid (GABA), increasing GABA concentration and decreasing CNS activity. **Effect:** Produces sedative effects. Also has anxiolytic, antidepressant, and anticonvulsant effects.

AVAILABILITY

Capsules.
Extract.
Tablets.
Tea.
Tincture.

INDICATIONS AND DOSAGES

▸ **Sleeping disorders associated with anxiety or restlessness**
PO (Extract)
Adults, Elderly. 400–900 mg 30–60 min before bedtime.
PO (Tea)
Adults, Elderly. 1 cup taken several times a day.

CONTRAINDICATIONS

Breast-feeding, hepatic disease, pregnancy

INTERACTIONS

Drug

Alcohol, barbiturates, benzodiazepines: May increase the CNS depressant effects of these drugs and increase the therapeutic and adverse effects of valerian.

Herbal

Chamomile, ginseng, kava kava, melatonin, St. John's wort: May enhance the therapeutic and adverse effects of valerian.

Food

None known.

DIAGNOSTIC TEST EFFECTS

None known.

SIDE EFFECTS

Headache, hangover, cardiac disturbances

SERIOUS REACTIONS

! Difficulty walking, excitability, hypothermia, increased muscle relaxation, hypersensitivity, and insomnia may occur.

NURSING CONSIDERATIONS

Baseline Assessment

- Determine if the patient is using other CNS depressants, especially a benzodiazepine.
- Assess the patient's liver function test results.

Lifespan Considerations

- Valerian use is contraindicated in breast-feeding and pregnant women.
- The safety and efficacy of valerian have not been established in children. Children should not use valerian.
- No age-related precautions have been noted in the elderly.

Precautions

- Use saw palmetto cautiously in patients with hepatic or renal disorders because the herb's safety has not been established in these patients.

Administration and Handling

- Store valerian in a cool, dry place.

Intervention and Evaluation

- Assess the patient for a hypersensitivity reaction.
- Monitor the patient's liver function test results.
- Assess the herb's effectiveness in decreasing the patient's insomnia.

Patient Teaching

- Inform the patient that it may take up to 4 weeks for this herb to relieve insomnia.
- Caution the patient to avoid performing tasks that require mental alertness or motor skills until his or her response to the herb has been established.
- Warn the female patient to avoid valerian use if she is breast-feeding, pregnant, or planning to become pregnant.
- Instruct the patient to taper valerian dosage slowly, not to abruptly stop taking the herb.

yohimbe

yo-**him**-bay

Also known as aphrodien, corynine, johimbi

CATEGORY AND SCHEDULE

Pregnancy Risk Category: N/A

OTC

MECHANISM OF ACTION

An herb that dilates genital blood vessels, increasing penile blood flow; also improves nerve impulse transmission to the genital area. **Effect:** Improves sexual vigor.

AVAILABILITY

Liquid: 5 mg/5 ml.

Tablets: 5 mg.

INDICATIONS AND DOSAGES

▸ **Impotence**

PO

Adults, Elderly. 15–30 mg/day in divided doses.

CONTRAINDICATIONS

Angina, benign prostatic hyperplasia (BPH), breast-feeding, depression, heart disease, hepatic disease, pregnancy (may have uterine relaxant effect and cause fetal toxicity), renal disease

INTERACTIONS

Drug

Antidiabetics, antihypertensives: May interfere with the effects of these drugs.

Clonidine: May antagonize the effects of clonidine.

MAOIs, sympathomimetics, tricyclic antidepressants: May increase the effects of these drugs.

Herbal

Ginkgo biloba, St. John's wort: May have additive therapeutic and adverse effects of yohimbe.

Food

Caffeine-containing products (such as coffee, tea, chocolate), tyramine-containing foods (such as aged cheese, chianti wine): May increase the risk of hypertensive crisis.

DIAGNOSTIC TEST EFFECTS

None known.

SIDE EFFECTS

Excitement, tremors, insomnia, anxiety, hypertension, tachycardia, dizziness, headache, irritability, salivation, dilated pupils, nausea, vomiting, hypersensitivity reaction

SERIOUS REACTIONS

! Paralysis, severe hypotension, arrhythmias, and heart failure may occur.

! Overdose may be fatal.

NURSING CONSIDERATIONS

Baseline Assessment

- Determine if the patient is breast-feeding or pregnant.
- Determine the patient's other medical conditions, especially angina, heart disease, and BPH, and medication history.
- Assess the patient's blood chemistry values, especially BUN and serum alkaline phosphatase, creatinine, AST (SGOT), and ALT (SGPT) levels to assess hepatic and renal function.

Lifespan Considerations

- Yohimbe use is contraindicated in breast-feeding and pregnant women.
- The safety and efficacy of yohimbe have not been established in children. Children should not use this herb.

- In the elderly, age-related hepatic and renal impairment may require discontinuation of yohimbe.

Precautions

- Use yohimbe cautiously in patients with anxiety, diabetes mellitus, hypertension, post-traumatic stress disorder, or schizophrenia.

Administration and Handling

- Store yohimbe in a cool, dry place.

Intervention and Evaluation

- Monitor the patient's BP and liver and renal function test results.
- Assess the patient for signs and symptoms of a hypersensitivity reaction.

Patient Teaching

- Instruct the patient not to take any other medications, including OTC drugs, without first notifying the physician.
- Warn the female patient to avoid using yohimbe if she is breast-feeding, pregnant, or planning to become pregnant.

76 Minerals and Electrolytes

aluminum hydroxide
calcium acetate, calcium carbonate, calcium chloride, calcium citrate, calcium glubionate, calcium gluconate
citrates (potassium citrate, potassium citrate and citric acid, sodium citrate and citric acid, tricitrates)
fluoride
lanthanum carbonate
magnesium
phosphates
potassium acetate, potassium bicarbonate/citrate, potassium chloride, potassium gluconate
sodium bicarbonate
sodium chloride
zinc oxide, zinc sulfate

Uses: Minerals and electrolytes are used as replacements to correct specific electrolyte imbalances, such as hypokalemia, hyponatremia, and hypermagnesemia. Additional uses vary greatly. *Aluminum* is used to treat hyperacidity and gastroesophageal reflux disease (GERD) and to prevent GI bleeding and phosphate calculi formation. *Calcium* is also prescribed to treat hyperacidity. *Citrates* treat metabolic acidosis. *Fluoride* prevents dental caries in children. *Lanthanum* is used to reduce serum phosphate in end-stage renal disease. *Magnesium* is also used to treat hypertension, torsades de pointes, encephalopathy, constipation, hyperacidity, and seizures from acute nephritis.

Phosphates are used to prevent and treat hypophosphatemia, to treat constipation, to evacuate the colon for examination, and to acidify the urine and reduce calcium calculi formation. *Sodium bicarbonate* is used to manage metabolic acidosis and hyperacidity, alkalinize urine, stabilize acid-base balance, and treat cardiac arrest. *Sodium chloride* is also used to promote hydration, assess renal function, and manage hyperosmolar diabetes; in addition, it has nasal and ophthalmic uses. *Zinc oxide* is used to protect the skin from mild irritation and abrasions and to promote the healing of chapped skin and diaper rash. *Zinc sulfate* helps prevent zinc deficiency and is used to promote wound healing.

Action: Minerals are needed for normal body function. Electrolytes are substances that carry a positive or negative charge. Their functions include transmission of nerve impulses to contract skeletal and smooth muscles. Additional specific actions vary with the agent. *Aluminum* reduces gastric acid, binds with phosphate, and may increase calcium absorption. (See the illustration *Sites of Action: Drugs Used to Treat GERD,* page 980.) *Calcium* neutralizes or reduces gastric acid. *Citrates* increase urinary pH and citrate level, decrease calcium activity, increase plasma bicarbonate, and buffer excess hydrogen ions. *Fluoride* increases tooth resistance to acid dissolution.

Lanthanum dissociates in the upper GI tract to lanthanum ions, which bind to dietary phosphate released from food during digestion, forming highly insoluble lanthanum phosphate complexes. This action reduces phosphate absorption. *Magnesium* neutralizes gastric acid, produces osmotic effects on the small intestine, and blocks neuromuscular transmission. *Phosphates* participate in bone deposition, calcium metabolism, B-complex vitamin use, and acid-base buffering. *Sodium bicarbonate* dissociates to provide bicarbonate ions, which raises the blood and urine pH. *Sodium chloride* controls water distribution and fluid and electrolyte balance; it also helps maintain acid-base balance. As an astringent, *zinc oxide* forms a protective coating for the skin. As a co-factor for enzymes important to protein and carbohydrate metabolism, *zinc sulfate* maintains normal growth and tissue repair as well as skin hydration.

COMBINATION PRODUCTS

GAVISCON (ORAL SUSPENSION): aluminum hydroxide/magnesium carbonate (an antacid) 31.7 mg/119.3 mg.
GAVISCON (TABLETS): aluminum hydroxide/magnesium trisilicate (an antacid) 80 mg/20 mg.
GELUSIL: aluminum hydroxide/magnesium hydroxide (an antacid)/simethicone (an antiflatulent) 200 mg/200 mg/25 mg.
HALEY'S M-O: magnesium/mineral oil (a laxative) 300 mg/1.25 ml.
MAALOX: aluminum hydroxide/magnesium hydroxide (an antacid) 200 mg/200 mg (oral suspension); 225 mg/200 mg (tablets).
MAALOX PLUS: aluminum hydroxide/magnesium hydroxide (an antacid)/simethicone (an antiflatulent) 200 mg/200 mg/25 mg.
MYLANTA: aluminum hydroxide/magnesium hydroxide (an antacid)/simethicone (an antiflatulent) 200 mg/200 mg/20 mg; 400 mg/400 mg/40 mg.
PEPCID COMPLETE: calcium chloride/magnesium hydroxide (an antacid)/famotidine (a histamine [H_2] antagonist) 800 mg/165 mg/10 mg.

aluminum hydroxide

a-**loo**-mi-num hye-**drox**-ide
(Alternagel, Alu-Tab, Amphojel[CAN], Basaljel[CAN])

CATEGORY AND SCHEDULE

Pregnancy Risk Category: C (Considered safe except for chronic, high-dose use).
OTC

MECHANISM OF ACTION

An antacid that reduces gastric acid by binding with phosphate in the intestine and is then excreted as aluminum carbonate in feces; decreased serum phosphate levels may result in increased absorption of calcium. The drug also has astringent and adsorbent properties. **Therapeutic Effect:** Neutralizes or increases gastric pH; reduces phosphate levels in urine, preventing formation of phosphate urinary calculi; reduces the serum phosphate level; decreases the fluidity of stools.

AVAILABILITY

Capsules: 475 mg.
Suspension: 320 mg/5 ml, 600 mg/5 ml.

INDICATIONS AND DOSAGES

▸ **Antacid**

PO

Adults, Elderly. 600–1200 mg between meals and at bedtime.

▸ **Hyperphosphatemia**

PO

Adults, Elderly. Initially, 300–600 mg 3 times a day with meals.
Children. 50–150 mg/kg/day in divided doses q4–6h.

CONTRAINDICATIONS

Children age 6 years or younger, intestinal obstruction

INTERACTIONS

Drug

Anticholinergics, quinidine: May decrease excretion of aluminum hydroxide.
Iron preparations, isoniazid, ketoconazole, quinolones, tetracyclines: May decrease absorption of aluminum hydroxide.
Methenamine: May decrease effects of the methenamine.
Salicylate: May increase salicylate excretion.

Herbal

None known.

Food

None known.

DIAGNOSTIC TEST EFFECTS

May increase the serum gastrin level and systemic and urinary pH. May decrease the serum phosphate level.

SIDE EFFECTS

Frequent

Chalky taste, mild constipation, abdominal cramps

Occasional

Nausea, vomiting, speckling or whitish discoloration of stools

SERIOUS REACTIONS

! Prolonged constipation may result in intestinal obstruction.
! Excessive or chronic use may produce hypophosphatemia manifested as anorexia, malaise, muscle weakness, or bone pain, which may result in osteomalacia and osteoporosis.
! Prolonged use may produce urinary calculi.

NURSING CONSIDERATIONS

Baseline Assessment

- Don't give other oral drugs within 1 to 2 hours of antacid administration.

Lifespan Considerations

- Aluminum hydroxide is contraindicated for children 6 years or younger.

Precautions

- Use aluminum hydroxide cautiously in elderly patients and patients with Alzheimer's disease, chronic diarrhea, constipation, dehydration, fecal impaction, fluid restrictions, gastric outlet obstruction, GI or rectal bleeding, impaired renal function, or symptoms of appendicitis.

Administration and Handling

PO

- The usual dose of aluminum hydroxide is 30 to 60 ml.
- Administer aluminum hydroxide 1 to 3 hours after meals and at bedtime.
- Expect the dosage to be individualized based on the antacid's neutralizing capacity.
- Instruct the patient to thoroughly chew chewable tablets (combination forms) before swallowing and then to drink a glass of water or milk.
- Shake the suspension well before use.

Intervention and Evaluation

- Assess the patient's pattern of daily bowel activity and stool consistency.
- Expect to monitor the patient's serum aluminum, calcium, phosphate, and uric acid levels.
- Evaluate and document the patient's relief from gastric distress.

Patient Teaching

- Instruct the patient to chew chewable tablets (combination forms) thoroughly before swallowing and to then drink a glass of water or milk.
- Inform the patient that stool discoloration may occur but will resolve when the drug is discontinued.
- Stress the need to drink plenty of fluids.

calcium acetate

kal-see-um

(PhosLo)

calcium carbonate

(Apo-Cal[CAN], Calsan[CAN], Cal-Sup[AUS], Caltrate, Dicarbosil, OsCal, Titralac, Tums)

calcium chloride

calcium citrate

(Citracal, Calcitrate)

calcium glubionate

(Calcione, Calciquid)

calcium gluconate

Do not confuse OsCal with Asacol, Citracal with Citrucel, or PhosLo with PhosChol.

CATEGORY AND SCHEDULE

Pregnancy Risk Category: C

OTC (acetate, carbonate, citrate, glubionate, gluconate [tablets only])

MECHANISM OF ACTION

An electrolyte that is essential for the function and integrity of the nervous, muscular, and skeletal systems. Calcium plays an important role in normal cardiac and renal function, respiration, blood coagulation, and cell membrane and capillary permeability. It helps regulate the release and storage of neurotransmitters and hormones, and it neutralizes or reduces gastric acid (increase pH). Calcium acetate combines with dietary phosphate to form insoluble calcium phosphate. **Therapeutic Effects:** Replaces calcium in deficiency states; controls hyperphosphatemia in end-stage renal disease.

PHARMACOKINETICS

Moderately absorbed from the small intestine (absorption depends on presence of vitamin D metabolites and patient's pH). Primarily eliminated in feces.

AVAILABILITY

Calcium Acetate
Gelcap (Phoslo): 667 mg (equivalent to 169 mg elemental calcium).
Tablet (Phoslo): 667 mg (equivalent to 169 mg elemental calcium).
Calcium Carbonate
Tablets: (Caltrate 600): equivalent to 600 mg elemental calcium.
Tablets (Os-Cal 500): equivalent to 500 mg elemental calcium.
Tablets (Chewable [Os-Call 500]): equivalent to 500 mg elemental calcium.
Tablets (Chewable [Tums]): equivalent to 200 mg elemental calcium.
Calcium Chloride
Injection: 10% (100 mg/ml) equivalent to 27.2 mg elemental calcium per ml.
Calcium Citrate
Tablets: (Cal-Citrate): 250 mg (equivalent to 53 mg elemental calcium).
Tablets (Citracal): 950 mg (equivalent to 200 mg elemental calcium).
Calcium Glubionate
Syrup: 1.8 g/5 ml (equivalent to 115 mg of elemental calcium per 5 ml).
Calcium Gluconate
Injection: 10% (equivalent to 9 mg elemental calcium per ml).

INDICATIONS AND DOSAGES

▸ Hyperphosphatemia
PO (calcium acetate)
Adults, Elderly. 2 tablets 3 times a day with meals.
▸ Hypocalcemia
PO (calcium carbonate)
Adults, Elderly. 1–2 g/day in 3–4 divided doses.
Children. 45–65 mg/kg/day in 3–4 divided doses.
PO (calcium glubionate)
Adults, Elderly. 6–18 g/day in 4–6 divided doses.
Children, Infants. 0.6–2 g/kg/day in 4 divided doses.
Neonates. 1.2 g/kg/day in 4–6 divided doses.
IV (calcium chloride)
Adults, Elderly. 0.5–1 g repeated q4–6h as needed.
Children. 2.5–5 mg/kg/dose q4–6h.
IV (calcium gluconate)
Adults, Elderly. 2–15 g/24 hr.
Children. 200–500 mg/kg/day.
▸ Antacid
PO (calcium carbonate)
Adults, Elderly. 1–2 tabs (5–10 ml) q2h as needed.
▸ Osteoporosis
PO (calcium carbonate)
Adults, Elderly. 1200 mg/day.
▸ Cardiac arrest
IV (calcium chloride)
Adults, Elderly. 2–4 mg/kg. May repeat q10min.
Children. 20 mg/kg. May repeat in 10 min.
▸ Hypocalcemia tetany
IV (calcium chloride)
Adults, Elderly. 1 g may repeat in 6 hours.
Children. 10 mg/kg over 5–10 min. May repeat in 6–8 hr.
IV (calcium gluconate)
Adults, Elderly. 1–3 g until therapeutic response achieved.
Children. 100–200 mg/kg/dose q6–8h.

OFF-LABEL USES

Treatment of hyperphosphatemia (calcium carbonate)

CONTRAINDICATIONS

Calcium renal calculi, digoxin toxicity, hypercalcemia, hypercalciuria, sarcoidosis, ventricular fibrillation
Calcium acetate: Decreased renal function, hypoparathyroidism

INTERACTIONS

Drug

Digoxin: May increase the risk of arrhythmias.

Etidronate, gallium: May antagonize the effects of these drugs.

Ketoconazole, phenytoin, tetracyclines: May decrease the absorption of these drugs.

Magnesium (parenteral), methenamine: May decrease the effects of these drugs.

Herbal

None known.

Food

None known.

DIAGNOSTIC TEST EFFECTS

May increase, blood pH, and serum gastrin and calcium levels. May decrease serum phosphate and potassium levels.

IV INCOMPATIBILITIES

Calcium chloride: amphotericin B complex (Abelcet, AmBisone, Amphotec), propofol (Diprivan), sodium bicarbonate

Calcium gluconate: amphotericin B complex (Abelcet, AmBisome, Amphotec), fluconazole (Diflucan)

IV COMPATIBILITIES

Calcium chloride: Amikacin (Amikin), dobutamine (Dobutrex), lidocaine, milrinone (Primacor), morphine, norepinephrine (Levophed)

Calcium gluconate: Ampicillin, aztreonam (Azactam), cefazolin (Ancef), cefepime (Maxipime), ciprofloxacin (Cipro), dobutamine (Dobutrex), enalapril (Vasotec), famotidine (Pepcid), furosemide (Lasix), heparin, lidocaine, magnesium sulfate, meropenem (Merrem IV), midazolam (Versed), milrinone (Primacor), norepinephrine (Levophed), piperacillin and tazobactam (Zosyn), potassium chloride, propofol (Diprivan)

SIDE EFFECTS

Frequent

PO: Chalky taste

Parenteral: Hypotension; flushing; feeling of warmth; nausea; vomiting; pain, rash, redness, or burning at injection site; diaphoresis

Occasional

PO: Mild constipation, fecal impaction, peripheral edema, metabolic alkalosis (muscle pain, restlessness, slow breathing, altered taste)

Calcium carbonate: Milk-alkali syndrome (headache, decreased appetite, nausea, vomiting, unusual tiredness)

Rare

Difficult or painful urination

SERIOUS REACTIONS

! Hypercalcemia is a serious adverse effect of calcium acetate use. Early signs include constipation, headache, dry mouth, increased thirst, irritability, decreased appetite, metallic taste, fatigue, weakness, and depression. Later signs include confusion, somnolence, hypertension, photosensitivity, arrhythmias, nausea, vomiting, and increased painful urination.

NURSING CONSIDERATIONS

Baseline Assessment

- Obtain the patient's BP; EKG; serum magnesium, potassium, and phosphate levels; and renal function test results.

Lifespan Considerations

- Calcium acetate is distributed in breast milk; it is unknown whether calcium chloride and gluconate are distributed in breast milk.
- Restrict IV use in children because their small vasculature increases the risk of developing extreme irritation

and possible tissue necrosis or sloughing.
• Oral absorption may be decreased in the elderly.

Precautions

• Use calcium cautiously in patients with chronic renal impairment, decreased cardiac function, dehydration, history of renal calculi, or ventricular fibrillation during cardiac resuscitation.

Administration and Handling

PO

• Give tablets with a full glass of water 30 minutes to 1 hour after meals.
• Dilute the syrup in juice or water and administer it before meals to increase absorption.
• Have the patient chew the chewable tablets thoroughly before swallowing them.

IV

• Store vials at room temperature.
• Calcium chloride may be given undiluted or may be diluted with an equal amount 0.9% NaCl or sterile water for injection.
• Calcium gluconate may be given undiluted or may be diluted in up to 1,000 ml 0.9% NaCl.
• Give calcium chloride by slow IV push (0.5 to 1 ml/minute). Rapid administration may produce bradycardia, hypotension, peripheral vasodilation, a chalky or metallic taste, and a feeling of warmth.
• Give calcium gluconate by IV push at a rate of 0.5 to 1 ml/minute. Rapid administration may produce arrhythmias, hypotension, MI, and vasodilation.
• When administering calcium gluconate by intermittent IV infusion, the maximum rate is 200 mg/minute.

Intervention and Evaluation

• Monitor the patient's BP; EKG; and serum magnesium, phosphate, and potassium levels; urine calcium concentrations; as well as renal function test results.
• Monitor the patient for signs and symptoms of hypercalcemia.

Patient Teaching

• Instruct the patient to take tablets with a full glass of water, 30 minutes to 1 hour after meals.
• Advise the patient to drink liquids before meals.
• Emphasize the importance of diet if the patient is receiving calcium as an antacid or a supplement.
• Advise the patient not to take calcium within 2 hours of consuming other oral drugs or fiber-containing foods.
• Urge the patient to avoid consuming excessive amounts of alcohol, caffeine, and tobacco.

citrates (potassium citrate, potassium citrate and citric acid, sodium citrate and citric acid, tricitrates)

sih-traits

(Bicitra, Oracit, Polycitra, Polycitra-K, Polycitra-LC, Urocit-K)

CATEGORY AND SCHEDULE

Pregnancy Risk Category: C (potassium citrate); other forms not expected to cause fetal harm.

MECHANISM OF ACTION

These alkalinizers increase the solubility of cystine in urine and the ionization of uric acid to urate ion. The increase in urinary pH and urinary citrate level decreases calcium ion activity and the saturation of calcium oxalate. Citrates also increase the plasma bicarbonate and buffer excess hydrogen ion concentration. **Therapeutic Effect:** Increase blood and urinary pH and reverse metabolic acidosis.

AVAILABILITY

Tablets: 5 mEq, 10 mEq.
Syrup (Polycitra): 550 mg potassium citrate, plus 500 mg sodium citrate, plus 334 mg citric acid per 5 ml.
Oral Solution (Bicitra): 500 mg sodium citrate and 334 mg citric acid per 5 ml.
Oral Solution (Oracit): 490 mg sodium citrate and 640 mg citric acid per 5 ml.
Oral Solution (Polycitra-K): 1,100 mg potassium citrate and 334 mg citric acid per 5 ml.
Oral Solution (Polycitra-LC): 550 mg potassium citrate, 500 mg sodium citrate, and 334 mg citric acid per 5 ml.

INDICATIONS AND DOSAGES

▸ Metabolic acidosis

PO
Adults, Elderly. 15–30 ml after meals and at bedtime or 30–60 mEq/day in 3–4 divided doses.
Children. 5–15 ml after meals and at bedtime or 2–3 mEq/kg/day in 3–4 divided doses.

CONTRAINDICATIONS

Acute dehydration, anuria, azotemia, heat cramps, hypersensitivity to citrates, severe myocardial damage, severe renal impairment, sodium-restricted diet, untreated Addison's disease
Urocit-K: Concurrent use of anticholinergics, delayed gastric emptying, intestinal obstruction or stricture, severe peptic ulcer disease

INTERACTIONS

Drug

ACE inhibitors, NSAIDs, potassium-containing medications, potassium-sparing diuretics: May increase the risk of hyperkalemia.
Antacids: May increase the risk of systemic alkalosis.
Methenamine: May decrease the effects of methenamine.
Quinidine: May increase the excretion of quinidine.

Herbal

None known.

Food

None known.

DIAGNOSTIC TEST EFFECTS

None known.

SIDE EFFECTS

Occasional

Diarrhea, mild abdominal pain, nausea, vomiting

SERIOUS REACTIONS

! Metabolic alkalosis, bowel obstruction or perforation, hyperkalemia, and hypernatremia occur rarely.

NURSING CONSIDERATIONS

Precautions

- Use citrates cautiously in patients with CHF, hypertension, or pulmonary edema.
- Use cautiously because citrate use may increase the risk of urolithiasis.

Administration and Handling

- Administer citrates after meals and at bedtime.

Intervention and Evaluation

- Assess the EKG and urinary pH of patients with cardiac disease.
- Assess the patient's CBC (particularly blood Hct and Hgb level), serum acid-base balance, and serum creatinine level.

Patient Teaching

- Instruct the patient to take citrates after meals and at bedtime.
- Teach the patient to mix citrates in water or juice and to drink additional liquids after taking the drug.

fluoride

flur-eyed

(Fluor-A-Day, Fluorigard, Fluotic[CAN], Flura-Drops, Flurets[AUS], Luride, NeutroGard, Pediaflor)

Do not confuse Fluor-A-Day with Fludara.

CATEGORY AND SCHEDULE

Pregnancy Risk Category: N/A

MECHANISM OF ACTION

A trace element that increases tooth resistance to acid dissolution. **Therapeutic Effect:** Promotes remineralization of decalcified enamel, inhibits dental plaque bacteria, increases resistance to development of caries, maintains bone strength.

AVAILABILITY

Lozenge: 2.2 mg.
Oral Solution Drops: 1.1 mg/ml.
Oral Solution Rinse: 0.05%, 0.2%, 0.44%.
Tablets (Chewable): 0.58 mg, 1.1 mg, 2.2 mg.
Topical Cream: 1.1%.
Topical Gel: 0.4%, 1.1%.
Topical Gel-Drops: 1.1%.

INDICATIONS AND DOSAGES

▸ **Dietary supplement for prevention of dental caries in children**

Fluoride level in water	Age	Dosage
less than 0.3 ppm*	younger than 2 yr	0.25 mg/day
	2–3 yr	0.5 mg/day
	4–13 yr	1 mg/day
0.3–0.7 ppm*	younger than 2 yr	None
	2–3 yr	0.25 mg/day
	4–13 yr	0.5 mg/day
greater than 0.7 ppm*	None	None

* ppm = parts per million

CONTRAINDICATIONS

Arthralgia, GI ulceration, severe renal insufficiency

INTERACTIONS

Drug

Aluminum hydroxide, calcium: May decrease the absorption of fluoride.

Herbal

None known.

Food

Dairy products: May decrease fluoride's absorption.

DIAGNOSTIC TEST EFFECTS

May increase serum alkaline phosphatase and AST (SGOT) levels.

SIDE EFFECTS

Rare

Oral mucous membrane ulceration

SERIOUS REACTIONS

! Hypocalcemia, tetany, bone pain (especially in ankles and feet), electrolyte disturbances, and arrhythmias occur rarely.

! Fluoride use may cause skeletal fluorosis, osteomalacia, and osteosclerosis.

NURSING CONSIDERATIONS

Patient Teaching

- Teach the patient to use gels and rinses at bedtime after brushing and flossing. Advise the patient to expectorate excess fluoride, not swallow it.
- Advise the patient not to drink, eat, or rinse the mouth after application.
- Instruct the patient not to take fluoride with dairy products, which may decrease fluoride's absorption.

lanthanum carbonate

lan-**thah**-num

(Fosrenol)

CATEGORY AND SCHEDULE

Pregnancy Risk Category: C

MECHANISM OF ACTION

A phosphate regulator that dissociates in the acidic environment of the upper GI tract to lanthanum ions, which bind to dietary phosphate released from food during digestion, forming highly insoluble lanthanum phosphate complexes. **Therapeutic Effect:** Reduces phosphate absorption.

PHARMACOKINETICS

Phosphate complexes are eliminated in urine.

AVAILABILITY

Tablets (Chewable): 250 mg, 500 mg.

INDICATIONS AND DOSAGES

▸ Reduce serum phosphate in end-stage renal disease

PO

Adults, Elderly. 750 mg–1,500 mg in divided doses, taken with or immediately after a meal. Dosage may be titrated in 750-mg increments q2-3wk based on serum phosphate levels.

CONTRAINDICATIONS

None known.

INTERACTIONS

Drug

Antacids: Interact with lanthanum; separate administration by 2 hours.

Herbal

None known.

Food

All foods: Enhance lanthanum's effect and reduce phosphate absorption.

DIAGNOSTIC TEST EFFECTS

None known.

SIDE EFFECTS

Frequent

Nausea (11%), vomiting (9%), dialysis graft occlusion (8%), abdominal pain (5%)

SERIOUS REACTIONS

! None known.

NURSING CONSIDERATIONS

Precautions

- Use lanthanum cautiously in patients with acute peptic ulcer disease, bowel obstruction, Crohn's disease, or ulcerative colitis.

Administration and Handling

PO

- Have the patient chew the tablets thoroughly before swallowing.
- Give the drug with or immediately after a meal.

Patient Teaching

- Instruct the patient to take lanthanum with or immediately after a meal.
- Tell the patient not to take lantha-

num within 2 hours of antacids.
• Explain that lanthanum's side effects of nausea and vomiting decrease over time.

magnesium

See Laxatives

phosphates

fos-fates
(Fleet Enema, Fleet Phospho-Soda, K-Phos ME, K-Phos Neutral, Neutra-Phos, Uro-KP-Neutral)

CATEGORY AND SCHEDULE

Pregnancy Risk Category: C

MECHANISM OF ACTION

Electrolytes that participate in bone deposition, calcium metabolism, and utilization of B complex vitamins and act as a buffer in maintaining acid-base balance. Also exert an osmotic effect in small intestine, producing distention and promoting peristalsis. **Therapeutic Effect:** Correct hypophosphatemia, acidify urine in UTIs, help prevent calcium deposits in urinary tract, and promote evacuation of the bowel.

PHARMACOKINETICS

Poorly absorbed after PO administration. PO form excreted in feces; IV form excreted in urine.

AVAILABILITY

Oral Solution (Fleet Phospho-Soda): 4 mmol phosphate per ml.
Powder (Neutra-Phos, Neutra-Phos K): 250 mg (8 mmol) phosphate.
Tablets (K-Phos ME): 125 mg (4 mmol) phosphate.
Tablets (K-Phos Neutral, Uro-KP-Neutral): 250 mg (8 mmol) phosphate.
Enema (Fleet Enema): 2.25 oz, 4.5 oz.
Injection (potassium phosphate): 3 mmol phosphate and 4.4 mEq potassium per ml.
Injection (sodium phosphate): 3 mmol phosphate and 4 mEq sodium per ml.

INDICATIONS AND DOSAGES

▸ **Hypophosphatemia**

PO (Neutra-Phos, Neutra-Phos K, K-Phos ME, K-Phos-Neutral, Uro-KP-Neutral)
Adults, Elderly. 50–150 mmol/day.
Children. 2–3 mmol/kg/day.
IV
Adults, Elderly. 50–70 mmol/day.
Children. 0.5–1.5 mmol/kg/day.

▸ **Laxative**

PO (Neutra-Phos, Neutra-Phos K, Uro-KP-Neutral)
Adults, Elderly, Children 4 yr and older. 1–2 capsules/packets 4 times a day.
Children younger than 4 yr. 1 capsule/packet 4 times a day.
Rectal
Adults, Elderly, Children 12 yr and older. 4.5-oz enema as single dose. May repeat.
Children younger than 12 yr. 2.25-oz enema as single dose. May repeat.

▸ **Urine acidification**

PO
Adults, Elderly. 8 mmol 4 times a day.

OFF-LABEL USES

Prevention of calcium renal calculi

CONTRAINDICATIONS

Abdominal pain or fecal impaction (from rectal dosage form), CHF, hyperkalemia, hypernatremia, hyperphosphatemia, hypocalcemia, hypomagnesemia, phosphate renal calculi, severe renal impairment

INTERACTIONS

Drug

ACE inhibitors, NSAIDs, potassium-containing medications, potassium-sparing diuretics, salt substitutes containing potassium phosphate: May increase potassium blood concentration.
Antacids: May decrease the absorption of phosphates.
Calcium-containing medications: May increase the risk of calcium deposition in soft tissues and decrease phosphate absorption.
Digoxin: May increase the risk of heart block caused by hyperkalemia when given with potassium phosphates.
Glucocorticoids: May cause edema when given with sodium phosphate.
Phosphate-containing medications: May increase the risk of hyperphosphatemia.
Sodium-containing medications: May increase the risk of edema when given with sodium phosphate.

Herbal

None known.

Food

None known.

DIAGNOSTIC TEST EFFECTS

None known.

IV INCOMPATIBILITIES

Dobutamine (Dobutrex)

IV COMPATIBILITIES

Diltiazem (Cardizem), enalapril (Vasotec), famotidine (Pepcid), magnesium sulfate, metoclopramide (Reglan)

SIDE EFFECTS

Frequent

Mild laxative effect (in first few days of therapy)

Occasional

Diarrhea, nausea, abdominal pain, vomiting

Rare

Headache; dizziness; confusion; heaviness of lower extremities; fatigue; muscle cramps; paraesthesia; peripheral edema; arrhythmias, weight gain; thirst

SERIOUS REACTIONS

! Hyperphosphatemia may produce extraskeletal calcification.

NURSING CONSIDERATIONS

Baseline Assessment

- Assess the patient for abdominal pain. Note its pattern, duration, quality, intensity, location, and areas of radiation, as well as factors that relieve or worsen it.
- If the patient is taking phosphates as a laxative, assess the pattern of daily bowel activity, including the amount, color, and consistency of stools, and auscultate bowel sounds for peristalsis.
- Determine if the patient has a history of recent abdominal surgery, nausea, vomiting, and weight loss.
- Obtain the results of baseline phosphate levels and urinary pH.

Lifespan Considerations

- It is unknown if phosphates cross the placenta or are distributed in breast milk.
- No age-related precautions have been noted in children or the elderly.

Precautions

- Use phosphates cautiously in patients with adrenal insufficiency, cirrhosis, or renal impairment and in those receiving potassium-sparing drugs concurrently.

Administration and Handling

PO
- Dissolve tablets in water.
- Give phosphates after meals or with food to decrease GI upset.
- Maintain high fluid intake to prevent renal calculi.

IV
- Store vials at room temperature.
- Dilute the drug before using.
- Infuse at a maximum rate of 0.06 mmol phosphate/kg/hour, as prescribed.

Intervention and Evaluation

- Routinely monitor the patient's serum alkaline phosphatase, bilirubin, calcium, phosphorus, potassium, sodium, AST (SGOT), and ALT (SGPT) levels.

Patient Teaching

- Advise the patient to notify the physician if he or she experiences diarrhea, nausea, or vomiting.

potassium acetate

poe-**tah**-see-um

potassium bicarbonate/citrate

(K-Lyte, Klor-Con EF, Effer K, K-Lyte DS)

potassium chloride

(Apo-K[CAN], Kaochlor, K-Dur, K-Lor, K-Lor-Con M 15, Kaon-Cl, KSR[AUS], KSR-600[AUS], Micro-K, Slow-K[AUS], Span-K[AUS])

potassium gluconate

(Kaon)

Do not confuse K-Dur with Cardura.

CATEGORY AND SCHEDULE

Pregnancy Risk Category: C (A for potassium chloride)

MECHANISM OF ACTION

An electrolyte that is necessary for multiple cellular metabolic processes. Primary action is intracellular. **Therapeutic Effect:** Is necessary for nerve impulse conduction and contraction of cardiac, skeletal, and smooth muscle; maintains normal renal function and acid-base balance.

PHARMACOKINETICS

Well absorbed from the GI tract. Enters cells by active transport from extracellular fluid. Primarily excreted in urine.

AVAILABILITY

Potassium Acetate
Injection: 2 mEq/ml.
Potassium Bicarbonate and Potassium Citrate
Tablet for Solution (Klor-Con EF, Effer-K, K-Lyte): 25 mEq.
Tablet for Solution (K-Lyte DS): 50 mEq.
Potassium Chloride
Capsules (Controlled-Release [Micro-K]): 8 mEq, 10 mEq.
Liquid (Kaochlor): 20 mEq/15 ml.
Liquid (Kaon-Cl): 40 mEq/15 ml.
Powder for Oral Solution (K-Lor): 20 mEq.
Injection: 2 mEq/ml.
Tablets (Extended-Release [Klor-Con, Micro-K]): 8 mEq, 10 mEq.
Tablets (Extended-Release [Kaon-Cl, K-Tab]): 10 mEq.
Tablets (Extended-Release [K-Dur]): 10 mEq, 20 mEq.
Potassium Gluconate
Elixir (Kaon): 20 mEq/15 ml.

INDICATIONS AND DOSAGES

▸ Prevention of hypokalemia (in patients on diuretic therapy)

PO

Adults, Elderly. 20–40 mEq/day in 1–2 divided doses.

Children. 1–2 mEq/kg/day in 1–2 divided doses.

▸ **Treatment of hypokalemia**

PO

Adults, Elderly. 40–80 mEq/day; further doses based on laboratory values.

Children. 2–5 mEq/day; further doses based on laboratory values.

IV

Adults, Elderly. 5–10 mEq/hr. Maximum: 400 mEq/day.

Children. 1 mEq/kg over 1–2 hr.

CONTRAINDICATIONS

Concurrent use of potassium-sparing diuretics, digitalis toxicity, heat cramps, hyperkalemia, postoperative oliguria, severe burns, severe renal impairment, shock with dehydration or hemolytic reaction, untreated Addison's disease

INTERACTIONS

Drug

ACE inhibitors, beta-adrenergic blockers, heparin, NSAIDs, potassium-containing medications, potassium-sparing diuretics, salt substitutes: May increase potassium blood concentration.

Anticholinergics: May increase the risk of GI lesions.

Herbal

None known.

Food

None known.

DIAGNOSTIC TEST EFFECTS

None known.

IV INCOMPATIBILITIES

Amphotericin B complex (Abelcet, AmBisome, Amphotec), methylprednisolone (Solu-Medrol), phenytoin (Dilantin)

IV COMPATIBILITIES

Aminophylline, amiodarone (Cordarone), atropine, aztreonam (Azactam), calcium gluconate, cefepime (Maxipime), ciprofloxacin (Cipro), clindamycin (Cleocin), dexamethasone (Decadron), digoxin (Lanoxin), diltiazem (Cardizem), diphenhydramine (Benadryl), dobutamine (Dobutrex), dopamine (Intropin), enalapril (Vasotec), famotidine (Pepcid), fluconazole (Diflucan), furosemide (Lasix), granisetron (Kytril), heparin, hydrocortisone (Solu-Cortef), insulin, lidocaine, lorazepam (Ativan), magnesium sulfate, methylprednisolone (Solu-Medrol), metoclopramide (Reglan), midazolam (Versed), milrinone (Primacor), morphine, norepinephrine (Levophed), ondansetron (Zofran), oxytocin (Pitocin), piperacillin and tazobactam (Zosyn), procainamide (Pronestyl), propofol (Diprivan), propranolol (Inderal)

SIDE EFFECTS

Occasional

Nausea, vomiting, diarrhea, flatulence, abdominal discomfort with distention, phlebitis with IV administration (particularly when potassium concentration of greater than 40 mEq/L is infused)

Rare

Rash

SERIOUS REACTIONS

! Hyperkalemia (more common in elderly patients and those with impaired renal function) may be manifested as paresthesia, feeling of heaviness in the lower extremities, cold skin, grayish pallor, hypotension, confusion, irritability, flaccid paralysis, and cardiac arrhythmias.

NURSING CONSIDERATIONS

Baseline Assessment

- Obtain the patient's serum potassium level.

Lifespan Considerations

- It is unknown if potassium crosses the placenta or is distributed in breast milk.
- No age-related precautions have been noted in children.
- The elderly may be at increased risk for hyperkalemia because of an impaired ability to excrete potassium.

Precautions

- Use potassium cautiously in patients with cardiac disease or tartrazine sensitivity (most common in those with aspirin hypersensitivity).

Administration and Handling

◀ALERT▶ Potassium dosage must be individualized.

PO

- Give potassium with or after meals and with full glass of water to decrease GI upset.
- Mix effervescent tablets, liquids, and powder with juice or water and let them dissolve before administering.
- Instruct the patient to swallow the tablets whole and not to chew or crush them.

IV

- Store vials at room temperature.
- Dilute the drug to a concentration of no more than 40 mEq/L and mix it well before IV infusion.
- Avoid adding potassium to a hanging IV line.
- Infuse the drug slowly at a rate not exceeding 20 mEq/hr.
- Check the patient's IV site closely during the infusion for evidence of phlebitis (hardness of vein; heat, pain, and red streaking of skin over vein) and extravasation (cool skin, little or no blood return, pain, and swelling).

Intervention and Evaluation

- Monitor the patient's serum potassium level, particularly those with renal impairment.
- If the patient experiences GI upset, dilute the IV preparation further or give oral forms with meals.
- Monitor the patient's intake and output diligently for diuresis. Be alert for decreased urine output, which may be an indication of renal insufficiency.
- Assess the patient's pattern of daily bowel activity and stool consistency.
- Be alert for signs and symptoms of hyperkalemia, including cold skin, feeling of heaviness in lower extremities, paraesthesia, and skin pallor.

Patient Teaching

- Give the patient a list of foods rich in potassium, including apricots, avocados, bananas, beans, beef, broccoli, brussel sprouts, cantaloupe, chicken, dates, fish, ham, lentils, milk, molasses, potatoes, prunes, raisins, spinach, turkey, watermelon, veal, and yams.
- Warn the patient to notify the physician if he or she experiences a feeling of heaviness in the lower extremities and paraesthesia.

sodium bicarbonate

sew-dee-um bye-**car**-bon-ate

CATEGORY AND SCHEDULE

Pregnancy Risk Category: C

OTC

MECHANISM OF ACTION

An alkalinizing agent that dissociates to provide bicarbonate ion. **Therapeutic Effect:** Neutralizes hydrogen ion concentration, raises blood and urinary pH.

PHARMACOKINETICS

Route	Onset	Peak	Duration
PO	15 min	N/A	1–3 hr
IV	Immediate	N/A	8–10 min

After administration, sodium bicarbonate dissociates to sodium and bicarbonate ions. With increased hydrogen ion concentrations bicarbonate ions combine with hydrogen ions to form carbonic acid, which then dissociates to CO_2, which is excreted by the lungs.

AVAILABILITY

Tablets: 325 mg, 650 mg.
Injection: 0.5 mEq/ml (4.2%), 0.6 mEq/ml (5%), 0.9 mEq/ml (7.5%), 1 mEq/ml (8.4%).

INDICATIONS AND DOSAGES

▸ **Cardiac arrest**
IV
Adults, Elderly. Initially, 1 mEq/kg (as 7.5%–8.4% solution). May repeat with 0.5 mEq/kg q10min during continued cardiopulmonary arrest. Use in the postresuscitation phase is based on arterial blood pH, partial pressure of carbon dioxide in arterial blood ($PaCO_2$) and base deficit calculation.
Children, Infants. Initially, 1 mEq/kg.

▸ **Metabolic acidosis (not severe)**
IV
Adults, Elderly, Children. 2–5 mEq/kg over 4–8 hr. May repeat based on laboratory values.

▸ **Metabolic acidosis (associated with chronic renal failure)**
PO
Adults, Elderly. Initially, 20–36 mEq/day in divided doses.

▸ **Renal tubular acidosis (distal)**
PO
Adults, Elderly. 0.5–2 mEq/kg/day in 4–6 divided doses.
Children. 2–3 mEq/kg/day in divided doses.

▸ **Renal tubular acidosis (proximal)**
PO
Adults, Elderly, Children. 5–10 mEq/kg/day in divided doses.

▸ **Urine alkalinization**
PO
Adults, Elderly. Initially, 4 g, then 1–2 g q4h. Maximum: 16 g/day.
Children. 84–840 mg/kg/day in divided doses.

▸ **Antacid**
PO
Adults, Elderly. 300 mg–2 g 1–4 times a day.

▸ **Hyperkalemia**
IV
Adults, Elderly. 1 mEq/kg over 5 minutes.

CONTRAINDICATIONS

Excessive chloride loss due to diarrhea, vomiting, or GI suctioning; hypocalcemia; metabolic or respiratory alkalosis

INTERACTIONS

Drug

Calcium-containing products: May result in milk-alkali syndrome.
Corticosteroids: May cause edema and hypertension.
Lithium, salicylates: May increase the excretion of these drugs.
Methenamine: May decrease the effects of methenamine.

Herbal

None known.

Food

Milk, other dairy products: May result in milk-alkali syndrome.

DIAGNOSTIC TEST EFFECTS

May increase serum and urinary pH.

IV INCOMPATIBILITIES

Ascorbic acid, diltiazem (Cardizem), dobutamine (Dobutrex), dopamine (Intropin), hydromorphone (Dilaudid), magnesium sulfate, midazolam (Versed), morphine, norepinephrine (Levophed)

IV COMPATIBILITIES

Aminophylline, calcium chloride, furosemide (Lasix), heparin, insulin, lidocaine, mannitol, milrinone (Primacor), morphine, phenylephrine (Neo-Synephrine), phenytoin (Dilantin), potassium chloride, propofol (Diprivan), vancomycin (Vancocin)

SIDE EFFECTS

Frequent

Abdominal distention, flatulence, belching

SERIOUS REACTIONS

! Excessive or chronic use may produce metabolic alkalosis (characterized by irritability, twitching, paraesthesias, cyanosis, slow or shallow respirations, headache, thirst, and nausea).

! Fluid overload results in headache, weakness, blurred vision, behavioral changes, incoordination, muscle twitching, elevated BP, bradycardia, tachypnea, wheezing, coughing, and distended neck veins.

! Extravasation may occur at the IV site, resulting in tissue necrosis and ulceration.

NURSING CONSIDERATIONS

Baseline Assessment

- Assess the patient for signs of metabolic acidosis, including disorientation, hyperventilation, and weakness.
- Assess the patient for GI symptoms, including flatulence and abdominal distention

Lifespan Considerations

- Sodium bicarbonate use may produce hypernatremia and increased deep tendon reflexes in the neonate or fetus whose mother is administered chronically high doses.
- Sodium bicarbonate may be distributed in breast milk.
- No age-related precautions have been noted in children; however, sodium bicarbonate should not be used as an antacid in children younger than 6 years.
- In the elderly, age-related renal impairment may require cautious use.

Precautions

- Use sodium bicarbonate cautiously in patients with CHF, renal insufficiency, or edema and in those receiving corticosteroid therapy concurrently.

Administration and Handling

◀ALERT▶ Sodium bicarbonate may be given by IV push, IV infusion, or orally. Dosage is individualized based on the patient's age, weight, clinical conditions, and laboratory values and on the severity of acidosis. Metabolic alkalosis may result if the bicarbonate deficit is fully corrected during the first 24 hours.

PO

- Give sodium bicarbonate 1 to 3 hours after meals.
- Don't give other oral drugs within 2 hours of sodium bicarbonate administration.

IV

- Store vials at room temperature.

◀ALERT▶ For patients with acidosis, administer sodium bicarbonate when the plasma bicarbonate level is less than 15 mEq/L.

- Sodium bicarbonate may be given undiluted.

◀ALERT▶ Use a 0.5 mEq/ml concentration for direct IV administration to neonates and infants.

• For IV push, give up to 1 mEq/kg over 1 to 3 minutes for cardiac arrest.
• Don't exceed an infusion rate of 50 mEq/hour. For children younger than 2 years, premature infants, and neonates, administer by slow infusion, up to 8 mEq/minute.

Intervention and Evaluation

• Monitor the patient's blood and urinary pH, $PaCO_2$ and CO_2, plasma bicarbonate, and serum electrolyte levels.
• Monitor the patient's serum calcium, phosphate, and uric acid levels.
• Observe the patient for signs and symptoms of fluid overload and metabolic alkalosis.
• Assess the patient for clinical improvement of metabolic acidosis, including relief from disorientation, hyperventilation, and weakness.
• Assess the patient's pattern of daily bowel activity and stool consistency.
• Assess the patient for relief of gastric distress.

Patient Teaching

• Advise the patient who is considering breast-feeding to consult her physician before taking sodium bicarbonate.
• Encourage the patient to check with the physician before taking any OTC drugs because they may contain sodium.

sodium chloride

sew-dee-um **klor**-eyed
(Muro 128, Nasal Mist, Nasal Moist, Ocean, SalineX, SeaMist, Slo-Salt)

CATEGORY AND SCHEDULE

Pregnancy Risk Category: C
OTC (Tablets, nasal solution, ophthalmic solution, ophthalmic ointment)

MECHANISM OF ACTION

Sodium is a major cation of extracellular fluid that controls water distribution, fluid and electrolyte balance, and osmotic pressure of body fluids; it also maintains acid-base balance.

PHARMACOKINETICS

Well absorbed from the GI tract. Widely distributed. Primarily excreted in urine.

AVAILABILITY

Tablets: 1 g
Injection (Concentrate): 23.4% (4 mEq/ml).
Injection: 0.45%, 0.9%, 3%.
Irrigation: 0.45%, 0.9%.
Nasal Gel (Nasal Moist): 0.65%.
Nasal Solution (OTC [SalineX]): 0.4%.
Nasal Solution (OTC [Nasal Moist, SeaMist]): 0.65%.
Ophthalmic Solution (OTC [Muro 128]): 5%.
Ophthalmic Ointment (OTC [Muro 128]): 5%.

INDICATIONS AND DOSAGES

▸ **Prevention and treatment of sodium and chloride deficiencies; source of hydration**
IV
Adults, Elderly. 1–2 L/day 0.9% or 0.45% or 100 ml 3% or 5% over 1

hr; assess serum electrolyte levels before giving additional fluid.

▸ **Prevention of heat prostration and muscle cramps from excessive perspiration**

PO

Adults, Elderly. 1–2 g 3 times a day.

▸ **Relief of dry and inflamed nasal membranes**

Intranasal

Adults, Elderly. Use as needed.

▸ **Diagnostic aid in ophthalmoscopic exam, treatment of corneal edema**

Ophthalmic Solution

Adults, Elderly. Apply 1–2 drops q3–4h.

Ophthalmic Ointment

Adults, Elderly. Apply once a day or as directed.

CONTRAINDICATIONS

Fluid retention, hypernatremia

INTERACTIONS

Drug

Hypertonic saline solution, oxytocics: May cause uterine hypertonus, ruptures, or lacerations.

Herbal

None known.

Food

None known.

DIAGNOSTIC TEST EFFECTS

None known.

SIDE EFFECTS

Frequent

Facial flushing

Occasional

Fever; irritation, phlebitis, or extravasation at injection site

Ophthalmic: Temporary burning or irritation

SERIOUS REACTIONS

! Too-rapid administration may produce peripheral edema, CHF, and pulmonary edema.

! Excessive dosage may cause hypokalemia, hypervolemia, and hypernatremia.

NURSING CONSIDERATIONS

Baseline Assessment

• Assess the patient's daily weight and intake and output; examine for edema; and auscultate breath sounds to determine fluid balance.

Lifespan Considerations

• No age-related precautions have been noted in children or the elderly.

Precautions

• Use sodium chloride cautiously in patients with cirrhosis, CHF, hypertension, or renal impairment.

• Don't administer sodium and chloride preserved with benzyl alcohol to neonates.

Administration and Handling

◂ **ALERT** ▸ Dosage is based on the patient's acid-base status, age, weight, clinical condition, and fluid and electrolyte status.

PO

• Do not crush or break enteric-coated or slow-release tablets.

• Administer tablets with a full glass of water.

IV

• Administer hypertonic solutions (3% or 5%) through a large vein at a rate not exceeding 100 ml/hr. Avoid infiltration.

• Dilute vials containing 2.5 to 4 mEq/ml (concentrated NaCl) with D_5W or $D_{10}W$ before administration.

Nasal

• Instruct the patient to begin inhaling slowly just before releasing the drug into nose.

• Teach the patient to inhale slowly and then release air gently through the mouth.

• Have the patient continue this technique for 20 to 30 seconds.
Ophthalmic
• Place a gloved finger on the patient's lower eyelid, and pull it out until a pocket is formed between the eye and lower lid.
• Hold the dropper above the pocket and instill the prescribed number of drops (or apply a thin strip of ointment) in the pocket.
• Instruct the patient to close the eyes gently so that the drug isn't squeezed out of the sac.
• After administering the solution, apply gentle finger pressure to the lacrimal sac for 1 to 2 minutes to reduce systemic absorption.
• Released the lower lid, and have the patient who has received the solution keep the affected eye open without blinking for at least 30 seconds; have the patient who has received the ointment close the affected eye and roll the eyeball to distribute the drug.

Intervention and Evaluation

• Assess the IV site for extravasation.
• Monitor the patient's fluid balance, acid-base balance, BP, and serum electrolyte levels.
• Assess the patient for signs and symptoms of hypernatremia (edema, hypertension, and weight gain) and hyponatremia (dry mucous membranes, muscle cramps, nausea, and vomiting).

Patient Teaching

• Inform the patient that he or she may experience temporary burning or irritation after instillation of the ophthalmic drug.
• Instruct the patient to discontinue the ophthalmic medication and notify the physician if he or she experiences acute redness of eyes, floating spots, severe eye pain or pain on exposure to light, a rapid change in vision (side and straight ahead), or headache.

zinc oxide

zink ox-eyed
(Balmex, Desitin)

zinc sulfate

zink sul-fate
(Orazinc, Zincaps[AUS])

CATEGORY AND SCHEDULE

Pregnancy Risk Category: C

MECHANISM OF ACTION

A mineral that acts as a co-factor for enzymes that are important for protein and carbohydrate metabolism. **Therapeutic Effect:** Zinc oxide acts as a mild astringent and skin protectant. Zinc sulfate helps maintain normal growth and tissue repair as well as skin hydration.

AVAILABILITY

Zinc Oxide
Ointment: 10%, 20%, 40%.
Zinc Sulfate
Capsules: 110 mg, 220 mg.
Tablets: 110 mg.
Injection: 1 mg/ml.

INDICATIONS AND DOSAGES

▸ **Mild skin irritations and abrasions (such as chapped skin, diaper rash)**
Topical (zinc oxide)
Adults, Elderly, Children. Apply as needed.

▸ **Treatment and prevention of zinc deficiency, wound healing.**
PO (zinc sulfate)
Adults, Elderly. 220 mg 3 times a day.

CONTRAINDICATIONS

None known.

INTERACTIONS

Drug

H blockers (such as famotidine): May decrease zinc absorption.
Quinolones (such as ciprofloxacin, tetracycline): May decrease the absorption of these drugs.

Herbals

None known.

Food

Coffee, dairy products: May decrease zinc sulfate (capsules, tablets) absorption.

DIAGNOSTIC TEST EFFECTS

None known.

SIDE EFFECTS

None known.

SERIOUS REACTIONS

! None known.

NURSING CONSIDERATIONS

Baseline Assessment

- Assess the skin for signs of infection before applying topical zinc.

Lifespan Considerations

- Pregnant women should avoid using zinc oxide and zinc sulfate, unless prescribed.

Precautions

- Don't exceed the prescribed dosage. Excessive zinc intake can cause impaired leukocyte function, a reduction in HDL levels, and vomiting.

Administration and Handling

PO

- Take zinc sulfate with food.

Topical

- Apply zinc oxide after cleaning and drying the affected area.
- Zinc oxide is for external use only. Avoid use in the eyes.

Intervention and Evaluation

- Monitor skin integrity for signs of improvement.

Patient Teaching

- Explain that coffee and dairy products may decrease the absorption of oral zinc sulfate capsules and tablets.
- If nausea occurs, instruct the patient to take zinc sulfate with food.
- Instruct the patient to notify the physician if the skin condition doesn't improve after 7 days of treatment.

77 Vitamins

ascorbic acid (vitamin C)
cyanocobalamin (vitamin B_{12})
flavocoxid
folic acid (vitamin B_9), sodium folate
leucovorin calcium (folinic acid, citrovorum factor)
niacin, nicotinic acid (vitamin B_3)
pyridoxine hydrochloride (vitamin B_6)
thiamine hydrochloride (vitamin B_1)
vitamin A
vitamin D
vitamin E
vitamin K

Uses: Vitamins are primarily used to supplement the diet to meet the body's need for the organic substances required for growth, reproduction, and maintenance of health. The need for vitamin supplementation may result from inadequate dietary intake, increased physiologic need (such as during pregnancy), or certain disorders or conditions, such as Crohn's disease, renal disease, and gastrectomy.

Some vitamins have additional uses. *Vitamin C* is used to prevent and treat scurvy. *Flavocoxid* is used to decrease the pain and inflammation associated with osteoarthritis. *Leucovorin* is used to prevent and treat methotrexate, pyrimethamine, and trimethoprim toxicity. As an adjunct, *niacin* is used to treat hyperlipidemias and peripheral vascular disease. *Pyridoxine* is used to treat isoniazid poisoning, seizures in neonates who don't respond to conventional therapy, and sideroblastic anemia caused by increased serum iron concentrations. *Thiamine* is helpful in treating alcoholic patients with altered sensorium. *Vitamin K* is used to prevent and treat hemorrhagic states in neonates and as the antidote for hemorrhage caused by oral anticoagulants.

Action: Vitamins are essential for energy transformation and regulation of metabolic processes. They're catalysts for all reactions using proteins, fats, and carbohydrates for energy, growth, and cell maintenance. *Water-soluble vitamins,* such as folic acid and vitamins C, B_1, B_3, B_6, and B_{12}, act as coenzymes for almost every cellular reaction in the body. B-complex vitamins differ from one another in structure and function, but are grouped together because they were first isolated from the same source (yeast and liver).

Fat-soluble vitamins, such as vitamins A, D, E, and K, are stored in body tissue and may be toxic when excessive quantities are consumed. Vitamin A is needed for normal retinal function, night vision, bone growth, gonadal function, embryonic development, and epithelial cell integrity. Vitamin D is essential for calcium absorption and use and for normal calcification of bone. Vitamin E prevents oxidation and protects fatty acids from free radicals. Vitamin K is required for hepatic formation of coagulation factors II, VII, IX, and X.

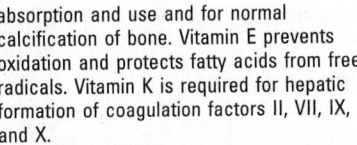

Flavocoxid inhibits prostaglandin synthesis and arachidonic acid metabolism, which reduces the production of leukotrienes and produces anti-inflammatory and analgesic effects.

ascorbic acid (vitamin C)

a-**skor**-bic

(Apo-C[CAN], Cecon, Cenolate, Pro-C[AUS], Redoxon[CAN])

CATEGORY AND SCHEDULE

Pregnancy Risk Category: A (C if used in doses above recommended daily allowance)

OTC

MECHANISM OF ACTION

Assists in collagen formation and tissue repair and is involved in oxidation reduction reactions and other metabolic reactions. **Therapeutic Effect:** Involved in carbohydrate use and metabolism, as eell as synthesis of carnitine, lipids, and proteins. Preserves blood vessel integrity.

PHARMACOKINETICS

Readily absorbed from the GI tract. Protein binding: 25%. Metabolized in the liver. Excreted in urine. Removed by hemodialysis.

AVAILABILITY

Capsules (Controlled-Release): 500 mg.
Liquid: 500 mg/5 ml.
Oral Solution: 500 mg/5 ml.
Tablets: 100 mg, 250 mg, 500 mg, 1 g.
Tablets (Chewable): 100 mg, 250 mg, 500 mg.
Tablets (Controlled-Release): 500 mg, 1 g, 1,500 mg.
Injection: 250 mg/ml, 500 mg/ml.

INDICATIONS AND DOSAGES

▸ **Dietary supplement**

PO

Adults, Elderly. 50–200 mg/day.
Children. 35–100 mg/day.

▸ **Acidification of urine**

PO

Adults, Elderly. 4–12 g/day in 3–4 divided doses.
Children. 500 mg q6–8h.

▸ **Scurvy**

PO

Adults, Elderly. 100–250 mg 1–2 times a day.
Children. 100–300 mg/day in divided doses.

▸ **Prevention and reduction of severity of colds**

PO

Adults, Elderly. 1–3 g/day in divided doses.

OFF-LABEL USES

Prevention of common cold, control

of idiopathic methemoglobinemia, urine acidifier

CONTRAINDICATIONS

None known.

INTERACTIONS

Drug

Deferoxamine: May increase iron toxicity.

Herbal

None known.

Food

None known.

DIAGNOSTIC TEST EFFECTS

May decrease serum bilirubin level and urinary pH. May increase urine uric acid and urine oxalate levels.

IV INCOMPATIBILITIES

No information available for Y-site administration.

IV COMPATIBILITIES

Calcium gluconate, heparin

SIDE EFFECTS

Rare

Abdominal cramps, nausea, vomiting, diarrhea, increased urination with doses exceeding 1 g
Parenteral: Flushing, headache, dizziness, sleepiness or insomnia, soreness at injection site.

SERIOUS REACTIONS

! Ascorbic acid may acidify urine, leading to crystalluria.
! Large doses of IV ascorbic acid may lead to deep vein thrombosis.
! Abrupt discontinuation after prolonged use of large doses may produce rebound ascorbic acid deficiency.

NURSING CONSIDERATIONS

Baseline Assessment

- Assess the patient's nutritional status with a focus on foods high in vitamin C. Before and during treatment, assess for signs and symptoms of vitamin C deficiency, including bleeding gums, digestive difficulties, gingivitis, poor wound healing, and arthralgia.

Lifespan Considerations

- Ascorbic acid crosses the placenta and is excreted in breast milk.
- Large doses of ascorbic acid taken during pregnancy may produce scurvy in neonates.
- No age-related precautions have been noted in children or the elderly.

Precautions

- Use ascorbic acid cautiously in patients with diabetes mellitus or a history of renal scalculi; those on sodium-restricted diet; and those receiving warfarin or daily doses of salicylate.

Administration and Handling

PO

- Give ascorbic acid without regard to food.

IV

- Refrigerate vials and protect them from freezing and sunlight.
- Ascorbic acid may be given undiluted or may be diluted in D_5W, 0.9% NaCl, or lactated Ringer's solution.
- For IV push, dilute with an equal volume of D_5W or 0.9% NaCl and infuse over 10 minutes. For IV solution, infuse over 4 to 12 hours.

Intervention and Evaluation

- Assess the patient for signs of clinical improvement, such as improved wound healing.
- Monitor for signs and symptoms of recurring vitamin C deficiency, including bleeding gums, digestive

difficulties, gingivitis, poor wound healing, and arthralgia.

Patient Teaching

- Instruct the patient to reduce ascorbic acid dosage gradually, as prescribed, because abrupt discontinuation may produce rebound deficiency.
- Encourage the patient to eat foods rich in vitamin C, including citrus fruits, green peppers, brussel sprouts, rose hips, spinach, strawberries, and watercress.

cyanocobalamin (vitamin B_{12})

sye-an-oh-koe-**bal**-a-min

(Bedoz[CAN], Cytamen[AUS])

CATEGORY AND SCHEDULE

Pregnancy Risk Category: A (C if used in doseas above recommended daily allowance)

MECHANISM OF ACTION

Acts as a coenzyme for various metabolic functions, including fat and carbohydrate metabolism and protein synthesis. **Therapeutic Effect:** Necessary for cell growth and replication, hematopoiesis, and myelin synthesis.

PHARMACOKINETICS

In the presence of calcium, absorbed systemically in lower half of ileum. Initially, bound to intrinsic factor; this complex passes down intestine, binding to receptor sites on ileal mucosa. Protein binding: High. Metabolized in the liver. Primarily eliminated unchanged in urine. ***Half-life:*** 6 days.

AVAILABILITY

Tablets: 50 mcg, 100 mcg, 250 mcg, 500 mcg, 1,000 mcg, 5000 mcg.
Tablet (Extended-Release): 1,500 mcg.
Injection: 1,000 mcg/ml.

INDICATIONS AND DOSAGES

▸ **Pernicious anemia**

IM, Subcutaneous

Adults, Elderly. 100 mcg/day for 7 days, then every other day for 7 days, then every 3–4 days for 2–3 wk. Maintenance: 100 mcg/mo (oral 1,000–2,000 mcg/day).

Children. 30–50 mcg/day for 2 or more wk. Maintenance: 100 mcg/mo.

Neonates. 1,000 mcg/day for 2 or more wk. Maintenance: 50 mcg/mo.

▸ **Uncomplicated vitamin B_{12} deficiency**

PO

Adults, Elderly. 1,000–2,000 mcg/day

IM, Subcutaneous

Adults, Elderly. 100 mcg/day for 5–10 days, followed by 100–200 mcg/mo.

▸ **Complicated vitamin B_{12} deficiency**

IM, Subcutaneous

Adults, Elderly. 1,000 mcg (with IM or IV folic acid 15 mg) as a single dose, then 1,000 mcg/day plus oral folic acid 5 mg/day for 7 days.

CONTRAINDICATIONS

Folic acid deficiency anemia, hereditary optic nerve atrophy, history of allergy to cobalamins

INTERACTIONS

Drug

Alcohol, colchicines: May decrease the absorption of cyanocobalamin.
Ascorbic acid: May destroy cyanocobalamin.

Folic acid (large doses): May decrease cyanocobalamin blood concentration.

Herbal

None known.

Food

None known.

DIAGNOSTIC TEST EFFECTS

None known.

SIDE EFFECTS

Occasional

Diarrhea, pruritus

SERIOUS REACTIONS

! Impurities in preparation may cause a rare allergic reaction.

! Peripheral vascular thrombosis, pulmonary edema, hypokalemia, and CHF may occur.

NURSING CONSIDERATIONS

Baseline Assessment

- Before and during therapy, assess the patient for signs and symptoms of vitamin B_{12} deficiency, including anorexia, ataxia, fatigue, hyporeflexia, insomnia, irritability, loss of positional sense, pallor, and palpitations on exertion.

Lifespan Considerations

- Cyanocobalamin crosses the placenta and is excreted in breast milk.
- No age-related precautions have been noted in children or the elderly.

Administration and Handling

PO

- Give cyanocobalamin with meals to increase absorption.

Intervention and Evaluation

- Assess the patient for CHF, hypokalemia, and pulmonary edema, especially in those receiving IM or subcutaneous cyanocobalamin.
- Monitor the patient's serum potassium level, which normally ranges from 3.5 to 5 mEq/L, and serum cyanocobalamin level, which normally ranges from 200 to 800 mcg/ml. Also watch for a rise in the blood reticulocyte count, which peaks in 5 to 8 days.
- Evaluate the patient for reversal of deficiency symptoms (anorexia, ataxia, fatigue, hyporeflexia, insomnia, irritability, loss of positional sense, pallor, and palpitations on exertion). A therapeutic response to treatment usually occurs within 48 hours.

Patient Teaching

- Inform the patient with pernicious anemia that lifetime treatment may be necessary.
- Instruct the patient to notify the physician if he or she experiences symptoms of an infection.
- Encourage the patient to eat foods rich in vitamin B_{12}, including clams, dairy products, egg yolks, fermented cheese, herring, muscle and organ meats, oysters, and red snapper.

flavocoxid

flay-**vox**-ah-sid

(Limbrel)

CATEGORY AND SCHEDULE

Pregnancy Risk Category: Not classified.

MECHANISM OF ACTION

An oral nutritional supplement that inhibits prostaglandin synthesis and arachidonic acid metabolism, reducing the production of leukotrienes. Also acts through an antioxidant mechanism. **Therapeutic Effect:** Produces anti-inflammatory and analgesic effects and increases mobility.

PHARMACOKINETICS
Undergoes hydrolysis at the gut mucosal border. Food decreases absorption. Little hepatic metabolism.

AVAILABILITY
Capsules: 250 mg.

INDICATIONS AND DOSAGES
▸ **Osteoarthritis**
PO
Adults 18 yr and older, Elderly. One 250-mg capsule q12h.

CONTRAINDICATIONS
History of peptic ulcer

INTERACTIONS
Drug
None known.
Herbal
None known.
Food
All foods: Decrease the absorption of flavocoxid.

DIAGNOSTIC TEST EFFECTS
None known.

SIDE EFFECTS
Rare (2%)
Increase in varicose veins, psoriasis, mild hypertension

SERIOUS REACTIONS
! GI bleeding, perforation, and ulceration occur rarely in patients currently or previously treated with NSAIDs or COX-2 inhibitors.

NURSING CONSIDERATIONS
Baseline Assessment
- Assess the duration, location, onset, and type of the patient's pain or inflammation.
- Inspect the patient's affected joints for deformities, immobility, and skin condition.

Lifespan Considerations
- It is unknown if flavocoxid crosses the placenta or is distributed in breast milk.
- Flavocoxid use is not recommended during pregnancy.
- The safety and efficacy of flavocoxid have not been established in children younger than 18 years.
- No age-related precautions have been noted in the elderly.

Administration and Handling
PO
- Don't administer flavocoxid within 1 hour of eating because food decreases the drug's absorption.

Intervention and Evaluation
- Assess the patient for a therapeutic response, including improved grip strength, increased joint mobility, reduced joint tenderness, and relief of pain, stiffness, and swelling.

Patient Teaching
- Instruct the patient to take flavocoxid at least 1 hour before or after eating because food decreases the drug's absorption.

folic acid (vitamin B_9)
foe-lik
(Apo-Folic[CAN], Folvite, Megafol[AUS])

sodium folate
(Folvite-parenteral)
Do not confuse Folvite with Florvite.

CATEGORY AND SCHEDULE
Pregnancy Risk Category: A (C if used in doses above the recommended daily allowance)
OTC (0.4-mg and 0.8-mg tablets only)

MECHANISM OF ACTION

A coenzyme that stimulates production of platelets, RBCs, and WBCs.
Therapeutic Effect: Essential for nucleoprotein synthesis and maintenance of normal erythropoiesis.

PHARMACOKINETICS

PO form almost completely absorbed from the GI tract (upper duodenum). Protein binding: High. Metabolized in the liver and plasma to active form. Excreted in urine. Removed by hemodialysis.

AVAILABILITY

Tablets: 0.4 mg, 0.8 mg, 1 mg.
Injection: 5 mg/ml.

INDICATIONS AND DOSAGES

▸ **Vitamin B_9 deficiency**

PO, IV, IM, Subcutaneous

Adults, Elderly, Children 12 yr and older. Initially, 1 mg/day. Maintenance: 0.5 mg/day.
Children 1–11 yr. Initially 1 mg/day. Maintenance: 0.1–0.4 mg/day.
Infants. 50 mcg/day.

▸ **Dietary supplement**

PO, IV, IM, Subcutaneous

Adults, Elderly, Children 4 yr and older. 0.4 mg/day.
Children 1–younger than 4 yr. 0.3 mg/day.
Children younger than 1 yr. 0.1 mg/day.
Pregnant women. 0.8 mg/day.

OFF-LABEL USES

To decrease the risk of colon cancer

CONTRAINDICATIONS

Anemias (aplastic, normocytic, pernicious, refractory)

INTERACTIONS

Drug

Analgesics, carbamazepine, estrogens: May increase folic acid requirements.
Antacids, cholestyramine: May decrease the absorption of folic acid.
Hydantoin anticonvulsants: May decrease the effects of these drugs.
Methotrexate, triamterene, trimethoprim: May antagonize the effects of folic acid.

Herbal

None known.

Food

None known.

DIAGNOSTIC TEST EFFECTS

May decrease vitamin B_{12} concentration.

SIDE EFFECTS

None known.

SERIOUS REACTIONS

! Allergic hypersensitivity occurs rarely with parenteral form. Oral folic acid is nontoxic.

NURSING CONSIDERATIONS

Baseline Assessment

- Expect the physician to rule out pernicious anemia with a Schilling test and vitamin B_{12} blood level before beginning folic acid therapy because the signs of pernicious anemia may be masked while irreversible neurologic damage progresses.
- Patients with alcoholism, decreased hematopoiesis, or deficiency of vitamin B_6, B_{12}, C, or E and those using antimetabolic drugs may develop a resistance to treatment.

Lifespan Considerations

- Folic acid is distributed in breast milk.
- No age-related precautions have been noted in children or the elderly.

Administration and Handling

◀ **ALERT** ▶ Parenteral folic acid is used in acutely ill patients, those receiving enteral or total parenteral nutrition, and patients with malabsorption syndrome who are unresponsive to the oral form. Folic acid dosages greater than 0.1 mg/day may conceal signs of pernicious anemia.

Intervention and Evaluation

• Assess the patient for evidence of therapeutic improvement, including improved sense of well-being and relief from iron deficiency symptoms, such as fatigue, headache, pallor, dyspnea, and sore tongue.

Patient Teaching

• Encourage the patient to eat foods rich in folic acid, including fruits, vegetables, and organ meats.

leucovorin calcium (folinic acid, citrovorum factor)

loo-koe-**vor**-in

(Calcium Leucovorin[AUS], Wellcovorin)

Do not confuse Wellcovorin with Wellbutrin or Wellferon.

CATEGORY AND SCHEDULE

Pregnancy Risk Category: C

MECHANISM OF ACTION

An antidote to folic acid antagonists that may limit methotrexate action on normal cells by competing with methotrexate for the same transport processes into the cells. **Therapeutic Effect:** Reverses toxic effects of folic acid antagonists. Reverses folic acid deficiency.

PHARMACOKINETICS

Readily absorbed from the GI tract. Widely distributed. Primarily concentrated in the liver. Metabolized in the liver and intestinal mucosa to active metabolite. Primarily excreted in urine. ***Half-life:*** 15 min; metabolite, 30–35 min.

AVAILABILITY

Tablets: 5 mg, 10 mg, 15 mg, 25 mg.
Injection: 10 mg/ml.
Powder for Injection: 50 mg, 100 mg, 200 mg, 350 mg.

INDICATIONS AND DOSAGES

▸ **Conventional rescue dosage in high-dose methotrexate therapy**

PO, IV, IM

Adults, Elderly, Children. 10 mg/m^2 IM or IV one time, then PO q6h until serum methotrexate level is less than 10^{-8} M. If 24-hr serum creatinine level increases by 50% or greater over baseline or methotrexate level exceeds 5×10^{-6} M or 48-hr level exceeds 9×10^{-7} M, increase to 100 mg/m^2 IV q3h until methotrexate level is less than 10^{-8} M.

▸ **Folic acid antagonist overdose**

PO

Adults, Elderly, Children. 2–15 mg/day for 3 days or 5 mg every 3 days.

▸ **Megaloblastic anemia**

IM

Adults, Elderly, Children. 3–6 mg/day.

▸ **Megaloblastic anemia secondary to folate deficiency**

IM

Adults, Elderly, Children. 1 mg/day.

▸ **Prevention of hematologic toxicity (for toxoplasmosis), with sulfadiazine**

PO, IV

Adults, Elderly, Children. 5–10 mg/day, repeat every 3 days.

▸ **Prevention of hematologic toxicity with pyrimethamine, PCP**

PO, IV

Adults, Children. 25 mg once weekly.

OFF-LABEL USES
Treatment of Ewing's sarcoma, gestational trophoblastic neoplasms, or non-Hodgkin's lymphoma; treatment adjunct for head and neck carcinoma

CONTRAINDICATIONS
Pernicious anemia, other megaloblastic anemias secondary to vitamin B_{12} deficiency

INTERACTIONS
Drug
Anticonvulsants: May decrease the effects of anticonvulsants.
Chemotherapeutic agents: May increase the effects and toxicity of these drugs when taken in combination.
Herbal
None known.
Food
None known.

DIAGNOSTIC TEST EFFECTS
None known.

IV INCOMPATIBILITIES
Amphotericin B complex (Abelcet, AmBisome, Amphotec), droperidol (Inapsine), foscarnet (Foscavir)

IV COMPATIBILITIES
Cisplatin (Platinol AQ), cyclophosphamide (Cytoxan), doxorubicin (Adriamycin), etoposide (VePesid), filgrastim (Neupogen), 5-fluorouracil, gemcitabine (Gemzar), granisetron (Kytril), heparin, methotrexate, metoclopramide (Reglan), mitomycin (Mutamycin), piperacillin and tazobactam (Zosyn), vinblastine (Velban), vincristine (Oncovin)

SIDE EFFECTS
Frequent
When combined with chemotherapeutic agents: Diarrhea, stomatitis, nausea, vomiting, lethargy or malaise or fatigue, alopecia, anorexia
Occasional
Urticaria, dermatitis

SERIOUS REACTIONS
! Excessive dosage may negate chemotherapeutic effects of folic acid antagonists.
! Anaphylaxis occurs rarely.
! Diarrhea may cause rapid clinical deterioration.

NURSING CONSIDERATIONS
Baseline Assessment
- For treatment of accidental overdosage of folic acid antagonists, give leucovorin as soon as possible (preferably within 1 hour), as prescribed.

Lifespan Considerations
- It is unknown if leucovorin crosses the placenta or is distributed in breast milk.
- Leucovorin use in children may increase the risk of seizures by counteracting the anticonvulsant effects of barbiturates and hydantoins.
- Age-related renal impairment may require a dosage adjustment for elderly patients receiving drug for rescue from effects of high-dose methotrexate therapy.

Precautions
- Use leucovorin cautiously in patients with bronchial asthma or a history of allergies.
- Use leucovorin with 5-fluorouracil cautiously in patients with GI toxicities.

Administration and Handling
◀ALERT▶ For rescue therapy in chemotherapy, refer to specific protocol being used for optimal dosage and sequence of leucovorin administration.
PO
- Scored tablets may be crushed.

IV

- Store vials for parenteral use at room temperature.
- The injection solution normally appears clear and yellowish.
- Reconstitute each 50-mg vial with 5 ml sterile water for injection or bacteriostatic water for injection (containing benzyl alcohol) to provide a concentration of 10 mg/ml. Reconstitute doses greater than 10 mg/m^2 with sterile water for injection.
- Further dilute with D_5W or 0.9% NaCl.
- Use the solution immediately if reconstituted with sterile water for injection and within 7 days if reconstituted with bacteriostatic water for injection.
- Don't exceed an infusion rate of 160 mg/minute (because of drug's calcium content).

Intervention and Evaluation

- Monitor the patient for vomiting, which may require a change from oral to parenteral therapy.
- Observe elderly and debilitated patients closely because of the risk of severe toxicities.
- Assess the patient's CBC and BUN and serum creatinine levels to assess renal function (important in leucovorin rescue).
- Assess electrolyte levels and liver function test results of patients receiving chemotherapeutic agents in combination with leucovorin.

Patient Teaching

- Encourage the patient with folic acid deficiency to eat foods high in folic acid, including dried beans, meat proteins, and green leafy vegetables.
- Urge the patient to notify the physician if he or she experiences an allergic reaction or vomiting.

niacin, nicotinic acid (vitamin B_3)

See Antihyperlipidemics

pyridoxine hydrochloride (vitamin B_6)

peer-i-**dox**-een

(Aminoxin, Beesix, Doxine, Nestrex, Pryi, Pyroxin[AUS], Rodex, Vitabee 6)

Do not confuse pyridoxine with paroxetine, pralidoxime, or Pyridium.

CATEGORY AND SCHEDULE

Pregnancy Risk Category: A

OTC

MECHANISM OF ACTION

Acts as a coenzyme for various metabolic functions, including metabolism of proteins, carbohydrates, and fats. Aids in the breakdown of glycogen and in the synthesis of gamma-aminobutyric acid in the CNS. **Therapeutic Effect:** Prevents pyridoxine deficiency. Increases the excretion of certain drugs, such as isoniazid, that are pyridoxine antagonists.

PHARMACOKINETICS

Readily absorbed primarily in jejunum. Stored in the liver, muscle, and brain. Metabolized in the liver. Primarily excreted in urine. Removed by hemodialysis. ***Half-life:*** 15–20 days.

AVAILABILITY

Capsules: 250 mg.

Tablets: 20 mg, 25 mg, 50 mg, 100 mg, 250 mg, 500 mg.

Injection: 100 mg/ml.

INDICATIONS AND DOSAGES

▸ **Pyridoxine deficiency**
PO
Adults, Elderly. Initially, 2.5–10 mg/day; then 2.5 mg/day when clinical signs are corrected.
Children. Initially, 5–25 mg/day for 3 wk, then 1.5–2.5 mg/day.

▸ **Pyridoxine dependent seizures**
PO, IV, IM
Infants. Initially,10–100 mg/day. Maintenance: PO: 50–100 mg/day.

▸ **Drug-induced neuritis**
PO (treatment)
Adults, Elderly. 100–300 mg/day in divided doses
Children. 10–50 mg/day.
PO (prophylaxis)
Adults, Elderly. 25–100 mg/day.
Children. 1–2 mg/kg/day.

CONTRAINDICATIONS

None known.

INTERACTIONS

Drug
Immunosuppressants, isoniazid, penicillamine: May antagonize pyridoxine, causing anemia or peripheral neuritis.
Levodopa: Reverses the effects of levodopa.
Herbal
None known.
Food
None known.

DIAGNOSTIC TEST EFFECTS

None known.

IV INCOMPATIBILITIES

Don't mix pyridoxine with any other medications.

SIDE EFFECTS

Occasional
Stinging at IM injection site
Rare
Headache, nausea, somnolence; sensory neuropathy (paraesthesia, unstable gait, clumsiness of hands) with high doses

SERIOUS REACTIONS

! Long-term megadoses (2–6 g over more than 2 mo) may produce sensory neuropathy (reduced deep tendon reflexes, profound impairment of sense of position in distal limbs, gradual sensory ataxia). Toxic symptoms subside when drug is discontinued.
! Seizures have occurred after IV megadoses.

NURSING CONSIDERATIONS

Baseline Assessment
• Before and during therapy, assess the patient for signs and symptoms of pyridoxine deficiency, including CNS abnormalities (anxiety, depression, insomnia, motor difficulty, peripheral numbness, tremors) and skin lesions (glossitis, seborrhea-like lesions around eyes, mouth, nose).
Lifespan Considerations
• Pyridoxine crosses the placenta and is excreted in breast milk.
• High doses of pyridoxine in pregnancy may produce seizures in neonates.
• No age-related precautions have been noted in children or the elderly.
Administration and Handling
◂**ALERT**▸ Give pyridoxine orally unless malabsorption, nausea, or vomiting occurs. Avoid IV use in cardiac patients.
PO
• Administer extended-release capsules and tablets whole without crushing or breaking them. Have the patient avoid chewing the capsule or tablet.
IV
• Pyridoxine may be given undiluted

or may be added to IV solutions and given as an infusion.

Intervention and Evaluation

- Observe the patient for improvement of deficiency symptoms, including CNS abnormalities (anxiety, depression, insomnia, motor difficulty, paraesthesia and tremors) and skin lesions (glossitis, seborrhea-like lesions around eyes, mouth, nose).
- Evaluate the patient for nutritional adequacy.

Patient Teaching

- Inform the patient that IM injection may cause discomfort.
- Encourage the patient to eat foods rich in pyridoxine, including avocados, bananas, bran, carrots, eggs, organ meats, tuna, shrimp, hazelnuts, legumes, soybeans, sunflower seeds, and wheat germ.

thiamine hydrochloride (vitamin B_1)

thy-a-min

(Beta-Sol[AUS], Betaxin[CAN], Thiamilate)

CATEGORY AND SCHEDULE

Pregnancy Risk Category: A (C if used in doses above recommended daily allowance)

OTC (tablets)

MECHANISM OF ACTION

A water-soluble vitamin that combines with adenosine triphosphate in the liver, kidneys, and leukocytes to form thiamine diphosphate, a coenzyme that is necessary for carbohydrate metabolism. **Therapeutic Effect:** Prevents and reverses thiamine deficiency.

PHARMACOKINETICS

Readily absorbed from the GI tract, primarily in duodenum, after IM administration. Widely distributed. Metabolized in the liver. Primarily excreted in urine.

AVAILABILITY

Tablets: 50 mg, 100 mg, 250 mg, 500 mg.

Injection: 100 mg/ml.

INDICATIONS AND DOSAGES

▸ **Dietary supplement**

PO

Adults, Elderly. 1–2 mg/day.

Children. 0.5–1 mg/day.

Infants. 0.3–0.5 mg/day.

▸ **Thiamine deficiency**

PO

Adults, Elderly. 5–30 mg/day, as a single dose or in 3 divided doses, for 1 mo.

Children. 10–50 mg/day in 3 divided doses.

▸ **Thiamine deficiency in patients who are critically ill or have malabsorption syndrome**

IV, IM

Adults, Elderly. 5–100 mg, 3 times a day.

Children. 10–25 mg/day.

▸ **Metabolic disorders**

PO

Adults, Elderly, Children. 10–20 mg/day; increased up to 4 g/day in divided doses.

CONTRAINDICATIONS

None known.

INTERACTIONS

Drug

None known.

Herbal

None known.

Food

None known.

DIAGNOSTIC TEST EFFECTS
None known.

IV INCOMPATIBILITIES
Sodium bicarbonate

IV COMPATIBILITIES
Famotidine (Pepcid), multivitamins

SIDE EFFECTS
Frequent
Pain, induration, and tenderness at IM injection site

SERIOUS REACTIONS
! IV administration may result in a rare, severe hypersensitivity reaction marked by a feeling of warmth, pruritus, urticaria, weakness, diaphoresis, nausea, restlessness, tightness in throat, angioedema, cyanosis, pulmonary edema, GI tract bleeding, and cardiovascular collapse.

NURSING CONSIDERATIONS
Baseline Assessment
• Before and during treatment, assess the patient for signs and symptoms of thiamine deficiency, including peripheral neuropathy, ataxia, hyporeflexia, muscle weakness, nystagmus, ophthalmoplegia, confusion, peripheral edema, bounding arterial pulse, and tachycardia.

Lifespan Considerations
• Thiamine crosses the placenta; it is unknown if it's excreted in breast milk.
• No age-related precautions have been noted in children or the elderly.

Precautions
• Use thiamine cautiously in patients with Wernicke's encephalopathy.

Administration and Handling
◀ALERT▶ IM and IV administration routes are used only in acutely ill patients and those who are unresponsive to the PO route, such as those with malabsorption syndrome. The IM route is preferred over the IV route. The solution may be given by IV push or may be added to most IV solutions and given as an IV infusion.

Intervention and Evaluation
• Monitor the patient's EKG and erythrocyte count.
• Assess the patient for signs and symptoms of improvement, including an improved sense of well-being and weight gain.
• Observe the patient for reversal of neurologic signs and symptoms of deficiency (such as peripheral neuropathy, ataxia, hyporeflexia, muscle weakness, nystagmus, ophthalmoplegia, and confusion) and cardiac signs and symptoms (such as peripheral edema, bounding arterial pulse, tachycardia, and venous hypertension).

Patient Teaching
• Inform the patient that IM injection may cause discomfort.
• Encourage the patient to consume foods rich in thiamine, including legumes, nuts, organ meats, pork, rice bran, seeds, wheat germ, whole grain and enriched cereals, and yeast.
• Advise the patient that urine may appear bright yellow during thiamine therapy.

vitamin A
vight-ah-myn **A**
(Aquasol A, Palmitate A)
Do not confuse Aquasol A with Anusol.

CATEGORY AND SCHEDULE
Pregnancy Risk Category: A
(X if used in doses above recommended daily allowance)

MECHANISM OF ACTION

A fat-soluble vitamin that may act as a cofactor in biochemical reactions. **Therapeutic Effect:** Is essential for normal function of retina, visual adaptation to darkness, bone growth, testicular and ovarian function, and embryonic development; preserves integrity of epithelial cells.

PHARMACOKINETICS

Rapidly absorbed from the GI tract if bile salts, pancreatic lipase, protein, and dietary fat are present. Transported in blood to the liver, where it's metabolized; stored in parenchymal hepatic cells, then transported in plasma as retinol, as needed. Excreted primarily in bile and, to a lesser extent, in urine.

AVAILABILITY

Capsules: 10,000 units, 25,000 units.
Injection (Aquasol A): 50,000 units/ml.
Tablets (Palmitate A): 5,000 units, 15,000 units.

INDICATIONS AND DOSAGES

▸ **Severe vitamin A deficiency**

PO

Adults, Elderly, Children 8 yr and older. 500,000 units/day for 3 days; then 50,000 units/day for 14 days, then 10,000–20,000 units/day for 2 mo.
Children 1–7 yr. 5,000 units/kg/day for 5 days, then 5,000–10,000 units/day for 2 mo.
Children younger than 1 yr. 5,000–10,000 units/day for 2 mo.

IM

Adults, Elderly, Children 8 yr and older. 100,000 units/day for 3 days; then 50,000 units/day for 14 days.
Children 1–7 yr. 17,500–35,000 units/day for 10 days.
Children younger than 1 yr. 7,500–15,000 units/day.

▸ **Malabsorption syndrome**

PO

Adults, Elderly, Children 8 yr and older. 10,000–50,000 units/day.

▸ **Dietary supplement**

PO

Adults, Elderly. 4,000–5,000 units/day.
Children 7–10 yr. 3,300–3,500 units/day.
Children 4–6 yr. 2,500 units/day.
Children 6 mo–3 yr. 1,500–2,000 units/day.
Neonates younger than 5 mos. 1,500 units/day.

CONTRAINDICATIONS

Hypervitaminosis A

INTERACTIONS

Drug

Cholestyramine, colestipol, mineral oil: May decrease the absorption of vitamin A.
Isotretinoin: May increase the risk of toxicity.

Herbal

None known.

Food

None known.

DIAGNOSTIC TEST EFFECTS

May increase BUN and serum cholesterol, calcium, and triglyceride levels. May decrease blood erythrocyte and leukocyte counts.

SIDE EFFECTS

None known.

SERIOUS REACTIONS

! Chronic overdose produces malaise, nausea, vomiting, drying or cracking of skin or lips, inflammation of tongue or gums, irritability, alopecia, and night sweats.
! Bulging fontanelles have occurred in infants.

NURSING CONSIDERATIONS

Baseline Assessment

- Before and during treatment, assess the patient for signs and symptoms of vitamin A deficiency, including night blindness, dry and brittle nails, alopecia, and drying of corneas.

Lifespan Considerations

- Vitamin A crosses the placenta and is distributed in breast milk.
- Use caution when administering high doses of vitamin A to children and the elderly.

Precautions

- Use vitamin A cautiously in patients with renal impairment.

Administration and Handling

◀ALERT▶ IM administration is used only in acutely ill patients or patients unresponsive to the oral route, such as those with malabsorption syndrome.

PO

- Do not crush, open, or break capsules.
- Give vitamin A without regard to food.

IM

- For adults, an IM injection dose of 1 ml (50,000 units) may given in the deltoid muscle; a dose greater than 1 ml should be given in a large muscle mass. The anterolateral thigh is the preferred site for infants younger than 7 months.

Intervention and Evaluation

- Be alert for symptoms of overdose in patients receiving prolonged administration of more than 25,000 units/day.
- Monitor the patient for therapeutic serum vitamin A levels (80 to 300 units/ml).

Patient Teaching

- Encourage the patient to consume foods rich in vitamin A, including cod, halibut, tuna, and shark. Explain to the patient that naturally occurring vitamin A is found only in animal sources.
- Instruct the patient to avoid taking cholestyramine (Questran), colestipol, and mineral oil during vitamin A therapy.

vitamin D

vight-a-myn **D**
(Calciferol, Drisdol, Ostoforet [CAN])

CATEGORY AND SCHEDULE

Pregnancy Risk Category: A (D if used in doses above recommended daily allowance)

MECHANISM OF ACTION

A fat-soluble vitamin that stimulates calcium and phosphate absorption from small intestine, promotes secretion of calcium from bone to blood, and promotes resorption of phosphate in renal tubules; also acts on bone cells to stimulate skeletal growth and on parathyroid gland to suppress hormone synthesis and secretion. **Therapeutic Effect:** Essential for absorption and utilization of calcium and phosphate and normal bone calcification. Reduces parathyroid hormone level. Improves phosphorus and calcium homeostasis in chronic renal failure.

PHARMACOKINETICS

Readily absorbed from small intestine. Concentrated primarily in liver and fat deposits. Activated in the liver and kidneys. Eliminated by biliary system; excreted in urine. ***Half-life:*** 19–48 hr for ergocalciferol.

AVAILABILITY

Capsules (Drisdol): 50,000 units (1.25 mg).

Injection (Calciferol): 500,000 units/ml (12.5 mg).
Oral Liquid Drops (Calciferol, Drisdol): 8,000 units/ml.

INDICATIONS AND DOSAGES

◀ **ALERT** ▶ Oral dosing is preferred. Administer the drug IM only in patients with GI, hepatic, or biliary disease associated with malabsorption of vitamin D.

▶ **Dietary supplement**
PO
Adults, Elderly, Children. 10 mcg (400 units)/day.
Neonates. 10–20 mcg (400–800 units)/day.

▶ **Renal failure**
PO
Adults, Elderly. 0.5 mg/day.
Children. 0.1–1 mg/day.

▶ **Hypoparathyroidism**
PO
Adults, Elderly. 625 mcg–5 mg/day (with calcium supplements).
Children. 1.25–5 mg/day (with calcium supplements).

▶ **Nutritional rickets, osteomalacia**
PO
Adults, Elderly, Children. 25–125 mcg/day for 8–12 wk.
Adults, Elderly (with malabsorption syndrome). 250–7,500 mcg/day.
Children (with malabsorption syndrome). 250–625 mcg/day.

▶ **Vitamin D–dependent rickets**
PO
Adults, Elderly. 250 mcg–1.5 mg/day.
Children. 75–125 mcg/day. Maximum: 1,500 mcg/day.

▶ **Vitamin D–resistant rickets**
PO
Adults, Elderly. 250–1,500 mcg/day (with phosphate supplements).
Children. Initially 1,000–2,000 mcg/day (with phosphate supplements). May increase in 250- to 600-mcg increments q3–4mo.

CONTRAINDICATIONS

Hypercalcemia, malabsorption syndrome, vitamin D toxicity

INTERACTIONS

Drug

Aluminum-containing antacids (long-term use): May increase aluminum blood concentration and risk of aluminum bone toxicity.
Calcium-containing preparations, thiazide diuretics: May increase the risk of hypercalcemia.
Magnesium-containing antacids: May increase magnesium blood concentration.
Mineral oil: Excessive use of mineral oil decreases vitamin D absorption.

Herbal

None known.

Food

None known.

DIAGNOSTIC TEST EFFECTS

May increase serum cholesterol, calcium, magnesium, and phosphate levels. May decrease serum alkaline phosphatase level.

SIDE EFFECTS

None known.

SERIOUS REACTIONS

! Early signs and symptoms of overdose are weakness, headache, somnolence, nausea, vomiting, dry mouth, constipation, muscle and bone pain, and metallic taste.

! Later signs and symptoms of overdose include polyuria, polydipsia, anorexia, weight loss, nocturia, photophobia, rhinorrhea, pruritus, disorientation, hallucinations, hyperthermia, hypertension, and cardiac arrhythmias.

NURSING CONSIDERATIONS

Baseline Assessment

• Vitamin D therapy should begin at the lowest possible dosage.

Lifespan Considerations

• It is unknown if vitamin D crosses the placenta or is distributed in breast milk.
• Children may be more sensitive to the effects of vitamin D.
• No age-related precautions have been noted in the elderly.

Precautions

• Use vitamin D cautiously in patients with contrary artery disease, renal calculi, or renal impairment.

Administration and Handling

◀ **ALERT** ▶ Be aware that 1 mcg of vitamin D = 40 units.

PO

• Give vitamin D without regard to food.
• Have the patient swallow the capsules whole and avoid crushing, chewing, or opening them.

Intervention and Evaluation

• Monitor the patient's BUN level; serum alkaline phosphatase, calcium, creatinine, magnesium, phosphate, and urinary calcium level. The therapeutic serum calcium level is 9 to 10 mg/dl.
• Estimate the patient's daily dietary calcium intake.

Patient Teaching

• Encourage the patient to consume foods rich in vitamin D, including milk, eggs, leafy vegetables, margarine, meats, and vegetable oils and shortening.
• Instruct the patient not to take mineral oil during vitamin D therapy.
• Advise the patient receiving chronic renal dialysis not to take magnesium-containing antacids during vitamin D therapy.
• Advise the patient to drink plenty of liquids.

vitamin E

vight-a-myn **E**
(Aqua Gem E, Aquasol E, E-Gems, Key-E, Key-E Kaps)
Do not confuse Aquasol E with Anusol.

CATEGORY AND SCHEDULE

Pregnancy Risk Category: A (C if used in doses above recommended daily allowance)
OTC

MECHANISM OF ACTION

An antioxidant that prevents oxidation of vitamins A and C, protects fatty acids from attack by free radicals, and protects RBCs from hemolysis by oxidizing agents. **Therapeutic Effect:** Prevents and treats vitamin E deficiency.

PHARMACOKINETICS

Variably absorbed from the GI tract (requires bile salts, dietary fat, and normal pancreatic function). Primarily concentrated in adipose tissue. Metabolized in the liver. Primarily eliminated by biliary system.

AVAILABILITY

Capsules (E-Gems): 100 units, 600 units, 800 units, 1,000 units, 1,200 units.
Capsules (Aqua-Gem E, Key-E Kaps): 200 units, 400 units.
Tablets (Key-E): 100 units, 200 units, 400 units, 800 units.

INDICATIONS AND DOSAGES

▸ **Vitamin E deficiency**

PO

Adults, Elderly. 60–75 units/day.
Children. 1 unit/kg/day.

OFF-LABEL USES
To decrease severity of tardive dyskinesia

CONTRAINDICATIONS
None known.

INTERACTIONS
Drug
Cholestyramine, colestipol, mineral oil: May decrease the absorption of vitamin E.
Iron (large doses): May increase vitamin E requirements.
Herbal
None known.
Food
None known.

DIAGNOSTIC TEST EFFECTS
None known.

SIDE EFFECTS
None known.

SERIOUS REACTIONS
! Chronic overdose may produce fatigue, weakness, nausea, headache, blurred vision, flatulence, and diarrhea.

NURSING CONSIDERATIONS
Baseline Assessment
- Before and during treatment, assess the patient for signs and symptoms of vitamin E deficiency, including peripheral neuropathy, irritability, and muscle weakness.

Lifespan Considerations
- It is unknown if vitamin E crosses the placenta or is distributed in breast milk.
- No age-related precautions have been noted with normal dosages in children or the elderly.

Precautions
- Vitamin E use may impair the hematologic response in patients with iron deficiency anemia.

Administration and Handling
PO
- Don't crush, open, or break capsules or tablets.
- Give vitamin E without regard to food.

Intervention and Evaluation
- Assess the patient for signs and symptoms of hypervitaminosis E, including headache, fatigue, nausea, weakness, and diarrhea.
- Ensure that the patient receives a diet high in vitamin E.

Patient Teaching
- Instruct the patient to swallow tablets and capsules whole, not to chew, open, or crush them.
- Urge the patient to notify the physician if he or she experiences signs and symptoms of toxicity including blurred vision, diarrhea, nausea, dizziness, flulike symptoms, or headache.
- Encourage the patient to consume foods rich in vitamin E, including eggs, meats, milk, leafy vegetables, margarine, and vegetable oils and shortening.

vitamin K
vight-a-myn **K**
(AquaMEPHYTON, Konakion [CAN], Mephyton)
Do not confuse Mephyton with melphalan or mephenytoin.

CATEGORY AND SCHEDULE
Pregnancy Risk Category: C

MECHANISM OF ACTION
A fat-soluble vitamin that promotes hepatic formation of coagulation

factors II, VII, IX, and X. **Therapeutic Effect:** Essential for normal clotting of blood.

PHARMACOKINETICS

Readily absorbed from the GI tract (duodenum) after IM or subcutaneous administration. Metabolized in the liver. Excreted in urine; eliminated by biliary system. Onset of action: with PO form, 6–10 hr; with parenteral form, hemorrhage controlled in 3–6 hr and PT returns to normal in 12–14 hr.

AVAILABILITY

Tablets (Mephyton): 5 mg.
Injection (AquaMephyton): 2 mg/ml, 10 mg/ml.

INDICATIONS AND DOSAGES

▸ **Oral anticoagulant overdose**

PO, IV, Subcutaneous
Adults, Elderly. 2.5–10 mg/dose. May repeat in 12–48 hr if given orally and in 6–8 hr if given by IV or subcutaneous route.
Children. 0.5–5 mg depending on need for further anticoagulation and severity of bleeding.

▸ **Vitamin K deficiency**

PO
Adults, Elderly. 2.5–25 mg/24 hr.
Children. 2.5–5 mg/24 hr.
IV, IM, Subcutaneous
Adults, Elderly. 10 mg/dose.
Children. 1–2 mg/dose.

▸ **Hemorrhagic disease of newborn**

IM, Subcutaneous
Neonate. Treatment: 1–2 mg/dose/day. Prophylaxis: 0.5–1 mg within 1 hr of birth; may repeat in 6–8 hr if necessary.

CONTRAINDICATIONS

None known.

INTERACTIONS

Drug

Broad-spectrum antibiotics, high-dose salicylates: May increase vitamin K requirements.
Cholestyramine, colestipol, mineral oil, sucralfate: May decrease the absorption of vitamin K.
Oral anticoagulants: May decrease the effects of these drugs.

Herbal

None known.

Food

None known.

DIAGNOSTIC TEST EFFECTS

None known.

IV INCOMPATIBILITIES

No known incompatibilities for Y-site administration.

IV COMPATIBILITIES

Heparin, potassium chloride

SIDE EFFECTS

Occasional

Pain, soreness, and swelling at IM injection site; pruritic erythema (with repeated injections); facial flushing; unusual taste

SERIOUS REACTIONS

! Newborns (especially premature infants) may develop hyperbilirubinemia.

! A severe reaction (cramplike pain, chest pain, dyspnea, facial flushing, dizziness, rapid or weak pulse, rash, diaphoresis, hypotension progressing to shock, cardiac arrest) occurs rarely just after IV administration.

NURSING CONSIDERATIONS

Baseline Assessment

• Before and during treatment, assess the patient for signs and symptoms of vitamin K deficiency, including hematuria and increased bruising and petechiae.

Lifespan Considerations

• Vitamin K crosses the placenta and is distributed in breast milk.
• No age-related precautions have been noted in children or the elderly.

Administration and Handling

◀ALERT▶ The subcutaneous route is preferred. IV or IM administration is restricted to emergency situations.

◀ALERT▶ The oral and subcutaneous routes of administration are less likely to produce side effects than the IM and IV routes.

PO

• Scored tablets may be crushed.

IV

• Store vials at room temperature.
• Vitamin K may be diluted with preservative-free 0.9% NaCl or D_5W immediately before use. Do not use other diluents. Discard unused portions.
• Administer by slow IV at rate of 1 mg/minute.
• Monitor the patient for signs and symptoms of hypersensitivity or of an anaphylactic reaction during and immediately after IV administration.

IM, Subcutaneous

• Inject the drug into the anterolateral aspect of thigh or the deltoid region.

Intervention and Evaluation

• Routinely monitor PT and international normalized ratio in patients taking anticoagulants.
• Examine the patient's skin for ecchymosis and petechiae and gums for erythema and gingival bleeding. Also be alert for hematuria, excessive bleeding from minor cuts and scratches, and increased menstrual flow.
• Assess the patient's blood Hct, platelet count, and stool and urine specimens for occult blood.
• Monitor the patient for abdominal or back pain, decrease in BP, increase in pulse rate, and severe headache, which may indicate hemorrhage.
• Assess the patient's peripheral pulses.

Patient Teaching

• Inform the patient that parenteral administration may cause discomfort.
• Warn the patient to notify the physician if he or she experiences black or red stool, coffee-ground vomitus, red or dark urine, or red-speckled mucus from a cough.
• Caution the patient against taking any other medications, including OTC preparations, without the physician's approval because they may interfere with platelet aggregation.
• Instruct adult patients to use an electric razor and soft toothbrush to prevent bleeding.
• Encourage the patient to consume foods rich in vitamin K, including milk, egg yolks, leafy green vegetables, meat, tomatoes, and vegetable oil.

78 Cholinergics

bethanechol chloride
cevimeline
neostigmine
physostigmine
pilocarpine hydrochloride
pyridostigmine bromide

Uses: Cholinergics are primarily used to treat urine retention and myasthenia gravis and to reverse non-depolarizing neuromuscular blockade. Additionally, *cevimeline* is used to treat dry mouth in Sjögren's syndrome. *Neostigmine* is used to prevent postoperative urine retention and to diagnose myasthenia gravis. *Physostigmine* is used to reverse the toxic CNS effects of anticholinergic drugs and tricyclic antidepressants. *Pilocarpine* is used to treat dry mouth from salivary gland hypofunction in patients receiving radiation therapy for head and neck cancer.

Action: Some cholinergics, such as *bethanechol* and *pilocarpine,* directly bind to cholinergic (muscarinic) receptors and activate them, mimicking the action of acetylcholine. Others, such as *neostigmine* and *physostigmine,* inhibit the enzyme acetylcholinesterase, preventing the destruction of acetylcholine. Cholinergic agents mainly affect the heart, exocrine glands, and smooth muscle. In the heart, they can lead to bradycardia. In the exocrine glands, they may increase sweating, salivation, and bronchial secretions. In smooth muscle, they promote contraction. Several also stimulate ciliary muscles, leading to miosis.

bethanechol chloride

be-**than**-e-kole
(Duvoid[CAN], Myotonachol[CAN], Urecholine, Urocarb[AUS])
Do not confuse bethanechol with betaxolol.

CATEGORY AND SCHEDULE
Pregnancy Risk Category: C

MECHANISM OF ACTION
A cholinergic that acts directly at cholinergic receptors in the smooth muscle of the urinary bladder and GI tract. Increases detrusor muscle tone.

Therapeutic Effect: May initiate micturition and bladder emptying. Improves gastric and intestinal motility.

AVAILABILITY
Tablets (Duvoid): 10 mg, 25 mg, 50 mg.

INDICATIONS AND DOSAGES
▸ **Postoperative and postpartum urine retention, atony of bladder**
PO
Adults, Elderly. 10–50 mg 3–4 times a day. Minimum effective dose determined by giving 5–10 mg

initially, then repeating same amount at 1-hr intervals until desired response is achieved, or maximum of 50 mg is reached.
Children. 0.6 mg/kg/day in 3–4 divided doses.

OFF-LABEL USES

Treatment of congenital megacolon, gastroesophageal reflux, postoperative gastric atony

CONTRAINDICATIONS

Active or latent bronchial asthma, acute inflammatory GI tract conditions, anastomosis, bladder wall instability, cardiac or coronary artery disease, epilepsy, hypertension, hyperthyroidism, hypotension, GI or urinary tract obstruction, parkinsonism, peptic ulcer, pronounced bradycardia, recent GI resection, vasomotor instability

INTERACTIONS

Drug

Cholinesterase inhibitors: May increase the effects and risk of toxicity of bethanechol.
Procainamide, quinidine: May decrease the effects of bethanechol.

Herbal

None known.

Food

None known.

DIAGNOSTIC TEST EFFECTS

May increase serum amylase, lipase, and AST (SGOT) levels.

SIDE EFFECTS

Occasional

Belching, blurred or changed vision, diarrhea, urinary urgency

SERIOUS REACTIONS

! Overdosage produces CNS stimulation (including insomnia, anxiety, and orthostatic hypotension), and cholinergic stimulation (such as headache, increased salivation diaphoresis, nausea, vomiting, flushed skin, abdominal pain, and seizures).

NURSING CONSIDERATIONS

Baseline Assessment

- Obtain vital signs before and regularly throughout therapy. Be alert for bradycardia and hypotension.
- Monitor and document the patient's intake and output, assessing for urine retention and urge incontinence.

Administration and Handling

◀ **ALERT** ▶ Avoid giving IM or IV route because doing so will precipitate a violent cholinergic reaction marked by bloody diarrhea, circulatory collapse, severe hypotension, and shock. The antidote is 0.6–1.2 mg atropine sulfate.

◀ **ALERT** ▶ Side effects are more noticeable with subcutaneous administration.

Intervention and Evaluation

- Assess the patient for cholinergic reaction manifested as blurred vision, excessive salivation, diaphoresis, facial warmth, GI cramping or discomfort, lacrimation, pallor, and urinary urgency.
- Observe the patient for difficulty chewing or swallowing and progressive muscle weakness.
- Measure and record fluid intake and output.

Patient Teaching

- Tell the patient to notify the physician if he or she experiences difficulty breathing, irregular heartbeat, muscle weakness, nausea and vomiting, diarrhea, severe abdominal pain, and increased salivation or sweating.

cevimeline

sev-**im**-el-ine
(Evoxac)
Do not confuse Evoxac with Eurax.

CATEGORY AND SCHEDULE

Pregnancy Risk Category: C

MECHANISM OF ACTION

A cholinergic agonist that binds to muscarinic receptors of effector cells, thereby increasing secretion of exocrine glands, such as salivary glands. **Therapeutic Effect:** Relieves dry mouth.

AVAILABILITY

Capsules: 30 mg.

INDICATIONS AND DOSAGES

▸ **Dry mouth**

PO

Adults. 30 mg 3 times a day.

CONTRAINDICATIONS

Acute iritis, angle-closure glaucoma, uncontrolled asthma

INTERACTIONS

Drug

Amiodarone, diltiazem, erythromycin, fluoxetine, itraconazole, ketoconazole, paroxetine, quinidine, ritonavir, verapamil: May increase the effects of cevimeline.

Atropine, phenothiazines, tricyclic antidepressants: May decrease the effects of cevimeline.

Beta blockers: May increase the risk of conduction disturbances.

Herbal

None known.

Food

All foods: Decreases the absorption rate of cevimeline.

DIAGNOSTIC TEST EFFECTS

None known.

SIDE EFFECTS

Frequent (19%–11%)

Diaphoresis, headache, nausea, sinusitis, rhinitis, upper respiratory tract infection, diarrhea

Occasional (10%–3%)

Dyspepsia, abdominal pain, cough, UTI, vomiting, back pain, rash, dizziness, fatigue

Rare (2%–1%)

Skeletal pain, insomnia, hot flashes, excessive salivation, rigors, anxiety

SERIOUS REACTIONS

! Cevimeline use may result in decreased visual acuity, especially at night, and impaired depth perception.

NURSING CONSIDERATIONS

Baseline Assessment

- Determine if the patient has a history of acute iritis, angle-closure glaucoma, or uncontrolled asthma before beginning therapy.

Precautions

- Use cevimeline cautiously in patients with cardiovascular disease, CHF, chronic bronchitis, COPD, cholelithiasis, or a history of nephrolithiasis.

Administration and Handling

- Give cevimeline without regard to food.

Intervention and Evaluation

- Assess patients with a history of a respiratory disorder, such as asthma, for increased wheezing, coughing, or sputum production.
- Monitor patients with a cardiovascular disease for an increase in the frequency, duration, or severity of angina or changes in BP or heart rate.

Patient Teaching

- Advise the patient to use caution

while driving at night or performing hazardous duties in reduced lighting because cevimeline use may decrease visual acuity or impair depth perception.
• Encourage the patient to drink extra fluids to prevent dehydration.

neostigmine

nee-oh-**stig**-meen
(Prostigmin)
Do not confuse neostigmine with physostigmine.

CATEGORY AND SCHEDULE
Pregnancy Risk Category: C

MECHANISM OF ACTION
A cholinergic that prevents destruction of acetylcholine by inhibiting the enzyme acetylcholinesterase, thus enhancing impulse transmission across the myoneural junction. **Therapeutic Effect:** Improves intestinal and skeletal muscle tone; stimulates salivary and sweat gland secretions.

AVAILABILITY
Tablets: 15 mg.
Injection: 0.5 mg/ml, 1 mg/ml.

INDICATIONS AND DOSAGES
▸ **Myasthenia gravis**
PO
Adults, Elderly. Initially, 15–30 mg 3–4 times a day. Increase as necessary. Maintenance: 150 mg/day (range of 15–375 mg).
Children. 2 mg/kg/day or 60 mg/m^2/day divided q3–4h.
IV, IM, Subcutaneous
Adults. 0.5–2.5 mg as needed.
Children. 0.01–0.04 mg/kg q2–4h.

▸ **Diagnosis of myasthenia gravis**
IM
Adults, Elderly. 0.022 mg/kg. If cholinergic reaction occurs, discontinue tests and administer 0.4–0.6 mg or more atropine sulfate IV.
Children. 0.025–0.04 mg/kg preceded by atropine sulfate 0.011 mg/kg subcutaneously.

▸ **Prevention of postoperative urinary retention**
IM, Subcutaneous
Adults, Elderly. 0.25 mg q4–6h for 2–3 days.

▸ **Postoperative abdomonial distention and urine retention**
IM, Subcutaneous
Adults, Elderly. 0.5–1 mg. Catheterize patient if voiding does not occur within 1 hr. After voiding, administer 0.5 mg q3h for 5 injections.

▸ **Reversal of neuromuscular blockade**
IV
Adults, Elderly. 0.5–2.5 mg given slowly.
Children. 0.025–0.08 mg/kg/dose.
Infants. 0.025–0.1 mg/kg/dose.

CONTRAINDICATIONS
GI or GU obstruction, peritonitis

INTERACTIONS
Drug
Anticholinergics: Reverse or prevent the effects of neostigmine.
Cholinesterase inhibitors: May increase the risk of toxicity.
Neuromuscular blockers: Antagonizes the effects of these drugs.
Procainamide, quinidine: May antagonize the action of neostigmine.
Herbal
None known.
Food
None known.

DIAGNOSTIC TEST EFFECTS
None known.

IV INCOMPATIBILITIES
None known.

IV COMPATIBILITIES
Glycopyrrolate (Robinul), heparin, ondansetron (Zofran), potassium chloride, thiopental (Pentothal)

SIDE EFFECTS
Frequent
Muscarinic effects (diarrhea, diaphoresis, increased salivation, nausea, vomiting, abdominal cramps or pain)
Occasional
Muscarinic effects (urinary urgency or frequency, increased bronchial secretions, miosis, lacrimation)

SERIOUS REACTIONS
! Overdose produces a cholinergic crisis manifested as abdominal discomfort or cramps, nausea, vomiting, diarrhea, flushing, facial warmth, excessive salivation, diaphoresis, lacrimation, pallor, bradycardia or tachycardia, hypotension, bronchospasm, urinary urgency, blurred vision, miosis, and fasciculation (involuntary muscular contractions visible under the skin).

NURSING CONSIDERATIONS
Baseline Assessment
- Before beginning therapy, determine if the patient has reduced GI motility or megacolon because these patients should not receive large doses.

Precautions
- Use neostigmine cautiously in patients with arrhythmias, asthma, bradycardia, epilepsy, hyperthyroidism, peptic ulcer disease, or recent coronary occlusion.

Administration and Handling
◀ALERT▶ Discontinue all anticholinesterase therapy at least 8 hours before testing, as prescribed. Plan to give 0.011 mg/kg atropine sulfate IV simultaneously with neostigmine or IM 30 minutes before administering neostigmine to prevent adverse effects.
- Expect to give larger doses when the patient is most tired.

Intervention and Evaluation
- Monitor the patient's muscle strength and vital signs.
- Monitor the patient for evidence of a therapeutic response to the drug, including decreased fatigue, improved chewing and swallowing, and increased muscle strength.
- Monitor the patient's fluid intake and output.
- Palpate the patient's bladder for signs of distention.

Patient Teaching
- Instruct the patient to notify the physician if he or she experiences diarrhea, difficulty breathing, increased salivation, irregular heartbeat, muscle weakness, nausea and vomiting, severe abdominal pain, or increased sweating.
- Tell the patient to keep a log of his or her energy level and muscle strength to help guide drug dosing.

physostigmine
fi-zoe-**stig**-meen
(Antilirium)
Do not confuse physostigmine with Prostigmin or pyridostigmine.

CATEGORY AND SCHEDULE
Pregnancy Risk Category: C

MECHANISM OF ACTION
A cholinergic that inhibits destruction of acetylcholine by enzyme acetylcholinesterase, thus enhancing impulse transmission across the

myoneural junction. **Therapeutic Effect:** Improves skeletal muscle tone, stimulates salivary and sweat gland secretions.

AVAILABILITY

Injection: 1 mg/ml.

INDICATIONS AND DOSAGES

▸ To reverse CNS effects of anticholinergic drugs and tricyclic antidepressants

IV, IM

Adults, Elderly. Initially, 0.5–2 mg. If no response, repeat q20min until response or adverse cholinergic effects occur. If initial response occurs, may give additional doses of 1–4 mg q30–60min as life-threatening signs, such as arrhythmias, seizures, and deep coma, recur.
Children. 0.01–0.03 mg/kg. May give additional doses q5–10min until response or adverse cholinergic effects occur or total dose of 2 mg given.

OFF-LABEL USES

Treatment of hereditary ataxia

CONTRAINDICATIONS

Active uveal inflammation, angle-closure glaucoma before iridectomy, asthma, cardiovascular disease, concurrent use of ganglionic-blocking agents, diabetes, gangrene, glaucoma associated with iridocyclitis, hypersensitivity to cholinesterase inhibitors or their components, mechanical obstruction of intestinal or urogenital tract, vagotonic state

INTERACTIONS

Drug

Cholinesterase agents, including bethanechol and carbachol: May increase the effects of these drugs.
Succinylcholine: May prolong the action of succinylcholine.

Herbal

None known.

Food

None known.

DIAGNOSTIC TEST EFFECTS

None known.

SIDE EFFECTS

Expected

Miosis, increased GI and skeletal muscle tone, bradycardia

Occasional

Marked drop in BP (hypertensive patients)

Rare

Allergic reaction

SERIOUS REACTIONS

! Parenteral overdose produces a cholinergic crisis manifested as abdominal discomfort or cramps, nausea, vomiting, diarrhea, flushing, facial warmth, excessive salivation, diaphoresis, urinary urgency, and blurred vision. If overdose occurs, stop all anticholinergic drugs and immediately administer 0.6–1.2 mg atropine sulfate IM or IV for adults, or 0.01 mg/kg for infants and children younger than 12 years.

NURSING CONSIDERATIONS

Baseline Assessment

- Before beginning therapy, establish the patient's baseline BP and heart rate and rhythm. Monitor the patient before and regularly during therapy for hypotension and bradycardia.

Precautions

- Use physostigmine cautiously in patients with bradycardia, bronchial asthma, epilepsy, GI disturbances, hypotension, parkinsonism, peptic ulcer disease, or disorders that may be adversely affected by drug's vagotonic effects and in those who have recently had an MI.

Administration and Handling

IV

- For adults, administer at a rate not exceeding 1 mg/minute.
- For children, administer no more than 0.02 mg/kg over at least 1 minute.

Intervention and Evaluation

- Assess the patient's vital signs immediately before and every 15 to 30 minutes after physostigmine administration.
- Monitor the patient for cholinergic reactions, such as abdominal pain, dyspnea, hypotension, arrhythmias, muscle weakness, and diaphoresis, after drug administration.

Patient Teaching

- Tell the patient that the drug's adverse effects usually subside after the first few days of therapy.
- Caution the patient to avoid driving at night and activities requiring visual acuity in dim light during physostigmine therapy.

pilocarpine hydrochloride

pye-loe-**kar**-peen

(Isopto Carpine[AUS], Ocusert Pilo-20[AUS], Ocusert Pilo-40[AUS], Pilopt Eye Drops[AUS], P.V. Carpine Liquifilm Ophthalmic Solution[AUS], Salagen)

CATEGORY AND SCHEDULE

Pregnancy Risk Category: C

MECHANISM OF ACTION

A cholinergic that increases exocrine gland secretions by stimulating cholinergic receptors. **Therapeutic Effect:** Improves symptoms of dry mouth in patients with salivary gland hypofunction.

PHARMACOKINETICS

Route	Onset	Peak	Duration
PO	20 min	1 hr	3–5 hr

Absorption decreased if taken with a high-fat meal. Inactivation of pilocarpine thought to occur at neuronal synapses and probably in plasma. Excreted in urine. ***Half-life:*** 4–12 hr.

AVAILABILITY

Tablets: 5 mg.

INDICATIONS AND DOSAGES

▸ **Dry mouth associated with radiation treatment for head and neck cancer**

PO

Adults, Elderly. 5 mg three times a day. Range: 15–30 mg/day. Maximum: 2 tablets/dose.

▸ **Dry mouth associated with Sjögren's syndrome**

PO

Adults, Elderly. 5 mg four times a day. Range: 20–40 mg/day.

▸ **Dosage in hepatic impairment**

Dosage decreased to 5 mg twice a day for adults and elderly with hepatic impairment.

CONTRAINDICATIONS

Conditions in which miosis is undesirable, such as acute iritis and angle-closure glaucoma; uncontrolled asthma

INTERACTIONS

Drug

Anticholinergics: May antagonize the effects of anticholinergics.

Beta blockers: May produce conduction disturbances.

Herbal

None known.

Food
High-fat meals: May decrease the absorption rate of pilocarpine.

DIAGNOSTIC TEST EFFECTS
None known.

SIDE EFFECTS
Frequent (29%)
Diaphoresis
Occasional (11%–05%)
Headache, dizziness, urinary frequency, flushing, dyspepsia, nausea, asthenia, lacrimation, visual disturbances
Rare (less than 4%)
Diarrhea, abdominal pain, peripheral edema, chills

SERIOUS REACTIONS
! Patients with diaphoresis who don't drink enough fluids may develop dehydration.

NURSING CONSIDERATIONS
Baseline Assessment
- Assess the patient's oral mucosa for evidence of dryness.

Lifespan Considerations
- Pilocarpine use may impair reproductive function.
- The safety and efficacy of pilocarpine have not been established in children.
- Elderly patients have an increased incidence of diarrhea, dizziness, and urinary frequency.

Precautions
- Use pilocarpine cautiously in patients with hepatic impairment, pulmonary disease, or significant cardiovascular disease.

Administration and Handling
PO
- Give pilocarpine without regard to food.

Intervention and Evaluation
- Assess the patient's pattern of daily bowel activity and stool consistency.
- Monitor the patient for signs of dehydration, such as decreased skin turgor, and dizziness.
- Monitor the patient's urinary frequency.

Patient Teaching
- Instruct the patient to drink plenty of fluids.
- Inform the patient that he or she may experience visual changes, especially at night.
- Warn the patient to avoid tasks that require mental alertness or motor skills until his or her response to the drug has been established.

pyridostigmine bromide
peer-id-oh-**stig**-meen
(Mestinon, Mestinon SR [CAN], Mestinon Timespan)
Do not confuse pyridostigmine with physostigmine, or Mesitonin with Mesantoin or Metatensin.

CATEGORY AND SCHEDULE
Pregnancy Risk Category: C

MECHANISM OF ACTION
A cholinergic that prevents destruction of acetylcholine by inhibiting the enzyme acetylcholinesterase, thus enhancing impulse transmission across the myoneural junction.
Therapeutic Effect: Produces miosis; increases tone of intestinal, skeletal muscle tone; stimulates salivary and sweat gland secretions.

AVAILABILITY
Syrup (Mestinon): 60 mg/5 ml.
Tablets (Mestinon): 60 mg.

Tablets (Extended-Release [Mestinon Timespan]): 180 mg.
Injection (Mestinon): 5 mg/ml.

INDICATIONS AND DOSAGES

▸ Myasthenia gravis

PO

Adults, Elderly. Initially, 60 mg 3 times a day. Dosage increased at 48 hr intervals. Maintenance: 60 mg–1.5 g a day.

PO (Extended-Release)

Adults, Elderly. 180–540 mg once or twice a day with at least a 6-hr interval between doses.

IV, IM

Adults, Elderly. 2 mg q2–3h.
Children, Neonates. 0.05–0.15 mg/kg/dose. Maximum single dose: 10 mg.

▸ Reversal of nondepolarizing neuromuscular blockade

IV

Adults, Elderly. 10–20 mg with, or shortly after, 0.6–1.2 mg atropine sulfate or 0.3–0.6 mg glycopyrrolate.
Children. 0.1–0.25 mg/kg/dose preceded by atropine or glycopyrrolate.

CONTRAINDICATIONS

Mechanical GI or urinary tract obstruction

INTERACTIONS

Drug

Anticholinergics: Prevent or reverse the effects of pyridostigmine.
Cholinesterase inhibitors: May increase the risk of toxicity.
Neuromuscular blockers: Antagonizes the effects of these drugs.
Procainamide, quinidine: May antagonize the action of pyridostigmine.

Herbal

None known.

Food

None known.

DIAGNOSTIC TEST EFFECTS

None known.

IV INCOMPATIBILITIES

Don't mix pyridostigmine with any other medications.

SIDE EFFECTS

Frequent

Miosis, increased GI and skeletal muscle tone, bradycardia, constriction of bronchi and ureters, diaphoresis, increased salivation

Occasional

Headache, rash, temporary decrease in diastolic BP with mild reflex tachycardia, short periods of atrial fibrillation (in hyperthyroid patients), marked drop in BP (in hypertensive patients)

SERIOUS REACTIONS

! Overdose may produce a cholinergic crisis, manifested as increasingly severe muscle weakness that appears first in muscles involving chewing and swallowing and is followed by muscle weakness of the shoulder girdle and upper extremities, respiratory muscle paralysis, and pelvis girdle and leg muscle paralysis. If overdose occurs, stop all cholinergic drugs and immediately administer 1–4 mg atropine sulfate IV for adults or 0.01 mg/kg for infants and children younger than 12 years.

NURSING CONSIDERATIONS

Baseline Assessment

- Assess the patient's muscle strength before and after drug administration.
- Before beginning therapy, determine if the patient has reduced GI motility or megacolon because these patients should not receive large doses.

Precautions

• Use pyridostigmine cautiously in patients with bradycardia, bronchial asthma, cardiac arrhythmias, epilepsy, hyperthyroidism, peptic ulcer disease, recent coronary occlusion, or vagotonia.

Administration and Handling

◀ **ALERT** ▶ Drug dosage and frequency of administration are dependent on the patient's daily clinical response, including exacerbations, physical and emotional stress, and remissions.

PO

• Crush tablets as needed.
• Give larger doses at times of increased fatigue, for example 30 to 45 minutes before meals for patients with difficulty chewing.

IV, IM

• Give large parenteral doses concurrently with 0.6 to 1.2 mg atropine sulfate IV, as prescribed, to minimize side effects.

Intervention and Evaluation

• Monitor the patient's respirations closely when dosage is increased.
• Be alert for signs of a cholinergic reaction, and for bradycardia in the patient with myasthenic crisis.
• Monitor the patient for evidence of a therapeutic response to the drug, such as decreased fatigue, improved chewing and swallowing, and increased muscle strength.
• Have tissues available at the patient's bedside.

Patient Teaching

• Inform the patient that he or she may crush regular tablets if needed and may break extended-release tablets but should not chew or crush them.
• Warn the patient to notify the physician if he or she experiences diarrhea, difficulty breathing, profuse salivation or sweating, irregular heartbeat, muscle weakness, severe abdominal pain, or nausea and vomiting.
• Tell the patient to keep a log of his or her energy level and muscle strength to help guide drug dosing.

79 Diuretics

amiloride hydrochloride
bumetanide
chlorthalidone
furosemide
hydrochlorothiazide
indapamide
mannitol
metolazone
spironolactone
torsemide
triamterene

Uses: The several subclasses of diuretics have slightly different indications. *Thiazide diuretics,* such as hydrochlorothiazide and metolazone, are used to manage edema caused by various disorders, including CHF and hepatic cirrhosis. They're also used alone or with other antihypertensives to control hypertension. *Loop diuretics,* such as bumetanide and furosemide, are prescribed to manage edema caused by CHF, hepatic cirrhosis, and renal disease. Furosemide is also used to treat hypertension, either alone or with other antihypertensives. *Potassium-sparing diuretics,* such as amiloride and spironolactone, are used as adjuncts to thiazide or loop diuretics in treating CHF and hypertension. *Osmotic diuretics,* such as mannitol, are used to prevent and treat the oliguric phase of acute renal failure, to reduce increased intracranial pressure, and to promote the urinary excretion of certain toxic substances.

Action: Diuretics act to increase the excretion of water, sodium, and other electrolytes by the kidneys. Although their exact mechanism in hypertension is unknown, these agents may act by decreasing plasma volume or peripheral vascular resistance. They're subclassified based on their mechanism and site of action. *Thiazide diuretics* act at the cortical diluting segment of the nephron, blocking sodium, chloride, and water reabsorption and promoting the excretion of sodium, chloride, potassium, and water. *Loop diuretics* act primarily at the thick ascending limb of the loop of Henle to inhibit sodium, chloride, and water absorption. Among the *potassium-sparing diuretics,* amiloride and triamterene act on the distal nephron, decreasing sodium reuptake and reducing potassium excretion; spironolactone blocks aldosterone from acting on the distal nephron, which causes potassium retention and sodium excretion. *Osmotic diuretics* work in the proximal convoluted tubule by increasing the osmotic pressure of the glomerular filtrate and inhibiting the passive reabsorption of water, sodium, and chloride. (See the illustration *Sites of Action: Diuretics,* page 1384.)

COMBINATION PRODUCTS

ACCURETIC: hydrochlorothiazide/quinapril (an ACE inhibitor) 12.5 mg/10 mg; 12.5 mg/20 mg; 25 mg/20 mg.
ALDACTAZIDE: hydrochlorothiazide/spironolactone 25 mg/25 mg; 50 mg/50 mg.
ALDORIL: hydrochlorothiazide/methyldopa (an antihypertensive) 15 mg/250 mg; 25 mg/250 mg; 30 mg/500 mg; 50 mg/500 mg.
APRESAZIDE: hydrochlorothiazide/hydralazine (a vasodilator) 25 mg/25 mg; 50 mg/50 mg; 50 mg/100 mg.
ATACAND HCT: hydrochlorothiazide/candesartan (an angiotensin II receptor antagonist) 12.5 mg/16 mg; 12.5 mg/32 mg.
AVALIDE: hydrochlorothiazide/irbesartan (an angiotensin II receptor antagonist) 12.5 mg/150 mg; 12.5 mg/300 mg.
BENICAR HCT: hydrochlorothiazide/olmesartan (an angiotensin II receptor antagonist) 12.5 mg/20 mg; 12.5 mg/40 mg; 25 mg/40 mg.
CAPOZIDE: hydrochlorothiazide/captopril (an ACE inhibitor) 15 mg/25 mg; 15 mg/50 mg; 25 mg/25 mg; 25 mg/50 mg.
COMBIPRES: chlorthalidone/clonidine (an antihypertensive) 15 mg/0.1 mg; 15 mg/0.2 mg; 15 mg/0.3 mg.
DIOVAN HCT: hydrochlorothiazide/valsartan (an angiotensin II receptor antagonist) 12.5 mg/80 mg; 12.5 mg/160 mg.
DYAZIDE: hydrochlorothiazide/triamterene 25 mg/37.5 mg; 25 mg/50 mg; 50 mg/75 mg.
HYZAAR: hydrochlorothiazide/losartan (an angiotensin II receptor antagonist) 12.5 mg/50 mg; 25 mg/100 mg.
INDERIDE: hydrochlorothiazide/propranolol (a beta blocker) 25 mg/40 mg; 25 mg/80 mg; 50 mg/80 mg; 50 mg/120 mg; 50 mg/160 mg.
INDERIDE LA: hydrochlorothiazide/propranolol (a beta blocker) 50 mg/80 mg; 50 mg/120 mg; 50 mg/160 mg.
LOPRESSOR HCT: hydrochlorothiazide/metoprolol (a beta-blocker) 25 mg/50 mg; 25 mg/100 mg; 50 mg/100 mg.
LOTENSIN HCT: hydrochlorothiazide/benazepril (an ACE inhibitor) 6.25 mg/5 mg; 12.5 mg/10 mg; 12.5 mg/20 mg; 25 mg/20 mg.
MAXZIDE: hydrochlorothiazide/triamterene 25 mg/37.5 mg; 25 mg/50 mg; 50 mg/75 mg.
MICARDIS HCT: hydrochlorothiazide/telmisartan (an angiotensin II receptor antagonist) 12.5 mg/40 mg; 12.5 mg/80 mg.
MODURETIC: hydrochlorothiazide/amiloride 50 mg/5 mg.
NORMOZIDE: hydrochlorothiazide/labetalol (a beta blocker) 25 mg/100 mg; 25 mg/300 mg.
PRINZIDE: hydrochlorothiazide/lisinopril (an ACE inhibitor) 12.5 mg/10 mg; 12.5 mg/20 mg; 25 mg/20 mg.
TENORETIC: chlorthalidone/atenolol (a beta blocker) 25 mg/50 mg; 25 mg/100 mg.
TEVETEN HCT: hydrochlorothiazide/eprosartan (an angiotensin II receptor antagonist) 12.5 mg/600 mg; 25 mg/600 mg.
TIMOLIDE: hydrochlorothiazide/timolol (a beta-blocker) 25 mg/10 mg.
UNIRETIC: hydrochlorothiazide/moexipril (an ACE inhibitor) 12.5 mg/7.5 mg; 25 mg/15 mg.
VASERETIC: hydrochlorothiazide/enalapril (an ACE inhibitor) 12.5 mg/5 mg; 25 mg/10 mg.
ZESTORETIC: hydrochlorothiazide/lisinopril (an ACE inhibitor) 12.5 mg/10 mg; 12.5 mg/20 mg; 25 mg/20 mg.
ZIAC: hydrochlorothiazide/bisoprolol

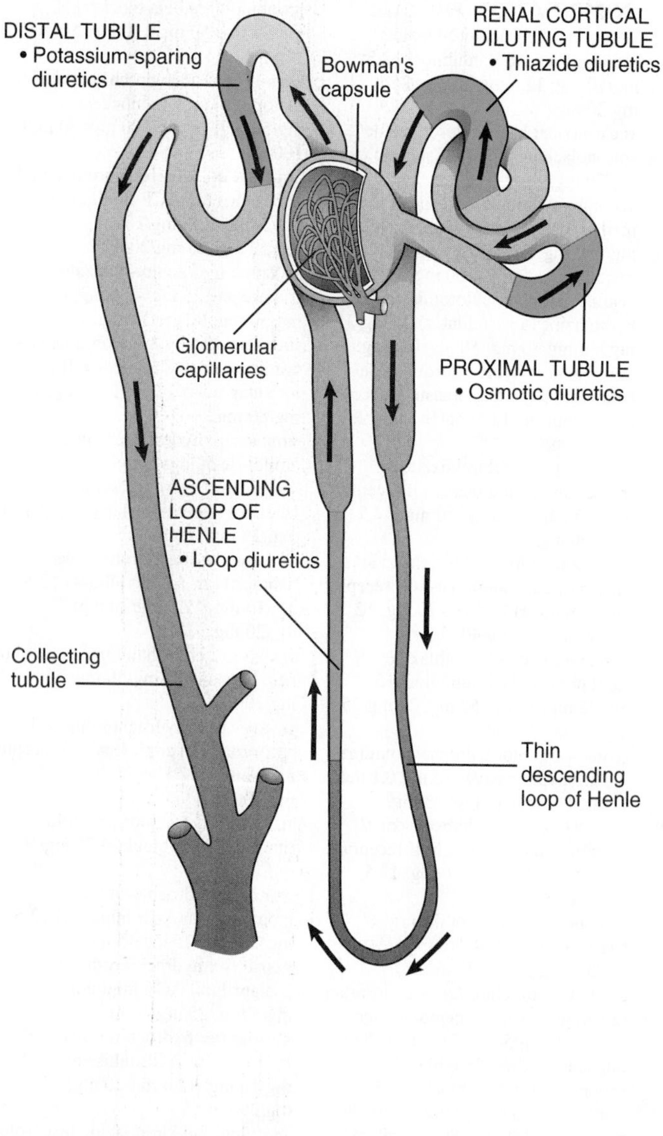
DISTAL TUBULE
• Potassium-sparing diuretics
Bowman's capsule
RENAL CORTICAL DILUTING TUBULE
• Thiazide diuretics
Glomerular capillaries
PROXIMAL TUBULE
• Osmotic diuretics
ASCENDING LOOP OF HENLE
• Loop diuretics
Collecting tubule
Thin descending loop of Henle

Sites of Action: Diuretics

Diuretics act primarily to increase water and sodium excretion by the kidneys, thereby increasing urine output. In the process, chloride, potassium, and other electrolytes may also be excreted. Most diuretics act by blocking sodium, water, and chloride reabsorption by peritubular capillaries in the nephrons. As a result, water and electrolytes remain in the convoluted tubules to be excreted as urine. The increased water and electrolyte excretion reduces blood volume—and ultimately blood pressure.

Diuretics belong to four major subclasses: thiazide, loop, potassium-sparing, and osmotic diuretics. Although similar in action, drugs in each subclass act at different sites along the nephron. Also, because the solute concentration decreases as the filtrate passes through the nephron's tubules, drugs that act earlier in the process can block more water and electrolytes, promoting greater diuresis.

Thiazide diuretics, such as hydrochlorothiazide, act in the early portion of the distal convoluted tubule, called the cortical diluting segment. These drugs block sodium, chloride, and water reabsorption and promote their excretion along with potassium.

Loop diuretics, such as furosemide, act primarily in the thick ascending limb of the loop of Henle, blocking sodium, water, and chloride reabsorption. Then these substances are excreted along with potassium.

Potassium-sparing diuretics, such as spironolactone, act in the late portion of the distal convoluted tubule and collecting tubule. Here, they inhibit the action of aldosterone, leading to sodium excretion and potassium retention. Although triamterene and amiloride, two other potassium-sparing diuretics, act at the same site, they don't affect aldosterone. Instead, these drugs directly block the exchange of sodium and potassium, leading to decreased sodium reabsorption and decreased potassium excretion.

Osmotic diuretics, such as mannitol, work in the proximal convoluted tubule. As their name implies, these diuretics increase the osmotic pressure of the glomerular filtrate, inhibiting the passive reabsorption of water, sodium, and chloride.

(a beta blocker) 6.25 mg/5 mg; 6.25 mg/10 mg.

amiloride hydrochloride

a-**mill**-oh-ride

(Kaluril[AUS], Midamor)

Do not confuse amiloride with amiodarone or amlodipine.

CATEGORY AND SCHEDULE

Pregnancy Risk Category: B (D if used in pregnancy-induced hypertension)

MECHANISM OF ACTION

A guanidine derivative that acts as a potassium-sparing diuretic, antihypertensive, and antihypokalemic by directly interfering with sodium reabsorption in the distal tubule. **Therapeutic Effect:** Increases sodium and water excretion and decreases potassium excretion.

PHARMACOKINETICS

Route	Onset	Peak	Duration
PO	2 hr	6–10 hr	24 hr

Incompletely absorbed from the GI tract. Protein binding: Minimal. Primarily excreted in urine; partially eliminated in feces. ***Half-life***: 6–9 hr.

AVAILABILITY

Tablets: 5 mg.

INDICATIONS AND DOSAGES

▸ To counteract potassium loss induced by other diuretics

PO

Adults, Children weighing more than 20 kg. 5–10 mg/day up to 20 mg.
Elderly. Initially, 5 mg/day or every other day.
Children weighing 6–20 kg. 0.625 mg/kg/day. Maximum: 10 mg/day.

▸ Dosage in renal impairment

Creatinine Clearance	Dosage
10–50 ml/min	50% of normal
less than 10 ml/min	avoid use

OFF-LABEL USES

Treatment of edema associated with CHF, liver cirrhosis, and nephrotic syndrome; treatment of hypertension; reduces lithium-induced polyuria, slows pulmonary function reduction in cystic fibrosis

CONTRAINDICATIONS

Acute or chronic renal insufficiency, anuria, diabetic nephropathy, patients on other potassium-sparing diuretics, serum potassium greater than 5.5 mEq/L

INTERACTIONS

Drug

ACE inhibitors, including captopril, and potassium-containing diuretics: May increase potassium levels.
Anticoagulants, including heparin: May decrease effect of anticoagulants, including heparin.
Lithium: May decrease lithium clearance and increase risk of amiloride toxicity.
NSAIDs: May decrease antihypertensive effect.

Herbal

None known.

Food

None known.

DIAGNOSTIC TEST EFFECTS

May increase BUN, calcium excretion, and glucose, serum creatinine, serum magnesium, serum potassium, and uric acid levels. May decrease serum sodium levels.

SIDE EFFECTS

Frequent (8%–3%)
Headache, nausea, diarrhea, vomiting, decreased appetite
Occasional (3%–1%)
Dizziness, constipation, abdominal pain, weakness, fatigue, cough, impotence
Rare (less than 1%)
Tremors, vertigo, confusion, nervousness, insomnia, thirst, dry mouth, heartburn, shortness of breath, increased urination, hypotension, rash

SERIOUS REACTIONS

! Severe hyperkalemia may produce irritability, anxiety, a feeling of heaviness in the legs, paresthesia of hands, face, and lips, hypotension, bradycardia, tented T waves, widening of QRS, and ST depression.

NURSING CONSIDERATIONS

Baseline Assessment

- As appropriate, assess the patient's serum electrolyte levels, especially for low potassium.
- Monitor the patient's renal function tests and serum hepatic enzyme levels.
- Determine the location and extent of edema and assess the patient's skin turgor. Note the skin temperature and moisture level.

• Check the patient's mucous membranes to determine his or her hydration status.
• Assess the patient's muscle strength and mental status.
• Determine the patient's baseline weight.
• Initiate strict intake and output procedures and document.
• Obtain a baseline 12-lead EKG.
• Assess the patient's pulse rate and rhythm.

Lifespan Considerations
• Be aware that it is unknown if amiloride crosses the placenta or is distributed in breast milk.
• There are no age-related precautions noted in children.
• In the elderly, age-related decreased renal function increases the risk of hyperkalemia and may require caution.

Precautions
• Use cautiously in patients with a BUN greater than 30 mg/dl or serum creatinine greater than 1.5 mg/dl.
• Use cautiously in the debilitated and elderly.
• Use cautiously in those with cardiopulmonary disease, diabetes mellitus, or liver insufficiency.

Administration and Handling
PO
• Give with food to avoid GI distress.

Intervention and Evaluation
• Expect to monitor the patient's BP, vital signs, electrolytes, intake and output, and weight. Note the extent of diuresis.
• Watch for changes from the initial assessment. Hyperkalemia may result in cardiac arrhythmias, a change in mental status, muscle cramps, muscle strength changes, or tremor.
• Monitor the patient's serum potassium level, particularly during initial therapy.
• Weigh the patient each day.
• Assess lung sounds for rales, rhonchi, or wheezing.

Patient Teaching
• Advise the patient to expect an increase in the volume and frequency of urination.
• Explain to the patient that the therapeutic effect of the drug takes several days to begin and can last for several days after the drug is discontinued.
• Warn the patient that a high-potassium diet and potassium supplements can be dangerous, especially if he or she has liver or kidney problems. Caution the patient to avoid foods high in potassium such as apricots, bananas, legumes, meat, orange juice, raisins, whole grains, including cereals, and white and sweet potatoes.
• Instruct the patient to notify the physician if he or she experiences the signs and symptoms of hyperkalemia: confusion, difficulty breathing, irregular heartbeat, nervousness, numbness of the hands, feet, or lips, unusual tiredness, and weakness in the legs.

bumetanide
byoo-**met**-a-nide
(Bumex, Burinex[CAN])

CATEGORY AND SCHEDULE
Pregnancy Risk Category: C (D if used in pregnancy-induced hypertension)

MECHANISM OF ACTION
A loop diuretic that enhances excretion of sodium, chloride, and to lesser degree, potassium, by direct action at the ascending limb of the loop of Henle and in the proximal

tubule. **Therapeutic Effect:** Produces diuresis.

PHARMACOKINETICS

Route	Onset	Peak	Duration
PO	30–60 min	60–120 min	4–6 hr
IV	Rapid	15–30 min	2–3 hr
IM	40 min	60–120 min	4–6 hr

Completely absorbed from the GI tract (absorption decreased in CHF and nephrotic syndrome). Protein binding: 94%–96%. Partially metabolized in the liver. Primarily excreted in urine. Not removed by hemodialysis. ***Half-life:*** 1–1.5 hr.

AVAILABILITY

Tablets: 0.5 mg, 1 mg, 2 mg.
Injection: 0.25 mg/ml.

INDICATIONS AND DOSAGES

▸ **Edema**

PO

Adults, Children older than 18 yr. 0.5–2 mg as a single dose in the morning. May repeat at q4–5hr.
Elderly. 0.5 mg/day, increased as needed.

IV, IM

Adults, Elderly. 0.5–2 mg/dose; may repeat in 2–3 hr. Or 0.5–1 mg/hr by continuous IV infusion.

▸ **Hypertension**

PO

Adults, Elderly. Initially, 0.5 mg/day. Range: 1–4 mg/day. Maximum: 5 mg/day. Larger doses may be given 2–3 doses/day.

▸ **Usual pediatric dosage**

PO, IV, IM

Children. 0.015–0.1 mg/kg/dose q6–24h.

OFF-LABEL USES

Treatment of hypercalcemia, hypertension

CONTRAINDICATIONS

Anuria, hepatic coma, severe electrolyte depletion

INTERACTIONS

Drug

Amphotericin B, nephrotoxic and ototoxic medications: May increase the risk of nephrotoxicity and ototoxicity.
Anticoagulants, heparin: May decrease the effects of these drugs.
Lithium: May increase the risk of lithium toxicity.
Other hypokalemia-causing medications: May increase the risk of hypokalemia.

Herbal

None known.

Food

None known.

DIAGNOSTIC TEST EFFECTS

May increase blood glucose, BUN, serum uric acid, and urinary phosphate levels. May decrease serum calcium, chloride, magnesium, potassium, and sodium levels.

IV INCOMPATIBILITIES

Midazolam (Versed)

IV COMPATIBILITIES

Aztreonam (Azactam), cefepime (Maxipime), diltiazem (Cardizem), dobutamine (Dobutrex), furosemide (Lasix), lorazepam (Ativan), milrinone (Primacor), morphine, piperacillin and tazobactam (Zosyn), propofol (Diprivan)

SIDE EFFECTS

Expected

Increased urinary frequency and urine volume

Frequent

Orthostatic hypotension, dizziness

Occasional

Blurred vision, diarrhea, headache,

anorexia, premature ejaculation, impotence, dyspepsia

Rare

Rash, urticaria, pruritus, asthenia, muscle cramps, nipple tenderness

SERIOUS REACTIONS

! Vigorous diuresis may lead to profound water and electrolyte depletion, resulting in hypokalemia, hyponatremia, dehydration, coma, and circulatory collapse.

! Ototoxicity—manifested as deafness, vertigo, or tinnitus—may occur, especially in patients with severe renal impairment and those taking other ototoxic drugs.

! Blood dyscrasias and acute hypotensive episodes have been reported.

NURSING CONSIDERATIONS

Baseline Assessment

• Check the patient's vital signs, especially BP for hypotension, before administering bumetanide.

• Assess the patient's baseline electrolyte levels, particularly for hypokalemia.

• Evaluate the patient for edema and determine the patient's hydration status.

Lifespan Considerations

• It is unknown if bumetanide is distributed in breast milk.

• The safety and efficacy of bumetanide have not been established in children.

• Elderly patients are at increased risk for circulatory collapse or thromboembolic episodes and may be more sensitive to the drug's hypotensive and electrolyte effects.

• Age-related renal impairment may require reduced dosage or an extended dosage interval in the elderly.

Precautions

• Use bumetanide cautiously in elderly and debilitated patients and patients with diabetes mellitus, hypersensitivity to sulfonamides, and hepatic or renal impairment.

Administration and Handling

PO

• Give bumetanide with food to avoid GI upset, preferably with breakfast to help prevent nocturia.

IV

• Store vials at room temperature.

• Bumetanide is compatible with D_5W, 0.9% NaCl, and lactated Ringer's solution, but it may also be given undiluted. The solution remains stable for 24 hours if diluted.

• Administer the drug by IV push over 1 to 2 minutes. Bumetanide may also be given as a continuous infusion.

Intervention and Evaluation

• Continue to monitor the patient's BP, electrolyte levels, fluid intake and output, vital signs, and weight.

• Note the extent of diuresis.

• Monitor the patient for electrolyte disturbances. Hypokalemia may result in arrhythmias, altered mental status, muscle cramps, asthenia, and tremor. Hyponatremia may result in cold and clammy skin, confusion, and thirst.

Patient Teaching

• Advise the patient to take bumetanide with food to avoid GI distress.

• Tell the patient to expect an increase in the frequency and volume of urination.

• Inform the patient that hearing abnormalities, such as a sense of fullness or ringing in ears, may occur.

• Encourage the patient to consume foods high in potassium, including apricots, bananas, orange juice, raisins, potatoes, legumes, meat, and whole grains (including cereals).

• Instruct the patient to rise slowly from a sitting or lying position.

chlorthalidone

klor-**thal**-i-doan
(Apo-Chlorthalidone[CAN], Hygroton[AUS], Thalitone)

CATEGORY AND SCHEDULE

Pregnancy Risk Category: B (D if used in pregnancy-induced hypertension)

MECHANISM OF ACTION

A thiazide diuretic that blocks reabsorption of sodium, potassium, and water at the distal convoluted tubule; also decreases plasma and extracellular fluid volume and peripheral vascular resistance. **Therapeutic Effect:** Produces diuresis; lowers BP.

PHARMACOKINETICS

Route	Onset	Peak	Duration
PO (diuretic)	2 hr	2–6 hr	Up to 36 hr

Rapidly absorbed from the GI tract. Excreted unchanged in urine. ***Half-life:*** 35–50 hr. Onset of antihypertensive effect: 3–4 days; optimal therapeutic effect: 3–4 wk.

AVAILABILITY

Tablets: 15 mg, 25 mg, 50 mg, 100 mg.

INDICATIONS AND DOSAGES

▸ **Hypertension, edema**

PO

Adults. 25–100 mg/day or 100 mg 3 times a week.

Elderly. Initially, 12.5–25 mg/day or every other day.

CONTRAINDICATIONS

Anuria, history of hypersensitivity to sulfonamides or thiazide diuretics, renal decompensation

INTERACTIONS

Drug

Cholestyramine, colestipol: May decrease the absorption and effects of chlorthalidone.

Digoxin: May increase the risk of digoxin toxicity associated with chlorthalidone-induced hyperkalemia.

Lithium: May increase the risk of lithium toxicity.

Herbal

None known.

Food

None known.

DIAGNOSTIC TEST EFFECTS

May increase blood glucose and serum cholesterol, LDL, bilirubin, calcium, creatinine, uric acid, and triglyceride levels. May decrease urinary calcium and serum magnesium, potassium, and sodium levels.

SIDE EFFECTS

Expected

Increase in urinary frequency and urine volume

Frequent

Potassium depletion (rarely produces symptoms)

Occasional

Anorexia, impotence, diarrhea, orthostatic hypotension, GI disturbances, photosensitivity

Rare

Rash

SERIOUS REACTIONS

! Vigorous diuresis may lead to profound water and electrolyte depletion, resulting in hypokalemia, hyponatremia, and dehydration.

! Acute hypotensive episodes may occur.

! Hyperglycemia may occur during prolonged therapy.
! Overdose can lead to lethargy and coma without changes in electrolytes or hydration.

NURSING CONSIDERATIONS

Baseline Assessment

- Assess the patient's BP for hypotension before administering chlorthalidone.
- Assess the patient's baseline electrolyte levels, particularly serum potassium level.
- Examine the patient for edema, and assess mucous membranes and skin turgor to determine hydration status.
- Evaluate the patient's mental status and muscle strength.

Lifespan Considerations

- Chlorthalidone crosses the placenta and a small amount is distributed in breast milk. Breast-feeding is not recommended for patients taking this drug.
- No age-related precautions have been noted in children.
- The elderly may be more sensitive to the drug's hypotensive and electrolyte effects.

Precautions

- Use chlorthalidone cautiously in elderly or debilitated patients and in patients with diabetes mellitus, gout, hypercholesterolemia, hepatic impairment, or severe renal disease.

Administration and Handling

PO

- Give chlorthalidone with food or milk if GI upset occurs, preferably with breakfast to help prevent nocturia.
- Crush scored tablets if needed.

Intervention and Evaluation

- Monitor the patient for electrolyte disturbances. Hypokalemia may result in altered mental status, muscle cramps, nausea, and vomiting, tachycardia, asthenia, and tremor; hyponatremia may result in cold and clammy skin, confusion, and thirst.
- For patients receiving prolonged therapy, periodically check the blood glucose level, as ordered, for hyperglycemia.

Patient Teaching

- Tell the patient to expect an increase in the frequency and volume of urination.
- Advise the patient to take chlorthalidone with food to avoid GI distress, preferably early in the morning to avoid nighttime urination.
- Instruct the patient to change positions slowly to reduce the drug's hypotensive effect.
- Encourage the patient to eat foods high in potassium, such as apricots, bananas, raisins, orange juice, potatoes, legumes, meat, and whole grains (including cereals).
- Urge the patient to avoid prolonged exposure to sunlight.

furosemide

fur-**oh**-se-mide
(Apo-Furosemide[CAN], Frusehexal[AUS], Frusid[AUS], Lasix, Uremide[AUS], Urex-M[AUS])
Do not confuse Lasix with Lidex, Luvox, or Luxiq; or furosemide with Torsemide.

CATEGORY AND SCHEDULE

Pregnancy Risk Category: C (D if used in pregnancy-induced hypertension)

MECHANISM OF ACTION

A loop diuretic that enhances excretion of sodium, chloride, and potassium by direct action at the ascending limb of the loop of Henle. **Therapeutic Effect:** Produces diuresis and lower BP.

PHARMACOKINETICS

Route	Onset	Peak	Duration
PO	30–60 min	1–2 hr	6–8 hr
IV	5 min	20–60 min	2 hr
IM	30 min	N/A	N/A

Well absorbed from the GI tract. Protein binding: 91%–97%. Partially metabolized in the liver. Primarily excreted in urine (nonrenal clearance increases in severe renal impairment). Not removed by hemodialysis. ***Half-life:*** 30–90 min (increased in renal or hepatic impairment, and in neonates).

AVAILABILITY

Oral Solution: 10 mg/ml, 40 mg/5 ml.
Tablets: 20 mg, 40 mg, 80 mg.
Injection: 10 mg/ml.

INDICATIONS AND DOSAGES

▸ **Edema, hypertension**

PO

Adults, Elderly. Initially, 20–80 mg/dose; may increase by 20–40 mg/dose q6–8h. May titrate up to 600 mg/day in severe edematous states.
Children. 1–6 mg/kg/day in divided doses q6–12h.

IV, IM

Adults, Elderly. 20–40 mg/dose; may increase by 20 mg/dose q1–2h.
Children. 1–2 mg/kg/dose q6–12h.
Neonates. 1–2 mg/kg/dose q12–24h.

IV Infusion

Adults, Elderly. Bolus of 0.1 mg/kg, followed by infusion of 0.1 mg/kg/hr; may double q2h. Maximum: 0.4 mg/kg/hr.
Children. 0.05 mg/kg/hr; titrate to desired effect.

OFF-LABEL USES

Hypercalcemia

CONTRAINDICATIONS

Anuria, hepatic coma, severe electrolyte depletion

INTERACTIONS

Drug

Amphotericin B, nephrotoxic and ototoxic medications: May increase the risk of nephrotoxicity and ototoxicity.
Anticoagulants, heparin: May decrease the effects of these drugs.
Lithium: May increase the risk of lithium toxicity.
Other hypokalemia-causing medications: May increase the risk of hypokalemia.
Probenecid: May increase furosemide blood concentration.

Herbal

None known.

Food

None known.

DIAGNOSTIC TEST EFFECTS

May increase blood glucose, BUN, and serum uric acid levels. May decrease serum calcium, chloride, magnesium, potassium, and sodium levels.

IV INCOMPATIBILITIES

Ciprofloxacin (Cipro), diltiazem (Cardizem), dobutamine (Dobutrex), dopamine (Intropin), doxorubicin (Adriamycin), droperidol (Inapsine), esmolol (Brevibloc), famotidine (Pepcid), filgrastim (Neupogen), fluconazole (Diflucan), gemcitabine (Gemzar), gentamicin (Garamycin), idarubicin (Idamycin), labetalol (Trandate), meperidine (Demerol), metoclopramide (Reglan), midazolam (Versed), milrinone (Primacor), nicardipine (Cardene), ondansetron (Zofran), quinidine, thiopental (Pentothal), vecuronium (Norcuron), vinblastine (Velban), vincristine (Oncovin), vinorelbine (Navelbine)

IV COMPATIBILITIES

Aminophylline, amiodarone (Cordarone), bumetanide (Bumex), calcium gluconate, cimetidine (Tagamet), heparin, hydromorphone (Dilaudid), lidocaine, morphine, nitroglycerin, norepinephrine (Levophed), potassium chloride, propofol (Diprivan)

SIDE EFFECTS

Expected

Increased urinary frequency and urine volume

Frequent

Nausea, dyspepsia, abdominal cramps, diarrhea or constipation, electrolyte disturbances

Occasional

Dizziness, light-headedness, headache, blurred vision, paresthesia, photosensitivity, rash, fatigue, bladder spasm, restlessness, diaphoresis

Rare

Flank pain

SERIOUS REACTIONS

! Vigorous diuresis may lead to profound water loss and electrolyte depletion, resulting in hypokalemia, hyponatremia, and dehydration.

! Sudden volume depletion may result in increased risk of thrombosis, circulatory collapse, and sudden death.

! Acute hypotensive episodes may occur, sometimes several days after beginning therapy.

! Ototoxicity—manifested as deafness, vertigo, or tinnitus—may occur, especially in patients with severe renal impairment.

! Furosemide use can exacerbate diabetes mellitus, systemic lupus erythematosus, gout, and pancreatitis.

! Blood dyscrasias have been reported.

NURSING CONSIDERATIONS

Baseline Assessment

- Monitor the patient's vital signs, especially temperature and BP (for hypotension), before giving furosemide.
- Assess the patient's baseline electrolyte levels, particularly for hypokalemia.
- Examine the patient for edema, and assess mucous membranes and skin turgor to determine hydration status.
- Evaluate the patient's mental status and muscle strength.
- Obtain the patient's baseline weight.
- Begin monitoring the patient's fluid intake and output.

Lifespan Considerations

- Furosemide crosses the placenta and is distributed in breast milk.
- Neonates may require an increased dosage interval because the drug's half-life is increased in this age-group.
- The elderly may be more sensitive to the drug's electrolyte and hypotensive effects, and are at increased risk for circulatory collapse and thromboembolic effects.
- Age-related renal impairment may require a dosage adjustment in the elderly.

Precautions

- Use furosemide cautiously in patients with hepatic cirrhosis.

Administration and Handling

PO

- Give furosemide with food to avoid GI upset, preferably with breakfast to help prevent nocturia.

IV

- The solution normally appears

clear and colorless. Discard yellow solutions.
- Furosemide is compatible with D_5W, 0.9% NaCl, and lactated Ringer's solution, but it may also be given undiluted.
- Administer each 40 mg or less by IV push over 1 to 2 minutes. Don't exceed an administration rate of 4 mg/minute in patients with renal impairment.

IM
- Monitor the patient for temporary pain at the injection site.

Intervention and Evaluation
- Monitor the patient's BP, serum electrolyte levels, fluid intake and output, vital signs, and weight. Note the extent of diuresis.
- Monitor the patient for electrolyte disturbances. Hypokalemia may result in cardiac arrhythmias, altered mental status, muscle cramps, asthenia, and tremor. Hyponatremia may result in clammy and cold skin, confusion, and thirst.

Patient Teaching
- Tell the patient to expect an increase in the frequency and volume of urination.
- Advise the patient to notify the physician if he or she experiences hearing abnormalities (ringing, roaring, or sense of fullness in the ears) or signs of an electrolyte imbalance (irregular heartbeat, muscle cramps or weakness, tremor).
- Encourage the patient to eat foods high in potassium, including apricots, bananas, orange juice, potatoes, raisins, legumes, meat, and whole grains (such as cereals).
- Urge the patient to avoid overexposure sunlight and artificial lights, such as sun lamps.

hydrochlorothiazide

hye-droe-klor-oh-**thye**-a-zide
(Apo-Hydro[CAN], Aquazide H, Dichlotride[AUS], Dithiazide[AUS], Esidrix, HydroDIURIL, Microzide, Oretic)

CATEGORY AND SCHEDULE

Pregnancy Risk Category: B
(D if used in pregnancy-induced hypertension)

MECHANISM OF ACTION

A sulfonamide derivative that acts as a thiazide diuretic and antihypertensive. As a diuretic blocks reabsorption of water, sodium, and potassium at the cortical diluting segment of the distal tubule. As an antihypertensive reduces plasma, extracellular fluid volume, and peripheral vascular resistance by direct effect on blood vessels. **Therapeutic Effect:** Promotes diuresis; reduces BP.

PHARMACOKINETICS

Route	Onset	Peak	Duration
PO (diuretic)	2 hr	4–6 hr	6–12 hr

Variably absorbed from the GI tract. Primarily excreted unchanged in urine. Not removed by hemodialysis. ***Half-life:*** 5.6–14.8 hr.

AVAILABILITY

Capsules (Microzide): 12.5 mg.
Oral Solution: 50 mg/5 ml.
Tablets (Aquazide, Oretic): 25 mg, 50 mg, 100 mg.

INDICATIONS AND DOSAGES

▸ **Edema, hypertension**

PO

Adults. 12.5–100 mg/day. Maximum: 200 mg/day.

▸ **Usual pediatric dosage**

PO

Children 6 mo–12 yr. 2 mg/kg/day in 2 divided doses. Maximum: 200 mg/day.

Children younger than 6 mo. 2–4 mg/kg/day in 2 divided doses. Maximum: 37.5 mg/day.

OFF-LABEL USES

Treatment of diabetes insipidus, prevention of calcium-containing renal calculi

CONTRAINDICATIONS

Anuria, history of hypersensitivity to sulfonamides or thiazide diuretics, renal decompensation

INTERACTIONS

Drug

Cholestyramine, colestipol: May decrease the absorption and effects of hydrochlorothiazide.

Digoxin: May increase the risk of digoxin toxicity associated with hydrochlorothiazide-induced hypokalemia.

Lithium: May increase the risk of lithium toxicity.

Herbal

None known.

Food

None known.

DIAGNOSTIC TEST EFFECTS

May increase blood glucose and serum cholesterol, LDL, bilirubin, calcium, creatinine, uric acid, and triglyceride levels. May decrease urinary calcium, and serum magnesium, potassium, and sodium levels.

SIDE EFFECTS

Expected

Increase in urinary frequency and urine volume

Frequent

Potassium depletion

Occasional

Orthostatic hypotension, headache, GI disturbances, photosensitivity

SERIOUS REACTIONS

! Vigorous diuresis may lead to profound water and electrolyte depletion, resulting in hypokalemia, hyponatremia, and dehydration.

! Acute hypotensive episodes may occur.

! Hyperglycemia may occur during prolonged therapy.

! Pancreatitis, blood dyscrasias, pulmonary edema, allergic pneumonitis, and dermatologic reactions occur rarely.

! Overdose can lead to lethargy and coma without changes in electrolytes or hydration.

NURSING CONSIDERATIONS

Baseline Assessment

- Monitor the patient's vital signs, especially BP for hypotension before giving hydrochlorothiazide.
- Assess the patient's baseline electrolyte levels, particularly serum potassium.
- Evaluate the patient's mucous membranes and skin turgor, and check for peripheral edema to determine hydration status.
- Evaluate the patient's mental status and muscle strength.
- Record the patient's hydration status and temperature.
- Obtain the patient's baseline weight.
- Begin monitoring the patient's fluid intake and output.

Lifespan Considerations

- Hydrochlorothiazide crosses the placenta and a small amount is distributed in breast milk. Breast-feeding is not recommended for patients taking this drug.
- No age-related precautions have

been noted in children, except that jaundiced infants may be at risk for hyperbilirubinemia.
• The elderly may be more sensitive to the drug's electrolyte and hypotensive effects.
• Age-related renal impairment may require cautious use in the elderly.

Precautions
• Use hydrochlorothiazide cautiously in debilitated or elderly patients and in patients with diabetes mellitus, thyroid disorders, hepatic impairment, or severe renal disease.

Administration and Handling
PO
• Give hydrochlorothiazide with food or milk if GI upset occurs, preferably with breakfast to help prevent nocturia.

Intervention and Evaluation
• Continue to monitor the patient's BP, electrolyte levels, fluid intake and output, vital signs, and daily weight.
• Record the extent of patient diuresis.
• Monitor the patient for electrolyte disturbances. Hypokalemia may result in altered mental status, muscle cramps, nausea and vomiting, tachycardia, asthenia, and tremor. Hyponatremia may result in cold and clammy skin, confusion, and thirst.
• Be especially alert for signs of potassium depletion, such as cardiac arrhythmias, in patients taking digoxin.
• Give the patient potassium supplements, if ordered.
• Assess the patient for constipation, which may occur with exercise diuresis.

Patient Teaching
• Tell the patient to expect an increase in the frequency and volume of urination.
• Instruct the patient to change positions slowly and to let legs dangle momentarily before standing to reduce the drug's hypotensive effect.
• Encourage the patient to eat foods high in potassium, including apricots, bananas, raisins, orange juice, potatoes, legumes, meat, and whole grains (such as cereals).
• Urge the patient to avoid prolonged exposure to sunlight and ultraviolet rays because a photosensitivity reaction may occur.

indapamide

in-**dap**-a-mide
(Dapa-tabs[AUS], Indahexal[AUS], Insig[AUS], Lozide[CAN], Lozol, Natrilix[AUS], Natrilix SR[AUS])
Do not confuse indapamide with iodamide or iopamidol.

CATEGORY AND SCHEDULE

Pregnancy Risk Category: B (D if used in pregnancy-induced hypertension)

MECHANISM OF ACTION

A thiazide-like diuretic that blocks reabsorption of water, sodium, and potassium at the cortical diluting segment of the distal tubule; also reduces plasma and extracellular fluid volume and peripheral vascular resistance by direct effect on blood vessels. **Therapeutic Effect:** Promotes diuresis and reduces BP.

AVAILABILITY

Tablets: 1.25 mg, 2.5 mg.

INDICATIONS AND DOSAGES

▸ **Edema**
PO
Adults. Initially, 2.5 mg/day, may increase to 5 mg/day after 1 wk.

▸ **Hypertension**
PO
Adults, Elderly. Initially, 1.25 mg, may increase to 2.5 mg/day after 4 wk or 5 mg/day after additional 4 wk.

CONTRAINDICATIONS
None known.

INTERACTIONS
Drug
Digoxin: May increase the risk of digoxin toxicity associated with indapamide-induced hypokalemia.
Lithium: May increase the risk of lithium toxicity.
Herbal
None known.
Food
None known.

DIAGNOSTIC TEST EFFECTS
May increase plasma renin activity. May decrease protein-bound iodine and serum calcium, potassium, and sodium levels.

SIDE EFFECTS
Frequent (5% and greater)
Fatigue, numbness of extremities, tension, irritability, agitation, headache, dizziness, light-headedness, insomnia, muscle cramps
Occasional (less than 5%)
Tingling of extremities, urinary frequency, urticaria, rhinorrhea, flushing, weight loss, orthostatic hypotension, depression, blurred vision, nausea, vomiting, diarrhea or constipation, dry mouth, impotence, rash, pruritus

SERIOUS REACTIONS
! Vigorous diuresis may lead to profound water and electrolyte depletion, resulting in hypokalemia, hyponatremia, and dehydration.
! Acute hypotensive episodes may occur.
! Hyperglycemia may occur during prolonged therapy.
! Pancreatitis, blood dyscrasias, pulmonary edema, allergic pneumonitis, and dermatologic reactions occur rarely.
! Overdose can lead to lethargy and coma without changes in electrolytes or hydration.

NURSING CONSIDERATIONS
Baseline Assessment
- Assess the patient's BP for hypotension before giving indapamide.
- Assess the patient's baseline electrolyte levels, particularly serum potassium.
- Examine the patient for edema, and assess the mucous membranes and skin turgor to determine hydration status.
- Evaluate the patient's mental status and muscle strength.
- Obtain the patient's baseline weight and temperature.
- Begin monitoring the patient's fluid intake and output.

Precautions
- Use indapamide cautiously in debilitated and elderly patients and in patients with anuria, diabetes mellitus, a history of hypersensitivity to sulfonamides or thiazide diuretics, hepatic impairment, severe renal disease, or thyroid disorders.

Administration and Handling
PO
- Give indapamide with food or milk if GI upset occurs, preferably with breakfast to help prevent nocturia.
- Do not crush or break tablets.

Intervention and Evaluation
- Continue to monitor the patient's BP and other vital signs.
- Note the extent of diuresis by

measuring intake and output and recording daily weight.
- Monitor the patient for electrolyte disturbances. Hypokalemia may result in altered mental status, muscle cramps, nausea and vomiting, tachycardia, tremor, and weakness. Hyponatremia may result in cold and clammy skin, confusion, and thirst.

Patient Teaching
- Advise the patient to take indapamide early in the day to avoid urination at night.
- Tell the patient to expect an increase in the frequency and volume of urination.
- Instruct the patient to change positions slowly to let legs dangle momentarily before standing to reduce the drug's hypotensive effect.
- Encourage the patient to eat foods high in potassium, including such as apricots, bananas, raisins, orange juice, potatoes, legumes, meat, and whole grains (such as cereals).

mannitol

man-i-tall
(Osmitrol)

CATEGORY AND SCHEDULE
Pregnancy Risk Category: C

MECHANISM OF ACTION
An osmotic diuretic, antiglaucoma, and antihemolytic agent that elevates osmotic pressure of the glomerular filtrate, inhibiting tubular reabsorption of water and electrolytes, resulting in increased flow of water into interstitial fluid and plasma. **Therapeutic Effect:** Produces diuresis; reduces IOP; reduces ICP and cerebral edema.

PHARMACOKINETICS

Route	Onset	Peak	Duration
IV (diuresis)	15–30 min	N/A	2–8 hr
IV (Reduced ICP)	15–30 min	N/A	3–8 hr
IV (Reduced IOP)	N/A	30–60 min	4–8 hr

Remains in extracellular fluid. Primarily excreted in urine. Removed by hemodialysis. ***Half-life:*** 100 min.

AVAILABILITY
Injection: 5%, 10%, 15%, 20%, 25%.

INDICATIONS AND DOSAGES
▸ **Prevention and treatment of oliguric phase of acute renal failure; to promote urinary excretion of toxic substances (such as aspirin, barbiturates, bromides, and imipramine); to reduce increased ICP due to cerebral edema or edema of injured spinal cord; to reduce increased IOP due to acute glaucoma**

IV

Adults, Elderly, Children. Initially, 0.5–1 g/kg, then 0.25–0.5 g/kg q4–6h.

CONTRAINDICATIONS
Dehydration, intracranial bleeding, severe pulmonary edema and congestion, severe renal disease

INTERACTIONS
Drug

Digoxin: May increase the risk of digoxin toxicity associated with mannitol-induced hypokalemia.

Herbal

None known.

Food

None known.

DIAGNOSTIC TEST EFFECTS

May decrease serum phosphate, potassium, and sodium levels.

IV INCOMPATIBILITIES

Cefepime (Maxipime), doxorubicin liposomal (Doxil), filgrastim (Neupogen)

IV COMPATIBILITIES

Cisplatin (Platinol), ondansetron (Zofran), propofol (Diprivan)

SIDE EFFECTS

Frequent

Dry mouth, thirst

Occasional

Blurred vision, increased urinary frequency and urine volume, headache, arm pain, backache, nausea, vomiting, urticaria, dizziness, hypotension or hypertension, tachycardia, fever, angina-like chest pain

SERIOUS REACTIONS

! Fluid and electrolyte imbalance may occur from rapid administration of large doses or inadequate urine output resulting in overexpansion of extracellular fluid.

! Circulatory overload may produce pulmonary edema and CHF.

! Excessive diuresis may produce hypokalemia and hyponatremia.

! Fluid loss in excess of electrolyte excretion may produce hypernatremia and hyperkalemia.

NURSING CONSIDERATIONS

Baseline Assessment

- Monitor the patient's vital signs, especially BP for hypotension before giving mannitol.
- Evaluate the patient for edema, and assess mucous membranes and skin turgor to determine hydration status.
- Obtain the patient's baseline weight.
- Begin monitoring the patient's fluid intake and output.

Lifespan Considerations

- It is unknown if mannitol crosses the placenta or is distributed in breast milk.
- The safety and efficacy of mannitol have not been established in children younger than 12 years.
- Age-related renal impairment may require cautious use in the elderly.

Administration and Handling

IV

◀ALERT▶ Assess the IV site for patency before administering each dose. Pain and thrombosis are noted with extravasation.

◀ALERT▶ For patients with suspected renal insufficiency or marked oliguria, a test dose should be given. The test dose is 12.5 g for adults (200 mg/kg for children) over 3 to 5 minutes to produce a urine flow of at least 30 to 50 ml/hour (1 ml/kg/hour for children) over 2 to 3 hours.

- Store the drug at room temperature.
- If the solution crystallizes, warm the bottle in hot water and shake it vigorously at intervals. Don't use the solution if crystals remain after the warming procedure.
- Cool the solution to body temperature before administration.
- Use an in-line filter (less than 5 microns) for drug concentrations greater than 20%.
- The test dose for oliguria is IV push over 3 to 5 minutes. The test dose for cerebral edema or elevated ICP is IV over 20 to 30 minutes. Maximum concentration is 25%.
- Don't add potassium chloride or sodium chloride to mannitol with a concentration of 20% or greater.
- Don't add mannitol to whole blood for transfusion.

Intervention and Evaluation

- Monitor the patient's urine output to ascertain a therapeutic response.

• Monitor the patient's BUN and serum electrolyte levels and liver function test results.
• Weigh the patient daily.
• Observe the patient for electrolyte disturbances. Hypokalemia may result in cardiac arrhythmias, altered mental status, muscle cramps, nausea and vomiting, tachycardia, tremor, and weakness; hyperkalemia may result in arrhythmias, colic, diarrhea, and muscle twitching followed by paralysis or weakness; hyponatremia may result in cold and clammy skin, confusion, drowsiness, and thirst.

Patient Teaching

• Tell the patient to expect an increase in the frequency and volume of urination.
• Inform the patient that mannitol may cause dry mouth.
• Tell the patient to weigh himself or herself daily.

metolazone

met-**tole**-a-zone
(Mykrox, Zaroxolyn)
Do not confuse metolazone with methazolamide or metoprolol, or Zaroxolyn with Zarontin.

CATEGORY AND SCHEDULE

Pregnancy Risk Category: B (D if used in pregnancy-induced hypertension)

MECHANISM OF ACTION

A thiazide-like diuretic and antihypertensive. As a diuretic, blocks reabsorption of sodium, potassium, and chloride at the distal convoluted tubule, increasing renal excretion of sodium and water. As an antihypertensive, reduces plasma and extracellular fluid volume and peripheral vascular resistance. **Therapeutic Effect:** Promotes diuresis and reduces BP.

PHARMACOKINETICS

Route	Onset	Peak	Duration
PO (diuretic)	1 hr	2 hr	12–24 hr

Incompletely absorbed from the GI tract. Protein binding: 95%. Primarily excreted unchanged in urine. Not removed by hemodialysis. ***Half-life:*** 14 hr.

AVAILABILITY

Tablets (Prompt-Release [Mykrox]): 0.5 mg.
Tablets (Extended-Release [Zaroxolyn]): 2.5 mg, 5 mg, 10 mg.

INDICATIONS AND DOSAGES

▸ **Edema**

PO (Zaroxolyn)
Adults, Elderly. 5–10 mg/day. May increase to 20 mg/day in edema associated with renal disease or heart failure.
Children. 0.2–0.4 mg/kg/day in 1–2 divided doses.

▸ **Hypertension**

PO (Zaroxolyn)
Adults, Elderly. 2.5–5 mg/day.
PO (Mydrox)
Adults, Elderly. Initially, 0.5 mg/day. May increase up to 1 mg/day.

CONTRAINDICATIONS

Anuria, hepatic coma or precoma, history of hypersensitivity to sulfonamides or thiazide diuretics, renal decompensation

INTERACTIONS

Drug

Cholestyramine, colestipol: May decrease the absorption and effects of metolazone.

Digoxin: May increase the risk of digoxin toxicity associated with metolazone-induced hypokalemia.
Lithium: May increase the risk of lithium toxicity.

Herbal

None known.

Food

None known.

DIAGNOSTIC TEST EFFECTS

May increase blood glucose and serum cholesterol, LDL, bilirubin, calcium, creatinine, uric acid, and triglyceride levels. May decrease urinary calcium, and serum magnesium, potassium, and sodium levels.

SIDE EFFECTS

Expected

Increase in urinary frequency and urine volume

Frequent (10%–9%)

Dizziness, light-headedness, headache

Occasional (6%–4%)

Muscle cramps and spasm, fatigue, lethargy

Rare (less than 2%)

Asthenia, palpitations, depression, nausea, vomiting, abdominal bloating, constipation, diarrhea, urticaria

SERIOUS REACTIONS

! Vigorous diuresis may lead to profound water and electrolyte depletion, resulting in hypokalemia, hyponatremia, and dehydration.
! Acute hypotensive episodes may occur.
! Hyperglycemia may occur during prolonged therapy.
! Pancreatitis, paresthesia, blood dyscrasias, pulmonary edema, allergic pneumonitis, and dermatologic reactions occur rarely.
! Overdose can lead to lethargy and coma without changes in electrolytes or hydration.

NURSING CONSIDERATIONS

Baseline Assessment

- Monitor the patient's BP for hypotension before giving metolazone.
- Assess the patient's baseline electrolyte levels, particularly for hypokalemia.
- Evaluate the patient for peripheral edema, and check mucous membranes and skin turgor to determine hydration status.
- Evaluate the patient's mental status and muscle strength.
- Obtain the patient's baseline weight and temperature.
- Begin monitoring the patient's fluid intake and output.

Lifespan Considerations

- Metolazone crosses the placenta and a small amount is distributed in breast milk. Breast-feeding is not recommended for patients taking this drug.
- No age-related precautions have been noted in children.
- The elderly may be more sensitive to the drug's electrolyte and hypotensive effects.
- Age-related renal impairment may require cautious use in the elderly.

Precautions

- Use metolazone cautiously in patients with diabetes, elevated cholesterol and triglyceride levels, gout, hepatic impairment, lupus erythematosus, or severe renal disease.

Administration and Handling

PO

- Give metolazone with food or milk if GI upset occurs, preferably with breakfast to help prevent nocturia.

Intervention and Evaluation

- Continue to monitor the patient's BP and other vital signs, electrolyte levels, and weight.
- Record the extent of patient diuresis.

• Monitor the patient for electrolyte disturbances. Hypokalemia may result in altered mental status, muscle cramps, nausea and vomiting, tachycardia, tremor, and weakness. Hyponatremia may result in cold and clammy skin, confusion, and thirst.

Patient Teaching

• Tell the patient to expect an increase in the frequency and volume of urination.

• Instruct the patient to change position slowly and to let legs dangle momentarily before standing to reduce the drug's hypotensive effect.

• Encourage the patient to eat foods high in potassium such as apricots, bananas, raisins, orange juice, potatoes, legumes, meat, and whole grains (such as cereals).

spironolactone

speer-on-oh-**lak**-tone

(Aldactone, Novospiroton[CAN], Spiractin[AUS])

Do not confuse Aldactone with Aldactazide.

CATEGORY AND SCHEDULE

Pregnancy Risk Category: C (D if used in pregnancy-induced hypertension)

MECHANISM OF ACTION

An potassium-sparing diuretic that interferes with sodium reabsorption by competitively inhibiting the action of aldosterone in the distal tubule, thus promoting sodium and water excretion and increasing potassium retention. **Therapeutic Effect:** Produces diuresis; lowers BP; diagnostic aid for primary aldosteronism.

PHARMACOKINETICS

Route	Onset	Peak	Duration
PO	24–48 hr	48–72 hr	48–72 hr

Well absorbed from the GI tract (absorption increased with food). Protein binding: 91%–98%. Metabolized in the liver to active metabolite. Primarily excreted in urine. Unknown if removed by hemodialysis. ***Half-life:*** 0–24 hr (metabolite, 13–24 hr).

AVAILABILITY

Tablets: 25 mg, 50 mg, 100 mg.

INDICATIONS AND DOSAGES

▸ **Edema**

PO

Adults, Elderly. 25–200 mg/day as a single dose or in 2 divided doses.

Children. 1.5–3.3 mg/kg/day in divided doses.

Neonates. 1–3 mg/kg/day in 1–2 divided doses.

▸ **Hypertension**

PO

Adults, Elderly. 25–50 mg/day in 1–2 doses/day.

Children. 1.5–3.3 mg/kg/day in divided doses.

▸ **Hypokalemia**

PO

Adults, Elderly. 25–200 mg/day as a single dose or in 2 divided doses.

▸ **Male Hirsutism**

PO

Adults, Elderly. 50–200 mg/day as a single dose or in 2 divided doses.

▸ **Primary aldosteronism**

PO

Adults, Elderly. 100–400 mg/day as a single dose or in 2 divided doses.

Children. 100–400 mg/m^2/day as a single dose or in 2 divided doses.

▸ **Dosage in renal impairment**
Dosage interval is modified based on creatinine clearance.

Creatinine Clearance	Interval
10–50 ml/min	Usual dose q12–24h
less than 10 ml/min	Avoid use.

OFF-LABEL USES
Treatment of female hirsutism, polycystic ovary disease

CONTRAINDICATIONS
Acute renal insufficiency, anuria, BUN and serum creatinine levels more than twice normal values, hyperkalemia

INTERACTIONS
Drug
ACE inhibitors (such as captopril), potassium-containing medications, potassium supplements: May increase the risk of hyperkalemia.
Anticoagulants, heparin: May decrease the effects of these drugs.
Digoxin: May increase the half-life of digoxin.
Lithium: May decrease the clearance and increase the risk of toxicity of lithium.
NSAIDs: May decrease the antihypertensive effect of spironolactone.
Herbal
None known.
Food
None known.

DIAGNOSTIC TEST EFFECTS
May increase urinary calcium excretion; BUN and blood glucose levels; serum creatinine, magnesium, potassium, and uric acid levels. May decrease serum sodium level.

SIDE EFFECTS
Frequent
Hyperkalemia (in patients with renal insufficiency and those taking potassium supplements), dehydration, hyponatremia, lethargy
Occasional
Nausea, vomiting, anorexia, abdominal cramps, diarrhea, headache, ataxia, somnolence, confusion, fever
Male: Gynecomastia, impotence, decreased libido
Female: Menstrual irregularities (including amenorrhea and postmenopausal bleeding), breast tenderness
Rare
Rash, urticaria, hirsutism

SERIOUS REACTIONS
! Severe hyperkalemia may produce arrhythmias, bradycardia, and EKG changes (tented T waves, widening QRS complex and ST segment depression). These may proceed to cardiac standstill or ventricular fibrillation.
! Cirrhosis patients are at risk for hepatic decompensation if dehydration or hyponatremia occurs.
! Patients with primary aldosteronism may experience rapid weight loss and severe fatigue during high-dose therapy.

NURSING CONSIDERATIONS
Baseline Assessment
• Monitor the patient's vital signs, including pulse rate and quality. Also expect to perform a baseline EKG.
• Assess the patient's BUN, serum creatinine, and serum electrolyte levels; liver function test results; and urinalysis results.
• Note the extent and location of edema, and evaluate mucous membranes and skin turgor to determine the patient's hydration status.

• Obtain the patient's baseline weight, and begin monitoring fluid intake and output.

Lifespan Considerations

• An active metabolite of spironolactone is excreted in breast milk. Breast-feeding is not recommended for patients taking this drug.
• No age-related precautions have been noted in children.
• The elderly may be more susceptible to hyperkalemia. In addition, age-related renal impairment may require cautious use in this age-group.

Precautions

• Use spironolactone cautiously in patients with hyponatremia or hepatic or renal impairment, dehydrated patients, and those who take potassium supplements.

Administration and Handling

PO

• Give spironolactone with food to enhance its absorption.
• Crush scored tablets as needed.
• Oral suspension containing crushed tablets in cherry syrup is stable for up to 30 days if refrigerated.

Intervention and Evaluation

• Monitor the patient's BP and electrolytes values. Be especially alert for evidence of hyperkalemia, such as arrhythmias, colic, diarrhea, and muscle twitching, followed by paralysis and weakness.
• Obtain an EKG, as ordered, if hyperkalemia is severe.
• Assess the patient for symptoms of hyponatremia, such as cold and clammy skin, confusion, drowsiness, dry mouth, and thirst.
• Weigh the patient every day.
• Record changes in the patient's edema and skin turgor.

Patient Teaching

• Tell the patient to expect an increase in the frequency and volume of urination.
• Inform the patient that the drug's therapeutic effect takes several days to begin and can last for several days once the drug is discontinued (unless he or she is taking a potassium-losing drug concomitantly).
• Caution the patient to avoid consuming potassium supplements and foods high in potassium, including apricots, bananas, raisins, orange juice, potatoes, legumes, meat, and whole grains (such as cereals).
• Warn the patient to notify the physician if he or she experiences an irregular heartbeat, diarrhea, muscle twitching, cold and clammy skin, confusion, drowsiness, dry mouth, or excessive thirst.
• Warn the patient to avoid performing tasks that require mental alertness or motor skills until his or her response to the drug has been established.

torsemide

tor-se-mide

(Demadex)

Do not confuse torsemide with furosemide.

CATEGORY AND SCHEDULE

Pregnancy Risk Category: B

MECHANISM OF ACTION

A loop diuretic that enhances excretion of sodium, chloride, potassium, and water at the ascending limb of the loop of Henle; also reduces plasma and extracellular fluid volume. **Therapeutic Effect:** Produces diuresis; lowers BP.

PHARMACOKINETICS

Route	Onset	Peak	Duration
PO	1 hr	1–2 hr	6–8 hr
IV	10 min	1 hr	6–8 hr

Rapidly and well absorbed from the GI tract. Protein binding: 97%–99%. Metabolized in the liver. Primarily excreted in urine. Not removed by hemodialysis. ***Half-life:*** 3.3 hr.

AVAILABILITY

Tablets: 5 mg, 10 mg, 20 mg, 100 mg.
Injection: 10 mg/ml.

INDICATIONS AND DOSAGES

▸ Hypertension

PO

Adults, Elderly. Initially, 5 mg/day. May increase to 10 mg/day if no response in 4–6 wk. If no response, additional antihypertensive added.

▸ CHF

PO, IV

Adults, Elderly. Initially, 10–20 mg/day. May increase by approximately doubling dose until desired therapeutic effect is attained. Doses greater than 200 mg have not been adequately studied.

▸ Chronic renal failure

PO, IV

Adults, Elderly. Initially, 20 mg/day. May increase by approximately doubling dose until desired therapeutic effect is attained. Doses greater than 200 mg have not been adequately studied.

▸ Hepatic cirrhosis

PO, IV

Adults, Elderly. Initially, 5 mg/day given with aldosterone antagonist or potassium-sparing diuretic. May increase by approximately doubling dose until desired therapeutic effect is attained. Doses greater than 40 mg have not been adequately studied.

CONTRAINDICATIONS

Anuria, hepatic coma, severe electrolyte depletion

INTERACTIONS

Drug

Amphotericin B, nephrotoxic medications, ototoxic medications: May increase the risk of nephrotoxicity and ototoxicity.
Anticoagulants, heparin, thrombolytics: May decrease the effects of these drugs.
Digoxin: May increase the risk of digoxin toxicity associated with torsemide-induced hypokalemia.
Lithium: May increase the risk of lithium toxicity.
NSAIDs, probenecid: May decrease the diuretic effect of torsemide.
Other antihypertensives: May increase the risk of hypotension.
Other hypokalemia-causing medications: May increase the risk of hypokalemia.

Herbal

None known.

Food

None known.

DIAGNOSTIC TEST EFFECTS

May increase BUN, serum creatinine, and serum uric acid levels. May decrease serum calcium, chloride, magnesium, potassium, and sodium levels.

IV INCOMPATIBILITIES

Don't mix torsemide with any other medications except for milrinone (Primacor).

IV COMPATIBILITIES

Milrinone (Primacor)

SIDE EFFECTS

Frequent (10%–4%)
Headache, dizziness, rhinitis
Occasional (3%–1%)
Asthenia, insomnia, nervousness, diarrhea, constipation, nausea, dys-

pepsia, edema, EKG changes, pharyngitis, cough, arthralgia, myalgia

Rare (less than 1%)

Syncope, hypotension, arrhythmias

SERIOUS REACTIONS

! Ototoxicity may occur with high doses or a too-rapid IV administration.

! Overdose produces acute, profound water loss; volume and electrolyte depletion; dehydration; decreased blood volume; and circulatory collapse.

NURSING CONSIDERATIONS

Baseline Assessment

- Monitor the patient's electrolyte levels, especially serum potassium.
- Record the patient's baseline weight.

Lifespan Considerations

- It is unknown if torsemide is excreted in breast milk.
- The safety and efficacy of this drug have not been established in children.
- No age-related precautions have been noted in the elderly.

Precautions

- Use torsemide extremely cautiously in patients with a hypersensitivity to sulfonamides.
- Use torsemide cautiously in cardiac and elderly patients and patients with ascites, hepatic cirrhosis, renal impairment, systemic lupus erythematosus, or a history of ventricular arrhythmias.
- Use this drug cautiously in pediatric patients because the safety of torsemide use in children is unknown.

Administration and Handling

PO

- Give torsemide with food to avoid GI upset, preferably with breakfast to prevent nocturia.

IV

◀ **ALERT** ▶ Flush IV line with 0.9% NaCl before and after torsemide administration.

- Store torsemide at room temperature.
- Torsemide may be given undiluted as IV push over 2 minutes.
- For continuous IV infusion, dilute with 0.9% or 0.45% NaCl or D_5W and infuse over 24 hours.
- Administer IV push slowly because too-rapid administration may cause ototoxicity.

Intervention and Evaluation

- Monitor the patient's BP, serum electrolyte levels (especially potassium), fluid intake and output, and weight.
- Assess the patient's lungs for crackles and rhonchi.
- Evaluate the patient for edema, particularly of dependent areas.
- Assess the patient for signs of hypokalemia, including cardiac arrhythmias, altered mental status, muscle cramps, weakness, or tremor. Know that less potassium is lost with torsemide than with furosemide.

Patient Teaching

- Instruct the patient to take torsemide in the morning to prevent nocturia.
- Tell the patient to expect an increase in the frequency and volume of urination.
- Advise the patient to notify the physician if he or she experiences cramps, dizziness, an irregular heartbeat, muscle weakness, nausea, or hearing abnormalities.
- Caution the patient against taking other medications, including OTC drugs, without first consulting the physician.
- Encourage the patient to eat foods high in potassium, including apricots, bananas, raisins, orange juice,

potatoes, legumes, meat, and whole grains (such as cereals).

triamterene

try-**am**-ter-een
(Dyrenium)
Do not confuse triamterene with trimipramine.

CATEGORY AND SCHEDULE

Pregnancy Risk Category: C (D if used in pregnancy-induced hypertension)

MECHANISM OF ACTION

A potassium-sparing diuretic that inhibits sodium, potassium, ATPase. Interferes with sodium and potassium exchange in distal tubule, cortical collecting tubule, and collecting duct. Increases sodium and decreases potassium excretion. Also increases magnesium, decreases calcium loss. **Therapeutic Effect:** Produces diuresis and lowers BP.

PHARMACOKINETICS

Route	Onset	Peak	Duration
PO	2–4 hr	N/A	7–9 hr

Incompletely absorbed from the GI tract. Widely distributed. Metabolized in the liver. Primarily eliminated in feces via biliary route. ***Half-life:*** 1.5–2.5 hr (increased in renal impairment).

AVAILABILITY

Capsules: 50 mg, 100 mg.

INDICATIONS AND DOSAGES

▸ **Edema, hypertension**

PO

Adults, Elderly. 25–100 mg/day as a single dose or in 2 divided doses. Maximum: 300 mg/day.

Children. 2–4 mg/kg/day as a single dose or in 2 divided doses. Maximum: 6 mg/kg/day or 300 mg/day.

OFF-LABEL USES

Treatment adjunct for hypertension, prevention and treatment of hypokalemia

CONTRAINDICATIONS

Drug-induced or pre-existing hyperkalemia, progressive or severe renal disease, severe hepatic disease

INTERACTIONS

Drug

ACE inhibitors (such as captopril), potassium-containing medications, potassium supplements: May increase the risk of hyperkalemia.
Anticoagulants, heparin: May decrease the effects of these drugs.
Lithium: May decrease the clearance and increase the risk of toxicity of lithium.
NSAIDs: May decrease the antihypertensive effect of triamterene.

Herbal

None known.

Food

None known.

DIAGNOSTIC TEST EFFECTS

May increase urinary calcium excretion; BUN and blood glucose levels; and serum calcium, creatinine, potassium, magnesium, and uric acid levels. May decrease serum sodium levels.

SIDE EFFECTS

Occasional

Fatigue, nausea, diarrhea, abdominal pain, leg cramps, headache

Rare

Anorexia, asthenia, rash, dizziness

SERIOUS REACTIONS

! Triamterene use may result in hyponatremia (somnolence, dry mouth, increased thirst, lack of energy) or severe hyperkalemia (irritability, anxiety, heaviness of legs, paresthesia, hypotension, bradycardia, EKG changes [tented T waves, widening QRS complex, ST segment depression]).

! Agranulocytosis, nephrolithiasis, and thrombocytopenia occur rarely.

NURSING CONSIDERATIONS

Baseline Assessment

- Assess the patient's baseline serum electrolyte levels, particularly for hypokalemia.
- Assess the patient's BUN and serum creatinine levels and liver function test results.
- Assess the patient's pulse rate and rhythm.
- Examine the patient for edema and note its extent and location.
- Evaluate the patient's mucous membranes and skin turgor to determine hydration status.
- Evaluate the patient's mental status and muscle strength.
- Obtain and record the patient's baseline weight and temperature.
- Begin monitoring the patient's fluid intake and output.

Lifespan Considerations

- Triamterene crosses the placenta and is distributed in breast milk. Breast-feeding is not recommended for patients taking this drug.
- The safety and efficacy of this drug have not been established in children.
- The elderly may be at increased risk for developing hyperkalemia.

Precautions

- Use triamterene cautiously in patients with diabetes mellitus, a history of renal calculi, or hepatic or renal impairment and in patients who take other potassium-sparing diuretics or potassium supplements.

Administration and Handling

PO

- Give triamterene with food if GI disturbances occur.
- Do not crush or break capsules.

Intervention and Evaluation

- Monitor the patient's BP, electrolyte levels (particularly potassium), fluid intake and output, vital signs, and daily weight.
- Monitor the patient for electrolyte disturbances. Hypokalemia may result in altered mental status, muscle cramps, nausea and vomiting, tachycardia, tremor, and weakness.
- Auscultate the patient's breath sounds for rhonchi and wheezing.

Patient Teaching

- Instruct the patient to take triamterene in the morning to help prevent nocturia.
- Inform the patient that the drug's therapeutic effect takes several days to begin and can last for several days after the drug is discontinued.
- Tell the patient to expect an increase in the frequency and volume of urination.
- Advise the patient to notify the physician if he or she experiences dry mouth, fever, headache, nausea and vomiting, persistent or severe weakness, sore throat, or unusual bleeding or bruising.
- Encourage the patient to avoid consuming salt substitutes and foods high in potassium.

darifenacin hydrobromide
flavoxate
oxybutynin
phenazopyridine hydrochloride
solifenacin succinate
tolterodine tartrate
trospium chloride

Uses: Spasmolytic agents are used to treat urinary frequency and urgency or urge incontinence. *Darifenacin, solifenacin,* and *trospium* are used to treat overactive bladder. *Flavoxate* also relieves other symptoms of cystitis, proctatitis, urethritis, and related disorders. *Oxybutynin* also minimizes other symptoms of neurogenic bladder. *Phenazopyridine* also relieves other symptoms of urinary mucosal irritation, which may be caused by infection, trauma, or surgery. *Tolterodine* also reduces other symptoms of overactive bladder.

Action: Most spasmolytics competitively block the actions of acetylcholine at muscarinic receptors. *Darifenacin, solifenacin,* and *trospium* act as direct antagonists at muscarinic receptor sites in cholinergically innervated organs, including the bladder. In the bladder, this blockade of receptors limits bladder contractions, reducing symptoms of bladder irritability and overactivity and improving bladder capacity. Because of this cholinergic blockade, *flavoxate, oxybutynin,* and *tolterodine* relax detrusor and other smooth muscles, counteracting muscle spasms in the urinary tract. *Phenazopyridine* exerts a topical analgesic effect on the urinary mucosa.

COMBINATION PRODUCTS

ZOTRIM: phenazopyridine/trimethoprim (an anti-infective)/sulfamethoxazole (a sulfonamide) 200 mg/160 mg/800 mg.

darifenacin hydrobromide

dare-ih-**fen**-ah-sin
(Enablex)

CATEGORY AND SCHEDULE

Pregnancy Risk Category: C

MECHANISM OF ACTION

A urinary antispasmodic agent that acts as a direct antagonist at muscarinic receptor sites in cholinergically innervated organs. Blockade of the receptors limits bladder contractions. **Therapeutic Effect:** Reduces symptoms of bladder irritability and overactivity; improves bladder capacity.

AVAILABILITY

Tablets (Extended-Release): 7.5 mg, 15 mg.

INDICATIONS AND DOSAGES

▸ **Overactive bladder**

PO

Adults, Elderly. Initially, 7.5 mg once daily. If response is not adequate after at least 2 wk, dosage may be increased to 15 mg once daily.

▸ **Dosage in hepatic impairment**

For patients with moderate hepatic impairment, maximum dosage is 7.5 mg once daily.

CONTRAINDICATIONS

GI or GU obstruction, paralytic ileus, severe hepatic impairment, uncontrolled angle-closure glaucoma, urine retention

INTERACTIONS

Drug

Aminoglutethimide, carbamazepine, nafcillin, nevirapine, phenobarbital, phenytoin, rifamycins: May decrease the effects and blood level of darifenacin.

Amphetamines, beta blockers (selected), dextromethorphan, fluoxetine, lidocaine, mirtazapine, nefazodone, paroxetine, risperidone, ritonavir, thioridazine, tricyclic antidepressants, venlafaxine: May increase the effects and blood levels of these drugs.

Azole antifungals, ciprofloxacin, clarithromycin, diclofenac, doxycycline, erythromycin, imatinib, isoniazid, nefazodone, nicardipine, propofol, protease inhibitors, quinidine, verapamil: May increase the effects and blood level of darifenacin.

Codeine, hydrocodone, oxycodone, tramadol: May decrease the effects and blood levels of these drugs.

Herbal

None known.

Food

None known.

DIAGNOSTIC TEST EFFECTS

None known.

SIDE EFFECTS

Frequent (35%–21%)

Dry mouth, constipation

Occasional (8%–4%)

Dyspepsia, headache, nausea, abdominal pain

Rare (3%–2%)

Asthenia, diarrhea, dizziness, dry eyes

SERIOUS REACTIONS

! UTI occurs occasionally.

NURSING CONSIDERATIONS

Precautions

- Use darifenacin cautiously in patients with bladder outflow obstruction, constipation, controlled angle-closure glaucoma, decreased GI motility, GI obstructive disorders, hiatal hernia, myasthenia gravis, nonobstructive prostatic hyperplasia, reflux esophagitis, ulcerative colitis, and urine retention.

Administration and Handling

PO

- Give darifenacin without regard to food.
- Have the patient swallow extended-release tablets whole; don't crush them.

flavoxate

fla-**vox**-ate

(Urispas)

Do not confuse Urispas with Urised.

CATEGORY AND SCHEDULE

Pregnancy Risk Category: B

MECHANISM OF ACTION
An anticholinergic that relaxes detrusor and other smooth muscle by cholinergic blockade, counteracting muscle spasm in the urinary tract.
Therapeutic Effect: Produces anticholinergic, local anesthetic, and analgesic effects, relieving urinary symptoms.

AVAILABILITY
Tablets: 100 mg.

INDICATIONS AND DOSAGES
▸ **To relieve symptoms of cystitis, prostatitis, urethritis, urethrocystitis, or urethrotrigonitis**
PO
Adults, Elderly, Adolescents. 100–200 mg 3–4 times a day.

CONTRAINDICATIONS
Duodenal or pyloric obstruction, GI hemorrhage or obstruction, ileus, lower urinary tract obstruction

INTERACTIONS
Drug
None known.
Herbal
None known.
Food
None known.

DIAGNOSTIC TEST EFFECTS
None known.

SIDE EFFECTS
Frequent
Somnolence, dry mouth and throat
Occasional
Constipation, difficult urination, blurred vision, dizziness, headache, increased light sensitivity, nausea, vomiting, abdominal pain
Rare
Confusion (primarily in elderly), hypersensitivity, increased IOP, leukopenia

SERIOUS REACTIONS
! Overdose may produce anticholinergic effects, including unsteadiness, severe dizziness, somnolence, fever, facial flushing, dyspnea, nervousness, and irritability.

NURSING CONSIDERATIONS
Baseline Assessment
- Assess the patient's urinary symptoms (dysuria, frequency, urgency, incontinence, suprapubic pain).
- Plan to obtain a urine specimen for culture and sensitivity testing and urinalysis.

Precautions
- Use flavoxate cautiously in patients with glaucoma.

Administration and Handling
- Expect to reduce the dosage of flavoxate as symptoms improve.

Intervention and Evaluation
- Monitor the patient for symptomatic relief.
- Observe elderly patients for confusion.

Patient Teaching
- Warn the patient to avoid performing tasks that require mental alertness or motor skills until his or her response to the drug has been established.
- Teach the patient about signs and symptoms of flavoxate overdose, including unsteadiness, severe dizziness, drowsiness, fever, flushed face, shortness of breath, nervousness, and irritability.

oxybutynin

ox-i-**byoo**-ti-nin
(Ditropan, Ditropan XL, Oxytrol)
Do not confuse oxybutynin with Oxycontin, or Ditropan with diazepam.

CATEGORY AND SCHEDULE

Pregnancy Risk Category: B

MECHANISM OF ACTION

An anticholinergic that exerts antispasmodic (papaverine-like) and antimuscarinic (atropine-like) action on the detrusor smooth muscle of the bladder. **Therapeutic Effect:** Increases bladder capacity and delays desire to void.

PHARMACOKINETICS

Route	Onset	Peak	Duration
PO	0.5–1 hr	3–6 hr	6–10 hr

Rapidly absorbed from the GI tract. Metabolized in the liver. Primarily excreted in urine. Unknown if removed by hemodialysis. ***Half-life:*** 1–2.3 hr.

AVAILABILITY

Syrup (Ditropan): 5 mg/5 ml.
Tablets (Ditropan): 5 mg.
Tablets (Extended-Release [Ditropan XL]): 5 mg, 10 mg, 15 mg.
Transdermal (Oxytrol): 3.9 mg.

INDICATIONS AND DOSAGES

▸ **Neurogenic bladder**

PO

Adults. 5 mg 2–3 times a day up to 5 mg 4 times a day.
Elderly. 2.5–5 mg twice a day. May increase by 2.5 mg/day every 1–2 days.
Children 5 yr and older. 5 mg twice a day up to 5 mg 4 times a day.
Children 1–4 yr. 0.2 mg/kg/dose 2–4 times a day.

PO (Extended-Release)

Adults. 5–10 mg/day up to 30 mg/day.

Transdermal

Adults. 3.9 mg applied twice a week. Apply every 3–4 days.

CONTRAINDICATIONS

GI or GU obstruction, glaucoma, myasthenia gravis, toxic megacolon, ulcerative colitis

INTERACTIONS

Drug

Medications with anticholinergic effects (such as antihistamines): May increase the anticholinergic effects of oxybutynin.

Herbal

None known.

Food

None known.

DIAGNOSTIC TEST EFFECTS

None known.

SIDE EFFECTS

Frequent

Constipation, dry mouth, somnolence, decreased perspiration

Occasional

Decreased lacrimation or salivation, impotence, urinary hesitancy and retention, suppressed lactation, blurred vision, mydriasis, nausea or vomiting, insomnia

SERIOUS REACTIONS

! Overdose produces CNS excitation (including nervousness, restlessness, hallucinations, and irritability), hypotension or hypertension, confusion, tachycardia, facial flushing, and respiratory depression.

NURSING CONSIDERATIONS

Baseline Assessment

- Assess the patient's symptoms (dysuria; urinary frequency, urgency, or incontinence).

Lifespan Considerations

- It is unknown if oxybutynin crosses the placenta or is distributed in breast milk.
- No age-related precautions have been noted in children older than 5 years.
- The elderly may be more sensitive to the drug's anticholinergic effects, such as dry mouth and urine retention.

Precautions

- Use oxybutynin cautiously in patients with cardiovascular disease, hypertension, hyperthyroidism, hepatic or renal impairment, neuropathy, benign prostatic hyperplasia, or reflux esophagitis.

Administration and Handling

PO

- Give oxybutynin without regard to food.

Intervention and Evaluation

- Monitor the patient for symptomatic relief.
- Monitor the patient's intake and output, and palpate the bladder for signs of urine retention.
- Assess the patient's pattern of daily bowel activity and stool consistency.

Patient Teaching

- Inform the patient that oxybutynin may cause drowsiness and dry mouth.
- Urge the patient to avoid alcohol during oxybutynin therapy.
- Warn the patient to avoid performing tasks requiring mental alertness or motor skills until his or her response to the drug has been established.

phenazopyridine hydrochloride

fen-**az**-o-**peer**-i-deen
(Azo-Gesic, Azo-Standard, Phenazo[CAN], Prodium, Pyridium, Uristat)

Do not confuse phenazopyridine with pyridoxine, or Prodium with Perdiem.

CATEGORY AND SCHEDULE

Pregnancy Risk Category: B

MECHANISM OF ACTION

An interstitial cystitis agent that exerts topical analgesic effect on urinary tract mucosa. **Therapeutic Effect:** Relieves urinary pain, burning, urgency, and frequency.

PHARMACOKINETICS

Well absorbed from the GI tract. Partially metabolized in the liver. Primarily excreted in urine.

AVAILABILITY

Tablets (Azo-Gesic, Azo-Standard, Prodium, Uristat): 100 mg, 200 mg.
Tablets (Pyridium): 95 mg.

INDICATIONS AND DOSAGES

▸ Urinary analgesic

PO

Adults. 100–200 mg 3–4 times a day.
Children 6 yr and older. 12 mg/kg/day in 3 divided doses for 2 days.

▸ Dosage in renal impairment

Dosage interval is modified based on creatinine clearance.

Creatinine Clearance	Interval
50–80 ml/min	Usual dose q8–16h
less than 50 ml/min	Avoid use.

CONTRAINDICATIONS

Hepatic or renal insufficiency

INTERACTIONS

Drug
None known.
Herbal
None known.
Food
None known.

DIAGNOSTIC TEST EFFECTS

May interfere with urinalysis tests based on color reactions, such as urinary glucose, ketones, protein, and 17-ketosteroids.

SIDE EFFECTS

Occasional
Headache, GI disturbance, rash, pruritus

SERIOUS REACTIONS

! Overdose may lead to hemolytic anemia, nephrotoxicity, or hepatotoxicity. Patients with renal impairment or severe hypersensitivity to the drug may also develop these reactions.
! A massive and acute overdose may result in methemoglobinemia.

NURSING CONSIDERATIONS

Precautions
- Notify the physician and expect to discontinue the drug if the patient's skin or sclera turns yellow because this signifies impaired renal excretion.

Lifespan Considerations
- It is unknown if phenazopyridine crosses the placenta or is distributed in breast milk.
- No age-related precautions have been noted in children older than 6 years.
- Age-related renal impairment may increase the risk of toxicity in the elderly.

Administration and Handling
PO
- Give phenazopyridine with food.
- Expect to discontinue the drug after 2 days because there's no evidence that it's effective after this time period.

Intervention and Evaluation
- Assess the patient for a therapeutic response: relief of urinary frequency, pain, and burning.

Patient Teaching
- Instruct the patient to take phenazopyridine with meals to reduce the risk of GI upset.
- Inform the patient that phenazopyridine will turn urine a reddish orange color.

solifenacin succinate

sol-ih-**fen**-ah-sin
(VESIcare)

CATEGORY AND SCHEDULE

Pregnancy Risk Category: C

MECHANISM OF ACTION

A urinary antispasmodic that acts as a direct antagonist at muscarinic acetylcholine receptors in cholinergically innervated organs. Reduces tonus (elastic tension) of smooth muscle in the bladder and slows parasympathetic contractions. **Therapeutic Effect:** Decreases urinary bladder contractions, increases residual urine volume, and decreases detrusor muscle pressure.

AVAILABILITY

Tablets: 5 mg, 10 mg.

INDICATIONS AND DOSAGES

▸ Overactive bladder

PO

Adults, Elderly. 5 mg/day; if tolerated, may increase to 10 mg/day.

▸ Dosage in renal or hepatic impairment

For patients with severe renal impairment or moderate hepatic impairment, maximum dosage is 5 mg/day.

CONTRAINDICATIONS

Breast-feeding, GI obstruction, uncontrolled angle-closure glaucoma, urine retention

INTERACTIONS

Drug

Aminoglutethimide, carbamazepine, nafcillin, nevirapine, phenobarbital, phenytoin: May decrease the effects and serum level of solifenacin.

Azole antifungals, ciprofloxacin, clarithromycin, diclofenac, doxycycline, erythromycin, imatinib, isoniazid, nefazodone, nicardipine, propofol, protease inhibitors, quinidine, verapamil: May increase the effects and serum level of solifenacin.

Ketoconazole: May increase the serum level of solifenacin

Herbal

St John's wort: May decrease the effects and serum level of solifenacin.

Food

Grapefruit, grapefruit juice: May increase the effects and serum level of solifenacin.

DIAGNOSTIC TEST EFFECTS

None known.

SIDE EFFECTS

Frequent (11%–5%)

Dry mouth, constipation, blurred vision

Occasional (5%–3%)

UTI, dyspepsia, nausea

Rare (2%–1%)

Dizziness, dry eyes, fatigue, depression, edema, hypertension, upper abdominal pain, vomiting, urine retention

SERIOUS REACTIONS

! Angioneurotic edema and GI obstruction occur rarely.

! Overdose can result in severe central anticholinergic effects.

NURSING CONSIDERATIONS

Precautions

- Use solifenacin cautiously in pregnant patients and patients with bladder outflow obstruction, congenital or acquired prolonged QT interval, controlled angle-closure glaucoma, decreased GI motility, GI obstructive disorders, or hepatic or renal impairment.

Administration and Handling

PO

- Give solifenacin without regard to food.
- Instruct the patient to swallow solifenacin tablets whole.

tolterodine tartrate

tol-**tare**-oh-deen

(Detrol, Detrol LA)

CATEGORY AND SCHEDULE

Pregnancy Risk Category: C

MECHANISM OF ACTION

An antispasmodic that exhibits potent antimuscarinic activity by interceding via cholinergic muscarinic receptors, thereby inhibiting urinary bladder contraction. **Therapeutic Effect:** Decreases urinary frequency, urgency.

PHARMACOKINETICS

Rapidly and well absorbed after PO administration. Protein binding: 96%. Extensively metabolized in the liver to active metabolite. Primarily excreted in urine. Unknown if removed by hemodialysis. ***Half-life:*** 1.9–3.7 hr.

AVAILABILITY

Tablets (Detrol): 1 mg, 2 mg.
Capsules (Extended-Release [Detrol LA]): 2 mg, 4 mg.

INDICATIONS AND DOSAGES

▸ Overactive bladder
PO
Adults, Elderly. 1–2 mg twice a day.

▸ Dosage in severe renal or hepatic impairment
PO
Adults, Elderly. 1 mg twice a day.
PO (Extended-Release)
Adults, Elderly. 2–4 mg once a day.

CONTRAINDICATIONS

Uncontrolled angle-closure glaucoma, urine retention

INTERACTIONS

Drug

Clarithromycin, erythromycin, itraconazole, ketoconazole, miconazole: May increase tolterodine blood concentration.
Fluoxetine: May inhibit tolterodine metabolism.

Herbal

None known.

Food

None known.

DIAGNOSTIC TEST EFFECTS

None known.

SIDE EFFECTS

Frequent (40%)
Dry mouth
Occasional (11%–4%)
Headache, dizziness, fatigue, constipation, dyspepsia (heartburn, indigestion, epigastric discomfort), upper respiratory tract infection, UTI, dry eyes, abnormal vision (accommodation problems), nausea, diarrhea
Rare (3%)
Somnolence, chest or back pain, arthralgia, rash, weight gain, dry skin

SERIOUS REACTIONS

! Overdose can result in severe anticholinergic effects, including abdominal cramps, facial warmth, excessive salivation or lacrimation, diaphoresis, pallor, urinary urgency, blurred vision, and prolonged QT interval.

NURSING CONSIDERATIONS

Lifespan Considerations

- It is unknown if tolterodine is distributed in breast milk. However, breast-feeding is not recommended for patients taking this drug.
- The safety and efficacy of this drug have not been established in children.
- No age-related precautions have been noted in the elderly.

Precautions

- Use tolterodine cautiously in patients with renal impairment, clinically significant bladder outflow obstruction (increases risk of urine retention), GI obstructive disorders such as pyloric stenosis (increases risk of gastric retention), or treated angle-closure glaucoma.

Administration and Handling

PO
- Give tolterodine without regard to food.

Intervention and Evaluation

- Assist the patient with ambulation if he or she experiences dizziness.

- Determine if the patient experiences a change in vision.
- Monitor the patient for incontinence and residual urine in the bladder.

Patient Teaching

- Inform patient that tolterodine use may cause blurred vision, GI upset or constipation, and dry eyes and mouth.

trospium chloride

trow-spee-um
(Sanctura)

CATEGORY AND SCHEDULE

Pregnancy Risk Category: C

MECHANISM OF ACTION

An anticholinergic that antagonizes the effect of acetylcholine on muscarinic receptors, producing parasympatholytic action. **Therapeutic Effect:** Reduces smooth muscle tone in the bladder.

PHARMACOKINETICS

Minimally absorbed after PO administration. Protein binding: 50%–85%. Distributed in plasma. Excreted mainly in feces and, to a lesser extent, in urine. ***Half life:*** 20 hr.

AVAILABILITY

Tablets: 20 mg.

INDICATIONS AND DOSAGES

▸ Overactive bladder

PO

Adults. 20 mg 2 times/day.
Elderly (75 yr and older). Titrate dosage down to 20 mg once a day, based on tolerance.

▸ Dosage in renal impairment

For patients with creatinine clearance less than 30 ml/min, dosage reduced to 20 mg once a day at bedtime.

CONTRAINDICATIONS

Decreased GI motility, gastric retention, uncontrolled angle-closure glaucoma, urine retention

INTERACTIONS

Drug

Other anticholinergic agents: Increases the severity and frequency of side effects and may alter the absorption of other drugs because of anticholinergic effects on GI motility.
Digoxin, metformin, morphine, pancuronium, procainamide, tenofovir, vancomycin: May increase trospium blood concentration.

Herbal

None known.

Food

High-fat meal: May reduce trospium absorption.

DIAGNOSTIC TEST EFFECTS

None known.

SIDE EFFECTS

Frequent (20%)
Dry mouth
Occasional (10%–4%)
Constipation, headache
Rare (less than 2%)
Fatigue, upper abdominal pain, dyspepsia, flatulence, dry eyes, urine retention

SERIOUS REACTIONS

! Overdose may result in severe anticholinergic effects, such as abdominal pain, nausea and vomiting, confusion, depression, diaphoresis, facial flushing, hypertension, hypotension, respiratory depression, irritability, lacrimation, nervousness, and restlessness.

! Supraventricular tachycardia and hallucinations occur rarely.

NURSING CONSIDERATIONS

Baseline Assessment

- Assess the patient for dysuria and urinary urgency, frequency, and incontinence.

Lifespan Considerations

- It is unknown if trospium crosses the placenta or is distributed in breast milk.
- The safety and efficacy of trospium have not been established in children.
- Patients age 75 and older have a higher incidence of constipation, dry mouth, dyspepsia, urine retention, and UTI.

Precautions

- Use trospium cautiously in patients with renal or hepatic impairment, intestinal atony, obstructive GI disorders, significant bladder obstruction, ulcerative colitis, myasthenia gravis, or angle-closure glaucoma.

Administration and Handling

PO

- Store trospium at room temperature.
- Don't break or crush the tablets.
- Give the drug at least 1 hour before meals or on an empty stomach.

Intervention and Evaluation

- Monitor the patient's intake and output, and palpate the bladder for urine retention.
- Assess the patient's pattern of daily bowel activity and stool consistency.
- Relieve dry mouth by offering sips of tepid water.
- Monitor the patient for symptomatic relief.

Patient Teaching

- Advise the patient not to take trospium with high-fat meals because they may reduce drug absorption.
- Instruct the patient to notify the health care provider if he or she experiences increased salivation or sweating, an irregular heartbeat, nausea and vomiting, or severe abdominal pain.

81 Miscellaneous Renal and Genitourinary Agents

sevelamer hydrochloride
sildenafil citrate
tadalafil
vardenafil

Uses: Miscellaneous renal and GU agents are used for two different disorders. *Sevelamer* is prescribed to reduce the serum phosphorus level in patients with end-stage renal disease. *Sildenafil, tadalafil,* and *vardenafil* are used to treat male erectile dysfunction.

Action: Miscellaneous renal and GU agents have distinct actions. *Sevelamer* binds with dietary phosphorus in the GI, allowing it to be removed by normal digestive processes. *Sildenafil, tadalafil,* and *vardenafil* selectively inhibit phosphodiesterase type 5, the enzyme that normally degrades cyclic guanosine monophosphate in the corpus cavernosum of the penis. This action relaxes smooth muscle and increases blood flow to the corpus cavernosum, facilitating an erection.

sevelamer hydrochloride

seh-**vel**-a-mer
(Renagel)
Do not confuse Renagel with Reglan or Regonol.

CATEGORY AND SCHEDULE

Pregnancy Risk Category: C

MECHANISM OF ACTION

An antihyperphosphatemia agent that binds with dietary phosphorus in the GI tract, thus allowing phosphorus to be eliminated through the normal digestive process and decreasing the serum phosphorus level. **Therapeutic Effect:** Decreases incidence of hypercalcemic episodes in patients receiving calcium acetate treatment.

PHARMACOKINETICS

Not absorbed systemically. Unknown if removed by hemodialysis.

AVAILABILITY

Capsules: 403 mg.
Tablets: 400 mg, 800 mg.

INDICATIONS AND DOSAGES

▸ **Hyperphosphatemia**

PO

Adults, Elderly. 800–1,600 mg with each meal, depending on severity of hyperphosphatemia.

CONTRAINDICATIONS

Bowel obstruction, hypophosphatemia

INTERACTIONS

Drug
None known.
Herbal
None known.
Food
None known.

DIAGNOSTIC TEST EFFECTS
None known.

SIDE EFFECTS
Frequent (20%–11%)
Infection, pain, hypotension, diarrhea, dyspepsia, nausea, vomiting
Occasional (10%–1%)
Headache, constipation, hypertension, thrombosis, increased cough

SERIOUS REACTIONS
! None known.

NURSING CONSIDERATIONS
Baseline Assessment
• Obtain the patient's baseline serum phosphorus level.
• Assess the patient for signs of bowel obstruction, including absent bowel sounds, abdominal distention, and pain.
Lifespan Considerations
• Sevelamer is not distributed in breast milk.
• The safety and efficacy of sevelamer have not been established in children.
• No age-related precautions have been noted in the elderly.
Precautions
• Use sevelamer cautiously in patients with dysphagia, severe GI tract motility disorders, or swallowing disorders and in those who have undergone major GI tract surgery.
Administration and Handling
PO
• Give sevelamer with food.
• Don't break capsules apart because the contents expand in water.
• Give other medications at least 1 hour before or 3 hours after sevelamer.
Intervention and Evaluation
• Monitor the patient's serum bicarbonate, chloride, calcium, and phosphorus levels.
Patient Teaching
• Instruct the patient to take sevelamer with food and to swallow capsules or tablets whole.
• Tell the patient to take other medications at least 1 hour before or 3 hours after sevelamer.
• Warn the patient to notify the physician if he or she experiences diarrhea, signs of hypotension (such as light-headedness), nausea or vomiting, or a persistent headache.

sildenafil citrate
sill-**den**-a-fill
(Viagra)
Do not confuse Viagra with Vaniqa.

CATEGORY AND SCHEDULE
Pregnancy Risk Category: B

MECHANISM OF ACTION
An erectile dysfunction agent that inhibits phosphodiesterase type 5, the enzyme responsible for degrading cyclic guanosine monophosphate in the corpus cavernosum of the penis, resulting in smooth muscle relaxation and increased blood flow. **Therapeutic Effect:** Facilitates an erection.

AVAILABILITY
Tablets: 25 mg, 50 mg, 100 mg.

INDICATIONS AND DOSAGES
▸ **Erectile dysfunction**
PO
Adults. 50 mg (30 min–4 hr before sexual activity). Range: 25–100 mg. Maximum dosing frequency is once daily.
Elderly older than 65 yr. Consider starting dose of 25 mg.

OFF-LABEL USES
Treatment of diabetic gastroparesis, sexual dysfunction associated with the use of selective serotonin re-uptake inhibitors

CONTRAINDICATIONS
Concurrent use of sodium nitroprusside or nitrates in any form

INTERACTIONS
Drug
Cimetidine, erythromycin, itraconazole, ketoconazole: May increase sildenafil plasma concentration.
Nitrates: Potentiates the hypotensive effects of nitrates.
Herbal
None known.
Food
High-fat meals: Delay drug's maximum effectiveness by 1 hour.

DIAGNOSTIC TEST EFFECTS
None known.

SIDE EFFECTS
Frequent
Headache (16%), flushing (10%)
Occasional (7%–3%)
Dyspepsia, nasal congestion, UTI, abnormal vision, diarrhea
Rare (2%)
Dizziness, rash

SERIOUS REACTIONS
! Prolonged erections (lasting over 4 hours) and priapism (painful erections lasting over 6 hours) occur rarely.

NURSING CONSIDERATIONS
Baseline Assessment
- Assess the patient's cardiovascular status before beginning sildenafil treatment.

Precautions
- Use sildenafil cautiously in patients with an anatomic deformity of the penis; cardiac, hepatic, or renal impairment; or conditions that increase the risk of priapism, including leukemia, multiple myeloma, and sickle cell anemia.

Administration and Handling
PO
- Sildenafil is usually taken 1 hour before sexual activity but may be taken anywhere from 4 hours to 30 minutes beforehand.

Patient Teaching
- Tell the patient that sildenafil is not effective without sexual stimulation.
- Warn the patient to seek treatment immediately if an erection lasts longer than 4 hours.
- Instruct the patient to avoid using nitrate drugs concurrently with sildenafil.
- Inform the patient that high-fat meals may effect the drug's absorption rate and effectiveness.

tadalafil
tah-**dal**-ah-fill
(Cialis)

CATEGORY AND SCHEDULE
Pregnancy Risk Category: B

MECHANISM OF ACTION
An erectile dysfunction agent that inhibits phosphodiesterase type 5, the enzyme responsible for degrading cyclic guanosine monophosphate in the corpus cavernosum of the penis, resulting in smooth muscle relaxation and increased blood flow. **Therapeutic Effect:** Facilitates an erection.

PHARMACOKINETICS

Route	Onset	Peak	Duration
PO	16 min	2 hr	36 hr

Rapidly absorbed after PO administration. Drug has no effect on penile blood flow without sexual stimulation. ***Half-life:*** 17.5 hr.

AVAILABILITY

Tablets: 5 mg, 10 mg, 20 mg.

INDICATIONS AND DOSAGES

▸ Erectile dysfunction

PO

Adults, Elderly. 10 mg 30 min before sexual activity. Dose may be increased to 20 mg or decreased to 5 mg, based on patient tolerance. Maximum dosing frequency is once daily.

▸ Dosage in renal impairment

For patients with a creatinine clearance of 31-50 ml/min, the starting dose is 5 mg before sexual activity once a day and the maximum dose is 10 mg no more frequently than once q48h.

For patients with a creatinine clearance of less than 31 ml/min, the starting dose is 5 mg before sexual activity once a day.

▸ Dosage in mild or moderate hepatic impairment

Patients with Child-Pugh class A or B hepatic impairment should take no more than 10 mg once a day.

CONTRAINDICATIONS

Concurrent use of alpha-adrenergic blockers (other than the minimum dose tamsulosin), concurrent use of sodium nitroprusside or nitrates in any form, severe hepatic impairment

INTERACTIONS

Drug

Alcohol: Increases the risk of orthostatic hypotension.

Alpha-adrenergic blockers, nitrates: Potentiates the hypotensive effects of these drugs.

Doxazosin: May produce additive hypotensive effects.

Erythromycin, indinavir, itraconazole, ketoconazole, ritonavir: May increase tadalafil blood concentration.

Herbal

None known.

Food

None known.

DIAGNOSTIC TEST EFFECTS

None known.

SIDE EFFECTS

Occasional

Headache, dyspepsia, back pain, myalgia, nasal congestion, flushing

SERIOUS REACTIONS

! Prolonged erections (lasting over 4 hours) and priapism (painful erections lasting over 6 hours) occur rarely.

NURSING CONSIDERATIONS

Baseline Assessment

• Assess the patient's cardiovascular status before beginning tadalafil treatment.

Lifespan Considerations

• No age-related precautions have been noted in the elderly.

• This drug is not indicated for use in women and children.

Precautions

• Use tadalafil cautiously in patients with an anatomical deformity of the penis; cardiac, hepatic, or renal impairment; or conditions that may increase the risk of priapism, such as leukemia, multiple myeloma, and sickle cell anemia.

Administration and Handling

PO

- Give tadalafil without regard to food.
- Don't crush or break film-coated tablets.

Patient Teaching

- Inform the patient that tadalafil has no effect without sexual stimulation.
- Warn the patient to seek treatment immediately if an erection lasts longer than 4 hours.
- Instruct the patient to avoid using nitrate drugs and alpha-adrenergic blockers concurrently with tadalafil.

vardenafil

var-**den**-ah-fill

(Levitra)

Do not confuse Levitra with Lexiva.

CATEGORY AND SCHEDULE

Pregnancy Risk Category: B

MECHANISM OF ACTION

An erectile dysfunction agent that inhibits phosphodiesterase type 5, the enzyme responsible for degrading cyclic guanosine monophosphate in the corpus cavernosum of the penis, resulting in smooth muscle relaxation and increased blood flow. **Therapeutic Effect:** Facilitates an erection.

PHARMACOKINETICS

Rapidly absorbed after PO administration. Extensive tissue distribution. Protein binding: 95%. Metabolized in the liver. Excreted primarily in feces; a lesser amount eliminated in urine. Drug has no effect on penile blood flow without sexual stimulation. ***Half-life:*** 4–5 hr.

AVAILABILITY

Tablets: 2.5 mg, 5 mg, 10 mg, 20 mg.

INDICATIONS AND DOSAGES

▸ **Erectile dysfunction**

PO

Adults. 10 mg approximately 1 hr before sexual activity. Dose may be increased to 20 mg or decreased to 5 mg, based on patient tolerance. Maximum dosing frequency is once daily.

Elderly older than 65 yr. 5 mg.

▸ **Dosage in moderate hepatic impairment**

PO

For patients with Child-Pugh class B hepatic impairment, dosage is 5 mg 60 min before sexual activity.

▸ **Dosage with concurrent ritonavir**

PO

Adults. 2.5 mg in a 72-hr period.

▸ **Dosage with concurrent ketoconazole or itraconazole (at 400 mg/day), or indinavir**

PO

Adults. 2.5 mg in a 24-hour period.

▸ **Dosage with concurrent ketoconazole or itraconazole (at 200 mg/day), or erythromycin**

PO

Adults. 5 mg in a 24-hr period.

CONTRAINDICATIONS

Concurrent use of alpha-adrenergic blockers, sodium nitroprusside, or nitrates in any form

INTERACTIONS

Drug

Alpha-adrenergic blockers, nitrates: Potentiates the hypotensive effects of these drugs.

Erythromycin, indinavir, itraconazole, ketoconazole, ritonavir: May increase vardenafil blood concentration.

Herbal

None known.

Food

High-fat meals: Delay drug's maximum effectiveness.

DIAGNOSTIC TEST EFFECTS

None known.

SIDE EFFECTS

Occasional

Headache, flushing, rhinitis, indigestion

Rare (less than 2%)

Dizziness, changes in color vision, blurred vision

SERIOUS REACTIONS

! Prolonged erections (lasting over 4 hours) and priapism (painful erections lasting over 6 hours) occur rarely.

NURSING CONSIDERATIONS

Baseline Assessment

- Assess the patient's cardiovascular status before beginning vardenafil treatment.

Lifespan Considerations

- No age-related precautions have been noted in the elderly, but their initial dose should be 5 mg.

Precautions

- Use vardenafil cautiously in patients with an anatomical deformity of the penis; cardiac, hepatic, or renal impairment; conditions that may increase the risk of priapism, including leukemia, multiple myeloma, and sickle cell anemia.

Administration and Handling

PO

- Administer vardenafil approximately 1 hour before sexual activity.
- Don't crush or break film-coated tablets.

Patient Teaching

- Inform the patient that the drug has no effect without sexual stimulation.
- Warn the patient to seek treatment immediately if an erection lasts longer than 4 hours.
- Instruct the patient to avoid using nitrate drugs and alpha-adrenergic blockers concurrently with vardenafil.
- Inform the patient that high-fat meals delay the drug's maximum effectiveness.

82 Antihistamines

azelastine
cetirizine
clemastine fumarate
desloratidine
diphenhydramine hydrochloride
epinastine
fexofenadine hydrochloride
hydroxyzine
loratadine
promethazine hydrochloride

Uses: Antihistamines are chiefly used to relieve symptoms of upper respiratory allergic disorders. They're also used to manage allergic reactions to other drugs as well as blood transfusion reactions. These agents are used as a second choice in treating angioneurotic edema. Some can be used to provide preoperative and postoperative sedation, to manage insomnia, to relieve anxiety and tension, and to control muscle spasms. They also may be used to treat acute urticaria, and other dermatologic conditions, motion sickness, and Parkinson's disease. In addition, an ophthalmic form of azelastine is used to treat conjunctivitis.

Action: As histamine (H_1) antagonists, antihistamines cause vasoconstriction, which helps decrease edema, bronchodilation, and mucus secretion. These agents also block the increased capillary permeability and formation of edema and wheals caused by histamine. Many antihistamines can bind to receptors in the CNS, causing primarily depression (with decreased alertness, slowed reaction times, and somnolence), but also stimulation (with restlessness, nervousness, and inability to sleep). Some may counter motion sickness. (See the illustration *Sites of Action: Respiratory Agents,* page 1426.)

COMBINATION PRODUCTS

ALLEGRA-D: fexofenadine/pseudoephedrine (a nasal decongestant) 60 mg/120 mg.
ALLEGRA-D 24 HOUR: fexofenadine/pseudoephedrine (a nasal decongestant) 180 mg/240 mg.
CALADRYL: diphenhydramine/calamine (an astringent)/camphor (a counterirritant).
CLARITIN-D: loratadine/pseudoephedrine (a nasal decongestant) 5 mg/120 mg; 10 mg/240 mg.
PHENERGAN WITH CODEINE: promethazine/codeine (a cough suppressant) 6.25 mg/10 mg per 5 ml.
PHENERGAN VC: promethazine/phenylephrine (a vasopressor) 6.25 mg/5 mg per 5 ml.
PHENERGAN VC WITH CODEINE: promethazine/phenylephrine (a vasopressor)/codeine (a cough suppressant) 6.25 mg/5 mg/10 mg per 5 ml.
ZYRTEC D-12 HOUR: cetirizine/pseudoephedrine (a nasal decongestant) 5 mg/120 mg.
HYDROXYZINE: See antianxiety agents

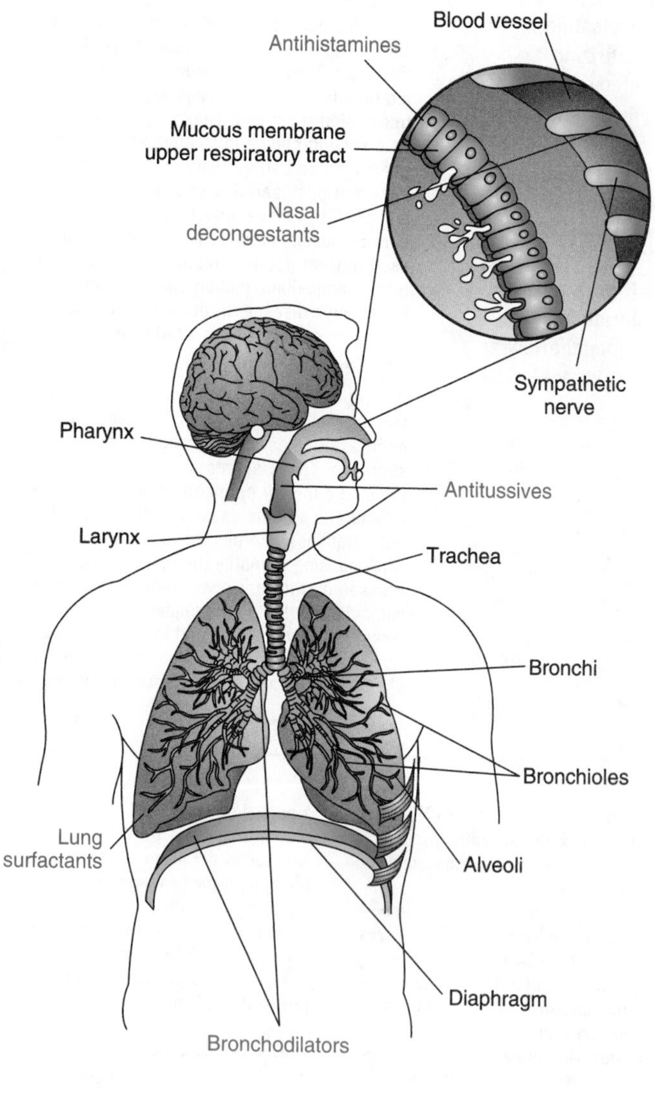
Blood vessel
Antihistamines
Mucous membrane
upper respiratory tract
Nasal
decongestants
Sympathetic
nerve
Pharynx
Antitussives
Larynx
Trachea
Bronchi
Bronchioles
Lung
surfactants
Alveoli
Diaphragm
Bronchodilators

Sites of Action: Respiratory Agents

Several clsses of drugs are used to manage respiratory disorders. Each class—and individual drugs within each class—can act at different sites in the respiratory tract.

Antihistamines, such as diphenhydramine, help relieve symptoms of upper respiratory allergic disorders by blocking the stimulation of histamine$_1$ (H_1) receptors primarily in the mucous membranes of the upper respiratory tract. Normally, stimulation of H_1 receptors results in vasodilation, increased capillary permeability and mucous secretion, and bronchoconstriction. Antihistamine's blocking of H_1 receptors results in vasoconstriction, which decreases edema, capillary permeability, and mucus secretion. The drugs also cause bronchodilation, improving airflow to and from the lungs. Unlike first-generation antihistamines, such as diphenhydramine, which cross the blood-brain barrier and cause sedation, second-generation antihistamines, such as loratadine, don't cross the blood-brain barrier and produce little or no sedation.

Non-narcotic antitussives, such as benzonatate, act on the stretch and cough receptors in the respiratory tract, including the pharynx, larynx, and tracheobronchial tree. Because benzonatate also has local anesthetic properties, it anesthetizes irritated tissues and suppresses cough. Another antitussive, guaifenesin, has an expectorant action that increases respiratory tract secretions by making mucus less viscous and adhesive and making the cough more productive.

All bronchodilators open the bronchioles to improve airflow. However, subclasses of bronchodilators work in different ways. Beta$_2$-adrenergic agonists may be short-acting, such as albuterol, or long-acting, such as salmeterol. Both types stimulate beta$_2$ receptors in the lungs, resulting in relaxation of bronchial smooth muscle, increased vital capacity, and decreased airway resistance. These agents also block histamine release from mast cells, decreasing capillary permeability and mucus secretion. Anticholinergics, such as ipratropium, block muscarinic cholinergic receptors in the bronchi, leading to bronchodilation. These drugs exert more action on larger airways, whereas beta$_2$-adrenergic agonists act primarily on smaller airways, Methylxanthines, such as aminophylline, relax bronchial smooth muscle and promote bronchodilation by inhibiting phosphodietsterase and adenosine. These drugs also increase the contractility of the diaphragm and may enhance mucus clearance.

Lung surfactants, such as beractant, restore pulmonary surfactant in infants who have a deficiency of it. They work by lowering the surface tension on alveoli. As a result, the alveoli become more stable and less likely to collapse. These actions lead to improved lung compliance and respiratory gas exchange.

Nasal decongestants, such as pseudoephedrine, constrict blood vessels in the nose by mimicking the actions of the sympathetic nervous system. They directly stimulate alpha$_1$-adrenergic receptors in the smooth muscle of nasal blood vessels, which shrinks swollen mucous membranes and decreases mucus production by reducing fluid exudation.

azelastine

a-zel-ah-steen
(Astelin, Optivar)
Do not confuse Optivar with Optiray.

CATEGORY AND SCHEDULE

Pregnancy Risk Category: C

MECHANISM OF ACTION

An antihistamine that competes with histamine for histamine receptor sites on cells in the blood vessels, GI tract, and respiratory tract. **Therapeutic Effect:** Relieves symptoms associated with seasonal allergic rhinitis such as increased mucus production and sneezing and symptoms associated with allergic conjunctivitis, such as redness, itching, and excessive tearing.

PHARMACOKINETICS

Route	Onset	Peak	Duration
Nasal spray	0.5–1 hr	2–3 hr	12 hr
Ophthalmic	N/A	3 min	8 hr

Well absorbed through nasal mucosa. Primarily excreted in feces. ***Half-life:*** 22 hr.

AVAILABILITY

Nasal Spray (Astelin): 137 mcg.
Ophthalmic Solution (Optivar): 0.05%.

INDICATIONS AND DOSAGES

▸ **Allergic rhinitis**

Nasal

Adults, Elderly, Children 12 yr and older. 2 sprays in each nostril twice a day.

Children 5–11 yr. 1 spray in each nostril twice a day.

▸ **Allergic conjunctivitis**

Ophthalmic

Adults, Elderly, Children 3 yr or older. 1 drop into affected eye twice a day.

CONTRAINDICATIONS

Breast-feeding women, history of hypersensitivity to antihistamines, neonates or premature infants, third trimester of pregnancy

INTERACTIONS

Drug

Alcohol, other CNS depressants: May increase CNS depression.

Cimetidine: May increase azelastine blood concentration.

Herbal

None known.

Food

None known.

DIAGNOSTIC TEST EFFECTS

May increase ALT (SGPT) levels. May suppress flare and wheal reactions to antigen skin testing unless drug is discontinued 4 days before testing.

SIDE EFFECTS

Frequent (20%–15%)

Headache, bitter taste

Rare

Nasal burning, paroxysmal sneezing
Ophthalmic: Transient eye burning or stinging, bitter taste, headache

SERIOUS REACTIONS

! Epistaxis occurs rarely.

NURSING CONSIDERATIONS

Baseline Assessment

• Determine if the patient has a hypersensitivity to antihistamines.

Lifespan Considerations

• It is unknown if azelastine crosses the placenta or is distributed in breast milk.
• Don't use azelastine during the third trimester of pregnancy.
• The safety and efficacy of azelastine have not been established in children younger than 12 years.
• No age-related precautions have been noted in the elderly.

Precautions

• Use azelastine cautiously in patients with renal impairment.

Administration and Handling

Nasal

• Clear the patient's nasal passages as much as possible before use.
• Tilt the patient's head slightly forward.
• Insert the applicator tip into one the nostril, pointing the tip toward the nasal passage and away from the nasal septum.
• While holding the other nostril closed, spray into the nostril and

have the patient inhale at the same time to deliver the drug as high into the nasal passages as possible.
- Repeat in the other nostril

Ophthalmic
- Tilt the patient's head back and instill the solution in the conjunctival sac of the affected eye.
- Have the patient close the eye; then press gently on the lacrimal sac for 1 minute.

Intervention and Evaluation
- Assess the patient's therapeutic response to the medication.

Patient Teaching
- Advise the patient to clear his or her nasal passages before using azelastine.
- Teach the patient to prime the pump with 4 sprays or until a fine mist appears before using the nasal spray the first time. After the first use and if the pump hasn't been used for 3 or more days, tell the patient to prime the pump with 2 sprays or until a fine mist appears.
- Instruct the patient to wipe the applicator tip with a clean, damp tissue and to replace the cap immediately after use.
- Warn the patient to avoid spraying the nasal drug into the eyes.
- Advise the patient to avoid drinking alcoholic beverages during azelastine therapy.

cetirizine

si-**tear**-a-zeen

(Reactine[CAN], Zyrtec)

Do not confuse Zyrtec with Zantac or Zyprexa.

CATEGORY AND SCHEDULE

Pregnancy Risk Category: B

MECHANISM OF ACTION

A second-generation piperazine that competes with histamine for H_1-receptor sites on effector cells in the GI tract, blood vessels, and respiratory tract. **Therapeutic Effect:** Prevents allergic response, produces mild bronchodilation, blocks histamine-induced bronchitis.

PHARMACOKINETICS

Route	Onset	Peak	Duration
PO	less than 1 hr	4–8 hr	less than 24 hr

Rapidly and almost completely absorbed from the GI tract (absorption not affected by food). Protein binding: 93%. Undergoes low first-pass metabolism; not extensively metabolized. Primarily excreted in urine (more than 80% as unchanged drug). ***Half-life:*** 6.5–10 hr.

AVAILABILITY

Syrup: 5 mg/5 ml.
Tablets: 5 mg, 10 mg.
Tablets (Chewable): 5 mg, 10 mg.

INDICATIONS AND DOSAGES

▸ **Allergic rhinitis, urticaria**

PO

Adults, Elderly, Children older than 5 yr. Initially, 5–10 mg/day as a single or in 2 divided doses.
Children 2–5 yr. 2.5 mg/day. May increase up to 5 mg/day as a single or in 2 divided doses.
Children 12–23 mo. Initially, 2.5 mg/day. May increase up to 5 mg/day in 2 divided doses.
Children 6–11 mo. 2.5 mg once a day.

▸ **Dosage in renal or hepatic impairment**

For adult and elderly patients with renal impairment (creatinine clearance of 11–31 ml/min), those receiving hemodialysis (creatinine clearance of less than 7 ml/min), and those with hepatic impairment, dosage is decreased to 5 mg once a day.

OFF-LABEL USES

Treatment of bronchial asthma

CONTRAINDICATIONS

Hypersensitivity to cetirizine or hydroxyzine

INTERACTIONS

Drug

Alcohol, other CNS depressants: May increase CNS depression.

Herbal

None known.

Food

None known.

DIAGNOSTIC TEST EFFECTS

May suppress wheal and flare reactions to antigen skin testing, unless drug is discontinued 4 days before testing.

SIDE EFFECTS

Occasional (10%–2%)

Pharyngitis; dry mucous membranes, nose, or throat; nausea and vomiting; abdominal pain; headache; dizziness; fatigue; thickening of mucus; somnolence; photosensitivity; urine retention

SERIOUS REACTIONS

! Children may experience paradoxical reactions, including restlessness, insomnia, euphoria, nervousness, and tremor.

! Dizziness, sedation, and confusion are more likely to occur in elderly patients.

NURSING CONSIDERATIONS

Baseline Assessment

- Auscultate the patient's breath sounds.
- Assess the severity of the patient's rhinitis, urticaria, or other symptoms.
- Expect to obtain the patient's liver function test results to assess hepatic function.

Lifespan Considerations

- Cetirizine use is not recommended during the early months of pregnancy.
- It is unknown if cetirizine is excreted in breast milk. Breast-feeding is not recommended for patients taking this drug.
- Cetirizine is less likely to cause anticholinergic effects in children.
- Elderly patients are more likely to experience anticholinergic effects, such as dry mouth and urine retention, as well as dizziness, sedation, and confusion.

Precautions

- Use cetirizine cautiously in patients with renal or hepatic impairment.
- Remember that cetirizine may cause drowsiness at dosages greater than 10 mg/day.

Administration and Handling

PO

- Give cetirizine without regard to food.

Intervention and Evaluation

- Ensure that the patient with upper respiratory allergies increases fluid intake to maintain thin secretions and offset thirst.
- Monitor the patient's symptoms for a therapeutic response.

Patient Teaching

- Warn the patient to avoid performing tasks that require alertness or motor skills until his or her response to the drug has been established. Inform the patient that cetirizine may cause drowsiness.

• Urge the patient to avoid alcohol during cetirizine therapy.
• Advise the patient to avoid prolonged exposure to sunlight.

clemastine fumarate

klem-as-teen
(Dayhistol Allergy, Tavist Allergy)

CATEGORY AND SCHEDULE

Pregnancy Risk Category: B

MECHANISM OF ACTION

An ethanolamine that competes with histamine on effector cells in the GI tract, blood vessels, and respiratory tract. **Therapeutic Effect:** Relieves allergy symptoms, including urticaria, rhinitis, and pruritus.

PHARMACOKINETICS

Route	Onset	Peak	Duration
PO	15–60 min	5–7 hr	10–12 hr

Well absorbed from the GI tract. Metabolized in the liver. Excreted primarily in urine.

AVAILABILITY

Syrup (Dayhist, Tavist): 0.67 mg/5 ml.
Tablets (Dayhist, Tavist): 1.34 mg, 2.68 mg.

INDICATIONS AND DOSAGES

▸ **Allergic rhinitis, urticaria**

PO

Adults, Children older than 11 yr. 1.34 mg twice a day up to 2.68 mg 3 times a day. Maximum: 8.04 mg/day.
Children 6–11 yr. 0.67–1.34 mg twice a day. Maximum: 4.02 mg/day.
Children younger than 6 yr. 0.05 mg/kg/day divided into 2–3 doses per day. Maximum: 1.34 mg/day.
Elderly. 1.34 mg 1–2 times a day.

CONTRAINDICATIONS

Angle-closure glaucoma, hypersensitivity to clemastine, use within 14 days of MAOIs

INTERACTIONS

Drug

Alcohol, other CNS depressants: May increase CNS depression.
MAOIs: May increase the anticholinergic and CNS depressant effects of clemastine.

Herbal

None known.

Food

None known.

DIAGNOSTIC TEST EFFECTS

May suppress wheal and flare reactions to antigen skin testing unless drug is discontinued 4 days before testing.

SIDE EFFECTS

Frequent

Somnolence, dizziness, urine retention, thickening of bronchial secretions, dry mouth, nose, or throat; in elderly, sedation, dizziness, hypotension

Occasional

Epigastric distress, flushing, blurred vision, tinnitus, paresthesia, diaphoresis, chills

SERIOUS REACTIONS

! A hypersensitivity reaction, marked by eczema, pruritus, rash, cardiac disturbances, angioedema, and photosensitivity, may occur.
! Overdose symptoms may vary from CNS depression, including sedation, apnea, cardiovascular collapse, and death, to severe

paradoxical reaction, such as hallucinations, tremor, and seizures.
! Children may experience paradoxical reactions, such as restlessness, insomnia, euphoria, nervousness, and tremors.
! Overdose in children may result in hallucinations, seizures, and death.

NURSING CONSIDERATIONS

Baseline Assessment

- For patients undergoing an allergic reaction, obtain a history of recently ingested drugs and foods, environmental exposure, and emotional stress.
- Monitor the patient's pulse rate and quality as well as respiratory rate, rhythm, and depth.
- Auscultate the patient's breath sounds for crackles, rhonchi, and wheezing.

Lifespan Considerations

- Clemastine is excreted in breast milk and should not be used in breast-feeding women.
- The safety and efficacy of clemastine have not been established in children younger than 6 years.
- Age-related renal impairment may require a dosage adjustment in the elderly.

Precautions

- Use clemastine cautiously in patients with asthma, GI or GU obstruction, peptic ulcer disease, or benign prostatic hyperplasia.

Administration and Handling

◀ALERT▶ Be aware that the fixed-combination form Tavist-D may produce mild CNS stimulation.
PO
- Give clemastine without regard to food.
- Crush scored tablets as needed.

Intervention and Evaluation

- Monitor the patient's BP, especially in elderly patients who are at increased risk for developing hypotension.
- Monitor children closely for paradoxical reaction.

Patient Teaching

- Inform the patient that dizziness, drowsiness, and dry mouth are expected side effects of clemastine but that he or she may develop a tolerance to the sedative effects. Explain that consuming coffee and tea may help reduce drowsiness.
- Warn the patient to avoid performing tasks that require mental alertness or motor skills until his or her response to the drug has been established.
- Urge the patient to avoid alcohol during clemastine therapy.

desloratidine

des-loer-**at**-ah-deen
(Aerius[CAN], Clarinex, Clarinex Redi-Tabs)
Do not confuse Clarinex with Claritin.

CATEGORY AND SCHEDULE

Pregnancy Risk Category: C

MECHANISM OF ACTION

A nonsedating antihistamine that exhibits selective peripheral histamine H_1 receptor blocking action. Competes with histamine at receptor sites. **Therapeutic Effect:** Prevents allergic responses mediated by histamine, such as rhinitis and urticaria.

PHARMACOKINETICS

Rapidly and almost completely absorbed from the GI tract. Distributed mainly in liver, lungs, GI tract, and bile. Metabolized in the liver to active metabolite and undergoes extensive first-pass metabolism. Eliminated in urine and feces. ***Half-life:*** 27 hr (increased in the elderly and in renal or hepatic impairment).

AVAILABILITY

Tablets: 5 mg.
Tablets (Orally Disintegrating [Reditabs]): 5 mg.
Syrup: 2.5 mg/5 ml.

INDICATIONS AND DOSAGES

▸ **Allergic rhinitis, urticaria**

PO

Adults, Elderly, Children older than 12 yr. 5 mg once a day.

▸ **Dosage in hepatic or renal impairment**

Dosage is decreased to 5 mg every other day.

CONTRAINDICATIONS

None known.

INTERACTIONS

Drug

Erythromycin, ketoconazole: May increase desloratadine blood concentration.

Herbal

None known.

Food

None known.

DIAGNOSTIC TEST EFFECTS

May suppress wheal and flare reactions to antigen skin testing unless the drug is discontinued 4 days before testing.

SIDE EFFECTS

Frequent (12%)
Headache
Occasional (3%)
Dry mouth, somnolence
Rare (less than 3%)
Fatigue, dizziness, diarrhea, nausea

SERIOUS REACTIONS

! None known.

NURSING CONSIDERATIONS

Baseline Assessment

- Auscultate the patient's breath sounds for wheezing.
- Examine the patient being treated for urticaria.
- Plan to discontinue the drug 4 days before antigen skin testing.

Lifespan Considerations

- Desloratadine is excreted in breast milk and should not be used by breast-feeding women.
- The safety and efficacy of desloratadine have not been established in children younger than 6 years.
- Children and the elderly are more sensitive to the drug's anticholinergic effects, such as dry mouth, nose, and throat.

Precautions

- Use desloratadine cautiously in patients with hepatic impairment.

Administration and Handling

PO

- Don't crush or break film-coated tablets.

◂ALERT▸ Desloratadine is 2.5–4 times more potent than its parent compound, loratadine.

Intervention and Evaluation

- Increase the fluid intake in patients with upper respiratory allergies to decrease the viscosity of secretions, offset thirst, and replace fluids lost from diaphoresis.
- Monitor the patient for a therapeutic response.

Patient Teaching

- Inform the patient that desloratadine does not cause drowsiness.
- Warn the patient to avoid performing tasks that require mental alertness or motor skills until his or her response to the drug has been established.

• Urge the patient to avoid consuming alcohol during desloratadine therapy.

diphenhydramine hydrochloride

dye-fen-**hye**-dra-meen
(Allerdryl[CAN], Banophen, Benadryl, Diphen, Diphenhist, Genahist, Nytol[CAN], Unisom Sleepgels[AUS])

Do not confuse diphenhydramine with dimenhydrinate; or Benadryl with benazepril, Bentyl, or Benylin; or Banophen with baclofen.

CATEGORY AND SCHEDULE

Pregnancy Risk Category: B
OTC (capsules, tablets, chewable tablets, syrup, elixir, cream, spray)

MECHANISM OF ACTION

An ethanolamine that competitively blocks the effects of histamine at peripheral H_1 receptor sites. **Therapeutic Effect:** Produces anticholinergic, antipruritic, antitussive, antiemetic, antidyskinetic, and sedative effects.

PHARMACOKINETICS

Route	Onset	Peak	Duration
PO	15–30 min	1–4 hr	4–6 hr
IV, IM	less than 15 min	1–4 hr	4–6 hr

Well absorbed after PO or parenteral administration.Protein binding: 98%–99%. Widely distributed. Metabolized in the liver. Primarily excreted in urine. ***Half-life:*** 1–4 hr.

AVAILABILITY

Capsules (Banophen, Diphen, Genahist): 25 mg.
Capsules (Nytol): 50 mg.
Syrup (Diphen, Diphenhist): 12.5 mg/5 ml.
Tablets (Banophen, Benadryl, Genahist, Nytol): 25 mg, 50 mg.
Injection (Benadryl): 50 mg/ml.
Cream (Benadryl): 1%, 2%.
Spray: 1%, 2%.

INDICATIONS AND DOSAGES

▸ **Moderate to severe allergic reaction, dystonic reaction**
PO, IV, IM
Adults, Elderly. 25–50 mg q4h. Maximum: 400 mg/day.
Children. 5 mg/kg/day in divided doses q6–8h. Maximum: 300 mg/day.

▸ **Motion sickness, minor allergic rhinitis**
PO, IV, IM
Adults, Elderly, Children 12 yr and older. 25–50 mg q4–6h. Maximum: 300 mg/day.
Children 6–11 yr. 12.5–25 mg q4–6h. Maximum: 150 mg/day.
Children 2–5 yr. 6.25 mg q4–6h. Maximum: 37.5 mg/day.

▸ **Antitussive**
PO
Adults, Elderly, Children 12 yr and older. 25 mg q4h. Maximum: 150 mg/day.
Children 6–11 yr. 12.5 mg q4h. Maximum: 75 mg/day.
Children 2–5 yr. 6.25 mg q4h. Maximum: 37.5 mg/day.

▸ **Nighttime sleep aid**
PO
Adults, Elderly, Children 12 yr and older. 50 mg at bedtime.
Children 2–11 yr. 1 mg/kg/dose. Maximum: 50 mg.

▸ **Pruritus**
Topical
Adults, Elderly, Children 12 yr and

older. Apply 1% or 2% cream or spray 3–4 times a day.
Children 2–11 yr. Apply 1% cream or spray 3–4 times a day.

CONTRAINDICATIONS

Acute exacerbation of asthma, use within 14 days of MAOIs

INTERACTIONS

Drug

Alcohol, other CNS depressants: May increase CNS depressant effects.
Anticholinergics: May increase anticholinergic effects.
MAOIs: May increase the anticholinergic and CNS depressant effects of diphenhydramine.

Herbal

None known.

Food

None known.

DIAGNOSTIC TEST EFFECTS

May suppress wheal and flare reactions to antigen skin testing unless the drug is discontinued 4 days before testing.

IV INCOMPATIBILITIES

Allopurinol (Aloprim), amphotericin B complex (Abelcet, AmBisome, Amphotec), cefepime (Maxipime), dexamethasone (Decadron), foscarnet (Foscavir)

IV COMPATIBILITIES

Atropine, cisplatin (Platinol), cyclophosphamide (Cytoxan), cytarabine (Ara-C), droperidol (Inapsine), fentanyl, glycopyrrolate (Robinul), heparin, hydrocortisone (Solu-Cortef), hydromorphone (Dilaudid), hydroxyzine (Vistaril), lidocaine, metoclopramide (Reglan), ondansetron (Zofran), promethazine (Phenergan), potassium chloride, propofol (Diprivan)

SIDE EFFECTS

Frequent
Somnolence, dizziness, muscle weakness, hypotension, urine retention, thickening of bronchial secretions, dry mouth, nose, throat, or lips; in elderly, sedation, dizziness, hypotension
Occasional
Epigastric distress, flushing, visual or hearing disturbances, paresthesia, diaphoresis, chills

SERIOUS REACTIONS

! Hypersensitivity reactions, such as eczema, pruritus, rash, cardiac disturbances, and photosensitivity, may occur.
! Overdose symptoms may vary from CNS depression, including sedation, apnea, hypotension, cardiovascular collapse, and death, to severe paradoxical reactions, such as hallucinations, tremor, and seizures.
! Children and neonates may experience paradoxical reactions, including restlessness, insomnia, euphoria, nervousness, and tremors.
! Overdosage in children may result in hallucinations, seizures, and death.

NURSING CONSIDERATIONS

Baseline Assessment

- If the patient is having an acute allergic reaction, obtain a history of recently ingested drugs and food, emotional stress, and environmental exposure.
- Monitor the patient's respiratory rate, depth, and rhythm and pulse rate and quality.
- Auscultate the patient's breath sounds for crackles, rhonchi, and wheezing.
- Plan to discontinue the drug 4 days before antigen skin testing.

Lifespan Considerations

- Diphenhydramine crosses the

placenta and appears in breast milk. Its use by breast-feeding women may inhibit lactation and produce irritability in breast-feeding infants.
• Use of the drug during the third trimester of pregnancy increases the risk of seizures in neonates and premature infants.
• Diphenhydramine is not recommended for children, neonates, or premature infants because they're at an increased risk for paradoxical reactions.
• The elderly are at increased risk for developing confusion, dizziness, hyperexcitability, hypotension, and sedation.

Precautions

• Use diphenhydramine cautiously in patients with asthma, cardiovascular disease, COPD, hypertension, hyperthyroidism, angle-closure glaucoma, increased IOP, peptic ulcer disease, benign prostatic hyperplasia, pyloroduodenal or bladder neck obstruction, or seizure disorders.

Administration and Handling

PO
• Give diphenhydramine without regard to food.
• Crush scored tablets as needed. Don't crush, break, or open capsules or film-coated tablets.

IM
• Inject diphenhydramine deep into a large muscle mass.

IV
• Diphenhydramine may be given undiluted.
• Administer IV injection over at least 1 minute.

Intervention and Evaluation

• Monitor the patient's BP, especially in the elderly because they have an increased risk of developing hypotension.
• Monitor children closely for paradoxical reactions.

Patient Teaching

• Inform the patient that dizziness, drowsiness, and dry mouth are expected side effects of diphenhydramine but that he or she may develop a tolerance to the drug's sedative effects.
• Warn the patient to avoid performing tasks that require mental alertness or motor skills until his or her response to the drug has been established.
• Urge the patient to avoid consuming alcohol during diphenhydramine therapy.

epinastine

eh-pin-**ass**-teen
(Elestat)

CATEGORY AND SCHEDULE

Pregnancy Risk Category: C

MECHANISM OF ACTION

An ophthalmic H_1 receptor antagonist that inhibits the release of histamine from the mast cell. **Therapeutic Effect:** Prevents pruritus associated with allergic conjunctivitis.

PHARMACOKINETICS

Low systemic exposure. Protein binding: 64%. Less than 10% is metabolized. Excreted primarily in urine and, to a lesser extent, in feces. ***Half-life:*** 12 hr.

AVAILABILITY

Ophthalmic Solution: 0.05%.

INDICATIONS AND DOSAGES

▸ **Allergic conjunctivitis**

Ophthalmic

Adults, Elderly, Children 3 yr and older. 1 drop in each eye twice a day. Continue treatment until period of exposure (pollen season, exposure to offending allergen) is over.

CONTRAINDICATIONS
None known.

INTERACTIONS
Drug
None known.
Herbal
None known.
Food
None known.

DIAGNOSTIC TEST EFFECTS
None known.

SIDE EFFECTS
Occasional
Ocular (10%–1%): Burning sensation in the eye, hyperemia, pruritus
Non-ocular (10%): Cold symptoms, upper respiratory tract infection
Rare (3%–1%)
Headache, rhinitis, sinusitis, increased cough, pharyngitis

SERIOUS REACTIONS
! None known.

NURSING CONSIDERATIONS
Baseline Assessment
- Assess the degree of eye inflammation, including redness, amount and color of discharge, and excessive tearing, before and regularly during therapy.

Lifespan Considerations
- It is not known if epinastine is distributed in breast milk.
- The safety and efficacy of epinastine have not been established in children younger than 3 years.
- No age-related precautions have been noted in the elderly.

Administration and Handling
Ophthalmic
- Don't let the applicator tip touch any surface.
- Place a gloved finger on the patient's lower eyelid, and pull it out until a pocket is formed between the eye and lower lid.
- Hold the dropper above the pocket, and place the prescribed number of drops in the pocket.
- Instruct the patient to close the affected eye gently so the medication won't squeeze out of the lacrimal sac.
- Apply gentle pressure to the lacrimal sac at the inner canthus for 1 minute after installation to lessen the risk of systemic absorption.

Intervention and Evaluation
- Monitor the patient for eye burning or stinging and headache.
- Assess the patient for a therapeutic response.

Patient Teaching
- Instruct the patient to remove contact lenses before instilling epinastine because the lenses may absorb the drug's preservatives. The lenses may be reinserted 10 minutes after administration unless the treated eye is red.
- Explain that epinastine is not for treatment of contact lens–related irritation.

fexofenadine hydrochloride
fex-oh-**fen**-eh-deen
(Allegra, Telfast[AUS])

CATEGORY AND SCHEDULE
Pregnancy Risk Category: C

MECHANISM OF ACTION
A piperidine that competes with histamine for H_1 receptor sites on effector cells. **Therapeutic Effect:** Relieves allergic rhinitis symptoms.

PHARMACOKINETICS

Rapidly absorbed after PO administration. Protein binding: 60%–70%. Does not cross the blood-brain barrier. Minimally metabolized. Eliminated in feces and urine. Not removed by hemodialysis. ***Half-life:*** 14.4 hr (increased in renal impairment).

AVAILABILITY

Tablets: 30 mg, 60 mg, 180 mg.

INDICATIONS AND DOSAGES

▸ Allergic rhinitis, urticaria

PO

Adults, Elderly, Children 12 yr and older. 60 mg twice a day or 180 mg once a day.

Children 6–11 yr. 30 mg twice a day.

▸ Dosage in renal impairment

For adults, elderly, and children 12 years and older, dosage is reduced to 60 mg once a day. For children 6–11 years, dosage is reduced to 30 mg once a day.

CONTRAINDICATIONS

None known.

INTERACTIONS

Drug

Antacids. May decrease fexofenadine absorption if given within 15 minutes of a fexofenadine dose.

Herbal

None known.

Food

None known.

DIAGNOSTIC TEST EFFECTS

May suppress wheal and flare reactions to antigen skin testing unless drug is discontinued at least 4 days before testing.

SIDE EFFECTS

Rare (less than 2%)

Somnolence, headache, fatigue, nausea, vomiting, abdominal distress, dysmenorrhea

SERIOUS REACTIONS

! None known.

NURSING CONSIDERATIONS

Baseline Assessment

- Obtain the history of recently ingested drugs and foods, emotional stress, and environmental exposure in patients undergoing an allergic reaction.
- Monitor the patient's respiratory rate, depth, and rhythm and pulse rate and quality.
- Auscultate the patient's breath sounds for crackles, rhonchi, and wheezing.
- Plan to discontinue the drug 4 days before antigen skin testing.

Lifespan Considerations

- It is unknown if fexofenadine crosses the placenta or is distributed in breast milk.
- The safety and efficacy of fexofenadine have not been established in children younger than 12 years.
- No age-related precautions have been noted in the elderly.

Precautions

- Use fexofenadine cautiously in patients with severe renal impairment.

Administration and Handling

PO

- Give fexofenadine without regard to food.

Intervention and Evaluation

- Assess the patient for relief of allergy symptoms including rhinorrhea, sneezing, itching, and red, watery eyes.

Patient Teaching

- Warn the patient to avoid performing tasks that require mental alertness or motor skills until his or her response to the drug has been established.

• Inform the patient that drinking coffee or tea may help reduce drowsiness.

• Urge the patient to avoid alcohol during antihistamine therapy.

hydroxyzine

See Antianxiety Agents

loratadine

loer-**at**-ah-deen

(Alavert, Claratyne[AUS], Claritin, Claritin RediTab, Dimetapp, Tavist ND)

CATEGORY AND SCHEDULE

Pregnancy Risk Category: B

MECHANISM OF ACTION

A long-acting antihistamine that competes with histamine for H_1 receptor sites on effector cells. **Therapeutic Effect:** Prevents allergic responses mediated by histamine, such as rhinitis, urticaria, and pruritus.

PHARMACOKINETICS

Route	Onset	Peak	Duration
PO	1–3 hr	8–12 hr	longer than 24 hr

Rapidly and almost completely absorbed from the GI tract. Protein binding: 97%; metabolite, 73%–77%. Distributed mainly to the liver, lungs, GI tract, and bile. Metabolized in the liver to active metabolite; undergoes extensive first-pass metabolism. Eliminated in urine and feces. Not removed by hemodialysis. ***Half-life:*** 8.4 hr; metabolite, 28 hr (increased in elderly and hepatic impairment).

AVAILABILITY

Syrup (Claritin): 10 mg/10 ml.
Tablets (Alavert, Claritin, Tavist ND): 10 mg.
Tablets (Rapid-Disintegrating [Alavert, Claritin RediTab]): 10 mg.

INDICATIONS AND DOSAGES

▸ **Allergic rhinitis, urticaria**

PO

Adults, Elderly, Children 6 yr and older. 10 mg once a day.
Children 2–5 yr. 5 mg once a day.

▸ **Dosage in hepatic impairment**

For adults, elderly, and children 6 years and older, dosage is reduced to 10 mg every other day.

OFF-LABEL USES

Adjunct treatment of bronchial asthma

CONTRAINDICATIONS

Hypersensitivity to loratadine or its ingredients

INTERACTIONS

Drug

Clarithromycin, erythromycin, fluconazole, ketoconazole: May increase the loratadine blood concentration.

Herbal

None known.

Food

All foods: Delay the absorption of loratadine.

DIAGNOSTIC TEST EFFECTS

May suppress wheal and flare reactions to antigen skin testing unless the drug is discontinued 4 days before testing.

SIDE EFFECTS

Frequent (12%–8%)
Headache, fatigue, somnolence
Occasional (3%)
Dry mouth, nose, or throat
Rare
Photosensitivity

SERIOUS REACTIONS

! None known.

NURSING CONSIDERATIONS

Baseline Assessment

- Assess the patient for allergy symptoms.
- Auscultate the patient's breath sounds for crackles, rhonchi, and wheezing. Examine the skin for urticaria.
- Expect to discontinue the drug 4 days before antigen skin testing.

Lifespan Considerations

- Loratadine is excreted in breast milk.
- Children and the elderly are more sensitive to the drug's anticholinergic effects, such as dry mouth, nose, and throat.

Precautions

- Use loratadine cautiously in breast-feeding women, children, and patients with hepatic impairment.

Administration and Handling

PO

- Give loratadine on an empty stomach because food delays its absorption.

Intervention and Evaluation

- Increase fluid intake patients with upper respiratory allergies to decrease the viscosity of secretions, offset thirst, and replace fluids lost from diaphoresis.
- Monitor the patient for relief of symptoms, including rhinorrhea, sneezing, and itching, red, watery eyes.

Patient Teaching

- Inform the patient that loratadine use may cause drowsiness.
- Warn the patient to avoid tasks requiring mental alertness or motor skills until his or her response to the drug has been established.
- Instruct the patient to drink plenty of water to help prevent dry mouth.
- Advise the patient to avoid direct exposure to sunlight and to wear sunscreen outdoors to prevent a photosensitivity reaction.
- Urge the patient to avoid alcohol during loratadine therapy.

promethazine hydrochloride

proe-**meth**-a-zeen
(Insomn-Eze[AUS], Phenadoz, Phenergan)
Do not confuse promethazine with promazine.

CATEGORY AND SCHEDULE

Pregnancy Risk Category: C

MECHANISM OF ACTION

A phenothiazine that acts as an antihistamine, antiemetic, and sedative-hypnotic. As an antihistamine, inhibits histamine at histamine receptor sites. As an antiemetic, diminishes vestibular stimulation, depresses labyrinthine function, and act on the chemoreceptor trigger zone. As a sedative-hypnotic, produces CNS depression by decreasing stimulation to the brain stem reticular formation. **Therapeutic Effect:** Prevents allergic responses mediated by histamine, such as rhinitis, urticaria, and pruritus. Prevents and relieves nausea and vomiting.

PHARMACOKINETICS

Route	Onset	Peak	Duration
PO	20 min	N/A	2–8 hr
IV	3–5 min	N/A	2–8 hr
IM	20 min	N/A	2–8 hr
Rectal	20 min	N/A	2–8 hr

Well absorbed from the GI tract after IM administration. Widely distributed. Metabolized in the liver. Primarily excreted in urine. Not removed by hemodialysis. ***Half-life:*** 16–19 hr.

AVAILABILITY

Syrup (Phenergan): 6.25 mg/ml.
Tablets (Phenergan): 12.5 mg, 25 mg, 50 mg.
Injection (Phenergan): 25 mg/ml, 50 mg/ml.
Suppositories (Phenergan): 12.5 mg, 25 mg, 50 mg.
Suppositories (Phenadoz): 25 mg.

INDICATIONS AND DOSAGES

▸ **Allergic symptoms**
PO
Adults, Elderly. 6.25–12.5 mg 3 times a day plus 25 mg at bedtime.
Children. 0.1 mg/kg/dose (maximum: 12.5 mg) 3 times a day plus 0.5 mg/kg/dose (maximum: 25 mg) at bedtime.
IV, IM
Adults, Elderly. 25 mg. May repeat in 2 hr.

▸ **Motion sickness**
PO
Adults, Elderly. 25 mg 30–60 min before departure; may repeat in 8–12 hr, then every morning on rising and before evening meal.
Children. 0.5 mg/kg 30–60 min before departure; may repeat in 8–12 hr, then every morning on rising and before evening meal.

▸ **Prevention of nausea, and vomiting**
PO, IV, IM, Rectal
Adults, Elderly. 12.5–25 mg q4–6h as needed.
Children. 0.25–1 mg/kg q4–6h as needed.

▸ **Preoperative and postoperative sedation; adjunct to analgesics**
IV, IM
Adults, Elderly. 25–50 mg.
Children. 12.5–25 mg.

▸ **Sedative**
PO, IV, IM, Rectal
Adults, Elderly. 25–50 mg/dose. May repeat q4–6h as needed.
Children. 0.5–1 mg/kg/dose q6h as needed. Maximum: 50 mg/dose.

CONTRAINDICATIONS

Angle-closure glaucoma, GI or GU obstruction, severe CNS depression or coma

INTERACTIONS

Drug

Alcohol, other CNS depressants: May increase CNS depressant effects.
Anticholinergics: May increase anticholinergic effects.
MAOIs: May intensify and prolong the anticholinergic and CNS depressant effects of promethazine.

Herbal

None known.

Food

None known.

DIAGNOSTIC TEST EFFECTS

May suppress wheal and flare reactions to antigen skin testing unless the drug is discontinued 4 days before testing.

IV INCOMPATIBILITIES

Allopurinol (Aloprim), amphotericin B complex (Abelcet, AmBisome, Amphotec), heparin, ketorolac

(Toradol), nalbuphine (Nubain), piperacillin and tazobactam (Zosyn)

IV COMPATIBILITIES

Atropine, diphenhydramine (Benadryl), glycopyrrolate (Robinul), hydromorphone (Dilaudid), hydroxyzine (Vistaril), meperidine (Demerol), midazolam (Versed), morphine, prochlorperazine (Compazine)

SIDE EFFECTS

Expected

Somnolence, disorientation; in elderly, hypotension, confusion, syncope

Frequent

Dry mouth, nose, or throat; urine retention; thickening of bronchial secretions

Occasional

Epigastric distress, flushing, visual disturbances, hearing disturbances, wheezing, paraesthesia, diaphoresis, chills

Rare

Dizziness, urticaria, photosensitivity, nightmares

SERIOUS REACTIONS

! Children may experience paradoxical reactions, such as excitation, nervousness, tremor, hyperactive reflexes, and seizures.

! Infants and young children have experienced CNS depression manifested as respiratory depression, sleep apnea, and sudden infant death syndrome.

! Long-term therapy may produce extrapyramidal symptoms, such as dystonia (abnormal movements), pronounced motor restlessness (most frequently in children), and parkinsonian symptoms (most frequently in elderly patients).

! Blood dyscrasias, particularly agranulocytosis, occur rarely.

NURSING CONSIDERATIONS

Baseline Assessment

- Assess the patient for dehydration, including dry mucous membranes, longitudinal furrows in the tongue, and poor skin turgor, before and regularly during therapy when promethazine is used as an antiemetic.
- Expect to discontinue the drug 4 days before antigen skin testing.

Lifespan Considerations

- Promethazine readily crosses the placenta and may produce extrapyramidal symptoms and jaundice in neonates if taken during pregnancy.
- It is unknown whether the drug is excreted in breast milk.
- Children are more likely to experience paradoxical reactions, such as increased excitement, nervousness, and tremor.
- Promethazine is not recommended for children younger than 2 years.
- The elderly are more sensitive to the drug's anticholinergic effects, such as dry mouth, confusion, dizziness, hypotension, syncope, and sedation.

Precautions

- Use promethazine cautiously in patients with asthma, history of seizures, cardiovascular disease, hepatic impairment, peptic ulcer disease, sleep apnea, or possible Reye's syndrome.

Administration and Handling

PO

- Give promethazine without regard to food.
- Crush scored tablets as needed.

IV

- Store vials at room temperature.
- Promethazine may be given undiluted or diluted with 0.9% NaCl; final dilution should not exceed 25 mg/ml.
- Inject the drug at a rate of 25

mg/minute through the tubing of an infusing IV solution, as prescribed.
- Injecting the drug too rapidly may cause a transient drop in BP, resulting in orthostatic hypotension and reflex tachycardia.

IM

◀ **ALERT** ▶ Avoid giving subcutaneously because significant tissue necrosis may occur. Inject the drug carefully because inadvertent intra-arterial injection may produce severe arteriospasm, possibly resulting in gangrene.
- Inject deep into a large muscle mass.

Rectal
- Refrigerate suppositories.
- Moisten the suppository with cold water before inserting it well into the rectum.

Intervention and Evaluation
- Assess BP and pulse rate if the patient receives the parenteral form of promethazine.
- Assist the patient with ambulation if he or she experiences drowsiness or light-headedness.
- Monitor serum electrolyte levels in patients with severe vomiting.

Patient Teaching
- Inform the patient that drowsiness and dry mouth are expected side effects of the drug. Tell the patient that drinking coffee or tea may help reduce drowsiness and sipping tepid water and chewing sugarless gum may relieve dry mouth.
- Warn the patient to avoid performing tasks that require mental alertness or motor skills until his or her response to the drug has been established.
- Instruct the patient to notify the physician if he or she experiences visual disturbances.
- Urge the patient to avoid alcohol and other CNS depressants during promethazine therapy.

83 Antitussives (Non-Narcotic)

benzonatate
guaifenesin

Uses: Antitussives are used to suppress cough. Specifically, *benzonatate* is used to relieve nonproductive cough, including acute cough caused by minor throat and bronchial irritation. *Guaifenesin* is used to relieve cough when mucus is present in the respiratory tract.

Action: Antitussives act in different ways to relieve cough. *Benzonatate* decreases the sensitivity of stretch receptors in the respiratory tract, which reduces cough production. *Guaifenesin* stimulates respiratory tract secretions by decreasing the adhesiveness and viscosity or phlegm, which promotes the removal of viscous mucus. (See the illustration *Sites of Action: Respiratory Agents,* page 1426.)

COMBINATION PRODUCTS

MUCINEX D: guaifenesin/pseudoephedrine (a sympathomimetic) 600 mg/60 mg; 1200 mg/120 mg.
MUCINEX DM: guaifenesin/dextromethorphan 600 mg/30 mg; 1200 mg/60 mg.
ROBITUSSIN AC: guaifenesin/codeine (a narcotic analgesic) 75 mg/2.5 mg per 5 ml;100 mg/10 mg per 5 ml.
ROBITUSSIN DM: guaifenesin/dextromethorphan (a cough suppressant) 100 mg/10 mg per 5 ml.

benzonatate

ben-**zoe**-na-tate
(Tessalon Perles)

CATEGORY AND SCHEDULE

Pregnancy Risk Category: C

MECHANISM OF ACTION

A non-narcotic antitussive that anesthetizes stretch receptors in respiratory passages, lungs, and pleura. **Therapeutic Effect:** Reduces cough production.

AVAILABILITY

Capsules: 100 mg, 200 mg.

INDICATIONS AND DOSAGES

▸ **Antitussive**

PO

Adults, Elderly, Children older than 10 yr. 100 mg 3 times a day or every 4 hours up to 600 mg/day.

CONTRAINDICATIONS

None known.

INTERACTIONS

Drug

CNS depressants: May increase the effects of benzonatate.

Herbal

None known.

Food

None known.

DIAGNOSTIC TEST EFFECTS

None known.

SIDE EFFECTS

Occasional

Mild somnolence, mild dizziness,

constipation, GI upset, skin eruptions, nasal congestion

SERIOUS REACTIONS

! Paradoxical reactions, including restlessness, insomnia, euphoria, nervousness, and tremor, have been noted.

NURSING CONSIDERATIONS

Baseline Assessment

• Assess the frequency, severity, and type of cough.
• Monitor the amount, color, and consistency of sputum.

Precautions

• Use benzonatate cautiously in patients with a productive cough.

Administration and Handling

PO

• Give benzonatate without regard to food.
• Have the patient swallow the capsules whole; chewing them or dissolving them in the mouth may produce temporary local anesthesia or choking.

Intervention and Evaluation

• Have the patient begin deep-breathing and coughing exercises, particularly if he or she has impaired pulmonary function.
• Monitor the patient for a paradoxical reaction.
• Increase environmental humidity and fluid intake to lower the viscosity of the patient's secretions.
• Assess the patient for clinical improvement, and record the onset of cough relief.

Patient Teaching

• Instruct the patient to swallow the capsules whole and not to chew them or let them dissolve in the mouth.
• Inform the patient that dizziness and drowsiness are common side effects.
• Warn the patient to avoid tasks that require mental alertness or motor skills until his or her response to the drug has been established.

guaifenesin

gwye-**fen**-e-sin
(Balminil[CAN], Benylin E[CAN], Guiatuss, Humibid LA, Mucinex, Organidin, Robitussin, Tussin)
Do not confuse guaifenesin with guanfacine.

CATEGORY AND SCHEDULE

Pregnancy Risk Category: C
OTC

MECHANISM OF ACTION

An expectorant that stimulates respiratory tract secretions by decreasing adhesiveness and viscosity of phlegm. **Therapeutic Effect:** Promotes removal of viscous mucus.

PHARMACOKINETICS

Well absorbed from the GI tract. Metabolized in the liver. Excreted in urine.

AVAILABILITY

Tablets (Organidin): 200 mg.
Tablets (Extended-Release [Humibid LA, Mucinex]): 600 mg.
Syrup (Guiatuss, Robitussin, Tussin): 100 mg/5 ml.

INDICATIONS AND DOSAGES

▸ **Expectorant**

PO

Adults, Elderly, Children older than 12 yr. 200–400 mg q4h.
Children 6–12 yr. 100–200 mg q4h. Maximum: 1.2 g/day.
Children 2–5 yr. 50–100 mg q4h.
Children younger than 2 yr. 12 mg/kg/day in 6 divided doses.

PO (Extended-Release)
Adults, Elderly, Children older than 12 yr. 600–1200 mg q12h. Maximum: 2.4 g/day.
Children 2–5 yr. 600 mg q12h. Maximum: 600 mg/day.

CONTRAINDICATIONS

None known.

INTERACTIONS

Drug

None known.

Herbal

None known.

Food

None known.

DIAGNOSTIC TEST EFFECTS

None known.

SIDE EFFECTS

Rare

Dizziness, headache, rash, diarrhea, nausea, vomiting, abdominal pain

SERIOUS REACTIONS

! Overdose may produce nausea and vomiting.

NURSING CONSIDERATIONS

Baseline Assessment

- Assess the frequency, severity, and type of cough.
- Ask about a history of cigarette smoking, asthma, emphysema, and chronic bronchitis because the drug is not recommended for coughs caused by these conditions.

Lifespan Considerations

- It is unknown if guaifenesin crosses the placenta or is distributed in breast milk.
- No age-related precautions have been noted in children or the elderly.
- Use guaifenesin cautiously in children younger than 2 years with a persistent cough.

Administration and Handling

PO

◀ALERT▶ Give extended-release tablets at 12-hour intervals, as prescribed.

- Store syrup, liquid, and capsules at room temperature.
- Give guaifenesin without regard to food.
- Don't crush or break extended-release capsules. Contents may be sprinkled on soft food and then swallowed without chewing or crushing.

Intervention and Evaluation

- Have the patient begin deep-breathing and coughing exercises, particularly if he or she has impaired pulmonary function.
- Increase environmental humidity and fluid intake to lower the viscosity of the patient's lung secretions.
- Assess the patient for clinical improvement, and record the onset of cough relief.

Patient Teaching

- Tell the patient not to take guaifenesin for chronic cough.
- Caution the patient to avoid performing tasks that require mental alertness or motor skills until his or her response to the drug has been established.
- Urge the patient to drink plenty of fluids.
- Advise the patient to notify the physician if the cough persists or is accompanied by fever, rash, headache, or sore throat.

albuterol
aminophylline, theophylline
formoterol fumarate
ipratropium bromide
levalbuterol
metaproterenol sulfate
salmeterol
terbutaline sulfate
tiotropium bromide

Uses: Bronchodilators are used to relieve bronchospasm that occurs during anesthesia and in bronchial asthma, bronchitis, emphysema, and COPD. Some may also be prescribed to prevent bronchospasm. Terbutaline is also used to delay premature labor.

Action: Each bronchodilator subclass works by a different mechanism of action. *Beta$_2$-adrenergic agonists,* such as albuterol and formoterol, stimulate beta receptors in the lungs, resulting in relaxed bronchial smooth muscle, increased vital capacity, and decreased airway resistance. Terbutaline also relaxes uterine muscle, inhibiting contractions during labor. *Anticholinergics,* such as ipratropium, inhibit cholinergic receptors on bronchial smooth muscle, blocking the action of acetylcholine. This causes bronchodilation and inhibits secretions from glands in the nasal mucosa. *Methylxanthines,* such as aminophylline, directly relax smooth muscle in the bronchial airways and pulmonary blood vessels, relieving bronchospasm and increasing vital capacity. They also produce cardiac and skeletal muscle stimulation. (See the illustration *Sites of Action: Respiratory Agents,* page 1426.)

COMBINATION PRODUCTS

ADVAIR: salmeterol/fluticasone (a corticosteroid) 50 mcg/100 mcg; 50 mcg/250 mcg; 50 mcg/500 mcg.
COMBIVENT: ipratropium/albuterol 18 mcg/103 mcg per actuation from mouthpiece.
DUONEB: ipratropium/albuterol base 0.5 mg/2.5 ml per 3 ml.

albuterol

al-**byoo**-ter-ole
(AccuNeb, Airomir[AUS], Asmol CFC-Free[AUS], Epaq Inhaler[AUS], Novosalmol[CAN], Proventil, Proventil Repetabs, Respax[AUS], Ventolin, Ventolin CFC-Free[AUS], Volmax, Vospire ER)
Do not confuse albuterol with Albutein or atenolol, or Proventil with Prinivil.

CATEGORY AND SCHEDULE

Pregnancy Risk Category: C

MECHANISM OF ACTION

A sympathomimetic that stimulates beta$_2$-adrenergic receptors in the lungs, resulting in relaxation of bronchial smooth muscle. **Therapeutic Effect:** Relieves bronchospasm and reduces airway resistance.

PHARMACOKINETICS

Route	Onset	Peak	Duration
PO	15–30 min	2–3 hr	4–6 hr
PO (extended-release)	30 min	2–4 hr	12 hr
Inhalation	5–15 min	0.5–2 hr	2–5 hr

Rapidly, well absorbed from the GI tract; gradually absorbed from the bronchi after inhalation. Metabolized in the liver. Primarily excreted in urine. ***Half-life:*** 2.7–5 hr (PO); 3.8 hr (inhalation).

AVAILABILITY

Syrup: 2 mg/5ml.
Tablet: 2 mg, 4 mg.
Tablet (Extended-Release [Proventil Repetabs]): 4 mg.
Tablets (Extended-Release [Volmax, VoSpire ER]): 4 mg, 8 mg.
Inhalation (Aerosol [Proventil, Ventolin]): 90 mcg/spray.
Inhalation (Solution [AccuNeb]): 0.75 mg/3 ml, 1.5 mg/3 ml.
Inhalation (Solution [Proventil]): 0.083%, 0.5%.

INDICATIONS AND DOSAGES

▸ Bronchospasm

PO

Adults, Children older than 12 yr. 2–4 mg 3–4 times a day. Maximum: 8 mg 4 times/day.
Elderly. 2 mg 3–4 times a day. Maximum: 8 mg 4 times a day.
Children 6–12 yr. 2 mg 3–4 times a day. Maximum: 24 mg/day.

PO (Extended-Release)

Adults, Children older than 12 yr. 4–8 mg q12h.

Inhalation

Adults, Elderly, Children older than 12 yr. 1–2 puffs by metered dose inhaler q4–6h as needed.
Children 4–12 yr. 1–2 puffs 4 times a day.

Nebulization

Adults, Elderly, Children older than 12 yr. 2.5 mg 3–4 times a day.
Children 2–12 yr. 0.63–1.25 mg 3–4 times a day.

▸ Exercise-induced bronchospasm

Inhalation

Adults, Elderly, Children 4 yr and older. 2 puffs 15–30 min before exercise.

CONTRAINDICATIONS

History of hypersensitivity to sympathomimetics

INTERACTIONS

Drug

Beta blockers: Antagonize effects of albuterol.
Digoxin: May increase the risk of arrhythmias.
MAOIs, tricyclic antidepressants: May potentiate cardiovascular effects.

Herbal

None known.

Food

None known.

DIAGNOSTIC TEST EFFECTS

May increase blood glucose level. May decrease serum potassium level.

SIDE EFFECTS

Frequent

Headache (27%); nausea (15%); restlessness, nervousness, tremors (20%); dizziness (less than 7%);

throat dryness and irritation, pharyngitis (less than 6%); BP changes, including hypertension (5%–3%); heartburn, transient wheezing (less than 5%)

Occasional (3%–2%)

Insomnia, asthenia, altered taste

Inhalation: Dry, irritated mouth or throat; cough; bronchial irritation

Rare

Somnolence, diarrhea, dry mouth, flushing, diaphoresis, anorexia

SERIOUS REACTIONS

! Excessive sympathomimetic stimulation may produce palpitations, extrasystole, tachycardia, chest pain, a slight increase in BP followed by a substantial decrease, chills, diaphoresis, and blanching of skin.

! Too-frequent or excessive use may lead to decreased bronchodilating effectiveness and severe, paradoxical bronchoconstriction.

NURSING CONSIDERATIONS

Baseline Assessment

- Auscultate breath sounds. Assess baseline behavior, such as nervousness.

Lifespan Considerations

- Albuterol appears to cross the placenta; it is unknown if albuterol is distributed in breast milk.
- Albuterol may inhibit uterine contractility.
- The safety and efficacy of this drug have not been established in children less than 2 years (syrup) or less than 6 years (tablets).
- The elderly may be more prone to tremors and tachycardia because of increased sensitivity to sympathomimetics.

Precautions

- Use albuterol cautiously in patients with cardiovascular disease, diabetes mellitus, hypertension, or hyperthyroidism.

Administration and Handling

PO

- Don't crush or break extended-release tablets.
- Give albuterol without regard to food.

Inhalation

- Shake the container well before inhalation.
- Have the patient wait 2 minutes before inhaling the second dose to allow for deeper bronchial penetration.
- Have the patient rinse his or her mouth with water immediately after inhalation to prevent mouth and throat dryness.

Nebulization

- Dilute 0.5 ml of 0.5% solution to a final volume of 3 ml with 0.9% NaCl to provide 2.5 mg.
- Administer over 5 to 15 minutes.
- The nebulizer should be used with compressed air or oxygen (O_2) at a rate of 6 to 10 L/minute.

Intervention and Evaluation

- Monitor the patient's 12-lead EKG; pulse rate and quality; respiratory rate, depth, rhythm, and type; and ABG and serum potassium levels.
- Auscultate the patient's breath sounds for wheezing (a possible sign of bronchoconstriction), and for crackles.
- Offer emotional support. The patient may become anxious because of difficulty breathing or the sympathomimetic response to the drug.

Patient Teaching

- Teach the patient how to use an inhaler properly.
- Advise the patient to take no more than 2 inhalations at any one time because excessive use may decrease the drug's effectiveness or produce paradoxical bronchoconstriction.
- Instruct the patient to rinse his or

her mouth with water immediately after inhalation to prevent mouth and throat dryness.

- Encourage the patient to drink plenty of fluids to decrease the thickness of lung secretions.
- Urge the patient to avoid excessive use of caffeinated products, such as chocolate, cocoa, cola, coffee, and tea.

aminophylline

am-in-**off**-i-lin
(Phyllocontin)

theophylline

(Elixophyllin, Nuelin[AUS], Nuelin SR[AUS], Quibron-T, Quibron-T/SR, Slo-Bid Gyrocaps, Theo-24, Thoechron, Theodur, Theolair, T-Phyl, Uniphyl).
Do not confuse aminophylline with amitriptyline or ampicillin, or Slo-Bid with Dolobid.

CATEGORY AND SCHEDULE

Pregnancy Risk Category: C

MECHANISM OF ACTION

A xanthine derivative that acts as a bronchodilator by directly relaxing smooth muscle of the bronchial airways and pulmonary blood vessels. **Therapeutic Effect:** Relieves bronchospasm and increases vital capacity.

AVAILABILITY

Capsules (Extended-Release [Theo-24]): 100 mg, 200 mg, 300 mg, 400 mg.
Elixir (Elixophyllin): 80 mg/15 ml.
Oral Solution: 80 mg/15 ml.
Tablets (Controlled-Release [Quibron-T/SR]): 300 mg.
Tablets (Controlled-Release [Theochron]): 100 mg, 200 mg, 300 mg.
Tablets (Controlled-Release [Theolair-SR]): 300 mg, 500 mg.
Tablets (Controlled-Release [T-Phyl]): 200 mg.
Tablets (Controlled-Release [Uniphyl]): 400 mg, 600 mg.
Infusion (theophylline): 0.8 mg/ml, 1.6 mg/ml, 2 mg/ml, 3.2 mg/ml, 4 mg/ml.
Injection (aminophylline): 25 mg/ml.

INDICATIONS AND DOSAGES

▸ **Chronic bronchospasm**
PO
Adults, Elderly, Children. 16 mg/kg or 400 mg/day (whichever is less) in 3–4 divided doses (8-hr intervals); may increase by 25% every 2–3 days. Maximum: 13 mg/kg/day (children 13–16 yr); 18 mg/kg/day (children 9–12 yr); 20 mg/kg/day (children 1–8 yr). Maximum dosages are based on serum theophylline concentrations, clinical condition, and presence of toxicity.

▸ **Acute bronchospasm in patients not currently taking theophylline**
PO
Adults, Children older than 1 yr. Initially, loading dose of 5 mg/kg (theophylline); then maintenance dosage of theophylline based on patient group (shown below).

Patient Group	Maintenance Theophylline Dosage
Healthy, nonsmoking adults	3 mg/kg q8h
Elderly patients, patients with cor pulmonale	2 mg/kg q8h
Patients with CHF or hepatic disease	1–2 mg/kg q12h
Children 9–16 yr, young adult smokers	3 mg/kg q6h
Children 1–8 yr	4 mg/kg q6h

IV
Adults, Children older than 1 yr. Initially, loading dose of 6 mg/kg (aminophylline); maintenance dosage of aminophylline based on patient group (shown below).

Patient Group	Maintenance Aminophylline Dosage
Healthy, nonsmoking adults	0.7 mg/kg/hr
Elderly patients, patients with cor pulmonale, CHF, or hepatic impairment	0.25 mg/kg/hr
Children 13–16 yr	0.7 mg/kg/hr
Children 9–12 yr, young adult smokers	0.9 mg/kg/hr
Children 1–8 yr	1–1.2 mg/kg/hr
Children 6 mo–1 yr	0.6–0.7 mg/kg/hr
Children 6 wk–6 mo	0.5 mg/kg/hr
Neonates	5 mg/kg q12h

▸ Acute bronchospasm in patients currently taking theophylline
PO, IV
Adults, children older than 1 yr. Obtain serum theophylline level. If not possible and patient is in respiratory distress and not experiencing toxic effects, may give 2.5 mg/kg dose. Maintenance: Dosage based on peak serum theophylline concentration, clinical condition, and presence of toxicity.

OFF-LABEL USES
Treatment of apnea in neonates

CONTRAINDICATIONS
History of hypersensitivity to caffeine or xanthine

INTERACTIONS
Drug
Beta blockers: May decrease the effects of aminophylline.
Cimetidine, ciprofloxacin, erythromycin, norfloxacin: May increase aminophylline blood concentration and risk of aminophylline toxicity.
Glucocorticoids: May produce hypernatremia.
Phenytoin, primidone, rifampin: May increase aminophylline metabolism.
Smoking: May decrease aminophylline blood concentration.
Herbal
None known.
Food
Charcoal-broiled foods; high-protein, low-carbohydrate diet: May decrease the theophylline blood level.

DIAGNOSTIC TEST EFFECTS
None known.

IV INCOMPATIBILITIES
Amiodarone (Cordarone), ciprofloxacin (Cipro), dobutamine (Dobutrex), ondansetron (Zofran)

IV COMPATIBILITIES
Aztreonam (Azactam), ceftazidime (Fortaz), fluconazole (Diflucan), heparin, morphine, potassium chloride

SIDE EFFECTS
Frequent
Altered smell (during IV administration), restlessness, tachycardia, tremor
Occasional
Heartburn, vomiting, headache, mild diuresis, insomnia, nausea

SERIOUS REACTIONS
! Too-rapid IV administration may produce marked hypotension with accompanying faintness, lightheadedness, palpitations, tachycardia, hyperventilation, nausea, vomit-

ing, angina-like pain, seizures, ventricular fibrillation, and cardiac standstill.

NURSING CONSIDERATIONS

Baseline Assessment

• Before and regularly during therapy, monitor the patient for anxiety due to difficulty breathing or the drug's sympathomimetic effects.

Lifespan Considerations

• Aminophylline crosses the placenta and small amounts of the drug may be distributed in breast milk and cause irritability in the breast-feeding infant.

• Use the drug cautiously in children less than 1 year.

Precautions

• Use aminophylline cautiously in patients with diabetes mellitus; glaucoma; hypertension; hyperthyroidism; cardiac, renal or hepatic impairment; peptic ulcer disease; or a seizure disorder.

Administration and Handling

◀ **ALERT** ▶ Aminophylline dosage is calculated based on lean body weight. It's also based on peak serum theophylline concentrations, the patient's clinical condition, and the absence of theophylline toxicity.

PO

• Give aminophylline with food to avoid GI distress.

• Don't crush or break sustained-release forms.

IV

• Store vials at room temperature.

• Discard the solution if it contains a precipitate.

• Give loading dose diluted in 100 to 200 ml of D_5W or 0.9% NaCl. Prepare maintenance dose in larger volume parenteral infusion.

• Don't exceed a flow rate of 1 ml/minute (25 mg/minute) for either piggyback or infusion.

• Administer loading dose over 20 to 30 minutes.

• Use an infusion pump or microdrip to regulate IV administration.

Intervention and Evaluation

• As ordered, obtain the peak serum concentration 1 hour after an IV dose, 1 to 2 hours after an immediate-release dose, and 3 to 8 hours after a sustained-release dose. Obtain the serum trough level just before the next dose.

• Monitor serum theophylline levels. The therapeutic serum level range is 10 to 20 mcg/ml.

• Monitor the pulse rate and quality as well as respiratory rate, depth, rhythm, and type. Auscultate breath sounds for rhonchi, wheezing, or crackles.

• Monitor the patient's ABG levels.

• Examine the patient's lips and fingernails for signs of hypoxemia, such as a blue or gray color in light-skinned patients and a gray color in dark-skinned patients.

• Assess the patient for clavicular retractions and hand tremor.

• Evaluate the patient for signs of clinical improvement such as cessation of clavicular retractions, quieter and slower respirations, and a relaxed facial expression.

Patient Teaching

• Encourage the patient to drink plenty of fluids to decrease the thickness of lung secretions.

• Urge the patient to avoid excessive use of caffeinated products, such as chocolate, cocoa, cola, coffee, and tea.

• Explain to the patient that smoking, charcoal-broiled foods, and a high-protein, low-carbohydrate diet may decrease the theophylline level.

formoterol fumarate

for-**moe**-ter-ol
(Foradil Aerolizer, Foradile[AUS], Oxis[AUS])

CATEGORY AND SCHEDULE

Pregnancy Risk Category: C

MECHANISM OF ACTION

A long-acting bronchodilator that stimulates $beta_2$-adrenergic receptors in the lungs, resulting in relaxation of bronchial smooth muscle. Also inhibits release of mediators from various cells in the lungs, including mast cells, with little effect on heart rate. **Therapeutic Effect:** Relieves bronchospasm, reduces airway resistance. Improves bronchodilation, nighttime asthma control, and peak flow rates.

PHARMACOKINETICS

Route	Onset	Peak	Duration
Inhalation	1–3 min	0.5–1 hr	12 hr

Absorbed from bronchi after inhalation. Metabolized in the liver. Primarily excreted in urine. Unknown if removed by hemodialysis. ***Half-life:*** 10 hr.

AVAILABILITY

Inhalation Powder in Capsules: 12 mcg.

INDICATIONS AND DOSAGES

▸ **Asthma, chronic obstructive pulmonary disease (COPD)**
Inhalation
Adults, Elderly, Children 5 yrs and older. 12 mcg capsule q12h.

▸ **Exercise-induced bronchospasm**
Inhalation
Adults, Elderly, Children 5 yr and older. 12 mcg capsule at least 15 min before exercise. Do not repeat for another 12 hours.

CONTRAINDICATIONS

None known.

INTERACTIONS

Drug

Beta blockers: May antagonize formoterol's bronchodilating effects.
Diuretics, steroids, xanthine derivatives: May increase the risk of hypokalemia.
Drugs that can prolong QT interval (including erythromycin, quinidine, and thioridazine), MAOIs, tricyclic antidepressants: May potentiate cardiovascular effects.

Herbal

None known.

Food

None known.

DIAGNOSTIC TEST EFFECTS

May decrease serum potassium level. May increase blood glucose level.

SIDE EFFECTS

Occasional

Tremor, muscle cramps, tachycardia, insomnia, headache, irritability, irritation of mouth or throat

SERIOUS REACTIONS

! Excessive sympathomimetic stimulation may produce palpitations, extrasystole, and chest pain.

NURSING CONSIDERATIONS

Baseline Assessment

• Determine if the patient has a history of cardiovascular disease,

hypertension, seizure disorder, or thyrotoxicosis.
• Check the patient's baseline EKG, QT interval, and peak flow readings.

Lifespan Considerations

• It is unknown if formoterol crosses the placenta or is distributed in breast milk.
• The safety and efficacy of formoterol have not been established in children younger than 5 years.
• The elderly may be more prone to tachycardia and tremor because of increased sensitivity to sympathomimetics.

Precautions

• Use formoterol cautiously in patients with cardiovascular disease, hypertension, a seizure disorder, or thyrotoxicosis.

Administration and Handling

Inhalation
• Keep capsules in individual blister packs until immediately before use. Don't let the patient swallow the capsules. Don't use with a spacer.
• Pull off the aerolizer inhaler cover, twisting the mouthpiece in the direction of the arrow to open.
• Place the capsule in the chamber, and twist the mouthpiece closed.
• Press both buttons on the side of the aerolizer only once. This action punctures the capsule.
• Have the patient exhale completely, then place his or her mouth on the mouthpiece and close the lips.
• Instruct the patient to inhale quickly and deeply through the mouth, which causes the capsule to spin and dispense the drug. Have the patient hold his or her breath for as long as possible before exhaling slowly.
• Check the capsule to make sure all the powder is gone. If not, instruct the patient to inhale again to receive the rest of the dose.
• Have the patient rinse his or her mouth with water immediately after inhalation to prevent mouth and throat dryness.

Intervention and Evaluation

• Monitor the pulse rate and quality and respiratory rate, depth, rhythm, and type.
• Auscultate the patient's breath sounds for rhonchi and wheezing, signs of bronchoconstriction.
• Monitor the patient's EKG and serum potassium and ABG levels.

Patient Teaching

• Teach the patient how to use the inhaler properly.
• Tell the patient that rinsing his or her mouth with water immediately after inhalation may prevent mouth and throat irritation.
• Encourage the patient to drink plenty of fluids to decrease the thickness of lung secretions.
• Teach the patient how to measure peak flow readings and keep a log of measurements.
• Urge the patient to avoid excessive use of caffeinated products, such as chocolate, cola, coffee, and tea.

ipratropium bromide

eye-pra-**troep**-ee-um
(Apo-Ipravent[CAN], Aproven[AUS], Atrovent, Atrovent Aerosol[AUS], Atrovent Nasal[AUS], Atrovent NPH, Novo-Ipramide[CAN], Nu-Ipratropium[CAN], PMS-Ipratropium[CAN])
Do not confuse Atrovent with Alupent.

CATEGORY AND SCHEDULE

Pregnancy Risk Category: B

MECHANISM OF ACTION

An anticholinergic that blocks the action of acetylcholine at parasympathetic sites in bronchial smooth muscle. **Therapeutic Effect:** Causes bronchodilation and inhibits nasal secretions.

PHARMACOKINETICS

Route	Onset	Peak	Duration
Inhalation	1–3 min	1–2 hr	4–6 hr

Minimal systemic absorption after inhalation. Metabolized in the liver (systemic absorption). Primarily eliminated in feces. ***Half-life:*** 1.5–4 hr.

AVAILABILITY

Oral Inhalation: 18 mcg/actuation.
Aerosol Solution for Inhalation: 0.02%.
Nasal Spray: 0.03%, 0.06%.

INDICATIONS AND DOSAGES

▸ Bronchospasm, acute treatment
Inhalation
Adults, Elderly, Children. 4–8 puffs as needed.
Nebulization
Adults, Elderly, Children 12 yr and older. 500 mcg q30min for 3 doses, then q2–4h as needed.
Children younger than 12 yr. 250 mcg q20min for 3 doses, then q2–4h as needed.

▸ Bronchospasm, maintenance treatment
Inhalation
Adults, Elderly, Children 12 yr and older. 2–3 puffs q6h.
Children younger than 12 yr. 1–2 puffs q6h.
Nebulization
Adults, Elderly, Children 12 yr and older. 500 mcg q6h.
Children younger than 12 yr. 250–500 mcg q6h.

▸ Rhinorrhea
Intranasal
Adults, Children older than 5 yr. 2 sprays of 0.06% solution 3–4 times a day.
Adults, Children older than 6 yr. 2 sprays of (0.03%) solution 2–3 times a day.

CONTRAINDICATIONS

History of hypersensitivity to atropine

INTERACTIONS

Drug

Cromolyn inhalation solution: Avoid mixing these drugs because they form a precipitate.

Herbal

None known.

Food

None known.

DIAGNOSTIC TEST EFFECTS

None known.

SIDE EFFECTS

Frequent

Inhalation (6%–3%): Cough, dry mouth, headache, nausea
Nasal: Dry nose and mouth, headache, nasal irritation

Occasional

Inhalation (2%): Dizziness, transient increased bronchospasm

Rare (less than 1%)

Inhalation: Hypotension, insomnia, metallic or unpleasant taste, palpitations, urine retention
Nasal: Diarrhea or constipation, dry throat, abdominal pain, stuffy nose

SERIOUS REACTIONS

! Worsening of angle-closure glaucoma, acute eye pain, and hypotension occur rarely.

NURSING CONSIDERATIONS

Baseline Assessment

- Auscultate breath sounds before and after treatment.

Lifespan Considerations

- It is unknown if ipratropium is distributed in breast milk.
- No age-related precautions have been noted in children or the elderly.

Precautions

- Use ipratropium cautiously in patients with bladder neck obstruction, angle-closure glaucoma, or benign prostatic hyperplasia.

Administration and Handling

Inhalation

- Shake the container well. Have the patient exhale completely through his or her mouth; then place the mouthpiece into the patient's mouth and have the patient close his or her lips, holding the inhaler upright.
- Instruct the patient to inhale deeply through the mouth while fully depressing the top of the canister. Have the patient hold his or her breath for as long as possible before exhaling slowly.
- Have the patient wait 2 minutes before inhaling the second dose to allow for deeper bronchial penetration.
- Have the patient rinse his or her mouth with water immediately after inhalation to prevent mouth and throat dryness.

Intervention and Evaluation

- Monitor pulse rate and quality and respiratory rate, depth, rate, rhythm, and type.
- Ausculatate the patient's breath sounds for crackles, rhonchi, and wheezing.
- Monitor the patient's ABG levels.
- Examine the patient's lips and fingernails for a blue or gray color in light-skinned patients and a gray color in dark-skinned patients, which are signs of hypoxemia.
- Observe the patient for clavicular, intercostal, and sternal retractions and a hand tremor.
- Offer emotional support. The patient may experience anxiety because of breathing difficulty or the sympathomimetic effects of the drug.
- Evaluate the patient for evidence of clinical improvement, such as cessation of retractions, quieter and slower respirations, and a relaxed facial expression.

Patient Teaching

- Instruct the patient not to take more than 2 inhalations at a time because excessive use decreases the drug's effectiveness and may cause paradoxical bronchoconstriction.
- Advise the patient to rinse his or her mouth with water immediately after inhalation to prevent mouth and throat dryness.
- Encourage the patient to drink plenty of fluids to decrease the thickness of lung secretions.
- Urge the patient to avoid excessive use of caffeinated products, such as chocolate, cocoa, cola, coffee, and tea.

levalbuterol

lee-val-**bwet**-err-all

(Xopenex)

Do not confuse Xopenex with Xanax.

CATEGORY AND SCHEDULE

Pregnancy Risk Category: C

MECHANISM OF ACTION

A sympathomimetic that stimulates beta$_2$-adrenergic receptors in the lungs resulting in relaxation of bronchial smooth muscle. **Therapeutic Effect:** Relieves bronchospasm and reduces airway resistance.

PHARMACOKINETICS

Route	Onset	Peak	Duration
Inhalation	10–17 min	1.5 hr	5–6 hr

Metabolized in the liver to inactive metabolite. ***Half-life:*** 3.3–4 hr.

AVAILABILITY

Solution for Nebulization: 0.31 in 3-ml vials, 0.63 mg in 3-ml vials, 1.25 mg in 3-ml vials.

INDICATIONS AND DOSAGES

▸ Treatment and prevention of bronchospasm

Nebulization

Adults, Elderly, Children 12 yr and older. Initially, 0.63 mg 3 times a day 6–8 hr apart. May increase to 1.25 mg 3 times a day with dose monitoring.

Children 3–11 yr. Initially 0.31 mg 3 times a day. Maximum: 0.63 mg 3 times a day

CONTRAINDICATIONS

History of hypersensitivity to sympathomimetics

INTERACTIONS

Drug

Beta blockers: Antagonize the effects of levalbuterol.

Digoxin: May increase the risk of arrhythmias.

MAOIs, tricyclic antidepressants: May potentiate cardiovascular effects.

Herbal

None known.

Food

None known.

DIAGNOSTIC TEST EFFECTS

May increase serum potassium level.

SIDE EFFECTS

Frequent

Tremor, nervousness, headache, throat dryness and irritation

Occasional

Cough, bronchial irritation

Rare

Somnolence, diarrhea, dry mouth, flushing, diaphoresis, anorexia

SERIOUS REACTIONS

! Excessive sympathomimetic stimulation may produce palpitations, extrasystoles, tachycardia, chest pain, a slight increase in BP followed by a substantial decrease, chills, diaphoresis, and blanching of skin.

! Too-frequent or excessive use may lead to decreased bronchodilating effectiveness and severe, paradoxical bronchoconstriction.

NURSING CONSIDERATIONS

Baseline Assessment

- Auscultate breath sounds before and after treatment.

Lifespan Considerations

- Levalbuterol crosses the placenta. It is unknown if the drug is distributed in breast milk.
- The safety and efficacy of levalbuterol have not been established in children younger than 12 years.
- A lower initial dosage is recommended for the elderly.

Precautions

- Use levalbuterol cautiously in patients with cardiovascular disorders (such as arrhythmias), diabetes mellitus, hypertension, or seizures.

Administration and Handling

Nebulization

- Protect the solution from light and

excessive heat. Store it at room temperature.
- Use the solution within 2 weeks of opening the foil.
- Discard the solution if it's not colorless.
- Don't dilute the solution.
- Don't mix levalbuterol with other medications.
- Administer levalbuterol over 5 to 15 minutes.

Intervention and Evaluation
- Monitor pulse rate and quality and respiratory rate, depth, rhythm, and type.
- Monitor the patient's EKG, and serum potassium and ABG levels.
- Auscultate the patient's breath sounds for crackles and wheezing, signs of bronchoconstriction.
- Offer emotional support. The patient may become anxious because of difficulty breathing or the sympathomimetic effects of the drug.

Patient Teaching
- Advise the patient to rinse his or her mouth with water immediately after inhalation to prevent mouth and throat dryness.
- Encourage the patient to drink plenty of fluids to decrease the thickness of lung secretions.
- Warn the patient to notify the physician if he or she experiences chest pain, dizziness, headache, palpitations, tachycardia, or tremors.
- Urge the patient to avoid excessive use of caffeinated products, such as chocolate, cocoa, cola, coffee, and tea.

metaproterenol sulfate

met-a-proe-**ter**-e-nole
(Alupent)
Do not confuse metaproterenol with metipranolol or metoprolol, or Alupent with Atrovent.

CATEGORY AND SCHEDULE

Pregnancy Risk Category: C

MECHANISM OF ACTION

A sympathomimetic that stimulates beta$_2$-adrenergic receptors, resulting in relaxation of bronchial smooth muscle. **Therapeutic Effect:** Relieves bronchospasm and reduces airway resistance.

AVAILABILITY

Syrup: 10 mg/5 ml.
Tablets: 10 mg, 20 mg.
Aerosol Oral Inhalation (Alupent): 0.65 mg/inhalation.
Solution for Oral Inhalation: 0.4%, 0.6%, 5%.

INDICATIONS AND DOSAGES

▸ Treatment of bronchospasm

PO
Adults, Children 10 yr and older. 20 mg 3–4 times a day.
Elderly. 10 mg 3–4 times a day. May increase to 20 mg/dose.
Children 6–9 yr. 10 mg 3–4 times a day.
Children 2–5 yr. 1.3–2.6 mg/kg/day in 3–4 divided doses.
Children younger than 2 yr. 0.4 mg/kg 3–4 times a day.

Inhalation
Adults, Elderly, Children 12 yr and older. 2–3 inhalations q3–4h. Maximum: 12 inhalations/24 hr.

Nebulization
Adults, Elderly, Children 12 yr and older. 10–15 mg (0.2–0.3 ml) of 5% q4–6h.
Children younger than 12 yr, Infants. 0.5–1 mg/kg (0.01–0.02 ml/kg) of 5% q4–6h.

CONTRAINDICATIONS

Angle-closure glaucoma, preexisting arrhythmias associated with tachycardia

INTERACTIONS

Drug

Beta blockers: May decrease the effects of beta blockers.
Digoxin, other sympathomimetics: May increase the risk of arrhythmias.
MAOIs: May increase the risk of hypertensive crisis.
Tricyclic antidepressants: May increase cardiovascular effects.

Herbal

None known.

Food

None known.

DIAGNOSTIC TEST EFFECTS

May decrease serum potassium level.

SIDE EFFECTS

Frequent (over 10%)
Rigors, tremors, anxiety, nausea, dry mouth
Occasional (9%–1%)
Dizziness, vertigo, asthenia, headache, GI distress, vomiting, cough, dry throat
Rare (less than 1%)
Somnolence, diarrhea, altered taste

SERIOUS REACTIONS

! Excessive sympathomimetic stimulation may cause palpitations, extrasystoles, tachycardia, chest pain, a slight increase in BP followed by a substantial decrease, chills, diaphoresis, and blanching of skin.

! Too-frequent or excessive use may lead to decreased drug effectiveness and severe, paradoxical bronchoconstriction.

NURSING CONSIDERATIONS

Baseline Assessment

- Auscultate breath sounds before and after treatment.

Precautions

- Use metaproterenol cautiously in patients with arrhythmias, CHF, ischemic heart disease, diabetes mellitus, hypertension, hyperthyroidism, or a seizure disorder.

Intervention and Evaluation

- Monitor pulse rate and quality and respiratory rate depth, rhythm, and type.
- Monitor the patient's ABG levels and pulmonary function test results.
- Auscultate the patient's breath sounds for rhonchi and wheezing, signs of bronchoconstriction.
- Observe the patient for evidence of cyanosis, a blue or a dusky color in light-skinned patients and a gray color in dark-skinned patients.
- Offer emotional support. The patient may become anxious because of difficulty breathing or the sympathomimetic effects of the drug.
- Evaluate the patient for signs of clinical improvement, such as cessation of retractions, quieter and slower respirations, and a relaxed facial expression.

Patient Teaching

- Instruct the patient not to exceed the recommended dosage.
- Encourage the patient to drink plenty of fluids to decrease the thickness of lung secretions.
- Inform the patient that metaproterenol may cause anxiety, insomnia, and restlessness.
- Warn the patient to notify the physician if he or she experiences

chest pain, difficulty breathing, dizziness, flushing, headache, palpitations, tachycardia, or tremors.
• Urge the patient to avoid excessive use of caffeine derivatives such as chocolate, cocoa, cola, coffee, and tea.

salmeterol

sal-**me**-te-rol
(Serevent Diskus, Serevent Inhaler and Disks[AUS])
Do not confuse Serevent with Serentil.

CATEGORY AND SCHEDULE

Pregnancy Risk Category: C

MECHANISM OF ACTION

An adrenergic agonist that stimulates $beta_2$-adrenergic receptors in the lungs, resulting in relaxation of bronchial smooth muscle. **Therapeutic Effect:** Relieves bronchospasm and reduces airway resistance.

PHARMACOKINETICS

Route	Onset	Peak	Duration
Inhalation	10–20 min	3 hr	12 hr

Low systemic absorption; acts primarily in the lungs. Protein binding: 95%. Metabolized by hydroxylation. Primarily eliminated in feces. ***Half-life:*** 3–4 hr.

AVAILABILITY

Powder for Oral Inhalation (Serevent Diskus): 50 mcg.

INDICATIONS AND DOSAGES

▸ Prevention and maintenance treatment of asthma
Inhalation (Diskus)
Adults, Elderly, Children 4 yr and older. 1 inhalation (50 mcg) q12h.
▸ Prevention of exercise-induced bronchospasm
Inhalation
Adults, Elderly, Children 4 yr and older. 1 inhalation at least 30 min before exercise.
▸ COPD
Inhalation
Adults, Elderly. 1 inhalation q12h.

CONTRAINDICATIONS

History of hypersensitivity to sympathomimetics

INTERACTIONS

Drug
Beta blockers: May decrease the effects of beta blockers.
Herbal
None known.
Food
None known.

DIAGNOSTIC TEST EFFECTS

May decrease serum potassium level.

SIDE EFFECTS

Frequent (28%)
Headache
Occasional (7%–3%)
Cough, tremor, dizziness, vertigo, throat dryness or irritation, pharyngitis
Rare (3%)
Palpitations, tachycardia, nausea, heartburn, GI distress, diarrhea

SERIOUS REACTIONS

! Salmeterol may prolong the QT interval, which may precipitate ventricular arrhythmias.

! Hypokalemia and hyperglycemia may occur.

NURSING CONSIDERATIONS

Baseline Assessment

- Ask the patient about a history of sensitivity to sympathomimetics.
- Obtain a baseline EKG and measure the QT interval.
- Check the patient's baseline peak flow readings.

Lifespan Considerations

- It is unknown if salmeterol is excreted in breast milk.
- No age-related precautions have been noted in children older than 4 years.
- Elderly may require a lower dosage because of increased sensitivity to sympathomimetics and increased susceptibility to tachycardia and tremors.

Precautions

- Use salmeterol cautiously in patients with cardiovascular disorders (such as coronary insufficiency, arrhythmias, and hypertension), seizure disorders, or thyrotoxicosis.
- Salmeterol is not for acute asthma symptoms and may cause paradoxical bronchospasm.

Administration and Handling

Inhalation

- Shake the container well. Instruct the patient to exhale completely through the mouth. Then place the mouthpiece in the patient's mouth and have the patient close his or her lips, holding the inhaler upright.
- Have the patient inhale deeply through the mouth while fully depressing the top of canister. Instruct the patient to hold his or her breath for as long as possible before exhaling slowly.
- Tell the patient to wait 1 minute before inhaling a second dose to allow for deeper bronchial penetration.
- Instruct the patient to rinse his or her mouth with water immediately after inhalation to prevent mouth and throat dryness.

Intervention and Evaluation

- Monitor the patient's BP, pulse rate and quality, and respiratory rate, depth, rhythm, and type.
- Auscultate the patient's breath sounds for crackles, rhonchi, and wheezing.
- Periodically evaluate the patient's serum potassium level.

Patient Teaching

- Inform the patient that salmeterol is not intended for relief of acute asthmatic episodes.
- Instruct the patient to keep the drug canister at room temperature because cold decreases the drug's effects.
- When the drug is used to prevent exercise-induced bronchospasm, direct the patient to administer the dose at least 30 to 60 minutes before exercising.
- Instruct the patient to wait at least 1 full minute before the second inhalation.
- Caution the patient against abruptly discontinuing the drug or exceeding the recommended dosage.
- Warn the patient to notify the physician if he or she experiences chest pain or dizziness.
- Urge the patient to avoid excessive consumption of caffeinated products, such as chocolate, cocoa, cola, coffee, and tea.
- Teach the patient how to measure peak flow readings and keep a log of measurements.

terbutaline sulfate

ter-**byoo**-te-leen

(Brethine, Bricanyl[CAN])

Do not confuse terbutaline with tolbutamide or terbinafine, or Brethine with Brethaire.

CATEGORY AND SCHEDULE

Pregnancy Risk Category: B

MECHANISM OF ACTION

An adrenergic agonist that stimulates $beta_2$-adrenergic receptors, resulting in relaxation of uterine and bronchial smooth muscle. **Therapeutic Effect:** Relieves bronchospasm and reduces airway resistance. Also inhibits uterine contractions.

AVAILABILITY

Tablets: 2.5 mg, 5 mg.
Injection: 1 mg/ml.

INDICATIONS AND DOSAGES

▸ **Bronchospasm**

PO

Adults, Elderly, Children 15 yr and older. Initially, 2.5 mg 3–4 times a day. Maintenance: 2.5–5 mg 3 times a day q6h while awake. Maximum: 15 mg/day.

Children 12–14 yr. 2.5 mg 3 times a day. Maximum: 7.5 mg/day.

Children younger than 12 yr. Initially, 0.05 mg/kg/dose q8h. May increase up to 0.15 mg/kg/dose. Maximum: 5 mg.

Subcutaneous

Adults, Children 12 yr and older. Initially, 0.25 mg. Repeat in 15–30 min if substantial improvement does not occur. Maximum: 0.5 mg/4 hr.

Children younger than 12 yr. 0.005–0.01 mg/kg/dose to a maximum of 0.4 mg/dose q15–20min for 2 doses.

▸ **Preterm labor**

PO

Adults. 2.5–10 mg q4–6h.

IV

Adults. 2.5–10 mcg/min. May increase gradually q15–20 min up to 17.5–30 mcg/min.

CONTRAINDICATIONS

History of hypersensitivity to sympathomimetics

INTERACTIONS

Drug

Beta blockers: May decrease the effects of beta blockers.

Digoxin, sympathomimetics: May increase the risk of arrhythmias.

MAOIs: May increase the risk of hypertensive crisis.

Tricyclic antidepressants: May increase cardiovascular effects.

Herbal

None known.

Food

None known.

DIAGNOSTIC TEST EFFECTS

May decrease serum potassium level.

SIDE EFFECTS

Frequent (23%–18%)

Tremor, anxiety

Occasional (11%–10%)

Somnolence, headache, nausea, heartburn, dizziness

Rare (3%–1%)

Flushing, asthenia, mouth and throat dryness or irritation (with inhalation therapy)

SERIOUS REACTIONS

! Too-frequent or excessive use may lead to decreased drug effectiveness and severe, paradoxical bronchoconstriction.

! Excessive sympathomimetic stimulation may cause palpitations, extrasystoles, tachycardia, chest pain, a slight increase in BP followed by a substantial decrease, chills, diaphoresis, and blanching of skin.

NURSING CONSIDERATIONS

Baseline Assessment

- For the patient taking terbutaline for preterm labor, assess the maternal BP and pulse, the duration and frequency of contractions, and the fetal heart rate.

Precautions

- Use terbutaline cautiously in patients with cardiovascular disorders, hypertension, diabetes mellitus, a history of seizures, or hyperthyroidism.

Administration and Handling

PO

- Give terbutaline with food if the patient experiences GI upset.
- Crush tablets as needed.

IV

- Increase the IV infusion slowly, as prescribed, until contractions stop.

Subcutaneous

- Don't use solution if it appears discolored.
- Inject the drug subcutaneously into the lateral deltoid region.

Intervention and Evaluation

- Monitor the patient's pulse rate and quality and respiratory rate, depth, rhythm, and type.
- Auscultate the patient's breath sounds for rhonchi and wheezing.
- Periodically evaluate the patient's serum potassium level.
- Monitor the patient's ABG levels.
- Observe the patient's fingernails and lips for a blue or dusky color in light-skinned patients and a gray color in dark-skinned patients, which are signs of hypoxemia.
- Observe the patient for clavicular retractions and hand tremor.
- Offer emotional support to the patient taking terbutaline for bronchospasm; these patients are prone to anxiety because of difficulty breathing and the sympathomimetic effects of the drug.
- Evaluate the patient for evidence of clinical improvement, such as cessation of clavicular retractions, quieter and slower respirations, and a relaxed facial expression.
- When the drug is used for preterm labor, monitor the duration and frequency of contractions and diligently monitor the fetal heart rate.

Patient Teaching

- Warn the patient to notify the physician if he or she experiences chest pain, difficulty breathing, dizziness, flushing, headache, muscle tremors, or palpitations.
- Tell the patient that terbutaline may cause anxiety, nervousness, and shakiness.
- Urge the patient to avoid excessive consumption of caffeinated products, such as chocolate, cocoa, cola, coffee, and tea.

tiotropium bromide

tee-oh-**trow**-pea-um
(Spiriva)

CATEGORY AND SCHEDULE

Pregnancy Risk Category: C

MECHANISM OF ACTION

An anticholinergic that binds to recombinant human muscarinic receptors at the smooth muscle, resulting in long-acting bronchial smooth-muscle relaxation. **Therapeutic Effect:** Relieves bronchospasm.

PHARMACOKINETICS

Route	Onset	Peak	Duration
Inhalation	N/A	N/A	24–36 hr

Binds extensively to tissue. Protein binding: 72%. Metabolized by oxidation. Excreted in urine. ***Half-life:*** 5–6 days

AVAILABILITY

Powder for Inhalation: 18 mcg/capsule (in blister packs containing 6 capsules with inhaler).

INDICATIONS AND DOSAGES

▸ COPD

Inhalation

Adults, Elderly. 18 mcg (1 capsule)/day via HandiHaler inhalation device.

CONTRAINDICATIONS

History of hypersensitivity to atropine or its derivatives, including ipratropium

INTERACTIONS

Drug

Ipratropium: Concurrent administration with this drug is not recommended.

Herbal

None known.

Food

None known.

DIAGNOSTIC TEST EFFECTS

None known.

SIDE EFFECTS

Frequent (16%–6%)

Dry mouth, sinusitis, pharyngitis, dyspepsia, UTI, rhinitis

Occasional (5%–4%)

Abdominal pain, peripheral edema, constipation, epistaxis, vomiting, myalgia, rash, oral candidiasis

SERIOUS REACTIONS

! Angina pectoris, depression, and flulike symptoms occur rarely.

NURSING CONSIDERATIONS

Baseline Assessment

- Perform baseline assessment of breath sounds, auscultating for adventitious sounds.
- Determine the patient's baseline exercise and activity tolerance.

Lifespan Considerations

- It is unknown if tiotropium is distributed in breast milk.
- The safety and efficacy of tiotropium have not been established in children.
- Elderly patients are more likely to experience constipation, dry mouth, and UTI.

Precautions

- Use tiotropium cautiously in patients with angle-closure glaucoma, benign prostatic hyperplasia, or bladder neck obstruction.

Administration and Handling

- Store tiotropium capsules at room temperature. Protect them from extreme temperatures and moisture.
- Don't store capsules in the HandiHaler device.

Inhalation

- Open the HandiHaler dustcap by pulling it up; then open the mouthpiece.
- Place the capsule in the center chamber and firmly close the mouthpiece until you hear a click, leaving the dustcap open.
- Holding the HandiHaler device with the mouthpiece up, press the piercing button completely once and then release it.
- Instruct the patient to exhale completely before inhaling slowly and deeply, at a rate sufficient to hear the capsule vibrate.
- Have the patient hold his or her

breath for as long as is comfortable and then exhale slowly.
- Instruct the patient to repeat this process a second time to ensure that he or she receives the full dose.

Intervention and Evaluation
- Monitor pulse rate and quality and respiratory rate, depth, rhythm, and type.
- Auscultate the patient's breath sounds for crackles, rhonchi, and wheezing.
- Monitor the patient's ABG levels.
- Examine the patient's lips and fingernails for signs of cyanosis, such as a blue or gray color in light-skinned patients and a gray color in dark-skinned patients.
- Observe the patient for clavicular retractions and hand tremor.
- Evaluate the patient for signs of clinical improvement, such as cessation of clavicular retractions, quieter and slower respirations, and a relaxed facial expression.
- Offer emotional support to the patient and family. Many patients with COPD experience anxiety from difficulty breathing and the sympathomimetic response to the drug.

Patient Teaching
- Instruct the patient to use only 1 capsule for inhalation at a time.
- Inform the patient that rinsing the mouth with water immediately after inhalation may prevent mouth and throat dryness and oral candidiasis.
- Instruct the patient to drink plenty of fluids to decrease the thickness of lung secretions.
- Urge the patient to avoid excessive consumption of caffeine products, such as chocolate, cocoa, cola, coffee, and tea.

85 Lung Surfactants

beractant
calfactant
poractant alfa

Uses: Lung surfactants are used to prevent and treat respiratory distress syndrome (RDS) in premature neonates, often improving oxygenation within minutes of administration.

Action: By replenishing pulmonary surfactant, which is deficient in premature neonates, lung surfactants lower the surface tension on alveolar surfaces during respiration. They also stabilize the alveoli to prevent the collapse that may occur with resting transpulmonary pressures. Their actions improve lung compliance and respiratory gas exchange. (See the illustration *Sites of Action: Respiratory Agents,* page 1426.)

beractant

ber-**akt**-ant
(Survanta)
Do not confuse Survanta with Sufenta.

CATEGORY AND SCHEDULE
Pregnancy Risk Category: This drug is not indicated for use in pregnant women.

MECHANISM OF ACTION
A natural bovine lung extract that reduces alveolar surface tension, stabilizing alveoli. **Therapeutic Effect:** Improves lung compliance and respiratory gas exchange.

PHARMACOKINETICS
Not absorbed systemically.

AVAILABILITY
Intratracheal Suspension for Inhalation: 25-mg/ml vials.

INDICATIONS AND DOSAGES
▸ Prevention and rescue treatment of respiratory distress syndrome (RDS) or hyaline membrane disease in premature infants
Intratracheal
Infants. 100 mg of phospholipids/kg birth weight (4 ml/kg). Give within 15 min of birth if infant weighs less than 1,250 g and has evidence of surfactant deficiency; give within 8 hr when RDS is confirmed by X-ray and requires mechanical ventilation. May repeat 6 hr or longer after preceding dose. Maximum: 4 doses in the first 48 hr of life.

CONTRAINDICATIONS
None known.

INTERACTIONS
Drug
None known.
Herbal
None known.
Food
None known.

DIAGNOSTIC TEST EFFECTS
None known.

SIDE EFFECTS

Frequent

Transient bradycardia, oxygen (O_2) desaturation, increased carbon dioxide (CO_2) retention

Occasional

Endotracheal tube reflux

Rare

Apnea, endotracheal tube blockage, hypotension or hypertension, pallor, vasoconstriction

SERIOUS REACTIONS

! Life-threatening nosocomial sepsis may occur.

NURSING CONSIDERATIONS

Baseline Assessment

• Administer beractant in a highly supervised setting. Clinicians caring for the neonate must be experienced with intubation and ventilator management.

Lifespan Considerations

• This drug is for use only in neonates. No age-related precautions have been noted.

Precautions

• Use beractant cautiously in patients at risk for circulatory overload.

Administration and Handling

Intratracheal

• Refrigerate vials. Unopened, unused vials may be returned to the refrigerator only once and within 8 hours after having been warmed to room temperature.
• Warm the vial by letting it stand at room temperature for 20 minutes or warming in your hand for 8 minutes.
• Gently swirl the vial, if needed, to redisperse contents. Do not shake it.
• The solution normally appears off-white to light brown.
• Enter each single-use vial only once; discard unused suspension.
• Instill the drug through a catheter inserted into the infant's endotracheal tube. Don't instill it into the main-stem bronchus.
• Monitor the infant for bradycardia and decreased arterial O_2 saturation during administration. Stop the procedure, as prescribed, if the infant experiences these effects, and take appropriate measures before reinstituting therapy.

Intervention and Evaluation

• Monitor the infant with arterial or transcutaneous measurement of systemic O_2 and CO_2.
• Auscultate the patient's breath sounds for crackles and rhonchi.
• Limit visitors during treatment, and monitor for hand washing and other infection control measures to minimize the risk of nosocomial infections.
• Offer emotional support to the patient's parents.

Patient Teaching

• Tell the parents the purpose of the treatment and the expected outcome.

calfactant

cal-**fac**-tant
(Infasurf)

CATEGORY AND SCHEDULE

Pregnancy Risk Category: This drug is not indicated for use in pregnant women.

MECHANISM OF ACTION

A natural lung extract that reduces alveolar surface tension, stabilizing the alveoli. **Therapeutic Effect:** Restores surface activity to infant lungs, improves lung compliance and respiratory gas exchange.

PHARMACOKINETICS

No studies have been performed.

AVAILABILITY

Intratracheal Suspension: 35-mg/ml vials.

INDICATIONS AND DOSAGES

▸ Respiratory distress syndrome (RDS)

Intratracheal

Neonates. 3 ml/kg of birth weight administered as soon as possible after birth in 2 doses of 1.5 ml/kg. Repeat 3-ml/kg doses, up to a total of 3 doses given 12 hr apart.

CONTRAINDICATIONS

None known.

INTERACTIONS

Drug

None known.

Herbal

None known.

Food

None known.

DIAGNOSTIC TEST EFFECTS

None known.

SIDE EFFECTS

Frequent

Cyanosis (65%), airway obstruction (39%), bradycardia (34%), reflux of surfactant into endotracheal tube (21%), need for manual ventilation (16%)

Occasional

Need for reintubation (3%)

SERIOUS REACTIONS

! None known.

NURSING CONSIDERATIONS

Baseline Assessment

- Administer calfactant in a highly supervised setting. Clinicians caring for the neonate must be experienced with intubation and ventilator management.

Lifespan Considerations

- This drug is for use only in neonates. No age-related precautions have been noted.

Precautions

- Use calfactant cautiously in patients with a hypersensitivity to calfactant.

Administration and Handling

Intratracheal

- Refrigerate vials. Unopened, unused vials may be returned to refrigerator only once after having been warmed to room temperature.
- Gently swirl the vial, if needed, to redisperse contents. Do not shake it.
- Enter each single-use vial only once; discard unused suspension.
- Instill the drug intratracheally through a side port adapter into the infant's endotracheal tube.
- Give each aliquot over 20–30 ventilatory breaths.
- Administer only during the inspiratory cycle.
- Between aliquot dosages, turn the infant so that the opposite lung is in the dependent position.

Intervention and Evaluation

- Monitor the neonate's oxygenation and ventilation using arterial or transcutaneous measurement of systemic oxygen (O_2) and carbon dioxide (CO_2).
- Auscultate the patient's breath sounds for crackles and rhonchi.
- Limit visitors during treatment, and monitor for hand washing and other infection control measures to minimize the risk of nosocomial infections.
- Offer emotional support to the patient's parents.

Patient Teaching

- Tell the parents the purpose of the treatment and the expected outcome.

poractant alfa

poor-**ak**-tant
(Curosurf)

CATEGORY AND SCHEDULE

Pregnancy Risk Category: This drug is not indicated for use in pregnant women.

MECHANISM OF ACTION

A pulmonary surfactant that reduces alveolar surface tension during ventilation and stabilizes the alveoli against collapse that may occur at resting transpulmonary pressures.
Therapeutic Effect: Improves lung compliance and respiratory gas exchange.

AVAILABILITY

Intratracheal Suspension: 1.5 ml (120 mg), 3 ml (240 mg).

INDICATIONS AND DOSAGES

▸ **Respiratory distress syndrome (RDS)**

Intratracheal
Infants. Initially, 2.5 ml/kg of birth weight. May give up to 2 subsequent doses of 1.25 ml/kg of birth weight at 12-hr intervals. Maximum: 5 ml/kg (total dose).

OFF-LABEL USES

Adult RDS due to viral pneumonia or near-drowning, *Pneumocystis carinii* pneumonia in HIV-infected patients, prevention of RDS

CONTRAINDICATIONS

None known.

INTERACTIONS

Drug
None known.
Herbal
None known.
Food
None known.

DIAGNOSTIC TEST EFFECTS

None known.

SIDE EFFECTS

Frequent
Transient bradycardia, oxygen (O_2) desaturation, increased carbon dioxide (CO_2) retention
Occasional
Endotracheal tube reflux
Rare
Apnea, endotracheal tube blockage, hypotension or hypertension, pallor, vasoconstriction

SERIOUS REACTIONS

! None known.

NURSING CONSIDERATIONS

Baseline Assessment

- Plan to correct acidosis, anemia, hypoglycemia, hypotension, and hypothermia before beginning poractant alfa administration.
- Change ventilator settings, as prescribed, to 40 to 60 breaths/minute, inspiratory time 0.5 sec, and supplemental O_2 sufficient to maintain arterial O_2 saturation (SaO_2) greater than 92% immediately before administering drug.
- Administer poractant in a highly supervised setting. Clinicians caring for the neonate must be experienced with intubation and ventilator management.

Lifespan Considerations

- This drug is for use only in neonates. No age-related precautions have been noted.

Precautions

- Use poractant cautiously in patients at risk for circulatory overload.

Administration and Handling

Intratracheal

- Refrigerate vials. Unopened, unused vials may be returned to the refrigerator only once after having been warmed to room temperature.
- Warm the vial by letting it stand at room temperature for 20 minutes or warming it in your hand for 8 minutes.
- Turn the vial upside down and gently swirl it, if needed, to obtain a uniform suspension. Do not shake the vial.
- Withdraw the entire contents of the vial into a 3- or 5-ml plastic syringe through a large-gauge needle (20 gauge or larger).
- Attach the syringe to a catheter that's inserted into the infant's endotracheal tube, and instill the solution through the catheter.
- Monitor the infant for bradycardia and decreased SaO_2 during administration. Stop the procedure if the infant experiences these effects, and take appropriate measures before reinstituting therapy.

Intervention and Evaluation

- Monitor the infant's oxygenation and ventilation using arterial or transcutaneous measurement of systemic O_2 and CO_2.
- Monitor the patient's heart rate and auscultate breath sounds for crackles and rhonchi.
- Limit visitors during treatment, and monitor for hand washing and other infection control measures to minimize the risk of nosocomial infections.
- Offer emotional support to the patient's parents.

Patient Teaching

- Tell the parents the purpose of the treatment and the expected outcome.

naphazoline
phenylephrine
pseudoephedrine
sodium chloride

Uses: Nasal decongestants are used to relieve stuffiness caused by such conditions as common cold, acute or chronic rhinitis, hay fever, and other allergies. Sodium chloride is administered nasally to restore moisture and relieve dry, inflamed nasal membranes.

Action: Most nasal decongestants stimulate $alpha_1$-adrenergic receptors on nasal blood vessels, causing vasoconstriction that shrinks swollen membranes and allows nasal drainage. As a major extracellular cation, sodium chloride soothes the nasal passages. (See the illustration *Sites of Action: Respiratory Agents,* page 1426.)

COMBINATION PRODUCTS

ADVIL COLD: pseudoephedrine/ibuprofen (an NSAID) 30 mg/200 mg; 15 mg/100 mg per 5 ml.
ALLEGRA-D: pseudoephedrine/fexofenadine (an antihistamine) 120 mg/60 mg.
ALLEGRA-D 24 HOUR: pseudoephedrine/fexofenadine (an antihistamine) 240 mg/180 mg.
CHILDREN'S ADVIL COLD: pseudoephedrine/ibuprofen (an NSAID) 15 mg/100 mg per 5 ml.
CLARITIN-D: pseudoephedrine/loratadine (an antihistamine) 120 mg/ 5 mg; 240 mg/10 mg.
MOTRIN COLD: pseudoephedrine/ibuprofen (an NSAID) 30 mg/200 mg; 15 mg/100 mg per 5 ml.
MUCINEX D: pseudoephedrine/guaifenesin (an antitussive) 60 mg/600 mg; 120 mg/1,200 mg.
NAPHCON-A: naphazoline/pheniramine (an antihistamine) 0.25%/0.3%.
PHENERGAN VC: phenylephrine/promethazine (an antihistamine) 5 mg/6.25 mg per 5 ml.
PHENERGAN VC WITH CODEINE: phenylephrine/promethazine (an antihistamine)/codeine (a narcotic analgesic) 5 mg/6.25 mg/10 mg per 5 ml.
ZYRTEC D-12 HOUR: pseudoephedrine/cetirizine (an antihistamine) 120 mg/5 mg.
PHENYLEPHRINE HYDROCHLORIDE: See vasopressors
SODIUM CHLORIDE: See minerals and electrolytes

naphazoline

naf-**az**-oh-leen
(AK-Con, Albalon Liquifilm[AUS], Clear Eyes[AUS], Naphcon, Naphcon Forte[AUS], Privine, Vasocon)

CATEGORY AND SCHEDULE

Pregnancy Risk Category: C

MECHANISM OF ACTION

A sympathomimetic that directly acts on alpha-adrenergic receptors in conjunctival arterioles and nasal blood vessels. **Therapeutic Effect:** Causes vasoconstriction, resulting in decreased congestion.

AVAILABILITY

Ophthalmic Solution: 0.012%, 0.1%.
Nasal Drops: 0.05%.
Nasal Spray: 0.05%.

INDICATIONS AND DOSAGES

▸ **Nasal congestion due to acute or chronic rhinitis, common cold, hay fever, or other allergies**

Intranasal

Adults, Elderly, Children older than 12 yr. 1–2 drops or sprays in each nostril q3–6h.

Children 6–12 yr. 1 spray or drop in each nostril q6h as needed.

▸ **Control of hyperemia in patients with superficial corneal vascularity; relief of congestion and inflammation; for use during ocular diagnostic procedures**

Ophthalmic

Adults, Elderly, Children older than 6 yr. 1–2 drops in affected eye q3–4h for 3–4 days.

CONTRAINDICATIONS

Angle-closure glaucoma, before peripheral iridectomy, patients with a narrow angle who do not have glaucoma

INTERACTIONS

Drug

Maprotiline, tricyclic antidepressants: May increase the effects of naphazoline.

Herbal

None known.

Food

None known.

DIAGNOSTIC TEST EFFECTS

None known.

SIDE EFFECTS

Occasional

Nasal: Burning, stinging, or drying of nasal mucosa; sneezing; rebound congestion

Ophthalmic: Blurred vision, dilated pupils, increased eye irritation

SERIOUS REACTIONS

! If naphazoline is systemically absorbed, the patient may experience tachycardia, palpitations, headache, insomnia, light-headedness, nausea, nervousness, and tremor.

! Large doses may produce tachycardia, palpitations, light-headedness, nausea, and vomiting.

! Overdose in patients older than 60 years may produce hallucinations, CNS depression, and seizures.

NURSING CONSIDERATIONS

Baseline Assessment

- Ask the patient if he or she takes tricyclic antidepressants before administering naphazoline.

Precautions

- Use naphazoline cautiously in patients with cerebral arteriosclerosis, diabetes, heart disease (including coronary artery disease), hypertension, hypertensive cardiovascular disease, hyperthyroidism, or long-standing bronchial asthma.

Administration and Handling

◂ **ALERT** ▸ Store nasal and ophthalmic drugs in a tightly closed container. Do not freeze.

Nasal

- Whenever possible, place the patient in an upright position to instill nasal spray.
- To minimize the risk of systemic absorption, tilt the patient's head slightly downward and avoid directing the spray towards the nasopharynx.

Intervention and Evaluation

- Monitor BP regularly for increases.
- Monitor for rebound nasal congestion in patients receiving long-term nasal naphazoline.

Patient Teaching

- Caution the patient not to use naphazoline for more than 72 hours without consulting a physician because too-frequent use may cause rebound congestion.
- Warn the patient who is using ophthalmic naphazoline to be cautious when performing tasks that require visual acuity.
- Tell the patient to discontinue the drug and contact the physician if he or she experiences acute eye redness or eye pain, floating spots, vision changes, headache, dizziness, insomnia, irregular heartbeat, tremor, or weakness.

phenylephrine

See Vasopressors

pseudoephedrine

soo-doe-e-**fed**-rin

(Balminil Decongestant[CAN], BioContac Cold 12 Hour Relief Non Drowsy[CAN], Decofed, Dimetapp 12 Hour Non Drowsy Extentabs, Dimetapp Decongestant, Dimetapp sinus liquid caps[AUS], Genaphed, PMS-Pseudoephedrine[CAN], Robidrine[CAN], Sudafed, Sudafed 12h[AUS], Sudafed 12 Hour, Sudafed 24 Hour)

CATEGORY AND SCHEDULE

Pregnancy Risk Category: C

OTC

MECHANISM OF ACTION

A sympathomimetic that directly stimulates alpha-adrenergic and beta-adrenergic receptors. **Therapeutic Effect:** Produces vasoconstriction of respiratory tract mucosa; shrinks nasal mucous membranes; reduces edema, and nasal congestion.

PHARMACOKINETICS

Route	Onset	Peak	Duration
PO (tablets, syrup)	15–30 min	N/A	4–6 hr
PO (extended-release)	N/A	N/A	8–12 hr

Well absorbed from the GI tract. Partially metabolized in the liver. Primarily excreted in urine. Not removed by hemodialysis. ***Half-life:*** 9–16 hr (children, 3.1 hr).

AVAILABILITY

Gelcaps (Dimetapp Decongestant): 30 mg.
Liquid (Sudafed): 15 mg/5 ml.
Oral Drops (Dimetapp Infant Drops): 7.5 mg/0.8 ml.
Syrup (Biofed, Decofed): 30 mg/5 ml.
Tablets (Genaphed, Sudafed): 30 mg.
Tablets (Chewable [Sudafed]): 15 mg.
Tablets (Extended-Release [Dimetapp 12 Hour Non Drowsy Extentabs, Sudafed 12 Hour]): 120 mg.
Tablets (Extended-Release [Sudafed 24 Hour]): 240 mg.

INDICATIONS AND DOSAGES

▸ **Decongestant**

PO

Adults, Children 12 yr and older. 60 mg q4–6h. Maximum: 240 mg/day.
Children 6–11 yr. 30 mg q6h. Maximum: 120 mg/day.
Children 2–5 yr. 15 mg q6h. Maximum: 60 mg/day.
Children younger than 2 yr. 4 mg/kg/day in divided doses q6h.
Elderly. 30–60 mg q6h as needed.

PO (Extended-Release)
Adults, Children 12 yr and older. 120 mg q12h.

CONTRAINDICATIONS

Breast-feeding women, coronary artery disease, severe hypertension, use within 14 days of MAOIs

INTERACTIONS

Drug

Antihypertensive, beta blockers, diuretics: May decrease the effects of these drugs.
MAOIs: May increase cardiac stimulant and vasopressor effects.

Herbal

None known.

Food

None known.

DIAGNOSTIC TEST EFFECTS

None known.

SIDE EFFECTS

Occasional (10%–5%)

Nervousness, restlessness, insomnia, tremor, headache

Rare (4%–1%)

Diaphoresis, weakness

SERIOUS REACTIONS

! Large doses may produce tachycardia, palpitations (particularly in patients with cardiac disease), light-headedness, nausea, and vomiting.
! Overdose in patients older than 60 years may result in hallucinations, CNS depression, and seizures.

NURSING CONSIDERATIONS

Baseline Assessment

- Ask the patient if he or she takes antihypertensives, beta blockers, diuretics, or MAOIs before administering pseudoephedrine.

Lifespan Considerations

- Pseudoephedrine crosses the placenta and is distributed in breast milk.
- The safety and efficacy of pseudoephedrine have not been established in children younger than 2 years.
- Age-related benign prostatic hyperplasia may require a dosage adjustment in the elderly.

Precautions

- Use pseudoephedrine cautiously in elderly patients and patients with diabetes, heart disease, hyperthyroidism, or benign prostatic hyperplasia.

Administration and Handling

PO
- Don't crush extended-release tablets; have the patient swallow them whole.

Patient Teaching

- Instruct the patient to swallow extended-release tablets whole, not to chew or crush them.
- Advise the patient to discontinue therapy and notify the physician if he or she experiences dizziness, insomnia, irregular or rapid heartbeat, tremors, or other side effects.

sodium chloride

See Minerals and Electrolytes

87 Respiratory Inhalants and Intranasal Steroids

acetylcysteine
beclomethasone dipropionate
budesonide
cromolyn sodium
flunisolide
fluticasone propionate
mometasone furoate monohydrate
nedocromil sodium
triamcinolone

Uses: Most respiratory inhalants and intranasal steroids are used to treat seasonal and perennial rhinitis, to prevent all major symptoms of rhinitis, and to manage bronchial asthma. Acetylcysteine is prescribed as an adjunct to treat bronchopulmonary disease and pulmonary complications of cystic fibrosis. It's also used in tracheostomy care and the treatment of acetaminophen overdose. Beclomethasone is also used to prevent nasal polyp recurrence after surgery.

Action: Several mechanisms of action account for the effects of respiratory inhalants and intranasal steroids. *Acetylcysteine* splits the disulfide linkages between mucoproteins, reducing the viscosity of pulmonary secretions. *Intranasal steroids,* such as beclomethasone and fluticasone, prevent the inflammatory response to allergens. *Cromolyn* and *nedocromil* prevent the release of inflammatory mediators from mast cells.

COMBINATION PRODUCTS

ADVAIR: fluticasone/salmeterol (a bronchodilator) 100 mcg/50 mcg; 250 mcg/50 mcg; 500 mcg/50 mcg.
MYCO-II: triamcinolone/nystatin (an antifungal) 0.1%/100,000 units/g.
MYCOLOG II: triamcinolone/nystatin (an antifungal) 0.1%/100,000 units/g.
MYCO-TRIACET: triamcinolone/nystatin (an antifungal) 0.1%/100,000 units/g.

acetylcysteine

a-see-til-**sis**-tay-een
(Acetadote, Mucomyst, Parvolex[CAN])
Do not confuse acetylcysteine with acetylcholine.

CATEGORY AND SCHEDULE

Pregnancy Risk Category: B

MECHANISM OF ACTION

An intratracheal respiratory inhalant that splits the linkage of mucoproteins, reducing the viscosity of pulmonary secretions. **Therapeutic Effect:** Facilitates the removal of pulmonary secretions by coughing, postural drainage, mechanical means. Protects against acetaminophen overdose–induced hepatotoxicity.

AVAILABILITY

Injection (Acedote): 20% (200 mg/ml).
Inhalation Solution (Mucomyst): 10% (100 mg/ml), 20% (200 mg/ml).

INDICATIONS AND DOSAGES

▸ **Adjunctive treatment of viscid mucus secretions from chronic bronchopulmonary disease and for pulmonary complications of cystic fibrosis**

Nebulization

Adults, Elderly, Children. 3–5 ml (20% solution) 3–4 times a day or 6–10 ml (10% solution) 3–4 times a day. Range: 1–10 ml (20% solution) q2–6h or 2–20 ml (10% solution) q2–6h.

Infants. 1–2 ml (20%) or 2–4 ml (10%) 3–4 times a day.

▸ **Treatment of viscid mucus secretions in patients with a tracheostomy**

Intratracheal

Adults, Children. 1–2 ml of 10% or 20% solution instilled into tracheostomy q1–4h.

▸ **Acetaminophen overdose**

PO (Oral solution 5%)

Adults, Elderly, Children. Loading dose of 140 mg/kg, followed in 4 hr by maintenance dose of 70 mg/kg q4h for 17 additional doses (unless acetaminophen assay reveals nontoxic level).

IV

Adults, Elderly, Children. 150 mg/kg infused over 15 minutes, then 50 mg/kg infused over 4 hr, then 100 mg/kg infused over 16 hr. See administration and handling. Repeat dose if emesis occurs within 1 hr of administration. Continue until all doses are given, until acetaminophen plasma level drops below toxic range.

▸ **Prevention of renal damage from dyes used during certain diagnostic tests**

PO (Oral solution 5%)

Adults, Elderly. 600 mg twice a day for 4 doses starting the day before the procedure.

OFF-LABEL USES

Prevention of renal damage from dyes given during certain diagnostic tests (such as CT scans)

CONTRAINDICATIONS

None known.

INTERACTIONS

Drug

None known.

Herbal

None known.

Food

None known.

DIAGNOSTIC TEST EFFECTS

None known.

SIDE EFFECTS

Frequent

Inhalation: Stickiness on face, transient unpleasant odor

Occasional

Inhalation: Increased bronchial secretions, throat irritation, nausea, vomiting, rhinorrhea

Rare

Inhalation: Rash

Oral: Facial edema, bronchospasm, wheezing

SERIOUS REACTIONS

! Large doses may produce severe nausea and vomiting.

NURSING CONSIDERATIONS

Baseline Assessment

- Assess respiratory rate, depth, and rhythm before treatment when this drug is used as a mucolytic.

Precautions

- Use acetylcysteine cautiously in patients with bronchial asthma and in elderly or debilitated patients with severe respiratory insufficiency.

Administration and Handling

PO

- To create the oral solution, dilute 20% solution with water or soft drinks to create a 5% concentration. Use within 1 hour.
- When administering the solution by nebulizer, avoid using equipment that contains copper, iron, or rubber because the drug will react with these materials on contact.

IV

- Give 3 infusions of different strengths: first dose (150 mg/kg) in 200 ml D_5W and infused over 15 minutes, second dose (50 mg/kg) in 500 ml D_5W and infused over 4 hours, third dose (100 mg/kg) in 1000 ml D_5W and infused over 16 hours.

Inhalation

- May administer either undiluted or diluted with 0.9% NaCl.

Intervention and Evaluation

- If bronchospasm occurs, discontinue treatment, notify the physician, and expect to administer a bronchodilator as needed.
- Monitor the respiratory rate, depth, rhythm, and type (such as abdominal or thoracic).
- Check the color, consistency, and amount of sputum.

Patient Teaching

- Inform the patient that a slight, disagreeable odor may emanate from the solution during initial administration but that it disappears quickly.
- Stress the importance of drinking plenty of fluids to maintain adequate hydration.
- Teach the patient proper coughing and deep breathing techniques.

beclomethasone dipropionate

be-kloe-**meth**-a-sone

(Aldecin[AUS], Aldecin Hayfever Aqueous Nasal Spray[AUS], Beclodisk[CAN], Becloforte inhaler[CAN], Beconase AQ, Becotide[AUS], Qvar)

Do not confuse Becloforte or Beconase with baclofen.

CATEGORY AND SCHEDULE

Pregnancy Risk Category: C

MECHANISM OF ACTION

An adrenocorticosteroid that prevents or controls inflammation by controlling the rate of protein synthesis; decreasing migration of polymorphonuclear leukocytes and fibroblasts; and reversing capillary permeability. **Therapeutic Effect:** Inhalation: Inhibits bronchoconstriction, produces smooth muscle relaxation, decreases mucus secretion. Intranasal: Decreases response to seasonal and perennial rhinitis.

PHARMACOKINETICS

Rapidly absorbed from pulmonary, nasal, and GI tissue. Undergoes extensive first-pass metabolism in the liver. Protein binding: 87%.

Primarily eliminated in feces. ***Half-life:*** 15 hr.

AVAILABILITY

Oral Inhalation (Qvar). 40 mcg/inhalation, 80 mcg/inhalation.
Nasal spray (Beconase AQ). 42 mcg/inhalation.

INDICATIONS AND DOSAGES

▸ **Long-term control of bronchial asthma, reduces need for oral corticosteriod therapy for asthma**
Oral Inhalation
Adults, Elderly Children 12 yr and older. 40–160 mcg twice a day. Maxiumum: 320 mcg twice a day.
Children 5–11 yr. 40 mcg twice a day. Maximum: 80 mcg twice a day.

▸ **Relief of seasonal or perennial rhinitis, prevention of nasal polyp recurrence after surgical removal, treatment of nonallergic rhinitis**
Nasal Inhalation
Adults, Children older than 12 yr. 1–2 sprays in each nostril twice a day.
Children 6–12 yr. 1 spray in each nostril twice a day. May increase up to 2 sprays in each nostril twice a day.

OFF-LABEL USES

Prevention of seasonal rhinitis (nasal form)

CONTRAINDICATIONS

Hypersensitivity to beclomethasone, status asthmaticus

INTERACTIONS

Drug
None known.

Herbal
None known.

Food
None known.

DIAGNOSTIC TEST EFFECTS

None known.

SIDE EFFECTS

Frequent
Inhalation (14%–4%): Throat irritation, dry mouth, hoarseness, cough
Intranasal: Nasal burning, mucosal dryness

Occasional
Inhalation (3%–2%): Localized fungal infection (thrush)
Intranasal: Nasal-crusting epistaxis, sore throat, ulceration of nasal mucosa

Rare
Inhalation: Transient bronchospasm, esophageal candidiasis
Intranasal: Nasal and pharyngeal candidiasis, eye pain

SERIOUS REACTIONS

! An acute hypersensitivity reaction, as evidenced by urticaria, angioedema, and severe bronchospasm, occurs rarely.

! A transfer from systemic to local steroid therapy may unmask previously suppressed bronchial asthma condition.

NURSING CONSIDERATIONS

Baseline Assessment
- Determine if the patient has hypersensitivity to corticosteroids.

Lifespan Considerations
- It is unknown if beclomethasone crosses the placenta or is distributed in breast milk.
- In children, prolonged treatment and high doses may decrease cortisol secretion and the short-term growth rate.
- No age-related precautions have been noted in the elderly.

Precautions
- Use beclomethasone cautiously in patients with cirrhosis, glaucoma,

hypothyroidism, osteoporosis, tuberculosis, or untreated systemic infections.

Administration and Handling

Inhalation

- Shake the container well. Instruct the patient to exhale completely and place the mouthpiece between the lips. Have the patient inhale and hold his or her breath for as long as possible before exhaling.
- Allow at least 1 minute between inhalations.
- Have the patient rinse his or her mouth after each use to decrease dry mouth and hoarseness.

Intranasal

- Have the patient clear his or her nasal passages as much as possible.
- Insert the spray tip into the patient's nostril, pointing toward the nasal passages, away from the nasal septum.
- Spray beclomethasone into the nostril while holding the patient's other nostril closed, and at the same time, have the patient inhale through the nose to deliver the medication as high into the nasal passages as possible.

Intervention and Evaluation

- During therapy, evaluate the patient for relief of symptoms, such as wheezing, congestion, and dyspnea.

Patient Teaching

- Advise the patient not to change the beclomethasone dosage schedule or stop taking the drug abruptly. Explain that he or she must taper the dosage gradually under medical supervision.
- Encourage the patient receiving beclomethasone by inhalation to maintain fastidious oral hygiene. Instruct the patient to rinse his or her mouth with water immediately after inhalation to prevent dryness and fungal infection of the mouth. Urge the patient to notify the physician or nurse if he or she develops a sore throat or mouth.
- Advise the patient receiving beclomethasone intranasally to clear the nasal passages before using the drug and to notify the physician if nasal irritation occurs or if symptoms, such as sneezing, fail to improve.
- If the patient is using a bronchodilator inhaler concomitantly with a steroid inhaler, advise him or her to use the bronchodilator several minutes before using the corticosteroid to help the steroid penetrate into the bronchial tree.
- Inform the patient that symptoms should improve in several days.

budesonide

bu-**dess**-ah-nide

(Burinex[AUS], Entocort EC, Pulmicort Respules, Pulmicort Turbuhaler, Rhinocort Aqua, Rhinocort Aqueous[AUS], Rhinocort Hayfever[AUS])

CATEGORY AND SCHEDULE

Pregnancy Risk Category: B

MECHANISM OF ACTION

A glucocorticoid that inhibits the accumulation of inflammatory cells and decreases and prevents tissues from responding to the inflammatory process. **Therapeutic Effect:** Relieves symptoms of allergic rhinitis or Crohn's disease.

PHARMACOKINETICS

Minimally absorbed from nasal tissue; moderately absorbed from inhalation. Protein binding: 88%. Primarily metabolized in the liver. ***Half-life:*** 2–3 hr.

AVAILABILITY

Capsules (Entocort EC): 3 mg.
Powder for oral inhalation (Pulmicort Turbuhaler): 200 mcg per inhalation.
Suspension for oral inhalation (Pulmicort Respules): 0.25 mg/2 ml; 0.5 mg/2 mg.
Nasal spray (Rhinocort Aqua): 32 mcg/spray.

INDICATIONS AND DOSAGES

▸ **Rhinitis**

Intranasal (Rhinocort Aqua)

Adults, Elderly, Children 6 yr and older. 1 spray in each nostril once a day. Maximum: 8 sprays/day for adults and children 12 yr and older; 4 sprays/day for children younger than 12 yr.

▸ **Bronchial asthma**

Nebulization

Children 6 mo–8 yr. 0.25–1 mg/day titrated to lowest effective dosage.

Inhalation

Adults, Elderly, Children 6 yr and older. Initially, 200–400 mcg twice a day. Maximum: Adults: 800 mcg twice a day. Children: 400 mcg twice a day.

▸ **Crohn's disease**

PO

Adults, Elderly. 9 mg once a day for up to 8 wk.

OFF-LABEL USES

Treatment of vasomotor rhinitis

CONTRAINDICATIONS

Hypersensitivity to any corticosteroid or its components, persistently positive sputum cultures for *Candida albicans*, primary treatment of status asthmaticus, systemic fungal infections, untreated localized infection involving nasal mucosa

INTERACTIONS

Drug

None known.

Herbal

None known.

Food

None known.

DIAGNOSTIC TEST EFFECTS

None known.

SIDE EFFECTS

Frequent (greater than 3%)

Nasal: Mild nasopharyngeal irritation, burning, stinging, or dryness; headache; cough

Inhalation: Flulike symptoms, headache, pharyngitis

Occasional (3%–1%)

Nasal: Dry mouth, dyspepsia, rebound congestion, rhinorrhea, loss of taste

Inhalation: Back pain, vomiting, altered taste, voice changes, abdominal pain, nausea, dyspepsia

SERIOUS REACTIONS

! An acute hypersensitivity reaction marked by urticaria, angioedema, and severe bronchospasm, occurs rarely.

NURSING CONSIDERATIONS

Baseline Assessment

- Determine if the patient is hypersensitive to any corticosteroids or their components.

Lifespan Considerations

- It is unknown if budesonide crosses the placenta or is distributed in breast milk.
- In children, prolonged treatment and high doses may decrease cortisol secretion and short-term growth rate.
- No age-related precautions have been noted in the elderly.

Precautions
- Use budesonide cautiously in patients with adrenal insufficiency, cirrhosis, glaucoma, hypothyroidism, osteoporosis, tuberculosis, or untreated infection.

Administration and Handling
Inhalation
- Shake the container well. Instruct the patient to exhale completely and place the mouthpiece between the lips. Have the patient inhale and hold his or her breath for as long as possible before exhaling.
- Allow at least 1 minute between inhalations.
- Have the patient rinse his or her mouth after each use to decrease dry mouth and hoarseness.

Intranasal
- Have the patient clear the nasal passages before using budesonide.
- Tilt the patient's head slightly forward.
- Insert the spray tip into the patient's nostril, pointing toward the nasal passages, away from the nasal septum.
- Spray the drug into the nostril while holding the other nostril closed, and at the same time have the patient inhale through the nose to deliver the drug as high into nasal passages as possible.

Intervention and Evaluation
- Monitor the patient for relief of symptoms.

Patient Teaching
- Inform the patient that symptoms may improve in 24 hours but the drug's full effect may take 3 to 7 days to appear.
- Advise the patient taking budesonide intranasally to notify the physician if nasal irritation occurs or if symptoms, such as sneezing, fail to improve.

cromolyn sodium

kroe-moe-lin
(Apo-Cromolyn[CAN], Crolom, Gastrocom, Intal, Nasalcrom, Opticrom, Rynacrom[AUS])

CATEGORY AND SCHEDULE
Pregnancy Risk Category: B

MECHANISM OF ACTION
An antiasthmatic and antiallergic agent that prevents mast cell release of histamine, leukotrienes, and slow-reacting substances of anaphylaxis by inhibiting degranulation after contact with antigens. **Therapeutic Effect:** Helps prevent symptoms of asthma, allergic rhinitis, mastocytosis, and exercise-induced bronchospasm.

PHARMACOKINETICS
Minimal absorption after PO, inhalation, or nasal administration. Absorbed portion excreted in urine or by biliary system. ***Half-life:*** 80–90 min.

AVAILABILITY
Oral Concentrate (Gastrocrom): 100 mg/5 ml.
Nasal Spray (Nasalcrom): 40 mg/ml.
Solution for Nebulization (Intal): 10 mg/ml.
Solution for Oral Inhalation (Intal): 800 mcg/inhalation.
Ophthalmic Solution (Crolom, Opticrom): 4%.

INDICATIONS AND DOSAGES
▸ Asthma
Inhalation (nebulization)
Adults, Elderly, Children older than 2 yr. 20 mg 3–4 times a day.
Aerosol Spray
Adults, Elderly, Children 12 yrs and older. Initially, 2 sprays 4 times a

day. Maintenance: 2–4 sprays 3–4 times a day.
Children 5–11 yr. Initially, 2 sprays 4 times a day, then 1–2 sprays 3–4 times a day.

▸ **Prevention of bronchospasm**
Inhalation (nebulization)
Adults, Elderly, Children older than 2 yr. 20 mg within 1 hr before exercise or exposure to allergens.
Aerosol Spray
Adults, Elderly, Children older than 5 yr. 2 sprays within 1 hr before exercise or exposure to allergens.

▸ **Food allergy, inflammatory bowel disease**
PO
Adults, Elderly, Children older than 12 yr. 200–400 mg 4 times a day.
Children 2–12 yr. 100–200 mg 4 times a day. Maximum: 40 mg/kg/day.

▸ **Allergic rhinitis**
Intranasal
Adults, Elderly, Children older than 6 yr. 1 spray each nostril 3–4 times a day. May increase up to 6 times a day.

▸ **Systemic mastocytosis**
PO
Adults, Elderly, Children older than 12 yr. 200 mg 4 times a day.
Children 2–12 yr. 100 mg 4 times a day. Maximum: 40 mg/kg/day.
Children younger than 2 yr. 20 mg/kg/day in 4 divided doses. Maximum: 30 mg/kg/day (children 6 mo–2 yr).

▸ **Conjunctivitis**
Ophthalmic
Adults, Elderly, Children older than 4 yr. 1–2 drops in both eyes 4–6 times a day.

CONTRAINDICATIONS

Status asthmaticus

INTERACTIONS

Drug
None known.

Herbal
None known.

Food
None known.

DIAGNOSTIC TEST EFFECTS

None known.

SIDE EFFECTS

Frequent
PO: Headache, diarrhea
Inhalation: Cough, dry mouth and throat, stuffy nose, throat irritation, unpleasant taste
Nasal: Nasal burning, stinging, or irritation; increased sneezing
Ophthalmic: Eye burning or stinging

Occasional
PO: Rash, abdominal pain, arthralgia, nausea, insomnia
Inhalation: Bronchospasm, hoarseness, lacrimation
Nasal: Cough, headache, unpleasant taste, postnasal drip
Ophthalmic: Lacrimation and itching of eye

Rare
Inhalation: Dizziness, painful urination, arthralgia, myalgia, rash
Nasal: Epistaxis, rash
Ophthalmic: Chemosis or edema of conjunctiva, eye irritation

SERIOUS REACTIONS

! Anaphylaxis occurs rarely when cromolyn is given by the inhalation, nasal, or oral route.

NURSING CONSIDERATIONS

Baseline Assessment
- Auscultate breath sounds for crackles, rhonchi, and wheezing.
- Determine the patient's baseline exercise and activity tolerance.
- Obtain baseline peak flow readings

and, if ordered, pulmonary function test results.

Lifespan Considerations

- It is unknown if cromolyn crosses the placenta or is distributed in breast milk.
- No age-related precautions have been noted in children.
- Age-related hepatic and renal impairment may require a dosage adjustment in the elderly.

Precautions

- Use cromolyn cautiously in patients with arrhythmias or coronary artery disease.
- When discontinuing the drug, taper the dosage cautiously because symptoms may recur.

Administration and Handling

PO

- Give cromolyn at least 30 minutes before meals.
- Pour contents of capsule into hot water and stir until completely dissolved; add an equal amount of cold water while stirring.
- Don't mix the drug with food, fruit juice, or milk.

Inhalation

- Shake the container well. Instruct the patient to exhale completely. Place the mouthpiece fully into the patient's mouth and have the patient inhale deeply and slowly while depressing the top of the canister. Instruct the patient to hold his or her breath for as long as possible before exhaling.
- Allow 1 to 10 minutes before inhaling a second dose to promote deeper bronchial penetration.
- Have the patient rinse his or her mouth with water immediately after inhalation to prevent mouth and throat dryness.

Nasal

- Have the patient clear the nasal passages before using the drug; a nasal decongestant may be required.
- Make sure the patient inhales through the nose.

Ophthalmic

- Place a gloved finger on the patient's lower eyelid and pull it down until a pocket is formed between the eye and lower lid.
- Hold the dropper above the pocket and instill the prescribed number of drops into the pocket.
- Instruct the patient to close the eyes gently so that the drug isn't squeezed out of the lacrimal sac.
- Apply gentle finger pressure to the patient's lacrimal sac at the inner canthus for 1 minute after instillation to lessen the risk of systemic absorption.

Intervention and Evaluation

- Monitor pulse rate and quality and respiratory rate, depth, rhythm, and type.
- Auscultate the patient's breath sounds for crackles, rhonchi, and wheezing.
- Observe the patient for cyanosis manifested as lips and fingernails with a blue or dusky color in light-skinned patients; a gray color in dark-skinned patients.

Patient Teaching

- Stress the importance of administering cromolyn at regular intervals to ensure its effectiveness.
- Teach the patient how to use a Spinhaler if he or she is to receive cromolyn by nebulization or inhalation capsules.
- Teach the patient to rinse his or her mouth with water immediately after inhalation to prevent mouth and throat dryness.
- Instruct the patient to drink plenty of fluids to decrease the thickness of lung secretions.

flunisolide

floo-**niss**-oh-lide
(AeroBid, Nasalide, Nasarel, Rhinalar[CAN])
Do not confuse flunisolide with fluocinonide, or Nasalide with Nasalcrom.

CATEGORY AND SCHEDULE

Pregnancy Risk Category: C

MECHANISM OF ACTION

An adrenocorticosteroid that controls the rate of protein synthesis, depresses migration of polymorphonuclear leukocytes, reverses capillary permeability, and stabilizes lysosomal membranes. **Therapeutic Effect:** Prevents or controls inflammation.

AVAILABILITY

Aerosol (AeroBid): 250 mcg/activation.
Nasal Spray (Nasalide, Nasarel): 25 mcg/activation.

INDICATIONS AND DOSAGES

▸ **Long-term control of bronchial asthma, assists in reducing or discontinuing oral corticosteroid therapy**

Inhalation

Adults, Elderly. 2 inhalations twice a day, morning and evening. Maximum: 4 inhalations twice a day.
Children 6–15 yr. 2 inhalations twice a day.

▸ **Relief of symptoms of perennial and seasonal rhinitis**

Intranasal

Adults, Elderly. Initially, 2 sprays each nostril twice a day, may increase at 4- to 7-day intervals to 2 sprays 3 times a day. Maximum: 8 sprays in each nostril daily.
Children 6–14 yr. Initially, 1 spray 3 times a day or 2 sprays twice a day. Maximum: 4 sprays in each nostril daily. Maintenance: 1 spray into each nostril each day.

OFF-LABEL USES

To prevent recurrence of nasal polyps after surgery

CONTRAINDICATIONS

Hypersensitivity to any corticosteroid, persistently positive sputum cultures for *Candida albicans,* primary treatment of status asthmaticus, systemic fungal infections

INTERACTIONS

Drug
None known.
Herbal
None known.
Food
None known.

DIAGNOSTIC TEST EFFECTS

None known.

SIDE EFFECTS

Frequent
Inhalation (25%–10%): Unpleasant taste, nausea, vomiting, sore throat, diarrhea, upset stomach, cold symptoms, nasal congestion
Occasional
Inhalation (9%–3%): Dizziness, irritability, nervousness, tremors, abdominal pain, heartburn, oropharynx candidiasis, edema
Nasal: Mild nasopharyngeal irritation or dryness, rebound congestion, bronchial asthma, rhinorrhea, altered taste

SERIOUS REACTIONS

! An acute hypersensitivity reaction, marked by urticaria, angioedema, and severe bronchospasm, occurs rarely.
! A transfer from systemic to local

steroid therapy may unmask previously suppressed bronchial asthma condition.

NURSING CONSIDERATIONS

Baseline Assessment

• Determine if the patient has a history of asthma or rhinitis.

Precautions

• Use flunisolide cautiously in patients with adrenal insufficiency.

Administration and Handling

◀ALERT▶ Expect to see improvement of the patient's symptoms within a few days and relief of symptoms within 3 weeks. Prepare to discontinue the drug after 3 weeks if the patient doesn't experience significant improvement.

Inhalation

• Shake the container well. Have the patient exhale as completely as possible. Place the mouthpiece fully into the patient's mouth; then, while holding the inhaler upright, have the patient inhale deeply and slowly while pressing the top of the canister. Instruct the patient to hold his or her breath for as long as possible before exhaling slowly.
• Allow 1 minute between inhalations to promote deeper bronchial penetration.
• Have the patient rinse his or her mouth with water immediately after inhalation to prevent mouth and throat dryness and oral candidiasis.

Intranasal

• Have the patient clear his or her nasal passages before using flunisolide. This may require the use of a topical nasal decongestant 5 to 15 minutes before flunisolide use.
• Tilt the patient's head slightly forward. Insert spray tip up into the nostril, pointing toward inflamed nasal turbinates, away from the nasal septum.
• Spray the drug into the nostril while holding the other nostril closed, and at the same time have the patient inhale through the nose.
• Discard opened nasal solution after 3 months.

Intervention and Evaluation

• Monitor pulse rate and quality and respiratory rate, depth, rhythm, and type.
• Monitor the patient's ABG levels.
• Auscultate the patient's breath sounds for rales, rhonchi, and wheezing.

Patient Teaching

• Inform the patient that symptoms should improve in several days.
• Caution the patient against discontinuing flunisolide abruptly or changing the dosage schedule. Explain that he or she must taper the dosage gradually under medical supervision.
• Urge the patient receiving the drug by inhalation to maintain fastidious oral hygiene. Instruct the patient to rinse his or her mouth with water immediately after inhalation to prevent mouth and throat dryness and a fungal infection.
• Instruct the patient to drink plenty of fluids to decrease the thickness of lung secretions.
• If the patient is using a bronchodilator inhaler concomitantly with a steriod inhaler, advise him or her to use the bronchodilator several minutes before using the corticosteroid to help the steroid penetrate into the bronchial tree.
• Teach patients taking flunisolide intranasally the proper use of the nasal spray. Instruct the patient to clear the nasal passages before use.
• Advise the patient to notify the physician if nasal irritation occurs or if symptoms, such as sneezing, fail to improve.

fluticasone propionate

flu-**tic**-a-zone

(Beconase Allergy 24 Hour[AUS], Beconase Hayfever[AUS], Cutivate, Flixotide Disks[AUS], Flixotide Inhaler[AUS], Flonase, Flovent, Flovent Diskus, Flovent HFA)

CATEGORY AND SCHEDULE

Pregnancy Risk Category: C

MECHANISM OF ACTION

A corticosteroid that controls the rate of protein synthesis, depresses migration of polymorphonuclear leukocytes, reverses capillary permeability, and stabilizes lysosomal membranes. **Therapeutic Effect:** Prevents or controls inflammation.

PHARMACOKINETICS

Inhalation/intranasal: Protein binding: 91%. Undergoes extensive first-pass metabolism in the liver. Excreted in urine. ***Half-life:*** 3–7.8 hr. Topical: Amount absorbed depends on affected area and skin condition (absorption increased with fever, hydration, inflamed or denuded skin).

AVAILABILITY

Aerosol for Oral Inhalation (Flovent, Flovent HFA): 44 mcg/inhalation, 110 mcg/inhalation, 220 mcg/inhalation.
Powder for Oral Inhalation (Flovent Diskus): 50 mcg, 100 mcg, 250 mcg.
Intranasal Spray (Flonase): 50 mcg/inhalation.
Topical Cream (Cutivate): 0.05%.
Topical Ointment (Cutivate): 0.005%.

INDICATIONS AND DOSAGES

▸ **Allergic Rhinitis**

Intranasal

Adults, Elderly. Initially, 200 mcg (2 sprays in each nostril once daily or 1 spray in each nostril q12h). Maintenance: 1 spray in each nostril once daily. Maximum: 200 mcg/day.
Children older than 4 yr. Initially, 100 mcg (1 spray in each nostril once daily). Maximum: 200 mcg/day.

▸ **Relief of inflammation and pruritus associated with steroid-responsive disorders, such as contact dermatitis and eczema**

Topical

Adults, Elderly, Children older than 3 mo. Apply sparingly to affected area once or twice a day.

▸ **Maintenance treatment for asthma for those previously treated with bronchodilators**

Inhalation Powder (Flovent Diskus)

Adults, Elderly, Children 12 yr and older. Initially, 100 mcg q12h. Maximum: 500 mcg/day.

Inhalation (Oral [Flovent])

Adults, Elderly, Children 12 yr and older. 88 mcg twice a day. Maximum: 440 mcg twice a day.

▸ **Maintenance treatment for asthma for those previously treated with inhaled steroids**

Inhalation Powder (Flovent Diskus)

Adults, Elderly, Children 12 yr and older. Initially, 100–250 mcg q12h. Maximum: 500 mcg q12h.

Inhalation (Oral [Flovent])

Adults, Elderly, Children 12 yr and older. 88–220 mcg twice a day. Maximum: 440 mcg twice a day.

▸ **Maintenance treatment for asthma for those previously treated with oral steroids**

Inhalation Powder (Flovent Diskus)

Adults, Elderly, Children 12 yr and older. 500–1,000 mcg twice a day.

Inhalation (Oral [Flovent])
Adults, Elderly, Children 12 yrs and older. 880 mcg twice a day.

CONTRAINDICATIONS

Primary treatment of status asthmaticus or other acute asthma episodes (inhalation); untreated localized infection of nasal mucosa

INTERACTIONS

Drug

None known.

Herbal

None known.

Food

None known.

DIAGNOSTIC TEST EFFECTS

None known.

SIDE EFFECTS

Frequent

Inhalation: Throat irritation, hoarseness, dry mouth, cough, temporary wheezing, oropharyngeal candidiasis (particularly if mouth is not rinsed with water after each administration)
Intranasal: Mild nasopharyngeal irritation; nasal burning, stinging, or dryness; rebound congestion; rhinorrhea; loss of taste

Occasional

Inhalation: Oral candidiasis
Intranasal: Nasal and pharyngeal candidiasis, headache
Topical: Skin burning, pruritus

SERIOUS REACTIONS

! None known.

NURSING CONSIDERATIONS

Baseline Assessment

- Establish the patient's history of asthma, rhinitis, and skin disorders.

Lifespan Considerations

- It is unknown if fluticasone crosses the placenta or is distributed in breast milk.
- The safety and efficacy of fluticasone have not been established in children younger than 4 years. Children 4 years and older may experience growth suppression with prolonged or high doses.
- No age-related precautions have been noted in the elderly.

Precautions

- Use fluticasone cautiously in patients with active or quiescent tuberculosis, ocular herpes simplex infection, or untreated systemic infections (including fungal, bacterial, or viral).

Administration and Handling

Inhalation

- Shake the container well. Have the patient exhale as completely as possible. Place the mouthpiece fully into the patient's mouth; then, while holding the inhaler upright, have the patient inhale deeply and slowly while pressing the top of the canister. Instruct the patient to hold his or her breath for as long as possible before exhaling slowly.
- Have the patient wait 1 minute between inhalations to allow for deeper bronchial penetration.
- Have the patient rinse his or her mouth with water immediately after inhalation to prevent mouth and throat dryness.

Intranasal

- Ensure that the patient clears the nasal passages before using fluticasone. The patient may need to use a topical nasal decongestant 5 to 15 minutes before using fluticasone.
- Tilt the patient's head slightly forward. Insert spray tip up into the nostril, pointing toward the inflamed nasal turbinates, away from nasal septum. Spray the drug into the nostril while holding the other nostril

closed, and at the same time have the patient inhale through the nose

Intervention and Evaluation

- Monitor pulse rate and quality and respiratory depth, rate, rhythm, and type.
- Monitor the patient's ABG levels.
- Auscultate the patient's breath sounds for rales, rhonchi, and wheezing.
- Evaluate the patient's oral mucous membranes for evidence of candidiasis.
- Monitor growth in pediatric patients.
- For patients using topical fluticasone, examine the affected area for a therapeutic response.

Patient Teaching

- Caution the patient against discontinuing the drug abruptly or changing the dosage schedule. Explain that the dosage must be tapered gradually under medical supervision.
- Instruct the patient to rinse his or her mouth with water immediately after inhalation to prevent mouth and throat dryness and oral candidiasis. Urge the patient to maintain careful oral hygiene.
- Instruct the patient to drink plenty of fluids to decrease the thickness of lung secretions.
- If the patient is using a bronchodilator inhaler concomitantly with a steroid inhaler, advise him or her to use the bronchodilator several minutes before using the corticosteroid to help the steroid penetrate into the bronchial tree.
- Teach the patient using intranasal fluticasone how to use the nasal spray. Instruct the patient to clear nasal passages before use. Warn the patient to notify the physician if nasal irritation occurs or if symptoms, such as sneezing, fail to improve.
- Tell the patient symptoms should improve in several days.
- Instruct the patient using topical fluticasone to rub a thin film gently on the affected area. Stress the importance of using the drug only on the prescribed area and for no longer than prescribed. Warn the patient to keep the preparation away from the eyes.

mometasone furoate monohydrate

mo-**met**-a-sone

(Allermax Aqueous[AUS], Elocon Cream[AUS], Elocon Ointment [AUS], Nasonex, Nasonex Nasal Spray[AUS], Novasone Cream [AUS], Novasone Lotion[AUS], Novasone Ointment[AUS])

CATEGORY AND SCHEDULE

Pregnancy Risk Category: C

MECHANISM OF ACTION

An adrenocorticosteroid that inhibits the release of inlammatory cells into nasal tissue, preventing early activation of the allergic reaction. **Therapeutic Effect:** Decreases response to seasonal and perennial rhinitis.

PHARMACOKINETICS

Undetectable in plasma. Protein binding: 98%–99%. The swallowed portion undergoes extensive metabolism. Excreted primarily through bile and, to a lesser extent, urine.

AVAILABILITY

Nasal Spray: 50 mcg/spray.

INDICATIONS AND DOSAGES

▸ Allergic rhinitis

Nasal Spray

Adults, Elderly, Children 12 yr and older. 2 sprays in each nostril once a day.

Children 2–11 yr. 1 spray in each nostril once a day.

CONTRAINDICATIONS

Hypersensitivity to any corticosteroid, persistently positive sputum cultures for *Candida albicans*, systemic fungal infections, untreated localized infection involving nasal mucosa

INTERACTIONS

Drug

None known.

Herbal

None known.

Food

None known.

DIAGNOSTIC TEST EFFECTS

None known.

SIDE EFFECTS

Occasional

Nasal irritation, stinging

Rare

Nasal or pharyngeal candidiasis

SERIOUS REACTIONS

! An acute hypersensitivity reaction, including urticaria, angioedema, and severe bronchospasm, occurs rarely.

! Transfer from systemic to local steroid therapy may unmask previously suppressed bronchial asthma condition.

NURSING CONSIDERATIONS

Baseline Assessment

- Determine if the patient is hypersensitive to any corticosteroids.

Lifespan Considerations

- It is unknown if mometasone crosses the placenta or is distributed in breast milk.
- In children, prolonged treatment and high dosages may decrease cortisol secretion and short-term growth rate.
- No age-related precautions have been noted in the elderly.

Precautions

- Use mometasone cautiously in patients with adrenal insufficiency, cirrhosis, glaucoma, hypothyroidism, osteoporosis, tuberculosis, or untreated infection.

Administration and Handling

Intranasal

- Shake the container well and have the patient clears his or her nasal passages before each use.
- Insert the spray tip into the nostril, pointing toward the inflamed nasal turbinates, away from the nasal septum.
- Spray the drug into the patient's nostril while holding the other nostril closed, and at the same time have the patient inhale through the nose to deliver the drug as high into the nasal passages as possible.

Patient Teaching

- Teach the patient the proper use of mometasone nasal spray.
- Instruct the patient to clear his or her nasal passages before using mometasone.
- Inform the patient tht symptoms should start to improve within 2 days of the first dose but that the drug's maximum benefit may take up to 2 weeks to appear.
- Caution the patient against abruptly discontinuing the drug or changing the drug's dose schedule. Explain that the dosage must be tapered gradually under medical supervision.
- Advise the patient to notify the

physician if he or she experiences nasal irritation or if symptoms, such as sneezing, fail to improve.

nedocromil sodium

ned-oh-**crow**-mil
(Alocril, Mireze[CAN], Tilade, Tilade CFC Free[AUS])

CATEGORY AND SCHEDULE

Pregnancy Risk Category: B

MECHANISM OF ACTION

A mast cell stabilizer that prevents the activation and release of inflammatory mediators, such as histamine, leukotrienes, mast cells, eosinophils, and monocytes. **Therapeutic Effect:** Prevents both early and late asthmatic responses.

AVAILABILITY

Aerosol for Inhalation (Tilade): 1.75 mg/activation.
Ophthalmic Solution (Alocril): 2%.

INDICATIONS AND DOSAGES

▸ **Mild to moderate asthma**
Oral Inhalation
Adults, Elderly, Children 6 yr and older. 2 inhalations 4 times a day. May decrease to 3 times a day then twice a day as asthma becomes controlled.

▸ **Allergic conjunctivitis**
Ophthalmic
Adults, Elderly, Children 3 yr and older. 1–2 drops in each eye twice a day.

OFF-LABEL USES

Prevention of bronchospasm in patients with reversible obstructive airway disease

CONTRAINDICATIONS

None known.

INTERACTIONS

Drug
None known.
Herbal
None known.
Food
None known.

DIAGNOSTIC TEST EFFECTS

None known.

SIDE EFFECTS

Frequent (10%–6%)
Cough, pharyngitis, bronchospasm, headache, altered taste
Occasional (5%–1%)
Rhinitis, upper respiratory tract infection, abdominal pain, fatigue
Rare (less than 1%)
Diarrhea, dizziness

SERIOUS REACTIONS

! None known.

NURSING CONSIDERATIONS

Baseline Assessment
- Auscultate breath sounds for crackles, rhonchi, and wheezing.
- Determine the patient's exercise and activity tolerance.
- Obtain peak flow readings and, if ordered, pulmonary function test results.

Precautions
- Nedocromil is not used to reverse acute bronchospasm.

Administration and Handling
- Shake the container well before each use.
- Protect the drug from direct exposure to light.

Intervention and Evaluation
- Evaluate the patient for a therapeutic response, such as less frequent or

severe asthmatic attacks or reduced dependence on antihistamines.

Patient Teaching

- Instruct the patient to administer nedocromil at regular intervals, even when he or she is symptom-free, to achieve optimal results.
- Inform the patient that rinsing his or her mouth with water immediately after inhalation may help relieve unpleasant taste.
- Instruct the patient to drink plenty of fluids to decrease the thickness of lung secretions.
- Teach the patient how to use a peak flow meter and record the values in a log.

triamcinolone

See Adrenocortical Steroids

88 Miscellaneous Respiratory Agents

dornase alfa
iloprost
montelukast
omalizumab
zafirlukast

Uses: Because they belong to separate subclasses, miscellaneous respiratory agents have different indications. Along with standard therapy, *dornase alfa* is used to reduce the frequency of respiratory infections and improve pulmonary function in patients with advanced cystic fibrosis. *Iloprost* is used to treat pulmonary hypertension in patients with NYHA Class III or IV symptoms. *Montelukast* and *zafirlukast* are used for prophylaxis and long-term treatment of asthma. *Omalizumab* is prescribed to treat moderate to severe persistent asthma triggered by year-round allergens.

Action: Miscellaneous respiratory agents act by various mechanisms. *Dornase alfa* selectively splits and hydrolyzed DNA in sputum, reducing the sputum's viscosity and elasticity. *Iloprost* is a prostaglandin that dilates systemic and pulmonary arterial vascular beds, alters pulmonary vascular resistance, and suppresses vascular smooth muscle proliferation. This action improves symptoms and exercise tolerance in patients with pulmonary hypertension and delays deterioration of the condition. *Montelukast* and *zafirlukast* block the effects of leukotrienes, which increase eosinophil migration, producing mucus and edema of the airway wall and causing bronchoconstriction. *Omalizumab* works by blocking immunoglobulin E, an underlying cause of allergic asthma.

dornase alfa

door-nace **al**-fa
(Pulmozyme)

CATEGORY AND SCHEDULE

Pregnancy Risk Category: B

MECHANISM OF ACTION

An enzyme that selectively splits and hydrolyzes DNA in sputum. **Therapeutic Effect:** Reduces sputum viscosity and elasticity.

AVAILABILITY

Inhalation: 2.5 mg ampules for nebulization.

INDICATIONS AND DOSAGES

▸ **To improve management of pulmonary function in patients with cystic fibrosis**

Nebulization

Adults, Children older than 5 yr. 2.5 mg (1 ampule) once daily by recommended nebulizer. May increase to 2.5 mg twice daily.

CONTRAINDICATIONS
Sensitivity to dornase alfa or epoetin alfa

INTERACTIONS
Drug
None known.
Herbal
None known.
Food
None known.

DIAGNOSTIC TEST EFFECTS
None known.

SIDE EFFECTS
Frequent (greater than 10%)
Pharyngitis, chest pain or discomfort, voice changes
Occasional (10%–3%)
Conjunctivitis, hoarseness, rash

SERIOUS REACTIONS
! None significant.

NURSING CONSIDERATIONS
Baseline Assessment
- Obtain the patient's ABG levels.
- Auscultate breath sounds and evaluate the amount, color, and viscosity of pulmonary secretions.
- Assess the patient for dyspnea and fatigue.

Administration and Handling
Nebulization
- Refrigerate unopened ampules and protect them from light. Don't expose them to room temperature longer than 24 hours.
- Don't mix any other medications in the nebulizer with dornase alfa.

Intervention and Evaluation
- Provide emotional support to the patient and family.
- Check for decreased viscosity of pulmonary secretions.
- Assess the patient for relief of dyspnea and fatigue.

Patient Teaching
- Instruct the patient to refrigerate dornase alfa and not to dilute or mix it with other drugs.
- Teach the patient how to use and clean the nebulizer.
- Inform the patient that he or she may have hoarseness, chest pain, or sore throat during dornase alfa therapy.
- Encourage the patient to drink plenty of fluids.

iloprost
eye-low-prost
(Ventavis)

CATEGORY AND SCHEDULE
Pregnancy Risk Category: C

MECHANISM OF ACTION
A prostaglandin that dilates systemic and pulmonary arterial vascular beds, alters pulmonary vascular resistance, and suppresses vascular smooth muscle proliferation. **Therapeutic Effect:** Improves symptoms and exercise tolerance in patients with pulmonary hypertension; delays deterioration of condition.

AVAILABILITY
Solution for Oral Inhalation: 10 mcg/ml (2-ml ampule).

INDICATIONS AND DOSAGES
▸ **Pulmonary hypertension in patients with NYHA Class III or IV symptoms**
Oral Inhalation
Adults. Initially, 2.5 mcg/dose; if tolerated, increased to 5 mcg/dose. Administer 6–9 times a day at intervals of 2 hr or longer while patient is awake. Maintenance: 5 mcg/dose. Maximum daily dose: 45 mcg.

CONTRAINDICATIONS
None known.

INTERACTIONS
Drug
Anticoagulants, antiplatelet agents: May increased the risk of bleeding.
Antihypertensives, other vasodilators: May increase the hypotensive effects of iloprost.
Herbal
None known.
Food
None known.

DIAGNOSTIC TEST EFFECTS
May increase serum alkaline phosphatase and GGT levels.

SIDE EFFECTS
Frequent (39%–27%)
Increased cough, headache, flushing
Occasional (13%–11%)
Flulike symptoms, nausea, lockjaw, jaw pain, hypotension
Rare (8%–2%)
Insomnia, syncope, palpitations, vomiting, back pain, muscle cramps

SERIOUS REACTIONS
! Hemoptysis and pneumonia occur occasionally.
! CHF, renal failure, dyspnea, and chest pain occur rarely.

NURSING CONSIDERATIONS
Precautions
• Use iloprost cautiously in patients with hepatic impairment and in those who are concurrently taking medications that may increase the risk of syncope.
Administration and Handling
Oral inhalation
• Iloprost is administered by inhalation only, using the Prodose ADD system.
• Transfer the entire contents of the ampule into the medication chamber. After use, discard the unused portion.

montelukast
mon-**te**-loo-kast
(Singulair)

CATEGORY AND SCHEDULE
Pregnancy Risk Category: B

MECHANISM OF ACTION
An antiasthmatic that binds to cysteinyl leukotriene receptors, inhibiting the effects of leukotrienes on bronchial smooth muscle. **Therapeutic Effect:** Decreases bronchoconstriction, vascular permeability, mucosal edema, and mucus production.

PHARMACOKINETICS

Route	Onset	Peak	Duration
PO	N/A	N/A	24 hr
PO (chewable)	N/A	N/A	24 hr

Rapidly absorbed from the GI tract. Protein binding: 99%. Extensively metabolized in the liver. Excreted almost exclusively in feces. ***Half-life:*** 2.7–5.5 hr (slightly longer in the elderly).

AVAILABILITY
Oral Granules: 4 mg.
Tablets: 10 mg.
Tablets (Chewable): 4 mg, 5 mg.

INDICATIONS AND DOSAGES
▸ **Bronchial asthma**
PO
Adults, Elderly, Adolescents older than 14 yr. One 10-mg tablet a day, taken in the evening.

Children 6–14 yr. One 5-mg chewable tablet a day, taken in the evening.
Children 1–5 yr. One 4-mg chewable tablet a day, taken in the evening.

CONTRAINDICATIONS

None known.

INTERACTIONS

Drug

Phenobarbital, rifampin: May decrease montelukast's duration of action.

Herbal

None known.

Food

None known.

DIAGNOSTIC TEST EFFECTS

May increase AST (SGOT) and ALT (SGPT) levels.

SIDE EFFECTS

Adults, Adolescents 15 years and older

Frequent (18%)
Headache

Occasional (4%)
Influenza

Rare (3%–2%)
Abdominal pain, cough, dyspepsia, dizziness, fatigue, dental pain

Children 6–14 years

Rare (less than 2%)
Diarrhea, laryngitis, pharyngitis, nausea, otitis media, sinusitis, viral infection

SERIOUS REACTIONS

! None known.

NURSING CONSIDERATIONS

Baseline Assessment

• Inform the parents of children with phenylketonuria that montelukast chewable tablets contain phenylalanine, a component of aspartame.

Lifespan Considerations

• Use montelukast during pregnancy only if necessary. It is unknown if montelukast is excreted in breast milk.
• No age-related precautions have been noted in children older than 6 years or the elderly.

Precautions

• Use montelukast cautiously in patients with hepatic impairment and those who are tapering systemic corticosteroid dosage during montelukast therapy.

Administration and Handling

PO
• Administer montelukast in the evening without regard to food.
• Don't abruptly substitute montelukast for inhaled or oral corticosteroids.

Intervention and Evaluation

• Monitor the patient's pulse rate and quality as well as respiratory depth, rate, rhythm, and type.
• Auscultate the patient's breatha sounds for crackles, rhonchi, and wheezing.
• Observe the patient's fingernails and lips for a blue or dusky color in light-skinned patients and a gray color in dark-skinned patients, which may be signs of hypoxemia.

Patient Teaching

• Teach the patient to take montelukast as prescribed, even during symptom-free periods and exacerbations.
• Caution the patient not to alter the dosage or abruptly discontinue other asthma medications.
• Explain to the patient that montelukast is not intended to treat acute asthma attacks.
• Instruct the patient to drink plenty of fluids to decrease the thickness of lung secretions.

• Tell patients with aspirin sensitivity to avoid aspirin and NSAIDs while taking montelukast.

omalizumab

oh-mah-**liz**-uw-mab
(Xolair)

CATEGORY AND SCHEDULE

Pregnancy Risk Category: B

MECHANISM OF ACTION

A monoclonal antibody that selectively binds to human immunoglobulin E (IgE) preventing it from binding to the surface of mast cells and basophiles. **Therapeutic Effect:** Prevents or reduces the number of asthmatic attacks.

PHARMACOKINETICS

Absorbed slowly after subcutaneous administration, with peak concentration in 7–8 days. Excreted in the liver, reticuloendothelial system, and endothelial cells. ***Half-life:*** 26 days.

AVAILABILITY

Powder for Injection: 202.5 mg/1.2 ml or 150 mg/1.2 ml after reconstitution.

INDICATIONS AND DOSAGES

▸ **Moderate to severe persistent asthma in patients who are reactive to a perennial allergen and whose asthma symptoms have been inadequately controlled with inhaled corticosteroids**

Subcutaneous

Adults, Elderly, Children 12 yr and older. 150–375 mg every 2 or 4 wk; dose and dosing frequency are individualized based on weight and pretreatment immunoglobulin E (IgE) level (as shown below).

▸ **4-week dosing table**

Pretreatment serum IgE levels (units/ml)	Weight 30–60 kg	Weight 61–70 kg	Weight 71–90 kg	Weight 91–150 kg
30 to 100	150 mg	150 mg	150 mg	300 mg
101–200	300 mg	300 mg	300 mg	See next table
201–300	300 mg	See next table	See next table	See next table

▸ **2-week dosing table**

Pretreatment serum IgE levels (units/ml)	Weight 30–60 kg	Weight 61–70 kg	Weight 71–90 kg	Weight 91–150 kg
101–200	See preceding table	See preceding table	See preceding table	225 mg
201–300	See preceding table	225 mg	225 mg	300 mg
301–400	225 mg	225 mg	300 mg	Do not dose
401–500	300 mg	300 mg	375 mg	Do not dose
501–600	300 mg	375 mg	Do not dose	Do not dose
601–700	375 mg	Do not dose	Do not dose	Do not dose

OFF-LABEL USES

Treatment of seasonal allergic rhinitis

CONTRAINDICATIONS

None known.

INTERACTIONS

Drug

None known.

Herbal

None known.

Food

None known.

DIAGNOSTIC TEST EFFECTS

May increase serum IgE levels.

SIDE EFFECTS

Frequent (45%–11%)

Injection site ecchymosis, redness, warmth, stinging, and urticaria; viral infections; sinusitis; headache; pharyngitis

Occasional (8%–3%)

Arthralgia, leg pain, fatigue, dizziness

Rare (2%)

Arm pain, earache, dermatitis, pruritus

SERIOUS REACTIONS

! Anaphylaxis occurs within 2 hours of the first dose or subsequent doses in 0.1% of patients.

! Malignant neoplasms occur in 0.5% of patients.

NURSING CONSIDERATIONS

Baseline Assessment

- Obtain the patient's serum total IgE levels before beginning omalizumab therapy because the drug dosage is based on these pretreatment levels.

Lifespan Considerations

- Since IgE is present in breast milk, omalizumab is also believed to be present in breast milk. Use omalizumab only if clearly needed.
- The safety and efficacy of omalizumab have not been established in children younger than 12 years.
- No age-related precautions have been noted in the elderly.

Precautions

- Omalizumab is not intended to reverse acute bronchospasm or status asthmaticus.

Administration and Handling

◀ ALERT ▶ Expect to base omalizumab dosage on serum IgE levels obtained before beginning treatment. Don't use serum IgE levels obtained during treatment to determine omalizumab dosage because IgE levels remain elevated for up to 1 year after the drug has been discontinued.

- Use only clear or slightly opalescent solution; the solution is slightly viscous.
- Store omalizumab in the refrigerator.
- The reconstituted solution is stable for 8 hours if refrigerated or 4 hours if stored at room temperature.
- Use only sterile water for injection to prepare for subcutaneous administration.
- Draw 1.4 ml sterile water for injection into a 3-ml syringe with a 1-inch, 18-gauge needle and inject contents into the vial of powder.
- Swirl the vial for approximately 1 minute; do not shake it. Then swirl the vial again for 5 to 10 seconds every 5 minutes until no gel-like particles appear in the solution. The drug takes 15 to 20 minutes to dissolve. Don't use the solution if the contents fail to dissolve completely in 40 minutes.
- Invert the vial for 15 seconds to allow the solution to drain toward the stopper.
- Using a new 3-ml syringe with a 1-inch, 18-gauge needle, withdraw the required 1.2-ml dose and replace the 18-gauge needle with a 25-gauge needle for subcutaneous administration.
- Subcutaneous administration may take 5 to 10 seconds because of omalizumab's viscosity.

Intervention and Evaluation

- Monitor the patient's pulse rate and quality as well as respiratory rate, depth, rhythm, and type.
- Auscultate the patient's breath sounds for rales, rhonchi, and wheezing.
- Observe the patient's fingernails and lips for cyanosis, characterized by a blue or dusky color in light-skinned patients or a gray color in dark-skinned patients.

Patient Teaching

- Warn the patient not to alter the drug dosage or discontinue other asthma medications.
- Instruct the patient to drink plenty of fluids to decrease the thickness of lung secretions.

zafirlukast

za-**feer**-loo-kast
(Accolate)
Do not confuse Accolate with Accupril or Aclovate.

CATEGORY AND SCHEDULE

Pregnancy Risk Category: B

MECHANISM OF ACTION

An antiasthmic that binds to leukotriene receptors, inhibiting bronchoconstriction due to sulfur dioxide, cold air, and specific antigens, such as grass, cat dander, and ragweed. **Therapeutic Effect:** Reduces airway edema and smooth muscle constriction; alters cellular activity associated with the inflammatory process.

PHARMACOKINETICS

Rapidly absorbed after PO administration (food reduces absorption). Protein binding: 99%. Extensively metabolized in the liver. Primarily excreted in feces. Unknown if removed by hemodialysis. ***Half-life:*** 10 hr.

AVAILABILITY

Tablets: 10 mg, 20 mg.

INDICATIONS AND DOSAGES

▸ **Bronchial asthma**

PO

Adults, Elderly, Children 12 yr and older. 20 mg twice a day.

Children 5–11 yr. 10 mg twice a day.

CONTRAINDICATIONS

None known.

INTERACTIONS

Drug

Aspirin: Increases zafirlukast blood concentration.

Erythromycin, theophylline: Decreases zafirlukast blood concentration.

Warfarin: Increases PT.

Herbal

None known.

Food

None known.

DIAGNOSTIC TEST EFFECTS

May increase ALT (SGPT) level.

SIDE EFFECTS

Frequent (13%)

Headache

Occasional (3%)

Nausea, diarrhea

Rare (less than 3%)

Generalized pain, asthenia, myalgia, fever, dyspepsia, vomiting, dizziness

SERIOUS REACTIONS

! Concurrent administration of inhaled corticosteroids increases the risk of upper respiratory tract infection.

NURSING CONSIDERATIONS

Baseline Assessment

- Obtain the patient's medication history.
- Assess the patient's liver function test results.

Lifespan Considerations

- Zafirlukast is distributed in breast milk. It is not recommended for breast-feeding women.
- The safety and efficacy of this drug have not been established in children younger than 5 years.
- No age-related precautions have been noted in the elderly.

Precautions

- Use zafirlukast cautiously in patients with impaired hepatic function.

Administration and Handling

PO

- Give zafirlukast 1 hour before or 2 hours after meals.
- Don't crush or break tablets.

Intervention and Evaluation

- Monitor the patient's pulse rate and quality and respiratory rate, depth, rhythm, and type.
- Monitor the patient's serum liver function test results.
- Auscultate the patient's breath sounds for crackles, rhonchi, and wheezing.
- Observe the patient's fingernails and lips for cyanosis, manifested as a blue or dusky color in light-skinned patients and a gray color in dark-skinned patients.

Patient Teaching

- Teach the patient to take zafirlukast as prescribed, even during symptom-free periods.
- Caution the patient not to alter the dosage or abruptly discontinue other asthma medications.
- Explain that zafirlukast is not intended to treat acute asthma episodes.
- Instruct the patient to drink plenty of fluids to decrease the thickness of lung secretions.
- Advise the patient to notify the physician if he or she experiences abdominal pain, nausea, flulike symptoms, jaundice, or worsening of asthma.
- Caution breast-feeding women not to breast-feed during zafirlukast therapy.

Appendixes

Appendix A

ANESTHETICS: GENERAL

USES	ACTION
IV anesthetic agents are used to induce general anesthesia. The general anesthetic state consists of unconsciousness, amnesia, analgesia, immobility, and attenuation of autonomic responses to noxious stimuli. *Volatile inhalation agents* produce all the components of the anesthetic state but are administered through the lungs via an anesthesia machine. Agents for use include desflurane, enflurane, halothane, isoflurane, and sevoflurane. They're used in practice to maintain general anesthesia.	*IV anesthetic agents* act on the gamma-aminobutyric acid (GABA) receptor complex to produce central nervous system (CNS) depression. GABA is the primary inhibitory neurotransmitter in the CNS. Ketamine produces dissociation between the thalamus and the limbic system. *Volatile inhalation agents* aren't fully understood, but may disrupt neuronal transmission throughout the CNS. These agents may either block excitatory or enhance inhibitory transmission through axons or synapses.

ANESTHETICS: GENERAL

Name	Availability	Uses	Dosage Range	Side Effects
Etomidate (Amidate)	**I:** 2 mg/ml	IV induction	0.2–0.6 mg/kg	Myoclonus, pain on injection, nausea, vomiting, respiratory depression
Ketamine (Ketalar)	**I:** 10 mg/ml, 50 mg/ml, 100 mg/ml	Analgesia, sedation, IV induction	1–4.5 mg/kg	Delirium, euphoria, nausea, vomiting
Methohexital (Brevital)	**Powder for injection:** 500 mg	IV induction, sedation	50–120 mg	Cardiovascular depression, myoclonus, nausea, vomiting, respiratory depression

Midazolam (Versed)	**I:** 1 mg/ml, 5 mg/ml	Anxiolytic, amnesic, sedation	1–5 mg titrated slowly	Respiratory depression
Propofol (Diprivan)	**I:** 10 mg/ml	Sedation IV induction Maintenance	0.5 mg/kg 2–2.5 mg/kg 100–200 mcg/kg/min	Cardiovascular depression, delirium, euphoria, pain on injection, respiratory depression
Thiopental (Pentothal)	**Powder for injection:** 2.5% (25 mg/ml)	IV induction	Titrate vs. pt response. **Average:** 50–75 mg	Cardiovascular depression, nausea, vomiting, respiratory depression

I, Injection.

ANESTHETICS: LOCAL

USES	ACTION
Local anesthetics suppress pain by blocking impulses along axons. Suppression of pain does not cause generalized depression of the entire nervous system. Local anesthetics may be given topically and by injection (local infiltration, peripheral nerve block [axillary], IV regional [bier block], epidural, and spinal).	Most local anesthetics fall into one of two groups: esters or amides. Both provide anesthesia and analgesia by reversibly binding to and blocking sodium (Na) channels. This slows the rate of depolarization of the nerve action potential, thus propagation of the electrical impulses needed for nerve conduction is prevented.

LOCAL ANESTHETICS

Name	Uses	Onset (minutes)	Duration (hours)	Side Effects
Esters				
Chloroprocaine (Nesacaine)	Local infiltrate Nerve block Spinal	6–12	0.25–0.5	Excitation (e.g., seizures) followed by decreased level of consciousness (drowsiness to unconsciousness), bradycardia, heart block, decreased myocardial contractile force, hypotension, hypersensitivity reaction
Procaine (Novocaine)	Local infiltrate Nerve block Spinal	2–5	0.25–1	Same as above
Tetracaine	Topical Spinal	15	2–3	Same as above

Amides

Bupivacaine (Marcaine, Sensorcaine)	Local infiltrate Nerve block Epidural Spinal	5	2–4	Same as above
Etidocaine (Duranest)	Local infiltrate Nerve block Epidural	3–5	5–10	Same as above
Levobupivacaine (Chirocaine)	Nerve block Epidural	–	–	Same as above
Lidocaine	Local infiltrate Nerve block Spinal Epidural Topical IV regional	Less than 2	0.5–1	Same as above
Mepivacaine (Carbocaine, Polocaine)	Local infiltrate Nerve block Epidural	3–5	0.75–1.5	Same as above
Ropivacaine (Naropin)	Local infiltrate Nerve block Epidural Spinal	1–15	2–6	Same as above

Note: Most side effects are manifestations of excessive plasma concentrations.

ANOREXIANTS

USES	ACTIONS
Adjunct to diet and physical activity in the treatment of chronic, relapsing obesity.	Two categories of medications are used for weight control: *Appetite suppressants:* Stimulate the central nervous system to decrease appetite and cause a feeling of fullness or satiety. *Digestion inhibitors:* Reversible lipase inhibitors that blocks the breakdown and absorption of dietary fats which reduces calorie intake.

ANOREXIANTS

Name	Type	Availability	Dosage	Side Effects
Benzphetamine (Didrex)	AS	**T:** 50 mg	25–50 mg 1–3 times a day	Headache, insomnia, nervousness, anxiety, irritability, dry mouth, constipation, euphoria, palpitations, hypertension
Diethylpropion (Tenuate)	AS	**T:** 25 mg, 75 mg	25 mg 3 times a day or 75 mg once daily	Headache, insomnia, nervousness, anxiety, irritability, dry mouth, constipation, euphoria, palpitations, hypertension
Mazindol (Sanorex)	AS	**T:** 1 mg, 2 mg	1–3 mg a day with meals	Palpitations, restlessness, dizziness, headache, depression, weakness, abdominal pain
Orlistat (Xenical)	DI	**C:** 120 mg	120 mg 3 times a day before meals	Flatulence, rectal incontinence, oily stools

Phendimetrazine (Bontril)	AS	**C:** 105 mg **T:** 35 mg	17.5–70 mg 2–3 times a day or 105 mg once daily	Headache, insomnia, nervousness, irritability, dry mouth, constipation, euphoria, palpitations, hypertension
Phenmetrazine (Preludin)	AS	**T:** 75 mg	75 mg once daily	Palpitations, hypertension, nervousness, anxiety, headache, dizziness, dry mouth, euphoria, constipation
Phenteramine (Ionamin)	AS	**C:** 15 mg, 30 mg, 37.5 mg	15–37.5 mg once daily	Headache, insomnia, nervousness, anxiety, irritability, dry mouth, constipation, euphoria, palpitations, hypertension
Sibutramine (Meridia)	AS	**C:** 5 mg, 10 mg, 15 mg	Initially, 10 mg, then increase to 15 mg/day or decrease to 5 mg/day	Hypertension, increased heart rate, headache, dry mouth, loss of appetite, insomnia, constipation

AS, Appetite suppressant; ***C,*** capsules; ***DI,*** digestion inhibitor; ***T,*** tablets.

Appendix C

CALCULATION OF DOSES

Frequently, dosages ordered do not correspond exactly to what is available and must be calculated.

RATIO/PROPORTION:
A patient is to receive 65 mg of a medication. It is available as 80 mg/2 ml. What volume (ml) needs to be administered to the patient?

STEP 1: Set up ratio.

$$\frac{80\text{ mg}}{2\text{ ml}} = \frac{65\text{ mg}}{x\text{ (ml)}}$$

STEP 2: Cross multiply and divide each side by the number with x to determine volume to be administered.

$$(80\text{ mg})(x\text{ ml}) = (65\text{ mg})(2\text{ ml})$$
$$80\,x = 130$$
$$x = 130/80 \text{ or } 1.625\text{ ml}$$

CALCULATIONS IN MICROGRAMS/KILOGRAM PER MINUTE (mcg/kg/min):
A 63-year-old patient (weight 165 lb) is to receive medication A at a rate of 8 mcg/kg/min. Given a solution containing medication A in a concentration of 500 mg/250 ml, at what rate (ml/hr) would you infuse this medication?

STEP 1: Convert to same units. In this problem, the dose is expressed in mcg/kg; therefore, convert weight to kg (2.2 lb = 1 kg) and drug concentration to mcg/ml (1 mg = 1,000 mcg)

165 lb divided by 2.2 = 75 kg

$$\frac{500\text{ mg}}{250\text{ ml}} = 2\text{ mg/ml} = 2{,}000\text{ mcg/ml}$$

STEP 2: Number of mcg/hr. (75 kg) × 8 mcg/kg/min = 600 mcg/min or 36,000 mcg/hr

STEP 3: Number of ml/hr. 36,000 mcg/hr divided by 2,000 mcg/ml = 18 ml/hr

Appendix D

COMBINATION DRUGS BY TRADE NAME

Many drugs are available in fixed combinations of two or more medications. Some of the most common trade names for combination drugs in the United States are listed below, along with their generic components and classifications.

Combination Product Name	Generic Components
AC Gel	cocaine (an anesthetic)/epinephrine (a vasopressor)
Accuretic	quinapril (an ACE inhibitor)/hydrochlorothiazide (a diuretic)
Activella	estradiol (an estrogen)/norethindrone (a hormone)
Advair	fluticasone (a corticosteroid)/salmeterol (a bronchodilator)
Advil Cold	pseudoephedrine (a sympathomimetic)/ibuprofen (an NSAID)
Aggrenox	aspirin (an antiplatelet and non-narcotic analgesic)/dipyridamole (an antiplatelet)
Aldactazide	spironolactone (a potassium-sparing diuretic)/hydrochlorothiazide (a diuretic)
Aldoril	methyldopa (an antihypertensive)/hydrochlorothiazide (a diuretic)
Allegra-D	fexofenadine (an antihistamine)/pseudoephedrine (a nasal decongestant)
Allegra-D 24 Hour	fexofenadine (an antihistamine)/pseudoephedrine (a sympathomimetic)
Anexsia	hydrocodone (a narcotic analgesic)/acetaminophen (a non-narcotic analgesic)
Apresazide	hydralazine (a vasodilator)/hydrochlorothiazide (a diuretic)
Arthrotec	diclofenac (an NSAID)/misoprostol (an antisecretory gastric protectant)
Atacand HCT	candesartan (an angiotensin II receptor antagonist)/hydrochlorothiazide (a diuretic)
Avalide	irbesartan (an angiotensin II receptor antagonist)/hydrochlorothiazide (a diuretic)
Avandamet	rosiglitazone (an antidiabetic)/metformin (an antidiabetic)
Bactrim	sulfamethoxazole (a sulfonamide)/trimethoprim (an anti-infective)
Bellergal-S	ergotamine (an antimigraine)/belladonna (an anticholinergic)/phenobarbital (an anticonvulsant)

(continued)

Combination Product Name	Generic Components
Benicar HCT	olmesartan (an angiotensin II receptor antagonist)/ hydrochlorothiazide (a diuretic)
Bicillin CR	penicillin G benzathine (a penicillin)/penicillin procaine (a penicillin)
Blephamide	sulfacetamide (an anti-infective)/prednisolone (an adrenocortical steroid)
Caduet	amlodipine (a calcium channel blocker)/ atorvastatin (an antihyperlipidemic)
Caladryl	calamine (an astringent)/ diphenhydramine (an antihistamine)/camphor (a counterirritant)
Capital with Codeine	acetaminophen (a non-narcotic analgesic)/codeine (a narcotic analgesic)
Capozide	captopril (an ACE inhibitor)/hydrochlorothiazide (a diuretic)
Children's Advil Cold	ibuprofen (an NSAID)/pseudoephedrine (a nasal decongestant)
CiproDex Otic	ciprofloxacin (an anti-infective)/dexamethasone (an adrenocortical steroid)
Cipro HC Otic	ciprofloxacin (an anti-infective)/hydrocortisone (and adrenocortical steroid)
Claritin-D	loratadine (an antihistamine)/pseudoephedrine (a nasal decongestant)
Combipatch	estradiol (an estrogen)/norethindrone (a hormone)
Combipres	clonidine (an antihypertensive)/chlorthalidone (a diuretic)
Combivent	ipratropium (a bronchodilator)/albuterol (a bronchodilator)
Combivir	lamivudine (an antiretroviral)/zidovudine (an antiretroviral)
Combunox	ibuprofen (an NSAID)/oxycodone (a narcotic analgesic)
Cortisporin	neomycin (and anti-infective)/polymyxin B (an anti-infective)/hydrocortisone (an adrenocortical steroid)
Corzide	nadolol (a beta-blocker)/bendroflumethiazide (a diuretic)
Cosopt	dorzolamide (a carbonic anhydrase inhibitor)/ timolol (a beta-blocker)
Darvocet A 500	propoxyphene (a narcotic analgesic)/ acetaminophen (a non-narcotic analgesic)
Darvocet-N	propoxyphene (a narcotic analgesic)/ acetaminophen (a non-narcotic analgesic)
Dexacidin	neomycin (an anti-infective)/polymyxin (an anti-infective)/dexamethasone (an adrenocortical steroid)

Dilantin with PB	phenobarbital (an anticonvulsant)/phenytoin (an anticonvulsant)
Diovan HCT	valsartan (an angiotensin II receptor antagonist)/hydrochlorothiazide (a diuretic)
Donnatal	atropine (an anticholinergic)/hyoscyamine (an anticholinergic)/phenobarbital (a sedative)/scopolamine (an anticholinergic)
Duocet	acetaminophen (a non-narcotic analgesic)/hydrocodone (a narcotic analgesic)
Duoneb	ipratropium (a bronchodilator)/albuterol base (a bronchodilator)
Dyazide	triamterene (a potassium-sparing diuretic)/hydrochlorothiazide (a diuretic)
EMLA	lidocaine (a local anesthetic)/prilocaine (an anesthetic)
Epzicom	abacavir (an antiretroviral)/lamivudine (an antiretroviral)
Eryzole	erythromycin (a macrolide)/sulfisoxazole (a sulfonamide)
Etrafon	perphenazine (an antipsychotic)/amitriptyline (an antidepressant)
Extra Strength Maalox	magnesium hydroxide (an antacid)/simethicone (an antiflatulent)
Femhrt	norethindrone (a hormone)/estradiol (an estrogen)
Ferro-Sequels	ferrous fumarate (a hematinic)/docusate (a laxative)
Fioricet	butabarbital (a sedative-hypnotic)/acetaminophen (a non-narcotic analgesic)/caffeine (a CNS stimulant)
Fiorinal	butabarbital (a sedative-hypnotic)/aspirin (a non-narcotic analgesic)/caffeine (a CNS stimulant)
Gaviscon (oral suspension)	aluminum hydroxide (an antacid)/magnesium carbonate (an antacid)
Gaviscon (tablets)	aluminum hydroxide (an antacid)/magnesium trisilicate (an antacid)
Gelusil	aluminum hydroxide (an antacid)/magnesium hydroxide (a laxative)/simethicone (an antiflatulent)
Gentlax-S	senna (a laxative)/docusate (a laxative)
Glucovance	glyburide (an antidiabetic)/metformin (an antidiabetic)
Haley's M-O	magnesium (a laxative)/mineral oil (a lubricant laxative)
Helidac	bismuth (an antidiarrheal)/metronidazole (an anti-infective)/ tetracycline (an anti-infective)

(continued)

Combination Product Name	Generic Components
Humalog Mix 75/25	insulin: lispro suspension 75% and lispro solution 25%
Humulin 50/50	insulin: NPH 50% and regular 50%
Humulin 70/30	insulin: NPH 70% and rapid-acting regular 30%
Hyzaar	losartan (an angiotensin II receptor antagonist)/ hydrochlorothiazide (a diuretic)
Imodium Advanced	loperamide (an antidiarrheal)/simethicone (an anti-flatulent)
Inderide	propranolol (a beta-blocker)/hydrochlorothiazide (a diuretic)
Inderide LA	propranolol (a beta-blocker)/hydrochlorothiazide (a diuretic)
Lexxel	enalapril (an ACE inhibitor)/felodipine (a calcium channel blocker)
Librax	chlordiazepoxide (an antianxiety agent)/clidinium (an anticholinergic)
Lidocaine with epinephrine	lidocaine (a local anesthetic)/epinephrine (a vasoconstrictor)
LidoSite	epinephrine (a sympathomimetic)/lidocaine (an anesthetic)
Limbitrol	chlordiazepoxide (an antianxiety agent)/ amitriptyline (an antidepressant)
Lomotil	diphenoxylate (an antidiarrheal)/atropine (an anti-cholinergic-antispasmodic)
Lopressor HCT	metoprolol (a beta-blocker)/hydrochlorothiazide (a diuretic)
Lorcet	acetaminophen (a non-narcotic analgesic)/ hydrocodone (a narcotic analgesic)
Lortab	hydrocodone (a narcotic analgesic)/ acetaminophen (a non-narcotic analgesic)
Lortab Elixir	hydrocodone (a narcotic analgesic)/ acetaminophen (a non-narcotic analgesic)
Lortab/ASA	hydrocodone (a narcotic analgesic)/aspirin (a non-narcotic analgesic)
Lotensin HCT	benazepril (an ACE inhibitor)/hydrochlorothiazide (a diuretic)
Lotrel	amlodipine (a calcium channel blocker)/benazepril (an ACE inhibitor)
Lotrisone	clotrimazole (an antifungal)/betamethasone (and adrenocortical steroid)
Lunelle	medroxyprogesterone (a progestin)/estradiol (an estrogen)
Maalox	aluminum hydroxide (an antacid)/magnesium hydroxide (an antacid)

Maalox Plus	aluminum hydroxide (an antacid)/magnesium hydroxide (an antacid)/simethicone (an anti-flatulent)
Maxitrol	neomycin (an anti-infective)/polymyxin (an anti-infective)/dexamethasone (an adrenocortical steroid)
Maxzide	triamterene (a potassium-sparing diuretic)/ hydrochlorothiazide (a diuretic)
Metaglip	glipizide (an antidiabetic)/metformin(an anti-diabetic)
Micardis HCT	telmisartan (an angiotensin II receptor antagonist)/ hydrochlorothiazide (a diuretic)
Minizide	prazosin (an antihypertensive)/polythiazide (a diuretic)
Moduretic	amiloride (a potassium-sparing diuretic)/ hydrochlorothiazide (a diuretic)
Motrin Cold	pseudoephedrine (a sympathomimetic)/ibuprofen (an NSAID)
Mucinex D	guaifenesin (an expectorant)/pseudoephedrine (a sympathomimetic)
Mucinex DM	guaifenesin (an expectorant)/dextromethorphan (an expectorant)
Mycitracin	neomycin (an aminoglycoside)/polymyxin B (an anti-infective)/ bacitracin (an anti-infective)
Myco II	nystatin (an antifungal)/triamcinolone (an adreno-cortical steroid)
Mycolog II	nystatin (an antifungal)/triamcinolone (an adreno-cortical steroid)
Myco-Triacet	nystatin (an antifungal)/triamcinolone (an adreno-cortical steroid)
Mylanta (oral suspension)	aluminum hydroxide (an antacid)/magnesium hydroxide (an antacid)/simethicone (an antiflatu-lent)
Mylanta (tablets)	calcium carbonate/magnesium hydroxide
Naphcon-A	naphazoline (a nasal decongestant/pheniramine (an antihistamine)
Neosporin GU Irrigant	neomycin (an aminoglycoside)/polymyxin B (an anti-infective)
Neosporin Ointment, Triple Antibiotic	neomycin (an aminoglycoside)/polymyxin B (an anti-infective)/bacitracin (an anti-infective)
Norco	hydrocodone (a narcotic analgesic)/ acetaminophen (a non-narcotic analgesic)
Normozide	labetalol (a beta-blocker)/hydrochlorothiazide (a diuretic)
Novolin 70/30	insulin: NPH 70% and rapid-acting regular 30%

(continued)

Combination Product Name	Generic Components
Novolog 70/30	insulin: aspart suspension 70% and aspart solution 30%
Pediazole	erythromycin (a macrolide)/sulfisoxazole (a sulfonamide)
Pepcid Complete	famotidine (an H_2 antagonist)/calcium chloride (an antacid)/magnesium hydroxide (an antacid)
Percocet	oxycodone (a narcotic analgesic)/acetaminophen (a non-narcotic analgesic)
Percodan	oxycodone (a narcotic analgesic)/aspirin (a non-narcotic analgesic)
Phenergan with Codeine	promethazine (an antihistamine)/codeine (a cough suppressant)
Phenergan VC	promethazine (an antihistamine)/phenylephrine (a vasopressor)
Phenergan VC with Codeine	promethazine (an antihistamine)/phenylephrine (a vasopressor)/codeine (a cough suppressant)
Polysporin	polymyxin B (an anti-infective)/bacitracin (an anti-infective)
Pravigard	aspirin (an antiplatelet)/pravastatin (an antihyperlipidemic)
Premphase	conjugated estrogens (an estrogen)/ medroxyprogesterone (an androgen)
Prempro	conjugated estrogens (an estrogen)/ medroxyprogesterone (an androgen)
Prevacid Napra-Pac	lansoprazole (a proton pump inhibitor)/naproxen (an NSAID)
Prinzide	lisinopril (an ACE inhibitor)/hydrochlorothiazide (a diuretic)
Rebetron	ribavirin (an antiviral)/interferon alpha-2b (an immunologic agent)
Reprexain CIII	ibuprofen (an NSAID)/hydrocodone (a narcotic analgesic)
Rifamate	rifampin (an antitubercular)/isoniazid (an antitubercular)
Rifater	rifampin (an antitubercular)/isoniazid (an antitubercular)/pyrazinamide (an antitubercular)
Robitussin AC	guaifenesin (an antitussive)/codeine (a narcotic analgesic)
Robitussin DM	dextromethorphan (a cough suppressant)/ guaifenesin (an antitussive)
Roxicet	oxycodone (a narcotic analgesic)/acetaminophen (a non-narcotic analgesic)
Senokot-S	senna (a laxative)/docusate (a laxative)

Septra	sulfamethoxazole (a sulfonamide)/trimethoprim (an anti-infective)
Silain-Gel	magnesium hydroxide (an antacid)/aluminum hydroxide (an antacid)/simethicone (an anti-flatulent)
Stalevo	carbidopa-levodopa (an antiparkinson agent)/ entacapone (an antiparkinson agent)
Suboxone	buprenorphine (a non-narcotic analgesic)/naloxone (a narcotic antagonist)
Symbax	fluoxetine (an antidepressant)/olanzapine (an antipsychotic)
TAC	tetracaine (an anesthetic)/epinephrine (a vasoconstrictor)/cocaine (an anesthetic)
Tarka	trandolapril (an ACE inhibitor)/verapamil (a calcium channel blocker)
Teczem	enalapril (an ACE inhibitor)/diltiazem (a calcium channel blocker)
Tenoretic	atenolol (a beta-blocker)/chlorthalidone (a diuretic)
Teveten HCT	eprosartan (an angiotensin II receptor antagonist)/ hydrochlorothiazide (a diuretic)
Thyrolar	liothyronine (a thyroid agent)/levothyroxine (a thyroid agent)
Timolide	timolol (a beta-blocker)/hydrochlorothiazide (a diuretic)
Tobradex	tobramycin (an aminoglycoside)/dexamethasone (an adrenocortical steroid)
Triavil	perphenazine (an antipsychotic)/amitriptyline (an antidepressant)
Trizivir	abacavir (an antiretroviral)lamivudine (an antiretroviral)/zidovudine (an antiretroviral)
Truvada	emtricitabine (an antiretroviral)/tenofovir (an antiretroviral)
Tylenol with Codeine	acetaminophen (a non-narcotic analgesic)/codeine (a narcotic analgesic)
Tylox	acetaminophen (a non-narcotic analgesic)/ oxycodone (a narcotic analgesic)
Ultracet	tramadol (a non-narcotic analgesic)/ acetaminophen (a non-narcotic analgesic)
Uniretic	moexipril (an ACE inhibitor)/hydrochlorothiazide (a diuretic)
Vaseretic	enalapril (an ACE inhibitor)/hydrochlorothiazide (a diuretic)
Vasocidin	sulfacetamide (an anti-infective)/prednisolone (an adrenocortical steroid)

(continued)

Combination Product Name	Generic Components
Vicodin	hydrocodone (a narcotic analgesic)/ acetaminophen (a non-narcotic analgesic)
Vicodin ES	hydrocodone (a narcotic analgesic)/ acetaminophen (a non-narcotic analgesic)
Vicodin HP	hydrocodone(a narcotic analgesic)/acetaminophen (a non-narcotic analgesic)
Vicoprofen	hydrocodone (a narcotic analgesic)/ibuprofen (an NSAID)
Vytorin	ezetimibe (an antihyperlipidemic)/simvastatin (an antihyperlipidemic)
Zestoretic	lisinopril (an ACE inhibitor)/hydrochlorothiazide (a diuretic)
Ziac	bisoprolol (a beta-blocker)/hydrochlorothiazide (a diuretic)
Zotrim	trimethoprim (an anti-infective)/sulfamethoxazole (a sulfonamide)/phenazopyridine (a spasmolytic)
Zydone	hydrocodone (a narcotic analgesic)/ acetaminophen (a non-narcotic analgesic)
Zyrtec D 12 hour tablets	cetirizine (an antihistamine)/pseudoephedrine (a nasal decongestant)

Appendix E

CONTROLLED DRUGS (UNITED STATES)

Schedule I: Medications having no legal medical use. These substances may be used for research purposes with proper registration (e.g., heroin, LSD).

Schedule II: Medications having a legitimate medical use but are characterized by a very high abuse potential and/or potential for severe physical and psychic dependency. Emergency telephone orders for limited quantities of these drugs are authorized, but the prescriber must provide a written, signed prescription order (e.g., morphine, amphetamines).

Schedule III: Medications having significant abuse potential (less than Schedule II). Telephone orders are permitted (e.g., opiates in combination with other substances such as acetaminophen).

Schedule IV: Medications having a low abuse potential. Telephone orders are permitted (e.g., benzodiazepines, propoxyphene).

Schedule V: Medications having the lowest abuse potential of the controlled substances. Some Schedule V products may be available without a prescription (e.g., certain cough preparations containing limited amounts of an opiate).

Appendix F

DRIP RATES FOR CRITICAL CARE MEDICATIONS

Dopamine

Dobutamine

Heparin

Nitroglycerin

Norepinephrine

Propofol

Sodium Nitroprusside

Dopamine (Intropin)
Mix 400 mg in 250 ml of D_5W (1,600 mcg/ml)

	Body Weight														
	lb	88	99	110	121	132	143	154	165	176	187	198	209	220	231
	kg	40	45	50	55	60	65	70	75	80	85	90	95	100	105
Dose ordered in mcg/kg/min	*Amount to infuse in mcgtts/min or ml/hr*														
2.5		4	4	5	5	6	6	7	7	8	8	8	9	9	10
5		8	8	9	10	11	12	13	14	15	16	17	18	19	20
7.5		11	13	14	15	17	18	20	21	23	24	25	27	28	30
10		15	17	19	21	23	24	26	28	30	32	34	36	38	39
12.5		19	21	23	26	28	30	33	35	38	40	42	45	47	49
15		23	25	28	31	34	37	39	42	45	48	51	53	56	59
20		30	34	38	41	45	49	53	56	60	64	68	71	75	79
25		38	42	47	52	56	61	66	70	75	80	84	89	94	98
30		45	51	56	62	67	73	79	84	90	96	101	107	113	118
35		53	59	66	72	79	85	92	98	105	112	118	125	131	138
40		60	68	75	83	90	98	105	113	120	128	135	143	150	158
45		68	76	84	93	101	110	118	127	135	143	152	160	169	177
50		75	84	94	103	113	122	131	141	150	159	169	178	188	197

- Administer 2.5–5 mcg/kg/min initially.
- Increase in increments of 5–10 mcg to 50 mcg/kg/min as needed.
- Do not mix with sodium bicarbonate.

Dobutamine (Dobutrex)
Mix 250 mg in 250 ml of D_5W (1,000 mcg/ml)

	Body Weight															
	lb	88	99	110	121	132	143	154	165	176	187	198	209	220	231	242
	kg	40	45	50	55	60	65	70	75	80	85	90	95	100	105	110
Dose ordered in mcg/kg/min	*Amount to infuse in mcgtts/min or ml/hr*															
2.5		6	7	8	8	9	10	11	11	12	13	14	14	15	16	17
5		12	14	15	17	18	20	21	23	24	26	27	29	30	32	33
7.5		18	20	23	25	27	29	32	34	36	38	41	43	45	47	50
10		24	27	30	33	36	39	42	45	48	51	54	57	60	63	66
12.5		30	34	38	41	45	49	53	56	60	64	68	71	75	79	83
15		36	41	45	50	54	59	63	68	72	77	81	86	90	95	99
20		48	54	60	66	72	78	84	90	96	102	108	114	120	126	132
25		60	68	75	83	90	98	105	113	120	128	135	143	150	158	165
30		72	81	90	99	108	117	126	135	144	153	162	171	180	189	198
35		84	95	105	116	126	137	147	158	168	179	189	200	210	221	231
40		96	108	120	132	144	156	168	180	192	204	216	228	240	252	264

- Administer 2.5–10 mcg/kg/min initially.
- Increase in increments of 5–10 mcg up to 40 mcg/kg/min as needed.
- Do not mix with sodium bicarbonate.

Heparin Drip Rate Chart

ACT (sec)	aPTT (sec)	Bolus Dose (ml)	Stop Infusion (min)	Rate Change (ml/hr)	Repeat PTT (hr)	Repeat aPTT (hr)
1–200	1–49	5,000	0	+3 ml/hr (increase by 150 units/hr)	4	4
201–239	50–59	0	0	+2 ml/hr (increase by 100 units/hr)	4	4
240–300	60–85	0	0	0 (no change)	8	8
301–400	86–95	0	0	–1 ml/hr (decrease by 50 units/hr)	8	8
401–500	96–120	0	30	–2 ml/hr (decrease by 100 units/hr)	4	4
500+	120+	0	60	–3 ml/hr (decrease by 150 units/hr)	4	4

Nitroglycerin (Tridil)

Dose ordered in mcg/min	50 mg/250 cc 100 mg/500 cc NTG/D_5W	100 mg/250 cc 200 mg/500 cc NTG/D_5W	Dose ordered in mcg/min	50 mg/250 cc 100 mg/500 cc NTG/D_5W	100 mg/250 cc 200 mg/500 cc NTG/D_5W
10	3	—	210	63	32
20	6	3	220	66	33
30	9	5	230	69	35
40	12	6	240	72	36
50	15	8	250	75	38
60	18	9	260	78	39
70	21	10	270	81	41
80	24	12	280	84	42
90	27	14	290	87	44
100	30	15	300	90	45
110	33	17	310	93	47
120	36	18	320	96	48
130	39	19	330	99	50
140	42	21	340	102	51
150	45	23	350	105	53
160	48	24	360	108	54
170	51	26	370	111	56
180	54	27	380	114	57
190	57	29	390	117	59
200	60	30	400	120	60
	Amt to infuse in mcgtts/min or ml/hr			***Amt to infuse in mcgtts/min or ml/hr***	

- Administer at 10–20 mcg/min initially.
- Increase at increments of 6–10 mcg/min every 5–10 min until desired response.

Norepinephrine (Levophed)

Mix: 4 mg in 250 ml D_5W

Norepinephrine 4 mg in 250 ml D_5W (rate is ml/hr)

	mcg/kg/min											
kg	0.01	0.02	0.03	0.04	0.05	0.06	0.07	0.08	0.09	0.10	0.20	0.30
50	1.9	3.8	5.7	7.6	9.5	11.4	13.3	15.2	17.1	19.0	38.0	57.0
55	2.1	4.2	6.3	8.4	10.5	12.6	14.7	16.8	18.9	21.0	42.0	63.0
60	2.3	4.6	6.9	9.2	11.5	13.8	16.1	18.4	20.7	23.0	46.0	69.0
65	2.4	4.8	7.2	9.6	12.0	14.4	16.8	19.2	21.6	24.0	48.0	72.0
70	2.6	5.2	7.8	10.4	13.0	15.6	18.2	20.8	23.4	26.0	52.0	78.0
75	2.8	5.6	8.4	11.2	14.0	16.8	19.6	22.4	25.2	28.0	56.0	84.0
80	3.0	6.0	9.0	12.0	15.0	18.0	21.0	24.0	27.0	30.0	60.0	90.0
85	3.2	6.4	9.6	12.8	16.0	19.2	22.4	25.6	28.8	32.0	64.0	96.0
90	3.4	6.8	10.2	13.6	17.0	20.4	23.8	27.2	30.6	34.0	68.0	102
95	3.6	7.2	10.8	14.4	18.0	21.6	25.2	28.8	32.4	36.0	72.0	108
100	3.8	7.6	11.4	15.2	19.0	22.8	26.6	30.4	34.2	38.0	76.0	114

Use: Hypotension, shock
Dose: 2–40 mcg/min or 0.05–0.25 mcg/kg/min doses of greater than 75 mcg/min or 1 mcg/kg/min have been used
Mechanism: Primary α_1 vasoconstriction effect (minor β_1 inotropic)
Elimination: Hepatic **Half-life:** Minutes
Adverse events: Tachyarrhythmias, hypertension at high doses

Propofol (Diprivan)

Mix: Undiluted (10 mg/ml) 100-ml vial

Propofol 10 mg/ml (premixed) (rate is ml/hr)

	mcg/kg/min											
kg	10	15	20	25	30	35	40	45	50	55	60	65
50	3	5	6	8	9	11	12	14	15	17	18	20
55	3	5	7	8	10	12	13	15	17	18	20	21
60	4	5	7	9	11	13	14	16	18	20	22	23
65	4	6	8	10	12	14	16	18	20	21	23	25
70	4	6	8	11	13	15	17	19	21	23	25	27
75	5	7	9	11	14	16	18	20	23	25	27	29
80	5	7	10	12	14	17	19	22	24	26	29	31
85	5	8	10	13	15	18	20	23	26	28	31	33
90	5	8	11	14	16	19	22	24	27	30	32	35
95	6	9	11	14	17	20	23	26	29	31	34	37
100	6	9	12	15	18	21	24	27	30	33	36	39

Use: Non-amnestic sedation

Dose: Load 1–2 mg/kg IV push; **do not load if patient is hypotensive or volume depleted**

Maintenance Initial dose of 5–20 mcg/kg/min, may titrate to effect (20–65 mcg/kg/min)

Mechanism: Di-isopropyl phenolic compound with intravenous general anesthetic properties unrelated to opiates, barbiturates, benzodiazepines

Elimination: Hepatic **Half-life:** 30 minutes

Adverse events: Hypotension, nausea, vomiting, seizures, hypertriglyceridemia, hyperlipidemia

Sodium Nitroprusside (Nipride)
Mix 50 mg in 250 ml of D_5W (200 mcg/ml)

	Body Weight														
lb	88	99	110	121	132	143	154	165	176	187	198	209	220	231	242
kg	40	45	50	55	60	65	70	75	80	85	90	95	100	105	110
Dose ordered in mcg/kg/min	*Amount to infuse in mcgtts/min or ml/hr*														
0.5	6	7	8	8	9	10	11	11	12	13	14	14	15	16	17
1	12	14	15	17	18	20	21	23	24	26	27	29	30	32	33
1.5	13	20	23	25	27	29	32	34	36	38	41	43	45	47	50
2	24	27	30	33	36	39	42	45	48	51	54	57	60	63	66
3	36	41	45	50	54	59	63	68	72	77	81	86	90	95	99
4	48	54	60	66	72	78	84	90	96	102	108	114	120	126	132
5	60	68	75	83	90	98	105	113	120	128	135	143	150	158	165
6	72	81	90	99	108	117	126	135	144	153	162	171	180	189	198
7	84	95	105	116	126	137	147	158	168	179	189	200	210	221	231
8	96	108	120	132	144	156	168	180	192	204	216	228	240	252	264
9	108	122	135	149	162	176	189	203	216	230	243	257	270	284	297
10	120	135	150	165	180	195	210	225	240	255	270	285	300	315	330

- Administer 0.5–10 mcg/kg/min initially.
- Increase in increments of 1 mcg/kg/min until desired response.
- Do not leave solution exposed to light.

Appendix G

DRUGS OF ABUSE

Name (Brand)	Class	Signs and Symptoms	Treatment
Acid (see LSD)			
Adam (see MDMA)			
Amphetamine (Adderall, Dexedrine)	Stimulant	Tachycardia, hypertension, diaphoresis, agitation, headache, seizures, dehydration, hypokalemia, lactic acidosis. Severe overdose: hyperthermia, dysrhythmia, shock, rhabdomyolysis, liver necrosis, acute renal failure.	Control agitation, reverse hyperthermia, support hemodynamic function. **Antidote:** No specific antidote.
Angel dust (see phencyclidine)			
Apache (see fentanyl)			
Barbiturates (Nembutal, Seconal)	Depressant	Hypotension, hypothermia, apnea, nystagmus, ataxia, hyporeflexia, somnolence, stupor, coma.	Airway management, decontamination, supportive care. **Antidote:** No specific antidote.
Barbs (see barbiturates)			
Benzodiazepines (Xanax, Valium, Librium, Halcion)	Depressant	Respiratory depression, hypothermia, hypotension, nystagmus, miosis, diplopia, bradycardia, nausea, vomiting, impaired speech and coordination, amnesia, ataxia, somnolence, confusion, depressed deep tendon reflexes.	**Antidote:** Flumazenil (Romazicon) is a specific antidote.
Black tar (see heroin)			
Horse (see heroin)			
Boomers (see LSD)			
Buttons (see mescaline)			
Cactus (see mescaline)			
Candy (see benzodiazepines)			
China girl (see fentanyl)			
China white (see heroin)			

Name (Brand)	Class	Signs and Symptoms	Treatment
Cocaine	Stimulant	Hypertension, tachycardia, mild hyperthermia, mydriasis, pallor, diaphoresis, psychosis, paranoid delusions, mania, agitation, seizures.	Control agitation, seizures, hyperthermia; support hemodynamic function. **Antidote:** No specific antidote.
Codeine	Opioid	Miosis, respiratory depression, decreased mental status, hypotension, cardiac dysrhythmia, hypoxia, bronchoconstriction, constipation, decreased intestinal motility, ileus, lethargy, coma.	Airway management, hemodynamic support. **Antidote:** Naloxone, nalmefene.
Coke (see cocaine)			
Crank (see amphetamine)			
Crank (see heroin)			
Crystal (see amphetamine)			
Crystal meth (see methamphetamine)			
Cubes (see LSD)			
Downers (see benzodiazepines)			
Ecstasy (see MDMA)			
Fentanyl (Sublimaze)	Opioid	Miosis, respiratory depression, decreased mental status, hypotension, cardiac dysrhythmia, hypoxia, bronchoconstriction, constipation, decreased intestinal motility, ileus, lethargy, coma.	Airway management, hemodynamic support. **Antidote:** Naloxone, nalmefene.
Flunitrazepam (Rohypnol)	Depressant	Drowsiness, slurred speech, impaired judgment and motor skills, hypothermia, hypotension, bradycardia, diplopia, blurred vision, nystagmus, respiratory depression, nausea, constipation, depression, lethargy, headache, ataxia, coma, amnesia, incoordination, tremors, vertigo.	Supportive care, airway control. **Antidote:** Flumazenil (Romazicon).

(continued)

Name (Brand)	Class	Signs and Symptoms	Treatment
Forget me pill (see flunitrazepam)			
GHB (gamma-hydroxybutyrate)	CNS depressant	Dose-related CNS depression, amnesia, hypotonia, drowsiness, dizziness, euphoria. Other effects: bradycardia, hypotension, hypersalivation, vomiting, hypothermia. Higher dosages: Cheyne-Stokes respiration, seizures, coma, death. Users may become highly agitated.	Supportive care. Severe intoxication may require airway support, including intubation. **Antidote:** No specific antidote.
Gib (see GHB)			
Goodfellas (see fentanyl)			
Grass (see marijuana)			
Hashish (see marijuana)			
Heroin	Opioid	Miosis, coma, apnea, pulmonary edema, bradycardia, hypotension, pinpoint pupils, CNS depression, seizures.	Airway management. **Antidote:** Naloxone, nalmefene.
Ice (see amphetamine)			
Ketamine (Ketalar)	Anesthetic	Feeling of dissociation from one's self (sense of floating over one's body), visual hallucinations, lack of coordination, hypertension, tachycardia, palpitations, respiratory depression, apnea, confusion, negativism, hostility, delirium, reduced awareness.	Supportive care, esp. respiratory and cardiac function. **Antidote:** No specific antidote.
Keets (see ketamine)			
Kit-kat (see ketamine)			
Liquid ecstasy (see GHB)			
Liquid X (see GHB)			

Name (Brand)	Class	Signs and Symptoms	Treatment
LSD	Hallucinogen	Diaphoresis, mydriasis, dizziness, twitching, flushing, hyperreflexia, hypertension, psychosis, behavioral changes, emotional lability, euphoria or dysphoria, paranoia, vomiting, diarrhea, anorexia, restlessness, incoordination, tremors, ataxia.	Airway management, control activity associated with hallucinations, psychosis, panic reaction. **Antidote:** No specific antidote.
Ludes (see methaqualone)			
Magic mushroom (see psilocybin)			
Marijuana	Cannabinoid	Increased appetite, reduced motility, constipation, urinary retention, seizures, euphoria, somnolence, heightened awareness, relaxation, altered time perception, short-term memory loss, poor concentration, mood alterations, disorientation, decreased strength, ataxia, slurred speech, respiratory depression, coma.	Airway management, supportive care. **Antidote:** No specific antidote.
MDMA (Methylene dioxymethamphetamine)	Stimulant	Euphoria, intimacy, closeness to others, loss of appetite, tachycardia, jaw tension, bruxism, diaphoresis.	**Antidote:** No specific antidote.
Mescaline	Hallucinogen	Diaphoresis, mydriasis, dizziness, twitching, flushing, hyperreflexia, hypertension, psychosis, behavioral changes, emotional instability, euphoria or dysphoria, paranoia, vomiting, diarrhea, anorexia, restlessness, incoordination, tremors, ataxia.	Airway management, control activity associated with hallucinations, psychosis, panic reaction. **Antidote:** No specific antidote.
Meth (see methamphetamine)			

(continued)

Name (Brand)	Class	Signs and Symptoms	Treatment
Methamphetamine (Desoxyn)	Stimulant	Hypertension, hyperthermia, hyperpyrexia, agitation, hyperactivity, fasciculation, seizures, coma, tachycardia, dysrhythmias, pale skin, diaphoresis, restlessness, talkativeness, insomnia, headache, coma, delusions, paranoia, aggressive behavior, visual, tactile, or auditory hallucinations.	Airway control, hyperthermia, seizures, dysrhythmias. **Antidote:** No specific antidote.
Methaqualone (Quaalude)	Depressant	Slurred speech, impaired judgment and motor skills, hypothermia, hypotension, bradycardia, diplopia, blurred vision, nystagmus, mydriasis, respiratory depression, depression, lethargy, headache, ataxia, coma, amnesia, incoordination, hypertonicity, myoclonus, tremors, vertigo.	Airway management, supportive care. **Antidote:** No specific antidote.
Methylphenidate (Ritalin)	Stimulant	Agitation, hypertension, tachycardia, hyperthermia, mydriasis, dry mouth, nausea, vomiting, anorexia, abdominal pain, agitation, hyperactivity, insomnia, euphoria, dizziness, paranoid ideation, social withdrawal, delirium, hallucinations, psychosis, tremors, seizures.	Control agitation, hyperthermia, seizures, support hemodynamic function. **Antidote:** No specific antidote.
Miss Emma (see morphine)			
Mister blue (see morphine)			

Name (Brand)	Class	Signs and Symptoms	Treatment
Morphine (MS-Contin, Roxanol)	Opioid	Miosis, respiratory depression, decreased mental status, hypotension, cardiac dysrhythmia, hypoxia, bronchoconstriction, constipation, decreased intestinal motility, ileus, lethargy, coma.	Airway management, hemodynamic support. **Antidote:** Naloxone, nalmefene.
Oxy (see oxycodone)			
Oxycodone (OxyContin)	Opioid	Miosis, respiratory depression, decreased mental status, hypotension, cardiac dysrhythmia, hypoxia, bronchoconstriction, constipation, decreased intestinal motility, ileus, lethargy, coma.	Airway management, hemodynamic support. **Antidote:** Naloxone, nalmefene.
OxyContin (see oxycodone)			
Peace pill (see phencyclidine)			
Phencyclidine (PCP)	Hallucinogen	Nystagmus, hypertension, tachycardia, agitation, hallucinations, violent behavior, impaired judgment, delusions, psychosis.	Support blood pressure, manage airway, control agitation. **Antidote:** No specific antidote.
Phennies (see barbiturates)			
Pot (see marijuana)			
Propoxyphene (Darvon)	Depressant	Respiratory depression, seizures, cardiac toxicity, miosis, dysrhythmias, nausea, vomiting, anorexia, abdominal pain, constipation, drowsiness, coma, confusion, hallucinations.	Maintain airway, seizures, cardiac toxicity. **Antidote:** Naloxone.

(continued)

Name (Brand)	Class	Signs and Symptoms	Treatment
Psilocybin	Hallucinogen	Diaphoresis, mydriasis, dizziness, twitching, flushing, hyperreflexia, hypertension, psychosis, behavioral changes, emotional lability, euphoria or dysphoria, paranoia, vomiting, diarrhea, anorexia, restlessness, incoordination, tremors, ataxia.	Manage airway, control activity associated with hallucinations, psychosis, panic reaction. **Antidote:** No specific antidote.
Purple passion (see psilocybin)			
Quay (see methaqualone)			
Reefer (see marijuana)			
Rock (see cocaine)			
Rocket fuel (see phencyclidine)			
Roofies (see flunitrazepam)			
Rope (see flunitrazepam)			
Rophies (see flunitrazepam)			
Salty water (see GHB)			
Schoolboy (see codeine)			
Scoop (see GHB)			
Snow (see cocaine)			
Special K (see ketamine)			
Speed (see amphetamine)			
STP (see MDMA)			
Super acid (see ketamine)			
Super K (see ketamine)			
Tranks (see benzodiazepines)			
Uppers (see amphetamine)			
White girl (see cocaine)			
Yellow jackets (see barbiturates)			
Yellow sunshine (see LSD)			

"CLUB DRUG" WEB SITES

www.drugfreeamerica.org	Partnership for a Drug-Free America
www.clubdrugs.org	Consumer-oriented site sponsored by the National Institute on Drug Abuse
www.health.org	Substance Abuse and Mental Health Services Administration
www.projectghb.org	Independent site devoted to risks and dangers of GHB use
www.nida.nih.gov	National Institute on Drug Abuse
www.dea.gov	Drug Enforcement Administration
www.whitehousedrugpolicy.org	Office of National Drug Control Policy

Appendix H

ENGLISH-SPANISH DRUG PHRASE TRANSLATOR

TAKING THE MEDICATION HISTORY

- Are you allergic to any medications? (If yes:)
¿Es alérgico a algún medicamento? (sí:)
(Ehs ah-lehr-hee-koh ah ahl-goon meh-dee-kah-mehn-toh) (see:)

—Which medications are you allergic to?
¿A cuál medicamento es alérgico?
(ah koo-ahl meh-dee-kah-mehn-toh ehs ah-lehr-hee-koh)

—What happens when you develop an allergic reaction?
¿Qué le pasa cuando desarrolla una reacción alérgica?
(Keh leh pah-sah koo-ahn-doh deh-sah-roh-yah oo-nah reh-ahk-see-ohn ah-lehr-hee-kah)

—What did you do to relieve or stop the allergic reaction?
¿Qué hizo para aliviar o detener la reacción alérgica?
(Keh ee-soh pah-rah ah-lee-bee-ahr oh deh-teh-nehr lah reh-ahk-see-ohn ah-lehr-hee-kah)

- Do you take any over-the-counter, prescription, or herbal medications? (If yes:)
¿Toma medicamentos sin receta, con receta, o naturistas (hierbas medicinales)? (sí:)
(Toh-mah meh-dee-kah-mehn-tohs seen reh-seh-tah, kohn reh-seh-tah, oh nah-too-rees-tahs [ee-ehr-bahs meh-dee-see-nah-lehs]) (see:)

—Why do you take each medication?
¿Porqué toma cada medicamento?
(Pohr-keh toh-mah kah-dah meh-dee-kah-mehn-toh)

—What is the dosage for each medication?
¿Cuál es la dosis de cada medicamento?
(Koo-ahl ehs lah doh-sees deh kah-dah meh-dee-kah-mehn-toh)

—How often do you take each medication?
¿Con qué frequencia toma cada medicamento?
(Kohn keh freh-koo-ehn-see-ah toh-mah kah-dah meh-dee-kah-mehn-toh)

Once a day?	¿Una vez por día; diariamente? (Oo-nah behs pohr dee-ah; dee-ah-ree-ah-mehn-teh)
Twice a day?	¿Dos veces por día? (dohs beh-sehs pohr dee-ah)
Three times a day?	¿Tres veces por día? (Trehs beh-sehs pohr dee-ah)
Four times a day?	¿Cuatro veces por día? (Koo-ah-troh beh-sehs pohr-dee-ah)
Every other day?	¿Cada tercer día? (Kah-dah tehr-sehr dee-ah)
Once a week?	¿Una vez por semana? (Oo-nah behs pohr seh-mah-nah)

- How does each medication make you feel?
¿Como le hace sentir cada medicamento?
(Koh-moh leh ah-seh sehn-teer kah-dah meh-dee-kah-mehn-toh)

—Does the medication make you feel better?
¿Le hace sentir mejor el medicamento?
(Heh ah-seh sehn-teer meh-hohr ehl meh-dee-kah-mehn-toh)

—Does the medication make you feel the same or unchanged?
¿Le hace sentir igual o sin cambio el medicamento?
(Leh ah-seh sehn-teer ee-goo-ahl oh seen kam-bee-oh ehl meh-dee-kah-mehn-toh)

—Does the medication make you feel worse? (If yes:)
¿Se siente peor con el medicamento? (si:)
(Seh see-ehn teh peh-ohr kohn ehl meh-dee-kah-mehn-toh) (see:)

What do you do to make yourself feel better?
¿Qué hace para sentirse mejor?
(Keh ah-seh pah-rah sehn-teer-seh meh-hohr)

PREPARING FOR TREATMENT TO MEDICATION THERAPY

Medication Purpose

This medication will help relieve:
Este medicamento le ayudará a aliviar:
(Ehs-teh meh-dee-kah-mehn-toh leh ah-yoo-dah-rah ah ah-lee-bee-ahr)

English	Spanish	Pronunciation
abdominal gas	gases intestinales	(gah-sehs een-tehs-tee-nah-lehs)
abdominal pain	dolor intestinal; dolor en el abdomen	(doh-lohr een-tehs-tee-nahl; doh-lohr ehn ehl ahb-doh-mehn)
chest congestion	congestión del pecho	(kohn-hehs-tee-ohn dehl peh-choh)
chest pain	dolor del pecho	(doh-lohr dehl peh-choh)
constipation	constipación; estreñimiento	(kohns-tee-pah-see-ohn; ehs-treh-nyee-mee-ehn-toh)
cough	tos	(tohs)
headache	dolor de cabeza	(doh-lohr-deh kah-beh-sah)
muscle aches and pains	achaques musculares y dolores	(ah-chah-kehs moos-koo-lah-rehs ee doh-loh-rehs)
pain	dolor	(doh-lohr)

This medication will prevent:
Este medicamento prevendrá:
(Ehs-teh meh-dee-kah-mehn-toh preh-behn-drah)

English	Spanish	Pronunciation
blood clots	coágulos de sangre	(koh-ah-goo-lohs deh sahn-greh)
constipation	constipación; estreñimiento	(kohns-tee-pah-see-ohn; ehs-treh-nyee-mee-ehn-toh)
contraception	contracepción; embarazo	(kohn-trah-sehp-see-ohn; ehm-bah-rah-soh)
diarrhea	diarrea	(dee-ah-reh-ah)
infection	infección	(een-fehk-see-ohn)
seizures	convulciónes; ataque epiléptico	(kohn-bool-see-ohn-ehs; ah-tah-keh eh-pee-lehp-tee-koh)
shortness of breath	respiración corta; falta de aliento	(rehs-pee-rah-see-ohn kohr-tah; fahl-tah deh ah-lee-ehn-toh)
wheezing	el resollar; la respiración ruidosa, sibilante	(ehl reh-soh-yahr; lah rehs-pee-rah-see-ohn roo-ee-doh-sah, see-bee-lahn-teh)

This medication will increase your:
Este medicamento aumentará su:
(Ehs-teh meh-dee-kah-mehn-toh ah-oo-mehn-tah-rah soo:)

English	Spanish	Pronunciation
ability to fight infections	habilidad a combatir infecciones	(ah-bee-lee-dahd ah kohm-bah-teer een-fehk-see-oh-nehs)
appetite	apetito	(ah-peh-tee-toh)
blood iron levels	nivel de hierro en la sargre	(nee-behl deh ee-eh-roh ehn lah sahn-greh)
blood sugar	azúcar en la sangre	(ah-soo-kahr ehn lah sahn-greh)
heart rate	pulso; latido	(pool-soh; lah-tee-doh)
red blood cell count	cuenta de células rojas	(koo-ehn-tah deh seh-loo-lahs roh-hahs)
thyroid hormone levels	niveles de hormona tiroide	(nee-beh-lehs deh ohr-moh-nah tee-roh-ee-deh)
urine volume	volumen de orina	(boh-loo-mehn deh oh-ree-nah)

This medication will decrease your:
Este medicamento reducirá su:
(Ehs-teh meh-dee-kah-mehn-toh reh-doo-see-rah soo:)

English	Spanish	Pronunciation
anxiety	ansiedad	(ahn-see-eh-dahd)
blood choles-terol level	nivel de colesterol en la sangre	(nee-behl deh koh-lehs-teh-rohl ehn lah sahn-greh)
blood lipid level	nivel de lípido en la sangre	(nee-behl deh lee-pee-doh ehn lah sahn-greh)
blood pressure	presión arterial; de sangre	(preh-see-ohn ahr teh-ree-ahl; deh sahn-greh)
blood sugar level	nivel de azúcar en la sangre	(nee-behl deh ah-soo-kahr ehn lah sahn-greh)
heart rate	pulso; latido	(pool-soh; lah-tee-doh)
stomach acid	ácido en el estómago	(ah-see-doh ehn ehl ehs-toh-mah-goh)
thyroid hormone levels	niveles de hormona tiroide	(nee-beh-lehs deh ohr-moh-nah tee-roh-ee-deh)
weight	peso	(peh-soh)

This medication will treat:
Este medicamento sirve para:
(Ehs-teh meh-dee-kah-mehn-toh seer-beh pah-rah)

English	Spanish	Pronunciation
cancer of your ______	cancer de su ______	(kahn-sehr deh soo)
depression	depresión	(deh-preh-see-ohn)
HIV infection	infección de VIH	(een-fehk-see-ohn deh beh ee ah-cheh)
inflammation	infamación	(een-flah-mah-see-ohn)
swelling	hinchazón	(een-chah-sohn)
the infection in your ______	la infección en su ______	(lah een-fehk-see-ohn ehn soo)
your abnormal heart rhythm	su ritmo anormal de corazón	(soo reet-moh ah-nohr-mahl deh koh-rah-sohn)
your allergy to ______	su alergia a ______	(soo eh-lehr-hee-ah ah)
your rash	su erupción; sarpullido	(soo eh-roop-see-ohn; sahr-poo-yee-doh)

ADMINISTERING MEDICATION

- Swallow this medication with water or juice.
  Tragüe este medicamento con agua o jugo
  (Trah-geh ehs-teh meh dee-kah-mehn-toh kohn ah-goo-ah oh hoo-goh)

- If you cannot swallow the medication whole, I can crush it and put it in food.
  Si no puede tragar el medicamento entero puedo aplastarlo (triturarlo) y ponerlo en el alimento.
  (See noh poo-eh-deh trah-gahr ehl meh-dee-kah-mehn-toh ehn-teh-roh poo-eh-doh ah-plahs-tahr-loh [tree-too-rahr-loh] ee poh-nehr-loh ehn ehl ah lee-mehn-toh)

- I need to mix this medication with water or juice before you drink it.
  Necesito mezclar este medicamento en agua o jugo antes de que lo tome.
  (Neh-seh-see-toh mehs-klahr ehs-teh meh-dee-kah-mehn-toh ehn ah-goo-ah oh hoo-goh ahn-tehs deh keh loh toh-meh)

- Do not chew this medication. Swallow it whole.
  No mastique este medicamento. Tragüelo entero.
  (Noh mahs-tee-keh ehs-teh meh-dee-kah-mehn-toh. Trah-geh-loh ehn-teh-roh)

- Gargle with this medication and then swallow it.
  Haga gargaras con este medicamento y luego tragüelo.
  (Ah-gah gahr-gah-rahs koh ehs-teh meh-dee-kah-mehn-toh ee loo-eh-goh trah-geh-loh)

- Place this medication under your tongue and let it dissolve.
  Ponga este medicamento bajo la lengua y deje que se disuelva
  (Pohn-gah ehs-teh meh-dee-kah-mehn-toh bah-hoh lah lehn-goo-ah ee deh-heh keh seh dee-soo-ehl-bah)

- I would like to give this injection in your:
  Quiero aplicar esta injección en su:
  (Kee-eh-roh ah-plee-kahr ehs-tah een-yehk-see-ohn ehn soo:)

  —abdomen
  abdomen
  (ahb-doh-mehn)

  —arm
  brazo
  (brah-soh)

—buttocks
nalga
(nahl-gah)

—hip
cadera
(kah-deh-rah)

—thigh
muslo
(moos-loh)

- I will give you this medication through your intravenous line.
  Le daré este medicamento por el tubo de suero intravenoso.
  (Leh dah-reh ehs-teh meh-dee-kah-mehn-toh pohr ehl too-boh deh soo-eh-roh een-trah-beh-noh-soh)

- Let me know if you feel burning or pain at the intravenous site.
  Digame si siente ardor o dolor en el sitio del suero intravenoso.
  (Dee-gah-meh see see-ehn-teh ahr-dohr oh doh-lohr ehn ehl see-tee-oh dehl soo-eh-roh een-trah-beh-noh-soh)

- I need to insert this suppository into your rectum (or vagina).
  Necesito meter este supositorio en el recto (o vagina).
  (Neh-seh-see-toh meh-tehr ehs-teh soo-poh-see-toh-ree-oh ehn ehl rehk-toh [oh bah-hee-nah])

- I need to put this medication into each ear; left ear; right ear.
  Necesito poner este medicamento en cada oreja; oreja izquierda; oreja derecha.
  (Neh-seh-see-toh poh-nehr ehs-teh meh-dee-kah-mehn-toh ehn kah-dah oh-reh-hah; oh-reh-hah ees-kee-ehr-dah; -oh-reh-hah deh-reh-chah)

- I need to put this medication into each eye; left eye; right eye.
  Necesito poner este medicamento en cada ojo; ojo izquierdo; ojo derecho.
  (Neh-seh-see-toh poh-nehr ehs-teh meh-dee-kah-mehn-toh ehn kah-dah oh-hoh; oh-hoh ees-kee-ehr-doh; oh-hoh deh-reh-choh)

PREPARING FOR DISCHARGE

- The generic name for this medication is ______ .
  El nombre genérico (sin marca) de este medicamento es ______ .
  (Ehl nohn-breh heh-neh-ree-koh [seen mahr-kah] deh ehs-teh meh-dee-kah-mehn-toh ehs ______)

- The trade name for this medication is ______ .
  El nombre comercial de este medicamento es ______ .
  (Ehs nohm-breh koh-mehr-see-ahl deh ehs-teh meh-dee-kah-mehn-toh ehs ______)

- Take the medication exactly as prescribed.
  Tome el medicamento exactamente como se receta.
  (Toh-meh ehl meh-dee-kah-mehn-toh ehx-ahk-tah-mehn-teh koh-moh seh reh-seh-tah)

- You can safely break a scored tablet in half.
  Puede partir por la mitad la tableta que tiene una muesca (marca).
  (Poo-eh-deh pahr-teer pohr lah mee-tahd lah tah-bleh-tah keh tee-eh-neh oo-nah moo-ehs-kah [mahr-kah])

- Do not crush or chew enteric-coated, extended-release, or sustained-release tablets or capsules.
  No aplaste (triture) o mastique una tableta con capa entérica, de acción prolongada o de mantenimiento.
  (Noh ah-plahs-teh [tree-too-reh] oh mahs-tee-keh oo-nah tah-bleh-tah kohn-kah-pah ehn-teh-ree-kah, deh ahk-see-ohn proh-lohn-gah-dah oh deh mahn-teh-nee-mee-ehn-toh)

- If you miss a dose:
  Si pierde una dosis:
  (See pee-ehr-deh oo-nah doh-sees:)

  —take it as soon as you remember it.
  tómela tan pronto se acuerde.
  (toh-meh-lah tahn prohn-toh seh ah-koo-ehr-deh)

  —wait until the next dose.
  espere hasta la siguiente dosis.
  (ehs-peh-reh ahs-tah lah see-ghee-ehn-teh doh-sees)

  —do not double the next dose.
  No doble la siguiente dosis.
  (noh doh-bleh lah see-ghee-ehn-teh doh-sees)

  —contact your physician.
  llame a su médico.
  (yah-meh ah soo meh-dee-koh)

- Do not stop taking your medication without first speaking with your physician.
  No deje de tomar su medicamento sin hablar primero con su médico.
  (Noh deh-heh deh toh-mahr soo meh-dee-kah-ehn-toh seen ah-blahr pree-meh-roh kohn soo meh-dee-koh)

- Do not drink alcohol while taking this medication.
  No tome alcohol cuando tome este medicamento.
  (Noh toh-meh ahl-kohl koo-ahn-doh toh-meh ehs-teh meh-dee-kah-mehn-toh)

- Do not drive or operate machinery while taking this medication.
  No maneje o use maquinaria cuando toma este medicamento.
  (Noh mah-neh-heh oh oo-seh mah-kee-nah-ree-ah koo-ahn-doh toh-mah ehs-teh meh-dee-kah-mehn-toh)

- Notify your physician right away if you experience a dangerous side effect.
  Llame a su médico inmediatamente si tiene efectos secundarios peligrosos.
  (Llah-meh ah soo meh-dee-koh een-meh-dee-ah-tah-mehn-teh see tee-eh-neh eh-fehk-tohs seh-koon-dah-ree-ohs peh-lee-groh-sohs)

- Check with your physician before taking any over-the-counter medications.
  Cheque con su médico antes de tomar medicamentos sin receta.
  (Cheh-keh kohn soo meh-dee-koh ahn-tehs deh toh-mahr meh-dee-kah-mehn-tohs seen reh-seh-tah)

- Notify your physician if you are pregnant or are planning to become pregnant while taking this medication.
  Dígale a su médico si está embarazada o planea el embarazo cuando toma este medicamento.
  (Dee-gah-leh ah soo meh-dee-koh see ehs-tah ehm-bah-rah-sah-dah oh plah-neh-ah ehl ehm-bah-rah-soh koo-ahn-doh toh-mah ehs-teh meh-dee-kah-mehn-toh)

- Notify your physician if you are breast-feeding while taking this medication.
  Dígale a su médico si está amamantando (dando de pecho) cuando toma este medicamento.
  (Dee-gah-leh ah soo meh-dee-koh see ehs-tah ah-mah-mahn-tahn-doh [dahn-doh deh peh-choh] koo-ahn-doh toh-mah ehs-teh meh-dee-kah-mehn-toh)

- Refill your prescription right away, unless you don't need it anymore.
  Rellene su receta inmediatamente, a menos que no la necesite.
  (Reh-yeh-neh soo reh-seh-tah een-meh-dee-ah-tah-mehn-teh, ah meh-nohs keh noh lah neh-seh-see-teh)

PROPER MEDICATION STORAGE

- Discard expired medications because they may become dangerous or ineffective.
  Tire los medicamentos con fecha vencida (caducados) porque pueden ser peligrosos o inefectivos.
  (Tee-reh lohs meh-dee-kah-mehn-tohs kohn feh-chah behn-see-dah [kah-doo-kah-dohs] pohr-keh poo-eh-dehn sehr peh-lee-groh-sohs oh een-eh-fehk-tee-bohs)

- Keep all medications out of the reach of children at all times.
  Guarde todos los medicamentos fuera del alcance de los niños todo el tiempo.
  (Goo-ahr-deh toh-dohs lohs meh-dee-kah-mehn-tohs foo-eh-rah dehl ahl-kahn-seh deh lohs nee-nyohs toh-doh ehl tee-ehm-poh)

- Store the medication:
  Almacene (guarde) el medicamento:
  (Ahl-mah-seh-neh [goo-ahr-deh] ehl meh-dee-kah-mehn-toh:)

  —in its original container.
  en su empaque original.
  (ehn-soo ehm-pah-keh oh-ree-hee-nahl)

  —in a cool, dry place.
  en un lugar fresco y seco.
  (ehn oon loo-gahr frehs-koh ee seh-koh)

  —away from heat.
  lejos del calor.
  (leh-hohs dehl kah-lohr)

  —at room temperature.
  a temperatura ambiente.
  (ah tehm-peh-rah-too-rah ahm-bee-ehn-teh)

  —out of direct sunlight.
  fuera de la luz directa del sol.
  (foo-eh-rah deh lah loos dee-rehk-tah dehl sohl)

  —in the refrigerator.
  en el refrigerador.
  (ehn ehl reh-free-heh-rah-dohr)

Selected Drug Classes
Clasificación de Drogas Selectas (Medicamentos Selectos)
(Klah see-fee-kah-see-ohn deh droh-gahs seh-lehk-tahs [Meh-dee-kah-mehn-tohs Seh-lehk-tohs])

English	Spanish	Pronunciation
Analgesic (narcotic, nonnarcotic)	Analgésico (narcótico, no narcótico)	(Ah-nahl-heh-see-koh [nahr-koh-tee-koh, noh nahr-koh-tee-koh])
Antacid	Antiácido	(Ahn-tee-ah-see-doh)
Antianginal	Antianginoso	(Ahn-tee-ahn-hee-noh-soh)
Antianxiety	Ansiolítico	(Ahn-see-oh-lee-tee-koh)
Antiarrhythmic	Antiarritmico	(Ahn-tee-ah-reet-mee-koh)
Antibiotic	Antibiótico	(Ahn-tee-bee-oh-tee-koh)
Anticoagulant	Anticoagulante	(Ahn-tee-koh-ah-goo-lahn-teh)
Anticonvulsant	Anticonvulsivo	(Ahn-tee-kohn-bool-see-boh)
Antidepressant	Antidepresivo	(Ahn-tee-deh-preh-see-boh)
Antidiarrheal	Antidiarréicos	(Ahn-tee-dee-ah-reh-ee-kohs)
Antifungal	Antimicótico	(Ahn-tee-mee-koh-tee-koh)
Antihistamine	Antihistamínico	(Ahn-tee-ees-tah-mee-nee-koh)
Antihyperlipemic	Antihiperlipémico	(Ahn-tee-ee-pehr-lee-peh-mee-koh)
Antihypertensive	Antihipertensivo	(Ahn-tee-ee-pehr-tehn-see-boh)
Anti-inflamatory	Antiinflamatorio; Contra la inflamación	(Ahn-tee-een-flah-mah-toh-ree-oh; kohn-trah lah een-flah-mah-see-ohn)
Antimigraine	Antimigrañoso	(Ahn-tee-mee-grah-nyoh-soh)
Antiparkinsonian	Contra el Parkinson	(Kohn-trah ehl Pahr-keen-sohn)
Antipsychotic	Medicamentos sicóticos	(Meh-dee-kah-mehn-tohs see-koh-tee-kohs)
Antipyretic	Antitérmicos	(Ahn-tee-tehr-mee-kohs)
Antiseptic	Antiséptico	(Ahn-tee-sehp-tee-koh)
Antispasmodic	Antiespasmódico	(Ahn-tee-ehs-pahs-moh-dee-koh)
Antithyroid	Antitiroideos	(Ahn-tee-tee-roh-ee-deh-ohs)
Antituberculosis	Antifímicos	(Ahn-tee-fee-mee-kohs)
Antitussive	Antitusígenos	(Ahn-tee-too-see-heh-nohs)
Antiviral	Antivirales	(Ahn-tee-bee-rah-lehs)

(continued)

English	Spanish	Pronunciation
Appetite suppressant	Antisupresivos del apetito	(Ahn-tee-soo-preh-see-bohs dehl ah-peh-tee-toh)
Appetite stimulant	Estimulantes del apetito	(Ehs-tee-moo-lahn-tehs dehl ah-peh-tee-toh)
Bronchodilator	Bronquiolíticos	(Brohn-kee-oh-lee-tee-kohs)
Cancer chemotherapy	Quimioterapia de cancer	(Kee-mee-oh teh-rah-pee-ah deh kahn-sehr)
Decongestant	Anticongestivo	(Ahn-tee-kohn-hehs-tee-boh)
Digestant	Digestible	(Dee-hehs-tee-bleh)
Diuretic	Diurético	(Dee-oo-reh-tee-koh)
Emetic	Emético	(Eh-meh-tee-koh)
Fertility	Inductor de la Ovulación	(Een-doohk-tohr deh lah Oh-boo-lah-see-ohn)
Herbal	Medicamentos Naturales; Hierbas Medicinales	(Meh-dee-kah-mehn-tohs Nah-too-rah-lehs, Ee-ehr-bhas Meh-dee-see-nah-lehs)
Hypnotic	Hipnótico	(Eep-noh-tee-koh)
Insulin	Insulina	(Een-soo-lee-nah)
Laxative	Laxante	(Lahx-ahn-teh)
Mineral	Mineral	(Mee-neh-rahl)
Muscle relaxant	Relajante muscular	(Reh-lah-hahn-teh moos-koo-lahr)
Oral contraceptive	Anticonceptivos orales	(Ahn-tee-kohn-sehp-tee-bohs oh-rah-lehs)
Oral hypoglycemic	Hipoglicémico oral	(Ee-poh-glee-seh-mee-koh oh-rahl)
Sedative	Sedantes	(Seh-dahn-tehs)
Steroid	Esteroide	(Ehs-teh-roh-ee-deh)
Thyroid hormone	Tiroideos, hormona tiroide	(Tee-roh-ee-deh-ohs, ohr-moh-nah tee-roh-ee-deh)
Vaccine	Vacuna	(Bah-koo-nah)

Administration Routes
Modo de Uso
(Moh-doh deh Oo-soh)

English	Spanish	Pronunciation
By mouth	Oral	(Oh-rahl)
Intradermal	Intradermica	(Een-trah-dehr-mee-kah)
Intramuscular	Intramuscular	(Een-trah-moos-koo-lahr)

English	Spanish	Pronunciation
Intravenous	Intravenosa	(Een-trah-beh-noh-sah)
Nasal	Nasal	(Nah-sahl)
Oral	Oral	(Oh-rahl)
Otic	Ótica	(Oh-tee-kah)
Patch	Parche	(Pahr-cheh)
Rectal	Rectal	(Rehk-tahl)
Subcutaneous	Subcutanea	(Soob-koo-tah-neh-ah)
Sublingual	Sublingual	(Soob-leen-goo-ahl)
Topical	Topical, Local	(Toh-pee-kahl, Loh-kahl)
Vaginal	Vaginal	(Bah-hee-nahl)

Drug Preparations
Presentación del Medicamento
(Preh-sehn-tah-see-ohn dehl Meh-dee-kah-mehn-toh)

English	Spanish	Pronunciation
Capsule	Cápsula	(Kahp-soo-lah)
Cream	Crema	(Kreh-mah)
Drops	Gotas	(Goh-tahs)
Elixir	Elixir, Jarabe	(Eh-leex-eer, Hah-rah-beh)
Fluid	Líquido	(Lee-kee-doh)
Gel	Gel, Jalea	(Hehl, Hah-leh-ah)
Inhaler	Inhalador*	(Een-ah-lah-dohr)
Injection	Inyección	(Een-yehk-see-ohn)
Liquid	Líquido	(Lee-kee-doh)
Lotion	Loción	(Loh-see-ohn)
Lozenge	Trocisco, pastilla	(Troh-sees-koh, Pahs-tee-yah)
Ointment	Ungüento	(Oon-goo-ehn-toh)
Pill	Píldora, Pastilla	(Peel-doh-rah, Pahs-tee-yah)
Powder	Polvo	(Pohl-boh)
Spray	Spray	(Sp-rah-ee)
Suppository	Supositorio	(Soo-poh-see-toh-ree-oh)
Syrup	Jarabe	(Hah-rah-beh)
Tablet	Tableta	(Tah-bleh-tah)

*The h is silent.

Administration Frequency
Frecuencia de la Administración
(Freh-koo-ehn-see-ah deh lah Ahd-mee-nees-trah-see-ohn)

English	Spanish	Pronunciation
Once a day	Una vez por día; diariamente	(Oo-nah behs pohr dee-ah; dee-ah-ree-ah-mehn-teh)
Twice a day	Dos veces por día	(Dohs beh-sehs pohr dee-ah)
Three times a day	Tres veces por día	(Trehs beh-sehs pohr dee-ah)
Four times a day	Cuatro veces por día	(Koo-ah-troh beh-sehs pohr dee-ah)
Every other day	Cada tercer día	(Kah-dah tehr-sehr dee-ah)
Once a week	Una vez por semana	(Oo-nah behs pohr seh-mah-nah)
Every 4 hours	Cada cuatro horas	(Kah-dah koo-ah-troh oh-rahs)
Every 6 hours	Cada seis horas	(Kah-dah seh-ees oh-rahs)
Every 8 hours	Cada ocho horas	(Kah-dah oh-choh oh-rahs)
Every 12 hours	Cada doce horas	(Kah-dah doh-seh oh-rahs)
In the morning	En la mañana	(Ehn lah mah-nyah-nah)
In the afternoon	En la tarde	(Ehn lah tahr-deh)
In the evening	En la noche	(Ehn lah noh-cheh)
Before bedtime	Antes de acostarse	(Ahn-tehs deh ah-kohs-tahr-seh)
Before meals	Antes de la comida; Antes del alimento	(Ahn-tehs deh lah koh-mee-dah; Ahn-tehs dehl ah-lee-mehn-toh)
With meals	Con los alimentos; Con la comida	(Kohn lohs ah-lee-mehn-tohs; Kohn lah koh-mee-dah)
After meals	Después de los alimentos; Después de la comida	(Dehs-poo-ehs deh lohs ah-lee-mehn-tohs; Dehs-poo-ehs deh lah koh-mee-dah)
Only when you need it	Solo cuando la necesite	(Soh-loh koo-ahn-doh lah neh-seh-see-teh)
When you have _______ (pain)	Cuando tiene _______ (dolor)	(Koo-ahn-doh tee-eh-neh _______) (doh-lohr)

50 Common Side Effects
Cincuenta Efectos Secundarios Comúnes
(Seen-koo-ehn-tah Eh-fehk-tohs Seh-koon-dah-ree-ohs Koh-moo-nehs)

English	Spanish	Pronunciation
Abdominal cramps	Retorcijón abdominal	(Reh-tohr-see-hohn ahb-doh-mee-nahl)
Abdominal pain	Dolor abdominal	(Doh-lohr ahb-doh-mee-nahl)
Abdominal swelling	Inflamación abdominal	(Een-flah-mah-see-ohn ahb-doh-mee-nahl)
Anxiety	Ansiedad	(Ahn-see-eh-dahd)
Blood in the stool	Sangre en el excremento	(Sahn-greh ehn ehl ehx-kreh-mehn-toh)
Blood in the urine	Sangre en la orina	(Sahn-greh ehn la oh-ree-nah)
Bone pain	Dolor de hueso*	(Doh-lohr deh oo-eh-soh)
Chest pain	Dolor de pecho	(Doh-lohr deh peh-choh)
Chest pounding	Palpitación; latidos fuertes en el pecho	(Pahl-pee-tah-see-ohn; lah-tee-dohs foo-ehr-tehs ehn ehl peh-choh)
Chills	Escalofrío	(Ehs-kah-loh-free-oh)
Confusion	Confusión	(Kohn-foo-see-ohn)
Constipation	Constipación, estreñimiento	(Kohns-tee-pah-see-ohn, ehs-treh-nyee-mee-ehn-toh)
Cough	Tos	(Tohs)
Mental depression	Depresión mental	(Deh-preh-see-ohn mehn-tahl)
Diarrhea	Diarrea	(Dee-ah-reh-ah)
Difficult urination	Dificultad al orinar	(Dee-fee-kool-tahd ahl oh-ree-nahr)
Difficulty breathing	Dificultad al respirar	(Dee-fee-kool-tahd ahl rehs-pee-rahr)
Difficulty sleeping	Dificultad al dormir	(Dee-fee-kool-tahd ahl dohr-meer)
Dizziness	Mareos; vahídos	(Mah-reh-ohs; bah-ee-dohs)
Dry mouth	Boca seca	(Boh-kah seh-kah)
Easy bruising	Fragilidad capilar; le salen moretones con facilidad	(Frah-hee-lee-dahd kah-pee-lahr; leh sah-lehn moh-reh-toh-nehs kohn fah-see-lee-dahd)
Faintness	Desvanecimiento; sintió un vahído	(Dehs-bah-neh-see-mee-ehn-toh; seen-tee-oh oon bah-ee-doh)
Fatigue	Fatiga, cansancio	(Fah-tee-gah, kahn-sahn-see-oh)

(continued)

English	Spanish	Pronunciation
Fever	Fiebre	(Fee-eh-breh)
Frequent urination	Orina frecuente	(Oh-ree-nah freh-koo-ehn-teh)
Headache	Dolor de cabeza	(Doh-lohr deh kah-beh-sah)
Impotence	Impotencia	(Eem-poh-tehn-see-ah)
Increased appetite	Aumento en el apetito	(Ah-oo-mehn-toh ehn ehl ah-peh-tee-toh)
Increased gas	Flatulencia	(Flah-too-lehn-see-ah)
Increased perspiration	Aumento en el sudor	(Ah-oo-mehn-toh ehn ehl soo-dohr)
Indigestion	Indigestión	(Een-dee-hehs-tee-ohn)
Itching	Comezón	(Koh-meh-sohn)
Loss of appetite	Pérdida en el apetito	(Pehr-dee-dah ehn ehl ah-peh-tee-toh)
Menstrual changes	Cambios en la menstruación; Cambio en el ciclo menstrual	(Kahm-bee-ohs ehn la mehns-truh-ah-see-ohn; Kahm-bee-oh ehn ehl see-kloh mehns-truh-ahl)
Mood changes	Cambio en el humor; Cambio en la disposición	(Kahm-bee-oh ehn ehl oo-mohr, Kahm-bee-oh ehn lah dees-poh-see-see-ohn)
Muscle pain	Dolores musculares	(Doh-loh-rehs moos-koo-lah-rehs)
Muscle aches	Achaques musculares	(Ah-chah-kehs moos-koo-lah-rehs)
Muscle cramps	Calambre muscular	(Kah-lahm-breh moos-koo-lahr)
Nasal congestion	Congestión nasal	(Kohn-hehs-tee-ohn nah-sahl)
Nausea	Nausea	(Nah-oo-seh-ah)
Ringing in the ears	Zumbido en los oidos	(Soom-bee-doh ehn lohs oh-ee-dohs)
Skin rash	Erupción en la piel	(Eh-roop-see-ohn ehn lah pee-ehl)
Swelling on the hands, legs or feet	Hinchazón en las manos, piernas, o pies	(Een-chah-sohn ehn lahs mah-nohs, pee-ehr-nahs, oh pee-ehs)
Vaginal bleeding	Sangrado vaginal	(Sahn-grah-doh bah-hee-nahl)
Vision changes	Cambios en la visión; cambios en la vista	(Kahm-bee-ohs ehn lah bee-see-ohn; cahm-bee-ohs ehn lah bees-tah)
Vomiting	Vomitando	(Boh-mee-tahn-doh)

English	Spanish	Pronunciation
Weakness	Debilidad	(Deh-bee-lee-dahd)
Weight gain	Aumento de peso	(Ah-oo-mehn-toh deh peh-soh)
Weight loss	Pérdida de peso	(Pehr-dee-day deh peh-soh)
Wheezing	Resollar; respiración sibilante	(Reh-soh-yahr; rehs-pee-rah-see-ohn see-bee-lahn-teh)

*The h is silent.

Appendix I

ENTERAL AND PARENTERAL NUTRITION

INDICATIONS: ENTERAL NUTRITION

Enteral nutrition (EN), also known as *tube feedings,* provides food and nutrients via the gastrointestinal (GI) tract, using special formulas, delivery techniques, and equipment. All EN routes consist of a tube through which liquid formula is infused.

Tube feedings are used in patients with major trauma or burns; those undergoing radiation or chemotherapy; and those with liver failure, severe renal impairment, or physical or neurologic impairment. They're also used preoperatively and postoperatively to promote anabolism. In addition, they're used to prevent cachexia and malnutrition.

ROUTES OF ENTERAL NUTRITION DELIVERY

NASOGASTRIC (NG):

INDICATIONS: This route is most common for short-term feeding in patients who can't or won't consume adequate nutrition by mouth. It requires at least a partially functioning GI tract. **ADVANTAGES:** NG tube placement doesn't require surgery, and the tube is fairly easily inserted. It allows full use of the digestive tract. It decreases the risk that hyperosmolar solutions may cause distention, nausea, and vomiting. **DISADVANTAGES:** This route is temporary, and the NG tube may be easily pulled out during routine nursing care. The patient is at risk for pulmonary aspiration of gastric contents, reflux esophagitis, and regurgitation.

NASODUODENAL (ND), NASOJEJUNAL (NJ):

INDICATIONS: These routes may be used in patients who can't or won't consume adequate nutrition by mouth. They require at least a partially functioning GI tract. **ADVANTAGES:** These tubes don't require surgical placement, are fairly easily inserted, and are preferred for patients at risk of aspiration. They're valuable for patients with gastroparesis. **DISADVANTAGES:** These routes are temporary. ND or NJ tubes may be pulled out during routine nursing care and may be dislodged by coughing or vomiting. Their small lumens increase the risk of clogging when drugs are given through them, and make them more susceptible to rupture when an infusion device is used. These tubes require x-rays for confirmation of placement and are frequently extubated.

GASTROSTOMY:

INDICATIONS: This route is used in patients with esophageal obstruction or impaired swallowing; those in whom the NG, ND, and NJ routes aren't feasible; and those who need long-term feeding. **ADVANTAGES:** Gastrostomy provides permanent feeding access. The tubing has a larger bore, allowing noncontinuous (bolus) feeding (300 to 400 ml over 30 to 60 min q 3 to 6 hr). It may be inserted endoscopically using local anesthetic (in a procedure called *percutaneous endoscopic gastrostomy* [PEG]). **DISADVANTAGES:** This route requires surgical placement, although the tubing may be inserted during other surgery or endoscopically (see **ADVANTAGES**). The tube may be inadvertently dislodged. Gastrostomy requires stoma care and increases the risk of aspiration, peritonitis, cellulitis, and leakage of gastric contents.

Jejunostomy:
INDICATIONS: This route is used for patients with stomach or duodenal obstruction or impaired gastric motility; those in whom the NG, ND, and NJ routes aren't feasible; and those who need long-term feeding. **ADVANTAGES:** Jejunostomy allows early postoperative feeding because small bowel function is least affected by surgery. It reduces the risk of aspiration, and its tubing is rarely pulled out inadvertently. **DISADVANTAGES:** This route requires surgical placement (laparotomy) and stoma care. It poses a risk of intraperitoneal leakage, and its tubing can be dislodged easily.

INTIATING ENTERAL NUTRITION

With continuous feeding, expect to begin feedings of isotonic (about 300 mOsm/L) or moderately hypertonic (up to 495 mOsm/L) formula at full strength, usually at a slow rate (30 to 50 ml/hr), and gradually increase it (25 ml/hr q 6 to 24 hr). Start formulas with an osmolality above 500 mOsm/L at half strength and gradually increase the rate and then the concentration. Tolerance increases when the rate and concentration aren't increased simultaneously.

SELECTION OF ENTERAL FORMULAS

Protein has many important physiologic roles and is the primary source of nitrogen in the body. It provides 4 kcal/g of protein. Sources of protein in enteral feedings include sodium caseinate, calcium caseinate, soy protein, and dipeptides.

Carbohydrate (CHO) provides energy for the body and heat to maintain the body temperature. It provides 3.4 kcal/g of carbohydrate. Sources of carbohydrate in enteral feedings include corn syrup, cornstarch, maltodextrin, lactose, sucrose, and glucose.

Fat provides a concentrated source of energy, referred to as *kilocalorie dense or protein sparing.* It provides 9 kcal/g of fat. Sources of fat in enteral feedings include corn oil, safflower oil, and medium chain triglycerides.

Electrolytes, vitamins, and trace elements are contained in formulas, but not in specialized products for patients with renal or hepatic insufficiency. All products containing protein, fat, carbohydrate, vitamins, electrolytes, and trace elements are nutritionally complete and designed to be used by patients for long periods.

COMPLICATIONS OF ENTERAL NUTRITION

MECHANICAL: These complications usually relate to some aspect of the feeding tube.

Aspiration pneumonia can result from delayed gastric emptying, gastroparesis, gastroesophageal reflux, or decreased gag reflex. To prevent or treat it, reduce the infusion rate, use lower fat formulas, feed beyond the pylorus, check residuals, use small-bore feeding tubes, elevate the head of the bed 30° to 45° during and for 30 to 60 minutes after each intermittent feeding, and regularly check tube placement.

Esophageal, mucosal, and pharyngeal irritation and otitis are caused by using a large-bore NG tube. To prevent these problems, use small-bore tubing whenever possible.

Irritation and leakage at the ostomy site can stem from digestive juice drainage from the site. To prevent them, provide frequent skin and stoma care.

Tube or lumen obstruction is caused by thickened formula residue and formation of formula-medication complexes. To prevent this, frequently irrigate the tube with clear water (also before and after giving formulas and medications) and avoid medication instillation if possible.

GASTROINTESTINAL: These complications usually relate to the formula, the delivery rate, or unsanitary handling of solutions or the delivery system.

Diarrhea may result from low-residue formulas, rapid delivery, hyperosmolar formulas, hypoalbuminemia, malabsorption, microbial contamination, or rapid GI transit time. To prevent it, use fiber-supplemented formulas, decrease the delivery rate, use dilute formula, and gradually increase its strength.

Cramping, gas, and abdominal distention are caused by nutrient malabsorption or rapid delivery of refrigerated formula. To prevent them, deliver formula by a continuous method, give formulas at room temperature, and decrease the delivery rate.

Nausea and vomiting can result from rapid delivery of formula and gastric retention. To prevent them, reduce the delivery rate, use dilute formulas, and select low-fat formulas.

Constipation is caused by inadequate fluid intake, reduced bulk, and inactivity. To prevent it, supplement the patient's fluid intake, use fiber-supplemented formula, and encourage ambulation.

METABOLIC: These complications require fluid and electrolyte monitoring. (See Monitoring of Enteral Nutrition section.) Very young and very old patients have a greater risk of developing such complications as dehydration or overhydration.

MONITORING OF ENTERAL NUTRITION

Daily: Estimate the patient's nutrient intake. Measure the patient's fluid intake and output and body weight and carefully monitor the patient's general health status.

Weekly: Evaluate the levels of serum electrolytes (potassium, sodium, magnesium, calcium, and phosphorus), blood glucose, blood urea nitrogen

(BUN), creatinine, liver enzymes (such as SGOT [AST] and alkaline phosphatase), 24-hr urea and creatinine excretion, total iron-binding capacity (TIBC) or serum transferrin, triglycerides, and cholesterol.

Monthly: Check the serum albumin level.

Other: Assess the urine glucose and acetone levels (when the blood glucose exceeds 250 mg/dl). Check vital signs (temperature, respirations, pulse, and blood pressure) every 8 hours.

ENTERAL NUTRITION DOSAGE FORM SELECTION AND ADMINISTRATION

Drug therapy should not have to be compromised in patients receiving enteral nutrition.

- Temporarily discontinue medications not immediately necessary.
- Consider an alternate route for administering medications (e.g., transdermal, rectal, intravenous).
- Consider alternate medications when the current medication is not available in alternate dosage forms.

Enteral Administration of Medications

Medications may be given via feeding tube with several considerations:

- Tube type
- Tube location in the GI tract
- Site of drug action
- Site of drug absorption
- Effects of food on drug absorption
- Use of liquid dosage forms is preferred whenever possible, many tablets may be crushed, and the contents of many capsules may be emptied and given through large-bore feeding tubes.
- Many oral products should not be crushed (e.g., sustained release, enteric coated)
- Some medications should not be given with enteral formulas because they form precipitates which may clog the feeding tube and reduce drug absorption.
- The feeding tube should be flushed with water before and after administration of medications to clear any residual medication.

INDICATIONS: PARENTERAL NUTRITION

Parenteral nutrition (PN), also known as *total parenteral nutrition* (TPN) or *hyperalimentation* (HAL), provides required nutrients to patients by the IV route of administration. The goal of PN is to maintain or restore nutritional balance, which may be upset by disease, injury, or inability to consume nutrients by other means.

PN is used in patients with conditions that preclude use of the alimentary tract by the oral, gastrostomy, or jejunostomy routes. Such conditions include impaired protein absorption due to obstruction, inflammation, or antineoplastic therapy; bowel rest after GI surgery or ileus, fistulas, or anastomotic leaks;

and conditions with increased metabolic requirements, such as burns, infection, and trauma. PN also is used to preserve tissue reserves (as in acute renal failure) and to provide adequate nutrition when tube-feeding methods can't.

COMPONENTS OF PARENTERAL NUTRITION

To meet IV nutritional requirements, PN needs six essential components for tissue synthesis and energy balance.

Protein takes the form of crystalline amino acids (CAA), which are primarily used for protein synthesis. Several products are designed to meet specific needs for patients with renal failure (such as NephrAmine), liver disease (such as HepatAmine), or stress and trauma (such as Aminosyn HBC) and for use in neonates and children (such as Aminosyn PF and TrophAmine). PN provides 4 kcal/g of protein.

Energy takes the form of dextrose, which is available in concentrations of 5% to 70%. Dextrose concentrations below 10% may be given peripherally; those above 10% must be given centrally. PN provides 3.4 kcal/g of dextrose.

IV fat emulsion comes in 10% or 20% concentrations and provides a concentrated source of energy (9 kcal/g of fat). It's also a source of essential fatty acids. It may be administered peripherally or centrally.

Electrolytes include calcium, magnesium, potassium, sodium, acetate, chloride, and phosphate. Electrolyte doses must be individualized, based on many factors, such as kidney function, liver function, and fluid status.

Vitamins are essential for maintaining metabolism and cellular function. They're widely used in PN.

Trace elements are needed in long-term PN. Trace elements include zinc, copper, chromium, manganese, selenium, molybdenum, and iodine.

Miscellaneous additives include insulin, albumin, heparin, and histamine$_2$ blockers, such as cimetidine, ranitidine, and famotidine. Other medications may be added on an individual basis, but admixture compatibility should be checked first.

ROUTES OF PARENTERAL NUTRITION DELIVERY

PN is administered by a peripheral or central vein.

Peripheral administration usually involves 2 to 3 L/day of 5% to 10% dextrose with 3% to 5% amino acid solution along with IV fat emulsion. Electrolytes, vitamins, and trace elements are added based on the patient's needs. Peripheral solutions provide about 2,000 kcal/day and 60 to 90 g protein/day. **ADVANTAGES:** Peripheral administration poses lower risks than central administration. **DISADVANTAGES:** Peripheral veins may not be suitable (especially in patients with long-term illness); may be more susceptible to phlebitis (because osmolality exceeds 600 mOsm/L); and may be viable for only 1 to 2 weeks. Also, large volumes of fluid are needed to meet nutritional requirements, which may be contraindicated in many patients.

Central administration usually uses hypertonic dextrose (in a concentration of 15% to 35%) and amino acid solution of 3% to 7% with IV fat emulsion. Electrolytes, vitamins, and trace elements are added based on patient needs. Central solutions provide 2,000 to 4,000 kcal/day. They must be given through a large central vein with high blood flow, allowing rapid dilution and avoiding phlebitis and thrombosis. Usually, a catheter is inserted percutaneously into the subclavian vein and then advanced to the superior vena cava. **ADVANTAGES:** Central administration allows more alternatives and flexibility in regimens and a greater ability to meet full nutritional requirements without the need for daily fat emulsion. It's useful in patients with fluid restrictions (because of increased solution concentration), in those with large nutritional requirements (such as from trauma or malignancy), and those for whom PN is indicated for more than 7 to 10 days. **DISADVANTAGES:** The insertion, use, and maintenance of a central line increase the risk of infection, catheter-induced trauma, and metabolic changes.

COMPLICATIONS OF PARENTERAL NUTRITION

MECHANICAL: Malfunction of the IV delivery system may include pump failure and problems with lines, tubing, administration sets, and catheters. Catheter placement may cause pneumothorax, catheter misdirection, arterial puncture, bleeding, and hematoma formation.

INFECTIOUS: Infections can occur because these patients are typically more susceptible to infection. Catheter sepsis can occur when no other site of infection is identified; it may cause fever, shaking chills, and glucose intolerance.

METABOLIC: These complications include hyperglycemia, elevated cholesterol and triglyceride levels, and abnormal liver function test results. They may also include altered potassium, sodium, phosphate, and magnesium levels and, therefore, require fluid and electrolyte monitoring.

NUTRITIONAL: Clinical effects may results from lack of adequate vitamins, trace elements, and essential fatty acids.

MONITORING OF PARENTERAL NUTRITION

Monitoring requirements may vary slightly among institutions.

Baseline: Document the CBC; blood platelet count; prothrombin time; body weight; body length and head circumference (in infants); levels of serum electrolytes, glucose, BUN, creatinine, uric acid, total protein, cholesterol, triglycerides, bilirubin, alkaline phosphatase, LDH, SGOT (AST), and albumin; and other test results as appropriate.

Daily: Measure the patient's body weight, vital signs (TPR), and nutritional intake (kcal, protein, fat). Check the levels of serum electrolytes (potassium, sodium, and chloride), glucose (serum, urine), acetone, and BUN. Evaluate osmolarity and the results of other tests as needed.

2 to 3 times/week: Record the CBC, acid-base status, results of coagulation studies (PT, PTT) and other tests, and levels of serum creatinine, calcium, magnesium, and phosphorus as needed.

Weekly: Evaluate the nitrogen balance; levels of total protein, albumin, prealbumin, transferrin, liver enzymes (SGOT [AST], SGPT [ALT]), alkaline phosphatase, LDH), bilirubin, hemoglobin, uric acid, cholesterol, and triglycerides; and results of other tests as needed.

PARENTERAL NUTRITION DOSAGE FORM SELECTION AND ADMINISTRATION

The compatibility of other intravenous medications patients may be administered while receiving parenteral nutrition is an important concern. Intravenous medications are usually given as a separate admixture via piggyback to the parenteral nutrition line, but in some instances they may be added directly to the parenteral nutrition solution. Because of the possibility of incompatibility when adding medication directly to the parenteral nutrition solution, specific criteria should be considered:

- Stability of the medication in the parenteral nutrition solution.
- Properties of the medication, including pharmacokinetics, which determines if the medication is appropriate for continuous infusion.
- Documented chemical and physical compatibility with the parenteral nutrition solution.

In addition, when medication is given via piggyback using the parenteral nutrition line, important criteria should include:

- Stability of the medication in the parenteral nutrition solution.
- Documented chemical and physical compatibility with the parenteral nutrition solution.

Appendix J

EQUI-ANALGESIC DOSING

Guidelines for equi-analgesic dosing of commonly used analgesics are presented in the following table. The dosages are equivalent to 10 mg of morphine intramuscularly. These guidelines are for the management of acute pain in the opioid naïve patient. Dosages may vary for the opioid tolerant patient and for the management of chronic pain. Clinical response is the criteria that must be applied for each patient with titration to desired response.

Name	Equi-analgesic Oral Dose	Equi-analgesic Parenteral Dose
Codeine	130 mg q3–4h	75 mg q3–4h
Morphine	30 mg q3–4h	10 mg q3–4h
Hydromorphone (Dilaudid)	7.5 mg q3–4h	1.5 mg q3–4h
Hydrocodone	5–10 mg q3–4h	Not available
Meperidine (Demerol)	300 mg q2–3h	75–100 mg q3h
Methadone (Dolophine)	10–20 mg q6–8h	10 mg q6–8h
Oxycodone (OxyContin)	20–30 mg q3–4h	Not available
Propoxyphene (Darvon)	65–130 mg q4–6h	Not available
Butorphanol (Stadol)	Not available	2 mg q3–4h
Nalbuphine (Nubain)	Not available	10 mg q3–4h

Appendix K

EYE AND TOPICAL AGENTS

ANTIGLAUCOMA AGENTS

USES	ACTION
Antiglaucoma agents are used to reduce elevated intraocular pressure (IOP) in patients with open-angle glaucoma and ocular hypertension.	Some antiglaucoma agents decrease IOP by increasing the outflow of aqueous humor: *Miotics (direct acting)* are cholinergic agents or miotics. They stimulate ciliary muscles, leading to increased contraction of the iris sphincter muscle. *Miotics (indirect acting)* primarily inhibit cholinesterase, allowing acetylcholine to accumulate, which prolongs parasympathetic activity. *Sympathomimetics* increase the rate of fluid flow out of the eyes and decrease the rate of aqueous humor production. Other antiglaucoma agents decrease IOP by decreasing aqueous humor production: *Alpha$_2$ agonists* activate receptors in the ciliary body, inhibiting aqueous secretion and increasing uveoscleral aqueous outflow. *Beta-blockers* reduce the production of aqueous humor. *Carbonic anhydrase inhibitors* reduce fluid flow into the eyes by inhibiting the enzyme carbonic anhydrase. *Prostaglandins* increase the outflow of aqueous fluid by the uveoscleral route.

Name	Availability	Dosage Range	Side Effects
Miotics			
Carbachol (Isopto-Carbachol)	**S:** 0.75%, 1.5%, 2.25%, 3%	1 drop 2 times/day	Ciliary or accommodative spasm, blurred vision, reduced night vision, diaphoresis, increased salivation, urinary frequency, nausea, diarrhea

Echothiophate (Phospholine Iodide)	**S**: 0.03%, 0.06%, 0.125%, 0.25%	1 drop 2 times/day	Headaches, accommodative spasm, diaphoresis, vomiting, nausea, diarrhea, tachycardia
Pilocarpine (Isopto Carpine)	**S**: 0.25%, 0.5%, 1%, 2%, 3%, 4%, 5%, 6%, 8%, 10%	1–2 drops 3–4 times/day	Same as carbachol
Physostigmine (Eserine)	**O**: 0.25%	Apply up to 3 times/day	Blurred vision, eye pain
Sympathomimetics			
Dipivefrin (Propine)	**S**: 0.1%	1 drop q12h	Ocular congestion, burning, stinging
Epinephrine (Epifrin, Epinal)	**S**: 0.5%, 1%, 2%	1 drop 1–2 times/day	Mydriasis, blurred vision, tachycardia, hypertension, tremors, headaches, anxiety
Alpha Agonists			
Apraclonidine (Iopidine)	**S**: 0.5%	1–2 drops 3 times/day	Hypersensitivity reaction, change in visual acuity, lethargy
Brimonidine (Alphagan)	**S**: 0.2%	1–2 drops 2–3 times/day	Headaches, hypersensitivity reaction, drowsiness, fatigue
Prostaglandins			
Bimatoprost (Lumigan)	**S**: 0.03%	1 drop daily in evening	Ocular hyperemia, eyelash growth, pruritus
Latanoprost (Xalatan)	**S**: 0.005%	1 drop daily in evening	Burning, stinging, iris pigmentation
Travoprost (Travatan)	**S**: 0.004%	1 drop daily in evening	Ocular hyperemia, eye discomfort, foreign body sensation, pain, pruritus
Unoprostone (Rescula)	**S**: 0.15%	1 drop 2 times/day	Iris pigmentation

(continued)

EYE AND TOPICAL AGENTS—cont'd

ANTIGLAUCOMA AGENTS—cont'd

Name	Availability	Dosage Range	Side Effects
Beta-Blockers			
Betaxolol (Betoptic)	**Suspension:** 0.25% **S:** 0.5%	1–2 drops 1–2 times/day	Transient irritation, burning, tearing, blurred vision
Carteolol (Ocupress)	**S:** 1%	1 drop 2 times/day	Mild, transient ocular stinging, burning, discomfort
Levobetaxolol (Betaxon)	**S:** 0.5%	1 drop 2 times/day	Transient irritation, burning, tearing, blurred vision
Levobunolol (Betagan)	**S:** 0.25%, 0.5%	1 drop 1–2 times/day	Local discomfort, conjunctivitis, brow ache, tearing, blurred vision, headache, anxiety
Metipranolol (OptiPranolol)	**S:** 0.3%	1 drop 2 times/day	Transient irritation, burning, stinging, blurred vision
Timolol (Istalol, Timoptic)	**S:** 0.25%, 0.5% **G:** 0.25%, 0.5%	**S:** 1 drop 2 times/day (Istalol): 1 drop daily. **G:** 1 drop daily	Same as betaxolol
Carbonic Anhydrase Inhibitors			
Acetazolamide (Diamox)	**T:** 125 mg, 250 mg **C:** 500 mg	0.25–1 g/day	Diarrhea, loss of appetite, metallic taste, nausea, tingling in hands and fingers
Brinzolamide (Azopt)	**Suspension:** 1%	1 drop 3 times/day	Blurred vision, bitter taste
Dorzolamide (Trusopt)	**S:** 2%	1 drop 2–3 times/day	Burning, stinging, blurred vision, bitter taste

C, Capsules; ***G,*** gel; ***O,*** ointment; ***S,*** solution; ***T,*** tablets.

MISCELLANEOUS OPHTHALMIC AGENTS

USES	ACTION
Miscellaneous ophthalmic agents are used to prevent and treat mild ophthalmic disorders, such as allergic conjunctivitis, keratitis, and dry eyes.	Miscellaneous ophthalmic agents act in various ways. For example, *hydroxypropyl methylcellulose* stabilizes and thickens precorneal tear film, protecting and lubricating the eyes. *Azelastine, emedastine,* and *levocabastine* antagonize histamine (H_1)-receptors, thus inhibiting histamine-stimulated responses in the conjunctiva, such as redness and itching. By stabilizing mast cells, *lodoxamide* prevents antigen-stimulated release of histamine, which inhibits Type 1 hypersensitivity reactions. A broad-spectrum anti-infective, *sulfacetamide* interferes with the synthesis of folic acid that bacteria require for growth. *Vidarabine* blocks deoxyribonucleic acid (DNA) polymerase, blocking viral DNA synthesis.

Name	Indications	Dosages	Side Effects
Azelastine (Optivar)	Relief of itching eyes caused by allergic conjunctivitis	1 drop 2 times/day	Transient eye burning or stinging, headache, bitter taste, eye pain, fatigue, flulike symptoms, pharyngitis, rhinitis, blurred vision
Emedastine (Emadine)	Treatment of signs and symptoms of allergic conjunctivitis	1–2 drops 2 times/day	Headache, bad taste, blurred vision, eye burning or stinging, dry eyes, tearing
Epinastine (Elestat)	Treatment of allergic conjunctivitis	1 drop 4 times/day	Headache, taste disturbance, drowsiness, blurred vision, eye burning or stinging, dry eyes, foreign body sensation, rhinitis

(continued)

EYE AND TOPICAL AGENTS—cont'd

MISCELLANEOUS OPHTHALMIC AGENTS—cont'd

Name	Indications	Dosages	Side Effects
Hydroxypropyl methylcellulose (Artificial Tears, Isopto Tears, Tears Naturale)	Relief of eye dryness and irritation caused by insufficient tear production	1–2 drops 3–4 times/day	Eye irritation, blurred vision, eyelash stickiness
Ketotifen (Zaditor)	Temporary relief of itching eyes caused by allergic conjunctivitis	1 drop every 8–12 hours	Conjunctival infection, headache, rhinitis, eye burning or stinging, ocular discharge, eye pain
Levocabastine (Livostin)	Treatment of signs and symptoms of seasonal allergic conjunctivitis	1 drop 4 times/day	Transient eye stinging, burning, or discomfort; headache; dry eyes; eyelid edema
Lodoxamide (Alomide)	Treatment of vernal keratoconjunctivitis and keratitis	1 drop 4 times/day	Transient eye stinging or burning, instillation discomfort, itching eyes, blurred vision, dry eyes, tearing, headache
Olopatadine (Patanol)	Treatment of signs and symptoms of allergic conjunctivitis	1–2 drops 2 times/day	Headache, drowsiness, eye burning or stinging, foreign body sensation, pharyngitis, rhinitis, pruritus

Pagaptanib (Macugen)	Treatment of neovascular (wet) age-related macular degeneration	For ophthalmic intravitreal injection only. 0.3 mg once every 6 weeks	Blepharitis, conjunctivitis, photopsia, bronchitis, headache, dizziness, nausea
Pemirolast (Alamast)	Prevention of itching eyes caused by allergic conjunctivitis	1–2 drops 3–4 times/day	Transient eye stinging or burning, instillation discomfort, itching eyes, blurred vision, tearing, headache
Sulfacetamide (Sulf-10)	Treatment of corneal ulcers, bacterial conjunctivitis, other superficial eye infections; prevention of infection after eye injury	1–3 drops every 2–3 hours; or 1.25- to 2.5-cm strip of ointment 4 times/day and at bedtime	Transient eye burning or stinging, headache, rash, itching eyes, eye swelling, photosensitivity
Vidarabine (Ara-A)	Treatment of keratitis or keratoconjunctivitis caused by herpes simplex virus, type 1 or 2	½″ 5 times/day at 3-hour intervals; after re-epithelialization, ½″ 2 times/day for 7 days	Eye burning or irritation, itching eyes, tearing, eye pain, photophobia

(continued)

EYE AND TOPICAL AGENTS—cont'd

TOPICAL ANTI-INFLAMMATORY AGENTS

USES	ACTION
Topical anti-inflammatory agents relieve inflammation and pruritus caused by corticosteroid-responsive disorders, such as contact dermatitis, eczema, insect bite reactions, first- and second-degree localized burns, and sunburn.	Topical anti-inflammatory agents diffuse across cell membranes and form complexes with cytoplasm. These complexes stimulate the synthesis of inhibitory enzymes that are responsible for the agents' anti-inflammatory effects, which include inhibition of edema, erythema, pruritus, capillary dilation, and phagocyte activity. Topical corticosteroids can be classified based on potency: *Low potency agents* provide modest anti-inflammatory effects. They're safest for long-term application, facial and intertriginous application, use with occlusive dressings, and for infants and young children. *Medium potency agents* are active against moderate inflammatory conditions, such as chronic eczematous dermatoses. They may be used for facial and intertriginous application for a limited time only. *High potency agents* are effective in more severe inflammatory conditions, such as lichen simplex chronicus and psoriasis. They may be used for facial and intertriginous application for a short time only and can be used on skin thickened by chronic conditions. *Very high potency agents* offer an alternative to systemic therapy for local effects, such as with chronic lesions caused by psoriasis. Because they pose an increased risk of skin atrophy, they should be used only for short periods on small areas without occlusive dressings.

TOPICAL CORTICOSTEROIDS

Name	Availability	Potency	Side Effects
Alclometasone (Aclovate)	**C, O:** 0.05%	Low	Skin atrophy, contact dermatitis, stretch marks on skin, enlarged blood vessels in the

			skin, hair loss, pigment changes, secondary infections
Amcinonide (Cyclocort)	**C, O, L:** 0.1%	High	Same as above
Betamethasone dipropionate (Diprosone)	**C, O, G, L:** 0.05%	High	Same as above
Betamethasone valerate (Valisone)	**C:** 0.01%, 0.05%, 0.1% **O:** 0.1% **L:** 0.1%	High	Same as above
Clobetasol (Temovate)	**C, O:** 0.05%	High	Same as above
Desonide (Tridesilon)	**C, O, L:** 0.05%	Low	Same as above
Desoximetasone (Topicort)	**C:** 0.25%, 0.5% **O:** 0.25% **G:** 0.05%	High	Same as above
Dexamethasone (Decadron)	**C:** 0.1%	Medium	Same as above
Fluocinolone (Synalar)	**C:** 0.01%, 0.025%, 0.2% **O:** 0.025%	High	Same as above
Fluocinonide (Lidex)	**C, O, G:** 0.05%	High	Same as above
Fluticasone (Cutivate)	**C:** 0.05% **O:** 0.005%	Medium	Same as above
Halobetasol (Ultravate)	**C, O:** 0.05%	High	Same as above
Hydrocortisone (Cort-Dome, Hytone)	**C, O:** 0.5%, 1%, 2.5%	Medium	Same as above
Mometasone (Elocon)	**C, O, L:** 0.1%	Medium	Same as above
Prednicarbate (Dermatop)	**C:** 0.1%	—	Same as above
Triamcinolone (Aristocort, Kenalog)	**C, O, L:** 0.025%, 0.1%, 0.5%	Medium	Same as above

C, Cream; ***G,*** gel; ***L,*** lotion; ***O,*** ointment.

(continued)

EYE AND TOPICAL AGENTS—cont'd

MISCELLANEOUS TOPICAL AGENTS

USES	ACTION
Miscellaneous topical agents are used to treat dermatologic disorders, such as acne, dermatitis, and infections. Some are also used to prevent certain dermatologic disorders and relieve localized pain.	Miscellaneous topical agents act in various ways. Some *anti-infectives,* such as *docosanol, mupirocin,* and *penciclovir,* prevent viral or bacterial replication; *silver sulfadiazine* acts on bacterial cell walls, producing bactericidal effects. *Becaplermin* is a platelet-derived growth factor that stimulates new tissue growth to heal open wounds. *Capsaicin* depletes and prevents the accumulation of substance P (a mediator of pain impulses) from peripheral sensory neurons to the central nervous system, relieving pain. *Pimecrolimus* is an anti-inflammatory agent that inhibits the release of cytokine, an enzyme that produces inflammatory reactions. *Tretinoin* decreases the cohesiveness of follicular epithelial cells and increases their turnover.

Name	Indications	Dosages	Side Effects
Azelaic acid (Azelex)	Treatment of mild to moderate acne vulgaris	Apply to affected area 2 times/day.	Pruritus, stinging, burning, tingling
Becaplermin (Regranex)	Treatment of lower leg diabetic neuropathic ulcers extending into subcutaneous tissue or beyond	Apply once daily. After 12 hours, rinse ulcer and recover with saline gauze.	Local rash near ulcer
Capsaicin (Zostrix)	Treatment of neuralgia, osteoarthritis, and rheumatoid arthritis	Apply directly to affected area 3–4 times/day.	Burning, stinging, erythema at application site
Collagenase (Santyl)	Debridement of necrotic tissue in chronic dermal ulcers and severe burns	Apply once daily, or more frequently if dressing becomes soiled.	Transient erythema

Docosanol (Abreva)	Treatment of cold sores or fever blisters caused by herpes simplex virus, type 1 or 2	Apply to lesions 5 times/day at onset of symptoms and until lesions are healed, up to a maximum of 10 days.	Headache, skin irritation
Eflornithine (Vaniqa)	Reduction of unwanted facial and chin hair	Apply to affected area 2 times/day at least 8 hours apart.	Anemia, leukopenia, thrombocytopenia, dizziness, alopecia, vomiting, diarrhea, hearing impairment
Imiquimod (Aldara)	Treatment of external genital and perianal warts (condylomata acuminata)	Apply 3 times/week before normal sleeping hours. Leave on skin for 6–10 hours, then remove. Continue for a maximum of 16 weeks.	Local skin reactions, erythema, itching, burning, excoriation, flaking, fungal infection
Mupirocin (Bactroban)	**Topical:** Treatment of impetigo and infected traumatic skin lesions **Nasal:** Reduction of spread of methicillin-resistant *S. aureus*	**Topical:** Apply 3 times/day. **Nasal:** Apply 2 times/day for 5 days.	**Topical:** Pain, burning, stinging, itching **Nasal:** Headache, rhinitis, upper respiratory congestion, pharyngitis, altered taste
Penciclovir (Denavir)	Treatment of recurrent herpes labialis (cold sores)	Apply every 2 hours while awake for 4 days.	Headache, mild erythema, altered taste, rash
Pimecrolimus (Elidel)	Treatment of mild to moderate atopic dermatitis (eczema)	Apply 2 times/day.	Upper respiratory tract infection, nasopharyngitis, burning, pyrexia, cough, nasal congestion, abdominal pain, sore throat, headache

(continued)

EYE AND TOPICAL AGENTS—cont'd

MISCELLANEOUS TOPICAL AGENTS—cont'd

Name	Indications	Dosages	Side Effects
Povidone iodine (Betadine)	External antiseptic action	Apply as needed.	Rash, pruritus, local edema
Sertaconazole (Ertaczo)	Treatment of superficial dermatophytic and candidal infections	Apply 2 times/day.	Headache, drowsiness, pruritus, erythema
Silver sulfadiazine (Silvadene)	Prevention and treatment of infection in second- and third-degree burns; protection against conversion from partial- to full-thickness wounds	Apply 1-2 times/day.	Burning feeling at application site, rash, itching, increased skin sensitivity to sunlight
Tretinoin (Retin-A)	Treatment of acne vulgaris	Apply once daily at bedtime.	Transient pigmentation changes, photosensitivity, local inflammatory reactions (peeling, dry skin, stinging, pruritus)

Appendix L

FDA PREGNANCY CATEGORIES

Alert: Medications should be used during pregnancy only if clearly needed.

A: Adequate and well-controlled studies have failed to show a risk to the fetus in the first trimester of pregnancy (also, no evidence of risk has been seen in later trimesters). Possibility of fetal harm appears remote.

B: Animal reproduction studies have failed to show a risk to the fetus, and there are no adequate/well-controlled studies in pregnant women.

C: Animal reproduction studies have shown an adverse effect on the fetus, and there are no adequate/well-controlled studies in humans. However, the benefits may warrant use of the drug in pregnant women despite potential risks.

D: There is positive evidence of human fetal risk based on data from investigational or marketing experience or from studies in humans, but the potential benefits may warrant use of the drug despite potential risks (e.g., use in life-threatening situations in which other medications cannot be used or are ineffective).

X: Animal or human studies have shown fetal abnormalities and/or there is evidence of human fetal risk based on adverse reaction data from investigational or marketing experience where the risks of using the medication clearly outweigh potential benefits.

Appendix M

LIFESPAN AND CULTURAL ASPECTS OF DRUG THERAPY

LIFESPAN

Drug therapy is unique to patients of different ages. Age-specific competencies involve understanding the development and health needs of the various age groups. Patients who are pregnant, children, and the elderly represent different age groups with important considerations during drug therapy.

CHILDREN

In pediatric drug therapy, drug administration is guided by the age of the child, weight, level of growth and development, and height. The dosage ordered is to be given either by kilogram of body weight or by square meter of body surface area, which is based on the height and weight of the child. Many dosages based on these calculations must be individualized based on pediatric response.

If the oral route of administration is used, often syrup or chewable tablets are given. Additionally, sometimes medication is added to liquid or mixed with foods. Remember to never force a child to take oral medications because choking or emotional trauma may ensue.

If an intramuscular injection is ordered, the vastus lateralis muscle in the mid-lateral thigh is used, because the gluteus maximus is not developed until walking occurs and the deltoid muscle is too small. For intravenous medications, administer very slowly in children. If given too quickly, high serum drug levels will occur with the potential for toxicity.

PREGNANCY

Women of childbearing years should be asked about the possibility of pregnancy before any drug therapy is initiated. Advise a woman who is either planning a pregnancy or believes she may be pregnant to inform her physician immediately. During pregnancy, medications given to the mother pass to the fetus via the placenta. Teratogenic (fetal abnormalities) effects may occur. Breast-feeding while the mother is taking certain medications may not be recommended due to the potential for adverse effects on the newborn.

The choice of drug ordered for the pregnant women is based on the stage of pregnancy, because the fetal organs develop during the first trimester. Cautious use of drugs in women of reproductive age who are sexually active and who are not using contraceptives is essential to prevent the potential for teratogenic or embryotoxic effects. Refer to the different pregnancy categories (found in Appendix F) to determine the relative safety of a medication during pregnancy.

ELDERLY

The elderly are more likely to experience an adverse drug reaction owing to physiologic changes (e.g., visual, hearing, mobility changes, chronic diseases) and cognitive changes (short-term memory loss or alteration in the thought process) that may lead to multiple medication dosing. In chronic disease states such as hypertension, glaucoma, asthma, or arthritis, the daily ingestion of multiple medications increases the potential for adverse reactions and toxic effects.

Decreased renal or hepatic function may lower the metabolism of medications in the liver and reduce excretion of medications, thus prolonging the half-life of the drug and the potential for toxicity. Dosages in the elderly should initially be smaller than for the general adult population and then slowly titrated based on patient response and therapeutic effect of the medication.

CULTURE

The term *ethnopharmacology* was first used to describe the study of medicinal plants used by indigenous cultures. More recently, it is being used as a reference to the action and effects of drugs in people from diverse racial, ethnic, and cultural backgrounds. Although there are insufficient data from investigations involving people from diverse backgrounds that would provide reliable information on ethnic-specific responses to all medications, there is growing evidence that modifications in dosages are needed for some members of racial and ethnic groups. There are wide variations in the perception of side effects by patients from diverse cultural backgrounds. These differences may be related to metabolic differences that result in higher or lower levels of the drug, individual differences in the amount of body fat, or cultural differences in the way individuals perceive the meaning of side effects and toxicity. Nurses and other health care providers need to be aware that variations can occur with side effects, adverse reactions, and toxicity so that patients from diverse cultural backgrounds can be monitored.

Some cultural differences in response to medications include the following:

African Americans: Generally, African Americans are less responsive to beta-blockers (e.g., propranolol [Inderal]) and angiotensin-converting enzyme (ACE) inhibitors (e.g., enalapril [Vasotec]).

Asian Americans: On average, Asian Americans have a lower percentage of body fat, so dosage adjustments must be made for fat-soluble vitamins and other drugs (e.g., vitamin K used to reverse the anticoagulant effect of warfarin).

Hispanic Americans: Hispanic Americans may require lower dosages and may experience a higher incidence of side effects with the tricyclic antidepressants (e.g., amitryptyline).

Native Americans: Alaskan Eskimos may suffer prolonged muscle paralysis with the use of succinylcholine when administered during surgery.

There has been a desire to exert more responsibility over one's health and, as a result, a resurgence of self-care practices. These practices are often influenced by folk remedies and the use of medicinal plants. In the United States, there are several major ethnic population subgroups (white, black, Hispanic,

Asian, and Native Americans). Each of these ethnic groups has a wide range of practices that influence beliefs and interventions related to health and illness. At any given time, in any group, treatment may consist of the use of traditional herbal therapy, a combination of ritual and prayer with medicinal plants, customary dietary and environmental practices, or the use of Western medical practices.

African Americans

Many African Americans carry the traditional health beliefs of their African heritage. Health denotes harmony with nature of the body, mind, and spirit, whereas illness is seen as disharmony that results from natural causes or divine punishment. Common practices to the art of healing include treatments with herbals and rituals known empirically to restore health. Specific forms of healing include using home remedies, obtaining medical advice from a physician, and seeking spiritual healing.

Examples of healing practices include the use of hot baths and warm compresses for rheumatism, the use of herbal teas for respiratory illnesses, and the use of kitchen condiments in folk remedies. Lemon, vinegar, honey, saltpeter, alum, salt, baking soda, and Epsom salt are common kitchen ingredients used. Goldenrod, peppermint, sassafras, parsley, yarrow, and rabbit tobacco are a few of the herbals used.

Hispanic Americans

The use of folk healers, medicinal herbs, magic, and religious rituals and ceremonies are included in the rich and varied customs of Hispanic Americans. This ethnic group believes that God is responsible for allowing health or illness to occur. Wellness may be viewed as good luck, a reward for good behavior, or a blessing from God. Praying, using herbals and spices, wearing religious objects such as medals, and maintaining a balance in diet and physical activity are methods considered appropriate in preventing evil or poor health.

Hispanic ethnopharmacology is more complementary to Western medical practices. After the illness is identified, appropriate treatment may consist of home remedies (e.g., use of vegetables and herbs), use of over-the-counter patent medicines, and use of physician-prescribed medications.

Asian Americans

For Asian Americans, harmony with nature is essential for physical and spiritual well-being. Universal balance depends on harmony among the elemental forces: fire, water, wood, earth, and metal. Regulating these universal elements are two forces that maintain physical and spiritual harmony in the body: the *yin* and the *yang.* Practices shared by most Asian cultures include meditation, special nutritional programs, herbology, and martial arts.

Therapeutic options available to traditional Chinese physicians include prescribing herbs, meditation, exercise, nutritional changes, or acupuncture.

Native Americans

The theme of total harmony with nature is fundamental to traditional Native

American beliefs about health. It is dependent on maintaining a state of equilibrium among the physical body, the mind, and the environment. Health practices reflect this holistic approach. The method of healing is determined traditionally by the medicine man, who diagnoses the ailment and recommends the appropriate intervention.

Treatment may include heat, herbs, sweat baths, massage, exercise, diet changes, or other interventions performed in a curing ceremony.

European Americans

Europeans often use home treatments as the front-line interventions. Traditional remedies practiced are based on the magical or empirically validated experience of ancestors. These cures are often practiced in combination with religious rituals or spiritual ceremonies.

Household products, herbal teas, and patent medicines are familiar preparations used in home treatments (e.g., salt water gargle for sore throat).

Appendix N

NORMAL LABORATORY VALUES

HEMATOLOGY/COAGULATION

Test	Specimen	Normal Range
Activated partial thromboplastin time (aPTT)	Whole blood	25–35 sec
Erythrocyte count (RBC count)	Whole blood	M: 4.3–5.7 million cells/mm^3 F: 3.8–5.1 million cells/mm^3
Hematocrit (HCT, Hct)	Whole blood	M: 39%–49% F: 35%–45%
Hemoglobin (Hb, Hgb)	Whole blood	M: 13.5–17.5 g/dl F: 12.0–16.0 g/dl
Leukocyte count (WBC count)	Whole blood	4.5–11.0 thousand cells/mm^3
Leukocyte differential count	Whole blood	
Basophils		0%–0.75%
Eosinophils		1%–3%
Lymphocytes		23%–33%
Monocytes		3%–7%
Neutrophils-bands		3%–5%
Neutrophils-segmented		54%–62%
Mean corpuscular hemoglobin (MCH)	Whole blood	26–34 pg/cell
Mean corpuscular hemoglobin concentration (MCHC)	Whole blood	31%–37% Hb/cell
Mean corpuscular volume (MCV)	Whole blood	80–100 fL
Partial thromboplastin time (PTT)	Whole blood	60–85 sec
Platelet count (thrombocyte count)	Whole blood	150–450 thousand/mm^3
Prothrombin time (PT)	Whole blood	11–13.5 sec
RBC count (see Erythrocyte count)		

CLINICAL CHEMISTRY (SERUM PLASMA, URINE)

Test	Specimen	Normal Range
Alanine aminotransferase (ALT, SGPT)	Serum	0–55 units/L
Albumin	Serum	3.5–5 g/dl
Alkaline phosphatase	Serum	M: 53–128 units/L F: 42–98 units/L
Anion gap	Plasma or serum	5–14 mEq/L
Aspartate aminotransferase (AST, SGOT)	Serum	0–50 units/L
Bilirubin (conjugated direct)	Serum	0–0.4 mg/dl

Test	Specimen	Normal Range
Bilirubin (total)	Serum	0.2–1.2 mg/dl
Calcium (total)	Serum	8.4–10.2 mg/dl
Carbon dioxide (CO_2) total	Plasma or serum	20–34 mEq/L
Chloride	Plasma or serum	96–112 mEq/L
Cholesterol (total)	Plasma or serum	Less than 200 mg/dl
C-Reactive protein	Serum	68–8,200 ng/ml
Creatine kinase (CK)	Serum	M: 38–174 units/L F: 26–140 units/L
Creatine kinase isoenzymes	Serum	Fraction of total: less than 0.04–0.06
Creatinine	Plasma or serum	M: 0.7–1.3 mg/dl F: 0.6–1.1 mg/dl
Creatinine clearance	Plasma or serum and urine	M: 90–139 ml/min/1.73 m^2 F: 80–125 ml/min/1.73 m^2
Free thyroxine index (FTI)	Serum	1.1–4.8
Glucose	Serum	Adults: 70–105 mg/dl Older than 60 yrs: 80–115 mg/dl
Hemoglobin A_{1c}	Whole blood	5.6%–7.5% of total Hgb
Homovanillic acid (HVA)	Urine, 24 hr	1.4–8.8 mg/day
17-Hydroxycorticosteroids (17-OHCS)	Urine, 24 hr	M: 3–10 mg/day F: 2–8 mg/day
Iron	Serum	M: 65–175 mcg/dl F: 50–170 mcg/dl
Iron-binding capacity, total (TIBC)	Serum	250–450 mcg/dl
Lactate dehydrogenase (LDH)	Serum	0–250 units/L
Magnesium	Serum	1.3–2.3 mg/dl
Oxygen (Po_2)	Whole blood, arterial	83–100 mm Hg
Oxygen saturation	Whole blood, arterial	95%–98%
pH	Whole blood, arterial	7.35–7.45
Phosphorus, inorganic	Serum	2.7–4.5 mg/dl
Potassium	Serum	3.5–5.1 mEq/L
Protein (total)	Serum	6–8.5 g/dl
Sodium	Plasma or serum	136–146 mEq/L
Specific gravity	Urine	1.002–1.030
Thyrotropin (hTSH)	Plasma or serum	2–10 mU/ml
Thyroxine (T_4) total	Serum	5–12 mcg/dl
Triglycerides (TG)	Serum, after 12-hr fast	20–190 mg/dl
Triiodothyronine resin uptake test (T_3RU)	Serum	22%–37%
Urea nitrogen	Plasma or serum	7–25 mg/dl
Urea nitrogen/creatinine ratio	Serum	12/1–20/1
Uric acid	Serum	M: 3.5–7.2 mg/dl F: 2.6–6 mg/dl
Vanillylmandelic acid (VMA)	Urine, 24 hr	2–7 mg/day

Appendix O

ORAL, VAGINAL, AND TRANSDERMAL CONTRACEPTIVES

ACTION	CLASSIFICATION
Oral contraceptives decrease fertility primarily by inhibiting ovulation. In addition, they can promote thickening of the cervical mucus, thereby creating a physical barrier to the passage of sperm. Also, they can modify the endometrium, making it less favorable for implantation. Contraception can also be achieved through the use of vaginal and transdermal agents.	Oral contraceptives may contain an estrogen and a progestin (combination oral contraceptives) or may contain only a progestin (progestin-only oral contraceptives). Combination oral contraceptives have four subgroups: *Monophasic contraceptives* have daily estrogen and progestin dosages that remain constant. *Biphasic contraceptives* have a constant estrogen dosage, and a progestin dosage that increases during the second half of the cycle. *Triphasic contraceptives* have a progestin dosage that changes for each phase of the cycle. *Estrophasic contraceptives* have a constant progestin dosage, and an estrogen dosage that gradually increases through the monthly cycle.

ORAL CONTRACEPTIVES

Brand Names	Estrogen (mcg)	Progestin (mg)	Brand Names	Estrogen (mcg)	Progestin (mg)
Monophasic			Monophasic		
Genora 1/50	50 mestranol	1 norethindrone	**Modicon**	35 ethinyl estradiol	0.5 norethindrone
Nelova 1/50M	50 mestranol	1 norethindrone	**Nelova 0.5/35E**	35 ethinyl estradiol	0.5 norethindrone

Norethin 1/50M	50 mestranol	1 norethindrone	**Ovcon-35**	35 ethinyl estradiol	0.4 norethindrone
Norinyl 1+ 50	50 mestranol	1 norethindrone	**Ortho-Cyclen**	35 ethinyl estradiol	0.25 norgestimate
Ortho-Novum 1/50	50 mestranol	1 norethindrone	**Demulen 1/35**	35 ethinyl estradiol	1 ethynodiol diacetate
Ovcon-50	50 ethinyl estradiol	1 norethindrone	**Loestrin 21 1.5/30**	30 ethinyl estradiol	1.5 norethindrone acetate
Demulen 1/50	50 ethinyl estradiol	1 ethynodiol diacetate	**Loestrin Fe 1.5/30**	30 ethinyl estradiol	1.5 norethindrone acetate
Ovral	50 ethinyl estradiol	0.5 norgestrel	**Lo/Ovral**	30 ethinyl estradiol	0.3 norgestrel
Genora 1/35	35 ethinyl estradiol	1 norethindrone	**Desogen**	30 ethinyl estradiol	0.15 desogestrel
Nelova 1/35E	35 ethinyl estradiol	1 norethindrone	**Ortho-Cept**	30 ethinyl estradiol	0.15 desogestrel
Norethin 1/35E	35 ethinyl estradiol	1 norethindrone	**Levlen**	30 ethinyl estradiol	0.15 levonorgestrel
Norinyl 1+35	35 ethinyl estradiol	1 norethindrone	**Levora**	30 ethinyl estradiol	0.15 levonorgestrel
Ortho-Novum 1/35	35 ethinyl estradiol	1 norethindrone	**Nordette**	30 ethinyl estradiol	0.15 levonorgestrel

(continued)

ORAL, VAGINAL, AND TRANSDERMAL CONTRACEPTIVES—cont'd

ORAL CONTRACEPTIVES—cont'd

Brand Names	Estrogen (mcg)	Progestin (mg)	Brand Names	Estrogen (mcg)	Progestin (mg)
Monophasic—cont'd			Monophasic—cont'd		
Brevicon	35 ethinyl estradiol	0.5 norethindrone	**Loestrin 21 1/20**	20 ethinyl estradiol	1 norethindrone acetate
Genora 0.5/35	35 ethinyl estradiol	0.5 norethindrone	**Yasmin**	30 ethinyl estradiol	3 drospirenone
Ortho Evra	0.02 ethinyl estradiol	0.15 norelgestromin			
NuvaRing	2.7 ethinyl estradiol	11.7 etonogestrel			

	Phase 1	Phase 2	
Biphasic			
Jenest-28	0.5 mg norethindrone 35 mcg ethinyl estradiol	1 mg norethindrone 35 mcg ethinyl estradiol	
Nelova 10/11	0.5 mg norethindrone 35 mcg ethinyl estradiol	1 mg norethindrone 35 mcg ethinyl estradiol	
Ortho-Novum 10/11	0.5 mg norethindrone 35 mcg ethinyl estradiol	1 mg norethindrone 35 mcg ethinyl estradiol	

Triphasic			
Tri-Norinyl	0.5 mg norethindrone 35 mcg ethinyl estradiol	1 mg norethindrone 35 mcg ethinyl estradiol	0.5 mg norethindrone 35 mcg ethinyl estradiol
Ortho-Novum 7/7/7	0.5 mg norethindrone 35 mcg ethinyl estradiol	0.75 mg norethindrone 35 mcg ethinyl estradiol	1 mg norethindrone 35 mcg ethinyl estradiol
Tri-Levlen Triphasil	0.05 mg levonorgestrel 30 mcg ethinyl estradiol	0.075 mg levonorgestrel 40 mcg ethinyl estradiol	0.125 mg levonorgestrel 30 mcg ethinyl estradiol
Ortho Tri-Cyclen	0.18 mg norgestimate 35 mcg ethinyl estradiol	0.215 mg norgestimate 35 mcg ethinyl estradiol	0.25 mg norgestimate 35 mcg ethinyl estradiol
Estrophasic			
Estrostep	1 mg norethindrone 20 mcg ethinyl estradiol	1 mg norethindrone 30 mcg ethinyl estradiol	1 mg norethindrone 35 mcg ethinyl estradiol
Progestin Only			
Micronor Nor Q D	0.35 mg norethindrone		
Ovrette	0.075 mg norgestrel		

(continued)

ORAL, VAGINAL, AND TRANSDERMAL CONTRACEPTIVES—cont'd

NEW CONTRACEPTIVE OPTIONS

Name	Ingredients	Cycle duration
Oral Contraceptive		
Yasmin 28	30 mcg ethinyl estradiol 3 mg drospirenone	28-day cycle (21 days active; 7 days placebo)
Micrette, Kariva	20 mcg ethinyl estradiol 0.15 mg desogestrel 10 mcg placebo, ethinyl estradiol	28-day cycle (21 days active, 2 days placebo, 5 days ethinyl estradiol 10 mcg)
Ortho Tri-Cyclen Lo	25 mcg ethinyl estradiol 180 mcg norgestimate (7 days); 215 mcg (7 days), 250 mcg (7 days), 7 days placebo	28-day cycle (21 days active; 7 days placebo)
Nortrel 7/7/7	35 mcg ethinyl estradiol norethindrone 0.5 mg (7 days), 0.75 mg (7 days), 1 mg (7 days), 7 days placebo	28-day cycle (21 days active; 7 days placebo)
Extended Contraceptive Regimen		
Seasonale	30 mcg ethinyl estradiol 150 mcg levonorgestrel	91-day cycle (84 days active; 7 days placebo)
Intrauterine System		
Mirena	52 mg levonorgestrel; total releasing 20 mcg/day	Device inserted into uterus once every 5 years

Vaginal Ring		
Nuva-Ring	15 mcg ethinyl estradiol 120 mcg/day etonogestrel	28-day cycle; self-inserted vaginal ring left in place for 21 days, then replaced after 7 days
Transdermal Patch		
Ortho-Evra	20 mcg ethinyl estradiol 150 mcg norelgestromin released per day	28-day cycle; one new patch applied and kept in place for 1 week and then replaced weekly for 3 weeks with a new patch. During week 4 a transdermal patch isn't used.
Injectable		
Lunelle	5 mg ethinyl cypionate 25 mg medroxyprogesterone	28-day cycle administered IM once q28 days

Appendix P

ORPHAN DRUGS

The term *orphan drug* refers to either a drug or a biologic that is intended for use in a rare disease or condition. A rare disease or condition is one that affects less than 200,000 people in the United States or, if greater than 200,000 people, in which there is no reasonable expectation that the cost of developing the drug or biologic and making it available would be recovered from the sales of that product.

A drug or biologic becomes an ''orphan drug'' when it is so designated from the Office of Orphan Products Development (OOPD) at the FDA. Orphan drug designation allows the sponsor of the drug or biologic to receive certain benefits from the government in exchange for developing the drug.

The drug or biologic must go through the FDA approval process like any other drug to evaluate it for both safety and efficacy. Since 1983, over 1,400 drugs and biologics have been designated orphan drugs, with over 250 products approved for marketing. After the orphan drug has been approved by the FDA for marketing, it becomes available through normal pharmaceutical supply channels. If not approved by the FDA, the product may be made available on a compassionate use basis. Contact information can be obtained from the OOPD at the FDA.

Office of Orphan Products Development
Food and Drug Administration
5600 Fishers Lane
Rockville, MD 20857
http://www.fda.gov/orphan/

Examples of orphan drugs include the following:

Drug Name	Proposed Use	Sponsor
90y-Hpama4 (Pan-cide)	Pancreatic cancer	Immunomedics, Inc.
Alpha-1-acid glycoprotein	Cocaine overdose, tricyclic antidepressant poisoning	Bio Products Laboratory
Ambrisentan	Pulmonary arterial hypertension	Maygen, Inc.
Aplidin	Acute lymphoblastic leukemia	PharmaMar USA, Inc.
Chenodeoxycholic acid (Chenofalk)	Cerebrotendinous xanthomatosis	Dr. Falk Pharma GmbH
Deferitrin	Iron overload	Genzyme Corporation
Depsipeptide	Cutaneous T-cell lymphoma	Glucester Pharmaceuticals, Inc.
Golimumab	Chronic sarcoidosis	Centocor, Inc.
Idebenone	Cardiomyopathy associated with Friedreich's ataxia	Santhera Pharmaceuticals LLC
Lenalidomide (Revimid)	Myelodysplastic syndromes	Celgene Corporation
Nelarabine	Acute lymphoblastic leukemia, lymphoblastic lymphoma	GlaxoSmithKline
Plitidepsin (Aplidin)	Multiple myeloma	PharmaMar USA, Inc.
Rufinamide	Lennox-Gastaut syndrome	Eisai Medical Research, Inc.
Sarsasapogenin	Amyotrophic lateral sclerosis (ALS)	Phytopharm
Sorafenib	Renal cell carcinoma	Bayer Pharmaceutical Corporation
Suberoylanilide hydroxamic acid	T-cell non-Hodgkin's lymphoma, mesothelioma	Merck & Co., Inc.
Tipifarnib (Zamestra)	Acute myeloid leukemia	Johnson & Johnson Pharmaceutical Research
Trabectedin (Yondelis)	Soft tissue sarcoma	Johnson & Johnson Pharmaceutical Research

Appendix Q

OVULATION STIMULANTS

Ovulation stimulants (medications that induce ovulation) are used to treat infertility (a decreased ability to reproduce), but not sterility (the inability to reproduce). Infertility may result from reproductive dysfunction of the male, female, or both.

Female infertility can be caused by disruption of any phase of the reproductive process. The most critical phases are follicular maturation, ovulation, ovum transport through the fallopian tubes, fertilization of the ovum, implantation, and growth and development of the conceptus. Female infertility can have a number of causes:

- ***Anovulation and failure of follicular maturation*** can result from lack of adequate hormonal stimulation. As a result, ovarian follicles don't ripen, and ovulation doesn't occur.
- ***Unfavorable cervical mucus*** may be scant, thick, or sticky. Normally, the cervical glands secrete large volumes of thin, watery mucus; if the mucus is unfavorable, sperm can't pass through to the uterus.
- ***Hyperprolactinemia*** causes excessive prolactin secretion, which may lead to amenorrhea, galactorrhea, and infertility.
- ***Luteal phase defect*** can occur in which progesterone secretion by the corpus luteum is insufficient to maintain endometrial integrity.
- ***Endometriosis*** (abnormal implantation of endometrial tissue, such as in the uterine wall and ovaries) can prevent normal implantation of the ovum.
- ***Androgen excess*** may decrease fertility, commonly by causing polycystic ovaries.

Male infertility may result from decreased density or motility of sperm or abnormal volume or quality of semen. The most obvious manifestation of male infertility is impotence (inability to achieve erection). Unlike female infertility, which usually stems from an identifiable endocrine disorder, most cases of male infertility have no identifiable endocrine cause.

Ovulation stimulants fall in several different categories:

- ***Antiestrogens*** are non-steroidal estrogen antagonists that increase FSH and LH levels by blocking estrogen negative feedback at the hypothalamus.
- ***Gonadotropins*** produce ovulation induction in women with hypogonadotropic hypogonadism and polycystic ovarian syndrome (PCOS). Ovaries must be able to respond normally to FSH and LH stimulation.
- ***Gonadotropin-releasing hormone (GnRH) agonists*** cause a down-regulation of endogenous FSH and LH levels. GnRH agonists stimulate release of pituitary gonadotropins. Suppression of endogenous LH can decrease the number of oocytes released prematurely, improve oocyte quality, and increase pregnancy rates.

Gonadotropin-releasing hormone (GnRH) antagonists suppress endogenous LH surges during ovarian stimulation. GnRH antagonists avoid initial flare-up seen with GnRH agonists, shortening the number of days needed for LH suppression and allowing ovarian stimulation to begin within the spontaneous cycle.

Name	Category	Availability	Indications	Side Effects
Cetrorelix (Cetrotide)	GnRH antagonist	**I:** 0.25 mg, 3 mg	Inhibition of premature LH surges in women undergoing ovarian hyperstimulation	OHSS: abdominal pain, indigestion, bloating, decreased urine output, nausea, vomiting, diarrhea, rapid weight gain, shortness of breath, peripheral/dependent edema. Headache, nausea, pain/redness at injection site.
Chorionic gonadotropin (APL, Pregnyl, Profasi, Profasi HP)	Gonadotropin	**I:** 5,000 units, 10,000 units, 20,000 units	In conjunction with clomiphene, human menotropins or urofollitropin to stimulate ovulation	OHSS: abdominal pain, indigestion, bloating, decreased urine output, nausea, vomiting, diarrhea, rapid weight gain, shortness of breath, peripheral/dependent edema. Ovarian enlargement, ovarian cyst formation.
Clomiphene (Clomid, Milophene, Serophene)	Antiestrogen	**T:** 50 mg	Anovulation, oligo-ovulation with intact pituitary/ovarian response and endogenous estrogen	Ovarian cyst formation, ovarian enlargement, visual disturbances, premenstrual syndrome, hot flashes.

(continued)

OVULATION STIMULANTS—cont'd

Name	Category	Availability	Indications	Side Effects
Follitropin alpha (Gonal-F)	Gonadotropin	**I:** 37.5 international units FSH, 75 international units FSH, and 150 international units FSH	In conjunction with human chorionic gonadotropin to stimulate ovarian follicular development in those with ovulatory dysfunction not due to primary ovarian failure (e.g., anovulation, olligo-ovulation)	OHSS: abdominal pain, indigestion, bloating, decreased urine output, nausea, vomiting, diarrhea, rapid weight gain, shortness of breath, peripheral/ dependent edema. Flulike symptoms, upper respiratory tract infections, bleeding between menstrual periods, nausea, ovarian enlargement, ovarian cysts, acne, breast pain/ tenderness.
Follitropin beta (Follistem)	Gonadotropin	**I:** 75 international units FSH	In conjunction with human chorionic gonadotropin to stimulate ovarian follicular development in those with ovulatory dysfunction not due to primary ovarian failure (e.g., anovulation, olligo-ovulation)	OHSS: abdominal pain, indigestion, bloating, decreased urine output, nausea, vomiting, diarrhea, rapid weight gain, shortness of breath, peripheral/ dependent edema. Flulike symptoms, breast tenderness, dry skin, rash, dizziness, fever, headache, nausea, unusual tiredness.
Ganirelex (Antagon)	GnRH antagonist	**I:** 250 mcg/ 0.5 ml	Inhibition of premature LH surges in women undergoing ovarian hyperstimulation	OHSS: abdominal pain, indigestion, bloating, decreased urine ouput, nausea, vomiting, diar-

				rhea, rapid weight gain, shortness of breath, peripheral/dependent edema. Headache, nausea, pain/redness at injection site.
Goserelin (Zoladex)	GnRH agonist	3.6 mg implant	Endometriosis, adjunct to menotropins for ovulation induction	Hot flashes, amenorrhea, blurred vision, edema, headache, nausea, vomiting, breast tenderness, increased weight.
Leuprolide (Lupron)	GnRH agonist	5 mg/ml for subcutaneous injection	Endometriosis, adjunct to menotropins/HCG for ovulation induction	Hot flashes, amenorrhea, blurred vision, edema, headache, nausea, vomiting, breast tenderness, increased weight.
Menotropins (Humegon, Pergonal)	Gonadotropin	75 units FSH, 75 units LH activity; 150 units FSH, 150 units LH activity	In conjunction with chorionic gonadotropin for ovulation stimulation in those with ovulatory dysfunction due to primary ovarian failure.	OHSS: abdominal pain, indigestion, bloating, decreased urine, nausea, vomiting, diarrhea, rapid weight gain, shortness of breath, peripheral/dependent edema. Ovarian enlargement, ovarian cyst formation.
Nafarelin (Synarel)	GnRH agonist	2 mg/ml nasal spray	Endometriosis, adjunct to menotropins/HCG for ovulation induction	Loss of bone mineral density, breast enlargement, bleeding between regular menstrual periods, acne, mood swings, seborrhea, hot flashes.

(continued)

OVULATION STIMULANTS—cont'd

Name	Category	Availability	Indications	Side Effects
Urofollitropin (Fertinex, Metrodin)	Gonadotropin	75 units FSH activity, 150 units FSH activity	In conjunction with human chorionic gonadotropin for stimulation ovulation in those with polycystic ovary syndrome who have elevated LH:FSH ratio and have failed clomiphene therapy	OHSS: abdominal pain, indigestion, bloating, decreased urine, nausea, vomiting, diarrhea, rapid weight gain, shortness of breath, peripheral/dependent edema. Ovarian enlargement, ovarian cyst formation, pain/redness at injection site, breast tenderness, nausea, vomiting, diarrhea.

FSH, Follicle-stimulating hormone; ***GnRM,*** gonadotropin-releasing hormone; ***HCG,*** human chorionic gonadotropin; ***I,*** injection; ***LM,*** luteinizing hormone; ***OHSS,*** ovarian hyperstimulation syndrome; ***T,*** tablets.

Appendix R

POISON ANTIDOTE CHART

Poisoning Agent	Antidote	Indication
Acetaminophen	Acetylcysteine (Acetadote, Mucomyst)	Acute ingestion (more than 7.5 g in adults, more than 150 mg/kg in children) serum level more than 150 mg/L 4 hr postingestion, chronic ingestion of toxic amounts
Anticholinergic agents	Physostigmine	Reverse severe effects, including hallucination, agitation, intractable seizures
Arsenic	Dimercaprol (BAL in oil)	Arsenic poisoning
Benzodiazepines	Flumazenil (Romazicon)	Complete or partial reversal of benzodiazepine effects
Beta blockers	Glucagon	Aid in improving arterial pressure and contractility
Calcium blockers	Glucagon	Aid in improving arterial pressure and contractility
Carbamate pesticides	Atropine	Treatment of cholinergic symptoms due to agents that inhibit acetylcholinesterase activity
Digoxin (Lanoxin)	Digoxin immune FAB (Digibind)	Potentially life-threatening digoxin intoxication (e.g., severe ventricular arrhythmias), ingestion of more than 10 mg in adults or more than 4 mg in children
Ethylene glycol	Fomepizole (Antizol)	Symptomatic patient with suspected ingestion of ethylene glycol
Extravasation of vasoconstrictive agents	Phentolamine (Regitine)	Extravasation of vasoconstrictive agents (e.g., epinephrine, norepinephrine)
Heparin	Protamine	Reversal of anticoagulant effect of heparin
Iron	Deferoxamine (Desferal)	Acute iron toxicity, chronic iron overload
Isoniazid	Pyridoxine (vitamin B_6)	Treatment of isoniazid overdose
Lead	Calcium EDTA	Acute and chronic lead poisoning, lead encephalopathy

(continued)

POISON ANTIDOTE CHART—cont'd

Poisoning Agent	Antidote	Indication
Lead	Dimercaprol (BAL in oil)	Acute lead poisoning of levels more than 70 mcg/dl when used with calcium EDTA
Lead	Succimer (Chemet)	Lead poisoning in patient with levels more than 45 mcg/dl
Methanol	Fomepizole (Antizol)	Symptomatic patient with suspected ingestion of methanol
Opioids	Naloxone (Narcan)	Complete or partial reversal of narcotic depression including respiratory depression
Organophosphate pesticides	Atropine	Treatment of cholinergic symptoms due to agents that inhibit acetylcholinesterase activity
Organophosphate pesticides	Pralidoxime (Protopam)	Treatment of severe poisoning in combination with atropine
Warfarin (Coumadin)	Phytonadione (vitamin K)	Excessive anticoagulation induced by warfarin

Appendix S

PREVENTING MEDICATION ERRORS AND IMPROVING MEDICATION SAFETY

Medication safety is a high priority for the health care professional. Prevention of medication errors and improved safety for the patient are important, especially in today's health care environment when today's patient is older and sometimes sicker and the drug therapy regimen can be more sophisticated and complex.

A medication error is defined by the National Coordinating Council for Medication Error Reporting and Prevention (NCC MERP) as "any preventable event that may cause or lead to inappropriate medication use or patient harm while the medication is in the control of the health care professional, patient, or consumer."

Most medication errors occur as a result of multiple, compounding events as opposed to a single act by a single individual.

Use of the wrong medication, strength, or dose; confusion over sound-alike or look-alike drugs; administration of medications by the wrong route; miscalculations (especially when used in pediatric patients or when administering medications intravenously); errors in prescribing and transcription all can contribute to compromising the safety of the patient. The potential for adverse events and medication errors is definitely a reality and is potentially tragic and costly in both human and economic terms.

Health care professionals must take the initiative to create and implement procedures to prevent medication errors from occurring and implement methods to reduce medication errors. The first priority in preventing medication errors is to establish a multidisciplinary team to improve medication use. The goal for this team would be to assess medication safety and implement changes that would make it difficult or impossible for mistakes to reach the patient. Some important criteria in making improved medication safety successful includes the following:

- Promote a nonpunitive approach to reducing medication errors
- Increase the detection and the reporting of medication errors, near misses, and potentially hazardous situations than may result in medication errors
- Determine root causes of medication errors
- Educate about the causes of medication errors and ways to prevent these errors
- Make recommendations to allow organization-wide, system-based changes to prevent medication errors
- Learn from errors that occur in other organizations and take measures to prevent similar errors

Some common causes and ways to prevent medication errors and improve safety include the following:

Handwriting: Poor handwriting can make it difficult to distinguish between two medications with similar names. Also, many drug names sound similar, especially when the names are spoken over the telephone, poorly enunciated, or mispronounced.

- Take time to write legibly.
- Keep phone or verbal orders to a minimum to prevent misinterpretation.
- Repeat back orders taken over the telephone.
- When ordering a new or rarely used medication, print the name.
- Always specify the drug strength, even if only one strength exists.
- Print generic and brand names of look-alike or sound-alike medications.

Zeros and decimal points: Hastily written orders can present problems even if the name of the medication is clear.

- Never leave a decimal point ''naked.'' Place a zero before a decimal point when the number is less than a whole unit (e.g., use 0.25 mg or 250 mcg, **not** .25 mg).
- Never have a trailing zero following a decimal point (e.g., use 2 mg, **not** 2.0 mg).

Abbreviations: Errors can occur because of a failure to standardize abbreviations. Establishing a list of abbreviations that should never be used is recommended.

- Never abbreviate unit as ''U,'' spell out ''unit.''
- Do not abbreviate ''once daily'' as OD or QD, or ''every other day'' as QOD; spell it out.
- Do not use D/C, as this may be misinterpreted as either discharge or discontinue.
- Do not abbreviate drug names; spell out the generic and/or brand names.

Ambiguous or incomplete orders: These types of orders can cause confusion or misinterpretation of the writer's intention. Examples include situations when the route of administration, dose, or dosage form has not been specified.

- Do not use slash marks—they are read as the number one (1).
- When reviewing an unusual order, verify the order with the person writing the order to prevent any misunderstanding.
- Read over orders after writing.
- Encourage that the drug's indication for use be provided on medication orders.
- Provide complete medication orders—do not use ''resume preop'' or ''continue previous meds.''

High-alert medications: Medications in this category have an increased risk of causing significant patient harm when used in error. Mistakes with these medications may or may not be more common but may be more devastating to the patient if an error occurs. A list of high-alert medications can be obtained from the Institute for Safe Medication Practices (ISMP) at www.ismp.org.

Technology available today that can be used to address and help to solve potential medication problems or errors include the following:

- Electronic prescribing systems—This refers to computerized prescriber order entry systems. Within these systems is the capability to incorporate medication safety alerts (e.g., maximum dose alerts, allergy screening). Additionally, these systems should be integrated or interfaced with pharmacy and laboratory systems to provide drug–drug and drug–disease interactions alerts and include clinical order screening capability.
- Bar codes—These systems are designed to use bar-code scanning devices to validate identity of patients, verify medications administered, document administration, and provide safety alerts.
- ''Smart'' infusion pumps—These pumps allow users to enter drug infusion protocols into a drug library along with predefined dosage limits. If a dosage is outside the limits established, an alarm is sounded and drug delivery is halted, informing the clinician that the dose is outside the recommended range.
- Automated dispensing systems–point of use dispensing system—These systems should be integrated with information systems, especially pharmacy systems.
- Pharmacy order entry system—This should be fully integrated with an electronic prescribing system with the capability of producing medication safety alerts. Additionally, the system should generate a computerized medication administration record (MAR), which would be used by a nursing staff while administering medications.

RECOMMENDED CHILDHOOD AND ADULT IMMUNIZATIONS

Recommended Childhood and Adolescent Immunization Schedule—United States, 2005

Vaccine ▼ / Age ▶	Birth	1 mo	2 mos	4 mos	6 mos	12 mos	15 mos	18 mos	24 mos	4–6 yrs	11–12 yrs	13–18 yrs
Hepatitis B[1]	HepB #1		HepB #2			HepB #3					HepB series	
Diphtheria, Tetanus, Pertussis[2]			DTaP	DTaP	DTaP			DTaP		DTaP	Td	Td
Haemophilus influenzae type b[3]			Hib	Hib	Hib	Hib						
Inactivated Polio			IPV	IPV		IPV				IPV		
Measles, Mumps, Rubella[4]						MMR #1				MMR #2	MMR #2	
Varicella[5]							Varicella				Varicella	
Pneumococcal[6]			PCV	PCV	PCV	PCV			PCV		PPV	
Influenza[7]						Influenza (yearly)					Influenza (yearly)	
- - - Vaccines below this line are for selected populations - - -												
Hepatitis A[8]											Hepatitis A series	

This schedule indicates the recommended ages for routine administration of currently licensed childhood vaccines, as of December 1, 2004, for children through age 18 yrs. Any dose not given at the recommemded age should be given at any subsequent visit when indicated and feasible.

▨ Indicates age groups that warrant special effort to administer those vaccines not previously given. Additional vaccines may be licensed and recommended during the year licensed combination vaccines may be used whenever any components of the combination are indicated and the vaccine's other components are not contraindicated. Providers should consult the manufacturers' package inserts for detailed recommendations. Clinically significant adverse events that follow immunization should be reported to the Vaccine Adverse Event Reporting System (VAERS). Guidance about how to obtain and complete a VAERS form can be found on the internet: **www.vaers.org** or by calling **800-822-7967.**

- **Range of recommended ages**
- **Preadolescent assessment**
- **Only if mother HBsAg(−)**
- **Catch-up immunization**

1. Hepatitis B (HepB) vaccine. All infants should receive the first dose of hepatitis B vaccine soon after birth and before hospital discharge; the first dose may also be given by age 2 mos if the infant's mother is hepatitis B surface antigen (HBsAg) negative. Only monovalent HepB can be used for the birth dose. Monovalent or combination vaccine containing HepB may be used to complete the series. Four doses of vaccine may be administered when a birth dose is given. The second dose should be given at least 4 wks after the first dose, except for combination vaccines, which cannot be administered before age 6 wks. The third dose should be given at least 16 wks after the first dose and at least 8 wks after the second dose. The last dose in the vaccination series (third or fourth dose) should not be administered before age 24 wks.

Infants born to HBsAg-positive mothers should receive HepB and 0.5 ml of Hepatitis B Immune Globulin (HBIG) within 12 hrs of birth at separate sites. The second dose is recommended at age 1–2 mos. The last dose in the immunization series should not be administered before age 24 wks. These infants should be tested for HBsAg and antibody to HBsAg (anti-HBs) at age 9–15 mos.

Infants born to mothers whose HBsAg status is unknown should receive the first dose of the HepB series within 12 hrs of birth. Maternal blood should be drawn as soon as possible to determine the mother's HBsAg status; if the HBsAg test is positive, the infant should receive HBIG as soon as possible (no later than age 1 wk). The second dose is recommended at age 1–2 mos. The last dose in the immunization series should not be administered before age 24 wks.

2. Diphtheria and tetanus toxoids and acellular pertusis (DTaP) vaccine. The fourth dose of DTaP may be administered as early as age 12 mos, provided 6 mos have elapsed since the third dose and the child is unlikely to return at age 15–18 mos. The final dose in the series should be given at age 4 yrs and older. **Tetanus and diphtheria toxoids (Td)** is recommended at age 11–12 yrs if at least 5 yrs have elapsed since the last dose of tetanus and diphtheria toxoid-containing vaccine. Subsequent routine Td boosters are recommended every 10 yrs.

3. *Haemophilus influenzae* type b (Hib) conjugate vaccine. Three Hib conjugate vaccines are licensed for infant use. If PRP-OMP (PedvaxHIB or ComVax [Merck]) is administered at ages 2 and 4 mos, a dose at age 6 mos is not required. DTaP/Hib combination products should not be used for primary immunization in infants at ages 2, 4 or 6 mos but can be used as boosters following any Hib vaccine. The final dose in the series should be given at age 12 mos and older.

4. Measles, mumps, and rubella vaccine (MMR). The second dose of MMR is recommended routinely at age 4–6 yrs but may be administered during any visit, provided at least 4 wks have elapsed since the first dose and both doses are administered beginning at or after age 12 mos. Those who have not previously received the second dose should complete the schedule by the visit at age 11–12 yrs.

5. Varicella vaccine. Varicella vaccine is recommended at any visit at or after age 12 mos for susceptible children (i.e., those who lack a reliable history of chickenpox). Susceptible persons aged 13 yrs and older should receive 2 doses, given at least 4 wks apart.

6. Pneumococcal vaccine. The heptavalent **pneumococcal conjugate vaccine (PCV)** is recommended for all children aged 2–23 mos. It is also recommended for certain children aged 24–59 mos. The final dose in the series should be given at age 12 mos and older. **Pneumococcal polysaccharide vaccine (PPV)** is recommended in addition to PCV for certain high-risk groups. See *MMWR* 2000;49(RR-9):1-35.

7. Influenza vaccine. Influenza vaccine is recommended annually for children aged 6 mos and older with certain risk factors (including but not limited to asthma, cardiac disease, sickle cell disease, HIV, and diabetes), health care workers, and other persons (including household members) in close contact with persons in groups at high risk (see *MMWR* 2004;53[RR-6]:1-40) and can be administered to all others wishing to obtain immunity. In addition, healthy children aged 6–23 mos and close contacts of healthy children aged 0–23 mos are recommended to receive influenze vaccine, because children in this age group are at substantially increased risk for influenza-related hospitalizations. For healthy persons aged 5–49 yrs, the intranasally administered live, attenuated influenza vaccine (LAIV) is an acceptable alternative to the intramuscular trivalent inactivated influenza vaccine (TIV). See *MMWR* 2004;53(RR-6):1-40. Children receiving TIV should be administered a dosage appropriate for their age (0.25 ml if 6–35 months or 0.5 ml if 3 yrs and older. Children aged 8 yrs and younger who are receiving influenza vaccine for the first time should receive 2 doses (separated by at least 4 weeks for TIV and at least 6 wks for LAIV).

8. Hepatitis A vaccine. Hepatitis A vaccine is recommended for children and adolescents in selected states and regions and for certain high-risk groups; consult your local public health authority. Children and adolescents in these states and regions and high-risk groups who have not been immunized against hepatitis A can begin the hepatitis A immunization series during any visit. The 2 doses in the series should be administered at least 6 mos apart. See *MMWR* 1999;48(RR-12):1–37.

For additional information about vaccines, including precautions and contraindications for immunization and vaccine shortages, please visit the National Immunization Program Website at www.cdc.gov/nip.

Approved by the Advisory Committee on Immunization Practices (ACIP) (www.cdc.gov/nip/acip), the American Academy of Pediatrics (www.aap.org), and the American Academy of Family Physicians (www.aafp.org).

Recommended Adult Immunization Schedule by Vaccine and Age Group

United States • October 2004–September 2005

Vaccine▼ Age Group▶	19–49	50–64	≥65
Tetanus, Diphtheria (Td)*		1 dose booster every 10 yrs[1]	
Influenza	1 dose annually[2]		1 dose annually[2]
Pneumococcal (polysaccharide)	1 dose[3,4]		1 dose[3,4]
Hepatitis B*		3 doses (0, 1–2, 4–6 mos)[5]	
Hepatitis A*		2 doses (0, 6–12 mos)[6]	
Measles, Mumps, Rubella (MMR)*	1 or 2 doses[7]		
Varicella*		2 doses (0, 4–8 wks)[8]	
Meningococcal (polysaccharide)		1 dose[9]	

* Covered by the Vaccine Compensation Program.
See footnotes for Recommended Adult Immunization Schedule.

- For all persons in this group
- For persons lacking documentation of vaccination or evidence of disease
- For persons at rick (i.e., with medical/exposure indications)

The Recommended Adult Immunization Schedule is Approved by the Advisory Commitee on Immunization Practices (ACIP), the American College of Obstetricians and Gynecologists (AGOB), and the American Academy of Family Physicians (AAFP)

This schedule indicates the recommended age groups for routine administration of currently licensed vaccines for persons aged 19 yrs and older. Licensed combination vaccines may be used whenever any components of the combination are indicated and when the vaccine's other components are not contraindicated. Providers should consult manufacturers' package inserts for detailed recommendations.

Report all clinically significant postvaccination reactions to the Vaccine Adverse Event Reporting System (VAERS). Reporting forms and instructions on filing a VAERS report are available by telephone at 800-822-7967 or from the VAERS website at http://www.vaers.org.

Information on how to file a Vaccine Injury Compensation Program claim is available at http://www.hrsa.gov/osp/vicp or by telephone at 800-338-2382. To file a claim for vaccine injury, contact the U.S. Court of Federal Claims, 717 Madison Place, N.W., Washington, D.C. 20005, telephone 202-219-9657.

Additional information about the vaccines listed above and contraindications for immunization is available at http://www.cdc.gov/nip or 800-CDC-INFO [800-232-4636] (English and Spanish).

Footnotes for Recommended Adult Immunization Schedule, United States, 2004–2005

1. Tetanus and diphtheria (Td). Adults, including pregnant women with uncertain history of a complete primary vaccination series, should receive a primary series of Td. A primary series for adults is 3 doses; administer the first 2 doses at least 4 wks apart and the 3rd dose 6–12 mos after the second. Administer 1 dose if the person received the primary series and if the last vaccination was received 10 yrs and longer previously. Consult recommendations for administering Td as prophylaxis in wound management (see *MMWR* 1991;40[No. RR-10]). The American College of Physicians Task Force on Adult Immunization supports a second option for Td use in adults: a single Td booster at age 50 yrs for persons who have completed the full pediatric series, including the teenage/young adult booster.

2. Influenza vaccination. The Advisory Committee on Immunization Practices (ACIP) recommends inactivated influenza vaccination for the following indications, when vaccine is available. *Medical indications:* chronic disorders of the cardiovascular or pulmonary systems, including asthma; chronic metabolic diseases, including diabetes mellitus, renal dysfunction, hemoglobinopathies, or immunosuppression (including immunosuppression caused by medications or by human immunodeficiency virus [HIV]); and pregnancy during the influenza season. *Occupational indications:* health care workers and employees of long-term–care and assisted living facilities. *Other indications:* residents of nursing homes and other long-term–care facilities; persons likely to transmit influenza to persons at high risk (i.e., in-home caregivers to persons with medical indications, household/close contacts and out-of-home caregivers of children aged 0–23 mos, household members and caregivers of elderly persons and adults with high-risk conditions); and anyone who wishes to be vaccinated. For healthy persons aged 5–49 yrs without high-risk conditions who are not contacts of severely immunocompromised persons in special care units, either the inactivated vaccine or the intranasally administered influenza vaccine (FluMist®) may be administered (see *MMWR* 2004;53[No. RR-6]).

Note: Because of the vaccine shortage for the 2004–2005 influenza season, CDC has recommended that vaccination be restricted to the following groups, which are considered to be of equal importance: all children aged 6–23 mos; adults aged 65 yrs and older; persons aged 2–64 yrs with underlying chronic medical conditions; all women who will be pregnant during the influenza season; residents of nursing homes and long-term–care facilities; children aged 6 mos–18 yrs on chronic aspirin therapy; health care workers involved in direct patient care; and out-of-home caregivers and household contacts of children aged younger than 6 mos. For the 2004–05 season, intranasally administered, live, attenuated influenza vaccine, if available, should be encouraged for healthy persons who are aged 5–49 yrs and are not pregnant, including health-care workers (except those who care for severely immunocompromised patients in special care units) and persons caring for children aged younger than 6 mos (see *MMWR* 2004;53:923–4).

3. Pneumococcal polysaccharide vaccination. *Medical indications:* chronic disorders of the pulmonary system (excluding asthma); cardiovascular diseases; diabetes mellitus; chronic hepatic diseases, including hepatic disease as a result of alcohol abuse (e.g., cirrhosis); chronic renal failure or nephrotic syndrome; functional or anatomic asplenia (e.g., sickle cell disease or splenectomy); immunosuppressive conditions (e.g., congenital immunodeficiency, HIV infection, leukemia, lymphoma, multiple myeloma, Hodgkin's disease, generalized malignancy, or organ or bone marrow transplantation); chemotherapy with alkylating agents, antimetabolites, or long-term systemic corticosteroids; or cochlear implants. *Geographic/other indications:* Alaska Natives and certain American Indian populations. *Other indications:* residents of nursing homes and other long-term–care facilities (see *MMWR* 1997;46[No. RR-8] and *MMWR* 2003;52:739–40).

4. Revaccination with pneumococcal polysaccharide vaccine. One-time revaccination after 5 yrs for persons with chronic renal failure of nephrotic syndrome; functional or anatomic asplenia (e.g., sickle cell disease or splenectomy); immunosuppressive conditions (e.g., congenital immunodeficiency, HIV infection, leukemia, lymphoma, multiple myeloma, Hodgkin's disease, generalized malignancy, or organ or bone marrow transplantation); or chemotherapy with alkylating agents, antimetabolites, or long-term systemic corticosteroids. For persons aged 65 yrs and older, one-time revaccination if they were vaccinated 5 yrs or longer previously and were aged younger than 65 years at the time of primary vaccination (see *MMWR* 1997;46[No. RR-8]).

5. Hepatitis B vaccination. *Medical indications:* hemodialysis patients or patients who receive clotting factor concentrates. *Occupational indications:* health care workers and public-safety workers who are exposed to blood in the workplace; and persons in training in schools of medicine, dentistry, nursing, laboratory technology, and other allied health professions. *Behavioral indications:* injection-drug users; persons with more than one sex partner during the previous 6 mos; persons with a recently acquired sexually transmitted disease (STD); all clients in STD clinics; and men who have sex with men. *Other indications:* household contacts and sex partners of persons with chronic hepatitis B virus (HBV) infection; clients and staff members of institutions for the developmentally disabled; inmates of correctional facilities; or international travelers who will be in countries with high or intermediate prevalence of chronic HBV infection for more than 6 mo. (http://www.cdc.gov/travel/diseases/hbv.htm) (see *MMWR* 1991;40[No. RR-13]).

6. Hepatitis A vaccination. *Medical indications:* persons with clotting factor disorders or chronic hepatic disease. *Behavioral indications:* men who have sex with men or users of illegal drugs. *Occupational indications:* persons working with hepatitis A virus (HAV)-infected primates or with HAV in a research laboratory setting. *Other indications:* persons traveling to or working in countries that have high or intermediate endemicity of hepatitis A. If the combined hepatitis A and hepatitis B vaccine is used, administer 3 doses at 0, 1, and 6 mos (http://www.cdc.gov/travel/diseases/hav.htm) (see *MMWR* 1999;48[No. RR-12]).

7. Measles, mumps, rubella (MMR) vaccination. *Measles component:* adults born before 1957 can be considered immune to measles. Adults born during or after 1957 should receive 1 dose or more of MMR unless they have a medical contraindication, documentation of 1 dose or more, or other acceptable evidence of immunity. A second dose of MMR is recommended for adults who (1) were recently exposed to measles or in an outbreak setting, (2) were previously vaccinated with killed measles vaccine, (3) were vaccinated with an unknown vaccine during 1963–1967, (4) are students in postsecondary educational institutions, (5) work in health care facilities, or (6) plan to travel internationally. *Mumps component:* 1 dose of MMR vaccine should be adequate for protection. *Rubella component:* Administer 1 dose of MMR vaccine to women whose rubella vaccination history is unreliable and counsel women to avoid becoming pregnant for 4 wks after vaccination. For women of childbearing age, regardless of birth year, routinely determine rubella immunity and counsel women regarding congenital rubella syndrome. Do not vaccinate pregnant women or those planning to become pregnant during the next 4 wks. For women who are pregnant and susceptible, vaccinate as early in the postpartum period as possible (see *MMWR* 1998;47[No. RR-8] and *MMWR* 2001;50:1117).

8. Varicella vaccination. Recommended for all persons lacking a reliable clinical history of varicella infection or serologic evidence of varicella zoster virus (VZV) infection who might be at high risk for exposure or transmission. This includes health care workers and family contacts of immunocompromised persons; persons who live or work in environments where transmission is likely (e.g., teachers of young children, child care employees, and residents and staff members in institutional settings); persons who live or work in environments where VZV transmission can occur (e.g., college students, inmates, and staff members of correctional institutions, and military personnel); adolescents aged 11–18 yrs and adults living in households with children; women who are not pregnant but who might become pregnant; and international travelers who are not immune to infection.

Note: Approximately 95% of U.S.-born adults are immune to VZV. Do not vaccinate pregnant women or those planning to become pregnant during the next 4 wks. For women who are pregnant and susceptible, vaccinate as early in the postpartum period as possible (see *MMWR* 1999;48[No. RR-6]).

9. Meningococcal vaccine (quadrivalent polysaccharide for serogroups A, C, Y, and W 135). *Medical indications:* adults with terminal complement component deficiencies or those with anatomic or functional asplenia. *Other indications:* travelers to countries in which meningococcal disease is hyperendemic or epidemic (e.g., the "meningitis belt" of sub-Saharan Africa and Mecca, Saudi Arabia). Revaccination after 3–5 yrs might be indicated for persons at high risk for infection (e.g., persons residing in areas where disease is epidemic). Counsel college freshmen, especially those who live in dormitories, regarding meningococcal disease and availability of the vaccine to enable them to make an educated decision about receiving the vaccination (see *MMWR* 2000;49[No. RR-7]). The American Academy of Family Physicians recommends that colleges should take the lead on providing education on meningococcal infection and availability of vaccination and offer it to students who are interested. Physicians need not initiate discussion of meningococcal quadrivalent polysaccharide vaccine as part of routine medical care.

Appendix U

SIGNS AND SYMPTOMS OF ELECTROLYTE IMBALANCE

HYPOGLYCEMIA (excessive insulin)

Tremors, cold/clammy skin, mental confusion, rapid/shallow respirations, unusual fatigue, hunger, drowsiness, anxiety, headache, muscular incoordination, paraesthesia of tongue/mouth/lips, hallucination, increased pulse/blood pressure, tachycardia, seizures, coma.

HYPERGLYCEMIA (insufficient insulin)

Hot/flushed/dry skin, fruity breath odor, excessive urination (polyuria), excessive thirst (polydipsia), acute fatigue, air hunger, deep/labored respirations, mental changes, restlessness, nausea, polyphagia (excessive appetite).

HYPOKALEMIA (potassium level less than 3.5 mEq/L)

Weakness/paraesthesia of extremities, muscle cramps, nausea, vomiting, diarrhea, hypoactive bowel sounds, absent bowel sounds (paralytic ileus), abdominal distention, weak/irregular pulse, postural hypotension, difficulty breathing, disorientation, irritability.

HYPERKALEMIA (potassium level greater than 5.0 mEq/L)

Diarrhea, muscle weakness, heaviness of legs, paraesthesia of tongue/hands/feet, slow/irregular pulse, decreased blood pressure, abdominal cramps, oliguria/anuria, respiratory difficulty, cardiac abnormalities.

HYPONATREMIA (sodium level less than 130 mEq/L)

Abdominal cramping, nausea, vomiting, diarrhea, cold/clammy skin, poor skin turgor, tremors, muscle weakness, leg cramps, increased pulse rate, irritability, apprehension, hypotension, headache.

HYPERNATREMIA (sodium level greater than 150 mEq/L)

Hot/flushed/dry skin, dry mucous membranes, fever, extreme thirst, dry/rough/red tongue, edema, restlessness, postural hypotension, oliguria.

HYPOCALCEMIA (calcium level less than 8.4 mg/dl)

Circumoral/peripheral numbness and tingling, muscle twitching; Chvostek's sign (facial muscle spasm; test by tapping of facial nerve anterior to earlobe, just below zygomatic arch), muscle cramping, Trousseau's sign (carpopedal spasm), seizures, arrhythmias.

HYPERCALCEMIA (calcium level greater than 10.2 mg/dl)

Muscle hypotonicity, incoordination, anorexia, constipation, confusion, impaired memory, slurred speech, lethargy, acute psychotic behavior, deep bone pain, flank pain.

Appendix V

SOUND-ALIKE AND LOOK-ALIKE DRUGS

Generic/Trade Name	Sounds or Looks Like
Accolate	Accutane
Accupril	Accolate, Accutane, Monopril
Acetazolamide	Acetohexamide
Adderall	Inderal
Adriamycin	Aredia, Idamycin
Aggrastat	Aggrenox
Akarpine	Atropine
Alkeran	Leukeran
Allegra	Viagra
Alprazolam	Lorazepam
Alupent	Atrovent
Amantadine	Ranitidine, Rimantadine
Ambien	Amen
Amicar	Amikin
Anaspaz	Antispas
Asparaginase	Pegaspargase
Atropine	Akarpine
Avapro	Anaprox
Azithromycin	Erythromycin
Benadryl	Benylin
Benylin	Ventolin
Bepridil	Prepidil
Bumex	Buprenex, Permax
Bupropion	Buspirone
Cafergot	Carafate
Calciferol	Calcitriol
Captopril	Carvedilol
Carbatrol	Carbitral
Cardura	Cardene, Ridaura
Carteolol	Carvedilol
Cefotan	Ceftin
Cefotaxime	Cefuroxime
Ceftazidime	Ceftizoxime

Generic/Trade Name	Sounds or Looks Like
Cefzil	Kefzol, Ceftin
Celebrex	Celexa, Cerebyx
Celexa	Zyprexa, Celebrex
Chlorpromazine	Chlorpropamide, Prochlorperzine
Chlorpropamide	Chlorpromazine
Cirtacal	Citrucel
Clinoril	Clozaril, Oruvail
Clomipramine	Desipramine
Clonazepam	Klonopin, Clorazepate, Lorazepam
Combivir	Epivir
Compazine	Chlorpromazine
Covera	Provera
Cozaar	Hyzaar, Zocor
Cycloserine	Cyclosporine
Cytotec	Cytoxan
Darvon	Diovan
Daunorubicin	Doxorubicin
Deferoxamine	Cefuroxime
Demerol	Detrol, Desyrel
Denavir	Indinavir
Desipramine	Clomipramine, Imipramine, Nortriptyline
DiaBeta	Zebeta
Diazepam	Ditropam, Lorazepam
Diovan	Darvon, Dioval, Zyban
Dobutamine	Dopamine
Doxorubicin	Daunorubicin
Dynabac	DynaCirc
Edecrin	Eulexin
Efudex	Eurax
Elavil	Eldepryl, Enalapril, Oruvail
Eldepryl	Enalapril
Elmiron	Imuran
Enalapril	Eldepryl
Erythromycin	Azithromycin
Esmolol	Osmitrol
Etidronate	Etomidate, Etretinate
Fioricet	Fiorinal

(continued)

Generic/Trade Name	Sounds or Looks Like
Flomax	Foxamax, Volmax
Fludarabine	Flumadine
Flumadine	Fludarabine, Flutamide
Folic Acid	Folinic Acid
Furosemide	Torsemide
Gengraf	Prograf
Glipizide	Glyburide
Glyburide	Glipizide, Glucotrol
Guaifenesin	Guanfacine
Herceptin	Perceptin
Humalog, Insulin Human	Humulin, Insulin Human
Hydralazine	Hydroxyzine
Hydroxyzine	Hydralazine
Imipramine	Desipramine
Inderal	Adderall, Isordil, Toradol
Indanavir	Denavir
Kefzol	Cefzil
Lamictal	Lamisil, Lomotil, Ludiomil
Lamivudine	Lamotrigine
Lanoxin	Levoxine, Lonox
Leucovorin	Leukine, Leukeran
Levbid	Lithobid, Lopid, Larabid
Lithobid	Levbid, Lithostat
Loniten	Lotensin
Lonox	Lanoxin
Lopid	Levbid, Lorabid
Lorabid	Lortab
Lorazapam	Alprazolam, Clonazepam, Diazepam
Lorsartan	Valsartan
Lotensin	Loniten, Lovastatin
Lovenox	Lotronex
Medroxyprogester-one	Methylprednisolone
Melphalan	Myleran
Metoprolol	Misoprostol
Miacalcin	Micatin
Micro-K	Micronase

Generic/Trade Name	Sounds or Looks Like
Minoxidil	Monopril
MiraLax	Mirapex
Monopril	Minoxidil, Monoket
Myleran	Melphalan
Naprelan	Naprosyn
Nasarel	Nizoral
Neoral	Neurontin, Nizoral
Nicardipine	Nifedipine, Nimodipine
Nicoderm	Nitroderm
Nizoral	Nasarel, Neoral
Ocufen	Ocuflox, Ocupress
Os-Cal	Asacol
Oxycodone	OxyContin
OxyContin	Oxybutynin, Oxycodone
Paclitaxel	Paxil
Parlodel	Pindolol
Paroxetine	Pyridoxine
Paxil	Paclitaxel, Plavix, Taxol
Penicillamine	Penicillin
Pentobarbital	Phenobarbital
Perceptin	Herceptin
Pindolol	Parlodel, Plendil
Plendil	Pindolol, Pletal, Prinivil
Pletal	Plendil
Pravachol	Prevacid, Prinivil, Propranolol
Prednisone	Prednisolone, Primidone
Prepidil	Bepridil
Prinivil	Plendil, Proventil
Prochlorperazine	Chlorpromazine
Propranolol	Pravachol, Propulsid
Proscar	ProSom, Prozac
Protonix	Lotronex
Pyridoxine	Paroxetine
Ranitidine	Amatadine, Rimantadine
Ratgam	Atgam
Remegel	Renagel
Remeron	Zemuron
Renagel	Remegel

(continued)

Generic/Trade Name	Sounds or Looks Like
Retrovir	Ritonavir
Risperidone	Reserpine, Risperdal
Ritonavir	Retrovir
Ropivacaine	Bupivacaine
Sarafem	Serophene
Selegiline	Sertraline
Slo-bid	Dolobid, Lopid, Lorabid
Sulfadiazine	Sulfasalazine
Sumatriptan	Zolmitriptan
Tegretol	Toradol
Tiagabine	Tizanidine
Tiazac	Ziac
Tobradex	Tobres
Toradol	Tegretol, Torecan, Tramadol
Torsemide	Furosemide
Trandate	Tridate
Ultram	Ultane
Valsartan	Losartan
Vancomycin	Vecuronium
Vantin	Ventolin
VePesid	Versed
Verelan	Virilon
Vexol	VoSol
Viracept	Viramune
Vistaril	Versed, Zestril
Xanax	Zantac, Zyrtec
Zantac	Xanax, Zyrtec, Zofran
Zebeta	DiBeta
Zemuron	Remeron
Zestril	Visteril
Ziac	Tiazac
Zocor	Cozaar, Yocon, Zoloft

Appendix W

TECHNIQUES OF MEDICATION ADMINISTRATION

OPHTHALMIC

Eye Drops

1. Wash hands.
2. Instruct patient to lie down or tilt head backward and look up.
3. Gently pull lower eyelid down until a pocket (pouch) is formed between eye and lower lid (conjunctival sac).
4. Hold dropper above pocket. Without touching tip of eye dropper to eyelid or conjunctival sac, place prescribed number of drops into the center pocket (placing drops directly onto eye may cause a sudden squeezing of eyelid, with subsequent loss of solution). Continue to hold the eyelid for a moment after the drops are applied (allows medication to distribute along entire conjunctival sac).
5. Instruct patient to close eyes gently so that medication is not squeezed out of sac.
6. Apply gentle finger pressure to the lacrimal sac at the inner canthus (bridge of the nose, inside corner of the eye) for 1–2 min (promotes absorption, mini-

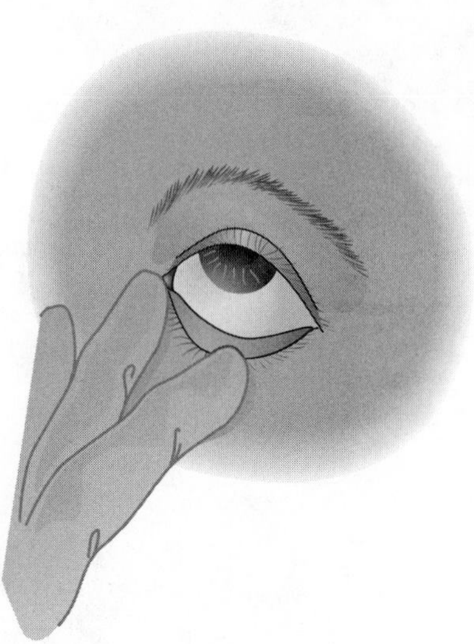

mizes drainage into nose and throat, lessens risk of systemic absorption).
7. Remove excess solution around eye with a tissue.
8. Wash hands immediately to remove medication on hands. Never rinse eye dropper.

Eye Ointment

1. Wash hands.
2. Instruct patient to lie down or tilt head backward and look up.
3. Gently pull lower eyelid down until a pocket (pouch) is formed between eye and lower lid (conjunctival sac).
4. Hold applicator tube above pocket. Without touching the applicator tip to eyelid or conjunctival sac, place prescribed amount of ointment (¼–½ inch) into the center pocket (placing ointment directly onto eye may cause discomfort).
5. Instruct patient to close eye for 1–2 min, rolling eyeball in all directions (increases contact area of drug to eye).
6. Inform patient of temporary blurring of vision. If possible, apply ointment just before bedtime.
7. Wash hands immediately to remove medication on hands. Never rinse tube applicator.

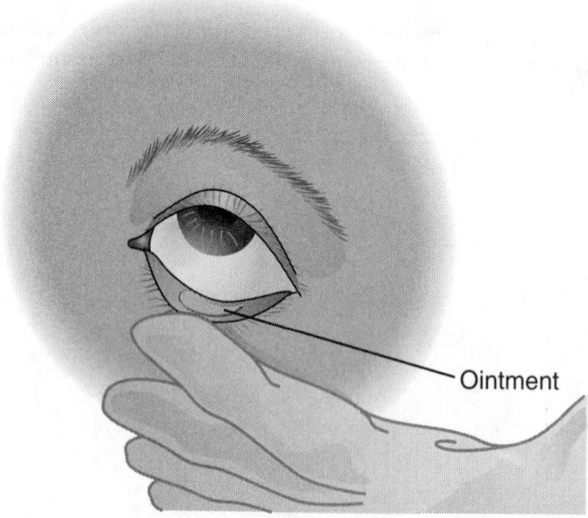

OTIC

1. Ear drops should be at body temperature (wrap hand around bottle to warm contents). Body temperature instillation prevents startling of patient.
2. Instruct patient to lie down with head turned so affected ear is upright (allows medication to drip into ear).
3. Instill prescribed number of drops toward the canal wall, not directly on eardrum.
4. To promote correct placement of ear drops, pull the auricle down and posterior in children (A) and pull the auricle up and posterior in adults (B).

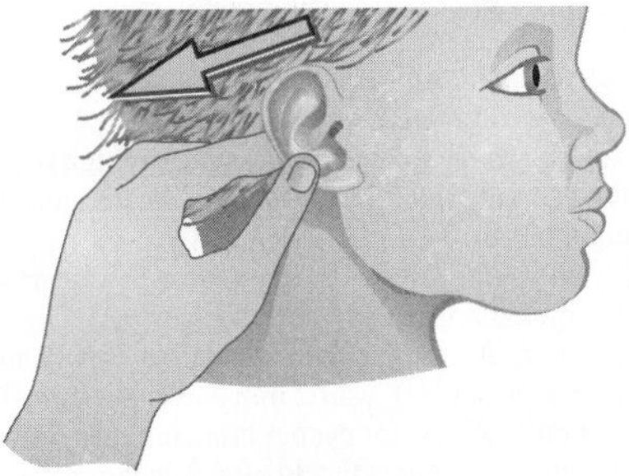

A

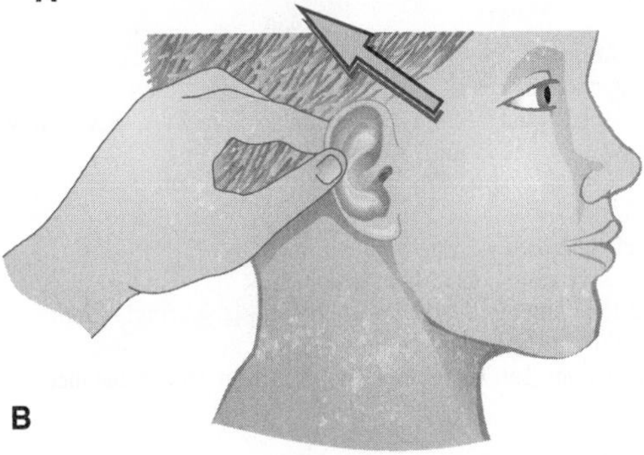

B

NASAL

Nose Drops and Sprays

1. Instruct patient to blow nose to clear nasal passages as much as possible.
2. Tilt head slightly forward if instilling nasal spray, slightly backward if instilling nasal drops.
3. Insert spray tip into 1 nostril, pointing toward inflamed nasal passages, away from nasal septum.
4. Spray or drop medication into 1 nostril while holding other nostril closed and concurrently inspire through nose to permit medication as high into nasal passages as possible.
5. Discard unused nasal solution after 3 mo.

INHALATION

Aerosol (Multidose Inhalers)

1. Shake container well before each use.
2. Exhale slowly and as completely as possible through the mouth.
3. Place mouthpiece fully into mouth, holding inhaler upright, and close lips fully around mouthpiece.
4. Inhale deeply and slowly through the mouth while depressing the top of the canister with the middle finger.
5. Hold breath as long as possible before exhaling slowly and gently.
6. When 2 puffs are prescribed, wait 2 min and shake container again before inhaling a second puff (allows for deeper bronchial penetration).
7. Rinse mouth with water immediately after inhalation (prevents mouth and throat dryness).

SUBLINGUAL

1. Administer while seated.
2. Dissolve sublingual tablet under tongue (do not chew or swallow tablet).
3. Do not swallow saliva until tablet is dissolved.

TOPICAL

1. Gently cleanse area prior to application.
2. Use occlusive dressings only as ordered.
3. Without touching applicator tip to skin, apply sparingly; gently rub into area thoroughly unless ordered otherwise.
4. When using aerosol, spray area for 3 sec from 15-cm distance; avoid inhalation.

TRANSDERMAL

1. Apply transdermal patch to clean, dry, hairless skin on upper arm or body (not below knee or elbow).
2. Rotate sites (prevents skin irritation).
3. Do not trim patch to adjust dose.

RECTAL

1. Instruct patient to lie in left lateral Sims position.
2. Moisten suppository with cold water or water-soluble lubricant.
3. Instruct patient to slowly exhale (relaxes anal sphincter) while inserting suppository well up into rectum.
4. Inform patient as to length of time (20–30 min) before desire for defecation occurs or less than 60 min for systemic absorption to occur, depending on purpose for suppository.

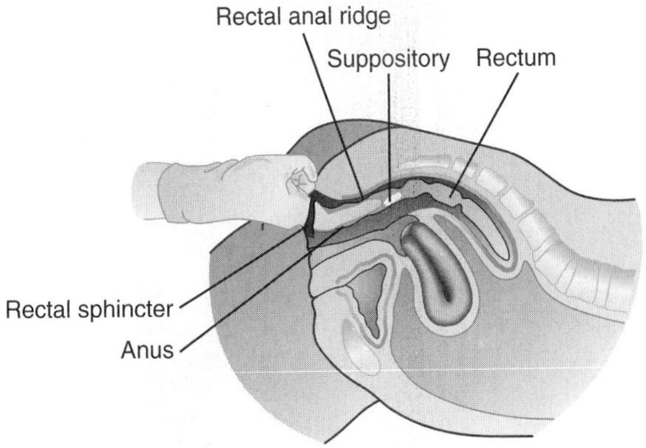

SUBCUTANEOUS

1. Use 25- to 27-gauge, ½- to ⅝-inch needle; 1–3 ml. Angle of insertion depends on body size: 90° if patient is obese. If patient is very thin, gather the skin at the area of needle insertion and administer also at a 90° angle. A 45° angle can be used in a patient with average weight.
2. Cleanse area to be injected with circular motion.
3. Avoid areas of bony prominence, major nerves, blood vessels.
4. Aspirate syringe before injecting (to avoid intra-arterial administration), except insulin, heparin.
5. Inject slowly; remove needle quickly.

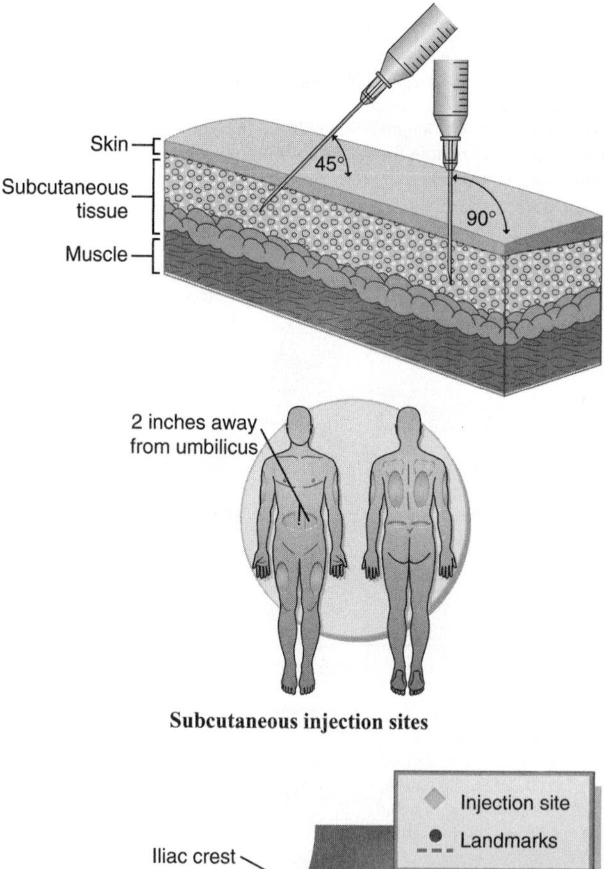

Subcutaneous injection sites

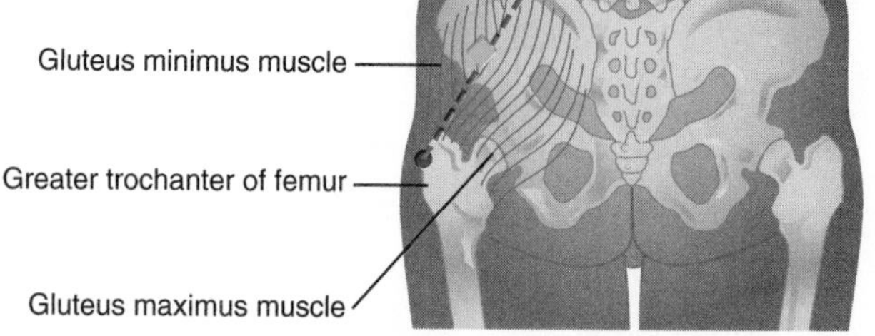

Dorsogluteal (upper outer quadrant)

IM

Injection Sites

1. Use this site if volume to be injected is 1–3 ml. Use 18- to 23-gauge, 1.25- to 3-inch needle. Needle should be long enough to reach the middle of the muscle.
2. Do not use this site in children younger than 2 yr or in those who are emaciated. Patient should be in prone position.
3. Using 90° angle, flatten the skin area using the middle and index fingers and inject between them.

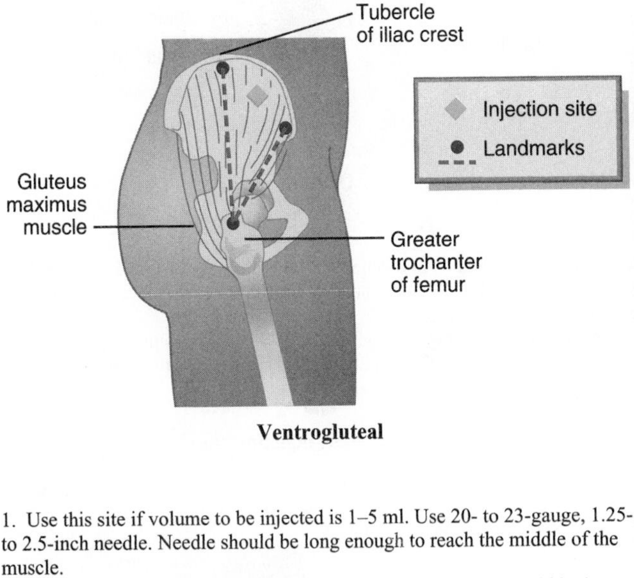

Ventrogluteal

1. Use this site if volume to be injected is 1–5 ml. Use 20- to 23-gauge, 1.25- to 2.5-inch needle. Needle should be long enough to reach the middle of the muscle.
2. Preferred site for adults, children older than 7 mo. Patient should be in supine lateral position.
3. Using 90° angle, flatten the skin area using the middle and index fingers and inject between them.

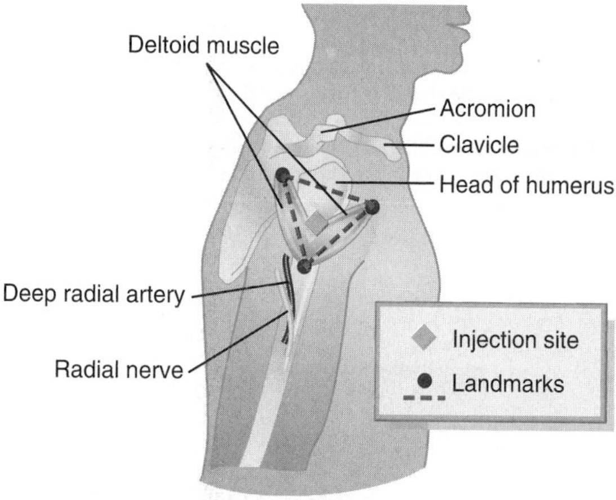

Deltoid

1. Use this site if volume to be injected is 0.5–1 ml. Use 23- to 25-gauge, ⅛- to ½-inch needle. Needle should be long enough to reach the middle of the muscle.
2. Patient may be in prone, sitting, supine, or standing position.
3. Using 90° angle or angled slightly toward acromion, flatten the skin area using the thumb and index finger and inject between them.

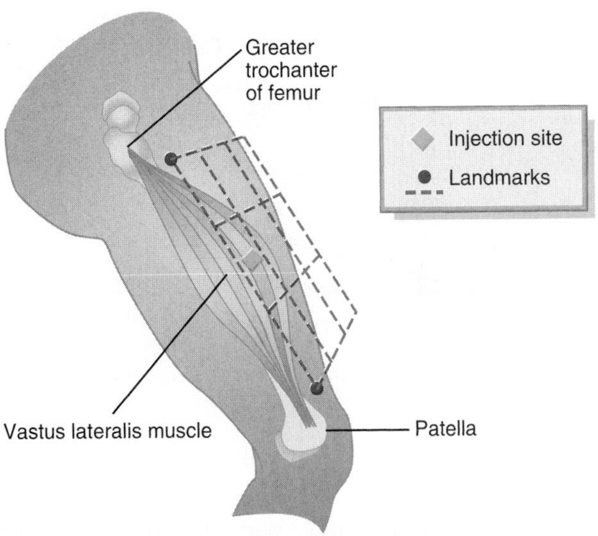

Anterolateral Thigh

1. Anterolateral thigh is site of choice for infants and children younger than 7 mo. Use 22- to 25-gauge, ⅝- to 1-inch needle.
2. Patient can be in supine or sitting position.
3. Using 90° angle, flatten the skin area using the thumb and index finger and inject between them.

Z-TRACK TECHNIQUE

1. Draw up medication with one needle, and use new needle for injection (minimizes skin staining).
2. Administer deep IM in upper outer quadrant of buttock only (dorsogluteal site).
3. Displace the skin lateral to the injection site before inserting the needle.
4. Withdraw the needle before releasing the skin.

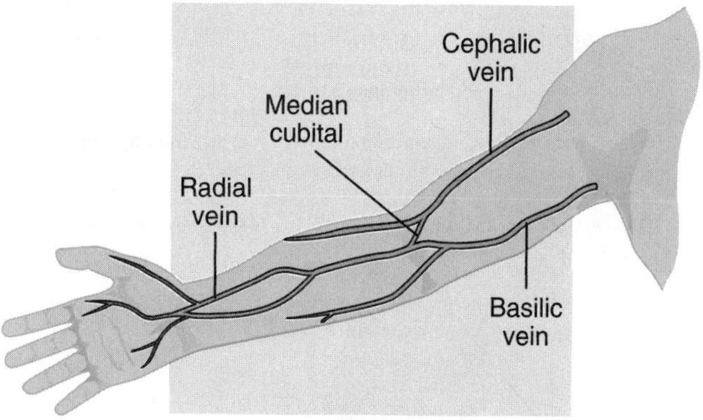

IV

1. Medication may be given as direct IV, intermittent (piggyback), or continuous infusion.
2. Ensure that medication is compatible with solution being infused (see IV compatibility chart in this drug handbook).
3. Do not use if precipitate is present or discoloration occurs.
4. Check IV site frequently for correct infusion rate, evidence of infiltration, extravasation.

Intravenous medications are administered by the following:

1. Continuous infusing solution.
2. Piggyback (intermittent infusion).
3. Volume control setup (medication contained in a chamber between the IV solution bag and the patient).
4. Bolus dose (a single dose of medication given through an infusion line or saline lock). Sometimes this is referred to as an IV push.

Adding medication to a newly prescribed IV bag:

1. Remove the plastic cover from the IV bag.
2. Cleanse rubber port with an alcohol swab.
3. Insert the needle into the center of the rubber port.
4. Inject the medication.
5. Withdraw the syringe from the port.
6. Gently rotate the container to mix the solution.
7. Label the IV, including the date, time, medication, and dosage. The label should be placed so that it is easily read when hanging.
8. Spike the IV tubing and prime the tubing.

Hanging an IV piggyback (IVPB):

1. When using the piggyback method, lower the primary bag at least 6 inches below the piggyback bag.
2. Set the pump as a secondary infusion when entering the rate of infusion and volume to be infused.
3. Most piggyback medications contain 50–100 cc and usually infuse in 20–60 min, although larger-volume bags take longer.

Administering IV medications through a volume control setup (Buretrol):

1. Insert the spike of the volume control set (Buretrol, Soluset, Pediatrol) into the primary solution container.
2. Open the upper clamp on the volume control set and allow sufficient fluid into volume control chamber.
3. Fill the volume control device with 30 cc of fluid by opening the clamp between the primary solution and the volume control device.

Administering an IV bolus dose:

1. If an existing IV is infusing, stop the infusion by pinching the tubing above the port.
2. Insert the needle into the port and aspirate to observe for a blood return.
3. If the IV is infusing properly with no signs of infiltration or inflammation, it should be patent.
4. Blood indicates that the intravenous line is in the vein.
5. Inject the medication at the prescribed rate.
6. Remove the needle and regulate the IV as prescribed.

GENERAL INDEX

Mosby's 2006 Drug Consult for Nurses

MINIMUM SYSTEM REQUIREMENTS

Windows®

Windows 98 SE, ME, 2000, and XP
800×600 pixels screen resolution
16.7 million colors
256 MB RAM
Pentium® III 1 GHz (Pentium IV recommended)
CD-ROM drive

Macintosh®

OS X and above
800×600 pixels screen resolution
Millions of colors
256 MB RAM
G3 800 MHz (G4 1 GHz recommended)
CD-ROM drive

INSTALLATION INSTRUCTIONS

For both Windows and Mac users:

1. Insert the CD into the CD-ROM drive.
2. The application should auto-start on your system.

Note:

i. For Mac users, if the application does not start automatically, double-click on "MDCN.osx" to launch the application from the open folder.
ii. For Windows users, if the application does not start automatically, then:
   a. Right-click on the "My Computer" icon on the Desktop and choose "Explore."
   b. Click once on the CD-ROM drive icon that appears on the screen.
   c. Double-click the "MDCN.exe" file to launch the application.

TECHNICAL SUPPORT

Technical support for this product is available between 7:30 AM and 7 PM CST, Monday through Friday. Before calling, make sure that your computer meets the minimum system requirements to run this software. Inside the United States, call (800) 692-9010. Outside the United States, call (314) 872-8370. You may also fax your questions to (314) 997-5080.

You may also contact Technical Support via e-mail at: *technical.support@elsevier.com*

For access to a list of *Frequently Asked Questions (FAQ)*, as well as trouble-shooting tips, please visit our website at *http://www.us.elsevierhealth.com/TechSupport*

Part Number: 9996011194

NANDA Nursing Diagnoses

Activity intolerance
Activity intolerance, Risk for
Adjustment, Impaired
Airway clearance, Ineffective
Allergy response, Latex
Allergy response, Risk for latex
Anxiety
Anxiety, Death
Aspiration, Risk for
Attachment, Risk for impaired parent/infant/child
Autonomic dysreflexia
Autonomic dysreflexia, Risk for

Body image, Disturbed
Body temperature, Risk for imbalanced
Bowel incontinence
Breastfeeding, Effective
Breastfeeding, Ineffective
Breastfeeding, Interrupted
Breathing pattern, Ineffective

Cardiac output, Decreased
Caregiver role strain
Caregiver role strain, Risk for
Communication, Impaired verbal
Communication, Readiness for enhanced
Conflict, Decisional
Conflict, Parental role
Confusion, Acute
Confusion, Chronic
Constipation
Constipation, Perceived
Constipation, Risk for
Coping, Compromised family
Coping, Defensive
Coping, Disabled family
Coping, Ineffective
Coping, Ineffective community
Coping, Readiness for enhanced
Coping, Readiness for enhanced community
Coping, Readiness for enhanced family

Denial, Ineffective
Dentition, Impaired
Development, Risk for delayed
Diarrhea
Disuse syndrome, Risk for
Diversional activity, Deficient

Energy field, Disturbed
Environmental interpretation syndrome, Impaired

Failure to thrive, Adult
Falls, Risk for
Family processes: Alcoholism, Dysfunctional
Family processes, Interrupted
Family processes, Readiness for enhanced
Fatigue
Fear
Fluid balance, Readiness for enhanced
Fluid volume, Deficient
Fluid volume, Excess
Fluid volume, Risk for deficient
Fluid volume, Risk for imbalanced

Gas exchange, Impaired
Grieving, Anticipatory
Grieving, Dysfunctional
Growth, Risk for disproportionate
Growth and development, Delayed

Health maintenance, Ineffective
Health-seeking behaviors
Home maintenance, Impaired
Hopelessness
Hyperthermia
Hypothermia

Identity, Disturbed personal
Incontinence, Functional urinary
Incontinence, Reflex urinary
Incontinence, Risk for urge urinary
Incontinence, Stress urinary
Incontinence, Total urinary
Incontinence, Urge urinary
Infant behavior, Disorganized
Infant behavior, Readiness for enhanced organized
Infant behavior, Risk for disorganized
Infant feeding pattern, Ineffective
Infection, Risk for
Injury, Risk for
Injury, Risk for perioperative-positioning
Intracranial adaptive capacity, Decreased

Knowledge, Deficient
Knowledge, Readiness for enhanced